Atlas of Interventional Orthopedics Procedures

Atlas of Interventional Orthopedics Procedures

Essential Guide for Fluoroscopy and Ultrasound-Guided Procedures

Chris J. Williams, MD

Adjunct Professor
Emory Rehabilitation Department
Emory University, Atlanta
Georgia
USA
CEO/Owner
Interventional Orthopedics of Atlanta, Atlanta
Georgia
USA

Walter I. Sussman, DO

Assistant Clinical Professor
Physical Medicine & Rehabilitation
Tufts University, Boston
Massachusetts
USA

John Pitts, MD

Fellowship Director
Interventional Orthopedics
Centeno- Schultz Clinic, Broomfield
Colorado
USA

ELSEVIER London New York Oxford Philadelphia St Louis Sydney 2023

Notices

ISBN: 978-0-323-75514-6

Content Strategist: Humayra Khan
Content Development Specialist: Kim Benson/Grace Onderlinde
Project Manager: Andrew Riley
Design: Patrick Ferguson
Illustration Manager: Muthukumaran Thangaraj
Illustrator: Dr Patrick Nguyen
Marketing Manager: Kate Bresnahan

Printed in India

Last digit is the print number: 9 8 7 6 5 4 3 2

Contents

Foreword

In the early 2000s, I was frustrated with interventional spine care. We were performing imaging-guided corticosteroid injections in the spine as well as radiofrequency ablation and could help many patients, but these were often "Band-aid" procedures. The same held true for the corticosteroid or hyaluronic acid injections we could offer in peripheral joints for osteoarthritis. Then a 2004 article was published showing that a rabbit disc could be regenerated with an injection of mesenchymal stem cells (MSCs) and my mind exploded. By 2005, we had begun an IRB-approved clinical trial using cultured bone marrow MSCs in the intervertebral disc and in various peripheral joints.

As we treated patients, we began to realize that what we had learned in interventional spine was only a small part of what was possible. For example, when tissue regeneration or healing is possible, placing stem cells or platelets using ultrasound or fluoroscopy into specific damaged structures of the musculoskeletal system is the goal. However, it soon became clear that there were several limitations to the possibilities of treating musculoskeletal injuries. For example, there were no interventional spine courses or texts that discussed how to inject a damaged knee anterior cruciate ligament (ACL), shoulder labrum, or ankle ligament.

Additionally, the diagnostic and therapeutic approach to these issues was entirely different than interventional spine or orthopedic surgery. For example, interventional spine had nothing to say about how to diagnose an ACL tear or which tears would be appropriate for injection-based regenerative medicine versus which ACL tears would be more appropriate for traditional surgical reconstruction. While orthopedic surgery had a diagnostic approach, it was focused on a binary decision, which is whether the damaged ACL should be surgically removed and replaced or not.

Hence, it was clear based on the techniques required and the different diagnostic and therapeutic approach that this was a new medical specialty. Consequently, the concept of interventional orthopedics was born. Our clinic soon set up a fellowship program to educate physicians as well as a non-profit organization, the Interventional Orthopedics Foundation (IOF). The primary goal of the IOF was to train physicians in the United States and abroad with a background in musculoskeletal care how to precisely inject structures under image guidance with hands-on didactic sessions.

Looking back, I realize that this textbook is the culmination of both the problem of a limited set of treatment options for musculoskeletal injuries and the dream of bridging non-operative and operative orthopedic care with precision-based interventional orthopedics. In other words, a new interventional specialty needs standard texts that describe the core procedures of that specialty. As radical as this concept may seem, *there is nothing new under the sun*, as the phrase goes. Medicine witnessed a similar specialty emergence and transition in paradigm from a more surgical model of cardiovascular care with the inception of interventional cardiology in the late 1980s.

This textbook includes contributions from many of the leaders in the field and several physicians that have completed a fellowship in interventional orthopedics and completed hundreds of didactic hours staying up to date on emerging techniques and new research. This willingness to be an innovator and disrupter in the field is necessary for laying the foundation of stones to the metaphorical building, which will continue to cement the legitimacy of this new medical specialty. I applaud and 100% support their efforts and happily pass the torch to that next generation.

Christopher J. Centeno, MD

Preface

Evolution

"The only constant in life is change"

—HERACLITUS

Musculoskeletal medicine is currently undergoing a paradigm shift as alternatives to the traditional approaches of care are being investigated vigorously by clinicians, scientists, and patients. Conventional methods utilizing anatomic landmarks for injection-based therapy have slowly been replaced by precision-guided injections at the point-of-care with high-definition ultrasound and fluoroscopy. Long-established surgical procedures are being substituted for minimally invasive techniques without having a negative impact on patient outcomes.

All the procedure techniques described in this book are image guided and we believe this to be the standard of care at this time. Topics covered range from simple ultrasound-guided joint injections, ligament and tendon injections, perineural hydrodissection, fluoroscopically guided spine procedures, and advanced microinvasive surgical procedures—such as minimally invasive carpal tunnel release, A1 pulley/trigger finger release, intraosseous subchondral injections, calcific tendinopathy debridement, and the TENEX procedure, to name a few.

Inception

"An Idea Is Like A Virus."

—CHRISTOPHER NOLAN

The idea of this book came about as the authors were collecting fluoroscopic and ultrasound-guided images of structures to perfect new injections techniques and for educating doctors in training as well. We began collecting images showing desired contrast flow patterns for structures such as the ACL, PCL, spine ligaments, shoulder labrum, and the hip ligamentum teres. During this process, we realized that the majority of the techniques are not widely known and only a handful of courses were offered to teach some of the advanced techniques sporadically throughout the year. The idea was then born to create an inclusive "atlas" incorporating both ultrasound- and fluoroscopy-guided musculoskeletal procedures. Additionally, we wanted to include an up-to-date resource on the current research and clinical outcomes for orthobiologics given the overwhelming utilization by many clinicians.

With the advent and growing evidence for the use of orthobiologics in orthopedic medicine, we realized these substances could be injected in far more tissue areas than the traditional steroids and local anesthetics. Because these substances can be used to treat joints, bursae, fibrocartilage structures, tendons, ligaments, muscles, bones, and perineurally, they open up a whole new world of procedures that were previously not described. Thus, the pioneers of these treatments had to discover or invent new ways to inject these substances safely and accurately into tissues one would not typically treat with steroids only.

Blueprint

"Reading is the foundation of learning but an artist drew up the blueprints."

—GEORGE E. MILLER

"Of what use is a dream if not a blueprint for courageous action."

—ADAM WEST

We have been fortunate to have the opportunity to learn, advance, and create many of these techniques we learned from pioneers in this field, such as Chris Centeno, John Schultz, and Kenneth Mautner to name a few.

This atlas provides a systematic approach for injecting all the relevant structures that are commonly encountered by non-operative sports medicine and interventional spine physicians. The primary goal was to provide a single text that an injectionist could utilize throughout the spectrum of learning and practicing.

Section I of the book introduces the basics of image guidance. Section II discusses the background and evidence for the most commonly used injectates and orthobiologics available at the time of writing this text. Section III is the bulk of the text and describes ultrasound- and fluoroscopy-guided procedures separated by body region. We provide relevant anatomy and pathology and describe a step-by-step guide for the injectionist to utilize as a supplemental learning tool for hands-on training. Section IV provides evidence and descriptions for more advanced procedures that can aide the more experienced interventional orthopedist and should not be attempted until significant hands-on experience has been completed. Finally, Section V starts with a chapter on postprocedure rehabilitation principles and current evidence. It concludes with a chapter on imaging, with visual examples demonstrating various degrees of tissue healing and regeneration.

Ideally, this text will serve as a fluid reference point as procedural techniques and injectate options continue to evolve.

Making this book has expanded our thought process and clinical knowledge, and we sincerely hope that the readers of this book experience the same. Our hope is to further advance the field of interventional orthopedics and regenerative medicine and inspire the next generation to take the field further.

Chris J. Williams, MD
Walter I. Sussman, DO
John Pitts, MD

Editor Biographies

Chris J. Williams, MD

Christopher J. Williams, MD, was born and raised in Jacksonville, Florida. After high school, Dr. Williams entered the US Air Force and worked as a public health technician in England, Kuwait, and Mississippi. After serving 4 years in the Air Force, he decided to get his undergraduate degree from the University of North Florida, where he graduated summa cum laude. He then opted to attend medical school at Emory University where he also completed his residency training in physical medicine and rehabilitation. During residency, he was awarded the Resident of Year award for all 3 years of his residency training and was Chief Resident his last year of training. During residency, Dr. Williams spearheaded the development of a musculoskeletal (MSK) ultrasound training curriculum and started a prosthetics and orthotics annual symposium in collaboration with Georgia Tech.

Dr. Williams is board certified in physical medicine and rehabilitation and completed fellowship training in interventional orthopedics and regenerative medicine for 1 year at the Centeno-Schultz Clinic in Broomfield, CO. After completing his training, he was an attending physician at the Centeno-Schultz Clinic prior to opening his practice in Atlanta, GA: Interventional Orthopedics of Atlanta. In collaboration with Ken Mautner at Emory, they started a joint non-accredited fellowship program in interventional orthopedics and graduated their first fellow in July 2020.

Education is one of his passions, as he was raised by a very hardworking single parent who was also a teacher and instilled in him the principles of humility, hard work, and dedication. Currently, Dr. Williams is an adjunct faculty member at Emory University in the Department of Rehabilitation Medicine, providing didactics annually and also allowing the residents to get hands-on training while rotating with him during their elective time. He is an instructor and the educational committee co-chair for the Interventional Orthobiologics Foundation, teaching several courses annually. He also has lectured at the annual conference for The Orthobiologics Institute (TOBI).

Dr. Williams has published over 10 peer-reviewed research articles and book chapters on the topics of orthobiologics and rehabilitation medicine. He achieved best-selling author status on Amazon for his book *Exercise 2.0* and was recognized by Emory University Alumni Association 40 Under 40 in 2019.

In his private practice at the Interventional Orthopedics of Atlanta, Dr. Williams specializes in the diagnosis and treatment of musculoskeletal conditions in athletes, weekend warriors, adolescents, the underserved, and the elderly. He strives to provide exceptional care to everyone he encounters.

Dr. Williams resides in Atlanta, Georgia with his wife Layla, who is an ObGyn physician; two children, Kemet and Egypt; and enjoys cooking, fitness activities, art, music, and traveling.

Walter I. Sussman, DO

Dr. Walter I. Sussman is board certified in physical medicine and rehabilitation with fellowship training in sports medicine. He completed his undergraduate studies at Colgate University and medical school at the University of New England College of Osteopathic Medicine in Biddeford, Maine. During medical school, he completed a 1-year fellowship in anatomy and osteopathic manipulative medicine. He completed his residency in physical medicine and rehabilitation at Emory University, where he served as chief resident. He then pursued a fellowship in sports medicine at Emory University, where he provided coverage for the Atlanta Dream WNBA team, Georgia Tech athletics, and Emory University athletics.

Dr. Sussman currently works in private practice outside of Boston and serves as the Head Team Physician for the University of Massachusetts Dartmouth and provides care for many of the local high schools. He is a clinical Assistant Professor at Tufts University and is engaged in resident education. Dr. Sussman has published multiple book chapters and peer-reviewed articles on regenerative medicine, chronic tendon injuries, diagnostic musculoskeletal ultrasound, and concussion management.

Dr. Sussman takes pride in promoting the patient experience and individualizing the treatment to fit each patient. Dr. Sussman has a clinical interest in the use of ultrasound to diagnose musculoskeletal injuries, in post-concussion syndrome, in orthobiologics, and in minimally invasive procedures. Dr. Sussman manages chronic musculoskeletal conditions, acute sports injuries, and sports-related concussions.

John Pitts, MD

John Pitts, MD, was born and raised on the south side of Chicago, IL. He received a BA in Mathematics/Economics at Emory University in Atlanta, Georgia. Dr. Pitts received his medical education at Vanderbilt School of Medicine in Nashville and then completed a physical medicine and rehabilitation residency back at Emory University. After residency he completed a 1-year fellowship (non-accredited) in regenerative medicine and interventional orthopedics at the Centeno - Schultz Clinic, where he works currently and is part of the Regenexx network of physicians. He serves as the fellowship director and helps to train new Regenexx physicians. He also regularly teaches procedural courses for the Interventional Orthopedics foundations and has given presentations at major conference for the American Academy of Physical Medicine and Rehabilitation (AAPMR), The Orthobiologics Institute (TOBI), and the American Association of Orthopedic Medicine (AAOM).

Dr. Pitts has been practicing regenerative Medicine and interventional orthopedics exclusively since 2013. He diagnoses and treats patients with a variety of orthopedic and musculoskeletal problems, including spine (cervical, thoracic, lumbar, sacroiliac joints), temporomandibular joint, upper extremity (shoulder, elbow, wrist, hand, fingers), lower extremity (hip, knee, ankle, foot, toes), and problems relating to peripheral nerves, joints, ligaments, tendons, bones, and muscle. He regularly uses orthobiologics such as prolotherapy, neuroprolotherapy, platelet-rich plasma (PRP), platelet lysate, bone marrow concentrate, micronized adipose tissue graft, and amniotic membrane. Additionally, he works in Grand Cayman Island several times per year, where he is able to treat patients with cultured expanded bone marrow mesenchymal stem cells (MSCs). He utilizes other devices to be used in interventional orthopedics and helps to pioneer and advance many of the procedures.

Dr. Pitts has co-authored several peer-reviewed articles relating to regenerative treatments. He also authored a book named *Nutrition 2.0, Guide to Eating and Living to Achieve a Higher Quality of Life Now and into Your Golden Years,* and gives this to all his patients.

Dr. Pitts resides in Denver, CO, with his wife, Ria, and two young children, Malcolm and Camila. He enjoys working out, playing sports, snowboarding, scuba diving, being outdoors, traveling, watching movies, and spending time with his family.

Contributors

Associate Editors

Marko Bodor, MD
Founder
Interventional Spine and Sports Medicine
Bodor Clinic
Napa, California
USA
Assistant Professor
Physical Medicine and Rehabilitation
University of California Davis
Sacramento, California
USA
Assistant Professor
Neurological Surgery
University of California San Francisco
San Francisco, California
USA

Don Buford, MD, RMSK
Orthopedic Surgeon
Sports Medicine
Texas Orthobiologic Institute
Dallas, Texas
USA

Rahul Naren Desai, MD
CEO
Musculoskeletal Radiology
Restore
PDX Spine & Sports Medicine
Beaverton, Oregon
USA
President
Interventional Orthopedic Foundation
Broomfield, Colorado
USA

Gerard Malanga, MD
Partner
New Jersey Sports Medicine, LLC
Cedar Knolls, New Jersey
USA
Clinical Professor
PM&R
Rutgers Medical School
Newark, New Jersey
USA

Jason Markle, DO
Interventional Orthopedic Physician
Orthopedics
The Centeno-Schultz Clinic
Broomfield, Colorado
USA

Ken Mautner, MD
Assistant Professor
Physical Medicine & Rehabilitation
Emory University, Atlanta
USA

Contributors

Wyatt Andersen, BS, ATC
Research Assistant
Physical Medicine & Rehabilitation
Sacramento, California
USA

Sairam Atluri, MD
Medical Director
ReGen
StemCures
Cincinnati, Ohio
USA

Allison C. Bean, MD, PhD
Department of Physical Medicine and Rehabilitation
University of Pittsburgh Medical Center
Pittsburgh, Pennsylvania
USA

David J. Berkoff, MD
Professor
Orthopedics and Emergency Medicine
UNC Chapel Hill
Chapel Hill, North Carolina
USA

Virlyn Bishop
Anesthesiology and Pain Medicine
Center for Spine Interventions
Acworth, GA
USA

Carolyn Black, MD, PhD
Resident Physician
Physical Medicine and Rehabilitation
Harvard Medical School/Spaulding Rehabilitation Hospital
Boston, Massachusetts
USA

Jason Ian Blaichman, MDCM, FRCPC
Adjunct Lecturer
Department of Medical Imaging
University of Toronto
Toronto, Ontario
Canada
Staff Radiologist
Department of Diagnostic Imaging
Scarborough Health Network
Scarborough, Ontario
Canada

Brice W. Blatz, MD, MS
Physician/Owner
Sports and Regenerative Medicine
Pacific Regenerative and Interventional Sports Medicine
San Jose, California
USA

Navneet Boddu, MD
Anesthesiologist
Anesthesiology
Anesthesia Service Medical Group
San Diego, California
USA

Marko Bodor, MD
Founder
Interventional Spine and Sports Medicine
Bodor Clinic
Napa, California
USA
Assistant Professor
Physical Medicine and Rehabilitation
University of California Davis
Sacramento, California
USA
Assistant Professor
Neurological Surgery
University of California San Francisco
San Francisco, California
USA

Zach Bohart, MD, MS
Associate Professor
Tufts University School of Medicine
Boston, Massachusetts
USA

Joanne Borg-Stein, MD
Associate Professor
Physical Medicine and Rehabilitation
Harvard Medical School
Boston, Massachusetts
USA

Jay E. Bowen, DO
Medical Director
New Jersey Regenerative Institute, LLC
Cedar Knolls, New Jersey
USA Clinical Assistant Professor PM&R, Rutgers Medical School, New Jersey
USA

Robert Bowers, DO, PhD
Assistant Professor
Department of Orthopaedics
Emory University School of Medicine
Atlanta, Georgia
USA
Assistant Professor
Department of Rehabilitation Medicine
Emory University School of Medicine
Atlanta, Georgia
USA

Don Buford, MD, RMSK
Orthopedic Surgeon
Sports Medicine
Texas Orthobiologic Institute
Dallas, Texas
USA

Christopher J. Centeno, MD
Research and Development
Regenexx, LLC
Broomfield, Colorado
USA
Centeno-Schultz Clinic
Broomfield, Colorado
USA

Otto Chan, MBBS, FRCS, FRCR
Doctor
Radiology Department
Whittington Hospital
London
United Kingdom

Ricardo E. Colberg, MD, RMSK
Sports Medicine Physician
Andrews Sports Medicine & Orthopaedic Center
Birmingham, Alabama
USA

Kevin Conley, MD
Fellow
Swedish Sports & Spine
Providence-Swedish Health Alliance
Seattle, Washington
USA

Di Cui, MD
Assistant Professor
Department of Rehabilitation
Emory University
Atlanta, Georgia
USA

Brian Davis, MD, FACSM
Volunteer Clinical Professor
Department of Physical Medicine & Rehabilitation
UC Davis Health System, Sacramento
California
USA

Arthur Jason De Luigi, DO
Chair
Physical Medicine & Rehabilitation
Mayo Clinic Arizona
Scottsdale, Arizona
USA
Professor of Rehabilitation Medicine
Rehabilitation Medicine
Georgetown University School of Medicine
Washington, District of Columbia
USA
Associate Professor of Physical Medicine & Rehabilitation
Physical Medicine & Rehabilitation
Mayo Clinic Alix School of Medicine
Scottsdale, Arizona
USA

Stephen Derrington, DO
President and Medical Director
Interventional Orthobiologics
Derrington Orthopedics – Interventional Sports and Spine
Oceanside and Laguna Hills, California
USA

Rahul Naren Desai, MD
CEO
Musculoskeletal Radiology
RestorePDX Spine & Sports Medicine
Beaverton, Oregon
USA
President
Interventional Orthopedic Foundation
Broomfield, Colorado
USA

Pierre D'Hemecourt, MD
Physician
Sports Medicine
Boston Children's Hospital
Boston, Massachusetts
USA

Nidal Elbaridi, MD, PT
Medical Director
Interventional Pain
Loop Medical Center
Chicago, Illinois
USA

Max H. Epstein, MD
Resident
Physical Medicine & Rehabilitation
Baylor College of Medicine
Houston, Texas
USA

Michael Erickson, MD
Swedish Sports Medicine Fellowship Director
Swedish Family Medicine Residency
Swedish Medical Center
Seattle, Washington
USA
Clinical Instructor
Family Medicine
University of Washington
Seattle, Washington
USA

Peter A. Everts, PhD, FRSM
Chief Scientific Officer EmCyte
Program Director Gulf Coast Biologics
Fort Myers. Florida
USA

Jonathan T. Finnoff, DO, FAMSSM, FACSM
Chief Medical Officer
United States Olympic and Paralympic Committee, Colorado Springs
Colorado
USA
Professor
Department of Physical Medicine and Rehabilitation
Mayo Clinic College of Science and Medicine, Rochester
Minnesota
USA

Lisa Foster, MD
Assistant Professor
Orthopedics
Emory University
Atlanta, Georgia
USA

Josh Hackel, MD, RMSK, CAQSM
Fellowship Director USA/Andrews Research and Education Foundation
Primary Care Sports Medicine
Andrews Institute
Gulf Breeze, Florida
USA

Mederic M. Hall, MD
Associate Professor
Orthopaedics and Rehabilitation
University of Iowa
Iowa City, Iowa
USA

Todd Hayano, DO
Sports Medicine Fellow
Orthopedics & Sports Medicine
Andrews Research & Education Foundation
Pensacola, Florida
USA

Romain Haym, MSc (MSK Ultrasound), MSc (Adv. Physiotherapy), MHCPC, MCSP, MMACPC
Tendon Clinic—Senior Physiotherapist
Physiotherapy
BMI The London Independent Hospital, London
United Kingdom
MSK Sonographer
Imaging
NHS Whittington Trust, London
United Kingdom

Phillip Henning, DO
Medical Director of Sports Medicine
Rehabilitation and Performance Medicine
Swedish Medical Center, Seattle,
Washington
USA

Alan M. Hirahara, MD, FRCSC
Owner
Private Practice
Sacramento, California
USA

Douglas Hoffman, MD
Director of Musculoskeletal Ultrasound
Orthopedics and Radiology
Essentia Health
Duluth, Minnesota
USA

Nicola Hyde
Sports Medicine and Family Medicine Physician
Seattle, Washington
USE

Katarzyna Iwan, MD
Doctor
Pain Medicine
RestorePDX
Beaverton, Oregon
USA

Amir A. Jamali, MD
Medical Director
Orthopaedic Surgery
Joint Preservation Institute
Walnut Creek, California
USA

Prathap Jayaram, MD
Director of Regenerative Sports Medicine
H. Ben Taub Physical Medicine & Rehabilitation
Department of Orthopedic Surgery
Baylor College of Medicine
Houston, Texas
USA

Mairin A. Jerome, MD
Fellow
Interventional Orthopedics
Centeno-Schultz Clinic
Broomfield, Colorado
USA

Jacob Jones, MD
Physician
Orthopedics and Sports Medicine
Boston Children's Hospital
Boston, Massachusetts
USA

Javier A. Jurado
Medical Student
The University of Alabama at Birmingham School of Medicine
Birmingham, Alabama
USA

Brian Hart Keogh Jr., MD
East Carolina Pain Consultants
Interventional Pain Management
Vidant Medical Center
Greenville, North Carolina
USA
Affiliate Clinical Faculty
Department of Physical Medicine and Rehabilitation
East Carolina University School of Medicine
Greenville, North Carolina
USA

Lee Kneer, MD FAAPMR
Assistant Professor
Department of Orthopaedics
Emory University School of Medicine, Atlanta
Georgia
USA
Assistant Professor
Department of Rehabilitation Medicine
Emory University School of Medicine, Atlanta
Georgia
USA

Ryan C. Kruse, MD, CAQSM, RMSK
Assistant Professor
Orthopedics and Rehabilitation
University of Iowa
Iowa City, Iowa
USA

Sonali Lal, MD
Assistant Professor, Columbia University
Attending Physician, New York
Presybyterian Hospital

Stanley K. H. Lam, MBBS, MScSEM, FHKIMM, RMSK, CIPS, FIPP, POCUS
President
Clinical Research
The Hong Kong Institute of Musculoskeletal Medicine
Kowloon Bay
Hong Kong
Clinical Associate Professor
Family Medicine
The Chinese University of Hong Kong
New Territory
Hong Kong
Clinical Assistant Professor
Family Medicine
The University of Hong Kong
Hong Kong

Orlando Landrum, MD, MBA
Physician CEO
Pain & Regenerative Medicine
Cutting Edge Integrative Pain Centers
Elkhart, Indiana
USA

Kenneth S. Lee, MD/MBA
Professor of Radiology
Section Chief of Musculoskeletal Imaging & Intervention
Fellowship Director
Musculoskeletal Imaging & Intervention
University of Wisconsin School of Medicine and Public Health
Madison, Wisconsin
USA

Justin R. Lockrem, MD
Sports Medicine Fellow
Sports Medicine
University of North Carolina
Chapel Hill, North Carolina
USA

Daniel Lueders, MD
Assistant Professor
Physical Medicine and Rehabilitation
University of Pittsburgh Medical Center
Pittsburgh, Pennsylvania
USA

Nicola Maffulli, MD, MS, PhD, FRCP, FRCS(Orth)
Full Professor
Medicine, Surgery and Dentistry
University of Salerno
Salerno
Italy

Gerard Malanga, MD
Partner
New Jersey Sports Medicine, LLC
Cedar Knolls, New Jersey
USA
Clinical Professor
PM&R
Rutgers Medical School
Newark, New Jersey
USA

Vivek Manocha, MD
Medical Director
Pain Management
Midwest Spine Interventionalist
Springboro, Ohio
USA
Clinical Assistant Professor
Surgery
Wright State University
Boonshoft School of Medicine
Dayton, Ohio
USA

Jason Markle, DO
Interventional Orthopedic Physician
Orthopedics
The Centeno-Schultz Clinic
Broomfield, Colorado
USA

Ken Mautner, MD
Assistant Professor
Physical Medicine & Rehabilitation
Emory University, Atlanta
USA

Catherine Mills, MD
Resident Physician
Physical Medicine & Rehabilitation
Harvard Medical School/Spaulding Rehabilitation Hospital
Boston, Massachusetts
USA

Hassan Monfared, MD
Assistant Professor
Physical Medicine and Rehabilitation
Emory University
Atlanta, Georgia
USA
Residency Program Director
Physical Medicine and Rehabilitation
Emory University
Atlanta, Georgia
USA

Giorgio A. Negron, MD
Resident Physician
Department of Rehabilitation Medicine
Emory University
Atlanta, Georgia
USA

Oluseun Olufade, MD
Assistant Professor
Department of Orthopedics
Emory School of Medicine
Atlanta, Georgia
USA
Assistant Professor
Department of Physical Medicine & Rehabilitation
Emory School of Medicine
Atlanta, Georgia
USA

Kentaro Onishi
Assistant Professor
Physical Medicine and Rehabilitation
University of Pittsburgh Medical Center, Pittsburgh
Pennsylvania
USA

Alberto J. Panero, DO
http://sacsportsmed.com
Sports Medicine
SAC Regenerative Orthopedics
Sacramento, California
USA

Jaymin Patel, MD
Assistant Professor
Orthopaedics
Emory University
Atlanta, Georgia
USA

Shiv J. Patel, MD
Resident
Orthopaedic Surgery
University of Texas Medical Branch, Galveston
Texas
USA

Shounuck I. Patel, DO
Functional & Interventional Orthopedics
Spine & Sports Physiatry
Regenexx Los Angeles
Los Angeles, California
USA
Clinical Assistant Professor
College of Osteopathic Medicine of the Pacific
Western University
Pomona, California
USA
Clinical Assistant Professor
College of Osteopathic Medicine
Touro University
Harlem, New York
USA

Abby Perone, DC
Love Health, Owner
Movement Therapy & Functional Medicine
St. Petersburg, Florida
USA

John Pitts, MD
Fellowship Director
Interventional Orthopedics
Centeno-Schultz Clinic
Broomfield, Colorado
USA

Luga Podesta, MD
Director
Regenerative Sports Medicine
Bluetail Medical Group-Naples
Naples, Florida
USA
Team Physician
Florida Everglades
Estero, Florida
USA

Adam M. Pourcho, DO
Instructor of Sports Medicine
Physical Medicine and Rehabilitation
Swedish Medical Group
Seattle, Washington
USA

David Rabago, MD
Associate Professor
Department of Family Medicine
University of Wisconsin School of Medicine and Public Health
Madison, Wisconsin
USA

Kenneth D. Reeves, BS, MD
Private Practice
Physical Medicine and Rehabilitation and Pain Management
Roeland Park, Kansas
USA
Formerly Clinical Assistant/Associate Professor 1986–2015
Physical Medicine and Rehabilitation
University of Kansas Medical Center
Kansas City, Kansas
USA

Jacob Reisner, DO
Primary Care Sports Medicine Fellow
Physical Medicine and Rehabilitation
Mayo Clinic
Minneapolis, Minnesota
USA

Heather Lynn Saffel, MD, MS
Primary Care Sports Medicine Fellow
Department of Orthopedics
Emory Sports Medicine Center
Atlanta, Georgia
USA

Natalie Sajkowicz, MD
Physician
Physical Medicine and Rehabilitation
Tufts Medical Center
Boston, Massachusetts
USA

Steven Sampson, DO
Founder
PM&R
The Orthohealing Center
Los Angeles, California
USA
Founder
The Orthobiologic Institute
Los Angeles, California
USA
Clinical Instructor
Medicine
David Geffen School of Medicine UCLA
Los Angeles, California
USA

Diya Sandhu, MD
Assistant Professor
Orthopaedics
Emory University
Atlanta, Georgia
USA
Assistant Professor
Physical Medicine and Rehabilitation
Emory University
Atlanta, Georgia
USA

Allison N. Schroeder, MD
Resident Physician
Physical Medicine and Rehabilitation
University of Pittsburgh Medical Center
Pittsburgh, Pennsylvania
USA

Jacob Sellon, MD
Associate Professor
Physical Medicine and Rehabilitation/Sports Medicine Center
Mayo Clinic
Rochester, Minnesota
USA

Matthew Sherrier, MD
Resident Physician
Physical Medicine and Rehabilitation
University of Pittsburgh Medical Center
Pittsburgh, Pennsylvania
USA

Brian J. Shiple, DO, CAQSM, RMSK
President AAOM
Board Certified Sports Medicine
The Center for Sports Medicine
Philadelphia, Pennsylvania
USA

Alyssa A. Smith, BSc
Medical Assistant
Joint Preservation Institute, Sacramento, California
USA

Jay Smith, MD
Professor
Physical Medicine & Rehabilitation
Mayo Clinic
Rochester, Minnesota
USA

Alyssa Neph Speciale, MD
Assistant Clinical Professor, PM&R Sports Medicine
UC Davis Health System
Sacramento, California
USA

Cleo D. Stafford II, MD, MS, CAQSM, RMSK, FAAPMR
Assistant Professor
Department of Orthopaedics
Emory University School of Medicine, Atlanta
Georgia
USA
Assistant Professor
Department of Rehabilitation Medicine
Emory University School of Medicine, Atlanta
Georgia
USA

Jeffrey A. Strakowski, MD
Clinical Professor
Physical Medicine and Rehabilitation
The Ohio State University
Columbus, Ohio
USA
Associate Director of Medical Education
Physical Medicine and Rehabilitation
Riverside Methodist Hospital
Columbus, Ohio
USA
Director of Musculoskeletal Research
The McConnell Spine, Sport and Joint Center
Columbus, Ohio
USA

Adam Street, BS, DO
Fellow
Emory Sports Medicine Center
Emory University
Atlanta, Georgia
USA

Walter I. Sussman, DO
Assistant Clinical Professor
Physical Medicine & Rehabilitation
Tufts University
Boston, Massachusetts
USA

Selorm L. Takyi, MD
Regenerative Orthopedics and Musculoskeletal Medicine Physician
Physical Medicine & Rehabilitation
Revive Spine and Pain Center, Marlton
New Jersey
USA

Yodit Tefera, MD
Physician
Swedish Spine, Sports, & Musculoskeletal Medicine
Swedish Medical Center
Seattle, Washington
USA

Hunter Vincent, DO
Pain Fellow
Physical Medicine and Rehabilitation
University of California: Los Angeles
Los Angeles, California
USA

Chris J. Williams, MD
Adjunct Professor
Emory Rehabilitation Department
Emory University
Atlanta, Georgia
USA
CEO/Owner
Interventional Orthopedics of Atlanta
Atlanta, Georgia
USA

John J. Wolfson, RT (R), ASRT, (ARRT)
Imaging and Interventional Coordinator
OR
Injury Solutions
Greenwood Village, Colorado
USA
Instructor
Pain Imaging Education
Englewood, Colorado
USA

Colton L. Wood, MD
Primary Care Sports Medicine Fellow
Family Medicine
University of North Carolina at Chapel Hill
Chapel Hill, North Carolina
USA

Peter Chia Yeh, MD
Chief Resident
Physical Medicine and Rehabilitation
Baylor College of Medicine
Houston, Texas
USA

Maria-Cristina Zielinski, MD, PGDip, PGCert, AECC
Centre for Sports and Exercise Medicine
Barts and The London School of Medicine
Queen Mary University of London
London, UK

Acknowledgments

A huge thank you is well deserved for my wife, who has been patient and very supportive during the completion of this atlas. My siblings and the community I grew up in continue to serve as major inspiration for me. Additionally, my fellow associate editors John Pitts and Walter Sussman have made an almost gargantuan task as seamless and tolerable as possible. The contributing authors have been great to work with and their expertise is appreciated. A special thank you to all of the associate editors as well; I consider all of you as leaders in the field and most of you have served as a mentor for me at some point. Prior to starting PM&R residency at Emory University, I had no idea orthobiologics existed. I definitely owe an additional huge thank you to John Pitts, who is largely responsible for introducing me to orthobiologics and providing excellent training during my Fellowship at the Centeno-Schultz Clinic, which served as ground zero for the development and fine tuning of many of these procedural techniques. Last but not least, thank you to Elsevier for seeing the vision for the atlas and definitely the readers, who will ultimately lead to the continued evolution of the field.

Chris Williams, MD

I would first like to thank my wife for allowing me the extra time required to edit this book. I surely could not accomplish much without the love and support of my wife, children, mother, and family. I would like to thank Dr. Kenneth Mautner for first introducing me to PRP in residency. I would like to thank Drs. Christopher Centeno and John Schultz for pioneering much of this field and serving as great mentors and colleagues. Also, thank you to Dr. Ron Hanson for teaching me many of these techniques as a fellow. Many thanks to all the contributing authors for their time and expertise. Thank you to my staff who helped me acquire so many pictures for the book. Thanks to my co-editors, colleagues, and friends, Dr. Christopher Williams and Dr. Walter Sussman. It has been an honor and privilege to tackle this monumental task with you. Thank you to my patients for humbling and teaching me daily. Additionally, thanks to our publishing team at Elsevier for all the hard work of bringing this to print. Lastly, thank you to all the readers who will see this book as you are the reason for this.

John Pitts, MD

I would like to thank my family, especially my wife and three children, for their patience and understanding over this past year, and my co-editors Dr. Chris Williams and Dr. John Pitts, whose clinical skill and time are reflected in the broad scope of this book. While at Emory, I had the benefit of training with so many talented musculoskeletal and spine physicians, whose focus on individualized patient care, minimally invasive image-guided treatments, and finding new and effective treatments influenced this text and continue to guide my practice. A special thank you to Dr. Ken Mautner. I wouldn't be where I am today without his mentorship and introduction to this innovative field. I would like to also recognize Drs. Hassan Monfared, Lee Kneer, and John Xerogeanes at Emory and Drs. John Lin and Eric Shaw at the Shepherd Center for their time and guidance. Thank you to all whose work, expertise, and support helped with this textbook, including all the contributing authors, publishing team Elsevier, and all the readers. Finally, a big thank you to my patients and colleagues who continue to teach me daily.

Walter Sussman, DO

1

Introduction to Interventional Orthopedics and Review of the Pathophysiology of Orthopedic Conditions

WALTER I. SUSSMAN, JOHN PITTS, AND CHRIS WILLIAMS

Interventional orthopedics is a developing field that attempts to bridge the gap between traditional non-operative orthopedics (e.g., sports medicine, interventional spine or pain medicine) and surgical interventions. This field expands the traditional approach to orthopedic problems, broadening the number of diagnoses and pathology that can be targeted with minimally invasive injections and procedures. For instance, instead of only evaluating orthopedic pathology as severe enough versus not severe enough for surgery, we offer alternative interventions for patients that have not responded to conservative therapy such as patients with partial tendon or ligament tears, ligament laxity, and nerve entrapment syndromes where surgical options are limited. The use of diagnostic ultrasound to complement the traditional orthopedic history and examination allows the clinician to more accurately diagnose and then target the underlying soft tissue and joint pathology.

Instead of traditional interventions being limited to unguided injections and surgery, interventional orthopedics utilizes interventional musculoskeletal ultrasound and fluoroscopy to guide injections to expand treatment options with the goal of precisely targeting and treating common orthopedic problems. The use of image guidance for procedures has increased over the past decades, largely driven by decreased equipment costs, patient safety initiatives, and higher-resolution imaging.[1–3] In many cases, "blind" injections have been supplanted by image guidance, which gives the clinician the ability to directly visualize the target tissues and more accurately target specific pathology.

Therapeutic injections may include corticosteroids, but there is a focus on understanding the appropriate role of alternative injectates, which can be utilized to more accurately address the underlying pathophysiology. With the advent and expansion of regenerative treatments and orthobiologics, there is an increasing emphasis on tissue preservation, restoration of tissue function, and healing rather than solely procedures that target "inflammation" and only provide temporary pain relief, or more invasive surgical procedures carrying increased cost and risk of complications.

The traditional approach to the management of musculoskeletal pathology has largely been driven by locating and treating the primary pain generator. A good example is the treatment of low back pain. Typically, the interventionalist would try and identify a primary pain (i.e., the nerve root, facet joint, sacroiliac joint dysfunction, myofascial pain, or intradiscal pathology) and construct a treatment plan to specifically address the area of the spine most likely responsible for the patient symptoms. Conversely, an interventional orthopedics approach would take an approach of addressing the entire spine as a "functional spinal unit" and consider the interplay of these structures and the biomechanical role of adjacent ligaments, tendons, and muscles. The overall goal extends beyond general pain management and looks to address the underlying etiology of musculoskeletal pathology for long-term improvements in functional outcomes. With this in mind, the treatment plan for low back pain may include treating the lumbar facets, corresponding level epidurals if there is myoneural dysfunction on examination (e.g., weakness or gluteal enthesopathy at the posterior iliac crest), supraspinous and interspinous ligaments for stability, and possibly the multifidus muscle if there is decreased activation on examination and atrophy on magnetic resonance imaging (MRI).

The convergence of advances in imaging, an evolving understanding of the pathophysiology of both acute and chronic degenerative pathology, and a growing interest in minimally invasive approaches to orthopedic pathology has fueled this field and has expanded the type of injections and procedures performed.[1] Some of the procedures discussed in this text did not exist before the widespread adoption of ultrasound. Many of these new procedures have become more common, including nerve hydrodissection, barbotage of calcific tendinosis, and percutaneous needle tenotomy procedures. Others are characterized by using specialized surgical tools or devices to duplicate surgical procedures using a percutaneous approach that will expand and continue to be adopted due to improved safety and morbidity.

The growth of regenerative injections, including but not limited to dextrose, platelet-rich plasma, and autologous stem cells, has also driven the emergence of new techniques and procedures. In some cases, the use of these treatments clinically has outpaced the scientific data. The scientific literature will undoubtedly evolve, and the field of interventional orthopedics will continue to mature and as we explore alternatives to many of the more traditional injectates and many surgical techniques that have limited evidence and efficacy.[4,5] Several studies have been published that question whether nonsurgical conservative measures, sham surgeries, or placebo therapy is as effective as management. In some cases, it is unclear if the traditional injections with corticosteroids or surgical interventions are better than non-operative management, placebo, or sham surgery, including the intermediate and long-term benefit of corticosteroids,[6–9] arthroscopic meniscectomy, and debridement in patients with arthritis,[9–17] or subacromial decompression surgery for rotator cuff impingement.[18–21]

This introductory chapter focuses on the composition and organization of different tissue types and the current concepts in the pathophysiology of orthopedic conditions and how our understanding of common musculoskeletal conditions has influenced current and future management strategies. Conventional nonoperative therapies have targeted inflammation, but inflammation is important to the healing process. Treatment strategies must be tailored to the underlying tissue involved (nerve, muscle, tendon, ligament, bone, and cartilage) and the underlying pathology.

Tendinopathy

Tendons come in various shapes and sizes and connect muscle to bone. The normal tendon structure is largely composed of collagen and proteoglycans. Type I collagen comprises approximately 65% to 80% of the dry mass of the tendon, with smaller amounts of type II, III, IV, V, IX, and X collagen also present.[22] Collagen molecules are cross-linked polypeptide chains, and their principal role is to resist tension, while proteoglycans are primarily responsible for the viscoelastic behavior of the tendon.[23] The tendon is organized in a helical architecture, comparable to man-made ropes.[24] This helical organization of the tendon components is present at various levels or organizations, including when collagen fibers are bundled together to form fascicles, and fascicles are bundled to form the tendon itself.

The cellular component of the tendon is made up of tenoblasts and tenocytes arranged in parallel rows among the collagen fibers. Tenoblasts are immature tendon cells and transform into tenocytes as they mature. Tenocytes function to synthesize collagen and other components of the extracellular matrix (ECM). Tenoblasts and tenocytes comprise 90% of the cellular component of the tendon, with the remaining 5% to 10% made up of chondrocytes, synovial cells, and vascular cells.[22,25]

A thin film of loose connective tissue (endotenon) is present between the fascicles, allowing the fascicles to slide independently against each other. The endotenon is continuous with the connective tissue (epitenon) that surrounds the tendon as a whole (Fig. 1.1). Some tendons, such as the Achilles tendon, have a paratenon that surrounds the tendon but separate from the tendon itself.[23] The paratenon is made up of type I and III collagen fibers, and the inner surface is lined by synovial cells. In some cases, the tendon is surrounded by a true synovial sheath. There is often great confusion when describing the tissue that surrounds the tendon.

The tendon inserts on bone in the form of a myo-enthesis or cartilaginous entheses. Myo-enthesis have superior blood supply and are less prone to degenerative pathology. Intrinsic blood supply to the tendon is located at the myotendinous and osteotendinous junction, with extrinsic blood supply coming from the paratenon and synovial sheath. The musculotendinous junctions and entheses are vulnerable sites, and increased age and mechanical loading can decrease vascular supply to these areas. Small afferent nerves throughout the paratenon form plexuses with penetrating branches innervating the tendon.

Areas of the tendon with poor blood supply are at increased risk of injury. While tendon injuries can occur in the mid-tendon (i.e., Achilles), most pathology and pain arise at the enthesis. Poor blood supply predisposes damaged tendons to tissue hypoxia. Tendinopathy is thought to develop from excessive loading and tensile strain. Although load is a major component in the development pathology, the etiology of tendinopathy is likely multifactorial and includes genetics,[26] age,[27] body composition,[28] comorbidities (e.g., dyslipidemias, rheumatoid disease, tumors, infections, heritable connective tissue diseases, endocrinopathies including thyroid disease, metabolic diseases including diabetes), and medication exposure (e.g., statin, fluoroquinolones).[29]

The interplay between structural change, dysfunction, and pain is still not fully understood. Historically, tendon pain has been described as tendinitis, implying that inflammation was the central pathologic process. At the cellular level in early and chronic tendinopathy, there are

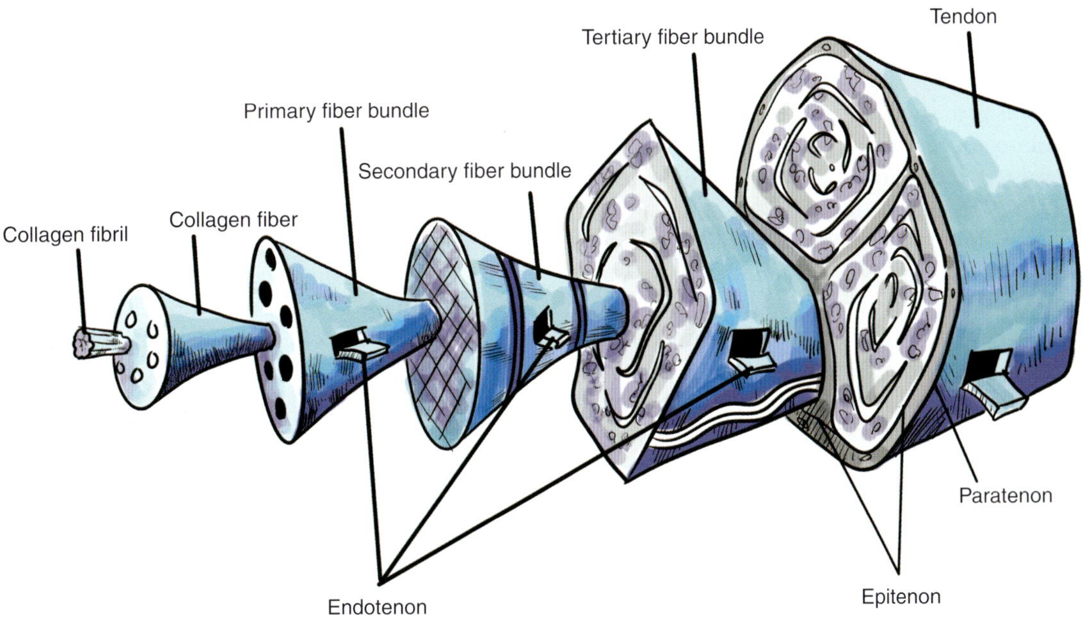

• **Fig. 1.1** Hierarchy of a Tendon.

an increased number of leukocytes (primarily macrophages and mast cells).[30–32] However, compared to rheumatoid arthritis and other immune-driven pathology, the number of leukocytes is small,[29] and there has been widespread recognition that the terminology of tendinitis, tendinosis, and paratenonitis should reflect the histopathologic feature of the tendon.[33]

Histopathologic studies have shown the progression from normal ECM to reactive response and tendon disrepair, characterized by greater tissue matrix breakdown, collagen separation, neovascularization, and proliferation of abnormal tenocytes. The new model of tendon pathology is of a continuum that has three stages: reactive tendinopathy, tendon disrepair (failed healing), and degenerative tendinopathy.[34–36] While these are described as three distinct stages for convenience, the idea of a continuum recognizes that the tendon can move forward or back along this continuum. This model highlights the need to tailor treatments to the specific tendon pathology and that a single intervention is unlikely to be efficacious in every case.

Ligament Injury

Similar to tendon tissue, ligaments are constructed from dense regular connective tissue and can vary in size, form, orientation, and location.[37] Skeletal ligaments stabilize the joint and guide the joint through a normal range of motion and provide proprioception to coordinate movements.[37,38] The orientation of collagen fibrils tends to be in the direction of applied force, and while tendon collagen fibrils tend to be in parallel, the ligament collagen fibrils are not uniformly oriented as forces are applied in more than one direction.[38] Type I collagen makes up 85% of the ligament, depending on the type of ligament, with the rest of the ligament composed of type III, VI,V, XI, and XIV collagen.[37] Collagen bundles within ligaments have a crimped appearance, and with stress, the ligament elongates as collagen fibers uncrimp. This allows the ligament to elongate without sustaining damage, contributing to the viscoelastic property of the ligament.[37]

In both tendons and ligaments, the major cell type is the fibroblast, or ligamentoblast and ligamentocytes.[37] Epiligamentous plexus forms a net-like branching anastomotic pattern on the surface of the ligament with branches that penetrate the ligament and become intraligamentous vessels distributed into longitudinal channels within the ligament.[39] The distribution of blood vessels varies among ligaments, and compared to the synovial tissue or bone, ligaments appear to be relatively hypovascular.[39]

Ligaments are most often injured in traumatic injuries and follow the three phases of healing (inflammation, proliferative, and remodeling).[40] Although the ligament may heal, the scar tissue that forms has major differences in collagen types,[41] failure of collagen crosslinking,[42] altered cell connections,[43] small collagen fibril diameter,[44] and increased vascularity.[45] Even after fully healing, the ligament matrix apparels grossly, histologically, and biomechanically different from normal ligament tissue.[46] The remodeled ligament can contain material other than collagen, including blood vessels, adipose cells, and inflammatory cells, resulting in weakness.[37,46,47] In studies of injured medial collateral ligaments (MCLs), the ligament typically remains weaker after healing and only regains 40% to 80% of the strength and stiffness compared to normal MCLs.[46,48] The viscoelastic property of an injured ligament has a somewhat better recovery, returning to within 10% to 20% of normal.[46]

Ligaments have a poor regenerative capacity due to the low cell density and lack of blood flow, and after an injury, the tissue is weaker, disorganized, and prone to reinjury.[40] These persistent collagen abnormalities can present as symptoms of instability, with 7% to 42% of subjects reporting symptoms even 1 year after injury.[49] Early resumption of activity can stimulate repair and restoration of function, while prolonged rest and immobilization delay or adversely affect recovery.[50–53] In chronic instability, traditional treatment strategies, including immobilization, rest, nonsteroidal antiinflammatory drugs (NSAIDs), and corticosteroid injections fail to address the underlying pathophysiology. In vitro studies have shown platelet-rich plasma (PRP) induces proliferation of fibroblasts and the production on type I collagen,[54] and there has been interest in the use of orthobiologics in the regeneration of ligaments.[55]

Cartilage Injury

There are two common types of cartilage: hyaline and fibrocartilage. Hyaline cartilage is present at the connection between the ribs and the sternum, in the trachea, and on the articular surfaces of synovial joints. Hyaline cartilage is composed of a rich ground substance, glycosaminoglycans (GAGs), and collagen fibers (mainly type II collagen). Unlike most tissues, articular cartilage is devoid of blood vessels, nerves, or lymphatics. Fibrocartilage is present in intervertebral discs and meniscal tissue.

Hyaline Cartilage

Articular cartilage is hyaline cartilage within synovial joints and functions as a shock-absorbing tissue that provides low friction movement during articulation. Chondrocytes are sparsely distributed throughout the dense ECM of the articular cartilage, and the ECM is primarily composed of collagen, proteoglycans, and water (Fig. 1.2). The composition of the ECM varies within different zones of the articular cartilage, and articular cartilage is typically divided into four zones: superficial, middle, deep, and calcified (Table 1.1).[56]

Injury to the articular cartilage can occur from a single traumatic event or repetitive microtrauma. Progressive cartilage injury can be accompanied by alteration in the underlying bone.

Articular cartilage has limited repair potential once damaged. In mature articular cartilage, chondrocytes are quiescent and no longer divide with very little turnover of the cartilage matrix.[57] The articular cartilage receives nutrition mainly through diffusion from the synovial membrane and cyclic loading.[58] The lack of a direct blood supply in articular cartilage, paucity of cells, and high matrix to cell ratio creates a challenging healing environment, and full-thickness articular cartilage defects rarely heal spontaneously.[56] Treatment approaches for focal cartilage defects or osteochondral lesions vary, and there is no uniform approach. Techniques to treat focal cartilage defects are usually divided into marrow-stimulating (reparative) and reconstructive techniques.

Isolated lesions to the cartilage should be differentiated from osteoarthritis (OA), where there is more diffuse damage to the articular surface. While impacting the same tissue, the pathophysiology differs. OA is characterized by the involvement of the cartilage, synovial membrane, and subchondral bone, making OA a disease of the whole joint.[57] The pathology is multifactorial but is driven by inflammatory mediators within the joint, resulting in pain, deformity, and loss of function.[59]

The earlier changes in the cartilage often appear at the joint surface in areas where mechanical and shear stress are the greatest.[60] In OA, chondrocytes go from being quiescent to becoming "activated," characterized by cell proliferation, matrix degradation and remodeling, and inappropriate hypertrophy-like maturation.[61] Degradation of the articular cartilage, thickening of the subchondral bone, osteophyte formation, and synovial inflammation. This proinflammatory environment can result in reduced chondrogenesis, as well as suppression of type II collagen synthesis.[62,63] These negative effects of inflammation on chondrogenic

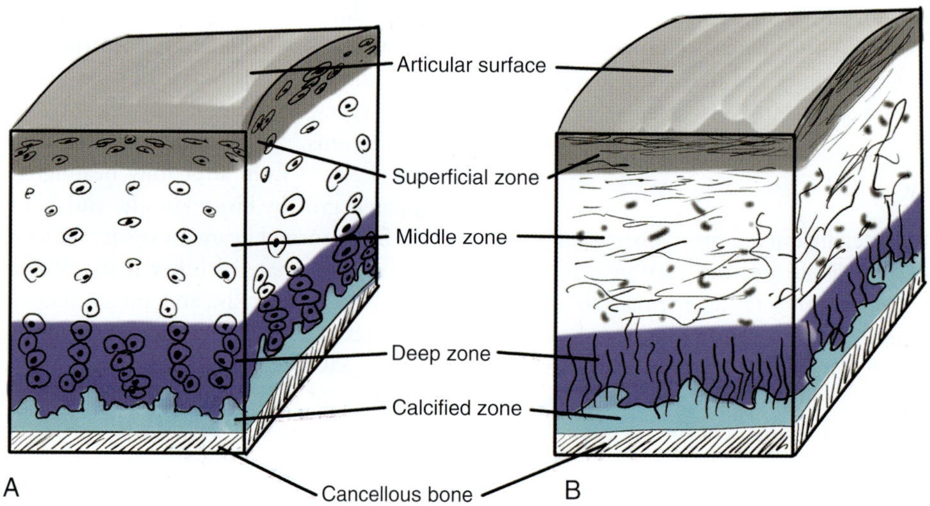

• **Fig. 1.2** Structure of articular cartilage with (A) schematic diagram of the cellular organization in the different zones and (B) diagram of the collagen fiber architecture.

TABLE 1.1 **Articular Cartilage Structure: Zones of the Extra-Cellular Matrix**

Zone	Cell	Thickness	Function
Superficial (STZ)	• High number of flattened chondrocytes • Tightly packed collagen (type II and IX) fibers, aligned parallel to the articular surface	10%–20%	Resists tensile forces and protects deeper layers from shear stresses
Middle	• Few chondrocytes • Thicker collagen fibrils, organized obliquely	40%–60%	Resists compressive forces
Deep	• Chondrocytes arranged in a columnar orientation • Largest collagen fibrils, aligned perpendicular to the joint surface • Highest proteoglycan content	30%	Resists compressive forces
Calcified	• Cell population is scarce		Anchors collagen fibrils to the subchondral bone

differentiation may have negative effects on cell-based therapy.

Treatment strategies for OA often involve behavioral (e.g., exercise and weight loss), pharmacologic (e.g., oral medications, injection therapy, and biologics), and in end stages, joint replacement surgery. Intra-articular injections are common in the management of OA; however, the dense articular cartilage is less permeable to injected medications penetrating the cartilage extracellular matrix, and the injectate can be rapidly cleared by the lymphatic system.[64,65] In recent years, there has been a growing interest in alternative approaches to injection therapy and altering joint homeostasis.[57] There has been increased interest in the treatment of the subchondral bone in patients with OA and focal lesions. The proposed mechanism is stimulating subchondral bone that influences the articular cartilage because of communication and cross-talk between both tissues.[66,67]

Fibrocartilage

Fibrocartilage contains high levels of type I and II collagen and is present between vertebral bodies, the pubic symphysis, menisci, labrum, and the tendon–bone interface.[68]

Intervertebral Disc

The intervertebral discs' major role is mechanical, transmitting load and forces through the spinal column.[69] Structurally, the intervertebral disc is composed of the inner nucleus pulposus (NP) and an outer annulus fibrosus. The NP is gelatinous and primarily formed from water, proteoglycans, and randomly organized type II collagen, and the intrinsic hydrostatic pressure of the NP resists compressive loads.[70] The outer fibrocartilaginous annulus fibrosus is composed of 15 to 25 concentric rings (lamellae), with elastin fibers and type I and II collagen fibers lying in parallel and provides the tensile strength of the disc.[71]

With age, the nucleus generally becomes more fibrotic and less gel-like,[72] and the collagen and elastin of the annular lamellae become irregular and disorganized.[69] It can be challenging to differentiate changes that occur due to aging and those that might be "pathologic." The most significant change that occurs in disc degeneration is the loss of proteoglycan (aggrecan), which is responsible for maintaining tissue hydration and impacts the disc load-bearing behavior.[73] The collagen population of the disc also changes with degeneration, but these changes are not as obvious as those of the proteoglycans.[74,75] The loss of proteoglycan and matrix disorganization leads to an inability to maintain hydration, and when loaded, they lose height, bulge, and subsequently lead to inappropriate stress along the endplate or the annulus.[76,77] The loss of disc height can also affect adjacent structures, resulting in spinal stenosis, apophyseal joint arthropathy, and ligamentum flavum hypertrophy.

The intervertebral disc is largely avascular and must rely on passive diffusion from adjacent endplate vessels for nutrition.[78] The limited vascular supply and indirect access to nutrition limit the discs' intrinsic capacity for remodeling and repair. Traditional therapies may provide symptomatic relief but do not target the underlying degenerative pathophysiology. Newer cell-based therapies aim to achieve cellular repair.[79]

Meniscus

Vascularization of the meniscus is from the lateral, medial, and middle genicular arteries, forming a perimeniscal capillary plexus. There is significant discrepancy in the vascularity of the meniscus, and the meniscus is often described as having three distinct zones characterized by the degree of vascularization. The outer zones with the greatest vascularity region are the red-red zone and the transitional red-white zone.[80] The inner or central avascular zone is the white-white zone. The healing capacity is directly related to blood circulation, with the peripheral meniscus (red-red and red-white zone) having the greatest potential for healing.[80,81]

The morphology of the meniscus cells also can be characterized by the zone in which the cells are found. There are three cell populations within the meniscus. The outer zone is mainly populated with fibroblast-like cells with an oval, fusiform shape and long cell extensions, which facilitate communication among cells and the extracellular matrix. These fibroblast-like cells are surrounded by dense connective tissue consisting of type I collagen, with a small percentage of glycoproteins and type III and V collagen present.[82] The main cell type in the inner zone is classified as fibrochondrocytes or chondrocyte-like cells, and they have a chondrocyte appearance (round or oval-shaped). These fibrochondrocytes are embedded in a fibrocartilage matrix consisting mainly of type I (60%) and II (40%) collagen and aggrecan.[83]

The superficial zone of the meniscus harbors progenitor cells.[84]

Meniscal injuries are classified depending on location, thickness, and resulting instability. The type of tear has a significant impact on the ability of the tear to heal and the most appropriate and effective therapy. Partial or total meniscectomy can lead to altered loading dynamics, leading to degeneration and OA on an average of 14 years following surgery.[4,85] A detailed discussion of surgical management is beyond the scope of this chapter, but in general, there is an increased emphasis on meniscal preservation whenever possible to preserve loading dynamics in the knee. Tears in the vascular region do have the potential to heal due to the existing blood supply and the possibility of progenitor cells in this region.[86–88]

Bone Pathology

The skeleton serves a variety of functions, providing support, permitting movement, and protecting vital internal organs. The skeleton also serves as a reservoir of hematopoietic stem cells, which give rise to blood cell lineages and mesenchymal stromal cells that are multipotent with the potential to differentiate into bone, cartilage, fat, or fibrous connective tissue.[89,90] In order to understand the mechanical properties of bone clinically, it is important to understand the component structure of bone.

At the macrostructure level, bone can be characterized as cancellous (trabecular) or cortical (compact) bone, with cortical bone forming a dense outer shell around the honeycomb-like structure of cancellous bone. Different bones have different ratios of cortical to cancellous bone. In long bones, the diaphysis is primarily composed of dense cortical bone, while the metaphysis and epiphysis are composed of cancellous bone surrounded by dense cortical bone. In general, cancellous bone is more metabolically active and remodeled more often than cortical bone.[91] Bone is surrounded by an inner endosteal and an outer periosteal surface. The periosteum is a fibrous connective tissue sheath surrounding cortical bone and is tightly attached to the bone by thick collagenous fibers (Sharpey's fibers). Unlike bone, the periosteum has nociceptive nerve endings and contains a store of bone-remodeling cells (osteoblasts) that play a role in healing fractures.[92]

The microstructure of bone is highly complex. In cortical bone, large vascular channels (Haversian canals and Volkmann canals) are oriented along the longitudinal direction of the bone and contain the blood supply to compact bone. These channels are surrounded by compact highly mineralized cylindrical rings (lamellae). The lamellae and Haversian canal form the osteon or Haversian systems, which is the chief structural unit of cortical bone.[93] Cancellous bone is spongy and fills the inside of many bones and has a rich vascular supply.[92,93]

Regarding the nanostructures, the mineral content of bone is mostly tiny mineral crystals (calcium phosphate–based hydroxyapatite), which provide rigidity and load-bearing strength to bone. The organic matrix is primarily composed of collagenous proteins, which crosslink to add stability to the bone matrix.[94,95] Collagenous proteins compose 85% to 90% of bone proteins, with bone matrix mainly composed of type I collagen.[91,94–96]

The primary cellular component of bone cells are osteocytes, osteoblasts, and osteoclasts. Osteoclasts are derived from a monocyte stem-cell lineage and carry out resorption of old bone, while osteoblasts are bone-forming cells and synthesize a new bone matrix. Osteoblasts are found in large numbers in the periosteum and endosteum, while osteocytes are osteoblasts that have become trapped in the calcified bone matrix. Together, osteoblasts and osteoclasts influence the remodeling of bone after trauma.[92]

Bone adapts to physical stimuli, dietary changes, or injury.[97] Bone is constantly undergoing remodeling to preserve bone strength. Remodeling occurs at sites that require repair but also occurs in a random manner throughout life.[98–100] Woven bone is put down rapidly during growth or repair, with fibers aligned at random. As a result, woven bone has lower strength than lamellar bone, which has its fibers oriented in parallel and in line with the axis of stress.[101]

Healing of cancellous bone with its rich vascular supply occurs more rapidly compared to the cortical bone that can be complicated by delay or nonunion. In normal fracture healing, osteoblasts form immature woven bone, resulting in early callus formation at the fracture margins. With remodeling, callus is replaced by lamellar bone.[92] Delayed union is when healing is slower than anticipated, and a nonunion of a fracture is defined as a fracture where healing has not occurred at 9 months.[102] There is a growing interest in orthobiologics for nonunion fractures, but there have been conflicting results in the literature.[103,104] Preclinical in vivo studies have suggested PRP may enhance bone regeneration with favorable results, but there are inherent limitations to the clinical translation of basic science studies and in the majority of studies PRP was used to augment surgery either at the time of surgery or a delayed injection.[103,105]

Fewer studies have examined autologous stem cells in nonunions,[106] and the real benefit of biologics for bone healing is unknown.[103,104]

Unlike fractures that are generally classified by mechanism of injury (i.e. traumatic, pathologic, stress), the events leading to avascular necrosis (AVN) are incompletely understood, have unclear causality, and have delayed diagnoses.[107,108] Ischemia or direct toxic effects on bone marrow and cells may contribute to AVN, and necrosis predominantly develops at sites composed predominantly of adipocytes (yellow marrow), such as the femoral head.[107] The natural history of AVN is better understood than the early triggering factors, with necrosis, inadequate remodeling, and eventually collapse of the necrotic segment and OA. Basic science and clinical trials of PRP may be more appropriate as an adjunct therapy, while autologous stem cells have shown promising results.[109,110]

Nerve Injury

Nervous tissue consists of two types of cells, neurons and glial cells.[111] Neurons are responsible for communication and are composed of the cell body (soma), dendrites, and axon. The dendrite receives information from other neurons, allowing the cell to integrate multiple impulses. Most cell bodies have multiple dendrites arising from the cell body, and dendrite-branching patterns are characteristic of each neuron. The axon arises from the cell body and propagates nerve impulses between cells, transporting nerve impulses along the axon, and the axon can branch repeatedly to communicate with many target cells. At the terminal end of the axon, synaptic junctions facilitate the transmission of the nerve impulse from one neuron to another or the target cell (muscle or gland cells) (Fig. 1.3).

Glial cells play a supporting role. The supporting glial cells differ in the central nervous system compared to the glial cells in the peripheral nervous system (PNS).[111] In the PNS, there are two types of glial cells: (1) satellite cells surrounding the cell bodies, and (2) Schwann cells ensheathing the axons with myelin. Myelin is a lipid-rich sheath that surrounds and insulates the axon and facilitates the transmission of electrical signals.[112,113]

Surrounding the peripheral nerve fibers and supporting the Schwann cell is connective tissue. Individual nerve fibers are embedded in the endoneurium, and each nerve fascicle is surrounded by the perineurium. The outermost connective tissue of the peripheral nerve is the epineurium.[114] A variety of mechanisms can injure the nerve. Systemic conditions include autoimmune inflammation or vasculitis, infectious, metabolic (i.e., diabetes mellitus), nutritional, toxin or drug-induced injury, or hereditary, and usually involve multiple nerves in multiple compartments or bilateral distributions.[115–122] Local pathology includes blunt or penetrating trauma, traction or stretch injury, or freezing injury.[123] Injury to the nerve can be divided into demyelinating and axonal pathology, involving a loss of the myelin sheath surrounding the axons or injury to the axon itself. Injury to the peripheral nerve can be classified according to the severity of injury, and different classification systems exist (Table 1.2).[124–126]

TABLE 1.2 Classification of Nerve Injury

Seddon	Sunderland	Nerve Injury
Neurapraxia	Grade I	Focal segment demyelination
Axonotemesis	Grade II	Axon damaged with intact endoneurium
Axonotemesis	Grade III	Axon and endoneurium damaged with intact perineurium
Axonotemesis	Grade IV	Axon, endoneurium, and perineurium damaged with intact epineurium
Neurotmesis	Grade V	Complete nerve transection

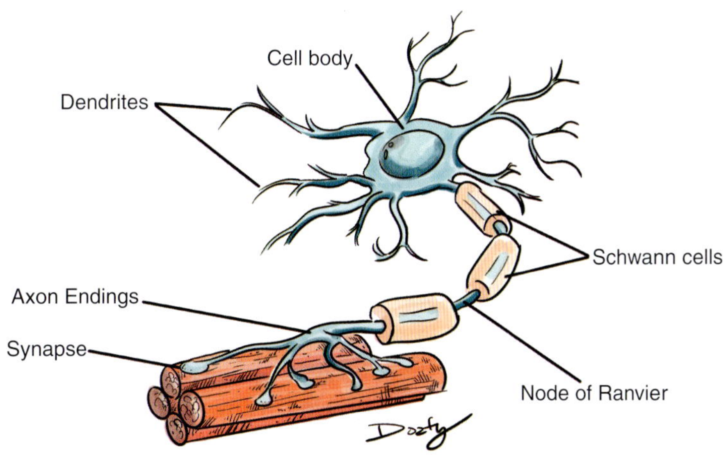

• **Fig. 1.3**

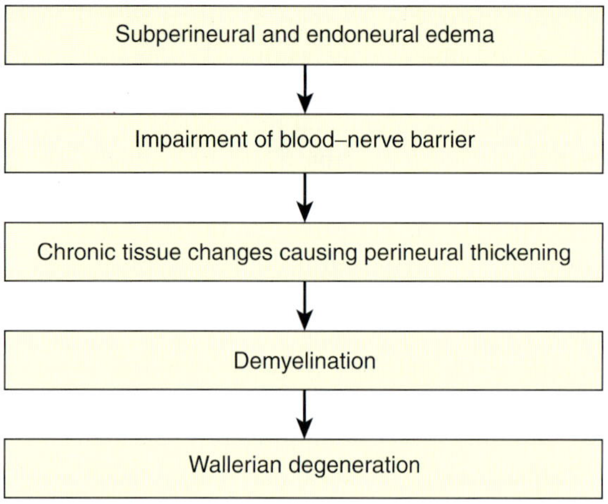

• **Fig. 1.4** Nerve Compression Pathology Cascade. (Modified from Barrett SL, Nickerson DS. *Pain Practice Management;* 2016.)

The type of trauma has a major influence on neurologic recovery, and injuries can vary from a mild injury due to compression resulting in mild or no pathologic changes to a traumatic stretch or penetrating injury with severely damaged and complete disruption of the normal nerve architecture. Compressive neuropathies can involve any peripheral nerve, are not always captured by the commonly used classification schemes, but generally fall under the general class of neuropraxia or Grade 1 nerve injuries. These are defined by focal demyelination at the site of compression and lack of axonal damage, although in later stages as the condition progresses, compression injuries can result in axonal damage.[123]

Chronic nerve compression injuries, such as carpal tunnel or cubital tunnel syndrome, are the most common peripheral nerve pathology.[127] The underlying pathophysiology of these focal entrapment neuropathies is primarily derived from animal models with bands or ligatures placed around the sciatic nerve.[128–133] While these models cannot reproduce in vivo nerve compression, the animal models have shown that physical compression with ligature or banding of the nerve can result in histologic changes and slowing of the nerve conduction velocity.[129,130,134] Increased pressure can compress the blood vessels that supply the nerve, impairing microcirculation and leading to epineural ischemia, venous stasis, and extraneural edema (Fig. 1.4).[135] This can result in fibroblast proliferation, connective tissue fibrosis and scaring around the nerve,[130] and late process focal demyelination and remyelination.[133,136,137] This process is distinct and different from traumatic crush injuries and results in Schwann cell proliferation in areas and thinner myelin following injury.[137,138] In many cases, compression or entrapment occurs in fibro-osseous structures formed by ligaments and bones but can also occur secondary to trauma and/or scar tissue.[139]

Treatment algorithms reflect the wide range of treatment options from medical to surgical management depending on the severity and duration of compression. Corticosteroid injections have a long history in managing carpal tunnel syndrome, but the role remains controversial with strong evidence only for short-term benefits.[140,141] Studies of corticosteroid injection for carpal tunnel syndrome have shown that the volume of the injectate does influence outcomes independent of the corticosteroid, with larger- volume injections significantly improving outcomes.[142] Hydrodissection of the surrounding constrictive tissue and flushing of inflammatory mediators has become more common clinically, but the literature on the hydrodissection of entrapment neuropathies is largely limited to case reports and retrospective studies.[139,143] Limited high-quality clinical data exist to determine the efficacy of these procedures. There is an increasing interest in biologics for nerve pathology, and a recent meta-analysis published in May 2020 of randomized trials comparing PRP to control groups (corticosteroid injection, saline injection, and splinting) for carpal tunnel syndrome demonstrated significant and similar improvement in visual analog score for pain and nerve conduction studies in the PRP group compared to controls.[144] In recalcitrant cases, peripheral nerve decompression procedures vary widely, and there has been increased interest in limiting incision size and minimally invasive approaches.[145]

Muscle Injury

The basic cellular unit of skeletal muscle is myocytes, or muscle fibers. A network of connective tissue (endomysium) surrounds each muscle fiber. Adjacent fibers are bundled together in a fasciculus and surrounded by the perimysium, and fasciculi are grouped together to form the complete muscle and are surrounded by epimysium (Fig. 1.5).[146] Each muscle fiber is composed of thousands of myofibrils, and the subunits are known as sarcomeres. The sarcomere is the basic contractile unit of a single muscle fiber and is composed of protein filaments that line up in parallel with overlapping sets of actin (thin filaments) and myosin (thick filaments).[147]

Myocytes are surrounded by a cell, or plasma membrane (plasmalemma), that along with various layers of the basement membrane for the sarcolemma provide external support and help maintain the shape of the muscle fiber.[146] In some texts, the plasmalemma and sarcolemma are used interchangeably. The sarcoplasmic reticulum and T system is a tubular system running parallel to the myofibrils and allows communication by relaying nerve impulses along the fibers and delivering calcium to the cells, which is necessary for muscle contraction.[146]

Nerve axon terminals interdigitate with the motor endplate of the muscle membrane, forming a neuromuscular junction (NMJ).[146] When an action potential reaches the axon terminal, acetylcholine (ACh) crosses the NMJ and binds to receptors on the plasmalemma, and this process is what is inhibited with botulinum toxin (for more, refer to Chapter 11). Having depolarized the muscle membrane,

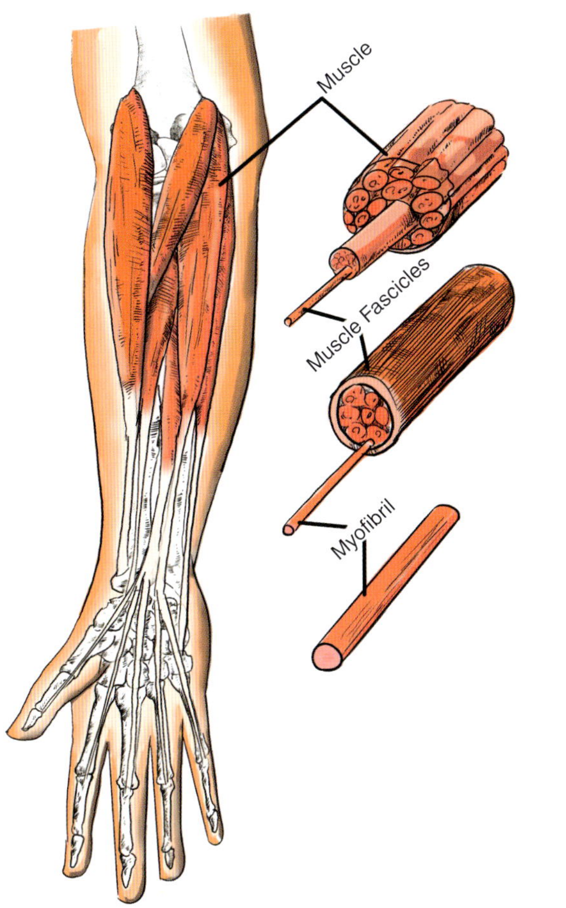

• **Fig. 1.5** The Hierarchical Structure of a Muscle. (2022). Used with permission of Elsevier.

the action potential spreads rapidly along the muscle fiber, releasing calcium from the sarcoplasmic reticulum and resulting in a muscle contraction as the actin and myosin fibers bind and slide in a ratchet-like fashion, shortening the muscle.[146]

Muscle fibers are classified into two groups, type I (slow-twitch) and type II (fast-twitch) fibers. Slow-twitch and fast-twitch fibers refer to the time taken for each type of fiber to reach peak tension, 110 milliseconds (ms) and 50 ms, respectively.[146] Fiber types differ in the form of myosin ATPase, structure of the sarcoplasmic reticulum, and neural innervation, with more fibers per motor neuron in type II fast-twitch fibers.[148] Type I fibers are used in low-intensity or endurance events, and type II fibers are used in short duration, high-intensity activities.

Skeletal muscle has a robust capacity for regeneration after focal injuries but is dependent on the type of injury and severity.[149–151] Muscle injuries caused by eccentric contraction typically damage the myofibrils, while other acute injuries (laceration, contusions, toxins, or thermal injury) largely damage the muscle cell membrane.[152] Skeletal muscle can compensate for up to a 20% loss in muscle mass, but beyond this, muscle injuries with significant volumetric loss typically will not heal without scar tissue formation and denervation of the muscle distal to the site of injury.[151,153] A loss of skeletal muscle mass (sarcopenia) occurs with aging, and aged muscles can also show an impaired response to injury.[149,154]

Tearing in muscle tissue creates a gap between the retracted fibers, and a hematoma will form at the site of injury. The interaction growth factor in muscle regeneration is a complex process, but there has been an interest in controlling the regenerative microenvironment.[150,151,155–158] The repair process has been described in detail in a number of articles. In brief, resident myogenic precursors (satellite cells) that are dormant in the periphery of healthy skeletal myofibers respond to signals coming from damaged myofibers and create new fibers. Over time, these nascent muscle fibers will continue to bridge the gap.[149,159]

The local milieu of certain growth factors can have varied effects on skeletal muscle cells. High concentrations of certain growth factors have been shown to promote myoblast proliferation and prevent differentiation, while low concentrations may induce myoblast differentiation and multinucleated cell formation.[160–162] PRP has shown a contradictory effect on myogenic differentiation and may even result in a fibrotic response, possibly due to variations in PRP preparation or dosing.[150] Recently platelet-poor plasma (PPP) preparations have shown a robust ability to induce human myoblast differentiation in vivo, and while PPP may hold promise, no consensus exists and additional investigation is needed.[155]

How to Use this Book

The primary objective of this text is to provide a reference to inject most areas of the musculoskeletal system safely and accurately. This text includes a comprehensive atlas section, which details techniques to safely approach ultrasound and fluoroscopically guided musculoskeletal and axial injections. It discusses the different types of injectates the practitioner should consider when approaching these structures and introduces new procedures and future trends. The text provides the most up-to-date literature on biologic injectates, techniques, indications, and supporting evidence for varying techniques. However, some of the newer techniques described may not be validated in the current literature, and many do not have a clear consensus on the appropriate injectates. Nevertheless, as more research emerges and our understanding of the role of orthobiolgics or other injectates emerges, this book will still be relevant as a comprehensive guided injection atlas. Additionally, we hope this text will also stimulate new research and innovation that helps advance the field of interventional orthopedics.

This text and atlas should serve as a reference tool and an adjunct to formal training. It is not meant to replace in-person instruction and hands-on training. This text does not seek to teach a comprehensive orthopedic history and physical examination, how to interpret imaging studies, or how to perform a diagnostic musculoskeletal ultrasound. Clinicians should also understand alternative treatments, including less-invasive options such as diet/weight loss, orthotics and bracing, acupuncture, manual techniques and physical/occupational therapy, and surgical indications to properly counsel patients and to review all the treatment options available.

References

1. Finnoff JT, Hall MM, Adams E, et al. American Medical Society for Sports Medicine (AMSSM) position statement: interventional musculoskeletal ultrasound in sports medicine. *PM R.* 2015;7(2):151–168.e112.
2. Smith J, Finnoff JT. Diagnostic and interventional musculoskeletal ultrasound: part 1. Fundamentals. *PM R.* 2009;1(1):64–75.
3. Valente CM, Wagner SM. History of the American Institute of Ultrasound in Medicine. *J Ultrasound Med.* 2005;24(2):131–142.
4. Lohmander LS, Englund PM, Dahl LL, Roos EM. The long-term consequence of anterior cruciate ligament and meniscus injuries: osteoarthritis. *Am J Sports Med.* 2007;35(10):1756–1769.
5. Louw A, Diener I, Fernandez-de-Las-Penas C, Puentedura EJ. Sham surgery in orthopedics: a systematic review of the literature. *Pain Med.* 2017;18(4):736–750.
6. Coombes BK, Bisset L, Vicenzino B. Efficacy and safety of corticosteroid injections and other injections for management of tendinopathy: a systematic review of randomised controlled trials. *Lancet.* 2010;376(9754):1751–1767.
7. Wernecke C, Braun HJ, Dragoo JL. The effect of intra-articular corticosteroids on articular cartilage: a systematic review. *Orthop J Sports Med.* 2015;3(5):2325967115581163.
8. Jayaram P, Kennedy DJ, Yeh P, Dragoo J. Chondrotoxic effects of local anesthetics on human knee articular cartilage: a systematic review. *PM R.* 2019;11(4):379–400.
9. Cohen SB, Short CP, O'Hagan T, Wu HT, Morrison WB, Zoga AC. The effect of meniscal tears on cartilage loss of the knee: findings on serial MRIs. *Phys Sportsmed.* 2012;40(3):66–76.
10. Katz JN, Shrestha S, Losina E, et al. Five-year outcome of operative and nonoperative management of meniscal tear in persons older than forty-five years. *Arthritis Rheumatol.* 2020;72(2):273–281.
11. Khan M, Evaniew N, Bedi A, Ayeni OR, Bhandari M. Arthroscopic surgery for degenerative tears of the meniscus: a systematic review and meta-analysis. *CMAJ (Can Med Assoc J).* 2014;186(14):1057–1064.
12. Sihvonen R, Paavola M, Malmivaara A, et al. Arthroscopic partial meniscectomy versus placebo surgery for a degenerative meniscus tear: a 2-year follow-up of the randomised controlled trial. *Ann Rheum Dis.* 2018;77(2):188–195.
13. Sihvonen R, Paavola M, Malmivaara A, et al. Arthroscopic partial meniscectomy versus sham surgery for a degenerative meniscal tear. *N Engl J Med.* 2013;369(26):2515–2524.
14. Lubowitz JH, Brand JC, Rossi MJ. Nonoperative management of degenerative meniscus tears is worth a try. *Arthroscopy.* 2020;36(2):327–328.
15. Netravali NA, Giori NJ, Andriacchi TP. Partial medial meniscectomy and rotational differences at the knee during walking. *J Biomech.* 2010;43(15):2948–2953.
16. Thorlund JB, Juhl CB, Roos EM, Lohmander LS. Arthroscopic surgery for degenerative knee: systematic review and meta-analysis of benefits and harms. *BMJ.* 2015;350:h2747.
17. Moseley JB, O'Malley K, Petersen NJ, et al. A controlled trial of arthroscopic surgery for osteoarthritis of the knee. *N Engl J Med.* 2002;347(2):81–88.
18. Karjalainen TV, Jain NB, Page CM, et al. Subacromial decompression surgery for rotator cuff disease. *Cochrane Database Syst Rev.* 2019;1:Cd005619.
19. Saltychev M, Virolainen P, Laimi K. Conservative treatment or surgery for shoulder impingement: updated meta-analysis. *Disabil Rehabil.* 2019:1–2.
20. Khan M, Alolabi B, Horner N, Bedi A, Ayeni OR, Bhandari M. Surgery for shoulder impingement: a systematic review and meta-analysis of controlled clinical trials. *CMAJ Open.* 2019;7(1):E149–e158.
21. Toliopoulos P, Desmeules F, Boudreault J, et al. Efficacy of surgery for rotator cuff tendinopathy: a systematic review. *Clin Rheumatol.* 2014;33(10):1373–1383.
22. Sharma P, Maffulli N. Tendon injury and tendinopathy: healing and repair. *J Bone Joint Surg Am.* 2005;87(1):187–202.
23. Benjamin M, Kaiser E, Milz S. Structure-function relationships in tendons: a review. *J Anat.* 2008;212(3):211–228.
24. Bozec L, van der Heijden G, Horton M. Collagen fibrils: nanoscale ropes. *Biophys J.* 2007;92(1):70–75.
25. Kirkendall DT, Garrett WE. Function and biomechanics of tendons. *Scand J Med Sci Sports.* 1997;7(2):62–66.
26. Kraemer R, Wuerfel W, Lorenzen J, Busche M, Vogt PM, Knobloch K. Analysis of hereditary and medical risk factors in Achilles tendinopathy and Achilles tendon ruptures: a matched pair analysis. *Arch Orthop Trauma Surg.* 2012;132(6):847–853.
27. Murrell GA. Understanding tendinopathies. *Br J Sports Med.* 2002;36(6):392–393.
28. Franceschi F, Papalia R, Paciotti M, et al. Obesity as a risk factor for tendinopathy: a systematic review. *Int J Endocrinol.* 2014;2014:670262.
29. Scott A, Backman LJ. Speed C. Tendinopathy: update on pathophysiology. *J Orthop Sports Phys Ther.* 2015;45(11):833–841.
30. Scott A, Lian O, Bahr R, Hart DA, Duronio V, Khan KM. Increased mast cell numbers in human patellar tendinosis: correlation with symptom duration and vascular hyperplasia. *Br J Sports Med.* 2008;42(9):753–757.
31. Millar NL, Hueber AJ, Reilly JH, et al. Inflammation is present in early human tendinopathy. *Am J Sports Med.* 2010;38(10):2085–2091.
32. Kragsnaes MS, Fredberg U, Stribolt K, Kjaer SG, Bendix K, Ellingsen T. Stereological quantification of immune-competent cells in baseline biopsy specimens from Achilles tendons: results from patients with chronic tendinopathy followed for more than 4 years. *Am J Sports Med.* 2014;42(10):2435–2445.
33. Maffulli N, Khan KM, Puddu G. Overuse tendon conditions: time to change a confusing terminology. *Arthroscopy.* 1998;14(8):840–843.
34. Cook JL, Purdam CR. Is tendon pathology a continuum? A pathology model to explain the clinical presentation of load-induced tendinopathy. *Br J Sports Med.* 2009;43(6):409–416.
35. Cook JL, Rio E, Purdam CR, Docking SI. Revisiting the continuum model of tendon pathology: what is its merit in clinical practice and research? *Br J Sports Med.* 2016;50(19):1187–1191.
36. McCreesh K, Lewis J. Continuum model of tendon pathology—where are we now? *Int J Exp Pathol.* 2013;94(4):242–247.

37. Frank CB. Ligament structure, physiology and function. *J Musculoskelet Neuronal Interact.* 2004;4(2):199–201.
38. Rumian AP, Wallace AL, Birch HL. Tendons and ligaments are anatomically distinct but overlap in molecular and morphological features—a comparative study in an ovine model. *J Orthop Res.* 2007;25(4):458–464.
39. Bray RC, Fisher AW, Frank CB. Fine vascular anatomy of adult rabbit knee ligaments. *J Anat.* 1990;172:69–79.
40. Molloy T, Wang Y, Murrell G. The roles of growth factors in tendon and ligament healing. *Sports Med.* 2003;33(5):381–394.
41. Amiel D, Frank CB, Harwood FL, Akeson WH, Kleiner JB. Collagen alteration in medial collateral ligament healing in a rabbit model. *Connect Tissue Res.* 1987;16(4):357–366.
42. Frank C, McDonald D, Wilson J, Eyre D, Shrive N. Rabbit medial collateral ligament scar weakness is associated with decreased collagen pyridinoline crosslink density. *J Orthop Res.* 1995;13(2):157–165.
43. Lo IK, Ou Y, Rattner JP, et al. The cellular networks of normal ovine medial collateral and anterior cruciate ligaments are not accurately recapitulated in scar tissue. *J Anat.* 2002;200(Pt 3):283–296.
44. Frank C, McDonald D, Bray D, et al. Collagen fibril diameters in the healing adult rabbit medial collateral ligament. *Connect Tissue Res.* 1992;27(4):251–263.
45. Bray RC, Rangayyan RM, Frank CB. Normal and healing ligament vascularity: a quantitative histological assessment in the adult rabbit medial collateral ligament. *J Anat.* 1996;188(Pt 1):87–95.
46. Plaas AH, Wong-Palms S, Koob T, Hernandez D, Marchuk L, Frank CB. Proteoglycan metabolism during repair of the ruptured medial collateral ligament in skeletally mature rabbits. *Arch Biochem Biophys.* 2000;374(1):35–41.
47. Jack EA. Experimental rupture of the medial collateral ligament of the knee. *J Bone Joint Surg Br.* 1950;32-b(3):396–402.
48. Shrive N, Chimich D, Marchuk L, Wilson J, Brant R, Frank C. Soft-tissue "flaws" are associated with the material properties of the healing rabbit medial collateral ligament. *J Orthop Res.* 1995;13(6):923–929.
49. Woo SL, Matthews JV, Akeson WH, Amiel D, Convery FR. Connective tissue response to immobility. Correlative study of biomechanical and biochemical measurements of normal and immobilized rabbit knees. *Arthritis Rheum.* 1975;18(3):257–264.
50. Bray RC, Shrive NG, Frank CB, Chimich DD. The early effects of joint immobilization on medial collateral ligament healing in an ACL-deficient knee: a gross anatomic and biomechanical investigation in the adult rabbit model. *J Orthop Res.* 1992;10(2):157–166.
51. Hart DP, Dahners LE. Healing of the medial collateral ligament in rats. The effects of repair, motion, and secondary stabilizing ligaments. *J Bone Joint Surg Am.* 1987;69(8):1194–1199.
52. Tipton CM, James SL, Mergner W, Tcheng TK. Influence of exercise on strength of medial collateral knee ligaments of dogs. *Am J Physiol.* 1970;218(3):894–902.
53. Goldstein WM, Barmada R. Early mobilization of rabbit medial collateral ligament repairs: biomechanic and histologic study. *Arch Phys Med Rehabil.* 1984;65(5):239–242.
54. Liu Y, Kalen A, Risto O, Wahlstrom O. Fibroblast proliferation due to exposure to a platelet concentrate in vitro is pH dependent. *Wound Repair Regen.* 2002;10(5):336–340.
55. Yilgor C, Yilgor Huri P, Huri G. Tissue engineering strategies in ligament regeneration. *Stem Cells Int.* 2012;2012:374676.
56. Armiento AR, Alini M, Stoddart MJ. Articular fibrocartilage—why does hyaline cartilage fail to repair? *Adv Drug Deliv Rev.* 2019;146:289–305.
57. Loeser RF, Goldring SR, Scanzello CR, Goldring MB. Osteoarthritis: a disease of the joint as an organ. *Arthritis Rheum.* 2012;64(6):1697–1707.
58. O'Hara BP, Urban JP, Maroudas A. Influence of cyclic loading on the nutrition of articular cartilage. *Ann Rheum Dis.* 1990;49(7):536–539.
59. Blagojevic M, Jinks C, Jeffery A, Jordan KP. Risk factors for onset of osteoarthritis of the knee in older adults: a systematic review and meta-analysis. *Osteoarthritis Cartilage.* 2010;18(1):24–33.
60. Andriacchi TP, Mundermann A, Smith RL, Alexander EJ, Dyrby CO, Koo S. A framework for the in vivo pathomechanics of osteoarthritis at the knee. *Ann Biomed Eng.* 2004;32(3):447–457.
61. Goldring MB, Marcu KB. Cartilage homeostasis in health and rheumatic diseases. *Arthritis Res Ther.* 2009;11(3):224.
62. Wehling N, Palmer GD, Pilapil C, et al. Interleukin-1beta and tumor necrosis factor alpha inhibit chondrogenesis by human mesenchymal stem cells through NF-kappaB-dependent pathways. *Arthritis Rheum.* 2009;60(3):801–812.
63. Shakibaei M, Schulze-Tanzil G, John T, Mobasheri A. Curcumin protects human chondrocytes from IL-l1beta-induced inhibition of collagen type II and beta1-integrin expression and activation of caspase-3: an immunomorphological study. *Ann Anat.* 2005;187(5–6):487–497.
64. Simkin PA. Synovial perfusion and synovial fluid solutes. *Ann Rheum Dis.* 1995;54(5):424–428.
65. Simkin PA, Bassett JE, Koh EM. Synovial perfusion in the human knee: a methodologic analysis. *Semin Arthritis Rheum.* 1995;25(1):56–66.
66. Delgado D, Garate A, Vincent H, et al. Current concepts in intraosseous Platelet-Rich Plasma injections for knee osteoarthritis. *J Clin Orthop Trauma.* 2019;10(1):36–41.
67. Sundaram K, Vargas-Hernandez JS, Sanchez TR, et al. Are subchondral intraosseous injections effective and safe for the treatment of knee osteoarthritis? A systematic review. *J Knee Surg.* 2019;32(11):1046–1057.
68. Benjamin M, Evans EJ. Fibrocartilage. *J Anat.* 1990;171:1–15.
69. Raj PP. Intervertebral disc: anatomy-physiology-pathophysiology-treatment. *Pain Pract.* 2008;8(1):18–44.
70. Inoue H. Three-dimensional architecture of lumbar intervertebral discs. *Spine (Phila Pa 1976).* 1981;6(2):139–146.
71. Marchand F, Ahmed AM. Investigation of the laminate structure of lumbar disc anulus fibrosus. *Spine (Phila Pa 1976).* 1990;15(5):402–410.
72. Buckwalter JA. Aging and degeneration of the human intervertebral disc. *Spine (Phila Pa 1976).* 1995;20(11):1307–1314.
73. Lyons G, Eisenstein SM, Sweet MB. Biochemical changes in intervertebral disc degeneration. *Biochim Biophys Acta.* 1981;673(4):443–453.
74. Antoniou J, Steffen T, Nelson F, et al. The human lumbar intervertebral disc: evidence for changes in the biosynthesis and denaturation of the extracellular matrix with growth, maturation, ageing, and degeneration. *J Clin Invest.* 1996;98(4):996–1003.
75. Hollander AP, Heathfield TF, Liu JJ, et al. Enhanced denaturation of the alpha (II) chains of type-II collagen in normal adult human intervertebral discs compared with femoral articular cartilage. *J Orthop Res.* 1996;14(1):61–66.
76. Frobin W, Brinckmann P, Kramer M, Hartwig E. Height of lumbar discs measured from radiographs compared with degeneration and height classified from MR images. *Eur Radiol.* 2001;11(2):263–269.

77. Adams MA, McNally DS, Dolan P. 'Stress' distributions inside intervertebral discs. The effects of age and degeneration. *J Bone Joint Surg Br*. 1996;78(6):965–972.
78. De Geer CM. Intervertebral disk nutrients and transport mechanisms in relation to disk degeneration: a narrative literature review. *J Chiropr Med*. 2018;17(2):97–105.
79. Monfett M, Harrison J, Boachie-Adjei K, Lutz G. Intradiscal platelet-rich plasma (PRP) injections for discogenic low back pain: an update. *Int Orthop*. 2016;40(6):1321–1328.
80. Arnoczky SP, Warren RF. Microvasculature of the human meniscus. *Am J Sports Med*. 1982;10(2):90–95.
81. Johnson D, Weiss B. Meniscal repair using the inside-out suture technique. *Sports Med Arthrosc Rev*. 2012;20(2):68–76.
82. Melrose J, Smith S, Cake M, Read R, Whitelock J. Comparative spatial and temporal localisation of perlecan, aggrecan and type I, II and IV collagen in the ovine meniscus: an ageing study. *Histochem Cell Biol*. 2005;124(3–4):225–235.
83. Cheung HS. Distribution of type I, II, III and V in the pepsin solubilized collagens in bovine menisci. *Connect Tissue Res*. 1987;16(4):343–356.
84. Muhammad H, Schminke B, Bode C, et al. Human migratory meniscus progenitor cells are controlled via the TGF-beta pathway. *Stem Cell Reports*. 2014;3(5):789–803.
85. Blackmore SA, McGee Jr AW, Gladstone JN, Strauss EJ, Davidson PA, Jazrawi LM. The management of meniscal pathology: from partial meniscectomy to transplantation. *Instr Course Lect*. 2015;64:511–520.
86. Seol D, Zhou C, Brouillette MJ, et al. Characteristics of meniscus progenitor cells migrated from injured meniscus. *J Orthop Res*. 2017;35(9):1966–1972.
87. Osawa A, Harner CD, Gharaibeh B, et al. The use of blood vessel-derived stem cells for meniscal regeneration and repair. *Med Sci Sports Exerc*. 2013;45(5):813–823.
88. Longo UG, Campi S, Romeo G, Spiezia F, Maffulli N, Denaro V. Biological strategies to enhance healing of the avascular area of the meniscus. *Stem Cells Int*. 2012;2012:528359.
89. Pittenger MF, Mackay AM, Beck SC, et al. Multilineage potential of adult human mesenchymal stem cells. *Science*. 1999;284(5411):143–147.
90. Taichman RS. Blood and bone: two tissues whose fates are intertwined to create the hematopoietic stem-cell niche. *Blood*. 2005;105(7):2631–2639.
91. Rho JY, Kuhn-Spearing L, Zioupos P. Mechanical properties and the hierarchical structure of bone. *Med Eng Phys*. 1998;20(2):92–102.
92. MacMahon P, Eustace SJ. General principles. *Semin Musculoskelet Radiol*. 2006;10(4):243–248.
93. Al-Rekabi Z, Fura AM, Juhlin I, Yassin A, Popowics TE, Sniadecki NJ. Hyaluronan-CD44 interactions mediate contractility and migration in periodontal ligament cells. *Cell Adh Migr*. 2019;13(1):138–150.
94. Ritchie RO. How does human bone resist fracture? *Ann N Y Acad Sci*. 2010;1192:72–80.
95. Unal M, Creecy A, Nyman JS. The role of matrix composition in the mechanical behavior of bone. *Curr Osteoporos Rep*. 2018;16(3):205–215.
96. Clarke B. Normal bone anatomy and physiology. *Clin J Am Soc Nephrol*. 2008;3 suppl 3(suppl 3):S131–S139.
97. Wohl GR, Boyd SK, Judex S, Zernicke RF. Functional adaptation of bone to exercise and injury. *J Sci Med Sport*. 2000;3(3):313–324.
98. Burr DB. Targeted and nontargeted remodeling. *Bone*. 2002;30(1):2–4.
99. Parfitt AM. Targeted and nontargeted bone remodeling: relationship to basic multicellular unit origination and progression. *Bone*. 2002;30(1):5–7.
100. Teitelbaum SL, Abu-Amer Y, Ross FP. Molecular mechanisms of bone resorption. *J Cell Biochem*. 1995;59(1):1–10.
101. Dalle Carbonare L, Valenti MT, Bertoldo F, et al. Bone microarchitecture evaluated by histomorphometry. *Micron*. 2005;36(7–8):609–616.
102. Calori GM, Mazza EL, Mazzola S, et al. Non-unions. *Clin Cases Miner Bone Metab*. 2017;14(2):186–188.
103. Roffi A, Di Matteo B, Krishnakumar GS, Kon E, Filardo G. Platelet-rich plasma for the treatment of bone defects: from preclinical rational to evidence in the clinical practice. A systematic review. *Int Orthop*. 2017;41(2):221–237.
104. Ghaffarpasand F, Dehghankhalili M, Shahrezaei M. Platelet rich plasma for traumatic non-union fractures: a novel but controversial bone regeneration strategy. *Bull Emerg Trauma*. 2013;1(3):99–101.
105. Wei LC, Lei GH, Sheng PY, et al. Efficacy of platelet-rich plasma combined with allograft bone in the management of displaced intra-articular calcaneal fractures: a prospective cohort study. *J Orthop Res*. 2012;30(10):1570–1576.
106. Ho-Shui-Ling A, Bolander J, Rustom LE, Johnson AW, Luyten FP, Picart C. Bone regeneration strategies: engineered scaffolds, bioactive molecules and stem cells current stage and future perspectives. *Biomaterials*. 2018;180:143–162.
107. Lafforgue P. Pathophysiology and natural history of avascular necrosis of bone. *Joint Bone Spine*. 2006;73(5):500–507.
108. Guerado E, Caso E. The physiopathology of avascular necrosis of the femoral head: an update. *Injury*. 2016;47(suppl 6):S16–s26.
109. Han J, Gao F, Li Y, et al. The use of platelet-rich plasma for the treatment of osteonecrosis of the femoral head: a systematic review. *BioMed Res Int*. 2020;2020:2642439.
110. Li R, Lin QX, Liang XZ, et al. Stem cell therapy for treating osteonecrosis of the femoral head: from clinical applications to related basic research. *Stem Cell Res Ther*. 2018;9(1):291.
111. Jessen KR. Glial cells. *Int J Biochem Cell Biol*. 2004;36(10):1861–1867.
112. Feltri ML, Poitelon Y, Previtali SC. How Schwann cells sort axons: new concepts. *Neuroscientist*. 2016;22(3):252–265.
113. Nave KA, Werner HB. Myelination of the nervous system: mechanisms and functions. *Annu Rev Cell Dev Biol*. 2014;30:503–533.
114. Thomas PK. The connective tissue of peripheral nerve: an electron microscope study. *J Anat*. 1963;97(Pt 1):35–44.
115. Cojocaru IM, Cojocaru M, Silosi I, Vrabie CD. Peripheral nervous system manifestations in systemic autoimmune diseases. *Maedica (Buchar)*. 2014;9(3):289–294.
116. Sampaio L, Silva LG, Terroso G, Nadais G, Mariz E, Ventura F. Vasculitic neuropathy. *Acta Reumatol Port*. 2011;36(2):102–109.
117. de Freitas MR. Infectious neuropathy. *Curr Opin Neurol*. 2007;20(5):548–552.
118. Eggermann K, Gess B, Häusler M, Weis J, Hahn A, Kurth I. Hereditary neuropathies. *Dtsch Arztebl Int*. 2018;115(6):91–97.
119. Weis S, Büttner A. Nutritional and systemic metabolic disorders. *Handb Clin Neurol*. 2017;145:167–173.
120. Vinik A, Casellini C, Nevoret ML. Diabetic neuropathies. In: Feingold KR, Anawalt B, Boyce A, et al., eds. *Endotext. South Dartmouth (MA)*. MDText.com, Inc. Copyright © 2000-2020, MDText.com, Inc.; 2000.
121. Weimer LH, Sachdev N. Update on medication-induced peripheral neuropathy. *Curr Neurol Neurosci Rep*. 2009;9(1):69–75.

122. Pratt RW, Weimer LH. Medication and toxin-induced peripheral neuropathy. *Semin Neurol.* 2005;25(2):204–216.
123. Menorca RM, Fussell TS, Elfar JC. Nerve physiology: mechanisms of injury and recovery. *Hand Clin.* 2013;29(3):317–330.
124. Sunderland S. A classification of peripheral nerve injuries producing loss of function. *Brain.* 1951;74(4):491–516.
125. Seddon HJ, Medawar PB, Smith H. Rate of regeneration of peripheral nerves in man. *J Physiol.* 1943;102(2):191–215.
126. Seddon HJ. A classification of nerve injuries. *Br Med J.* 1942;2(4260):237–239.
127. Shiri R. The prevalence and incidence of carpal tunnel syndrome in US working populations. *Scand J Work Environ Health.* 2014;40(1):101–102.
128. Bennett GJ, Xie YK. A peripheral mononeuropathy in rat that produces disorders of pain sensation like those seen in man. *Pain.* 1988;33(1):87–107.
129. Liu ZY, Chen ZB, Chen JH. A novel chronic nerve compression model in the rat. *Neural Regen Res.* 2018;13(8):1477–1485.
130. O'Brien JP, Mackinnon SE, MacLean AR, Hudson AR, Dellon AL, Hunter DA. A model of chronic nerve compression in the rat. *Ann Plast Surg.* 1987;19(5):430–435.
131. Mackinnon SE, Dellon AL, Hudson AR, Hunter DA. Chronic nerve compression—an experimental model in the rat. *Ann Plast Surg.* 1984;13(2):112–120.
132. Gupta R, Steward O. Chronic nerve compression induces concurrent apoptosis and proliferation of Schwann cells. *J Comp Neurol.* 2003;461(2):174–186.
133. Pham K, Gupta R. Understanding the mechanisms of entrapment neuropathies. Review article. *Neurosurg Focus.* 2009;26(2):E7.
134. Tapadia M, Mozaffar T, Gupta R. Compressive neuropathies of the upper extremity: update on pathophysiology, classification, and electrodiagnostic findings. *J Hand Surg Am.* 2010;35(4):668–677.
135. Rydevik B, Lundborg G, Bagge U. Effects of graded compression on intraneural blood blow. An in vivo study on rabbit tibial nerve. *J Hand Surg Am.* 1981;6(1):3–12.
136. Mackinnon SE. Pathophysiology of nerve compression. *Hand Clin.* 2002;18(2):231–241.
137. Mackinnon SE, Dellon AL, Hudson AR, Hunter DA. Chronic human nerve compression—a histological assessment. *Neuropathol Appl Neurobiol.* 1986;12(6):547–565.
138. Ludwin SK, Maitland M. Long-term remyelination fails to reconstitute normal thickness of central myelin sheaths. *J Neurol Sci.* 1984;64(2):193–198.
139. Trescot A, Brown M. Peripheral nerve entrapment, hydrodissection, and neural regenerative strategies. *Tech Reg Anesth Pain Manag.* 2015;19(1):85–93.
140. Marshall S, Tardif G, Ashworth N. Local corticosteroid injection for carpal tunnel syndrome. *Cochrane Database Syst Rev.* 2007;(2):Cd001554.
141. Huisstede BM, Hoogvliet P, Randsdorp MS, Glerum S, van Middelkoop M, Koes BW. Carpal tunnel syndrome. Part I: effectiveness of nonsurgical treatments—a systematic review. *Arch Phys Med Rehabil.* 2010;91(7):981–1004.
142. Evers S, Bryan AJ, Sanders TL, Gunderson T, Gelfman R, Amadio PC. Influence of injection volume on rate of subsequent intervention in carpal tunnel syndrome over 1-year follow-up. *J Hand Surg Am.* 2018;43(6):537–544.
143. Cass SP. Ultrasound-guided nerve hydrodissection: what is it? A review of the literature. *Curr Sports Med Rep.* 2016;15(1): 20–22.
144. Catapano M, Catapano J, Borschel G, Alavinia SM, Robinson LR, Mittal N. Effectiveness of platelet-rich plasma injections for nonsurgical management of carpal tunnel syndrome: a systematic review and meta-analysis of randomized controlled trials. *Arch Phys Med Rehabil.* 2020;101(5):897–906.
145. Ducic I, Endara M, Al-Attar A, Quadri H. Minimally invasive peripheral nerve surgery: a short scar technique. *Microsurgery.* 2010;30(8):622–626.
146. Exeter D, Connell DA. Skeletal muscle: functional anatomy and pathophysiology. *Semin Musculoskelet Radiol.* 2010;14(2):97–105.
147. Squire J. Special issue: the actin-myosin interaction in muscle: background and overview. *Int J Mol Sci.* 2019;20(22).
148. Bottinelli R, Reggiani C. Human skeletal muscle fibres: molecular and functional diversity. *Prog Biophys Mol Biol.* 2000;73(2–4):195–262.
149. Ehrhardt J, Morgan J. Regenerative capacity of skeletal muscle. *Curr Opin Neurol.* 2005;18(5):548–553.
150. Chellini F, Tani A, Zecchi-Orlandini S, Sassoli C. Influence of platelet-rich and platelet-poor plasma on endogenous mechanisms of skeletal muscle repair/regeneration. *Int J Mol Sci.* 2019;20(3).
151. Turner NJ, Badylak SF. Regeneration of skeletal muscle. *Cell Tissue Res.* 2012;347(3):759–774.
152. Tidball JG. Mechanisms of muscle injury, repair, and regeneration. *Compr Physiol.* 2011;1(4):2029–2062.
153. Liu J, Saul D, Böker KO, Ernst J, Lehman W, Schilling AF. Current methods for skeletal muscle tissue repair and regeneration. *BioMed Res Int.* 2018;2018:1984879.
154. Rosenberg IH. Sarcopenia: origins and clinical relevance. *J Nutr.* 1997;127(suppl 5):990s–991s.
155. Miroshnychenko O, Chang WT, Dragoo JL. The use of platelet-rich and platelet-poor plasma to enhance differentiation of skeletal myoblasts: implications for the use of autologous blood products for muscle regeneration. *Am J Sports Med.* 2017;45(4):945–953.
156. Huard J, Li Y, Fu FH. Muscle injuries and repair: current trends in research. *J Bone Joint Surg Am.* 2002;84(5):822–832.
157. Järvinen TA, Järvinen TL, Kääriäinen M, Kalimo H, Järvinen M. Muscle injuries: biology and treatment. *Am J Sports Med.* 2005;33(5):745–764.
158. Garrett Jr WE, Seaber AV, Boswick J, Urbaniak JR, Goldner JL. Recovery of skeletal muscle after laceration and repair. *J Hand Surg Am.* 1984;9(5):683–692.
159. Hurme T, Kalimo H. Activation of myogenic precursor cells after muscle injury. *Med Sci Sports Exerc.* 1992;24(2): 197–205.
160. Allen RE, Boxhorn LK. Inhibition of skeletal muscle satellite cell differentiation by transforming growth factor-beta. *J Cell Physiol.* 1987;133(3):567–572.
161. Liu D, Black BL, Derynck R. TGF-beta inhibits muscle differentiation through functional repression of myogenic transcription factors by Smad3. *Genes Dev.* 2001;15(22):2950–2966.
162. Mendias CL, Gumucio JP, Davis ME, Bromley CW, Davis CS, Brooks SV. Transforming growth factor-beta induces skeletal muscle atrophy and fibrosis through the induction of atrogin-1 and scleraxis. *Muscle Nerve.* 2012;45(1):55–59.
163. Barrett SL, Nickerson DS. Nerve decompression surgery can reverse neuropathy of the foot pain practice management. https://www.practicalpainmanagement.com/pain/neuropathic/diabetic-neuropathy/nerve-decompression-surgery-can-reverse--neuropathy-foot. Published 2016. Updated April 15, 2016. Accessed May 25, 2020

2 Ultrasound Basics

MATTHEW SHERRIER, ALLISON N. SCHROEDER, KENTARO ONISHI, AND DANIEL LUEDERS

Introduction

Ultrasound guidance can be applied to assist in a multitude of interventional orthopedic procedures. This chapter provides a review of ultrasound physics, image optimization, common artifacts, and fundamentals of ultrasound-guided interventions.

Ultrasound Principles

Diagnostic ultrasound knowledge complements interventional ultrasound skills. Understanding ultrasound physics, image optimization, and artifacts are key components of diagnostic ultrasound. Mastery of diagnostic ultrasound serves as the foundation for safe and effective ultrasound-guided interventions. Awareness of sonographic artifacts and why these occur is imperative to distinguish those artifacts from pathology and to effectively prevent or mitigate artifacts that could make an intervention unsafe or more challenging.

Ultrasound Physics

A comprehensive description of the pertinent physics of ultrasound mechanics and the resulting imaging output is beyond the scope of this chapter. Briefly, electric current is transmitted from a wall-plug or an affixed battery through the ultrasound processor and, ultimately, to the ultrasound transducer. The head of an ultrasound transducer contains an array of piezoelectric crystals, which convert the electric current into pulses of ultrasonic waves. The piezoelectric crystal array within a transducer head can vary in the alignment, shape, thickness, and width, which influence quality of spatial resolution, the depth of ultrasound wave penetration, and signal-to-noise ratio. The transducer is coupled to the skin of the patient through a sonoconductive gel for sound waves to conduct through the target tissue.

Once the sound wave travels through patient's skin, the energy of the waves can be reflected by a tissue, absorbed by a tissue, or penetrate through a tissue. More dense tissues will reflect more ultrasound energy, and less dense tissues will permit greater penetration of ultrasound energy. As the sound waves penetrate deeper, energy is lost to refracted and absorbed sound waves and the ultrasound signal becomes attenuated or weaker in strength. Reflected sound waves travel retrograde to return to the transducer where they interact with the piezoelectric crystal array of the transducer head. Those reflected sound waves are converted back to an electrical signal, by a reverse piezoelectric effect, and are transmitted to the central processor of the ultrasound machine. The processor knows the pulse velocity of the anterograde ultrasound waves that were transmitted and can calculate the depth of reflecting structures from the measured echo time to create an ultrasound image. Bright, hyperechogenic-appearing structures result from the reflection of greater amounts of ultrasound energy by more dense tissues, which have higher impedance, such as bone. Conversely, dark, hypoechogenic-appearing structures result from the reflection of less amount of ultrasound energy by less dense tissues with lower impedance, such as fibrocartilage.

Image Optimization

Image optimization requires selection of the most appropriate ultrasound transducer and skillful manipulation of ultrasound probe and ultrasound machine settings such as depth, focal zone number and location, gain, and dynamic range. This is imperative to best visualize the targeted structure, to permit the most complete visualization of the needle or tool, and to ensure the safety and avoidance of neurovascular structures.

Transducer Selection

Ultrasound transducers vary by the range of ultrasound frequencies (labeled on the body of the transducer in megahertz [MHz]) that they transmit and the size of the transducer head footprint (Fig. 2.1). In general, a linear array transducer can transmit higher-frequency, lower-amplitude ultrasound waves. The higher-frequency transducer will transmit more ultrasound waves and thus receive more returning ultrasound waves, facilitating the production of

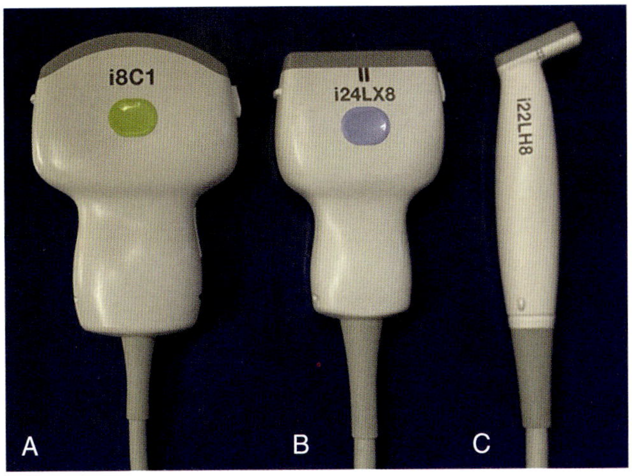

• **Fig. 2.1** Common Transducers From left to right, (A) 8-1 MHz curvilinear array transducer, (B) 24-8 MHz linear array transducer, and (C) 22-8 MHz small-footprint linear array transducer (commonly referred to as "hockey-stick" transducer).

greater detail and spatial resolution in the image produced. However, the lower-amplitude waves have less energy and will become attenuated and lose strength more quickly, so deeper objects are not as well visualized. In contrast, a curvilinear array transducer will transmit lower-frequency, higher-amplitude waves. The lower-frequency transducer will transmit fewer ultrasound waves, but those waves will have a higher amplitude and more energy; thus they are less susceptible to attenuation as they penetrate to deeper tissues. As a result, more sound waves return from deeper tissues and deeper objects are better visualized, but there is less detail and spatial resolution of superficial tissues.

In general, a lower-frequency curvilinear array transducer is preferable for tissues targeted at 4 to 5 cm and deeper and a higher-frequency linear array transducer will be preferable for tissues more superficial than that. The convex transmission of ultrasound waves from a curvilinear array transducer can improve visualization of a needle directed at a steep angle. The curvilinear array directs more ultrasound waves perpendicular to that needle that are reflected at an angle of incidence that facilitates return to the transducer, improving needle visualization. This same benefit can be obtained in beam-steering mode on linear array transducers, which is described later in this chapter.

Specialized small-footprint linear array transducers (commonly referred to as "hockey-stick" transducers because of their shape) will have a smaller footprint of approximately 15 to 20 mm (vs. 45+ mm for a standard linear transducer), which can facilitate improved skin contact and beam coupling on the sharp contours of the hands and feet. The smaller footprint also decreases the size of the field of view, which must also be considered when performing interventional procedures.

Knobology

The layout of knobs, switches, and touch screen interfaces will vary by ultrasound platform manufacturer and by different models within a manufacturer's range of platforms. It is essential for each individual operator to familiarize himself or herself with the layout of the control panel of each platform that might be used. The depth of the ultrasound image should be adjusted, often by turning a dial or adjusting a switch up or down, to ensure that the targeted structure and any "at-risk" structures are captured but also that the image does not have unnecessary depth beyond those structures (Fig. 2.2).

Focal zone depth can be adjusted and their number increased or decreased on most platforms. Focal zones represent the narrowest segments of the ultrasound beam where the ultrasound processor is directed to optimize the ultrasound waves and processing power so as to produce the best temporal and spatial resolution (Fig. 2.3). The number and positioning of focal zones should be modified according to the depth and size of the targeted structure. Minimization of the number of focal zones reduces processing demands by reducing the frame rate and improves image resolution.

Gain increases or decreases the overall brightness of the raw returned echoes and is most often adjusted and increased to account for beam attenuation resulting in image hypoechogenicity. Increasing or decreasing gain with the dial or switch does so uniformly and modifies the entire image. Time gain compensation (TGC) involves the individual manipulation of one of a vertically oriented stack of sliding switches which correlate to different image depths. Modification of the TGC permits focal manipulation of gain at specific image depths (Fig. 2.4). Typically, the TGC is used to focally increase gain in the far field to account for beam attenuation and relatively hypoechogenic imaging at increasing depths.

Sonographic Appearance of Normal Structures

An ultrasound image is produced by the return and processing of ultrasound waves by the transducer, which is affected by how the ultrasound waves penetrate, reflect, or are absorbed by different tissues. Different image echogenicities represent the reflection of waves at the interface of structures of relatively different density and orientation within a single tissue type or between different adjacent structures (Fig. 2.5).[1] The interface between structures with a wide difference in impedance (e.g., that seen between soft tissue and bone) results in more reflected sound waves and producing a relatively bright, or *hyperechoic,* structure on the ultrasound image. Structures that are less dense or sit adjacent to a very dense structure will reflect fewer sound waves or waves with smaller amplitude, resulting in a less bright, or hypoechogenic-appearing, structure. Adjacent structures of similar impedance are termed *isoechoic* to each other. Regions where all ultrasound waves are absorbed and no echo returns to the transducer appear black on an ultrasound image and are termed *anechoic.*

Comprehensive knowledge of local and regional musculoskeletal and neurovascular anatomy is essential. Tendon,

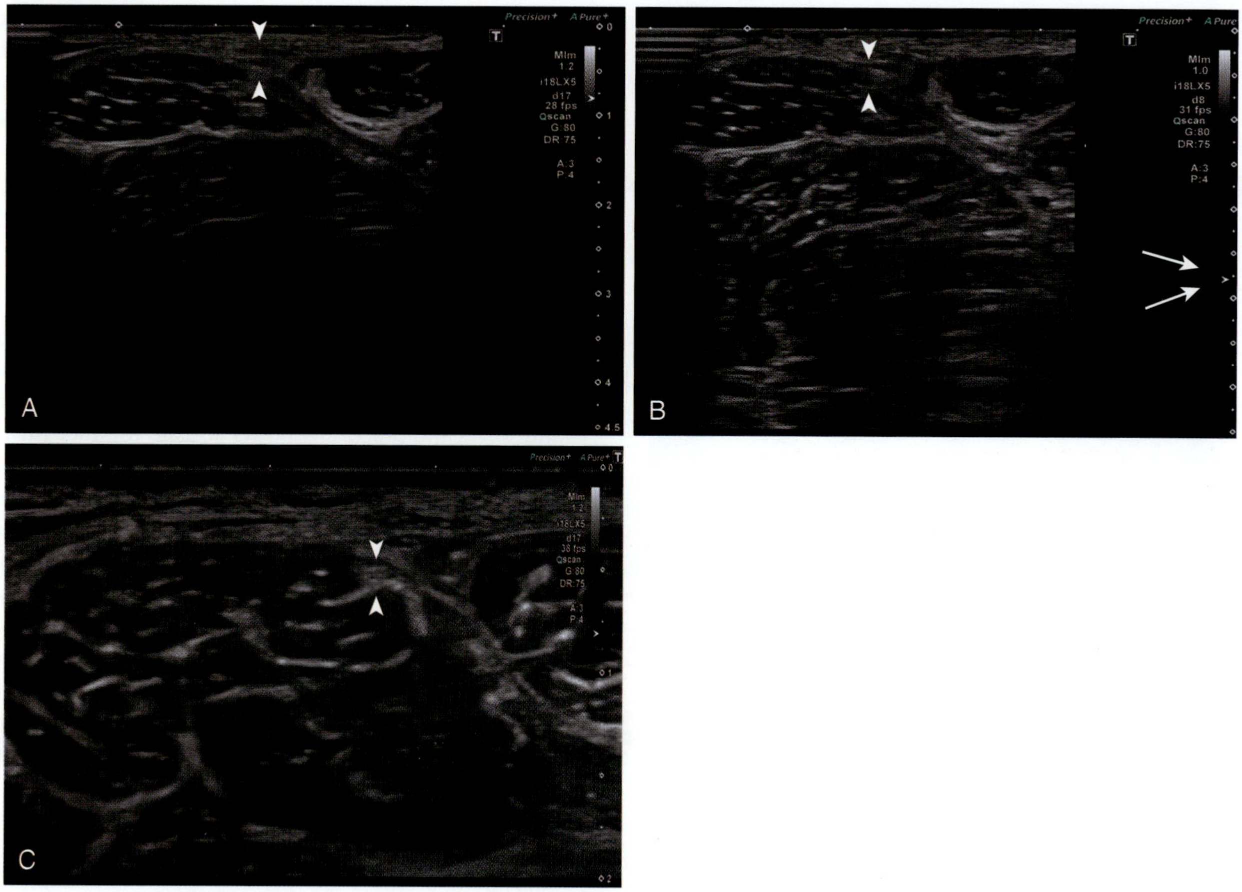

• **Fig. 2.2** Poorly optimized ultrasound images of the lateral femoral cutaneous nerve *(arrowheads)* demonstrating (A) excessive depth and (B) Suboptimal focal zone location *(arrows)* for such a superficial structure. (C) Ultrasound image of the lateral femoral cutaneous nerve *(arrowheads)* with an optimized depth and focal zone.

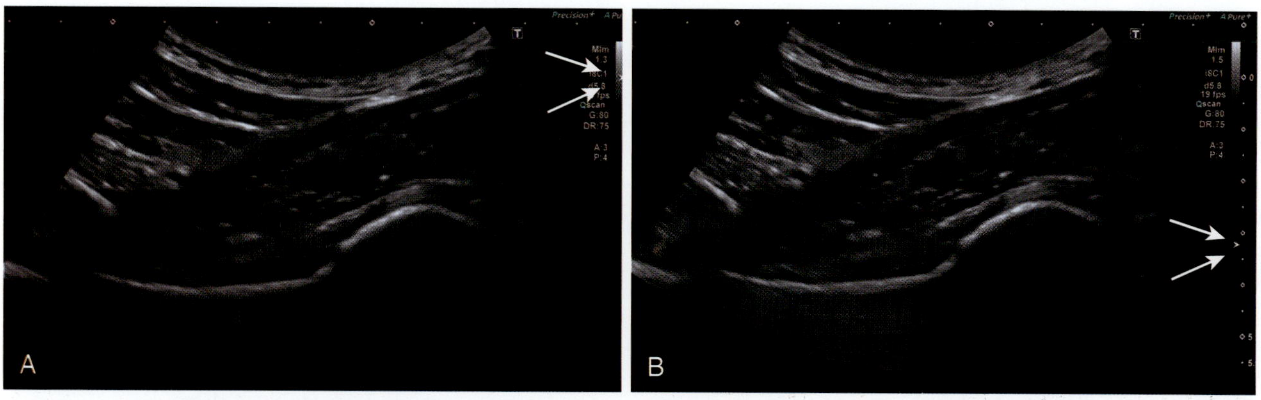

• **Fig. 2.3** Ultrasound image of the anterior femoroacetabular joint in long axis with the femoral neck contrasting the effect of focal zone location *(arrows)*. (A) Superficial focal zone, poorly optimized for the deep hip joint. (B) Deep focal zone which is better optimized for visualization of deep target structure.

ligament, muscle, bone, cartilage, bursa, and peripheral nerve have distinct sonographic appearances (Table 2.1). A thorough understanding of the normal sonographic appearance and surrounding anatomy of pertinent structures in both short-axis and long-axis imaging planes is critical to identify potentially at-risk structures, recognize congenital variation or absence of a structure, and diagnose pathology.[2,3] A comprehensive description of the sonographic appearance of pathologic tissues and anatomic variations is beyond the scope of this text.

Sonographic Artifacts

Ultrasound imaging is inherently susceptible to image artifacts because the sonographic character of normal tissue can change based on the angle of insonation of the ultrasound

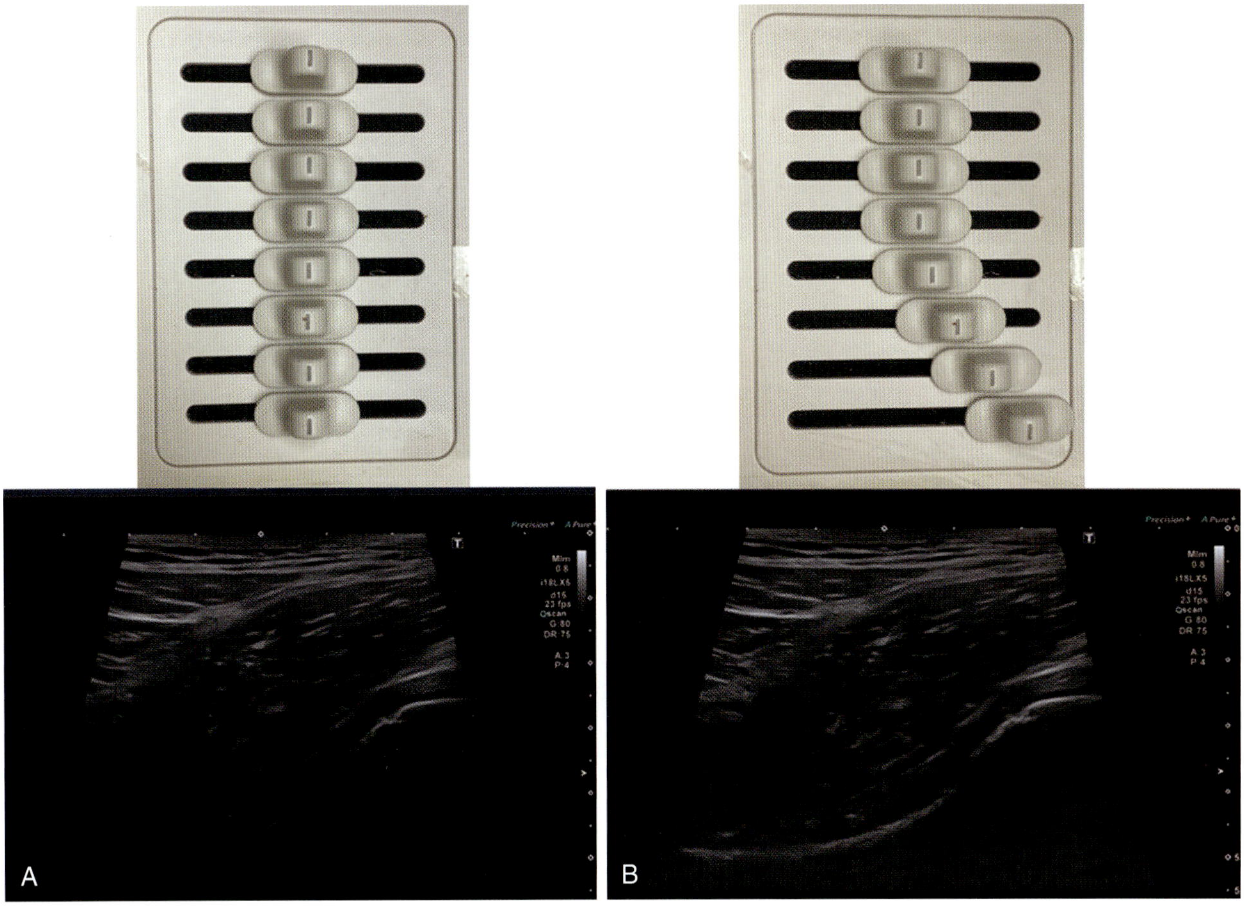

• **Fig. 2.4** Ultrasound image of the anterior femoroacetabular joint in long axis with the femoral neck demonstrating image optimization through manipulation of time gain compensation (TGC) at depth. (A) demonstrates neutral TGC settings, whereas (B) demonstrates increased gain at depth to better visualize the femoral neck.

beam and the relative sonographic characteristics of adjacent tissues. A thorough awareness of such artifacts and an understanding of why they occur is essential to avoid erroneous diagnosis of pathology and unnecessary and unproductive procedures.[5] Common artifacts include anisotropy, shadowing, posterior acoustic enhancement, posterior reverberation, and beam-width artifact.

Anisotropy

Anisotropy is the artifactually hypoechoic or anechoic appearance of a structure that occurs when a structure is imaged at an angle of incidence. The angle of incidence is the angle at which the ultrasound waves encounter the surface of a structure. If the angle is perpendicular, or close to 90 degrees, more waves will be reflected back to the transducer. If the ultrasound waves are more parallel, waves will be reflected or "scattered," resulting in a failure of the anticipated ultrasound waves returning to the transducer head. Anisotropy will occur when imaging structures in both long and short axes. Tendons and ligaments are most susceptible, specifically when curving around a bony prominence or quickly changing depth to become more deep or superficial (Fig. 2.7). Anisotropy produces an artifactually hypoechoic appearance that can mimic pathology.

Anisotropy can be minimized or eliminated in short-axis visualization by angulating or "wagging the tail" of the transducer to ensure that the ultrasound beam is perpendicular to the structure (face of the probe is parallel to the structure), approximating the angle of incidence as close to 90 degrees as possible. When visualizing a structure in long axis, anisotropy is addressed by heel-toeing or "rocking" one end of the transducer to ensure that the ultrasound beam is perpendicular to the structure, again, approximating the angle of incidence as close to 90 degrees as possible.

Posterior Acoustic Shadowing

Posterior acoustic shadowing results when ultrasound waves are reflected or attenuated by a structure resulting in little, to no, waves penetrating through to deeper structures (Fig. 2.8A).[6] This results in a relatively hypoechoic appearance of all tissues deep to the structure. Dense structures, such as bone, calcifications, and foreign bodies, are most likely to cast a posterior acoustic shadow.

Posterior Acoustic Enhancement

Posterior acoustic enhancement, or increased through-transmission, occurs deep to structures that are hypoechoic relative to adjacent tissues, resulting in less ultrasound beam

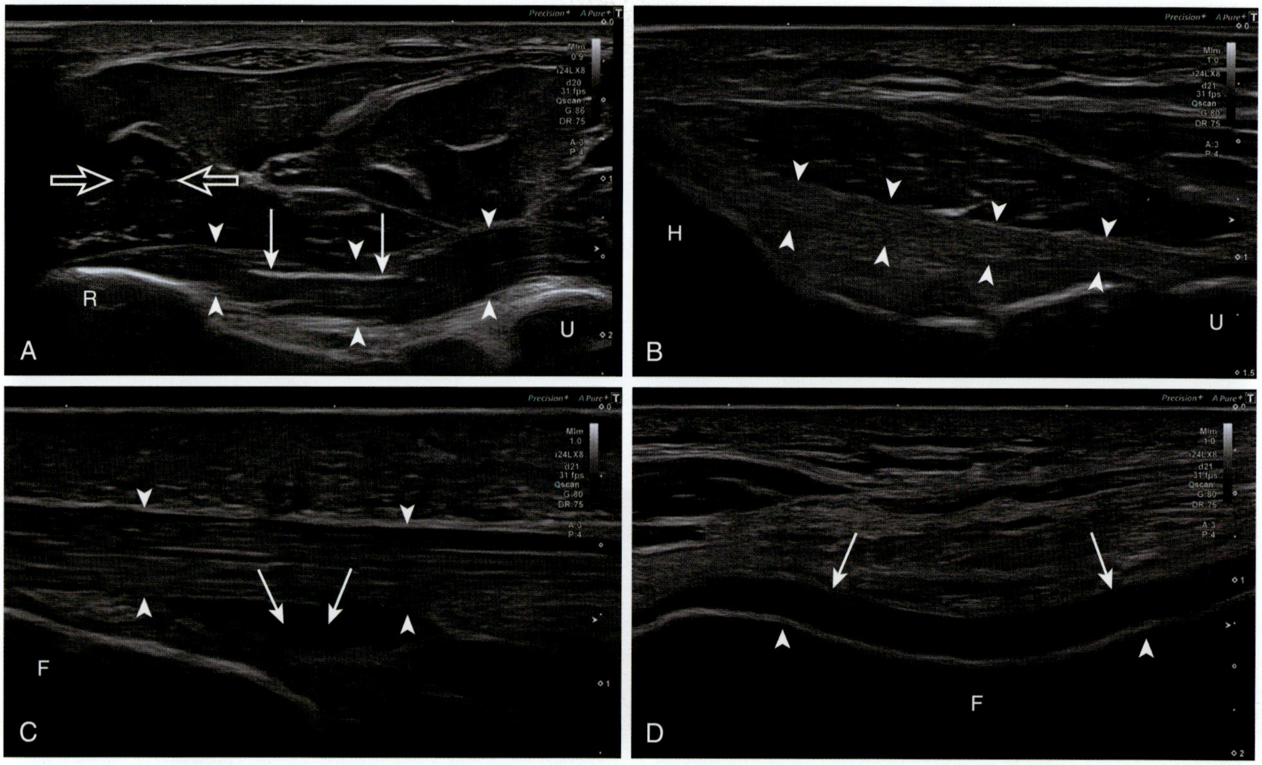

• **Fig. 2.5** (A) Pronator quadratus muscle *(arrowheads)* in long axis shows demonstrating hypoechoic myocytes and interspersed hyperechoic fibroadipose septae *(arrows)*. More superficially, the wrist and finger flexor musculature *(open arrows)* is demonstrated in anatomic short axis with the intramuscular fibroadipose septae appearing as punctate hyperechogenicities. (B) Ulnar collateral ligament of the elbow in long axis demonstrating compact fibrillar echotexture *(arrowheads)*. (C) Patellar tendon in long axis *(arrowheads)* demonstrating an even-appearing hyperechoic fibrillar echotexture. Deep to the tendon is hypoechoic fluid within the deep infrapatellar bursa *(arrows)*. (D) Transverse image of the femoral trochlea demonstrating the homogeneous, hypoechoic hyaline cartilage *(arrows)* overlying hyperechoic cortical bone *(arrowheads)*. *F*, Femur; *H*, humerus; *R*, radius; *U*, ulna.

attenuation or reflection (see Fig. 2.8B). Tissues deep to the less dense structure will appear relatively hyperechoic compared with adjacent soft tissues because relatively more of the ultrasound waves penetrate through the more superficial and less absorptive structure to the deeper tissues.[6] This artifact can be used to advantageously image structures deep to vasculature and cystic or fluid-filled structures.

Reverberation Artifacts

Reverberation appears as a series of hyperechoic, linear artifacts deep to dense structures and results from a series of ultrasound wave reflections between two parallel, highly reflective surfaces. The single reflection will be displayed at the proper location but the artifactual late return of attenuated, reflected ultrasound waves are interpreted by the ultrasound processor as deeper, hypoechoic structures. This commonly occurs with bone and with metal surfaces, such as a needle or orthopedic implant (Fig. 2.9). Ring-down artifact appears as a solid streak or series of parallel bands which result from the resonant vibration of air bubbles. Comet-tail artifact appears as a series of multiple closely spaced reverberation echoes deep to a more focal or punctate structure which results from sequential echoes from two closely spaced, highly reflective interfaces.

Beam-Width Artifact

Beam-width artifact results when the ultrasound beam is too wide relative to a small object being imaged and is similar to volume averaging in magnetic resonance imaging (MRI). For example, shadowing from a small calcification may not be visualized due to a wide beam width. This artifact can be eliminated by adjusting the focal zone to the level of the object of interest or changing to a probe with a smaller footprint.

Visualization of Blood Flow

Color and power Doppler imaging detect motion toward or away from the transducer by detecting the delay between frequencies of the transmitted and received ultrasound waves (Fig. 2.10).[7,8] Color Doppler displays differences in flow direction, red color representing flow toward the transducer and blue color representing flow away from the transducer. Power Doppler does not discriminate direction of flow but is more sensitive to low flow and provides superior detection of small vessels and slow flow rates. Power Doppler is sensitive to transducer movement and susceptible to flash artifact. Increased blood flow on Doppler imaging may occur with greater perfusion, inflammation, and neovascularization and can assist in differentiating complex fluid

TABLE 2.1 Distinct Sonographic Appearance of Neuromusculoskeletal Structures

Structure	Appearance on Ultrasound
Tendon	Linearly oriented between a muscle body and osseous insertion. Homogeneously and densely oriented fibers produce a dense, linear hyperechoic structure in long-axis imaging with distinct superficial and deep tenosynovial borders. In short axis, tendon appears as a regular-bordered ovoid structure with homogeneously echogenic and sized internal tendon fibers, often referred to as a "broomstick" viewed on end (Fig. 2.6)
Ligament	Linearly oriented between two osseous structures. Ligament is composed of homogeneously and densely oriented fibers and visualized as echogenic fibrillar fibers, which tend to be less echogenic than tendons but echogenicity also depends on anisotropy and contrast with surrounding structures.[4] Although the echotexture of nonpathological ligaments has not been well described, they are often visualized as a linear hyperechoic structure in long-axis imaging. In short axis, ligament will appear as a more irregularly bordered, flattened structure
Muscle	Composed of relatively hypoechoic muscle fibers and interspersed hyperechoic intramuscular stromal connective tissue of the endomysium and perimysium. In short axis, its appearance is often referred to as a "starry night"
Bone	Densely hyperechoic relative to all surrounding tissues because of the inherent high acoustic impedance mismatch. Cortical bone appears as a continuous, regular, brightly hyperechoic line with deep reverberation artifact and posterior acoustic shadowing which precludes visualization of any deeper structures
Hyaline cartilage	Densely and evenly hypoechoic secondary to its high water content and the high acoustic impedance mismatch with the deep bone
Fibrocartilage	Homogeneously hyperechoic relative to more superficial connective tissue or muscle. It has the same appearance in both long- and short-axis orientations
Bursa	When distended with fluid, anechoic-to-mixed-echogenic fluid and debris can fill the bursa. Firm transducer pressure will compress and displace the fluid
Peripheral nerve	Hyperechoic perineurium and endoneurium, which surrounds numerous small, round, and hypoechoic nerve fascicles. All of this is contained within a hyperechoic epineurium, giving a "honeycomb" appearance when visualized in short axis (see Fig. 2.6)[4]

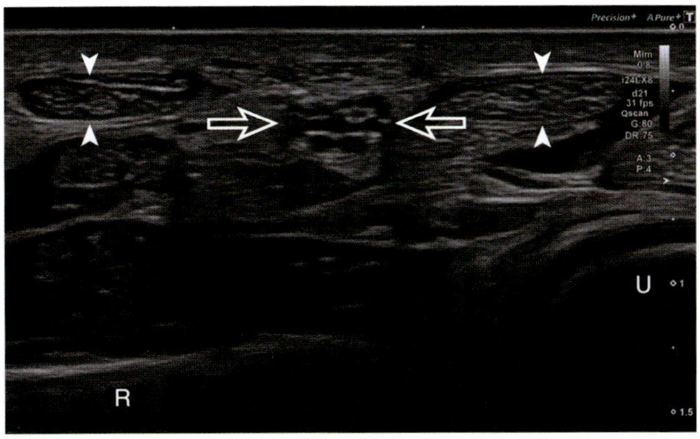

• **Fig. 2.6** Transverse Ultrasound Image of Distal Volar Forearm. Observe the "honeycomb" appearance of the median nerve in this short-axis view *(open arrows)* adjacent to the more hyperechoic and more densely packed fibrillar-appearing flexor tendons *(arrowheads)*. *R*, Radius; *U*, ulna.

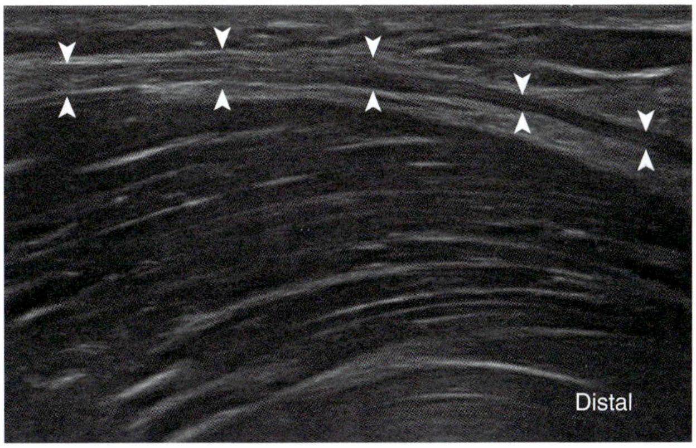

• **Fig. 2.7** The distal biceps brachii tendon *(arrowheads)* demonstrates anisotropy as it descends from superficial plane parallel to the transducer *(left of image)* toward its distal radial insertion in a deep plane oblique relative to the transducer *(right of image)*.

and synovitis because the former will often lack blood flow whereas the latter demonstrates increased flow.[9]

Microvascular imaging mode, such as superb microvascular imaging (SMI), has been demonstrated to have greater sensitivity for the identification of microvessels at a high frame rate.[10–12] This technology facilitates detailed visualization of microvessels and lower-velocity blood flow without the use of contrast medium.[13]

Role for Ultrasound Guidance in Interventional Orthopedic Procedures

General indications for needle placement into or about a soft tissue or joints include, but are not limited to, the removal of fluid for diagnostic evaluation or symptom palliation and the delivery of diagnostic or therapeutic agents. When considering the use of image guidance for a procedure, one should understand the indications and contraindications.

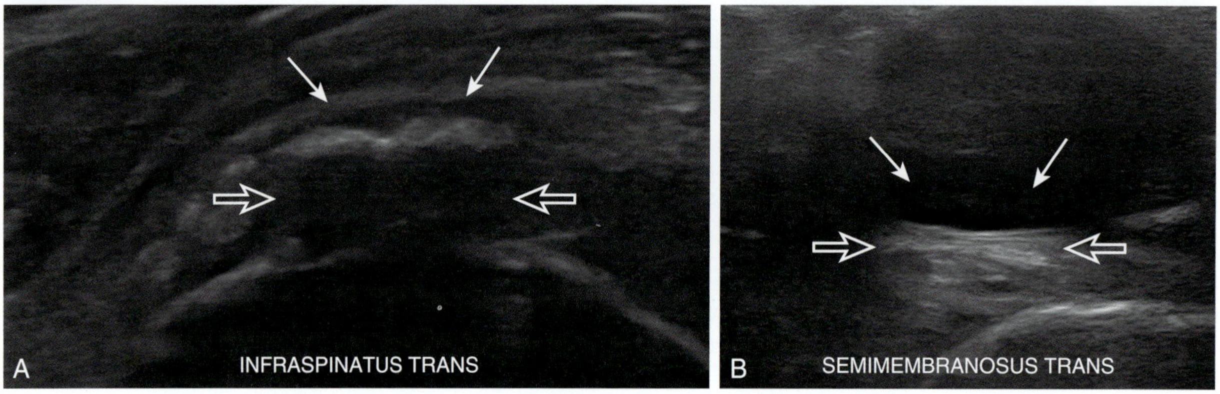

• **Fig. 2.8** (A) Posterior acoustic shadowing. A hyperechoic intratendinous calcification within infraspinatus *(arrows)* casts a posterior acoustic shadow, which results in an artifactually hypoechoic-appearing humerus deep to the calcification *(open arrows)*. (B) Posterior acoustic enhancement. A fluid-filled hypoechoic parameniscal cyst *(arrows)* attenuates less ultrasound energy than the adjacent musculature, which results in a relative hyperechogenic appearance of the joint capsule *(open arrows)* deep to the cyst.

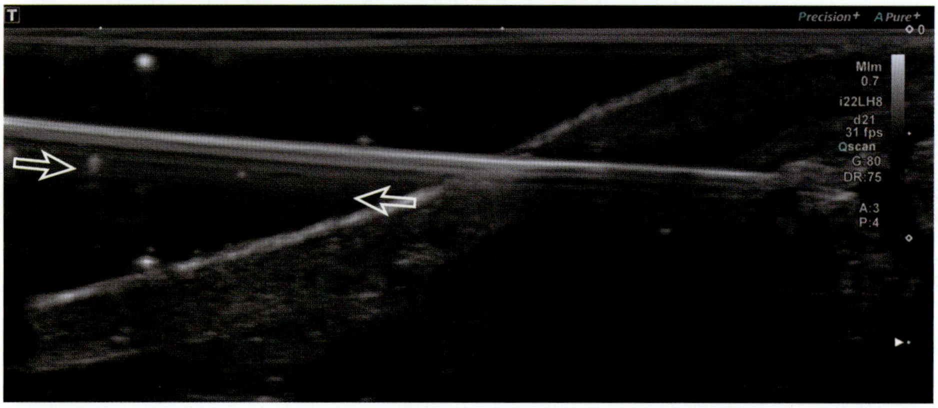

• **Fig. 2.9** Reverberation *(open arrows)* is seen as a series of linear reflective echoes extending deep as the sound beam reflects back and forth between the smooth surface of the needle shaft and the transducer.

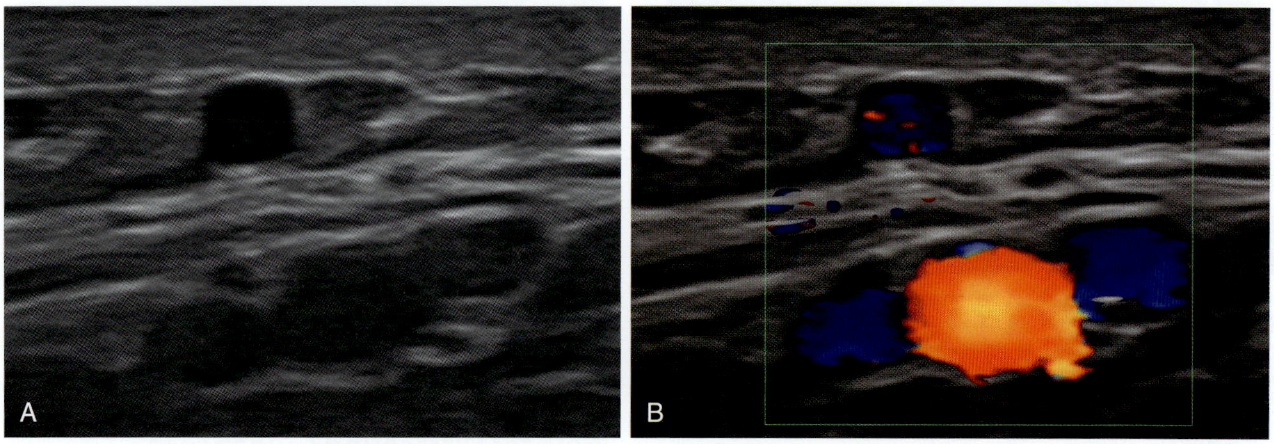

• **Fig. 2.10** Radial artery and veins without (A) and with (B) color Doppler.

Ultrasound affords many distinct advantages as an imaging modality for procedure guidance, but clinicians should be able to discern when the inherent limitations of ultrasound may make another imaging modality a safer or more effective tool for the procedure.

Advantages of Ultrasound

The use of ultrasound as an imaging modality to assist in the guidance of musculoskeletal interventions has the potential to improve accuracy, efficacy, and safety when compared

TABLE 2.2 Advantages of Ultrasound Over Other Imaging Modalities

Relative portability
Superior spatial resolution of superficial soft tissue and neurovascular structures
Relative low cost
Continuous needle/device visualization
No exposure to ionizing radiation
No metallic artifact on imaging allows for prosthetic imaging

with palpation guidance.[14,15] When used for procedural guidance, ultrasound also affords multiple distinct advantages over x-ray, MRI, and computed tomography (CT) that make it an ideal diagnostic and interventional imaging tool (Table 2.2). Ultrasound can be used at the point of care to identify tendinosis/tendinopathy, ligamentous injury, muscular injury, bony pathology and joint pathology (i.e., effusion, hemarthrosis, loose body, meniscal injury). Clinical evaluation, diagnostic ultrasound evaluation, and progression to an ultrasound-guided intervention are possible to complete in a single outpatient clinic visit.

Accuracy

Injection accuracy is defined as placement of the injectate or needle tip into or about the intended structure.[14] There is strong evidence that image-guided injections are more accurate than palpation-guided injections into joints of all sizes.[15] Most soft tissue and intrabursal injections are also more accurate when performed with ultrasound guidance.[16,17]

Efficacy

Assessments of the effectiveness of a procedure, whether palpation or ultrasound guided, vary based on different outcome measures used. For the purposes of this discussion, positive efficacy will be defined as studies that describe a positive change in an outcome measure such as pain, range of motion, mobility, function, or patient satisfaction.[14]

One would logically anticipate improved efficacy with more accurate injectate placement, but studies to date have demonstrated mixed outcomes with regards to improvements in efficacy with ultrasound guidance.[15] Multiple studies have demonstrated that ultrasound guidance for musculoskeletal conditions contributes to improved efficacy and quality of life when compared with palpation-guided injections.[18–23]

One important consideration is that most studies comparing palpation versus ultrasound-guided corticosteroid injections, except cortisone, will have some systemic effects of pain reduction no matter the specific location of the injection.[19,24] However, the mechanisms of action of medications other than corticosteroids, such as viscosupplementation injections and orthobiologic agents, may be dependent upon their accurate placement into or about a structure or joint. More research is needed to compare whether ultrasound guidance may improve the effectiveness of such interventions as compared with palpation guidance.

Safety

Ultrasound guidance of an intervention affords continuous visualization of the at-risk neurovascular structures, the target structure, and the needle or device, which can decrease the incidence of adverse events such as hematomas/hemarthrosis, postinjection pain, and neurovascular injuries.[25,26]

Indications for Use of Ultrasound-Guided Intervention

Use of ultrasound for guidance of an injection or procedural intervention is indicated when a palpation-guided injection has failed to have positive therapeutic effect or when the diagnostic or therapeutic injection depends upon precise visualization of the pathologic structure. In procedures with relatively high risk of injury to nearby neurovascular structures or unintended soft tissue structures, ultrasound guidance can be used to avoid injury. Furthermore, ultrasound is useful to monitor for postprocedure hematoma formation in anticoagulated patients.[27,28] Another common indication for ultrasound guidance is when palpation of bony anatomic landmarks and confident target identification are compromised by body habitus or pannus, postsurgical or posttraumatic changes and deformities, or deep location of the target.

Contraindications for Use of Ultrasound-Guided Intervention

Once the indications have been identified, contraindications must be assessed. Similar to palpation-guided injections, ultrasound-guided procedures should not be performed in patients with known allergy to injectate or in the location of an active infection, rash, or skin breakdown. Another important contraindication is the skill limitations of the proceduralist. Substantial training, practice, and time commitment are necessary to obtain competency; one must not perform an intervention that one does not feel comfortable performing.

Relative contraindications include interventions on patients with coagulopathy or who are on anticoagulation/antiplatelet therapy, given the increased risk of bleeding complications. Additional relative contraindications include underlying medical conditions that may be affected by the injectate, such as diabetics who receive corticosteroid injections.

Contraindications specific to ultrasound guidance relate to an inability to sufficiently or clearly visualize a targeted pathologic structure because of inherent imaging limitations. Specifically, ultrasound does not penetrate through bones and other dense or metallic structures. This can preclude visualization of structures deep to bone and needle visualization deep to bone or within an obliquely oriented joint, such as the sacroiliac (SI) joint or lumbar facet joint.

Ultrasound Compared With Other Imaging Modalities for Procedure Guidance

Ultrasound, MRI, CT, and fluoroscopy can each be used to guide interventional orthopedic procedures. Relative to other imaging modalities, ultrasound has the benefits of improved portability, lower cost, absence of exposure to ionizing radiation or gadolinium contrast, and unparalleled spatial resolution of superficial soft tissue structures. Even the largest platform-based ultrasound machine will have a smaller footprint and is more portable than other imaging hardware. Ultrasound can be moved between different procedure rooms, unlike other modalities which can require a large, dedicated room and outfitting with extensive electrical and computer wiring or leaded protection. Ultrasound also affords continuous, real-time visualization of the needle or device as it is advanced or redirected, unlike other modalities which require repeating a cycle of advancing a needle or device, taking an image, and image analysis.

Magnetic Resonance Imaging

MRI is often the imaging reference standard for musculoskeletal disorders because of its unparalleled global detail of osseous, articular, and musculotendinous structures. When compared with MRI, ultrasound is more accessible at the point-of-care, less expensive, and more cost-effective, has superior superficial spatial resolution, and provides dynamic anatomic detail in real time.[29–31] To the authors' knowledge, there are no studies that directly compare MRI versus ultrasound guidance for procedures performed on the musculoskeletal system.

Computed Tomography

CT provides cross-sectional imaging of bone, soft tissues, and blood vessels, making it a useful modality for procedural guidance. Limitations of CT relative to ultrasound are its requirement of a specialized and dedicated room for large machinery, exposure of the operator, staff, and patient to ionizing radiation, and lack of real-time visualization of the needle or device. CT guidance is most commonly used for spinal injections and implements cycles of needle/device advancement, image capture, and image analysis to confirm accurate needle/device placement and medication delivery; it does not allow for continuous real-time visualization of the needle or device that is possible with ultrasound. The cycle of needle/device advancement and image gathering used with CT guidance increases the length of time for the intervention and comparison studies have been mixed as to whether CT or ultrasound is more time efficient for image guidance for facet joint injections.[29,30]

Fluoroscopy

Fluoroscopy uses radiography to visualize detailed bony anatomy. However, relative to ultrasound, fluoroscopy exposes the operator, staff, and patient to ionizing radiation, requires contrast to confirm needle placement and injectate flow, and is much less portable. Fluoroscopy provides no detail of neurovascular structures, musculature, and tendons. Relative to ultrasound, fluoroscopy does afford superior visualization deep to and between bony prominences, and allows confirmation of placement with flow of injected radiopaque contrast into such joints.

Axial injections are believed to be safer and more effective when performed with fluoroscopic guidance compared with ultrasound guidance. However, in recent years, this opinion has been challenged in the literature. Ultrasound-guided cervical medial branch blocks take less time to perform and use fewer needle passes with no difference in preblock and postblock pain scores or complication rate when compared with fluoroscopic guidance.[31,32] In the lumbar spine, a recent systematic review of nine randomized controlled trials comparing ultrasound to fluoroscopic guidance for the management of lower back pain, including transforaminal and caudal steroid injections, found no difference in pain reduction, procedure time, complications and adverse events, patient satisfaction, or postprocedure opioid consumption.[33] These findings are similar to those reported in a meta-analysis of randomized and nonrandomized lumbar facet joint injections, which did not find significant differences in pain or function in the ultrasound-guided cohorts when compared to fluoroscopy.[34] Although the research for ultrasound guidance is promising, the accuracy and safety of fluoroscopy-guided neuraxial injections is well established and currently remains the standard of care for axial injections.

In addition to spine procedures, fluoroscopy has traditionally been the imaging modality of choice for SI joint injections.[35–37] Ultrasound has been demonstrated to have similar accuracy and improvements in pain scores and disability measures when compared with fluoroscopy for SI joint injections,[38] although some studies show superior accuracy of fluoroscopy when compared with ultrasound.[36,39]

Fluoroscopic guidance has historically been the imaging modality of choice for intra-articular hip joint injections and aspirations, but a growing body of evidence demonstrates equivalent accuracy, efficacy, and decreased cost with ultrasound guidance.[40–44] Ultrasound-guided intra-articular hip injections are less painful than fluoroscopically guided injections, which is likely attributable to its ability to visualize and to avoid painful contact or injury to periarticular structures.[45]

Cost

There is an 8% reduction in cost per patient per year and a 33% reduction in cost per responder per year with the use of ultrasound guidance compared with palpation guidance for intra-articular injections in patients with inflammatory arthritis.[23] In the knee joint specifically, ultrasound guidance achieves a 13% reduction in cost per patient per year and a 58% reduction in cost per responder per year when compared with palpation guidance in patients with osteoarthritis.[46] Ultrasound guidance has also been shown to be more cost-effective than palpation or fluoroscopic guidance for glenohumeral joint injections in patients with adhesive capsulitis.[47]

It is important to note that the cost-effectiveness of sonographic guidance for musculoskeletal interventions can be less impactful in the hands of a less-experienced operator who may be less efficient or less accurate. Additional studies are also needed to determine whether the improved accuracy from ultrasound guidance translates into improved outcomes and cost savings.

Technical Considerations

Prior to performing any procedure, the physician should: review prior imaging, confirm an accurate diagnosis, obtain the informed consent of the patient, use site marking and local anesthetic as appropriate, and apply aseptic technique. Specific to the ultrasound guidance of a procedure, the physician should ensure optimization of patient comfort, the ergonomics of the procedural setup, including arrangement of the procedure table, ultrasound platform, and screen.

Patient Information and Labeling

Patient identifier information should be entered to allow for proper documentation. This will usually consist of the patient's name, birth date, and an identifying medical record number. Specific standards for labeling of target tissue and orientation can vary but generally must include the structure of interest and its orientation, when appropriate. Labeling must also include an identifier of anatomic orientation. Conventionally, the proximal or right side of the patient corresponds with the right side of the ultrasound screen. However, when performing musculoskeletal ultrasound, the label should be appropriately placed on the ultrasound image, to accurately indicate medial/lateral, anterior/posterior, cephalad/caudal, or proximal/distal and allow the sonographer and anyone reviewing images to easily determine image orientation.

Ergonomics

Optimization of the physician, patient, and ultrasound platform ergonomics can minimize fatigue and work-related injuries.[48] Optimal comfort of the sonographer and patient are essential. To reduce fatigue, the height and placement of the examination table should allow the scanning hand to be lower than the ipsilateral shoulder. The elbow should be close to the sonographer's body with ample contact between the scanning hand and the patient to provide secure transducer positioning. A chair with wheels and back support can improve comfort and maximize maneuverability. Screen location should be adjusted to enable full visualization of the procedure site and the ultrasound image throughout the procedure to minimize head or neck movement. The transducer should be held with the nondominant hand, with the other hand performing the procedure. A supply tray should be within reach of the operator's dominant hand. An assistant may be required to help with image modification to ensure optimal visualization of the targeted structure and the needle/device, image storage, and modification of image labeling if orientation is changed. Lighting should be dimmed for optimal screen viewing and appreciation of black/white contrast.

The patient is positioned to facilitate reproducible and effective access to the procedural site while optimizing the orientation of the ultrasound platform for viewing and image manipulation. Patient comfort must also be considered. Ultimately, positioning is an interplay between physician access to the procedure site and minimization of patient discomfort and may require small compromises in both variables to effectively and efficiently complete the procedure.

Preprocedural Scan

The ultimate utility of the preprocedural scan is to make the procedure as efficient as possible after cleaning the procedural site and donning sterile equipment, so that no further modification of the ultrasound imaging and labeling is needed. The following should be completed in the preprocedural ultrasound scan: optimization of probe selection based on target depth, contour and access or limitations of the procedure site, optimization of the ultrasound image to visualize the target structure, location of any at-risk structures, determination of the most appropriate orientation of approach, and needle gauge and length. The skin at the procedural site can be marked with a surgical marking pen to ensure that the optimal image can be quickly and accurately located during the procedure and to minimize the possibility of skin contamination from rescanning from an area of uncleansed skin into the procedural site.

Anatomic variations of musculotendinous structures, anomalous neurovascular structures, and previously unidentified pathology can be encountered during the preprocedural ultrasound scan.[49,50] The physician must determine whether such variations would make an injection or procedure unsafe. However, with a comprehensive understanding of the specific anatomic variation and how it introduces risk to the procedure, adequate visualization of at-risk structures in the preprocedural scan and during the procedure, and calculation of a modified or an alternate approach for the procedure as needed, the injection/procedure can still be completed in most cases. All significant finding of pathology and anatomic variation should be documented in detail in the procedural report.

Direct Versus Indirect Guidance

Ultrasound-guided procedures can be separated into indirect and direct techniques. With the indirect approach, ultrasound is used to identify the target and determine its depth. The overlying skin is marked, the transducer is removed, and the procedure is performed without real-time guidance. The needle is typically directed perpendicular to the skin into the target. This technique has the obvious disadvantage of not being able to visualize the needle in real time. Although the use of either technique may be appropriate in specific clinical circumstances, the preferred modality of ultrasound guidance for interventional orthopedic procedures is the direct approach. In this approach, the needle tip is continuously visualized approaching and encountering the target throughout the procedure.

Needle Selection

Needle selection may vary per clinician preference and patient factors. Selection of the smallest-gauge needle with the appropriate length for the desired injection is recommended. Selection of needle type, gauge, and length will depend on the procedure at hand, but, in general, the smallest-gauge needle possible, while permitting adequate length and needle visualization, is preferable for patient comfort. Larger needles (e.g., 22 gauge or larger) are necessary for aspiration and for injection of viscous medications. When advancing the needle, it is important to keep in mind that smaller-gauge needles will be more prone to bending and more challenging to visualize.

Aseptic Technique

After adequate sonographic visualization of the target tissue, selection of the most appropriate transducer and needle gauge and length, and optimization of the ultrasound image settings, the skin overlying the location of transducer placement and needle entry can be marked and sterilized. A sterile field prepared by the operator or assistant should contain aseptic cleaning solution, sterile needles and syringes with medications prepared in a sterile manner, sterile probe cover and gel, sterile gauze, and a sterile bandage. Physicians performing the procedure should wash their hands and don sterile gloves before using an appropriate skin cleansing solution, such as iodine or chlorhexidine. These are available as a single-use swab or applicator. Sterile drapes or towels can be used to cover the surrounding areas, creating a sterile field surrounding the procedure site that allows the operator to easily set the transducer while exchanging equipment and minimizing contamination during the procedure. Nonsterile gel is applied to the probe, which is next draped with a sterile cover and secured, usually with supplied rubber bands. Sterile ultrasound gel can then be applied to the now-sterile ultrasound probe or directly to the skin at the procedure site.

The preprocedural technique detailed previously provides the best means by which to mitigate the risk of contamination and infection during an injection/procedure, but clinicians may prefer to use alternative or individualized techniques. The choice of infection management is dictated by specific practice or institution guidelines and may include nonsterile sheaths, gel, and gloves. Clinicians who use the "no-touch" technique place the uncovered transducer over the target region but remote from the prepared skin entry site. The needle is passed through the prepared skin region and passes under the transducer within the body but does not pass through unprepped skin, nor do the uncovered transducer and nonsterile gel contact the procedure site or needle. It is recommended that this technique be used only by experienced clinicians due to the risk of procedure site contamination. Specific detail of the aseptic technique used during the ultrasound-guided procedure should be documented in the procedure report.

Local Anesthesia

The injection of local anesthetic can reduce procedural discomfort. If used, it is best to start with a thinner, higher-gauge needle (e.g., 30- or 27-gauge) to minimize pain from the needle. This may limit the length of needle available and require a second skin entry with a longer, larger-gauge needle to get the therapeutic injectate to the target. If the operator is able to reach the target structure with the same needle used to administer local anesthetic, that needle can be left in place at the target structure, the anesthetic syringe removed, and one containing the therapeutic injectate affixed to obviate the need for a second needle entry. In addition, injection of local anesthetic with a smaller-gauge and shorter needle can provide the physician with an estimate of the appropriate needle trajectory to the target tissue and make the direction of the therapeutic injectate with a larger gauge and longer needle more accurate and efficient.

Needle Approach

In-Plane and Out-of-Plane Techniques

The targeted structure can be approached in two ways relative to the ultrasound transducer. In an "in-plane" approach the needle is parallel to the long axis of the ultrasound transducer, and the entire needle shaft is visualized during the procedure. An "out-of-plane" approach involves the needle being placed perpendicular to the ultrasound transducer, and the needle shaft and tip are visualized in short axis as a single punctate, hyperechoic dot. In the hands of those with greater technical ultrasounds skills, these approaches can both be used within the same single procedure by rotating the transducer to ensure accurate and safe direction of the needle to the target structure. The optimal approach includes the safest approach to the target structure that avoids injury to blood vessels, nerves, and surrounding structures. The operator should consider not only how to best orient the transducer to visualize the target and surrounding structures but also the needle trajectory relative to the transducer.

In an in-plane approach, also known as long-axis or longitudinal approach, the needle is directed co-linear to the long axis of the transducer, allowing for continuous visualization of the entire needle shaft throughout the procedure, including the needle tip and target. This method is preferable because it allows for real-time visualizations of needle angle and depth modifications during needle advancement.

In an out-of-plane technique, also known as short-axis or transverse approach, the needle is directed perpendicular to the long axis of the transducer. The target structure is centered on the ultrasound screen with the needle passed under the middle of the transducer. In this view, the needle manifests as a single, punctate, hyperechoic "dot" rather than a linear structure. The out-of-plane approach may be used in procedures where the target is superficial with minimal surrounding soft tissues, such as the acromioclavicular joint and small joints of the hand and foot. Many ultrasound machines can project a centerline on the display and will have indicator of the center point of the transducer head. Placing the centerline marker directly over the targeted structure and directing the skin entry site at the center point indicator on the transducer head can improve accuracy of needle direction to the target structure.

Disadvantages of the out-of-plane approach are that only a short segment of the needle is visualized at a single time as it passes through the sound beam plane. A common, and potentially dangerous, error is to pass the needle tip beyond the plane of the transducer because it can be challenging to distinguish the needle shaft from the needle tip in this view. When using the out-of-plane approach, one can consider the walk-down maneuver. In this technique, the needle enters superficially, the tip is identified, and then the needle is drawn back slightly, angled more steeply and advanced toward the target depth. This is repeated until the target is reached and ensures that the tip of the needle or structures in the needle trajectory are continuously visualized.

Alternation between in-plane and out-of-plane views facilitates identification of the entire needle shaft and tip location relative to the targeted structure and at-risk structures to ensure safety and accuracy.

Needle Trajectory

It is important to triangulate the depth of the target structure and to determine a needle entry point and trajectory that will allow for visualization of the needle tip during the entire procedure. A needle trajectory that is parallel to the face of the transducer will allow for improved needle visualization. This can be accomplished by choosing a needle entry point below the transducer when convex anatomy permits (Fig. 2.11). This is not always possible with very deep structures and when the overlying superficial anatomy is flat or concave. In those instances, an approach must be selected that best accounts for the depth of a structure, the anticipated subcutaneous distance needed to be traversed by the needle, superficial anatomy, and how it may limit or affect the trajectory (e.g., at-risk structures, abdominal pannus, large musculature). A curvilinear array transducer will usually be optimal for these instances as it affords better resolution of structures deeper than 4 to 5 cm and the curvilinear array of the transmitted ultrasound waves will be more co-linear to an injectate needle advanced at a steep angle with the skin.

Optimizing Needle Visualization

When directing a needle in the long axis of the ultrasound transducer (in-plane injection), the needle will be best visualized when it passes directly under the transducer without deviation. Leftward or rightward deviation of the needle from under the transducer will result in incomplete visualization of the needle and the loss of the needle tip as it advances out-of-plane from the transducer. If needle visualization is compromised, moving the transducer in small increments to the needle is preferred while maintaining the needle in the same location. The needle should not be advanced until the tip is again visualized to ensure the safety of any at-risk neurovascular structures. It can be helpful to look down at the procedure site from the ultrasound screen to visually reconfirm that the needle is indeed directly beneath and parallel to the transducer. As the needle enters deeper tissues, maneuverability is limited and may result in bending of the needle, which makes it difficult to visualize the tip and shaft in one image.

Transducer Manipulation

Manipulation of the ultrasound transducer will modify how the ultrasound waves are transmitted and return to the transducer, which will result in changes to the image that is produced. It is essential to understand how, and when, to use specific maneuvers to eliminate unwanted artifacts and to optimize visualization of the target tissue and the needle during a procedure. Nomenclature for these maneuvers can vary slightly. Frequently used transducer movements are described in Table 2.3 and Fig. 2.12, with their most common names listed.

Continuous Visualization of Needle Tip

The capacity for continuous visualization of a needle during a procedure and its relation to the target tissue and at-risk structures is a unique benefit of ultrasound. It is imperative that the operator is proficient in the skills of needle guidance during the procedure to ensure that these benefits are indeed realized. A general principle of ultrasound-guided procedures is that the operator must not continue to advance a needle or device if the tip is not visualized during an in-plane approach. Needle visualization can be improved by maintaining a steady hand on the transducer, specifically by firmly holding the transducer with three to four fingers and anchoring the hypothenar eminence of the hand on the skin. A thicker, larger-gauge needle will be more easily visualized because of the increased diameter. A needle trajectory parallel to the long axis of a linear ultrasound transducer head or convexity of a curvilinear probe will increase the return of ultrasound waves to the transducer and improve visualization of the needle. This can be modified by either withdrawing and redirecting a needle, by performing a heel-toe transducer maneuver, or by using a gel stand-off.

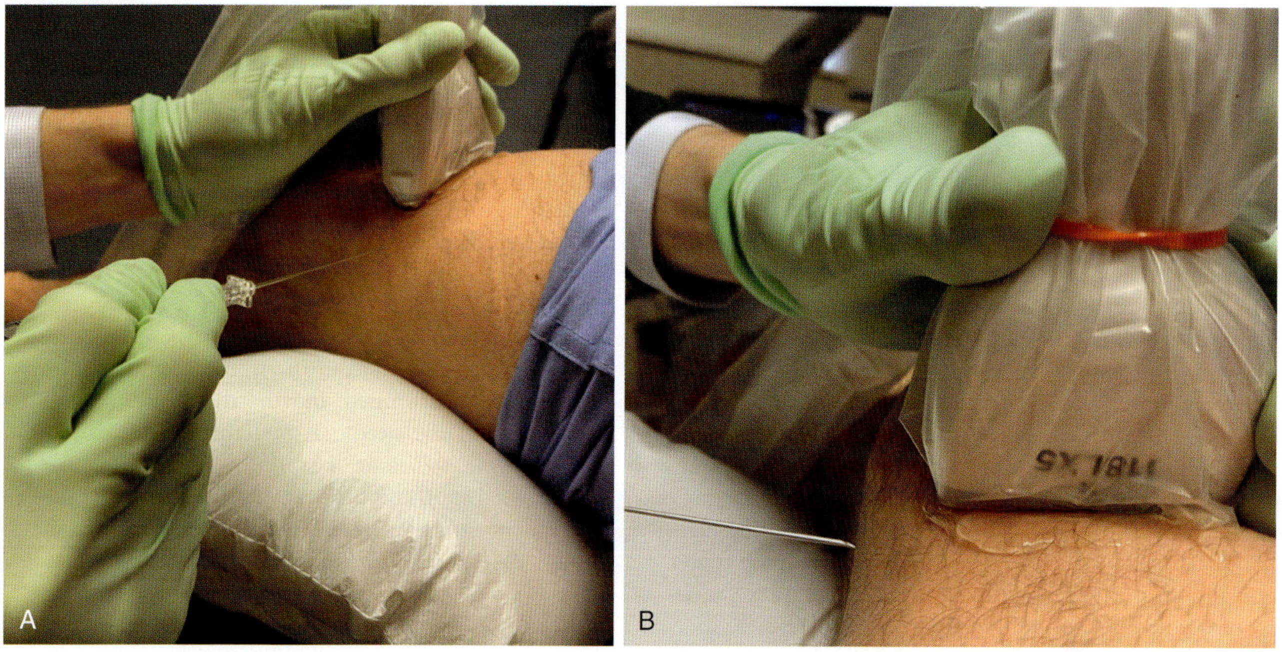

• **Fig. 2.11** Demonstration of a suprapatellar recess injection taking advantage of the convexity of the distal thigh to insert the needle at the depth of the targeted tissue at a trajectory parallel to the transducer, to best optimize needle visualization in figures (A) and (B).

TABLE 2.3 Frequently Used Transducer Movements

Transducer Movement	Description	Use for Image Optimization During Procedures
Translate, slide	Movement of the entire transducer in the direction of the long axis of the probe	Used to locate the needle or target structure
Sweep	Movement of the entire transducer in the direction of the short axis of the probe	Used to locate the needle or target structure
Rotate	Rotation of the transducer around a center point/axis	This can facilitate alternation between the short-axis and long-axis views of a structure or a needle
Rock, heel-toe	Angling the transducer along the long axis of the probe to change the angle of insonation by applying more or less pressure on one side of the probe while maintaining the same skin location	Modification of the angle of incidence when attempting to optimize tissue or needle visualization or eliminate anisotropy
Angulate, fan, toggle, tilt, wag	Angling the transducer along its short axis by moving the transducer its convex short-axis plane while maintaining the same skin location	Modification of the angle of incidence when attempting to optimize tissue or needle visualization or eliminate anisotropy
Compression	Increasing or decreasing the manual pressure of the transducer at the skin	Used to displace fluid, compress blood vessels, or aid in dynamic visualization of fascial planes

Gel Stand-off

A gel stand-off involves using a thick layer of gel under the transducer so that part of, or all of, the transducer does not directly contact the skin (Fig. 2.13). This facilitates sonocoupling from the transducer, through gel, to the underlying skin on convex anatomic surfaces. That sonocoupling maintains a continuous image. Conversely, lack of direct skin contact by the probe or sonocoupling through a continuous gel medium results in loss of all ultrasound waves and a completely anechoic image at that location. When performing an in-plane procedure, a gel stand-off under one side of the transducer can be combined with a heel-toe maneuver to facilitate entry of the needle at a steeper trajectory under the transducer, better capacity to maintain the

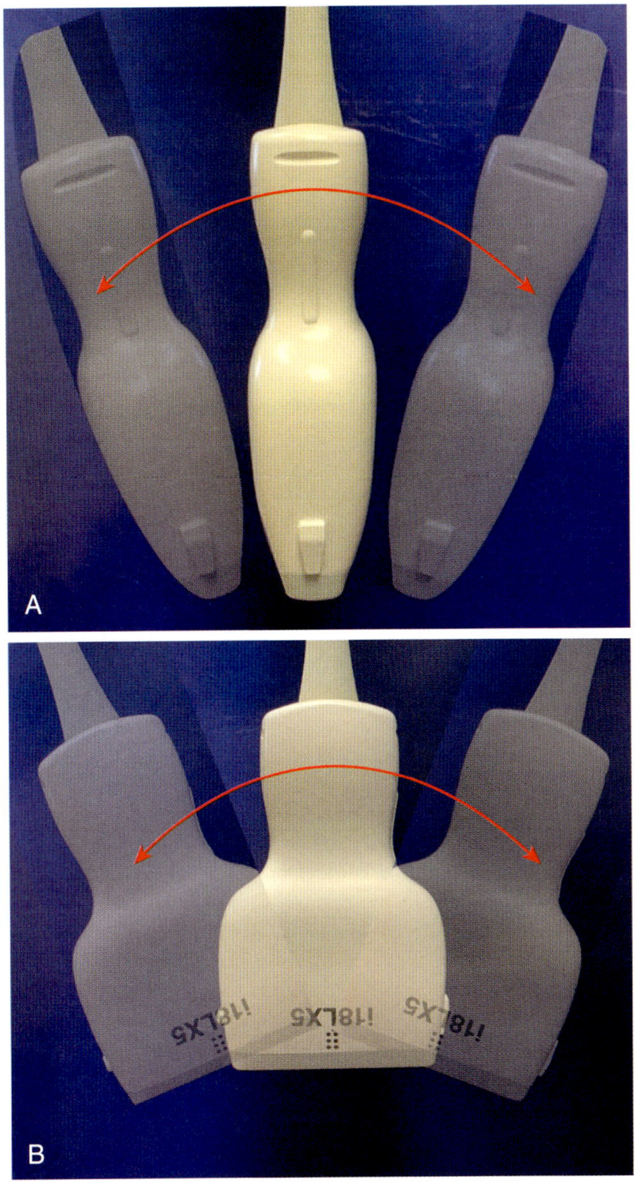

• **Fig. 2.12** (A) Transducer fan/wag. (B) Rock/heel-toe.

needle at a perpendicular to the angle of insonation to the ultrasound beam, and for continuous gel contact and visualization of the needle prior to puncture through the skin.

Needle Tracking Techniques

Identification of the needle and visualization throughout the procedure can be improved by different maneuvers and image modifications (Table 2.4).

Postprocedure Protocol

After completion of the procedure, the needle is withdrawn. The area should be scanned after the procedure to confirm that the injectate was placed in the intended location, indicated by sonographic visualization of injectate about the targeted tendon or soft tissue structure and within the targeted joint space. This postprocedure scan also allows for evaluation of hematoma formation. Injectate flow can also be confirmed in real time during the injection procedure with the use of Doppler imaging ahead of the needle tip. Following the procedure, a dressing is applied, and procedure-specific instructions are reviewed with the patient. Probes and ultrasound equipment should be disinfected between each procedure.

Conclusion

There is strong evidence to support improved accuracy, efficacy, and safety of musculoskeletal injection procedures with the utilization of ultrasound guidance when compared with palpation guidance. In addition, ultrasound provides many advantages over CT and fluoroscopy for procedural guidance, including lower cost, absence of ionizing radiation, greater portability and flexibility in setting up a procedure room, and real-time visualization of neurovasculature.

The skills required to effectively and efficiently use ultrasound for the guidance of musculoskeletal interventions requires extensive practice and training to develop

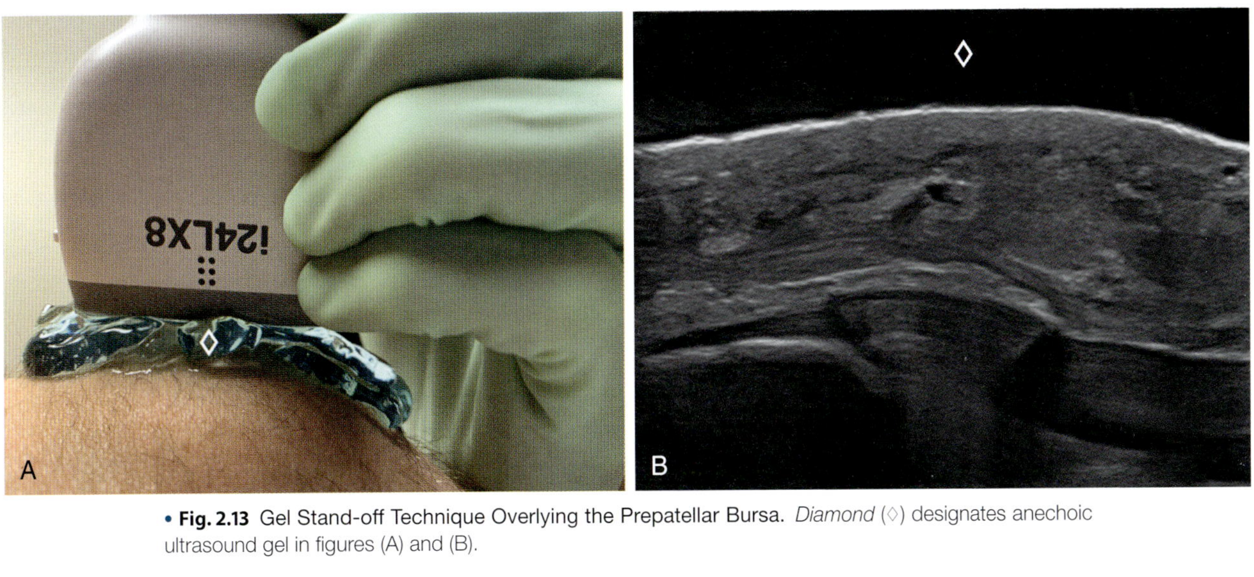

• **Fig. 2.13** Gel Stand-off Technique Overlying the Prepatellar Bursa. *Diamond* (◊) designates anechoic ultrasound gel in figures (A) and (B).

TABLE 2.4 Common Techniques to Improve Needle Tracking

Needle Tracking Technique	Action	Benefit
Needle perturbation	Needle is moved back and forth in a low-amplitude, high-velocity motion	Small degree of needle motion can make it more conspicuous and make the needle tip easier to visualize
Bevel rotation	Rotation of the needle bevel to alternately face up or down	The angled bevel at the needle tip can be easier to visualize when facing upward toward the transducer
Stylet movement	Advancing and withdrawing the stylet	Motion of the stylet can be visualized
Low volume injection	Injection of hypoechoic fluid can be visualized	Contrast between the hyperechoic needle tip and the hypoechoic surrounding fluid
Needle size and echogenicity[51]	Use of larger-gauge needle	Larger-gauge needle is easier to visualize
Compound imaging[52]	Uses beam steering to rapidly acquire overlapping views of a target from different angles	Needle is easier to visualize due to improved contrast resolution and tissue differentiation
Beam steering	Ultrasound beams are emitted at a 45-degree angle to the transducer, rather than perpendicular	Even if the transducer cannot be parallel to the needle, needle can be perpendicular to the angle of insonation of the ultrasound beam allowing for better visualization of the needle

sufficient understanding of normal sonographic anatomy and the technical skills of needle visualization and guidance under ultrasound. Training and education may be acquired through a structured residency or fellowship with a musculoskeletal ultrasound didactic curriculum. Didactic conferences, courses, books, online learning, and mentoring programs can also facilitate such learning. When diagnostic ultrasound knowledge and procedural skills are mastered by the skilled clinician, ultrasound-guided procedures are a valuable tool in the treatment of various musculoskeletal pathologies. As ultrasound technology and techniques advance, ultrasound will continue to play an increasingly important role in the clinical management of musculoskeletal conditions.

References

1. Dendy PP, Heaton B. *Physics for Diagnostic Radiology*. 3rd ed. London: CRC Press; 2011.
2. Smith J, Finnoff JT. Diagnostic and interventional musculoskeletal ultrasound: part 2. Clinical applications. *PM R*. 2009;1(2):162–177.
3. Smith J, Finnoff JT. Diagnostic and interventional musculoskeletal ultrasound: part 1. Fundamentals. *PM R*. 2009;1(1):64–75.
4. Silvestri E, Martinoli C, Derchi LE, Bertolotto M, Chiaramondia M, Rosenberg I. Echotexture of peripheral nerves: correlation between US and histologic findings and criteria to differentiate tendons. *Radiology*. 1995;197(1):291–296.
5. Gimber LH, Melville DM, Klauser AS, Witte RS, Arif-Tiwari H, Taljanovic MS. Artifacts at musculoskeletal US: resident and fellow education feature. *Radiographics*. 2016;36(2):479–480.
6. Scanlan KA. Sonographic artifacts and their origins. *AJR Am J Roentgenol*. 1991;156(6):1267–1272.
7. Boote EJ. AAPM/RSNA physics tutorial for residents: topics in US: Doppler US techniques: concepts of blood flow detection and flow dynamics. *Radiographics*. 2003;23(5):1315–1327.
8. Bude RO, Rubin JM. Power Doppler sonography. *Radiology*. 1996;200(1):21–23.
9. Breidahl WH, Stafford Johnson DB, Newman JS, Adler RS. Power Doppler sonography in tenosynovitis: significance of the peritendinous hypoechoic rim. *J Ultrasound Med*. 1998;17(2):103–107.
10. Chen J, Chen L, Wu L, et al. Value of superb microvascular imaging ultrasonography in the diagnosis of carpal tunnel syndrome: compared with color Doppler and power Doppler. *Medicine (Baltimore)*. 2017;96(21):e6862.
11. Ishikawa M, Ota Y, Nagai M, Kusaka G, Tanaka Y, Naritaka H. Ultrasonography monitoring with superb microvascular imaging technique in brain tumor surgery. *World Neurosurg*. 2017;97:749.e711–749.e720.
12. Ohno Y, Fujimoto T, Shibata Y. A New era in diagnostic ultrasound, superb microvascular imaging: preliminary results in pediatric hepato-gastrointestinal disorders. *Eur J Pediatr Surg*. 2017;27(1):20–25.
13. Toshiba Medical System JH. *Seeing the Unseen New Techniques in Vascular Imaging, Superb Micro-Vascular Imaging*. Toshiba Medical System Corporation; 2014.
14. Finnoff JT, Hall MM, Adams E, et al. American Medical Society for Sports Medicine (AMSSM) position statement: interventional musculoskeletal ultrasound in sports medicine. *PM R*. 2015;7(2):151–168. e112.
15. Hall MM. The accuracy and efficacy of palpation versus image-guided peripheral injections in sports medicine. *Curr Sports Med Rep*. 2013;12(5):296–303.
16. Dogu B, Yucel SD, Sag SY, Bankaoglu M, Kuran B. Blind or ultrasound-guided corticosteroid injections and short-term response in subacromial impingement syndrome: a randomized, double-blind, prospective study. *Am J Phys Med Rehabil*. 2012;91(8):658–665.

17. Rutten MJ, Maresch BJ, Jager GJ, de Waal Malefijt MC. Injection of the subacromial-subdeltoid bursa: blind or ultrasound-guided? *Acta Orthop*. 2007;78(2):254–257.
18. Chen MJ, Lew HL, Hsu TC, et al. Ultrasound-guided shoulder injections in the treatment of subacromial bursitis. *Am J Phys Med Rehabil*. 2006;85(1):31–35.
19. Ekeberg OM, Bautz-Holter E, Tveita EK, Juel NG, Kvalheim S, Brox JI. Subacromial ultrasound guided or systemic steroid injection for rotator cuff disease: randomised double blind study. *BMJ*. 2009;338:a3112.
20. Lee HJ, Lim KB, Kim DY, Lee KT. Randomized controlled trial for efficacy of intra-articular injection for adhesive capsulitis: ultrasonography-guided versus blind technique. *Arch Phys Med Rehabil*. 2009;90(12):1997–2002.
21. Naredo E, Cabero F, Beneyto P, et al. A randomized comparative study of short term response to blind injection versus sonographic-guided injection of local corticosteroids in patients with painful shoulder. *J Rheumatol*. 2004;31(2):308–314.
22. Ucuncu F, Capkin E, Karkucak M, et al. A comparison of the effectiveness of landmark-guided injections and ultrasonography guided injections for shoulder pain. *Clin J Pain*. 2009;25(9):786–789.
23. Sibbitt Jr WL, Band PA, Chavez-Chiang NR, Delea SL, Norton HE, Bankhurst AD. A randomized controlled trial of the cost-effectiveness of ultrasound-guided intraarticular injection of inflammatory arthritis. *J Rheumatol*. 2011;38(2):252–263.
24. Valtonen EJ. Double acting betamethasone (Celestone Chronodose) in the treatment of supraspinatus tendinitis: a comparison of subacromial and gluteal single injections with placebo. *J Int Med Res*. 1978;6(6):463–467.
25. Bhatia A, Gofeld M, Ganapathy S, Hanlon J, Johnson M. Comparison of anatomic landmarks and ultrasound guidance for intercostal nerve injections in cadavers. *Reg Anesth Pain Med*. 2013;38(6):503–507.
26. Leopold SS, Battista V, Oliverio JA. Safety and efficacy of intraarticular hip injection using anatomic landmarks. *Clin Orthop Relat Res*. 2001;391:192–197.
27. Malloy PC, Grassi CJ, Kundu S, et al. Consensus guidelines for periprocedural management of coagulation status and hemostasis risk in percutaneous image-guided interventions. *J Vasc Interv Radiol*. 2009;20(suppl 7):S240–249.
28. Taninishi H, Morita K. Ultrasound-guided peripheral nerve blocks for a patient receiving four kinds of anticoagulant and antiplatelet drugs: a case report. *J Anesth*. 2011;25(2):318–320.
29. Loizides A, Gruber H, Peer S, Galiano K, Bale R, Obernauer J. Ultrasound guided versus CT-controlled pararadicular injections in the lumbar spine: a prospective randomized clinical trial. *AJNR Am J Neuroradiol*. 2013;34(2):466–470.
30. Obernauer J, Galiano K, Gruber H, et al. Ultrasound-guided versus Computed Tomography-controlled facet joint injections in the middle and lower cervical spine: a prospective randomized clinical trial. *Med Ultrasonography*. 2013;15(1):10–15.
31. Finlayson RJ, Etheridge JP, Tiyaprasertkul W, Nelems B, Tran DQ. A randomized comparison between ultrasound- and fluoroscopy-guided c7 medial branch block. *Reg Anesth Pain Med*. 2015;40(1):52–57.
32. Park KD, Lim DJ, Lee WY, Ahn J, Park Y. Ultrasound versus fluoroscopy-guided cervical medial branch block for the treatment of chronic cervical facet joint pain: a retrospective comparative study. *Skeletal Radiol*. 2017;46(1):81–91.
33. Hofmeister M, Dowsett LE, Lorenzetti DL, Clement F. Ultrasound- versus fluoroscopy-guided injections in the lower back for the management of pain: a systematic review. *Eur Radiol*. 2019;29(7):3401–3409.
34. Wu T, Zhao WH, Dong Y, Song HX, Li JH. Effectiveness of ultrasound-guided versus fluoroscopy or computed tomography scanning guidance in lumbar facet joint injections in adults with facet joint syndrome: a meta-analysis of controlled trials. *Arch Phys Med Rehabil*. 2016;97(9):1558–1563.
35. De Luigi AJ, Saini V, Mathur R, Saini A, Yokel N. Assessing the accuracy of ultrasound-guided needle placement in sacroiliac joint injections. *Am J Phys Med Rehabil*. 2019;98(8):666–670.
36. Jee H, Lee JH, Park KD, Ahn J, Park Y. Ultrasound-guided versus fluoroscopy-guided sacroiliac joint intra-articular injections in the noninflammatory sacroiliac joint dysfunction: a prospective, randomized, single-blinded study. *Arch Phy Med Rehabil*. 2014;95(2):330–337.
37. Klauser A, De Zordo T, Feuchtner G, et al. Feasibility of ultrasound-guided sacroiliac joint injection considering sonoanatomic landmarks at two different levels in cadavers and patients. *Arthritis Rheum*. 2008;59(11):1618–1624.
38. Soneji N, Bhatia A, Seib R, Tumber P, Dissanayake M, Peng PW. Comparison of fluoroscopy and ultrasound guidance for sacroiliac joint injection in patients with chronic low back pain. *Pain Practice*. 2016;16(5):537–544.
39. Stelzer W, Stelzer D, Stelzer E, et al. Success rate of intra-articular sacroiliac joint injection: fluoroscopy vs ultrasound guidance – a cadaveric study. *Pain Med*. 2019;20(10):1890–1897.
40. Levi DS. Intra-articular hip injections using ultrasound guidance: accuracy using a linear array transducer. *PM R*. 2013;5(2):129–134.
41. Martinez-Martinez A, Garcia-Espinosa J, Ruiz-Santiago F, Guzman-Alvarez L, Castellano-Garcia MM. Comparison of ultrasound and fluoroscopic guidance for injection in CT arthrography and MR arthrography of the hip. *Radiologia*. 2016;58(6):454–459.
42. Micu MC, Bogdan GD, Fodor D. Steroid injection for hip osteoarthritis: efficacy under ultrasound guidance. *Rheumatology (Oxford)*. 2010;49(8):1490–1494.
43. Pourbagher MA, Ozalay M, Pourbagher A. Accuracy and outcome of sonographically guided intra-articular sodium hyaluronate injections in patients with osteoarthritis of the hip. *J Ultrasound Med*. 2005;24(10):1391–1395.
44. Smith J, Hurdle MF, Weingarten TN. Accuracy of sonographically guided intra-articular injections in the native adult hip. *J Ultrasound Med*. 2009;28(3):329–335.
45. Byrd JW, Potts EA, Allison RK, Jones KS. Ultrasound-guided hip injections: a comparative study with fluoroscopy-guided injections. *Arthroscopy*. 2014;30(1):42–46.
46. Sibbitt Jr WL, Band PA, Kettwich LG, Chavez-Chiang NR, Delea SL, Bankhurst AD. A randomized controlled trial evaluating the cost-effectiveness of sonographic guidance for intra-articular injection of the osteoarthritic knee. *J Clin Rheumatol*. 2011;17(8):409–415.
47. Gyftopoulos S, Abballe V, Virk MS, Koo J, Gold HT, Subhas N. Comparison between image-guided and landmark-based glenohumeral joint injections for the treatment of adhesive capsulitis: a cost-effectiveness study. *AJR Am J Roentgenol*. 2018;210(6):1279–1287.

48. Harrison G, Harris A. Work-related musculoskeletal disorders in ultrasound: can you reduce risk? *Ultrasound.* 2015;23(4):224–230.
49. Sites BD, Macfarlane AJ, Sites VR, et al. Clinical sonopathology for the regional anesthesiologist: part 2: bone, viscera, subcutaneous tissue, and foreign bodies. *Reg Anesth Pain Med.* 2010;35(3):281–289.
50. Sites BD, Macfarlane AJ, Sites VR, et al. Clinical sonopathology for the regional anesthesiologist: part 1: vascular and neural. *Reg Anesth Pain Med.* 2010;35(3):272–280.
51. Deam RK, Kluger R, Barrington MJ, McCutcheon CA. Investigation of a new echogenic needle for use with ultrasound peripheral nerve blocks. *Anaesth Intensive Care.* 2007;35(4):582–586.
52. Wiesmann T, Borntrager A, Zoremba M, Neff M, Wulf H, Steinfeldt T. Compound imaging technology and echogenic needle design: effects on needle visibility and tissue imaging. *Reg Anesth Pain Med.* 2013;38(5):452–455.

3

Principles of Fluoroscopy Imaging in Spine and Musculoskeletal Interventional Orthopedics

KATARZYNA IWAN, RAHUL NAREN DESAI, AND JOHN J. WOLFSON

Introduction

Fluoroscopy has played a central role for injection therapies of the spine and peripheral joints, for both interventional pain management and orthopedics. In this chapter, we focus on the principles and the use of fluoroscopy regarding both spinal and peripheral interventions as it applies to the emerging field of regenerative medicine. Fields such as interventional radiology, sports medicine, physiatry, and orthopedics rely on fluoroscopy to enhance the accuracy and effectiveness of procedures.[1–5] As these fields have incorporated regenerative injectates, it is a natural progression to use fluoroscopic guidance for more precise delivery of the biologic treatment to the injured tissue. Fluoroscopy allows providers to precisely, efficiently, and safely direct the needle and literally "pinpoint" the target location while minimizing damage to unintended structures. By using bony landmarks and confirmation with contrast, there is a very high degree of certainty that injectates reach the target tissues and give the best possible chance of therapeutic success. In addition, fluoroscopy allows for precision injection of materials, be it cement or orthobiologics into bone. Simply placing a needle into bone does not ensure placement and retention of the material into bone, and one can frequently see venous vascular flow of contrast out of the bone and away from the intended targets. Small adjustments of the needle tip can make a substantial difference in the deposition of the treatment injectate.

A keen sense of anatomy, trajectory, and understanding of vital structures is a crucial and required skill set for any interventionalist performing these therapies. Although it may be inferred, these procedures should only be performed by well-qualified physicians who have completed adequate postdoctoral training. Many injections, including joint injections, require experience, spatial awareness, and anatomic understanding so as not to puncture nerves, vessels, or critical structures that may be in the needle path. In the setting of fluoroscopic guidance, the superficial anatomy, manual palpation, and bony landmarks on the images serve as guides for the needle's pathway. The developing field of regenerative orthopedics relies on the knowledge and techniques of traditional diagnostic and therapeutic injections of the spine, joints, nerves, and soft tissues. In this chapter, we discuss the principles of fluoroscopy as it applies to diagnosis and treatment of musculoskeletal conditions.

Radiation Terminology and Measurement

There are numerous terms and units of measurement used in radiology, and one must be familiar with their value and relationship to each other. Radiation can be described in terms of radioactivity, exposure, absorbed dose, and dose equivalent (Table 3.1). In general:

- 1 R (exposure) = 1 rad (absorbed dose) = 1 rem or 1000 mrem (dose equivalent)

Fluoroscopy History and Background

Fluoroscopy is an imaging technique that uses real-time x-rays to create images of a patient. The history of fluoroscopy dates back over a century.[1–3] In 1895, physicist Wilhelm Conrad Roentgen (1845–1923) discovered and coined the term "x-ray." His discovery was accidental; he noticed a glow when attempting to pass cathode rays through glass. Later, he discovered that x-rays penetrate soft tissue but not

TABLE 3.1 **Measuring Radiation**

	Definition	Unit Measurements	Relationships
Radioactivity	Amount of radiation released by a material	Curie (Ci) Becquerel (Bq)	1 Ci = 3.7×10^{10} Bq
Exposure	Amount of radiation exiting the x-ray tube, traveling through the air	Roentgen (R) Coulomb/kilogram (C/kg)	1 R = 2.58×10^{-4} C/kg
Absorbed dose	Amount of radiation absorbed by an object/person	Rad (r) Gray (Gy)	I Gy = 100 r
Dose equivalent	Amount of radiation absorbed as it relates to the radiation type and subsequent biologic impact	Roentgen-equivalent-man (rem) Sievert (Sv)	1/1000th rem is known as millirem (mrem); commonly used for biologic dose equivalent 1 Sv = 100 rem

Created with information from the United States Nuclear Regulatory Commission. https://www.nrc.gov/about-nrc/radiation/health-effects/measuring-radiation.html

metal or bone, and he captured the first x-ray image of his wife's hand. In 1897, x-rays were used to identify broken bones during the Balkan War. In 1901, Roentgen won the Nobel Prize in Physics for his discovery. Following Roentgen's work on x-rays in 1895, Thomas Edison's assistant, glassblower Clarence Dally, worked on development of the Edison x-ray focus tube, resulting in a fluoroscope that produced sharper images than the Roentgen fluoroscope.

Unfortunately, the potential harmful effects of x-rays were identified more slowly. In 1904, Dally died from skin cancer. He is considered the first documented radiation fatality, but it was not until the 1950s that x-rays were determined to carry significant risk. In the subsequent decades, engineering and computing advances made fluoroscopy capable of high-resolution imaging using minimal radiation. Currently, the technique of fluoroscopy is practiced in most hospitals, surgery centers, and outpatient clinics and is readily available.

In general, fluoroscopes are considered fixed (permanent) or mobile (portable). Fixed fluoroscopes are either a vertical fluoroscope or fixed C-arm fluoroscope. Mobile fluoroscopes use a C-arm system on wheels and are commonly implemented in outpatient interventional pain practices. The C-arm system moves the x-ray tube and image intensifier in any axis, thereby allowing image acquisition from nearly any angle.[1–5]

Two categories of fluoroscopic units are currently available for mainstream medical use, traditional image-intensifier, and flat-panel detector systems. The more traditional image-intensifier television camera-based systems have been in use since the 1950s. The traditional image-intensifier based C-arm fluoroscopy system (Fig. 3.1) consists of the following components (from bottom to top):

- X-ray generator and tube: generates x-rays
- Collimator: restricts the x-ray field and focuses the beam
- Image intensifier: allows visualization of the image in a brightly lit room and reduces the radiation dose when compared with standard screen-film cassette
  - Input phosphor—cesium iodide: converts x-ray photons to light photons
  - Photocathode—antimony and alkali metals: converts light photons to electrons
  - Electrostatic focusing lens (electrode focusing plates): guides electrons to the anode
  - Accelerating anode: accelerates electrons and gives them electronic gain
  - Output phosphor—zinc cadmium sulfide: converts electrons back to light photons, creating magnification and a thousand times increase in brightness or intensity
- Lens/aperture: focuses the light
- Video camera (new technology) or television camera (older technology): displays the image

More recently, flat-panel detector systems have been available and have many advantages, most importantly reduction in radiation dose. Flat-panel digital fluoroscopy, derived from thin film transistor technology, emerged in the 1990s and is replacing the image intensifier and video camera. Thin film transistor technology, best known for its use in modern television, avoids motion or image distortion and improves dynamic range, allowing for improved image quality.[6,7,8–10] However, some concerns remain about its potentially poor image quality at low exposure levels, technology replacement costs, and equipment durability.[4,5]

There are significant benefits with flat-panel display (FPD) systems when compared with the image intensifier–based units. Solid-state FPD image receptors generally have better stability, lower radiation dose rates, and improved dynamic range, and they eliminate glare and geometric distortions such as vignetting and defocusing effects.[6] Costs for units appropriate for interventional pain procedures have dramatically reduced, which had been a major limiting factor for prior generations of the technology. Based upon the reduced exposure to radiation for both the patient and physician, this technology should be seriously considered by anyone purchasing new units for implementation.

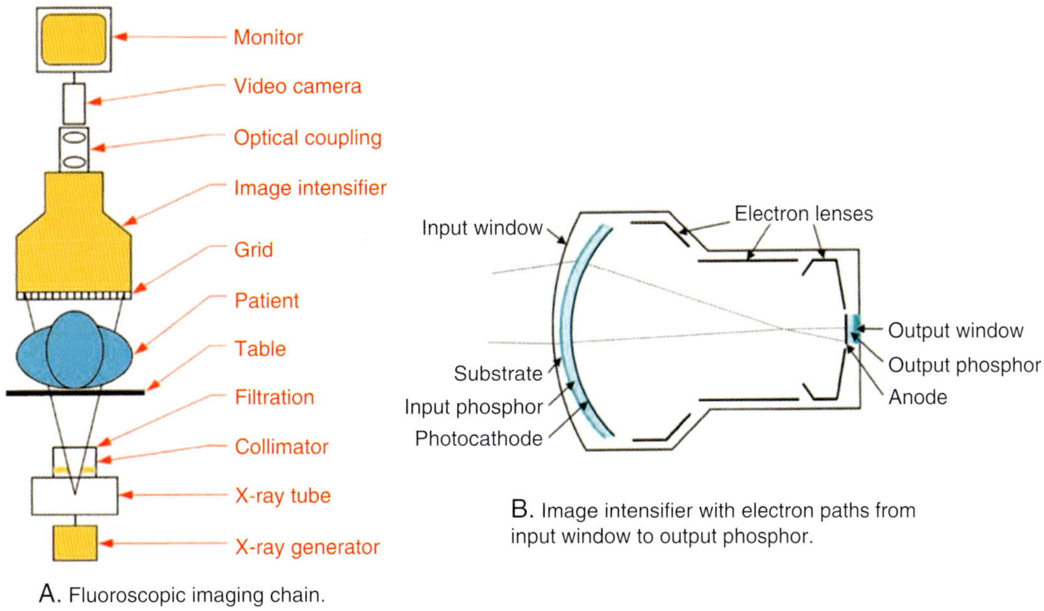

• **Fig. 3.1** The traditional image intensifier–based C-arm fluoroscopy system.

Disadvantages include a different appearance than the traditional image intensified units, and lower spatial resolution with very large or very small field of view (FOV).

Three-dimensional (3D) fluoroscopy, the newest innovation to modern fluoroscopy systems, is rotational 3D imaging in which the gantry of a fluoroscopy system rapidly rotates through 180 degrees while continuously acquiring images.[10] The resultant cine display resembles a volume-rendered computed tomographic image and may be used by physicians to better understand the geometric location of various structures, and precision delivery of biologics into bone, disc, and tissue.[9]

Precautions: As Low As Reasonably Achievable

Fluoroscopic guidance involves channeling beams of high-energy, ionized particles (x-rays) through the human body. The x-rays that do not follow this path are scattered into the surrounding environment and create occupational hazard concerns.[1–5,11] The resultant patient and staff exposure to radiation necessitates safety equipment and guidelines to minimize the risk of skin injury or cancer. ALARA (as low as reasonably achievable) is a radiation reduction concept that should be used and enforced in all fluoroscopic settings. It aims to minimize radiation exposure to patients and staff by implementing guidelines around exposure time, shielding, and distance (Table 3.2).

The annual individual radiation dose limits were set in 1990 and reconfirmed in 2007 by the International Commission on Radiological Protection and are currently as follows: 20 mSv (5000 mrem/year) for whole body, 150 mSv for thyroid, and 500 mSv for hands.[11] However, protective equipment is imperfect. It is estimated that approximately 0.6% to 6.8% of x-rays are transmitted through protective aprons.[12] Finally, the x-ray generator should be as far and the image intensifier as close to the patient as possible. The scatter of x-rays is greatest between the patient and the x-ray generator, and positioning the x-ray generator below the patient will concentrate scatter to the operator's feet rather than head. Placing the x-ray generator twice the distance from the patient reduces the scatter of x-rays by one-fourth.[13] As the demonstrated efficacy and ease of access of fluoroscopy increases, and thus the frequency of fluoroscopic use increases, it is imperative that practitioners prioritize radiation safety. Pain management interventionalists and regenerative specialists must appreciate the unwelcome fallout of improperly managed radiography, develop safety protocols to limit both patient and provider exposure, and follow the principle of ALARA.[14]

Radiation Dose

Most interventional pain medicine procedures performed under fluoroscopic guidance result in total radiation exposure time in seconds, not minutes. Regenerative medicine procedures should follow the benchmark guidelines of standard procedures and the average radiation dose delivered (Table 3.3). Studies show that doses less than 2 Gy should not result in any observable effects over the span of 400 days.[13] Assuming a 0.02 to 0.05 Gy/min skin absorption rate, this would take nearly an hour of constant fluoroscopic guidance to reach. There is contemporary discourse revolving around the wisdom of using peak skin dose or concentration in place of fluoroscopy time as a safety measure. This should be considered, particularly when a patient undergoes multiple consecutive injections, such as is commonly done with prolotherapy or platelet-rich plasma.[14] Furthermore, due to the necessary increase in dose and exposure, obese

TABLE 3.2 Reducing Risk from Fluoroscopic X-rays

Important actions for reducing exposure time and risk to patient and provider when using fluoroscopy	
1.	Obtain adequate and appropriate training
2.	Wear a dosimeter and know your own dose
3.	Use personal protective equipment including aprons, thyroid collar, eyewear, and shielding when appropriate
4.	Use good imaging-chain geometry; do not overuse geometric or electronic magnification
5.	Use collimation, and always collimate to the area of interest
6.	Position yourself in a low-scatter area
7.	Plan the intervention in advance to minimize number of acquired images
8.	Obese patients will require and receive higher doses, and you will too
9.	Keep beam-on time to a minimum
10.	Keep the image intensifier as close to the patient as possible and keep the patient as far from the x-ray tube as possible
11.	Use last-imaged-stored viewing
12.	Incorporate variable frame rate pulsed practices rather than continuous or "live" fluoroscopy when possible
13.	If image quality is not compromised, remove the grid during procedures on small patients or when the image intensifier cannot be placed close to the patient
14.	A single step away from the patient will decrease provider exposure by a factor of four

Adapted and modified from Miller DL, Van˜o´ E, Bartal G, et al. Occupational radiation protection in interventional radiology: a joint guideline of the Cardiovascular and Interventional Radiology Society of Europe and the Society of Interventional Radiology. *Cardiovasc Intervent Radiol*. 2010;33:230–239; and Wagner LK, Archer BR. *Minimizing Risks from Fluoroscopic X-rays*. 3rd ed. The Woodlands, TX: RM Partnership; 2000.

patients—and those present for their procedure—are at significantly greater risk of skin injury and possibly cancer due to fluoroscopy.[15]

Regarding radiation exposure, it is imperative to consider both stochastic and nonstochastic effects. Stochastic effects, such as cancer or genetic changes, are effects that take place by chance. The likelihood of a stochastic effect increases with the individual's radiation dose (e.g., occupational exposure or repeated fluoroscopic exams); however, there is not a single threshold dose that guarantees the effect to occur. The effects usually present years after exposure, and the severity does not correlate to the degree of exposure. In contrast, nonstochastic (or deterministic) effects, such as radiation burns or hair loss, are those that take place only when a threshold dose has occurred, usually as a large, single radiation dose. This is a consideration most notably in radiation oncology and radioactive spills. In this case, a clear cause and effect relationship is identified, and the degree of effect is dependent on the magnitude of exposure.

Although the relative simplicity of interventional procedures protects patients against the longer exposure times found with other fluoroscopic procedures, patient dose and exposure should not be taken lightly.[16] Of equal concern is practitioner exposure. It is significantly difficult to negate scatter radiation in interventional pain management and regenerative medicine procedure setting due to the proximity the interventionist must maintain with the injection (and the imaging) site; accordingly, this suggests reducing patient exposure would reduce occupational exposure. Cumulative dose and the risk of cancer becomes concerning when interventionalists regularly perform high volumes of interventional procedures, as is often done in a regenerative medicine practice.

Radiation Protection Services oversees the public's health and safety as it pertains to radiation exposure. The organization governs appropriate use and maintenance of fluoroscopes. Although national and statewide regulations vary widely, the following is an approximate list of the required documentation, taken from Oregon Radiation Protection Services (author's state of licensure and practice). Please see state-specific documents for a complete list.

Fluoroscope Inspection Required Documentation:

1. Dosimetry Records
2. Licenses for all qualified operators
3. Annual Physics Survey for each fluoroscope
4. Written procedures regarding the setup and operation of each fluoroscopic machine registered to the facility
5. Written radiation safety procedures pertaining to the use and operation of fluoroscopy
6. Benchmarks defining procedural exposure times
7. Fluoroscopy logs—documentation of procedure performed
8. Annual Program Review—benchmark review, quality assurance, and corrective actions
9. Patient ESE (entrance skin exposure)
10. Gonadal Shielding Policy
11. Annual lead apron check

Contrast Media

Contrast media are used to enhance or outline anatomic boundaries of a target area to help ensure proper needle placement prior to injection of a diagnostic or therapeutic agent and avoid inadvertent intravascular placement. When performed intentionally, this is referred to as an angiogram (arteriogram or venogram). Fluoroscopy may be superior for targeting soft tissue structures that are routinely difficult to visualize with ultrasound such as anterior cruciate ligament, posterior cruciate ligament, and iliolumbar ligament injections. Contrast can be injected into these ligaments, tendons, and other soft tissues to illustrate the lesion and

TABLE 3.3 Dose (mGy) Per Injection and Time (s) Per Injection by Procedure

				Radiation Dose (mGy)				
Procedure	**Number of Studies**	**Mean Dose**	**Standard Deviation**	**10th Percentile With 95% CI**	**25th Percentile With 95% CI**	**50th Percentile With 95% CI**	**75th Percentile With 95% CI**	**95th Percentile With 95% CI**
Transforaminal lumbar	3590	10.4	11.9	2.0 (1.9–2.2)	3.5 (3.3–3.6)	6.7 (6.5–7.0)	12.5 (11.9–13.1)	32.4 (30.6–34.2)
Transforaminal cervical	157	5.6	6.5	1.0 (0.8–1.1)	1.8 (1.4–2.2)	3.3 (3.0–3.7)	5.7 (3.3–6.5)	21.8 (18.0–27.6)
Caudal epidural	658	10.0	12.4	1.6 (1.3–1.7)	3.1 (2.8–3.6)	6.0 (5.5–6.4)	11.0 (9.6–12.4)	32.8 (27.3–36.3)
Facet joint cervical	62	2.6	2.8	0.5 (0.4–0.8)	0.7 (0.3–0.9)	1.5 (0.9–1.7)	3 (1.3–4)	8.4 (6.8–12.1)
Facet joint lumbar	410	6.45	6.41	1.1 (0.7–1.2)	2.2 (2.1–2.5)	4.1 (3.3–4.5)	8.7 (7.9–10)	19 (15.2–22.1)
Interlaminar (translaminar)	446	11.2	14.7	1.4 (1.2–1.6)	2.7 (2.2–3.0)	6.4 (5.8–7.4)	12.4 (9.3–13.6)	42.2 (26.7–52.5)
Radiofrequency denervation (lumbar)	318	4.7	6.6	0.5 (0.4–0.6)	1.3 (1.1–1.5)	2.7 (2.3–3.1)	6.3 (5.7–7.5)	15.8 (13.0–20.1)
Lumbar sympathetic block	296	15.4	16.2	2.5 (2.0–2.8)	4.5 (3.1–5.3)	9.9 (7.9–10.9)	19.2 (15.3–21.9)	49.9 (40.1–62.8)
Medial branch block cervical	41	2.2	2.1	0.4 (0.2–0.5)	0.7 (0.3–1)	1.7 (0.8–2.4)	2.8 (1.4–3.4)	6.4 (2.7–8.9)
Medial branch block lumbar	169	3.4	4.4	3.9 (3–4.1)	5.2 (4.6–5.5)	7.9 (6.8–8.5)	12.1 (10.6–13.8)	21.8 (14.8–25.7)
Sacroiliac joint	87	9.9	8.2	2.0 (1.4–2.5)	3.7 (1.9–4.9)	7.0 (5.9–7.7)	15.0 (11.8–21.3)	27.4 (22.6–33.9)
				Procedure Time (s)				
Procedure	**Number of Studies**	**Mean Time**	**Standard Deviation**	**10th Percentile With 95% CI**	**25th Percentile With 95% CI**	**50th Percentile With 95% CI**	**75th Percentile With 95% CI**	**95th Percentile With 95% CI**
Transforaminal lumbar	3590	24.3	15.4	10.4 (10.1–10.6)	14.3 (14.0–14.6)	20.3 (19.7–20.8)	29.9 (29.2–30.9)	52.7 (50.9–55.2)
Transforaminal cervical	157	40.4	28.6	18.2 (17.3–20.5)	21.1 (18.6–22.6)	31.2 (27.0–35.7)	46.3 (37.7–52.0)	105.0 (84.5–122.6)
Caudal epidural	658	18.9	13.9	7.3 (6.7–7.9)	10.1 (9.6–10.5)	14.8 (13.8–15.6)	22.6 (20.7–23.8)	44.8 (34.9–49.4)
Facet joint cervical	62	27.0	18.5	11.2 (9.7–13.5)	13.6 (10.3–15)	22.1 (17.8–26.7)	35.2 (28.3–43.6)	52.3 (19.8–61.2)

Continued

TABLE 3.3 Dose (mGy) Per Injection and Time (s) Per Injection by Procedure—Cont'd

	Procedure Time (s)							
Procedure	Number of Studies	Mean Time	Standard Deviation	10th Percentile With 95% CI	25th Percentile With 95% CI	50th Percentile With 95% CI	75th Percentile With 95% CI	95th Percentile With 95% CI
Facet joint lumbar	410	16.5	9.1	7.3 (6.7–7.7)	10.3 (9.3–11.1)	14.4 (13.5–14.9)	20.5 (18.9–21.8)	33.5 (31.2–37.2)
Interlaminar (translaminar)	446	29.5	20.7	11.6 (10.8–12.1)	15.4 (14.3–16.5)	23.5 (20.9–25.4)	37.3 (34.9–40.1)	64.2 (54.7–70.3)
Radiofrequency denervation (lumbar)	318	13.5	10.4	4.8 (3.7–5.5)	7.3 (6.6–8.0)	11.5 (10.9–12.4)	16.2 (14.8–17.8)	28.2 (21.4–30.6)
Lumbar sympathetic block	296	32.3	14.0	19.1 (17.8–20.6)	23.9 (22.9–24.7)	29.1 (27.2–30.5)	37.5 (35.8–39.7)	59.1 (48.9–67.8)
Medial branch block cervical	41	19.1	10.0	6.9(1.8–8.4)	12.3 (9.4–16.6)	16.9 (11.3–19.6)	25.4 (21.1–29.6)	35 (18.4–41.4)
Medial branch block lumbar	169	9.8	7.3	3.9 (3–4.1)	5.2 (4.6–5.5)	7.9 (6.8–8.5)	12.1 (10.6–13.8)	21.8 (14.8–25.7)
Sacroiliac joint	87	28.6	14.5	13.3 (12.4–15.1)	16.6 (13.5–19.4)	27.8 (23.7–33.8)	36.1 (30.1–38.6)	54.7 (46.7–63.8)

CI, Confidence interval.
Adapted from Cohen SL, Schneider R, Carrino JA, et al. Radiation dose practice audit of 6,234 fluoroscopically-guided spinal injections. *Pain Physician*. 2019;22:E119–E125.

ensure intralesional placement and accurate delivery of the biologic. Meniscal or labral lesions are often visualized and accessible via ultrasound; however, in cases such as meniscal root tears or glenoid labral tears in larger patients, fluoroscopy may be a superior modality.

When the needle is placed in a joint and direct contrast media is injected, this is referred to as an arthrogram. Similarly, if the contrast media is injected into an intervertebral disc, the fluoroscopic image is referred to as a discogram. When confirming epidural needle placement, injection of contrast media into the epidural space is referred to as an epidurogram. Differing imaging modalities may require one of many possible contrast media classes, yet the class of contrast media indicated for x-ray (and thus fluoroscopic) imaging is iodinated contrast agents (ICAs).

ICAs are broadly classified as either ionic or nonionic. Ionic ICAs such as diatrizoate (Hypaque) and ioxaglate (Hexabrix) are hyperosmolar relative to blood. These ionic agents are associated with a risk of neurotoxicity; therefore they should not be injected into the spinal cord or bronchial tree.[17,18,19] Nonionic ICAs, such as iohexol (Omnipaque) and iodixanol (Visipaque), are generally low osmolar or iso-osmolar, respectively. There are three general administration routes of a given contrast agent: intravascular, enteric, or direct injection. For the interventionalist performing fluoroscopic-guided procedures, direct injection is the indicated administration route. When considering risks associated with either contrast agent or route of administration, ionic ICAs delivered intravascularly pose the highest risk of adverse reaction. The incidence of adverse reaction to a high-osmolarity ionic agent is approximately 15% and only approximately 3% for low-osmolarity nonionic agents.[20] This is one of several reasons why low-osmolarity nonionic agents such as Omnipaque or Visipaque are the contrast agents of choice.

An ICA administered by direct injection is not metabolized locally or systemically.[21] Instead it is postulated that the ICA is slowly absorbed into the body via the lymphatic system and then cleared by the kidneys. Adverse reactions to a low-osmolar ICA delivered by direct injection is very rare, yet it is best practice to try to prevent possible acute adverse reactions by screening patients for the most common risk factors for an acute reaction to an ICA. These three risk factors are a history of asthma, a prior reaction to an ICA, and atopy.[22] For patients who have one of these risk factors, be sure to avoid ionic high-osmolar ICAs and consider whether an ultrasound-guided injection may be adequate. Recent literature review has shown that the relationship between shellfish allergies and iodine allergies does not increase the likelihood to contrast allergic reactions.[23,24] Moreover, common interventional procedures using ICAs expose the patient to very small volumes of contrast, unlike intravascular administration; therefore the risk is further diminished. Patients can be premedicated with diphenhydramine if there is any concern by the physician. All gadolinium-based contrast agents are chelated with the intention of making the agents less toxic or nontoxic while allowing for renal excretion. Adverse reactions to ICAs range from mild to severe and life threatening. If interventionalists are going to administer an ICA, they should be sure that they are trained and equipped to handle anaphylaxis and anaphylactoid reactions. Because the interventionalist will be administering the ICA by direct injection, the risk of contrast-induced nephropathy is negated. The most common adverse reactions reported in relation to direct ICA administration are swelling of the associated joint and injection site hematoma.

Contrast Media and Orthobiologics

To our knowledge, there are very little data on the effects of fluoroscopy and contrast media on biologics such as plasma-rich protein (PRP). A study using human intervertebral disc cells in vitro found contrast media to be cytotoxic to the cells. The cytotoxic effects were greater with ionic contrast media when compared with nonionic, dimeric contrast media and was dose dependent.[25] A more recent study from Wu et al. evaluated potential cytotoxic effects of iohexol (Omnipaque 300) on human adipose-derived mesenchymal stem cells (MSCs). Wu et al. demonstrated that there was toxicity to MSCs in a time- and concentration-dependent manner; however, a brief 30-minute exposure did not affect MSC function or viability.[26] Another study by McKee et al. studied the effects of contrast on human umbilical stem cells in vitro. It showed that contrast had cytotoxic effects in a concentration- and time-dependent manner, with iopamidol (Isovue-300) being significantly more toxic than iohexol.[27] One must consider the risks and benefits of placing the biologics in the incorrect location versus the possible effect of contrast media on the biologic injectate itself. As a general recommendation, as little contrast as needed for accurate and safe injection of cells should be used and one can consider diluting the contrast where appropriate to reduce the concentration. Avoid ionic agents and iopamidol (Isovue-300) for use with cellular therapies.

Practical Fluoroscopy Bullets

Protective Equipment, Shielding, Monitoring

Key Points

- Radiation safety can be accomplished with the use of widely available protective equipment, shielding, distances from the x-ray source to the pertinent anatomy, and awareness of personnel distances from the x-ray source.

Pertinent Information

- During fluoroscopic interventional spine procedures, the use of lead aprons with a lead equivalency of at least 0.25 mm should be worn by all staff members within the room and any personnel who may enter the room during procedures. Lead protective aprons with a 0.50-mm lead equivalent are preferred. This is especially true for the interventionalist and any staff members who would be at the patient's head during procedures.

- Lead aprons attenuate between 90% and 95% of scattered radiation.[28]

- During fluoroscopic orthopedic extremity procedures, it is recommended that lead aprons with at least 0.25-mm lead equivalent be worn by the interventionalist.
  - This is a recommendation only when using smaller, lower-output exposure fluoroscopic units that may commonly be termed as "mini C-arms."
- The use of additional lead transparent shielding is encouraged where available.
- Thyroid shields that meet a 0.50-mm lead equivalency should be worn in conjunction with lead aprons.
- Lead protective eye wear should also be used by the interventionalist and anesthesia provider whenever possible.
- The use of protective lead gloves is dependent upon the practices of the interventionalist. Interventionalists who practice techniques that keep their hands within the area of the imaging field should not wear protective lead gloves. The reasons for this are as follows:
  - The automatic exposure control used by most newer-generation C-arm fluoroscopy units will detect an increase in the density of the required imaging field. This density is created by now adding two layers of a lead protective glove into the imaging field.
  - The fluoroscopy unit will respond to any increase in detected density by increasing the overall output exposure to sufficiently penetrate the added density. The x-ray machine will try to penetrate two layers of lead protective gloves if the interventionalist's hands are in the imaging field.
  - The increased output exposure will cause the interventionalist's hands to become overradiated in addition to increasing the absorbed patient dose and the scatter dose that exposes other staff in the room.
- Interventionalists who regularly remove their hands to just beyond the area of the imaging field are encouraged to wear lead protective gloves. The x-ray beam attenuation properties of most commonly available lead protective gloves will decrease the scatter radiation exposure to the hands.
- Active radiation dosimetry monitoring should be used in every interventional procedure environment. The use of cumulative dosimetry badges that are analyzed, at least on a quarterly basis by an accredited dosimetry entity, is highly encouraged.
  - Care should be taken to remove the dosimeters from the procedure suite at the end of each procedure day.
  - Storing dosimeters within the lead protective aprons on a regular basis is discouraged because these may end up being left in the procedure suite, thereby producing falsely increased dose readings.
  - A secondary type of active radiation dosimetry monitoring is the use of real-time dosimeters. This type of dosimeter can be turned off or reset at the end of each day, and each dose reading can be logged daily.
  - For real-time dosimeters, it is common to wear the devices inside of the lead apron.
- Each facility should have a dedicated radiation or medical physicist who oversees the radiation safety program. The physicist will determine whether radiation dosimeters should be worn outside or inside of the lead protective aprons. If your facility does not have a physicist, then consult with your radiation dosimetry entity.

Dose Reduction During Interventional Orthopedic Procedures

Key Points

- There are many controllable techniques and machine features that can be used to decrease the x-ray radiation dose that the patient, interventionalist, and staff are exposed to.
- Use of good exposure practices can serve to decrease radiation exposure to the patient and staff.

Pertinent Information

- Most modern fluoroscopic C-arm units have dose-limiting and x-ray beam–limiting capabilities. The most common dose-limiting capabilities are the "low-dose" mode and pulsed fluoroscopy modes. Use of either of these capabilities will degrade image quality in exchange for lower radiation exposures. The interventionalist must weigh the risks of radiation exposure versus the need for image quality when using these dose-limiting modes.
- Fluoroscopic C-arms have beam limiting capabilities in the form of collimating the size and shape of the x-ray beam. Using proper collimation that allows visualization of the pertinent anatomy and the reference anatomy will decrease the overall output x-ray exposure of the machine.
- Distance from the x-ray source allows for the use of the inverse square law to reduce the radiation exposure to staff. When the distance from an x-ray source is doubled, the amount of exposure is decreased by a factor of 4.
- The use of high-level fluoroscopy or boosted fluoroscopy mode should be minimized (normally indicated by an icon that looks like an "eye" with a plus sign next to it). Although the amount of increased radiation exposure from using this mode will vary depending upon the fluoroscopy machine manufacturer, it is recommended that the use of this mode should be limited to intermittent spot visualization. The use of high-level fluoroscopy may also be needed due to patient body habitus or anatomic part thickness. Nonetheless, it is recommended that such use remains limited. Final documentation of needle or device positioning can be accomplished in normal or low-dose mode, depending upon patient body habitus. Care should be taken to limit constant exposure of the x-ray beam while in the high-level or boosted fluoroscopy mode.

Technique and Use of Good Exposure Practices

- The fluoroscopic C-arm consists of an image intensifier ("the receptor"), which is the larger rounded end, and on some newer models the flat-panel end. This receives

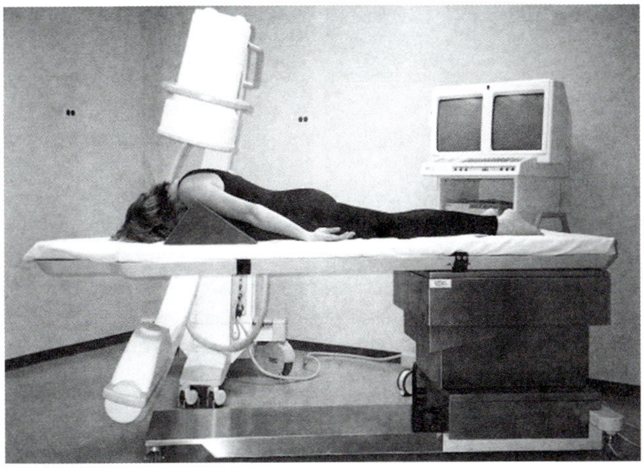

• **Fig. 3.2** Demonstration of correct C-arm orientation with the emitter underneath the procedure table and the receptor above the patient. (From Wagner LK. Radiation management for patients and protection of staff. In: Manchikanti L, Singh V, eds. *Interventional Techniques in Chronic Spinal Pain*. Paducah, KY: ASIPP Publishing; 2007:113–124.)

the x-ray beam and processes it into a video image that is seen on the displays. The opposite end of the C-arm is the emitter ("the tube"), where x-ray radiation is emitted from.

- The typical configuration when performing interventional orthopedic or pain management procedures is to keep the emitter below the surface of the procedure table (Fig. 3.2).
- Scatter radiation production is primarily generated from the area of the patient that is within the closest proximity to the x-ray radiation source.[29]
- Interventionalist and staff exposure rates will increase as they get closer to the side of the patient where the x-ray beam enters first.[29]
- Using a "best practice habit" of keeping the emitter below the table and patient will decrease the overall radiation exposure to the patient and staff.

- The interventionalist should direct the C-arm operator to adjust the C-arm to the angles needed, based upon how the target anatomy is positioned within the patient, before taking any exposures.[30]
  - This will facilitate a closer alignment of the x-ray beam to the target anatomy, thereby decreasing the usage of what is termed as "scout-fluoro."
  - Less "scout-fluoro" (continuous or rapidly intermittent exposure of the fluoroscopy beam to localize the target anatomy) utilization, will facilitate a decrease in the amount of overall x-ray exposure for each procedure.
  - The interventionalist should support the use of x-ray beam collimation whenever anatomic reference imaging is not required.
- The receptor should be as close to the patient as the procedure will allow. This will create increased distance between the emitter and the patient. As a result, the patient dose will decrease along with the amount of scatter radiation.
- Using the pulsed mode on fluoroscopy systems that are equipped with this feature significantly decreases radiation exposure during procedures. Systems that can pulse the x-ray beam at less than 10 pulses per second can result in up to 90% less exposure compared with nonpulsed systems.[31,32]
- Most modern day fluoroscopy units will have a "low-dose" feature that decreases the radiation output by as much as 50% when used.
- Proper collimation is the standard of care for technicians who operate fluoroscopic units, regardless of whether the technician is initiating each exposure or the interventionalist is using a foot pedal for exposure.
  - The use of both iris (sometimes referred to as "circle-cone") and shutter collimators is recommended. This will significantly reduce the amount of scatter radiation exposure to the patient and personnel.
  - Note: for older model fluoroscopic machines typically manufactured before 1999, some manufacturers used shutter collimators made primarily of copper. The use of shutter collimation on the older model machines is not advised, because the copper collimators will cause the machine to "average-in" the incorrect amount of contrasting. This may degrade the ability of visualize necessary detail. Therefore only iris collimation is recommended when using the older model machines.
- In addition to collimation, centering of pertinent anatomy within the fluoroscopic display is important. Centering anatomy will allow for a better overall averaging of the contrast and density by the fluoroscopic machine. Proper centering also serves to preserve the ability of "spatial acuity" (the visual reference points of the image) for the interventionalist each time that the interventionalist views the fluoroscopic display. These practices can serve to decrease the amount of repeat fluoroscopic exposure needed to visualize the same anatomic detail, which in turn, will lead to a decrease in overall exposed radiation to the patient and staff.

Conclusion

Fluoroscopic imaging will continue to play a very significant role in the precision delivery of biologics and regenerative materials for treatment of joint and spine pathology. In fact, as regenerative therapies become more prevalent, more sophisticated, and more comprehensive, there likely will be an increase in utilization of fluoroscopic guidance. It provides a level of precision and safety that, for many structures of the spine, cannot be replicated with ultrasound guidance. This is especially relevant to spine and neural axis-based therapies. There will also be increased use of mixed modality imaging in which both fluoroscopic and ultrasound guidance will be used to safely and comprehensively treat our patients. Real-time 3D fluoroscopy is an intriguing new technology that could greatly aid precision delivery of biologic materials into deep and complex structures, such as regions of avascular necrosis of bone, bone marrow lesions, disc herniations, annular tears, and other deep tissue structures. Radiation exposure will continue to be an area of concern, and proper education about exposure-limiting technique, increased availability, and decreased cost of flat-panel detector technology will provide for improved safety and less risk of stochastic and nonstochastic effects of radiation exposure.

References

1. Wagner LK. Foundations of safety in fluoroscopy. In: Manchikanti L, Singh V, eds. *Interventional Techniques in Chronic Spinal Pain*. Paducah, KY: ASIPP Publishing; 2007:89–100.
2. Wagner LK. Production, nature, and effects in fluoroscopy. In: Manchikanti L, Singh V, eds. *Interventional Techniques in Chronic Spinal Pain*. Paducah, KY: ASIPP Publishing; 2007:101–112.
3. Wagner LK. Radiation management for patients and protection of staff. In: Manchikanti L, Singh V, eds. *Interventional Techniques in Chronic Spinal Pain*. Paducah, KY: ASIPP Publishing; 2007:113–124.
4. Schultz DM. Fluoroscopy in the interventional pain unit: a physician perspective. In: Manchikanti L, Singh V, eds. *Interventional Techniques in Chronic Spinal Pain*. Paducah, KY: ASIPP Publishing; 2007:125–142.
5. Trescot AM. Fluoroscopy in the interventional pain center. In: Manchikanti L, Singh V, eds. *Interventional Techniques in Chronic Non-Spinal Pain*. Paducah, KY: ASIPP Publishing; 2009:27–34.
6. Edward LN. Physics tutorial for residents: physics of flat-panel fluoroscopy systems, survey of modern fluoroscopy imaging: flat-panel detectors. *RadioGraphics*. 2011;31:591–692.
7. Monfett M, Harrison J, Boachie-Adjei K, et al. Intradiscal platelet-rich plasma (PRP) injections for discogenic low back pain: an update. *Int Orthop*. 2016;40:1321–1328.
8. Bushberg J, Seibert J, Leidholdt E, et al. *The Essential Physics of Medical Imaging*. 2nd ed. Philadelphia: Lippincott, Williams & Wilkins; 2002:231–254.
9. ICRP, 2007. *The 2007 Recommendations of the International Commission on Radiological Protection*. ICRP Publication 103. Ann. ICRP 37.
10. Christodoulou EG, Goodsitt MM, Larson SC, et al. Evaluation of the transmitted exposure through lead equivalent aprons used in a radiology department, including the contribution from backscatter. *Med Phys*. 2003;30:1033–1038.
11. Kaplan DJ, Patel JN, Liporace FA, et al. Intraoperative radiation safety in orthopaedics: a review of the ALARA (as low as reasonably achievable) principle. *Patient Saf Surg*. 2016;10:27.
12. Giordano BD, Grauer JN, Miller CP, et al. Radiation exposure issues in orthopaedics. *J Bone Joint Surg Am*. 2011;93:e69.
13. Gibson TR, Bevill B, Foster M, Spohrer MA. *Technical White Paper: Monitoring and Tracking of Fluoroscopic Dose*. Conference of Radiation Control Directors; 2010.
14. Nicol AL, Benzon HT, Liu BP. Radiation exposure in interventional pain management: we still have much to learn. *Pain Pract*. 2015;15:389–392.
15. Giordano BD1, Baumhauer JF, Morgan TL, et al. Cervical spine imaging using standard C-arm fluoroscopy: patient and surgeon exposure to ionizing radiation. *Spine (Phila Pa 1976)*. 2008;33:1970–1976.
16. Makhesh M. Fluoroscopy: patient radiation exposure issues. *RadioGraphics*. 2001;21:1033–1045.
17. Cohen SL, et al. Radiation dose practice audit of 6,234 fluoroscopically guided spinal injections. *Pain Phys*. 2019;22:E119–E125.
18. Hakan I. *Radiographic Contrast Agents and Contrast Reactions*. Merck Manuals Professional Special Topics; 2015.
19. Newmark JL, Mehra A, Singla AK. Radiocontrast media allergic reactions and interventional pain practice—a review. *Pain Phys*. 2012;15:E665–E675.
20. Dickinson MC, Kam PC. Intravascular iodinated contrast media and the anaesthetist. *Anaesthesia*. 2008;63:626–634.
21. Katzberg RW. Urography into the 21st century: new contrast media, renal handling, imaginary characteristics, and nephrotoxicity. *Radiology*. 1997;204:297–312.
22. Pasternak JJ, Williamson EE. Clinical pharmacology, uses, and adverse reactions of iodinated contrast agents: a primer for the non-radiologist. *Mayo Clin Proc*. 2012;87:390–402.
23. Schabelman E, Witting M. The relationship of radiocontrast, iodine, and seafood allergies: a medical myth exposed. *J Emerg Med*. 2010;39(5):701–707.
24. Beaty AD, et al. Seafood allergy and radiocontrast media: are physicians propagating a myth? *Am J Med*. 2008;121(12):158.e1–e4.
25. Kim K, Park J, Park H, et al. Which iodinated contrast media is the least cytotoxic to human disc cells? *Spine J*. 2015;15:1021–1027.
26. Wu, Tao et al. Cytotoxic effects of nonionic iodinated contrast agent on human adipose-derived mesenchymal stem cells. *PM&R: the Journal of Injury, Function, and Rehabilitation*. 2018; S1934-1482(18):30294–30296.
27. McKee C, et al. Cytotoxicity of radiocontrast dyes in human umbilical cord mesenchymal stem cells. *Toxicol Appl Pharmacol*. 2018;349:72–82.
28. Manchikanti L, et al. Radiation exposure to the physician in interventional pain management. *Pain Physician*. 2002; 5(4):385–393.
29. Young, C. Fluoroscopy: Mobile Unit Operation and Safety. American Society of Radiologic Technologists web article. www.asrt.org/SelfDirectedLearning/10203.
30. McKay-Best T. *Fluoroscopy Manual for Pain Management*. American Society of Radiologic Technologists; 2000: ISBM-10: 0967817609.
31. Johnson M. *Fluoroscopy: Regulation and Radiation Protection*. American Society of Radiologic Technologists; 2017. Self-directed Learning article www.asrt.org.
32. Seeram E, Travis EL. *Radiation Protection*. Philadelphia, PA: Lippincott, Williams & Wilkins; 1997:171–176.

4

Principles of Injection Therapy

LEE KNEER, ROBERT BOWERS, AND CLEO D. STAFFORD II

Musculoskeletal injections are common procedures across various medical specialties. The evidence for musculoskeletal injections is varied and is complicated by differing injection techniques, injectates, and landmark versus image guidance. When performed for the proper indication and with correct technique, musculoskeletal injections can be beneficial and rewarding for both patients and physicians. Before proceeding with an injection, it is critical to obtain a proper diagnosis and rule out relevant contraindications. Absolute contraindications include injectate hypersensitivity, infection, uncontrolled bleeding disorder, and fracture. Relative contraindications include corrected bleeding disorder, anticoagulant use, hemarthrosis, diabetes, immunosuppression, prosthetic joint, high risk of tendon rupture, and psychogenic pain.[1,2]

This chapter addresses the most common nonbiologic injectates used in clinical practice including corticosteroids, local anesthetics, ketorolac, and hyaluronic acid (HA), as well as the evidence for and against their use.

Corticosteroids

Corticosteroid injections (CSIs) first gained popularity in the 1950s and were used to treat patients with joint pain associated with rheumatoid arthritis. Benefits included delivery of a lower dose of steroid compared with oral options, resulting in a lower systemic risk profile.[3] Risks associated with CSIs include infection, flushing, a transient increase in pain, skin hypopigmentation in superficial injections, allergic reaction, and transient hyperglycemia, among other less common complications.[4,5]

Corticosteroids are small hydrocarbon molecules. At the cellular level, once the amphipathic corticosteroid arrives in the synovial fluid it crosses the lipid bilayer of the cellular membrane and binds to the glucocorticoid receptor before being translocated into the nucleus and binding to the glucocorticoid response element (a short sequence of DNA that binds transcription factors and regulates gene transcription).[6] Corticosteroids affect cellular transcription in two ways: (1) inflammation is suppressed through the inhibition of tumor necrosis factor α and other proinflammatory mediators; and (2) antiinflammatory gene transcription is enhanced while inflammatory gene transcription is suppressed.[6,7]

When administered orally, these hydrophobic compounds are small enough to be transported via diffusion across the capillary wall; however, diffusion leads to low overall bioavailability in the synovial fluid. Thus the need to provide high doses to achieve an adequate therapeutic effect, and while the effects of oral steroids are theoretically beneficial to the targeted structure they are nonspecific and can have systemic side effects. Short-term systemic corticosteroid use is generally associated with mild side effects, including cutaneous effects, electrolyte abnormalities, hypertension, hyperglycemia, pancreatitis, hematologic, immunologic, and neuropsychologic effects. Long-term systemic corticosteroid use may be associated with more serious sequalae, including osteoporosis, avascular necrosis, adrenal insufficiency, gastrointestinal, hepatic, and ophthalmologic effects, hyperlipidemia, growth suppression, and possible congenital malformations.[8,9] Thus practitioners sought a more directed means of delivering corticosteroids into the joint space.

Intra-articular Injections

Intra-articular injection of corticosteroids not only improves the concentration within the joint and minimizes systemic effects but also allows for delivery of polymers or salts molecules complexed with the corticosteroid in aqueous solution to improve drug stability and extend the therapeutic window. Despite this, and due to their very low molecular weight (<700 Da), corticosteroids routinely exhibit a half-life of 12 hours or less.[10,11]

Corticosteroids have a long track record of use in intra-articular inflammatory processes. Matzkin and colleagues showed improvements in pain and function at all time points (3 weeks, 6 weeks, 3 months, and 6 months) after one CSI, with obesity and severity of disease associated with less improvement and duration of response.[12] Several organizations have deemed CSIs safe and temporarily efficacious, including the Osteoarthritis Research Society International, the US National Institute of Health, the American College of Rheumatology, the Arthroscopy Association of Canada, and the American Academy of Orthopaedic Surgeons.[13–16] An initial Cochrane review of the efficacy of intra-articular CSIs concluded temporary benefit.[17] However, an updated review of the literature suggested the heterogeneity in trial design and variability of studies limit the ability to assess the benefit of these injections and that there is a low likelihood of meaningful benefit 6 months post injection.[17,18] Despite the poor data quality, the Cochrane review did find that injected corticosteroids improved pain scores by 1 cm on a standard 10-cm visual analog scale compared with control, with a number needed to treat of 8.

More recently, the potential negative long-term effects of intra-articular CSIs have been highlighted. Cartilage exposure to corticosteroids has been associated with such deleterious outcomes as decreased extracellular matrix production, decreased type 1 collagen synthesis, and induction of chondrocyte apoptosis.[19,20] In a study by McAlindon and colleagues, repeated exposure to CSIs over 2 years for symptomatic knee osteoarthritis was associated with increased cartilage loss compared with control subjects injected with saline.[21]

Klocke and colleagues subsequently showed a decrease in the concentration of serum biomarkers for cartilage and bone metabolism at 3 weeks post injection, and Lu and colleagues demonstrated protective effects of steroids on glycosaminoglycan loss after a mechanical injury to the cartilage and proinflammatory cytokine exposure.[22,23] A systematic review from Wernecke and colleagues in 2015 determined that corticosteroids have a time- and dose-dependent effect on articular cartilage, with beneficial effects occurring at low doses and durations and detrimental effects at high doses and durations.[24] Therefore it seems prudent to use the lowest efficacious dose and to limit repeat injections based on current data. More research into the longer-term effects of these changes and clinical implications is warranted.

There is no consensus regarding the volume of injectate or choice of injected corticosteroid. A comparison study showed similar efficacy between injected triamcinolone hexacetonide (40 mg) and methylprednisolone acetate (40 mg).[25] There are data to suggest improved benefit from triamcinolone hexacetonide over triamcinolone acetonide, and the authors prefer the combined effectiveness with mitigation of risk in using 40 mg rather than 80 mg.[26] In addition, the authors prefer the use of ultrasonographic guidance because it is associated with improved accuracy of intra-articular injections.[27] Wyles and colleagues also demonstrated that corticosteroids are cytotoxic to human mesenchymal stem cells in a dose-dependent fashion, with betamethasone being most toxic and dexamethasone being the least toxic.[28] Again, current data suggest that use of the lowest efficacious dose of corticosteroid should be favored.

Management of pain associated with intra-articular inflammatory processes requires an individualized approach, taking into account the patient's personal goals, medical history, tolerance of risk, and extent of disability. Any intra-articular injection for such an inflammatory process, corticosteroid or otherwise, should only be pursued as part of a multimodal approach that includes mitigating other risk factors for recurrent pain and dysfunction.

Axial Spine Injections

Fluoroscopy-guided CSIs have been used for radicular pain, both diagnostically and therapeutically.[29,30] There are several options of corticosteroids for epidural steroid injections, and corticosteroids are divided between particulate (triamcinolone, methylprednisolone, betamethasone) and nonparticulate (dexamethasone) preparations. There is limited evidence to support the superiority of particulate or nonparticulate steroids for epidural CSIs, but there is a concern that particulate formulations pose an increased risk of embolism after inadvertent intravascular injection. The US Food and Drug Administration (FDA) has produced a risk assessment of serious neurologic events after epidural glucocorticoid injections and stated that "although many experts believe the risk is greatest with suspensions [or particulate steroids], the available data do not support comparative safety labeling implying that solutions are safer."[31] Given the lack of strong data favoring the efficacy of particulate steroids and the risk of catastrophic adverse events, the authors prefer nonparticulate corticosteroids for epidural CSIs.[32,33]

Irrespective of the choice of injectate, the cost-effectiveness and clinical benefit of epidural CSIs are debated.[34,35] Many reviews and meta-analyses have been written on the topic of epidural CSIs. A 2015 meta-analysis in *Annals of Internal Medicine* from Chou and colleagues determined that epidural CSIs provided immediate improvements in pain and function. However, the improvements were small and not sustained. Epidural CSIs also did not affect long-term surgery risk.[36] Furthermore, in a retrospective follow-up performed by Jang and colleagues, a small minority of those who underwent a remote lumbar transforaminal epidural CSI achieved complete relief with one injection, while nearly half had relied on repeat epidural CSIs and oral pain medications, and approximately 25% of patients had progressed to surgery.[37] Of note, outcomes from surgery in the cohort were relatively poor, leading the authors to recommend consideration of epidural CSIs as a viable presurgical intervention despite the lack of definitive relief in the majority of cases. In addition to the lack of expected permanent relief, repeat epidural CSIs expose the patient to the risk of significant adverse events including epidural hematoma, infection, and strokes, among others, and repeat epidural CSIs have been associated with adrenal suppression due to systemic uptake.[38,39]

Soft Tissue Corticosteroid Injections

CSIs have been used for decades to treat the pain and discomfort associated with soft tissue pathology, including injections into the bursae and tendon sheaths. In the upper extremity, CSIs directed at the common extensor tendon for the treatment of lateral epicondylalgia have been shown to lead to short-term pain relief but have been associated with worse outcomes at 1 year compared with placebo.[40–43] Other potential targets for ultrasound-guided CSIs have better data to support their use and include the first dorsal compartment of the wrist, trigger finger, median nerve in the carpal tunnel in the distal upper extremity, subacromial bursitis, and shoulder impingement when used in conjunction with an active home exercise program focusing on scapular stabilization.[44–48]

In the lower extremity, CSIs for patellar and insertional Achilles tendinopathy have not reliably shown benefit.[49,50] There are more data for the treatment of iliopsoas bursitis at the hip, trochanteric bursitis in the lateral hip, and pes anserine bursitis.[51–54] The use of CSIs in the setting of plantar fasciitis has shown mixed results in comparison with autologous blood-derived products and inferiority to dry needling.[55–57]

Despite widespread use, the rationale for use of CSIs is contentious. Chronic systemic steroid use in the etiology of tendon rupture is well established.[58,59] These negative effects have been shown to extend to injected corticosteroids as well.[60] In animal models, intratendinous injections have been shown to cause tendon necrosis at the site of injection and a delayed healing response compared with a saline injection.[61] Collagen degeneration and an increase in matrix metalloproteinase-3 (MMP3) have been identified in histologic analysis of tendons exposed to steroid injections. In contrast, other studies have shown a decrease in inflammatory mediators such as MMP2 and substance P.[62,63]

Potential complications of CSIs include infection, subcutaneous atrophy, skin depigmentation, and tendon rupture. The use of ultrasound guidance for these procedures has resulted in improved accuracy compared with palpation- or landmark-guided injections.[27] The authors encourage image guidance given the increased risk of tendon damage and risk of rupture with intratendinous CSIs. Further studies are certainly warranted to continue to evaluate the effects of corticosteroids on soft tissues and the efficacy of CSIs.

Local Anesthetics

Amide local anesthetics (lidocaine, bupivacaine, ropivacaine, etc.) are commonly used in musculoskeletal injections to relieve pain.[64,65] All local anesthetics are membrane-stabilizing drugs that decrease the rate of depolarization and repolarization of the cellular membranes of neurons by inhibiting sodium influx through ion channels in the cell membrane, thus inhibiting action potentials and blocking signal conduction.[66] All nerve fibers are sensitive to local anesthetics; however, type C pain fibers are some of the most sensitive.[67]

Beyond membrane-stabilizing effects, local anesthetics are known to have antiinflammatory actions due to their structural similarity to steroid agents.[68] Lidocaine is the most well-studied local anesthetic and is thought to have antiinflammatory effects by inhibiting sympathetic postganglionic neuron–mediated inflammation. Specifically, lidocaine inhibits the release of inflammatory mediators such as leukotriene B_4, interleukin (IL)-1α, and histamine and has direct inhibitory effects on proinflammatory SPGN-mediated plasma extravasations through inhibiting synovial EP1 receptors.[69] Thus mechanisms of local anesthetics, such as lidocaine, include stabilizing nerve cell membranes, inhibiting nociceptive signaling, and decreasing the inflammatory response.[67] Treatment with local anesthetics may also provide longer-term benefit beyond the immediate pain relief. Eker and colleagues showed that treatment of knee osteoarthritis with intra-articular injection of 0.5% lidocaine provided improvements in pain and function that continued at the 3-month follow-up.[67] They postulated that this may be due to decreasing neural cell metabolism and stabilizing the neural membrane.

However, it is important to note that local anesthetics are known to have chondrotoxic effects on human cartilage. Jayaram and colleagues published an elegant review on this topic, noting variable chondrotoxic potential of different local anesthetics and that a single injection can result in chondrocyte death.[70] Local anesthetics reviewed were lidocaine, bupivacaine, ropivacaine, levobupivacaine, and mepivacaine. The chondrotoxic effects are dose and duration dependent and are influenced by the type of local anesthetic used. Chondrotoxicity also seems to be exacerbated by co-administration with corticosteroid.[71] Of the local anesthetics studied, ropivacaine was the least chondrotoxic and bupivacaine the most chondrotoxic. The mechanisms leading to chondrotoxicity appear to be increased apoptosis, caspase inhibition, necrosis, mitochondrial dysfunction, extracellular matrix damage, and decreased DNA-normalized glycosaminoglycan expression. Local anesthetics have also been demonstrated to be toxic to human mesenchymal stem cells, which are crucial for healing.[72–74] Here too, ropivacaine is the least cytotoxic.[73,74] Furthermore, Zink and colleagues have shown local anesthetics to be toxic to muscle tissue, with bupivacaine causing significantly more tissue damage than ropivacaine.[75,76]

In summary, amide local anesthetics have general dose- and duration-dependent cytotoxic effects, with ropivacaine having the least toxicity, bupivacaine the most toxicity to chondrocytes and muscle tissue, and lidocaine the most toxicity to mesenchymal stem cells.[70,72–74]

Ketorolac

Ketorolac is a nonsteroidal antiinflammatory drug (NSAID) that inhibits the inflammatory cyclooxygenase and lipoxygenase enzyme systems, and the synthesis of prostaglandins and leukotrienes.[77] Ketorolac provides a reasonable alternative to corticosteroids and HA because it has fewer side effects than corticosteroid, has a faster onset of action than HA, and is more economical than both HA and corticosteroid.[78]

In patients with knee and first carpometacarpal joint osteoarthritis, the addition of ketorolac to HA injection provided more rapid onset of pain relief without any added complications when compared with HA alone.[79,80] In addition, when compared head-to-head with corticosteroid in patients with knee and hip osteoarthritis, ketorolac provided similar improvements in pain and function for up to 6 months.[78,81] Ketorolac has also been shown to be safe and more effective than corticosteroids in the treatment of shoulder impingement and adhesive capsulitis.[82,83]

In a 2018 review, Sardana and colleagues concluded that NSAID injections had a less severe side-effect profile compared with corticosteroids and provided equivalent, if not better, pain relief for musculoskeletal pathology.[84] Ketorolac has demonstrated no detrimental effects on chondrocytes and tenocytes in animal models.[85,86] Beitzel and colleagues reported no toxic effects on human chondrocytes and tenocytes; however, other studies have indicated a dose-dependent cytotoxic effect of ketorolac on human articular chondrocytes.[87,88] In Abrams and colleagues, the methods more closely reflect the exposure duration of a single-dose injection, but the authors note their methods potentially overestimated the chondrotoxicity of ketorolac.[88] Nonetheless, there is no consensus on the cytotoxicity of ketorolac and the risk of ketorolac intra-articular injections. There is a theoretical association between ketorolac injections and bleeding risk; however, there have been no studies documenting a bleeding complication after a ketorolac injection in contact or collision sport athletes.[89]

Hyaluronic Acid

HA is a polysaccharide consisting of repeating units of the disaccharide *N*-acetylglucosamine and sodium glucuronate.[90] This glycosaminoglycan structure is found within the extracellular matrix of a variety of soft tissue structures and is synthesized by type B synoviocytes, fibroblasts, and chondrocytes.[90,91] Namiki and colleagues were one of the first groups to evaluate its use of HA for knee osteoarthritis more than 30 years ago.[92] The injection was later approved by the FDA in 1997 for the treatment of knee osteoarthritis.

The term 'viscosupplementation' was coined for this injection based on the initial work of Namiki and colleagues, where the proposed mechanism of action was thought to be improving the viscosity of the arthritic joint.[92] However, since that time there have been several studies that have uncovered several possible mechanisms, including the decrease of inflammatory mediators, improvement in the viscosity of the microenvironment, immunomodulation of catabolic enzymes, and downregulation of nociceptors.[93,94]

Exogenous HA has been shown to decrease inflammation through the suppression of proinflammatory mediators; specifically, IL-β and tumor necrosis factor α.[94,95] HA has displayed the ability to immunomodulate catabolic processes by downregulating matrix MMP3 expression and inhibiting MMP synthesis, potentially reducing cartilage destruction.[5,7] Exogenous HA also has the capability of improving viscosity by stimulating the production of endogenous HA in the synovial fluid and restoring homeostasis.[96,97] Lastly, exogenous HA is able to decrease pain by binding neuropeptides, creating a boundary layer around nociceptors and not allowing the receptors to transmit pain signals.[98]

There are several exogenous HA products currently on the market that differ in their molecular properties, single- or multi-injection therapies, and whether they are derived from animal products or using a genetically modified bacterial source (Table 4.1). These differences have been shown to affect clinical outcomes, and thus all exogenous HA products should not be evaluated as a group.[99] Molecularly, the most significant difference between products is their molecular weight, with products either being low molecular weight (<1500 kilodaltons [kDa]), moderate molecular weight (>1500 kDa and <3000 kDa), or high molecular weight (>3000 kDa). A meta-analysis performed by Altman and colleagues has suggested that high-molecular-weight HA is more efficacious than moderate- or low-molecular-weight products.[99]

In addition to differences in molecular weight, exogenous HA products can also differ in the number of injections from single- to multi-injection formulations. A systematic review proposed that single-injection therapy has similar efficacy to multi-injection formulations, with less patient inconvenience.[100] The last major difference between exogenous HA products is if they are derived from bacterial processes of biologic fermentation or through extraction of avian-derived molecules. Based on the available data compiled by Vincent and colleagues, biologically fermented formulations tend to be more efficacious and have a better safety profile than avian-derived formulations.[100]

HA has been shown to be effective and safe in the treatment of knee osteoarthritis based on the most recent Cochrane review of the subject.[101] However, caution should be taken when attempting to apply this recommendation to all HA products, given the variability in formulations and molecular properties as stated earlier. Overall, given the available data, exogenous HA is a viable alternative in early to moderate osteoarthritis with the potential to delay the time until knee arthroplasty.[102,103]

Exogenous HA has been used for symptomatic ankle osteoarthritis with promising results.[104] Multiple systematic reviews have elucidated that HA is safe, decreases pain scores, and improves functional outcome measures for ankle osteoarthritis.[105,106] There have also been a number

TABLE 4.1 **Hyaluronic Acid Products Currently on the Market.**

Product Name	High, Moderate, or Low Molecular Weight (kDa)	Source	Dosing (mg/mL)	Number of Injections
Synvisc-one	High	Avian derived	48 mg/6 mL	Single
Gel-one	Unknown	Avian derived	30 mg/3 mL	Single
Monovisc	Moderate	Bacterial derived	88 mg/4 mL	Single
Durolane	High	Bacterial derived	60 mg/3 mL	Single
Hymovis	Unknown	Bacterial derived	24 mg/3 mL	Two
Synvisc	High	Avian derived	48 mg/2 mL	Three
Orthovisc	Moderate	Bacterial derived	30 mg/2 mL	Three
Euflexxa	High	Bacterial derived	20 mg/2 mL	Three
Gelsyn-3	Low	Bacterial derived	16.8 mg/2 mL	Three
Hyalgan	Low	Avian derived	20 mg/2 mL	Three or five
Supartz FX	Low	Avian derived	25 mg/2.5 mL	Three or five

of studies showing favorable results for the use of HA in glenohumeral osteoarthritis.[107–110] HA has been shown to be superior to physical therapy with treating glenohumeral osteoarthritis and has a numeric but not statistically significant advantage when compared with other injectables.[108,109] A meta-analysis and systematic review by Zhang and colleagues concluded that HA has the capability of improving pain scores and functional outcomes in glenohumeral osteoarthritis; however, more randomized controlled trials are needed to evaluate the optimal dosing and efficacy.[111] With the lack of high-quality and comparative studies with other commonly used intra-articular therapies for glenohumeral osteoarthritis, a definitive recommendation cannot be reached at this time. More high-level studies are warranted and needed to further uncover the potential of HA in this scenario.

HA is currently indicated (on-label) only for knee osteoarthritis by the FDA; however, it has been approved for ankle and shoulder osteoarthritis by the European Medicines Agency.[70] Given the unpredictability of coverage for this product by insurance companies in the United States, combined with the favorable evidence mentioned earlier, an off-label, out-of-pocket expense option could be discussed with patients when considering treatment options for degenerative pathology in the ankle and shoulder.

Lastly, there is some evidence that HA may have benefit in tendinopathies. A review by Abate and colleagues concluded that HA can be effective to prevent adhesions after flexor tendon surgery and that there are promising data on beneficial HA effects for the rotator cuff, trigger finger, patella tendinopathy, and elbow common extensors.[112] The mechanisms of effects are likely antiinflammatory, enhanced cell proliferation, collagen deposition, and lubricating the tendon sliding surface. In most of the studies, HA was injected intra-articularly or in the synovial sheath rather than the tendon itself. More rigorous study is needed to make robust conclusions on the efficacy of HA for tendinopathies, but early studies show promise.

Summary

In summary, a consensus does not exist regarding the use of traditional injectates corticosteroid, local anesthetic, ketorolac, or HA in musculoskeletal pathology. Emerging evidence suggests that there is dose- and time-dependent cytotoxicity associated with corticosteroid and local anesthetic. Therefore it seems prudent to use the lowest possible dose to exert clinical benefit. There are some data that ketorolac may be less toxic than corticosteroids yet provides similar improvements in pain and function. Thus ketorolac may be a safer alternative for use in musculoskeletal injections. HA is safe, has chondroprotective properties, and may have a positive effect on tendons; however, the onset of action is slow. To this point, the decision of when to use any of these injectates in clinical practice is based on specific pathology as well as patient and physician goals.

References

1. Stephens MB, Beutler AI, O'Connor FG. Musculoskeletal injections: a review of the evidence. *Am Fam Physician*. 2008;78(8):971–976.
2. Monseau AJ, Nizran PS. Common injections in musculoskeletal medicine. *Prim Care*. 2013;40(4):987–1000. ix-x.
3. Hollander JL, Brown Jr EM, Jessar RA, Brown CY. Hydrocortisone and cortisone injected into arthritic joints; comparative effects of and use of hydrocortisone as a local antiarthritic agent. *J Am Med Assoc*. 1951;147(17):1629–1635.
4. Charalambous CP, Tryfonidis M, Sadiq S, Hirst P, Paul A. Septic arthritis following intra-articular steroid injection of the

knee—a survey of current practice regarding antiseptic technique used during intra-articular steroid injection of the knee. *Clin Rheumatol.* 2003;22(6):386–390.

5. Smuin DM, Seidenberg PH, Sirlin EA, Phillips SF, Silvis ML. Rare adverse events associated with corticosteroid injections: a case series and literature review. *Curr Sports Med Rep.* 2016;15(3):171–176.
6. Hayashi R, Wada H, Ito K, Adcock IM. Effects of glucocorticoids on gene transcription. *Eur J Pharmacol.* 2004;500(1–3):51–62.
7. Miller WL, Auchus RJ. The molecular biology, biochemistry, and physiology of human steroidogenesis and its disorders. *Endocr Rev.* 2011;32(1):81–151.
8. Buchman AL. Side effects of corticosteroid therapy. *J Clin Gastroenterol.* 2001;33(4):289–294.
9. Stanbury RM, Graham EM. Systemic corticosteroid therapy—side effects and their management. *Br J Ophthalmol.* 1998;82(6):704–708.
10. Derendorf H, Mollmann H, Gruner A, Haack D, Gyselby G. Pharmacokinetics and pharmacodynamics of glucocorticoid suspensions after intra-articular administration. *Clin Pharmacol Ther.* 1986;39(3):313–317. f.
11. Armstrong RD, English J, Gibson T, Chakraborty J, Marks V. Serum methylprednisolone levels following intra-articular injection of methylprednisolone acetate. *Ann Rheum Dis.* 1981;40(6):571–574.
12. Matzkin EG, Curry EJ, Kong Q, Rogers MJ, Henry M, Smith EL. Efficacy and treatment response of intra-articular corticosteroid injections in patients with symptomatic knee osteoarthritis. *J Am Acad Orthop Surg.* 2017;25(10):703–714.
13. McAlindon TE, Bannuru RR, Sullivan MC, et al. OARSI guidelines for the non-surgical management of knee osteoarthritis. *Osteoarthritis Cartilage.* 2014;22(3):363–388.
14. Jevsevar DS. Treatment of osteoarthritis of the knee: evidence—based guideline, 2nd edition. *J Am Acad Orthop Surg.* 2013;21(9):571–576.
15. Hochberg MC, Altman RD, April KT, et al. American College of Rheumatology 2012 recommendations for the use of nonpharmacologic and pharmacologic therapies in osteoarthritis of the hand, hip, and knee. *Arthritis Care Res (Hoboken).* 2012;64(4):465–474.
16. Arthroscopy Association of Canada, Kopka M, Sheehan B, et al. Arthroscopy Association of Canada position statement on intra-articular injections for knee osteoarthritis. *Orthop J Sports Med.* 2019;7(7). 2325967119860110.
17. Bellamy N, Campbell J, Robinson V, Gee T, Bourne R, Wells G. Intraarticular corticosteroid for treatment of osteoarthritis of the knee. *Cochrane Database Syst Rev.* 2006;(2):CD005328.
18. Juni P, Hari R, Rutjes AW, et al. Intra-articular corticosteroid for knee osteoarthritis. *Cochrane Database Syst Rev.* 2015;10:CD005328.
19. Nakazawa F, Matsuno H, Yudoh K, Watanabe Y, Katayama R, Kimura T. Corticosteroid treatment induces chondrocyte apoptosis in an experimental arthritis model and in chondrocyte cultures. *Clin Exp Rheumatol.* 2002;20(6):773–781.
20. Dean BJ, Carr AJ. The effects of glucocorticoid on tendon and tendon derived cells. *Adv Exp Med Biol.* 2016;920:239–246.
21. McAlindon TE, LaValley MP, Harvey WF, et al. Effect of intra-articular triamcinolone vs saline on knee cartilage volume and pain in patients with knee osteoarthritis: a randomized clinical trial. *JAMA.* 2017;317(19):1967–1975.
22. Klocke R, Levasseur K, Kitas GD, Smith JP, Hirsch G. Cartilage turnover and intra-articular corticosteroid injections in knee osteoarthritis. *Rheumatol Int.* 2018;38(3):455–459.
23. Lu YC, Evans CH, Grodzinsky AJ. Effects of short-term glucocorticoid treatment on changes in cartilage matrix degradation and chondrocyte gene expression induced by mechanical injury and inflammatory cytokines. *Arthritis Res Ther.* 2011;13(5):R142.
24. Wernecke C, Braun HJ, Dragoo JL. The effect of intra-articular corticosteroids on articular cartilage: a systematic review. *Orthop J Sports Med.* 2015;3(5):2325967115581163.
25. Buyuk AF, Kilinc E, Camurcu IY, Camur S, Ucpunar H, Kara A. Compared efficacy of intra-articular injection of methylprednisolone and triamcinolone. *Acta Ortop Bras.* 2017;25(5):206–208.
26. Zulian F, Martini G, Gobber D, Plebani M, Zacchello F, Manners P. Triamcinolone acetonide and hexacetonide intra-articular treatment of symmetrical joints in juvenile idiopathic arthritis: a double-blind trial. *Rheumatology (Oxford).* 2004;43(10):1288–1291.
27. Daniels EW, Cole D, Jacobs B, Phillips SF. Existing evidence on ultrasound-guided injections in sports medicine. *Orthop J Sports Med.* 2018;6(2). 2325967118756576.
28. Wyles CC, Houdek MT, Wyles SP, Wagner ER, Behfar A, Sierra RJ. Differential cytotoxicity of corticosteroids on human mesenchymal stem cells. *Clin Orthop Relat Res.* 2015;473(3):1155–1164.
29. Lewandrowski KU. Successful outcome after outpatient transforaminal decompression for lumbar foraminal and lateral recess stenosis: the positive predictive value of diagnostic epidural steroid injection. *Clin Neurol Neurosurg.* 2018;173:38–45.
30. Rivera CE. Lumbar Epidural steroid injections. *Phys Med Rehabil Clin N Am.* 2018;29(1):73–92.
31. Racoosin JA, Seymour SM, Cascio L, Gill R. Serious neurologic events after epidural glucocorticoid injection—the FDA's risk assessment. *N Engl J Med.* 2015;373(24):2299–2301.
32. Bensler S, Sutter R, Pfirrmann CWA, Peterson CK. Particulate versus non-particulate corticosteroids for transforaminal nerve root blocks: comparison of outcomes in 494 patients with lumbar radiculopathy. *Eur Radiol.* 2018;28(3):946–952.
33. Mehta P, Syrop I, Singh JR, Kirschner J. Systematic review of the efficacy of particulate versus nonparticulate corticosteroids in epidural injections. *PM R.* 2017;9(5):502–512.
34. Pennington Z, Swanson MA, Lubelski D, et al. Comparing the short-term cost-effectiveness of epidural steroid injections and medical management alone for discogenic lumbar radiculopathy. *Clin Neurol Neurosurg.* 2020;191:105675.
35. Manchikanti L, Nampiaparampil DE, Candido KD, et al. Do cervical epidural injections provide long-term relief in neck and upper extremity pain? A systematic review. *Pain Physician.* 2015;18(1):39–60.
36. Chou R, Hashimoto R, Friedly J, et al. Epidural corticosteroid injections for radiculopathy and spinal stenosis: a systematic review and meta-analysis. *Ann Intern Med.* 2015;163(5):373–381.
37. Jang SH, Chang MC. At least 5-year follow up after transforaminal epidural steroid injection due to lumbar radicular pain caused by spinal stenosis. *Pain Pract.* 2020.
38. Epstein NE. Major risks and complications of cervical epidural steroid injections: an updated review. *Surg Neurol Int.* 2018;9:86.

39. Shin WS, Ahn DK, Kim MJ, Cho KJ, Go YR. Influence of epidural steroid injection on adrenal function. *Clin Orthop Surg.* 2019;11(2):183–186.
40. Sorani A, Campbell R. Image-guided elbow interventions: a literature review of interventional treatment options. *Br J Radiol.* 2016;89(1057):20150368.
41. Branson R, Naidu K, du Toit C, et al. Comparison of corticosteroid, autologous blood or sclerosant injections for chronic tennis elbow. *J Sci Med Sport.* 2017;20(6):528–533.
42. Coombes BK, Bisset L, Brooks P, Khan A, Vicenzino B. Effect of corticosteroid injection, physiotherapy, or both on clinical outcomes in patients with unilateral lateral epicondylalgia: a randomized controlled trial. *JAMA.* 2013;309(5):461–469.
43. Coombes BK, Bisset L, Vicenzino B. Efficacy and safety of corticosteroid injections and other injections for management of tendinopathy: a systematic review of randomised controlled trials. *Lancet.* 2010;376(9754):1751–1767.
44. Orlandi D, Corazza A, Silvestri E, et al. Ultrasound-guided procedures around the wrist and hand: how to do. *Eur J Radiol.* 2014;83(7):1231–1238.
45. Salim N, Abdullah S, Sapuan J, Haflah NH. Outcome of corticosteroid injection versus physiotherapy in the treatment of mild trigger fingers. *J Hand Surg Eur Vol.* 2012;37(1):27–34.
46. Huisstede BM, Randsdorp MS, van den Brink J, Franke TPC, Koes BW, Hoogvliet P. Effectiveness of oral pain medication and corticosteroid injections for carpal tunnel syndrome: a systematic review. *Arch Phys Med Rehabil.* 2018;99(8):1609–1622. e1610.
47. Lee DH, Hong JY, Lee MY, Kwack KS, Yoon SH. Relation between subacromial bursitis on ultrasonography and efficacy of subacromial corticosteroid injection in rotator cuff disease: a prospective comparison study. *Arch Phys Med Rehabil.* 2017;98(5):881–887.
48. Gasparre G, Fusaro I, Galletti S, Volini S, Benedetti MG. Effectiveness of ultrasound-guided injections combined with shoulder exercises in the treatment of subacromial adhesive bursitis. *Musculoskelet Surg.* 2012;96(suppl 1):S57–61.
49. Everhart JS, Cole D, Sojka JH, et al. Treatment options for patellar tendinopathy: a systematic review. *Arthroscopy.* 2017;33(4):861–872.
50. Hart L. Corticosteroid and other injections in the management of tendinopathies: a review. *Clin J Sport Med.* 2011;21(6):540–541.
51. Agten CA, Rosskopf AB, Zingg PO, Peterson CK, Pfirrmann CW. Outcomes after fluoroscopy-guided iliopsoas bursa injection for suspected iliopsoas tendinopathy. *Eur Radiol.* 2015;25(3):865–871.
52. Han JS, Sugimoto D, McKee-Proctor MH, Stracciolini A, d'Hemecourt PA. Short-term effect of ultrasound-guided iliopsoas peritendinous corticosteroid injection. *J Ultrasound Med.* 2019;38(6):1527–1536.
53. Mitchell WG, Kettwich SC, Sibbitt Jr WL, et al. Outcomes and cost-effectiveness of ultrasound-guided injection of the trochanteric bursa. *Rheumatol Int.* 2018;38(3):393–401.
54. Lee JH, Lee JU, Yoo SW. Accuracy and efficacy of ultrasound-guided pes anserinus bursa injection. *J Clin Ultrasound.* 2019;47(2):77–82.
55. Tseng WC, Uy J, Yi-Hsiang Chiu MD, Chen WS, Vora A. The comparative effectiveness of autologous blood-derived products vs steroids injection in plantar fasciitis: a systematic review and meta-analysis of randomized controlled trials. *PM R.* 2020.
56. Rastegar S, Baradaran Mahdavi S, Hoseinzadeh B, Badiei S. Comparison of dry needling and steroid injection in the treatment of plantar fasciitis: a single-blind randomized clinical trial. *Int Orthop.* 2018;42(1):109–116.
57. Peerbooms JC, Lodder P, den Oudsten BL, Doorgeest K, Schuller HM, Gosens T. Positive effect of platelet-rich plasma on pain in plantar fasciitis: a double-blind multicenter randomized controlled trial. *Am J Sports Med.* 2019;47(13):3238–3246.
58. Ge Z, Tang H, Chen W, et al. Downregulation of type I collagen expression in the Achilles tendon by dexamethasone: a controlled laboratory study. *J Orthop Surg Res.* 2020;15(1):70.
59. Kotnis RA, Halstead JC, Hormbrey PJ. Atraumatic bilateral Achilles tendon rupture: an association of systemic steroid treatment. *J Accid Emerg Med.* 1999;16(5):378–379.
60. Hugate R, Pennypacker J, Saunders M, Juliano P. The effects of intratendinous and retrocalcaneal intrabursal injections of corticosteroid on the biomechanical properties of rabbit Achilles tendons. *J Bone Joint Surg Am.* 2004;86(4):794–801.
61. Balasubramaniam P, Prathap K. The effect of injection of hydrocortisone into rabbit calcaneal tendons. *J Bone Joint Surg Br.* 1972;54(4):729–734.
62. Dinhane KGI, Godoy-Santos AL, Fabro AT, Moretto MR, Depra I, Yoshida WB. Short-term changes after corticosteroid injections into the normal tendons of rabbits: a controlled randomized study. *Am J Sports Med.* 2019;47(3):721–728.
63. Mousavizadeh R, Backman L, McCormack RG, Scott A. Dexamethasone decreases substance P expression in human tendon cells: an in vitro study. *Rheumatology (Oxford).* 2015;54(2):318–323.
64. Rothfuss J, Mau W, Zeidler H, Brenner MH. Socioeconomic evaluation of rheumatoid arthritis and osteoarthritis: a literature review. *Semin Arthritis Rheum.* 1997;26(5):771–779.
65. Yang Y, Zeng C, Wei J, et al. Single-dose intra-articular bupivacaine plus morphine versus bupivacaine alone after arthroscopic knee surgery: a meta-analysis of randomized controlled trials. *Knee Surg Sports Traumatol Arthrosc.* 2017;25(3):966–979.
66. Eng HC, Ghosh SM, Chin KJ. Practical use of local anesthetics in regional anesthesia. *Curr Opin Anaesthesiol.* 2014;27(4):382–387.
67. Eker HE, Cok OY, Aribogan A, Arslan G. The efficacy of intra-articular lidocaine administration in chronic knee pain due to osteoarthritis: a randomized, double-blind, controlled study. *Anaesth Crit Care Pain Med.* 2017;36(2):109–114.
68. Seeman P. The membrane actions of anesthetics and tranquilizers. *Pharmacol Rev.* 1972;24(4):583–655.
69. Pietruck C, Grond S, Xie GX, Palmer PP. Local anesthetics differentially inhibit sympathetic neuron-mediated and C fiber-mediated synovial neurogenic plasma extravasation. *Anesth Analg.* 2003;96(5):1397–1402, table of contents.
70. Jayaram P, Kennedy DJ, Yeh P, Dragoo J. Chondrotoxic effects of local anesthetics on human knee articular cartilage: a systematic review. *PM R.* 2019;11(4):379–400.
71. Seshadri V, Coyle CH, Chu CR. Lidocaine potentiates the chondrotoxicity of methylprednisolone. *Arthroscopy.* 2009;25(4):337–347.
72. Dregalla RC, Lyons NF, Reischling PD, Centeno CJ. Amide-type local anesthetics and human mesenchymal stem cells: clinical implications for stem cell therapy. *Stem Cells Transl Med.* 2014;3(3):365–374.
73. Rahnama R, Wang M, Dang AC, Kim HT, Kuo AC. Cytotoxicity of local anesthetics on human mesenchymal stem cells. *J Bone Joint Surg Am.* 2013;95(2):132–137.

74. Breu A, Eckl S, Zink W, Kujat R, Angele P. Cytotoxicity of local anesthetics on human mesenchymal stem cells in vitro. *Arthroscopy*. 2013;29(10):1676–1684.
75. Zink W, Seif C, Bohl JR, et al. The acute myotoxic effects of bupivacaine and ropivacaine after continuous peripheral nerve blockades. *Anesth Analg*. 2003;97(4):1173–1179, table of contents.
76. Zink W, Bohl JR, Hacke N, Sinner B, Martin E, Graf BM. The long term myotoxic effects of bupivacaine and ropivacaine after continuous peripheral nerve blocks. *Anesth Analg*. 2005;101(2):548–554, table of contents.
77. Vadivelu N, Gowda AM, Urman RD, et al. Ketorolac tromethamine—routes and clinical implications. *Pain Pract*. 2015;15(2):175–193.
78. Bellamy JL, Goff BJ, Sayeed SA. Economic impact of ketorolac vs corticosteroid intra-articular knee injections for osteoarthritis: a randomized, double-blind, prospective study. *J Arthroplasty*. 2016;31(suppl 9):293–297.
79. Koh SH, Lee SC, Lee WY, Kim J, Park Y. Ultrasound-guided intra-articular injection of hyaluronic acid and ketorolac for osteoarthritis of the carpometacarpal joint of the thumb: a retrospective comparative study. *Medicine (Baltimore)*. 2019;98(19):e15506.
80. Lee SC, Rha DW, Chang WH. Rapid analgesic onset of intra-articular hyaluronic acid with ketorolac in osteoarthritis of the knee. *J Back Musculoskelet Rehabil*. 2011;24(1):31–38.
81. Park KD, Kim TK, Bae BW, Ahn J, Lee WY, Park Y. Ultrasound guided intra-articular ketorolac versus corticosteroid injection in osteoarthritis of the hip: a retrospective comparative study. *Skeletal Radiol*. 2015;44(9):1333–1340.
82. Ahn JK, Kim J, Lee SJ, Park Y, Bae B, Lee W. Effects of Ultrasound-guided intra-articular ketorolac injection with capsular distension. *J Back Musculoskelet Rehabil*. 2015;28(3):497–503.
83. Min KS, St Pierre P, Ryan PM, Marchant BG, Wilson CJ, Arrington ED. A double-blind randomized controlled trial comparing the effects of subacromial injection with corticosteroid versus NSAID in patients with shoulder impingement syndrome. *J Shoulder Elbow Surg*. 2013;22(5):595–601.
84. Sardana V, Burzynski J, Hasan K, Zalzal P. Are non-steroidal anti-inflammatory drug injections an alternative to steroid injections for musculoskeletal pain? A systematic review. *J Orthop*. 2018;15(3):812–816.
85. Dogan N, Erdem AF, Gundogdu C, Kursad H, Kizilkaya M. The effects of ketorolac and morphine on articular cartilage and synovium in the rabbit knee joint. *Can J Physiol Pharmacol*. 2004;82(7):502–505.
86. Shapiro PS, Rohde RS, Froimson MI, Lash RH, Postak P, Greenwald AS. The effect of local corticosteroid or ketorolac exposure on histologic and biomechanical properties of rabbit tendon and cartilage. *Hand (N Y)*. 2007;2(4):165–172.
87. Beitzel K, McCarthy MB, Cote MP, et al. The effect of ketorolac tromethamine, methylprednisolone, and platelet-rich plasma on human chondrocyte and tenocyte viability. *Arthroscopy*. 2013;29(7):1164–1174.
88. Abrams GD, Chang W, Dragoo JL. In vitro chondrotoxicity of nonsteroidal anti-inflammatory drugs and opioid medications. *Am J Sports Med*. 2017;45(14):3345–3350.
89. Matava MJ. Injectable nonsteroidal anti-inflammatory drugs in sport. *Clin J Sport Med*. 2018;28(5):443–450.
90. Stitik TP, Issac SM, Modi S, Nasir S, Kulinets I. Effectiveness of 3 weekly injections compared with 5 weekly injections of intra-articular sodium hyaluronate on pain relief of knee osteoarthritis or 3 weekly injections of other hyaluronan products: a systematic review and meta-analysis. *Arch Phys Med Rehabil*. 2017;98(5):1042–1050.
91. McElheny K, Toresdahl B, Ling D, Mages K, Asif I. Comparative effectiveness of alternative dosing regimens of hyaluronic acid injections for knee osteoarthritis: a systematic review. *Sports Health*. 2019;11(5):461–466.
92. Namiki O, Toyoshima H, Morisaki N. Therapeutic effect of intra-articular injection of high molecular weight hyaluronic acid on osteoarthritis of the knee. *Int J Clin Pharmacol Ther Toxicol*. 1982;20(11):501–507.
93. Reid MC. Viscosupplementation for osteoarthritis: a primer for primary care physicians. *Adv Ther*. 2013;30(11):967–986.
94. Moreland LW. Intra-articular hyaluronan (hyaluronic acid) and hylans for the treatment of osteoarthritis: mechanisms of action. *Arthritis Res Ther*. 2003;5(2):54–67.
95. Cole BJ, Karas V, Hussey K, Pilz K, Fortier LA. Hyaluronic acid versus platelet-rich plasma: a prospective, double-blind randomized controlled trial comparing clinical outcomes and effects on intra-articular biology for the treatment of knee osteoarthritis. *Am J Sports Med*. 2017;45(2):339–346.
96. Goldberg VM, Buckwalter JA. Hyaluronans in the treatment of osteoarthritis of the knee: evidence for disease-modifying activity. *Osteoarthritis Cartilage*. 2005;13(3):216–224.
97. Goldberg VM, Goldberg L. Intra-articular hyaluronans: the treatment of knee pain in osteoarthritis. *J Pain Res*. 2010;3:51–56.
98. Gotoh S, Onaya J, Abe M, et al. Effects of the molecular weight of hyaluronic acid and its action mechanisms on experimental joint pain in rats. *Ann Rheum Dis*. 1993;52(11):817–822.
99. Altman RD, Bedi A, Karlsson J, Sancheti P, Schemitsch E. Product differences in intra-articular hyaluronic acids for osteoarthritis of the knee. *Am J Sports Med*. 2016;44(8):2158–2165.
100. Vincent P. Intra-articular hyaluronic acid in the symptomatic treatment of knee osteoarthritis: a meta-analysis of single-injection products. *Curr Ther Res Clin Exp*. 2019;90:39–51.
101. Bellamy N, Campbell J, Robinson V, Gee T, Bourne R, Wells G. Viscosupplementation for the treatment of osteoarthritis of the knee. *Cochrane Database Syst Rev*. 2006;2:CD005321.
102. Rosen J, Niazi F, Dysart S. Cost-effectiveness of treating early to moderate stage knee osteoarthritis with intra-articular hyaluronic acid compared to conservative interventions. *Adv Ther*. 2019.
103. Turajane T, Chaveewanakorn U, Fongsarun W, Aojanepong J, Papadopoulos KI. Avoidance of total knee arthroplasty in early osteoarthritis of the knee with intra-articular implantation of autologous activated peripheral blood stem cells versus hyaluronic acid: a randomized controlled trial with differential effects of growth factor addition. *Stem Cells Int*. 2017;2017:8925132.
104. Witteveen AG, Hofstad CJ, Kerkhoffs GM. Hyaluronic acid and other conservative treatment options for osteoarthritis of the ankle. *Cochrane Database Syst Rev*. 2015;(10):CD010643.
105. Faleiro TB, Schulz Rda S, Jambeiro JE, Tavares A, Delmonte FM, Daltro Gde C. Viscosupplementation in ankle osteoarthritis: a systematic review. *Acta Ortop Bras*. 2016;24(1):52–54.

106. Vannabouathong C, Del Fabbro G, Sales B, et al. Intra-articular injections in the treatment of symptoms from ankle arthritis: a systematic review. *Foot Ankle Int*. 2018;39(10):1141–1150.
107. Kwon YW, Eisenberg G, Zuckerman JD. Sodium hyaluronate for the treatment of chronic shoulder pain associated with glenohumeral osteoarthritis: a multicenter, randomized, double-blind, placebo-controlled trial. *J Shoulder Elbow Surg*. 2013;22(5):584–594.
108. Di Giacomo G, de Gasperis N. The role of hyaluronic acid in patients affected by glenohumeral osteoarthritis. *J Biol Regul Homeost Agents*. 2015;29(4):945–951.
109. Di Giacomo G, de Gasperis N. Hyaluronic acid intra-articular injections in patients affected by moderate to severe glenohumeral osteoarthritis: a prospective randomized study. *Joints*. 2017;5(3):138–142.
110. McKee MD, Litchfield R, Hall JA, Wester T, Jones J, Harrison AJ. NASHA hyaluronic acid for the treatment of shoulder osteoarthritis: a prospective, single-arm clinical trial. *Med Devices (Auckl)*. 2019;12:227–234.
111. Zhang B, Thayaparan A, Horner N, Bedi A, Alolabi B, Khan M. Outcomes of hyaluronic acid injections for glenohumeral osteoarthritis: a systematic review and meta-analysis. *J Shoulder Elbow Surg*. 2019;28(3):596–606.
112. Abate M, Schiavone C, Salini V. The use of hyaluronic acid after tendon surgery and in tendinopathies. *Biomed Res Int*. 2014;2014:783632.

5

Autologous Tissue Harvesting Techniques: Bone Marrow Aspirate and Adipose Tissue

GERARD MALANGA, JAY E. BOWEN, AND SELORM L. TAKYI

Introduction

Regenerative medicine has become an increasingly popular field of interest over the last several decades. Its potential application for treating various disease pathologies is promising and much research is currently being conducted across the globe.[1] Its application for orthopedic conditions has a place in the treatment paradigm for many conditions. There is a growing interest in the proper use of biologic treatments by clinicians and a desire for these services by patients. With this heightened level of interest comes the need to understand when and how best to apply biologics to musculoskeletal conditions.

We will focus this chapter on how to perform tissue harvesting for autologous use of bone marrow and adipose tissue. The techniques, materials, and pearls required to successfully perform these procedures are paramount. While obtaining these cells and tissues, it is important to recall that while practicing in the United States one must comply with Food and Drug Administration (FDA) regulations concerning minimal manipulation and intention for homologous use of the HCT/P (human cells, tissues, and cellular and tissue-based products). In addition, these tissues cannot be expanded.[2] The reader should be familiar with their regional regulations, which is beyond the scope of this chapter. It is also necessary to consider the potential adverse effects from performing these procedures: infection, hematoma, and anemia.[3]

Risks

Before performing bone marrow aspirate or adipose tissue harvesting it is imperative to obtain informed verbal and written consent. A patient must fully understand the potential risks of the procedure, anticipated benefits, and alternatives. The risks include but are not limited to infection, skin necrosis, hematoma, seroma, skin deformity, soreness at the graft site and donor site, or pulmonary embolism.

Contraindications

Contraindications to performing a bone marrow procedure are severe anemia, active systemic or local infection at the site of harvest or injection, and active cancer, including but not limited to myelodysplastic syndromes. Contraindications for an adipose procedure would be active cancer and infection at harvest or injection site. Relative contraindications include pregnancy. Low body mass index (BMI) individuals require additional investigation for adipose procedures.

Medications

After obtaining consent for an orthobiologic procedure, reviewing any medications, supplements, or habits that may interfere with good cell acquisition or potential therapeutic effect is crucial. Medicines can have deleterious effects on adipose and bone marrow procedures. Most have not been studied for their effects on healing. Therefore, it is important for patients to take only medications that are necessary, which helps reduce polypharmacy. It is in the best interest of the patient to avoid certain medications in order to optimize the harvest. Such medications include: systemic steroids, inhaled steroids or steroid injections, fluoroquinolone antibiotics, HMG-CoA (3-hydroxy-3-methylglutaryl-CoenzymeA) reductase inhibitors or statins, and nonsteroidal antiinflammatory drugs (NSAIDs).

Corticosteroids can have deleterious effects on stem cells and healing[4] and should be avoided for at least 6 weeks prior to the procedure. Fluoroquinolones can increase the risk of Achilles tendinitis and Achilles tendon rupture.[5] Statins have a negative effect on stem cells and muscle cells. They have been found to impair the chondrogenic and osteogenic potential of Medicinal Signaling Cells (MSC, formerly Mesenchymal Stem Cells) and they increase cell senescence and apoptosis.[6] If the patient is on a statin, they should supplement with coenzyme Q_{10}, which can help prevent some of the deleterious effects of statins on muscle cells.[7] NSAIDs can inhibit bone healing, increase the risk of bone fractures,[8] and increase bleeding. They should be held for at least 5 days prior to the procedure, and aspirin for at least 7 days prior. Holding of other antiplatelet medications and statin medications depends on the pharmacokinetics of the particular drug. If patients are on any anticoagulant medications, physicians should discuss with their prescribing doctors the procedure they will perform and determine if they can safely hold these medications.

Preparation

Patients should be instructed to hydrate in the days leading up to the procedure, especially for bone marrow aspiration. The patient should avoid eating solid food 4 to 6 hours prior to the procedure as a precaution against nausea but may continue to drink clear liquids. A review of the patient's past medical history should be performed to determine if there are risk factors for anemia, and obtaining a hemoglobin/hematocrit on patients prior to a bone marrow aspiration should be considered. Results may impact the clinician's decision to perform the procedure or how much bone marrow to extract.

The procedures to be discussed should be performed in a clean manner, using a sterile technique with the provider wearing sterile gloves, a facemask, and hair covering; consider using sterile sleeves or a gown. Baseline and post-procedure vital signs (blood pressure, heart rate, respiratory rate, oxygen saturation, and temperature) should be obtained; based on the vital signs, decisions can be made to proceed with the procedure. Patient monitoring with a pulse oximeter that includes heart rate monitoring is generally sufficient. Supplemental oxygen, blood pressure, automated external defibrillator (AED), and Crash Cart AED supplies should be available.

Anesthesia

Nonexperienced providers and patients may think that bone marrow procedures are very painful; however, in our experience, the procedure is well tolerated when adequate pre-procedure local anesthesia is provided. These procedures are routinely performed in the office setting outside of the hospital or surgical center and usually cause more anxiety than pain. Anxiety can lead to the patient having more muscular tension, which can increase discomfort, so relaxation is paramount. Less is more, and preferably music therapy is all that is necessary to control for anxiety.[9,10] In cases where patients have elevated levels of anxiety or other psychiatric diagnoses, the physician may recommend an oral anxiolytic of choice. The use of controlled substances may require more diligent monitoring. Patients with more extreme anxiety, minors, or patients with central sensitization may require the assistance of an anesthesiologist or certified registered nurse anesthetist (CRNA).

Bone Marrow Aspiration Techniques

Site and Positioning

Extracting red bone marrow is usually best performed at the iliac crest. This region has been shown to have a higher yield of osteogenic progenitor cells compared to the tibia and calcaneus.[11] Knowledge of the pertinent anatomy is important and the goal is to stay within the inner and outer tables of the iliac crest throughout the aspiration.[12] The two typical approaches when aspirating from the iliac crest are the parallel and perpendicular approaches (Fig. 5.1A and B).[13] For the perpendicular approach, you can access the posterior superior iliac spine (PSIS) with the patient in a prone or lateral decubitus position. For the parallel approach through the iliac crest, the patient may be supine for an anterior approach or prone for a posterior approach.

Bain and colleagues surveyed hematologists from 1995 to 2001. A total of 26 out of 54,890 reported adverse events from the perpendicular bone marrow biopsy approach for a rate of 0.05%. Of the 26 adverse events, 14 were reported as hemorrhage complications, with 6 requiring blood transfusions and 1 leading to death. Risk factors most often associated with these hemorrhaging events were aspirin use, myeloproliferative disorders, or both. Additional risk factors seen included warfarin use, disseminated intravascular coagulation, and obesity.[14] This population likely has a greater risk of complications than a typical patient who will have a cellular treatment.

Our preferred approach is harvesting in a perpendicular approach from the PSIS with the patient prone. The posterior region of the iliac crest has been shown to have one of the thickest regions of bone. The average distance of the iliac crest is 24 cm. When determining which area to best access along the iliac crest, the concept of dividing the iliac crest into six different sectors (Fig. 5.2A and B)[15] has been established to bring awareness of the anatomic differences in sector thickness and to help prevent violating neurovascular structures (Fig. 5.3A–C).[12]

Anesthetic

A local anesthetic is required to control pain from the larger needle/trocar used in bone marrow aspiration. The typical anesthetic used is 1% lidocaine without epinephrine and up to 10 mL total per side. Alternatively, 0.25% to 0.5% ropivacaine can be used as well. This may be guided by the same imaging modality used for harvesting. A 22- to 27-gauge, 2 inch to 3.5 inch needle is typically used, depending on the chosen approach. Local anesthetic should be applied to skin at the needle entry site, soft tissue trajectory of the needle, and the surface of the bone/periosteum. The needle used to anesthetize the bone should never be longer than the needle used to harvest the bone

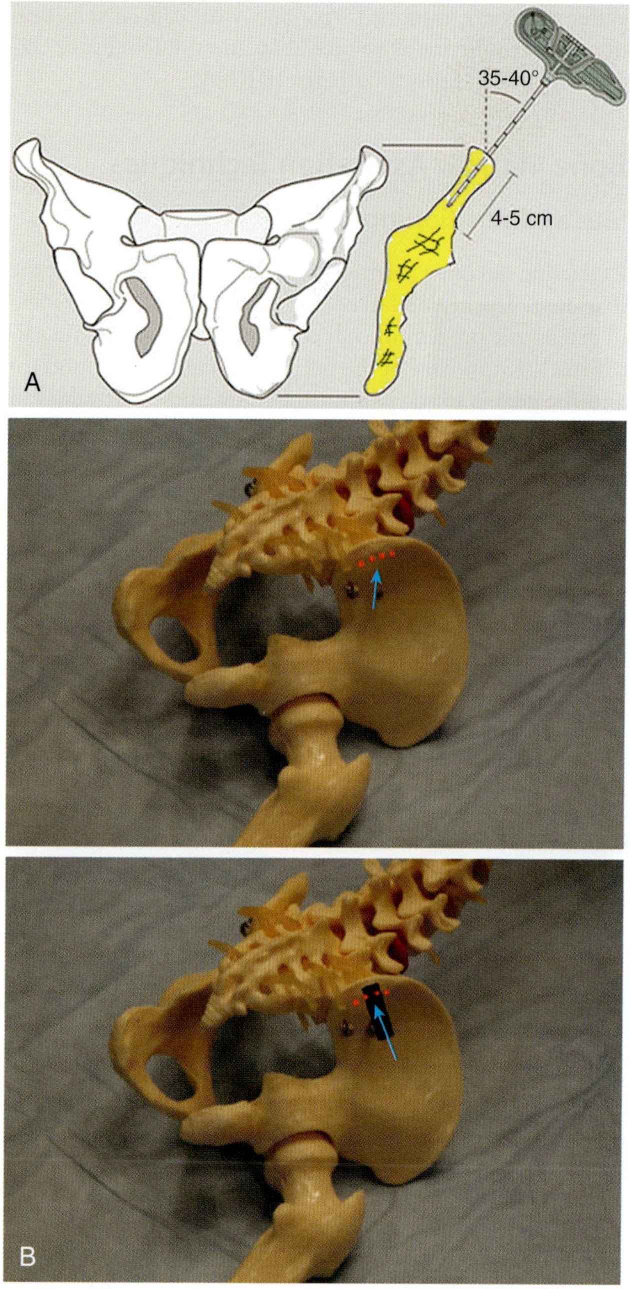

• **Fig. 5.1** (A) Bone marrow aspiration in parallel to the ilium. (B) Bone marrow aspiration in perpendicular. *Black box* represents the ultrasound probe footprint and *blue arrow* represents the needle for aspiration. (A, From Hernigou J, Alves A, Homma Y, et al. Anatomy of the ilium for bone marrow aspiration: map of sectors and implication for safe trocar placement. *Int Orthop*. 2014;38[12]:2585–2590. https://doi.org/10.1007/s00264-014-2353-7. B, From Bowen JE. Technical issues in harvesting and concentrating stem cells (bone marrow and adipose). *PM&R*. 2015;7:S8–S18. https://doi.org/10.1016/j.pmrj.2015.01.025)

marrow. This helps to avoid needle length mismatch in reaching the bone for harvesting. Never inject anesthetic through the trocar or needle used to aspirate marrow, as this can have a deleterious effect on cell viability. After the anesthetic is administered, the physician should wait at least 3 to 5 minutes until adequate anesthesia is achieved. Doing so greatly improves patient comfort.

Anticoagulation

Anticoagulant is necessary to prevent clotting of the marrow when performing an aspiration. If a proper anticoagulant protocol is not used, clots will form, preventing the acquisition, adequate isolation, and concentration of the desired buffy coat of the aspirate. Heparin is the desired anticoagulant. To calculate the proper dose, identify the amount of marrow desired and the syringes to be used for aspiration. Draw a ratio of 500 to 1000 IU of heparin per 1 mL of desired marrow amount. For example, if planning on aspirating 20 mL in a 30 mL syringe, draw 10,000 IU of heparin in the smallest-available volume. If planning on drawing 10 mL in a 10 mL syringe, draw 0.5 mL of heparin (10,000 IU/mL). An additional heparin mixture will be required for anticoagulation prior to bone marrow aspiration at each site. This will consist of a 5 mL syringe with 1 mL of heparin (5000 IU/mL) and 4 mL of normal saline or a 10 mL syringe with 1 mL of heparin (10,000 IU/mL) and 9 mL of normal saline. After each marrow aspiration, gently rock the syringe back and forth to ensure adequate anticoagulation.

Needles

Bone marrow aspiration can be obtained by manually placing a cannula (Fig. 5.4) into the iliac crest, which requires a larger gauge due to the axial load needed. This is usually 11 gauge and can be placed by hand with a clockwise/counterclockwise maneuver while applying axial force or placement of the cannula/trocar against the bone and use of a mallet to force the cannula through the cortex. If performing a manual needle aspiration, typically an 11-gauge 4 inch trocar is used. Rarely, in some larger patients a larger trocar may be needed. We prefer a diamond-tipped needle as opposed to a slanted tip, which may have a greater tendency to slip off of the periosteum. Alternatively, when using a rotary-powered device to guide the aspiration, a smaller gauge needle, such as a 15-gauge 2.7 inch to 3.5 inch, may be used. Additionally, a needle assisted with a rotary drill has been shown to decrease procedure time and residual pain for the patient.[16–18] Rotary devices decrease the stress on the wrist of the physician, especially when harvesting from multiple sites. Please refer to rotary device instructions on how to properly engage and disengage the needle for harvesting. It is important to have a good kinesthetic sense of how it feels to enter the marrow space. Adequate training including mentoring should occur prior to attempting bone marrow aspirations in live patients.

Syringe

Harvesting bone marrow from one site will likely result in a lower MSC count due to dilution with peripheral blood.[19] Therefore, multiple samples from different areas should be acquired while harvesting. MSCs adhere to the trabeculae of bone at low volume pressures, resulting in minimal nucleated cells. Therefore, it is important to obtain the best-quality

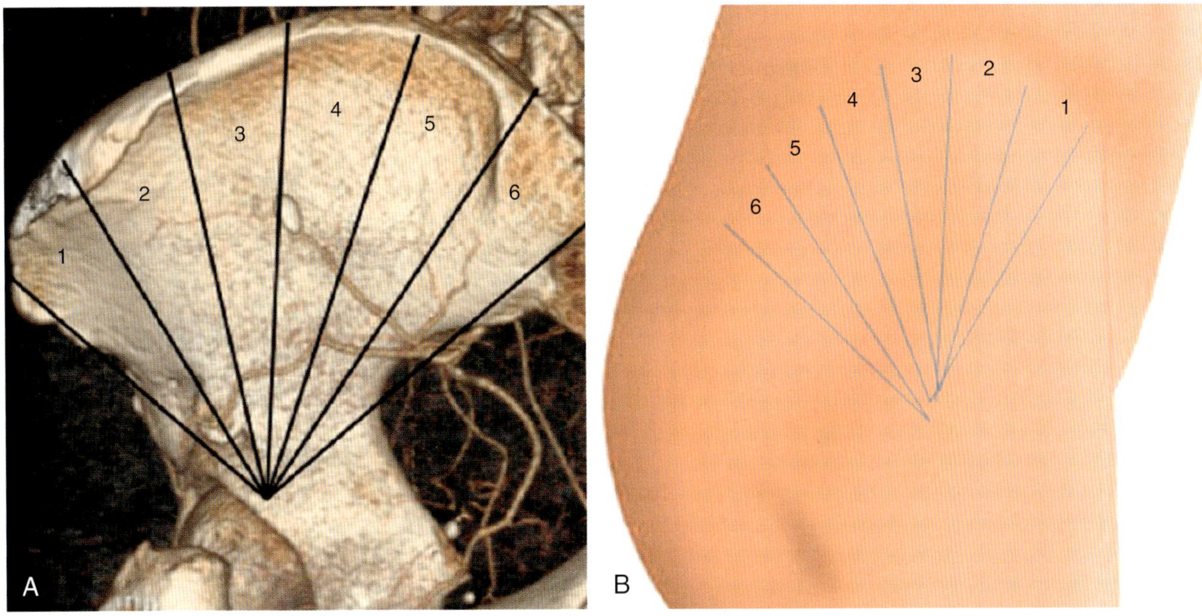

• **Fig. 5.2** Iliac Sectors for Bone Marrow Aspiration. (A) The iliac crest divided into six sectors has variability in sector thickness that must be understood when performing bone marrow aspiration. The iliac wing (three-dimensional reconstruction) was divided by drawing lines from equidistant points spaced along the rim of the iliac crest to the center of the hip. These lines were approximately perpendicular to the curve of the iliac crest. Six sectors were defined by these lines. Sectors 1 and 2, anterior part of the iliac bone; sectors 3 and 4, center part of the iliac bone; sectors 5 and 6, posterior part of the iliac bone. (B) The corresponding sectors can be found and marked on the patient by using the same technique and correspond in clinical practice to different zones of bone marrow aspiration according to the position of the patient. Three different approaches can be used to harvest bone marrow from the iliac crest: patient supine and anterior crest approach (sectors 1, 2, and 3), patient prone and posterior iliac crest approach (sectors 4, 5, and 6) and patient in the left or right lateral position allowing easier middle iliac crest approach (sectors 3 and 4). (From Hernigou J, Picard L, Alves A, et al. Understanding bone safety zones during bone marrow aspiration from the iliac crest: the sector rule. *Int Orthop*. 2014;38[11]:2377–2384. https://doi.org/10.1007/s00264-014-2343-9)

draws by not completely filling the syringes as you aspirate bone marrow. Hernigou and colleagues found that filling the syringe to 10% to 20% of its total volume resulted in an improved yield of MSCs and a better-quality harvest, and smaller-volume syringes resulted in a higher concentration of progenitor cells. Using 10 mL syringes yielded on average a 300% higher concentration of progenitor cells compared to a 50 mL syringe.[20]

Techniques

For these procedures, other medical staff members should prepare the procedure tray prior to the patient entering the room. Please refer to the previous sections for consideration of needle choice, syringe size, anesthetic, and manual or rotary-powered needle advancement. Our preferred technique consists of 20 mL aspirations at each site using 30 mL syringes.

Fluoroscopy Perpendicular

- The patient is placed prone on a firm surface such as the fluoroscopy table.
- The C-arm is then positioned to obtain an A-P scout view of the harvest site, followed by 20 to 30 degree ipsilateral oblique and caudal tilt to view the iliac crest, ilium, and PSIS.
- Identify the skin entry site by placing a radiopaque 18-gauge needle marker on the skin.
- Move the marker until you view your target entry image.
- The marker identifies your single entry point. Utilize a small-gauge needle to create a skin wheal of anesthetic at the skin entry site about 1 cm lateral to the PSIS.
- Next, anesthetize the soft tissue down to the periosteum, as detailed in the aforementioned anesthetic section. Redirect and aim for 3 to 5 different sites along the targeted area, depending on the total desired marrow.
- Allow sufficient time for the anesthetic to work (3 to 5 minutes). Confirm the heparin syringes and other equipment are ready per the above protocol with the procedure tray.
- Next, under intermittent fluoroscopy, guide the trocar from the skin entry site to the desired region on the ilium about 1 cm lateral to the PSIS that has been anesthetized and obtain a hub view (Fig. 5.5).
- Rotate the trocar back and forth while applying axial pressure until a loss of resistance is appreciated or the needle has advanced less than a 1 cm, which likely represents entrance into the marrow cavity. Alternatively, a rotary-powered device may be used to advance the needle, as detailed in the needle section, for less than 1 cm or until a loss of resistance is appreciated.

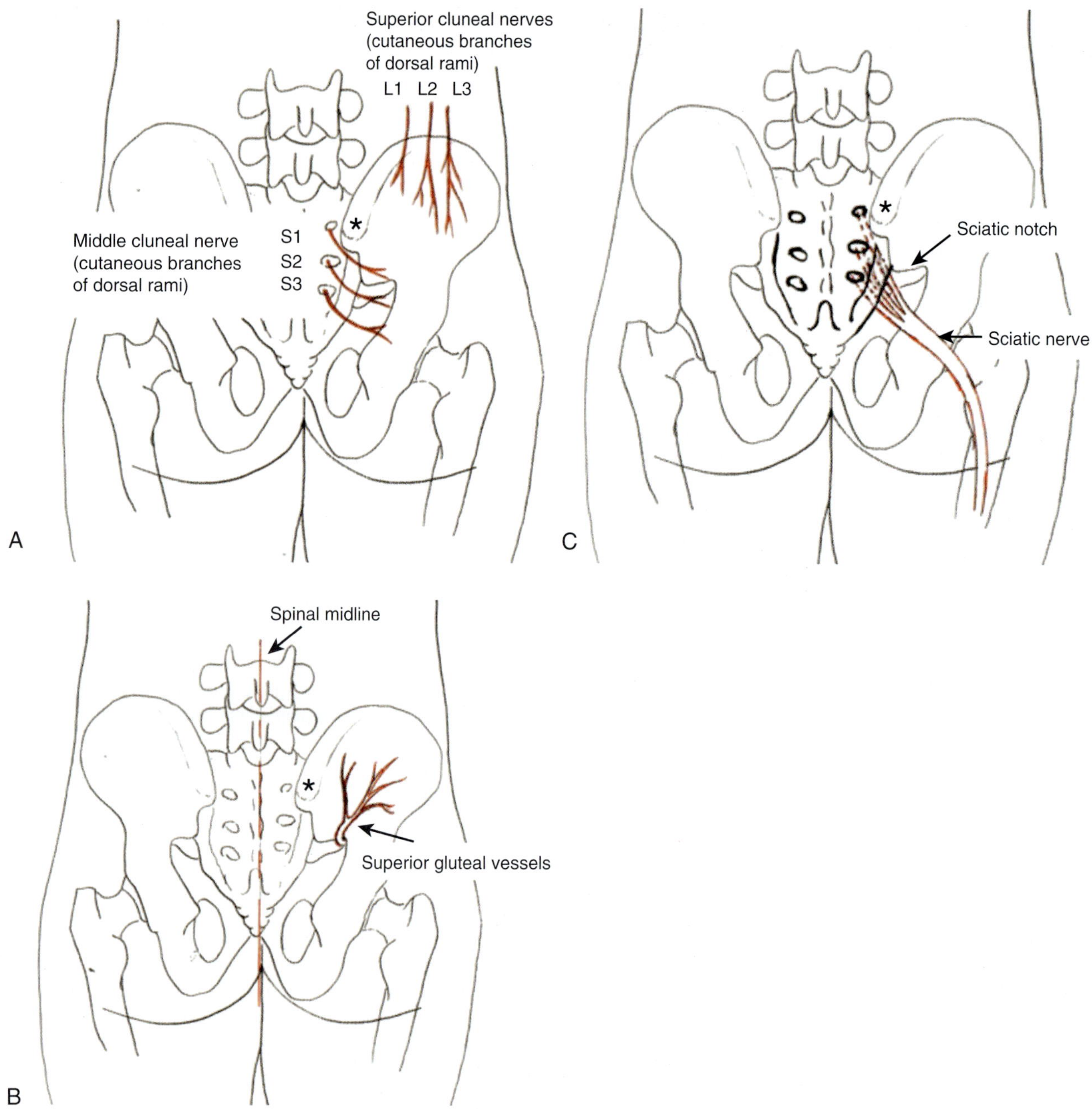

• **Fig. 5.3** (A) Diagrammatic representation of the sensory distribution for right posterior iliac crest. Procurement including the superior (L1 to L3) and middle (S1 to S3) cluneal nerves. Asterisk marks the posterior superior iliac spine. (B) Diagrammatic representation of the superior gluteal vessels. *Asterisk* marks the posterior superior iliac spine. (C) Diagrammatic representation of the course of the sciatic nerve. *Asterisk* marks the posterior superior iliac spine. (From Sittitavornwong S, Falconer DS, Shah R, et al. Anatomic considerations for posterior iliac crest bone procurement. *J Oral Maxillofac Surg*. 2013;71[10]:1777–1788. https://doi.org/10.1016/j.joms.2013.03.008)

- Remove the stylet and inject 0.5 mL of the heparin flush (1000 IU per mL of heparin solution with 9 mL of saline).
- Then attach a heparinized syringe and pull with a constant quick force to aspirate the desired volume of marrow.
- Replace the stylet and rotate the needle to barely withdraw from the bone. Redirect the trocar to the next aspiration site.
- Repeat this procedure for three to five sites depending on the desired volume of bone marrow aspirate.
- If necessary, repeat the procedure on the contralateral side to obtain the desired bone marrow volume.

Fluoroscopy Parallel

- The patient is positioned prone on a firm fluoroscopy table.
- The physician should be positioned on the patient's side.

- The C-arm is then positioned to obtain an A-P scout view of the harvest site, followed by 20- to 30-degree contralateral oblique to view the iliac crest and PSIS until the medial and lateral borders of the iliac crest are clearly defined.
- Identify the skin entry site by placing a radiopaque (18-gauge needle) marker on the skin.
- Move the marker and intermittently take pictures until you view your target entry image.
- Utilize a small-gauge needle to create a skin wheal of anesthetic at the skin entry site.
- Next anesthetize the skin and soft tissue down to the periosteum using a similar-size needle as the one you will aspirate with.
- Allow sufficient time for the anesthetic to work (3 to 5 minutes). Confirm the heparin syringes and other equipment are ready per the above protocol with the procedural tray.

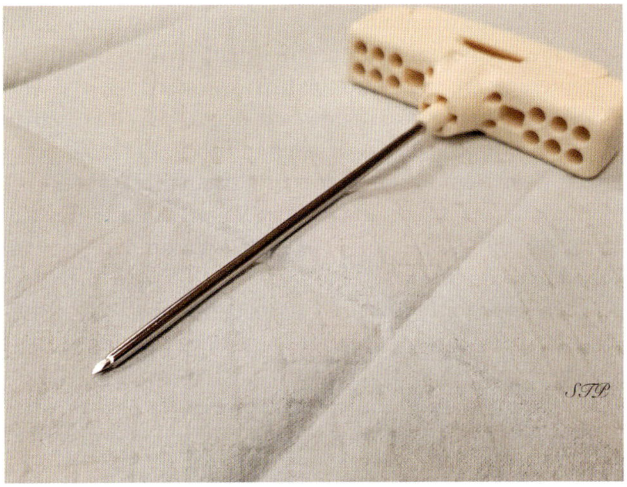

• **Fig. 5.4** J-style bone marrow manual aspiration needle (11 gauge × 4 inches).

- Manually advance the needle to the periosteum and confirm placement between the medial and lateral borders of the iliac crest with image guidance.
- Advance your needle until you just access the bone marrow cavity, as described above, pointing anterolateral along the plane of the ilium in your hub view.
- Remove the stylet and inject 0.5 mL of the heparin flush (1000 IU per mL of heparin solution with 9 mL of saline).
- Attach a heparinized syringe and pull with a constant quick force to aspirate the desired volume of marrow.
- Replace the stylet and rotate the needle to barely withdraw from the bone. Redirect the trocar to the next aspiration site.
- Redirect and aim for 2 to 4 different sites along the targeted area until obtaining the total desired marrow.

Ultrasound-guided Perpendicular (Author Preferred)

- The patient is positioned prone on a firm table.
- A 1 ultrasound probe is used to scan for the PSIS. The probe is perpendicular to the sagittal plane of the patient and to the posterior ilium. Identify the rounded PSIS.
- Keep the probe in the same orientation and scan cephalad 2 cm until the ilium has the appearance of a mountain peak. The bone should be in the middle of your screen or slightly further away from the needle entry site, which will be lateral. Rotate probe to be perpendicular to the face of the ilium.
- Make a skin wheal with local anesthetic 1 cm lateral to the PSIS adjacent to the footprint of the probe.
- Then in-plane anesthetize the soft tissue down to the periosteum. The needle should touch bone at a depth of 1 cm below (lateral to the PSIS) the peak or most superficial aspect of the bone (Fig. 5.6A and B).

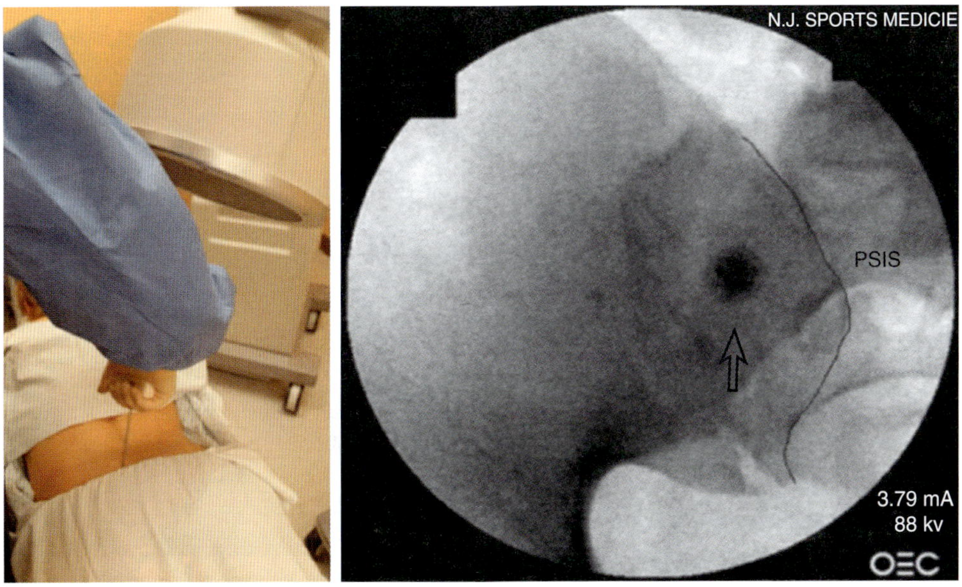

• **Fig. 5.5** Hub view of needle for bone marrow aspiration under fluoroscopic guidance. The arrow identifies the bone marrow aspiration needle which is in parallel to the x-ray.

- From the same needle entry on the skin redirect the probe inferiorly around the PSIS for 1 to 2 more locations and superior for 1 to 2 more locations. Pivot the proximal portion of the probe lateral along the iliac crest.
- Be sure you pivot the probe from the single needle entry site.
- When scanning inferiorly, avoid going too inferior where you lose the round superficial PSIS and see a drop in the bone as this is the sacrum and SI joint. When scanning inferior, the probe should only pivot 5 to 15 degrees to obtain a new area.
- When scanning superior, the probe should pivot 30 to 40 degrees for a new area and 70 to 80 degrees for a second new area. Note that the superior aspect of the ilium is deeper and usually requires a steeper angle. Do not pivot more than 90 degrees to avoid bringing the probe closer to the cluneal nerves.
- No matter the angle of the probe or the depth of the bone, the target should be 1 cm inferior to the most superficial aspect of the bone. This ensures you are staying in a thick area of bone and not so close to the surface that the needle risks sliding off. Do not go deeper than 1 to 2 cm, especially inferiorly, as this risks injury to the gluteal neurovascular structures.
- Allow sufficient time for the anesthetic to work (3 to 5 minutes). Confirm the heparin syringes and other equipment are ready per the above protocol with the procedure tray.
- Under ultrasound guidance guide the trocar to the sites that were anesthetized in the same technique described above.
- The needle should be as close to perpendicular to the bone angle as possible. This ensures a shorter distance to travel to the marrow space and less likelihood for the needle to slide off of the bone (Fig. 5.7).
- Advance the trocar until a loss of resistance is appreciated or the needle has advanced less than 1 cm, which likely represents entrance into the marrow cavity.
- Alternatively, a rotary-powered device may be used to advance the needle, as detailed in the needle section, for less than 1 cm or until a loss of resistance is appreciated.
- Remove the stylet and inject 0.5 mL of the heparin flush (1000 IU per mL of heparin solution with 9 mL of saline) (Fig. 5.8).
- Then attach a heparinized syringe and pull with a constant quick force to aspirate the desired volume of marrow (Fig. 5.9A and B).
- Replace the stylet and rotate the needle to barely withdraw from the bone. Redirect the trocar to the next aspiration site.
- Repeat this procedure for 3 to 5 sites depending on the desired volume of bone marrow aspirate.

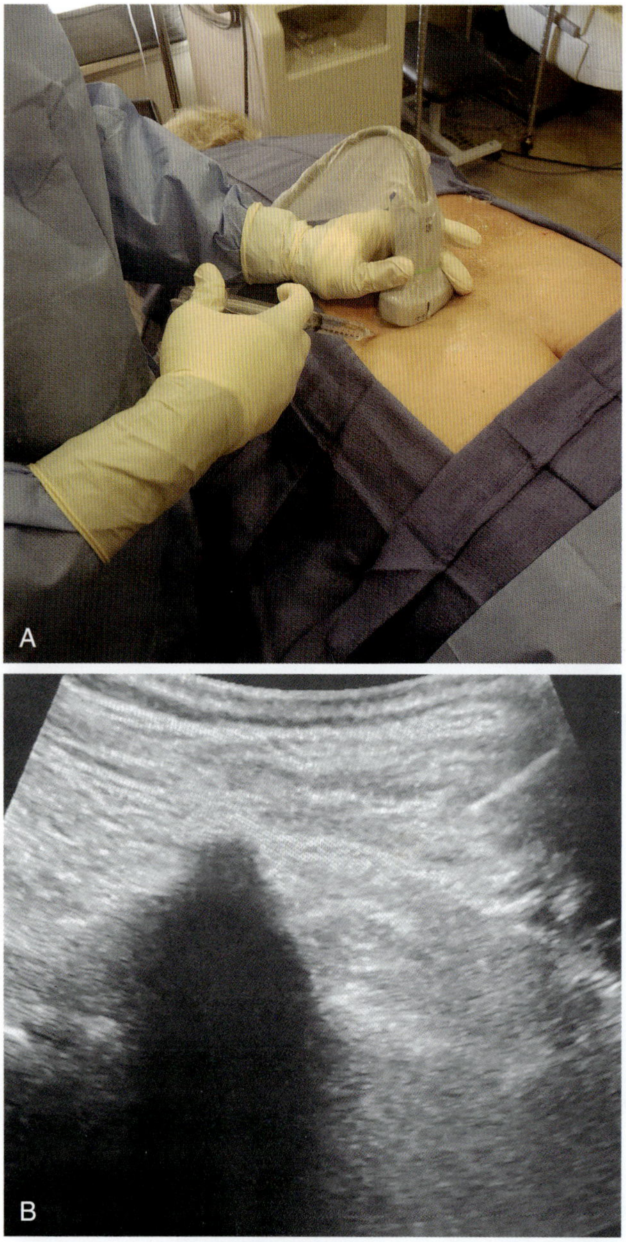

• **Fig. 5.6** (A) Bone marrow aspiration anesthetic setup. (B) Ultrasound-guided in-plane anesthetic injection of the soft tissue trajectory of the needle and the surface of the bone/periosteum.

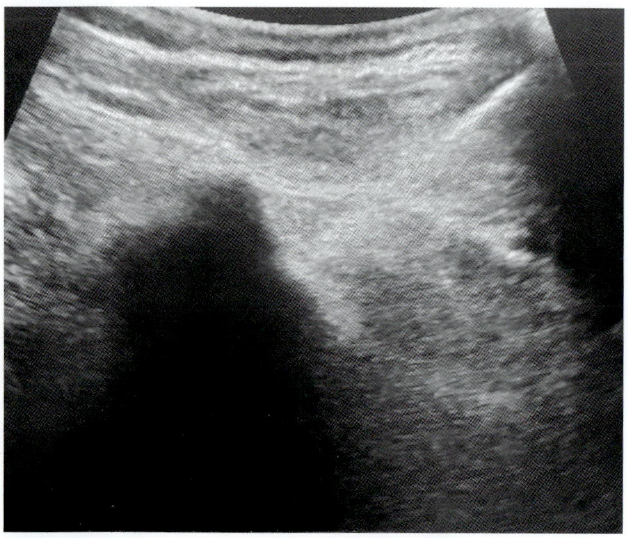

• **Fig. 5.7** Ultrasound image of a trocar in-plane for perpendicular bone marrow aspiration.

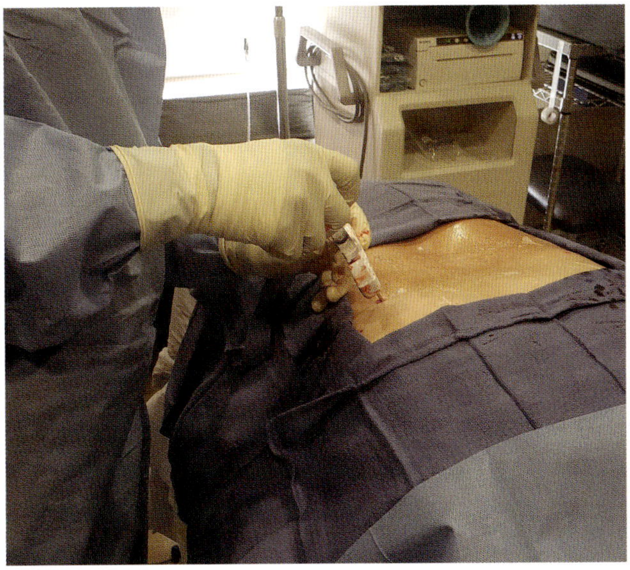

• **Fig. 5.8** Injection of 0.5 mL of heparin mixture prior to bone marrow aspiration.

- If necessary, repeat the procedure on the contralateral side to obtain the desired bone marrow volume.

Ultrasound-assisted Parallel

- The patient is positioned prone on a firm table.
- Using an ultrasound transducer identify the PSIS.
- Using ultrasound, identify the inferior (Fig. 5.10), medial, and lateral portion of the PSIS on the skin.
- Mark the medial border of the iliac crest, moving the ultrasound from a midline to lateral direction (Fig. 5.11).
- Mark the lateral border of the iliac crest, moving in a lateral to medial direction (Fig. 5.12).
- The needle entry site will be within the borders within the US marked regions.
- Mark the desired skin entry site with a surgical marker.
- Utilize a small-gauge needle to create a skin wheal of anesthetic at the skin entry site.
- Next, anesthetize the skin and soft tissue down to the periosteum using a needle similar in size to the one you will aspirate with.
- Allow sufficient time for the anesthetic to work (3 to 5 minutes). Confirm the heparin syringes and other equipment are ready per the above protocol with the procedure tray.
- Angle the needle 30 degrees directed anterolaterally along the plane of the iliac crest between the medial and lateral borders and advance to the bone (Fig. 5.13).
- Advance the trocar until you just access the bone marrow cavity, as described above, pointing anterolateral along the plane of the ilium.
- Remove the stylet and inject 0.5 mL of the heparin flush (1000 IU per mL of heparin solution with 9 mL of saline).
- Attach a heparinized syringe and pull with a constant quick force to aspirate the desired volume of marrow.
- Replace the stylet and rotate the needle to barely withdraw from the bone. Redirect the trocar to the next aspiration site.

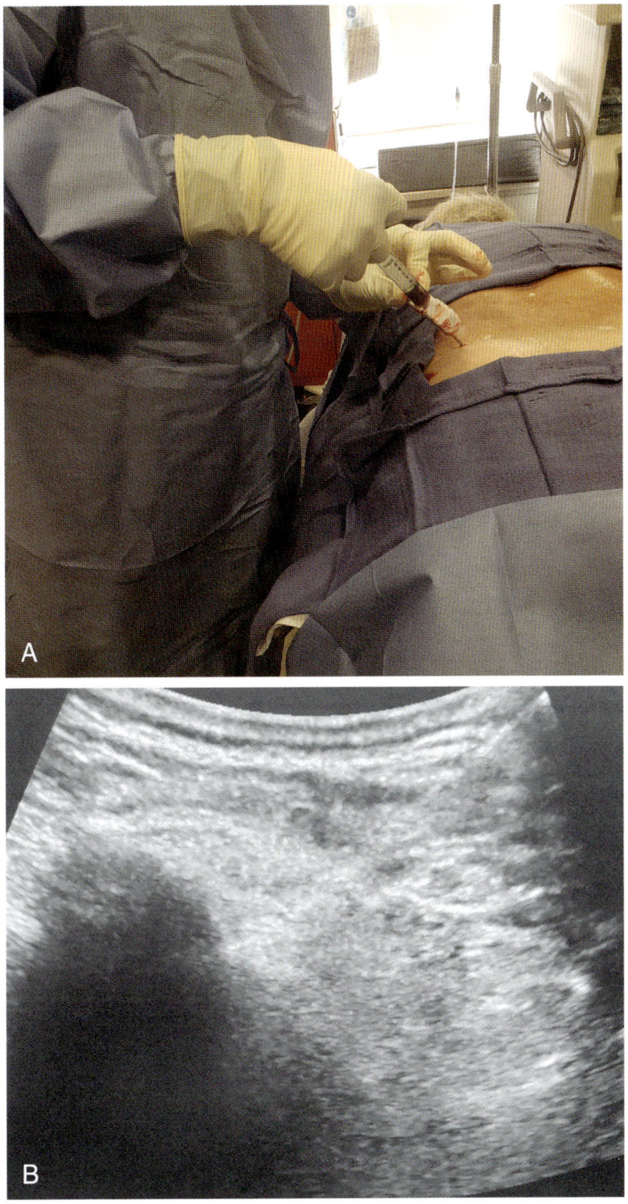

• **Fig. 5.9** (A) Bone marrow aspiration with a quick constant force. (B) Bone marrow aspiration under ultrasound guidance.

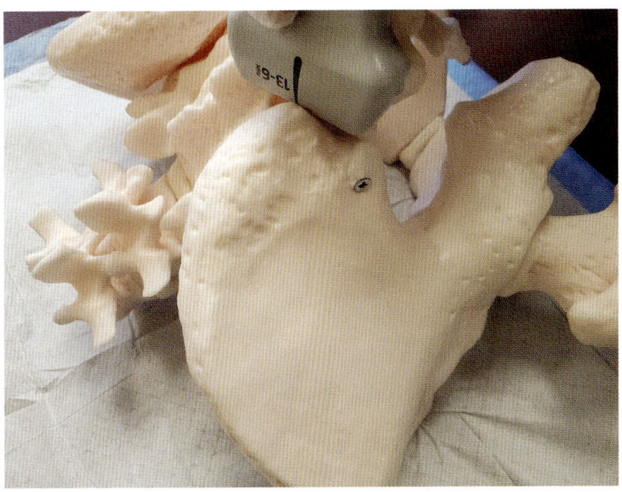

• **Fig. 5.10** Ultrasound scanning from inferior to superior to demarcate the PSIS.

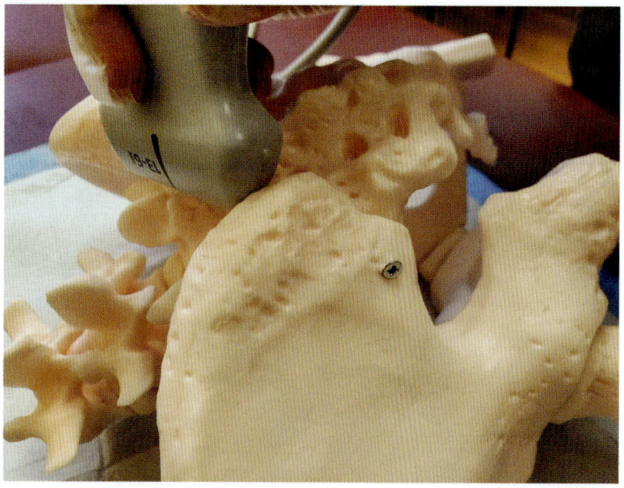

• **Fig. 5.11** Ultrasound scanning midline to lateral to demarcate the iliac crest.

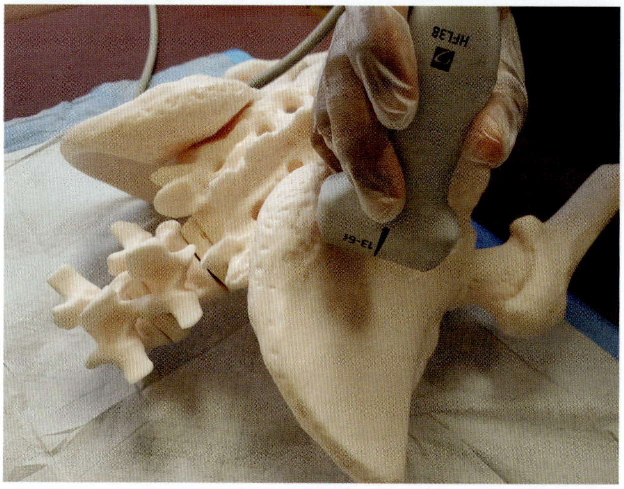

• **Fig. 5.12** Ultrasound scanning lateral to medial to demarcate the iliac crest.

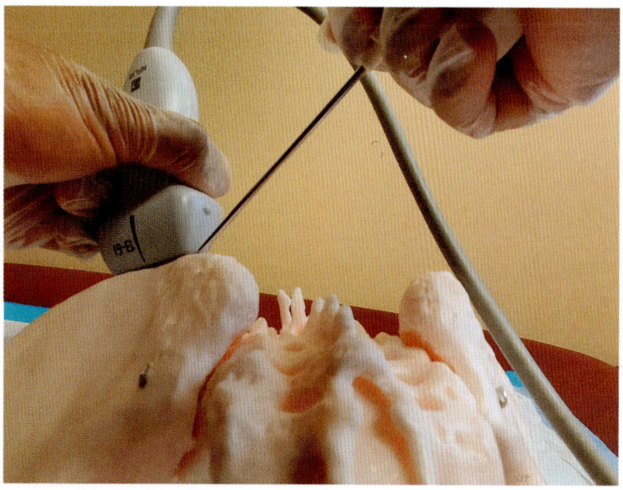

• **Fig. 5.13** Ultrasound-assisted parallel bone marrow aspiration along the iliac crest.

- Redirect and aim for 2 to 4 different sites along the targeted area until you have obtained the total desired marrow.

Processing

This varies depending upon the bone marrow aspiration kit and is beyond the scope of this chapter.

Adipose Harvesting Techniques

Positioning

Prior to a lipoaspiration, one must consider where the adipose tissue will be harvested. This is usually the area that contains the most adipose tissue on the individual and is dependent on body habitus. These areas include but are not limited to the lower abdomen, lateral thigh, flank, or buttock region. When harvesting from the lower abdomen the patient is supine. The lateral thigh is best accessed in the lateral decubitus position. While the patient is prone, adipose tissue can be harvested from the flank or buttock region.

Pearl: Choose a position that permits the patient to be most comfortable and stationary in order to tolerate the length of the procedure. Additionally, this position should easily allow the physician to acquire the tissue with minimal to no repositioning of the patient during the harvest.

Anesthetic

For adipose harvesting, it is important to consider the type of anesthetic used. Anesthetics can be toxic to the viability of the cells, particularly adipocytes, and a list of anesthetics and their maximum recommended doses can be seen in Table 5.1.[21] Generally, ropivacaine is the least toxic anesthetic available.[22–24] For adipose procedures, use a mixture of tumescent anesthetic which contains lidocaine with epinephrine to help control bleeding and provide pain relief. A typical tumescent anesthetic mixture would consist of 500 mL of normal saline, 25 mL of 2% lidocaine, two ampules of epinephrine 1:1000, and 10 mL of 8.4% sodium bicarbonate. If the patient has a lidocaine allergy you may consider ropivacaine as a tumescent; it has been used in both animal and human studies[25,26]; however, further studies are necessary to determine optimal concentrations.

Imaging

In patients with a very low body fat percentage, scanning with an ultrasound may be useful to identify sufficient quantities of adipose tissue for harvest. However, in our experience, the mid-buttock a few inches superior to the gluteal cleft is an adequate entry point even in some of the leanest or most fit individuals. With experience, the harvesting of adipose tissue will not require the use of an ultrasound.

TABLE 5.1 **Dose Recommendations for Commonly Used Local Anesthetics.**

Local Anesthetic	Concentration (%)	Maximum Dose (mg/kg)	Maximum Dose With Epinephrine (mg/kg)	Onset Time (min)	Duration (h)
Lidocaine	0.5–2	4–6	6–8	10–20	0.75–2
Bupivacaine	0.125–0.5	2	3	15–30	2.5–8
Ropivacaine	0.2–1	2–3	–	10–20	2.5–8
Mepivacaine	0.5–1.5	6–8	10	5–10	1–1.5
2-Chloroprocaine	2–3	10	15	5	1

Used with permission from Dillane D. Local Anesthetic Toxicity: Prevention and Management. Complications of Regional Anesthesia: Principles of Safe Practice in Local and Regional Anesthesia. 3rd ed. In Finucane BT, Tsui BCH, eds. Springer International Publishing;2017.

Technique

- Once the patient is sterilely draped and the harvest site cleansed in the normal aseptic fashion, a skin wheal of tumescent anesthesia is administered at the entry site of harvest.
- A superficial skin nick is required with an 18-gauge needle or scalpel to allow penetration through the skin with a blunt tip cannula that will ultimately deliver the rest of the tumescent anesthetic.
- A volume of 200 to 300 mL of the anesthetic is delivered to each harvest region. It is delivered in a fan-like distribution and the region should become tense and exhibit a tumescence toward the end of completion.
- After its delivery, at least 15 minutes is required for the anesthesia to take effect.
- **Pearl:** Adequate volume of tumescent anesthetic and time should allow for an easy harvest.
- When this time has passed, a blunt tip cannula can be introduced at the harvest entry site.
- Initially, this blunt tip cannula may be used to penetrate and break up the adipose tissue.
- Next, the lipoaspiration cannula with a vacuum lock syringe is attached.
- A vacuum locking syringe (20 to 60 mL) is typically supplied in the lipoaspirate kits.
- Aspirate by using back and forth movements in the areas that were anesthetized.
- Perform this technique until sufficient volume is obtained for the injectate.
- During the procedure, remember to talk to your patient as needed and encourage them to provide feedback if there are any sensitive areas throughout the harvest.
- In our experience, there is usually a 3:1 to 4:1 ratio of what is harvested to the final product after decanting and processing.
- Aspiration to final product ratio may vary depending on the chosen method of processing.

Adipose Processing

Processing adipose tissue to micro-fragmented adipose tissue (MFAT) depends on the specific device that is used. All devices must comply with FDA regulations so that less than minimal manipulation is achieved. One should not solely rely on a commercial representative of a company to determine whether a device is FDA-compliant prior to using it. Most processing for consists of washing the fat tissue to remove red blood cells, tumescent anesthesia, and oil from broken adipocytes. The remaining product is resized in different manners to leave intact tissue in small clusters that can be delivered through a small needle. FDA-compliant devices and methods such as Lipogems, PureGraft, or IntelliFat work within a closed system and allow for the final product to be delivered percutaneously. These systems do not extract cells from the adipose tissue (i.e., stromal vascular fraction [SVF]) and are compliant with the FDA's regulation of minimum manipulation.

At the time of publication, processing of adipose tissue and bone marrow must use minimal manipulation and be intended for homologous use for compliance with FDA regulations. Following processing, the adipose tissue may be transferred to additional syringes via Luer lock connectors for therapeutic use (Fig. 5.14).

Post Procedure

Once the tissue harvest is complete, the entry site can be cleansed and covered. A clear occlusive dressing, such as Tegaderm, with sterile gauze with or without antibiotic ointment may be used. Ice packs may be used temporarily, and a compressive garment may be applied to the harvest site. The compressive garment may be worn for a week, which can help to prevent post-procedural complications of a seroma and/or hematoma. NSAIDs should be avoided post-injection. The application of topical arnica to the harvesting site can help prevent bruising as well.

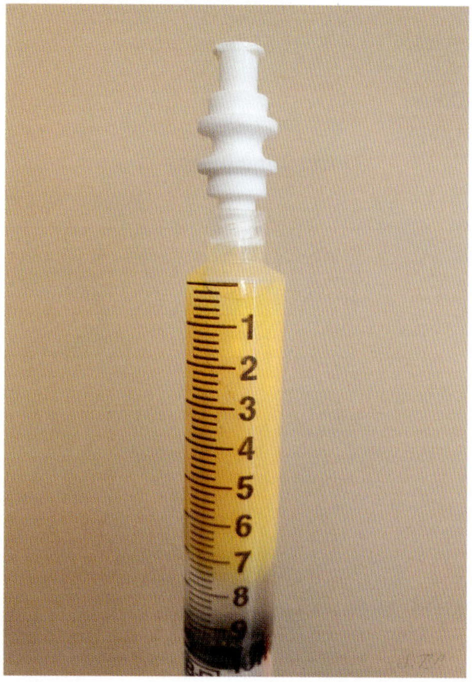

• **Fig. 5.14** Micro-fragmented Adipose Tissue. Micro-fragmented adipose tissue in a 10 mL syringe with a female–female Luer lock connector attached.

After the harvest and deployment of the orthobiologics, post-procedural vitals should be checked to ensure they are within normal limits. The patient should be reminded that the risk of bleeding is highest postprocedure when heparin is utilized for the first several hours. Strenuous activity and heavy lifting should be avoided for at least the first day following the procedure. It is normal for soreness to occur in the first day to a week following the procedure. The patient should monitor for any signs of increased puncture/incision site pain or discharge, fever, and/or erythema and inform the physician if these occur to prompt further evaluation. The harvest site should be kept dry and clean for at least 24 hours. Afterwards, the patient should not bath or submerge in fluids for 3 days (or until the skin incision is closed) but may shower. Written post-procedural instructions may be provided to the patient. There should be someone available to drive them from the office following the procedure.

Deployment

Various methods of deploying injectates, bone marrow aspirate concentrate (BMAC) or MFAT, to different regions will be discussed throughout this book. In general, one should not give these products systemically, such as intravenously, as it would not be compliant with homologous use. The products should be intended for the autologous treatment of orthopedic conditions. One should ensure delivery of the product to its intended destination as accurately as possible. Therefore, the deployment of these orthobiologics should be done with image guidance, such as ultrasound and/or fluoroscopy. The specific region being addressed and the provider's proficiency will determine which is optimal. Generally, ultrasound is preferred for most soft tissue structures and has the advantage over fluoroscopy of avoiding radiation exposure and providing the ability to visualize neurovascular structures.[27] Therefore, training and familiarity with these techniques are of utmost importance.

Rehabilitation

Rehabilitation after these procedures will be discussed in another chapter within this text. Generally, it is best to adhere to relative rest for the first 1 to 2 days, with a clear and comprehensive rehabilitation plan discussed with the treating provider.

References

1. Sheykhhasan M, Wong JKL, Seifalian AM. Human adipose-derived stem cells with great therapeutic potential. *Curr Stem Cell Res Ther*. 2019;14(7):532–548. https://doi.org/10.2174/1574888X14666190411121528.
2. Center for Biologics Evaluation and Research and Center for Devices and Radiological Health. Regulatory Considerations for Human Cells, Tissues, and Cellular and Tissue-Based Products: Minimal Manipulation and Homologous Use. US Food and Drug Administration. Published June 13, 2019. Accessed January 2, 2020. http://www.fda.gov/regulatory-information/search-fda-guidance-documents/regulatory-considerations-human-cells-tissues-and-cellular-and-tissue-based-products-minimal
3. Bowen JE. Technical issues in harvesting and concentrating stem cells (bone marrow and adipose). *PM&R*. 2015;7:S8–S18. https://doi.org/10.1016/j.pmrj.2015.01.025.
4. Wyles CC, Houdek MT, Wyles SP, Wagner ER, Behfar A, Sierra RJ. Differential cytotoxicity of corticosteroids on human mesenchymal stem cells. *Clin Orthop*. 2015;473(3):1155–1164. https://doi.org/10.1007/s11999-014-3925-y.
5. Stephenson AL, Wu W, Cortes D, Rochon PA. Tendon injury and fluoroquinolone use: a systematic review. *Drug Saf*. 2013;36(9):709–721. https://doi.org/10.1007/s40264-013-0089-8.
6. Izadpanah R, Schächtele DJ, Pfnür AB, et al. The impact of statins on biological characteristics of stem cells provides a novel explanation for their pleiotropic beneficial and adverse clinical effects. *Am J Physiol Cell Physiol*. 2015;309(8):C522–531. https://doi.org/10.1152/ajpcell.00406.2014.
7. Lee B-J, Tseng Y-F, Yen C-H, Lin P-T. Effects of coenzyme Q10 supplementation (300 mg/day) on antioxidation and anti-inflammation in coronary artery disease patients during statins therapy: a randomized, placebo-controlled trial. *Nutr J*. 2013;12(1):142. https://doi.org/10.1186/1475-2891-12-142.
8. van Esch RW, Kool MM, van As S. NSAIDs can have adverse effects on bone healing. *Med Hypotheses*. 2013;81(2):343–346. https://doi.org/10.1016/j.mehy.2013.03.042.
9. Graff V, Cai L, Badiola I, Elkassabany NM. Music versus midazolam during preoperative nerve block placements: a prospective randomized controlled study. *Reg Anesth Pain Med*. 2019. https://doi.org/10.1136/rapm-2018–100251. Published online July 18.
10. Packyanathan JS, Lakshmanan R, Jayashri P. Effect of music therapy on anxiety levels on patient undergoing dental extractions. *J Fam Med Prim Care*. 2019;8(12):3854–3860. https://doi.org/10.4103/jfmpc.jfmpc_789_19.

11. Hyer CF, Berlet GC, Bussewitz BW, Hankins T, Ziegler HL, Philbin TM. Quantitative assessment of the yield of osteoblastic connective tissue progenitors in bone marrow aspirate from the iliac crest, tibia, and calcaneus. *J Bone Joint Surg Am.* 2013;95(14):1312–1316. https://doi.org/10.2106/JBJS.L.01529.
12. Sittitavornwong S, Falconer DS, Shah R, Brown N, Tubbs RS. Anatomic considerations for posterior iliac crest bone procurement. *J Oral Maxillofac Surg.* 2013;71(10):1777–1788. https://doi.org/10.1016/j.joms.2013.03.008.
13. Hernigou J, Alves A, Homma Y, Guissou I, Hernigou P. Anatomy of the ilium for bone marrow aspiration: map of sectors and implication for safe trocar placement. *Int Orthop.* 2014;38(12):2585–2590. https://doi.org/10.1007/s00264-014-2353-7.
14. Bain BJ. Bone marrow biopsy morbidity and mortality. *Br J Haematol.* 2003;121(6):949–951. https://doi.org/10.1046/j.1365-2141.2003.04329.x.
15. Hernigou J, Picard L, Alves A, Silvera J, Homma Y, Hernigou P. Understanding bone safety zones during bone marrow aspiration from the iliac crest: the sector rule. *Int Orthop.* 2014;38(11):2377–2384. https://doi.org/10.1007/s00264-014-2343-9.
16. Swords RT, Anguita J, Higgins RA, et al. A prospective randomised study of a rotary powered device (OnControl) for bone marrow aspiration and biopsy. *J Clin Pathol.* 2011;64(9):809–813. https://doi.org/10.1136/jclinpath-2011-200047.
17. Reed LJ, Raghupathy R, Strakhan M, et al. The OnControl bone marrow biopsy technique is superior to the standard manual technique for hematologists-in-training: a prospective, randomized comparison. *Hematol Rep.* 2011;3(3). https://doi.org/10.4081/hr.2011.e21.
18. Berenson JR, Yellin O, Blumenstein B, et al. Using a powered bone marrow biopsy system results in shorter procedures, causes less residual pain to adult patients, and yields larger specimens. *Diagn Pathol.* 2011;6(1):23. https://doi.org/10.1186/1746-1596-6-23.
19. Li J, Wong WH-S, Chan S, et al. Factors affecting mesenchymal stromal cells yield from bone marrow aspiration. *Chin J Cancer Res.* 2011;23(1):43–48. https://doi.org/10.1007/s11670-011-0043-1.
20. Hernigou P, Homma Y, Flouzat Lachaniette CH, et al. Benefits of small volume and small syringe for bone marrow aspirations of mesenchymal stem cells. *Int Orthop.* 2013;37(11):2279–2287. https://doi.org/10.1007/s00264-013-2017-z.
21. Dillane D. Local Anesthetic Toxicity: Prevention and Management. *Complications of Regional Anesthesia: Principles of Safe Practice in Local and Regional Anesthesia*, 3rd edn. Brendan T. Finucane, Ban C.H. Tsui (Editors). Springer International Publishing, 2017, Kwofie MK. Complications of regional anesthesia: principles of safe practice in local and regional anesthesia.
22. Cai X-Y, Xiong L-M, Yang S-H, et al. Comparison of toxicity effects of ropivacaine, bupivacaine, and lidocaine on rabbit intervertebral disc cells in vitro. *Spine J.* 2014;14(3):483–490. https://doi.org/10.1016/j.spinee.2013.06.041.
23. Sung C-M, Hah Y-S, Kim J-S, et al. Cytotoxic effects of ropivacaine, bupivacaine, and lidocaine on rotator cuff tenofibroblasts. *Am J Sports Med.* 2014;42(12):2888–2896. https://doi.org/10.1177/0363546514550991.
24. Rahnama R, Wang M, Dang A, Kim H, Kuo A. Cytotoxicity of local anesthetics on human mesenchymal stem cells. *J Bone Jt Surg.* 2013;95(2):132–137. https://doi.org/10.2106/JBJS.K.01291.
25. Breuninger H, Hobbach PS, Schimek F. Ropivacaine: an important anesthetic agent for slow infusion and other forms of tumescent anesthesia. *Dermatol Surg.* 1999;25(10):799–802. https://doi.org/10.1046/j.1524-4725.1999.99087.x.
26. Abimussi CJX, Menegheti TM, Wagatsuma JT, et al. Tumescent local anesthesia with ropivacaine in different concentrations in bitches undergoing mastectomy: plasma concentration and postoperative analgesia. *Vet Anaesth Analg.* 2014;41(5):516–525. https://doi.org/10.1111/vaa.12178.
27. Smith J, Hurdle M-F, Locketz AJ, Wisniewski SJ. Ultrasound-guided piriformis injection: technique description and verification. *Arch Phys Med Rehabil.* 2006;87(12):1664–1667. https://doi.org/10.1016/j.apmr.2006.08.337.

6

Autologous Tissue Harvesting Techniques: Platelet-Rich Plasma

PETER A. EVERTS

Introduction

Whole Blood and Platelets

Platelet-rich plasma (PRP) was first used in cardiac surgery by Ferrari and colleagues in 1987 as an autologous blood transfusion after open heart procedures to avoid homologous blood product transfusions.[1] The use of PRP to treat musculoskeletal disorders (MSK-D) was noted in the mid-1990s for tendinosis and tendinitis. Currently PRP is being utilized by providers in multiple specialties, including maxillofacial surgery, spinal disorders, orthopedics, chronic wounds, and more.[2] During the physiologic cascades of soft tissue regeneration, a variety of cellular, hormonal, and growth factors play pivotal roles and are stored in the alpha and dense granules of platelets.

Platelets are formed from megakaryocytes in the bone marrow by pinching off from their progenitor cells before being released into the peripheral circulation. Platelets are small, anucleate, discoid blood cells (1 to 3 μm), with an in vivo half-life of 7 days, and the average platelet count in adults ranges from 150 to 350 × 10^6/mL of circulating blood.[3]

Since platelets are an integrated part of whole blood, mimicking and accelerating physiologic tissue healing and regeneration, harvesting a calculated amount of fresh blood is mandatory to acquire platelets and eventually other whole blood constituents.

Medical and US Food and Drug Administration (FDA)-approved point-of-care devices can fractionate a unit of autologous whole blood into various components and formulations, consisting of platelet-poor plasma, platelets, leukocytes, and red blood cells (RBCs).

Phlebotomy Procedure

Administrative duties, proper patient identification, and informed consent precede a blood harvesting procedure, with proper labeling of syringes. Patients can be placed in a comfortable seated or recumbent position. Sterile and single-use needles and syringes are used, and blood is generally drawn by phlebotomy with a venous catheter ranging from 18 to 21 gauge in adults. The practitioner responsible for harvesting blood should maintain proper local guidelines and use personal protective equipment (PPE). Several PRP manufacturers produce complete PRP kits that include processing devices, syringes (Fig. 6.1) and in most kits an anticoagulant and a phlebotomy kit (including tourniquet, butterfly assembly, gauzes, alcohol pad, labels) (Fig. 6.2).

The whole blood collection syringe should contain an anticoagulant to avoid blood clotting during blood harvesting and PRP preparation, thus preventing platelet activation prior to its use. Manufacturer instructions provide guidelines on loading sufficient anticoagulant in the harvesting syringe.

Vein Assessment

Assessment of the patient prior to phlebotomy to locate an adequate vein is advised. In most instances the median antecubital vein is preferred by practitioners, but care should be taken in this area due to the close proximity of the median nerve. For the blood draw, it is important to select a large and stable vein in the antecubital fossa, with the cephalic and basilic vein connected by the median antecubital vein (Fig. 6.3). Another common option is the base of the cephalic vein, located over the wrist joint proximal to the thumb (note that the superficial radial nerve is close to this area). In muscular patients, the cephalic vein is more superficial near the elbow in the antecubital fossa, presenting as the median antebrachial vein. Veins at the back of the hand (Fig. 6.4) are more peripheral veins and are more suitable for intravenous access to inject medication than for blood harvest. Supportive technology such as ultrasound devices or vein visualization systems can be used to map and access veins when not clearly visible/palpable on visual inspection.

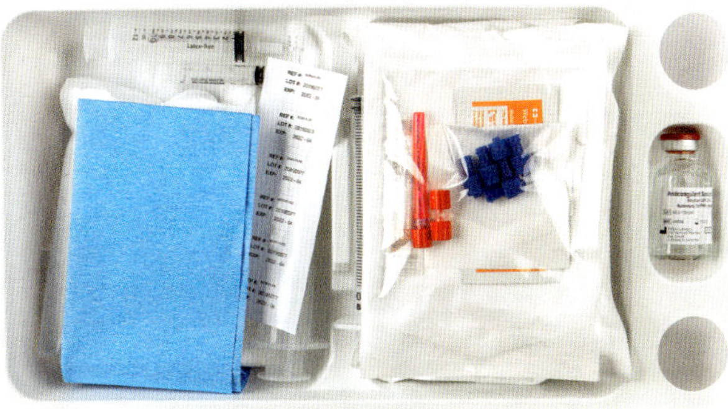

• **Fig. 6.1** Platelet-Rich Plasma Preparation Kit. Multiple platelet-rich plasma manufacturers produce complete preparation kits, including anticoagulant, drapes, concentrating system, syringes, phlebotomy set, and so on. (Shown is the Pure PRP II kit, EmCyte Corporation, Fort Myers, FL, USA.)

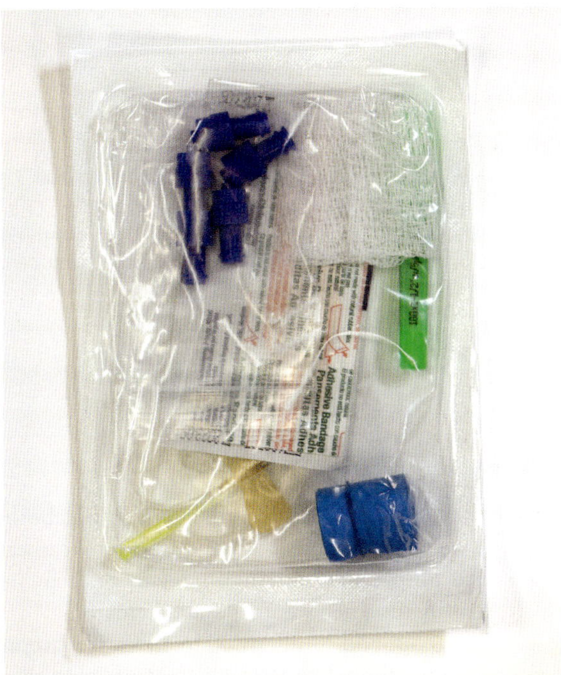

• **Fig. 6.2** Phlebotomy Kit. A complete phlebotomy set is included in the platelet-rich plasma preparation kit as shown in Fig. 6.1.

Tourniquet and Aseptic Technique

A tourniquet is placed to fill the patient's venous vascular system. Prior to venipuncture, aseptic techniques are used for skin preparation. Single stick draws are preferred to decrease chances of activation and patient discomfort. PRP systems that minimize exposure of blood and cellular components to open air, allowing for minimal manipulation of tissue, are mandatory as per FDA guidance.

Venipuncture

Before performing the venipuncture, flush the butterfly assembly with the anticoagulant in the syringe to avoid clotting. Pull the skin taut to anchor the vein, and insert the needle bevel up, entering the skin at a shallow angle of 5 to 15 degrees. Direct the needle into the vein from its top or side surface (Fig. 6.5). A slight resistance is felt as the needle passes through the dense skin tissue and vein wall. A slight ease in resistance is noted when the needle enters the lumen of the vein. If the blood does not flow, reposition the needle; if the blood is flowing slowly, adjust the angle of the needle, as it may be sitting against the wall of the vein.

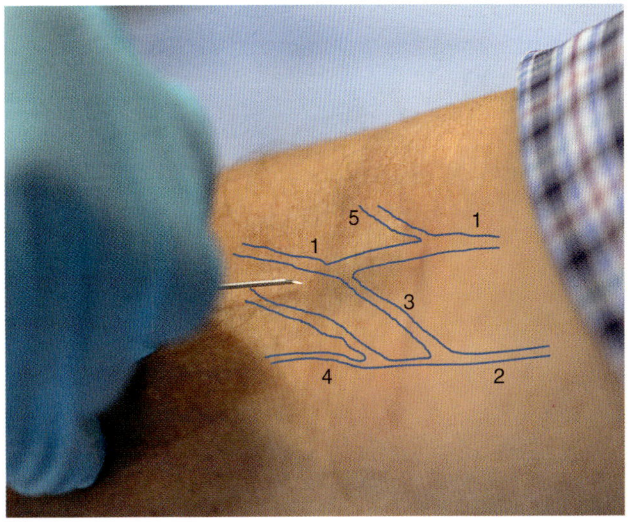

• **Fig. 6.3** Anterior view of the cubital fossa: *1,* cephalic vein; *2,* basilic vein; *3,* median cubital vein; *4,* median antebrachial vein; *5,* accessory cephalic vein.

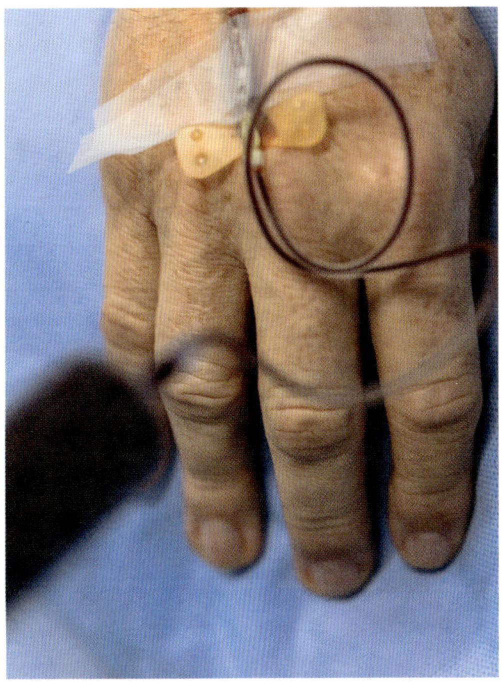

• **Fig. 6.4** Butterfly needle system injected in one of the dorsal metacarpal veins.

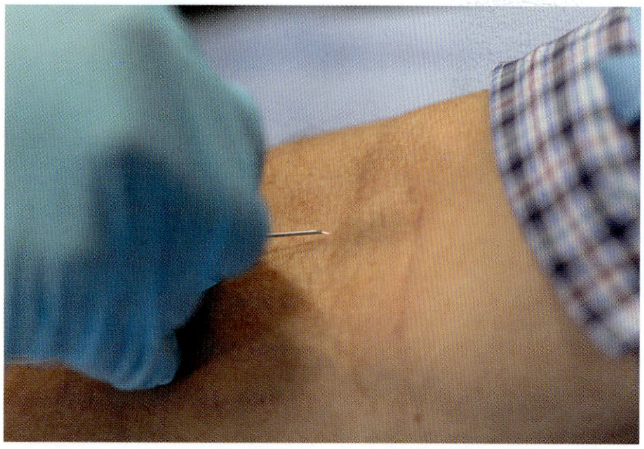

• **Fig. 6.5** Inserting the butterfly needle, directing the needle bevel up.

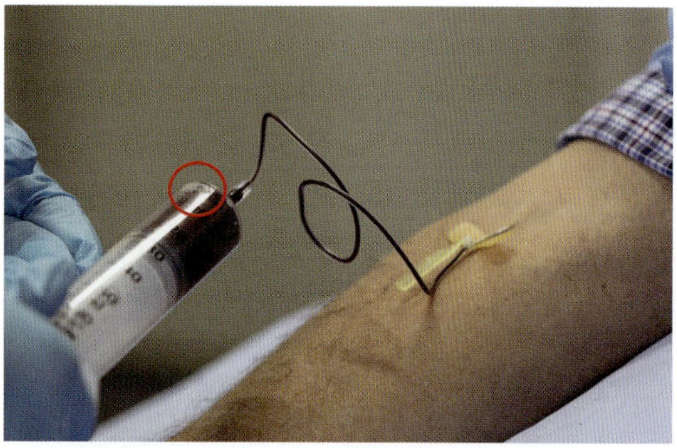

• **Fig. 6.6** Agitate the blood in the collection syringe during the blood draw period sufficiently to avoid central clotting in the syringe by inverting the syringe in order to move the air bubble as indicated in the red circle.

Blood Aspiration

Pull *slowly* back on the plunger of the collection syringe in a controlled fashion at a rate of approximately 1 mL/s to prevent the vein from collapsing and inducing too much negative pressure, which can cause cell damage. During aspiration, agitate the blood in the syringe with the anticoagulant twice (by moving an air bubble backward and forward) to assure proper mixing, as the whole blood is more dense than the anticoagulant and will not be properly anticoagulated otherwise during the blood draw, potentially initiating clotting within the central part of the syringe (Fig. 6.6).

When the required amount of blood is obtained the tourniquet can be released, the syringe is disconnected, and a sterile cap is placed. Remove the butterfly, or other needle assembly, and apply a folded gauze to the site as a pressure bandage. Invert the syringe clockwise-to-counterclockwise five times to mix the anticoagulant and blood more completely (Fig. 6.7).

Contaminated Materials

Dispose of sharps and contaminated materials in designated medical waste containers.

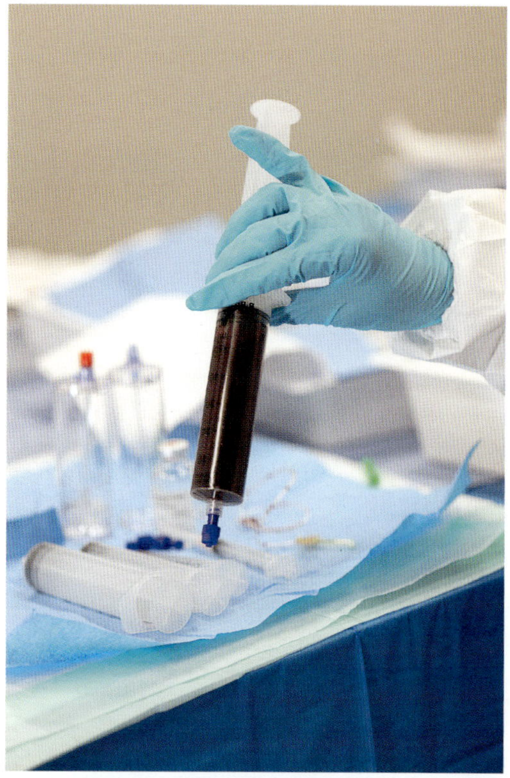

• **Fig. 6.7** After collecting the whole blood and removal of the butterfly (needle), agitate the blood in the collection syringe clockwise-to-counterclockwise to prevent the blood from clotting and enable proper and effective platelet-rich plasma processing.

Adverse Events and Complications Following Phlebotomy

Pain and Ecchymosis

Adverse events and complications following a phlebotomy are rare. However, a poorly executed phlebotomy can cause adverse effects for patients, ranging from pain or ecchymosis at the site of puncture, nerve damage, and hematoma.[4] Transient localized pain and localized ecchymosis are common and improve with time. Occasionally, patients may experience a vaso-vagal reaction with associated light-headedness, hypotension, nausea, and sweating. This is treated with laying the patient back, oral fluids, and the passage of time with reassurance of the patient. Pulse and blood pressure should be checked until they normalize and then the patient should be slowly brought to a seated, and then upright, position. The more severe adverse events that have been documented in blood transfusion services usually involve poor venipuncture practice or the presence of anatomic variants resulting in hematoma and injury to anatomic structures in the vicinity of the needle entry.

Infection

Poor infection-control practices can lead to bacterial infection at the site where the needle was inserted into the skin.[5] This is an extremely rare event. Such an infection could

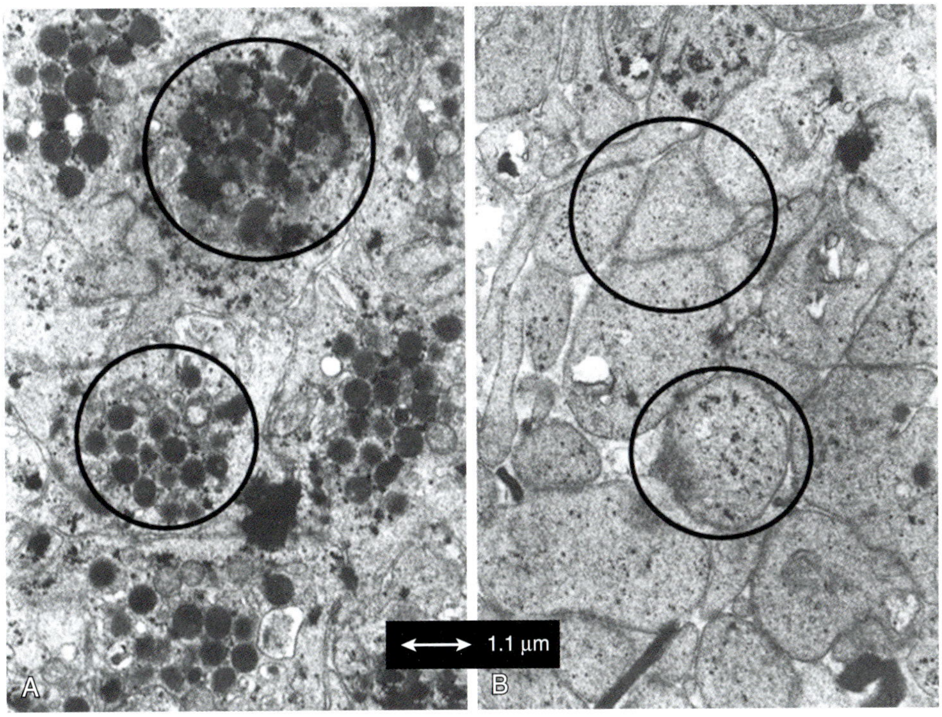

• **Fig. 6.8** Electron Microscopic Scanning of Platelet-Rich Plasma Platelets. (A) Electron microscopic image of single platelets in the circles. The platelet cell membranes are intact, and platelets contain platelet alpha granules and dense granules (*black* and *grey* structures, respectively) and lysosomes. (B) The platelet membranes are ruptured from the blood drawn from hand vein, and the granular content is no longer visible.

ascend more proximally in the venous vascular system and develop into a septic thrombophlebitis, which needs to be managed according to local protocols, potentially with culture-directed antibiotics. Furthermore, healthcare workers can be exposed to bloodborne pathogens from needlestick injuries.[6]

Paresthesia

In rare cases post-venipuncture paresthesias are observed, mainly due to edema at the site of the needlestick rather than a nerve injury. This should resolve within 3 weeks. Patients with longer-lasting paresthesia can be referred to a neurologist or electromyographer for further assessment.

Arterial Puncture

Another potential complication is an arterial puncture. This would be apparent by the spontaneous appearance, or withdrawal, of bright red blood in the syringe. This is managed by quick and direct pressure on the area and monitoring for any local expansion and/or change in pulse distally.

Possible Factors Influencing the Quality of Platelet-Rich Plasma

Blood Draw Anatomic Site and Time

Waters and Roberts discussed several possible factors that have an effect on the quantity and quality of platelets in aspirated whole blood intended for PRP preparation.[7] The authors concluded that the duration of the blood draw and manner in which the blood was drawn shows a relationship between the platelet count in the PRP prepared. Furthermore, the PRP platelet concentrations were also influenced by the whole blood harvesting site. Optimal platelet counts were obtained when blood was drawn from a peripheral vein as compared to an arterial collection site or a central venous line.

Shear Stress

The use of small-gauge harvesting needles, excessive pull force, and venipuncture of small blood vessels increase shear forces applied to blood components and will result in platelet activation and RBC lysis, resulting in plasma-free hemoglobin. Under normal operational procedures and avoiding high shear forces, PRP-platelet function is preserved (Fig. 6.8A). Intact platelets maintain the alpha granules integrity, containing a variety of platelet-derived growth factors. Blood draw from small hand veins that have tendency to collapse during aspiration and the use of small needles lead to high shear forces at the point of the needle, resulting in premature platelet activation (Fig. 6.8B). The release of platelet contents, including the alpha granules platelet growth factors, result in the platelets losing functionality.

Hemolysis

Shear stress can cause RBC cell membranes to rupture (hemolysis) with the subsequent release of heme and iron

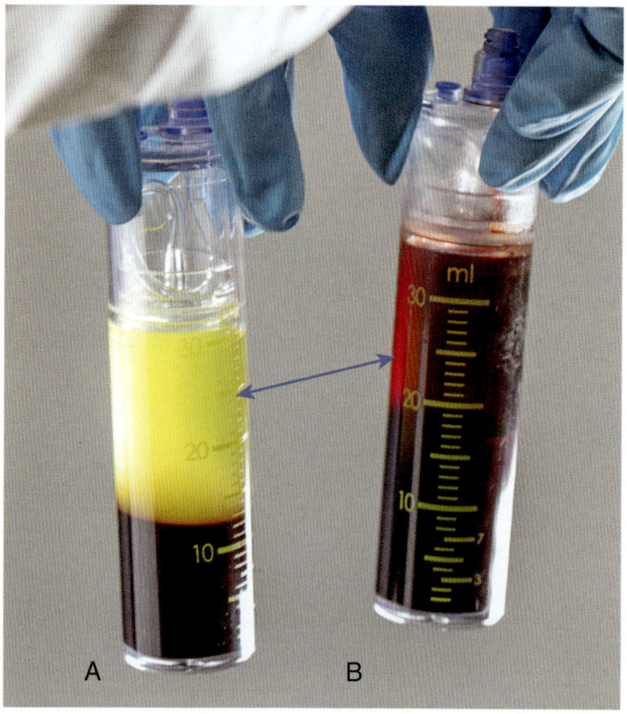

• **Fig. 6.9** (A) After the first spin of a concentration device, the plasma-poor fraction is showing a clear *yellow* aspect. (B) The same container has been used to process blood drawn from a metatarsal vein with a forceful extraction of the blood. After the first spin, the upper plasma part is clearly *red* colored, indicating ruptured red blood cell membranes. (Devices used are PurePRP II concentration system, EmCyte Corporation, Fort Myers, FL, USA.)

from hemoglobin. In a PRP syringe containing hemolyzed RBCs, free heme and iron cannot be cleared by natural scavenger mechanisms and will therefore be injected in tissues. This will lead to a significant inflammatory tissue response and might induce cellular dysfunction.[8] In Fig. 6.9A, a nonhemolytic and clear yellow platelet-poor plasma fraction on top of the RBC layer is visible after the first spin. In Fig. 6.9B, whole blood aspirated from a hand vein utilizing excessive force to fill the collection syringe (Fig. 6.10) was processed. After the first spin, the platelet-poor plasma fraction is colored red, indicating severe RBC hemolysis. RBC damage may signify platelet damage as well, as the platelet cell membranes are more fragile than the cell membrane from RBCs. Transferring the whole blood from the collection syringe to the concentration container for processing should be done in an unrushed fashion, to avoid causing damage to the cellular contents and allowing air in the device, possibly inducing hemolysis in this final step (Fig. 6.11).

Chemical Composition of Blood Anticoagulants

Manufactures of PRP systems may provide an anticoagulant in the kits. The most commonly used anticoagulants for blood draws are:

- citrate dextrose solution–formula A (ACD-A)

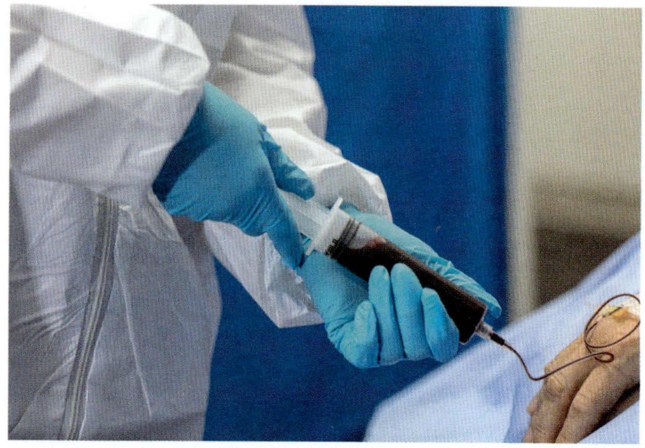

• **Fig. 6.10** A forceful blood draw from the hand is shown to extract blood from the vein.

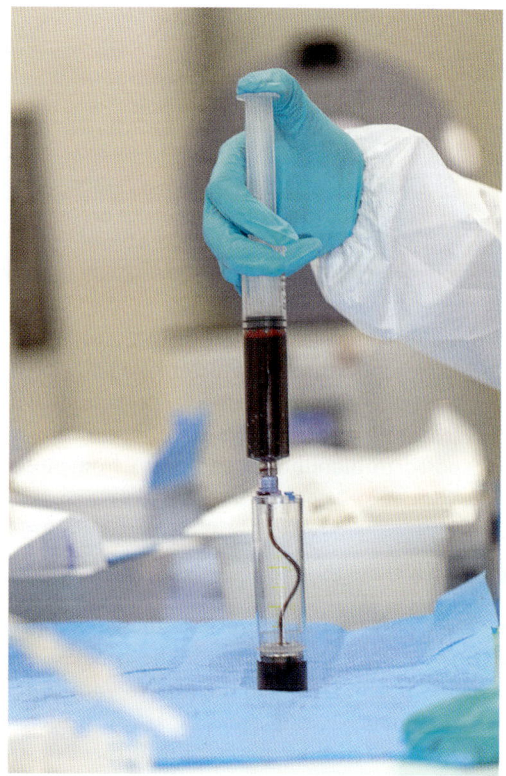

• **Fig. 6.11** **Transferring the Collected Whole Blood to a Concentration Device.** The transfer of the collected blood to the concentration device should be performed meticulously, avoiding squirting air and blood in the device.

- sodium citrate (SC)
- ethylenediaminetetraacetic acid (EDTA).

In clinical cases, heparin has also been used as an anticoagulant. Currently, ACD-A is present in the majority of commercially available PRP kits; EDTA is more frequently used in hematologic studies. The use of an anticoagulant to collect blood for PRP applications in MSK-D is a major issue and has impacts on the healing of tissues, platelet yields, and preservation following centrifugation, as well as platelet morphology. Different anticoagulants have different chemical compositions and pH. Several groups investigated whether the chemical composition of anticoagulants modulates PRP characteristics with regard to pH, platelet recovery, glucose concentration, growth factor release, and mesenchymal stem cell differentiation.[9,10]

Glucose Concentration

Fitzpatrick and colleagues concluded that the glucose concentration in PRP prepared with ACD-A was four to six times the baseline value when compared to the glucose levels of the donors. This PRP concentration was found to be a significant higher glucose concentration than used in prolotherapy.[9] Although the significance of these high glucose levels is yet unclear, it might be of clinical importance, as animal studies indicate that high glucose levels affect tendon homeostasis.[11]

Mesenchymal Stem Cell (MSC) Proliferation

From another study it was concluded that PRP obtained using SC presented the smallest variation in mesenchymal stem cell gene expression, with a larger amount of platelets and potential for better mesenchymal stem cell proliferation, without phenotype changes.[10]

Platelet Dosing and Blood Volume

PRP can be characterized as a complex composition of autologous multicellular components in a small volume of plasma with a substantial clinical dose of concentrated platelets, compared to baseline values. Marx[12] and Giusti and colleagues[13] concluded that 1 to 1.5 × 10^9 platelets/mL are needed to induce a functional angiogenic response in tissue repair mechanisms to stimulate (neo)angiogenesis and stimulate in the healing of MSK-D. Interestingly, Lopez-Vidriero and associates indicated that specific tissue structures and MSK pathologies with a poor healing tendency should be ideally treated with PRP preparations capable of increasing angiogenesis.[14] A PRP platelet count of at least 1 to 1.5 × 10^9/mL has become the working definition for therapeutic PRP, and subtherapeutic doses may explain negative clinical results, which may simply be due to platelet concentration.[15] In order to use a PRP product with therapeutic platelet numbers, practitioners have to acquire a sufficient amount of whole blood from their patients to yield high platelet concentrations after a dual spin processing. It is important to understand that not all PRP products are the same and that the therapeutic platelet concentrations cannot be achieved by many devices currently available on the market.

Blood Draw Volume and Platelet-Rich Plasma Protocols

Platelet-Rich Plasma Device Grouping

Many PRP systems are commercially available, with the intention to produce a "ready to go" PRP suspension. However, point-of-care PRP devices and centrifuges differ dramatically in the quality of PRP they produce. PRP systems operate on a relatively small volume of drawn blood (10 to 60 mL) and on the principle of density whole blood separation, by using a variety of centrifugation protocols and proprietary design. Based on specific design characteristics of the PRP collection device, methods of centrifugation, and processing time, the PRP composition and concentration of platelets and leukocytic cells differs widely. Ultimately, this influences the concentration of growth factors and other cytokines. Without addressing PRP classification strategies, PRP devices can be coarsely divided into:

- plasma type PRP (P-PRP) (0.5 to 1.25 times baseline concentration),
- low platelet content PRP (Lo-PRP) (1.5 to 3 times baseline concentration), and
- high platelet content PRP (Hi-PRP) (5 to 9 times baseline concentration) systems.[16]

The P-PRP systems require only 8 to 10 mL of whole blood. Several test-tube containers are used to perform a single-spin centrifugation of 8 to 10 mL of whole blood to acquire "some" acellular PRP, excluding RBCs and leukocytes, while collecting as many platelets as possible from the plasma layer.[9] It is noteworthy that some of these test-tube containers that are being used to process whole blood for PRP therapies (for example, BD Vacutainer CPT) are not intended for clinical human use, and according to their instructions for use these systems contain chemical additives and endotoxins that are not controlled.

The Lo-PRP producing devices need approximately 10 to 20 mL of whole blood. Both the P-PRP and Lo-PRP devices can be labeled as single-spin devices, as the harvested whole blood is spun only once in a centrifuge in order to accomplish whole blood separation. The platelet fraction after a single spin is collected as PRP. The Hi-PRP devices require a blood draw varying between 25 and 55 mL of whole blood and are dual-spin devices. These dual-spin devices are more effective in whole blood density separation and cellular and platelet concentration to create a so-called buffy-coat cellular stratum. It is important to understand that the platelet concentrate is located on top of the RBC layer (Fig. 6.12). Therefore, in order to collect as many platelets as possible, it is essential to make contact with the RBC layer during PRP collection. Unfortunately, there is no consensus on standardizing PRP techniques,[17] which has contributed to the large variation in PRP devices and produces variability in platelet concentrations and cellular compositions.[18,19]

Some offices prepare PRP using homemade protocols, with multiple modifications of plasma-based and buffy-coat-based preparation protocols.[20] Knowledge of proper laboratory techniques, the availability of proper and validated equipment, including a fume hood, are prerequisites in order to produce a reproducible PRP vial. Homemade PRP products should at a minimum meet the currently accepted clinical PRP formulations to treat patients according to the current standards of care.

Of substantial importance is that in the United States the collection, transport, preparation, and storage of blood

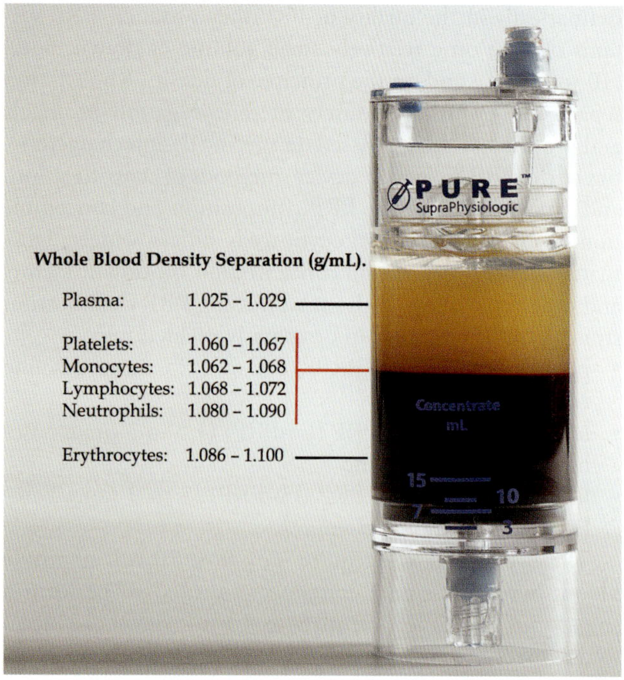

• **Fig. 6.12** Cellular Density Separation of Whole Blood by Centrifugation. After the first-spin centrifugation procedure, blood is separated in two layers. The first layer is the platelet-poor plasma fraction with a multicomponent buffy coat layer, containing platelets, monocytes, lymphocytes, and neutrophils. The second layer consists of the red blood cell pack. The range of the specific cell densities varies among individual cells as a result of the different cellular densities. (The device shown is the PurePRP. SP, EmCyte Corporation, Fort Myers, FL, USA.)

and blood components is governed by FDA regulations and specific guidance documents (http://www.aabb.org/advocacy/regulatorygovernment/bloodcomponents/Pages/default.aspx).

The basic characteristics for a minimal PRP product for efficacy in orthopedic conditions has been described, and this should be the goal for any practitioner providing PRP to patients.

Factors Determining the Need for Blood

In general, before harvesting a particular volume of blood to prepare PRP, the physician should ideally consider in each individual patient:

- the number of treatment sites
- the PRP volume per treatment site
- the need for a specific platelet dosing (formulation)
- the need, or absence, of specific leukocytic cells (neutrophil-monocyte poor/rich).

This detailed information will assist in deciding how much blood is required during the blood draw for that individual patient.

Remarkably, Marques and co-workers found that inferior PRP treatment outcomes correlated directly with poor quality and inconsistent PRP products.[21] Therefore, it is the authors' opinion that PRP devices should be versatile and compliant to enable the production of different PRP formulations. In addition, consideration should be made for cell counting following the production of a PRP product provided to patients to best *quantify* the amount of platelets and the presence of RBCs and white blood cells, which have been previously noted to affect outcomes.

References

1. Ferrari M, Zia S, Valbonesi M, et al. A new technique for hemodilution, preparation of autologous platelet-rich plasma and intraoperative blood salvage in cardiac surgery. *Int J Artif Organs.* 1987;10(1):47–50.
2. Everts PAM, Knape JTA, Weibrich G, Hoffmann J, Overdevest EP, Box HAM, et al. Platelet-rich plasma and platelet gel: a review. *J Extra Corpor Technol.* 2006 Jun;38(2):174–87.
3. Everts PA. Autologous platelet-rich plasma and mesenchymal stem cells for the treatment of chronic wounds. In: Hakan Dogan K, ed. *Wound Healing—Current Perspectives [Internet].* 2019. IntechOpen; [cited 2019 Oct 4]. Available from: https://www.intechopen.com/books/wound-healing-current-perspectives/autologous-platelet-rich-plasma-and-mesenchymal-stem-cells-for-the-treatment-of-chronic-wounds.
4. Daugherty K. Best practices in phlebotomy... in an ACO environment. *MLO Med Lab Obs.* 2012;44(4):20–22.
5. Bae M, In Kim H, Park JH, et al. Improvement of blood culture contamination rate, blood volume, and true positive rate after introducing a dedicated phlebotomy team. *Eur J Clin Microbiol Infect Dis.* 2019;38(2):325–330.
6. Wagner SJ, Leiby DA, Roback JD. Existing and emerging blood-borne pathogens: impact on the safety of blood transfusion for the hematology/oncology patient. *Hematol Clin.* 2019;33(5):739–748.
7. Waters JH, Roberts KC. Database review of possible factors influencing point-of-care platelet gel manufacture. *J Extra Corpor Technol.* 2004 Sep;36(3):250–4.
8. Everts PA, Malanga GA, Paul RV, Rothenberg JB, Stephens N, Mautner KR. Assessing clinical implications and perspectives of the pathophysiological effects of erythrocytes and plasma free hemoglobin in autologous biologics for use in musculoskeletal regenerative medicine therapies. A review. *Regen Ther.* 2019;11:56–64.
9. Fitzpatrick J, Bulsara MK, McCrory PR, Richardson MD, Zheng MH. Analysis of platelet-rich plasma extraction: variations in platelet and blood components between 4 common commercial kits. *Orthop J Sports Med.* 2017;5(1):232596711667527.
10. do Amaral RJFC, da Silva NP, Haddad NF, et al. Platelet-rich plasma obtained with different anticoagulants and their effect on platelet numbers and mesenchymal stromal cells behavior in vitro. *Stem Cells Int.* 2016;2016:1–11.
11. Snedeker JG. How High glucose levels affect tendon homeostasis. *Adv Exp Med Biol.* 2016;920:191—198.
12. Marx R. Platelet-rich plasma (PRP): what is PRP and what is not PRP? *Implant Dent.* 2001;10(4):225—228.
13. Giusti I, D'Ascenzo S, Mancò A, et al. Platelet concentration in platelet-rich plasma affects tenocyte behavior in vitro. *BioMed Res Int.* 2014;2014:1–12.
14. Lopez-Vidriero E, Goulding KA, Simon DA, Sanchez M, Johnson DH. The use of platelet-rich plasma in arthroscopy and sports medicine: optimizing the healing environment. *Arthrosc J Arthrosc Relat Surg.* 2010;26(2):269–278.

15. Dhurat R, Sukesh M. Principles and methods of preparation of platelet-rich plasma: a review and author's perspective. *J Cutan Aesthetic Surg*. 2014;7(4):189.
16. Dhurat R, Sukesh M. Principles and methods of preparation of platelet-rich plasma: a review and author's perspective. *J Cutan Aesthetic Surg*. 2014;7(4):189–197.
17. Chahla J, Cinque ME, Piuzzi NS, et al. A call for standardization in platelet-rich plasma preparation protocols and composition reporting: a systematic review of the clinical orthopaedic literature. *J Bone Jt Surg*. 2017;99(20):1769–1779.
18. Mazzucco L, Balbo V, Cattana E, Guaschino R, Borzini P. Not every PRP-gel is born equal evaluation of growth factor availability for tissues through four PRP-gel preparations: fibrinet®, RegenPRP-Kit®, Plateltex® and one manual procedure. *Vox Sang*. 2009;97(2):110–118.
19. Everts PAM, Hoffmann J, Weibrich G, et al. Differences in platelet growth factor release and leucocyte kinetics during autologous platelet gel formation. *Transfus Med*. 2006;16(5):363–368.
20. Mariani E, Pulsatelli L. Platelet concentrates in musculoskeletal medicine. *Int J Mol Sci*. 2020;21(4):1328.
21. Marques FP, Ingham SJM, Forgas A, Franciozi CE da S, Sasaki PH, Abdalla RJ. A manual method to obtain platelet rich plasma. *Acta Ortopédica Bras*. 2014;22(2):75–77.

7

Autologous Orthobiologics

PRATHAP JAYARAM, PETER CHIA YEH, MAX EPSTEIN, AND SHIV J. PATEL

Introduction

The delivery of cell- and non-cell-based therapies can generally be classified as either autologous or allogenic. Autologous treatments involve a procedure in which the patient's own tissues are collected and subsequently reintroduced into the patient's own body. Some benefits of using autologous products over allografts include the innate decrease in immunologic side effects and tissue rejection, transfusion reaction, and reduced possibility of disease transmission. Autologous products include platelet-rich plasma (PRP), platelet lysate (PL), alpha-2 macroglobulin, interleukin-1 (IL-1) receptor antagonist, bone marrow aspirate (BMA) and concentrate, adipose tissue, and cultured cellular injectates.

Platelet-Rich Plasma

PRP is an autologous preparation of concentrated platelets isolated from whole blood by centrifugation, defined as having a plasma product with total platelet count greater than normal physiologic levels. PRP therapy is currently being used in musculoskeletal medicine as an injectable therapy for bone, joint, and connective tissue pathology. Platelets are an abundant source of growth factors that when released are available to aid in tissue repair.[1] While the science behind PRP continues to evolve, there is a need for optimizing and characterizing PRP formulations.

PRP is formulated using various amounts of whole blood, with the final volume being around 10% of the original whole blood volume. The general process is outlined below, though it should be noted that each commercial kit will have differing protocols, including starting volume, varying speeds of centrifugation, and duration of the spin protocol, among others.[2] There are at least 33 commercial PRP systems available on the market at the time of publication of this textbook.[3,4] Each system varies in collecting tubes utilized, centrifugation speed, single versus double spin, use (or lack) of activating agents, leukocyte and red blood cell inclusion, and final platelet volume and total number.[3–5] There is significant variability across commercial kits. A 2017 study assessed platelet count, red blood cell count (RBC), leukocyte count, pH, and glucose in four commercially available PRP kits. The study revealed variation in platelet and other blood component concentrations, and lack of standardization of PRP preparation between kits.[6] Proponents of these systems cite internal consistency in platelet concentration and ease of use as reasons to use them; however, laboratory protocol can also produce precise PRP formulations without specialized commercial equipment.[7]

Another variable in PRP preparation is the use of an exogenous activator. While used more commonly in surgical applications, these activators promote platelet clotting for surgical scaffold applications, degranulation, and subsequent growth factor release.[8] Exogenous activators are commonly calcium (i.e., calcium chloride and calcium gluconate) or thrombin based. The majority of reported studies in the literature use 10% calcium chloride. Thrombin and arachidonic acid are other activators that have been used. There has been increasing interest in activator selection as some in vivo studies have found that they may variably release growth factors.[7] Exogenous activator may extend the growth factor release period to 7 to 10 days beyond the initial injection, in addition to the platelet clot providing a surgical scaffold.[3,9–12] A more detailed discussion of scaffolding applications is beyond the scope of this chapter.

Given the diversity in PRP preparation systems and formulations, characterizing PRP is important to optimizing formulations and interpreting the literature. There have been more than 10 proposed classifications for PRP since 1999.[13,14] Most call for characterization of platelet count, presence of cell lines besides platelets, and nuances of preparation such as the use of an exogenous activator. For example, the PAW system is based on absolute **P**latelet count, method of platelet **A**ctivation, and presence or absence of **W**hite blood cells (WBCs).[15] The PLRA classification by Mautner and colleagues. was one of the first classification systems to expand its characterization by including red blood cell and white blood cell counts.[16] Newer classification systems such as MARSPILL aim to address parameters such as concentration folds over baseline, amount of spins, and spin speed, but classification systems have not caught on widely due to the fragmented nature of PRP research.[13,14]

There are ongoing efforts to optimize PRP formulations, with a focus on platelet concentration. Current commercial systems vary widely in their platelet concentrations, ranging from 0.52 to 9× the baseline in some studies.[3] It is important to note that the positive effects of PRP can be dose dependent, and proliferation of tendon stem/progenitor cells cultured in various concentration of PRP has been shown to increase in a dose-dependent manner in up to a 10% PRP dose.[17] At high concentrations, PRP may begin to exhibit anti-chondrogenic activity and impair healing.[9,18] However this is largely dependent on which growth factors are being degranulated, i.e., chondrotoxic or chondroprotective mediators and may not be platelet concentration dependent. Conversely, a 2019 study suggests a dose-dependent response to higher PL concentrations in promoting tenocyte proliferation in vitro in the aged population (>50 years old) but not young donors.[19]

The presence and absence of leukocytes in PRP is another common area of discussion. Leukocyte infiltration of tissues has been linked to both muscle injury and repair and, as such, the argument can be made for or against included leukocytes in PRP formulations.[20–22] Leukocyte-poor (LP) PRP is generally defined as any PRP formulation containing fewer WBCs than baseline and leukocyte-rich (LR) PRP conversely contains more WBCs than baseline.[13]

Mechanism of Action and Clinical Applications

Currently, there are no guidelines on PRP dosing and the use of specific formulations for different pathologies. However, some studies have reported LP-PRP may be beneficial for cartilaginous injuries and LR-PRP for tendinous injuries. However, other studies report that LR-PRP should be avoided in osteoarthritis and tendinopathies because WBCs release proteases and reactive oxygen species that may harm remaining cartilage or tendinous tissue, respectively.[10] One study noted that compared to treatment with LP-PRP and phosphate-buffered saline (PBS), synovial cells treated with LR-PRP resulted in significantly greater cell death and some proinflammatory mediator production.[23] While the exact dosing and preparation are unknown, some studies have recommended that the platelet concentration for knee osteoarthritis and tendinopathies should target close to 3 to 4× and be leukocyte free.[10,24]

There is no clear in vivo mechanism for the therapeutic effects of PRP and its subtypes; however, PRP's therapeutic effects are often attributed to bioactive factors and high concentration of growth factors. The true biologic response to PRP is poorly understood and likely pleiotropic, and can have positive benefits on one tissue and deleterious effects on other. In vitro, platelets play important roles in wound healing including re-epithelialization, granulation tissue formation, cartilage and bone matrix formation/remodeling, chemotaxis, and angiogenesis.[2,25] Platelets accomplish this through their alpha granules that contain the necessary growth factors for these processes, such as platelet-derived growth factor (PDGF), vascular endothelial growth factor (VEGF), epidermal growth factor (EGF), and fibroblast growth factor-2 (FGF-2) (Table 7.1). They also produce tissue growth factor-β1 (TGF-β1)—one of the most important mediators in connective tissue regeneration and potent inhibitors of matrix metalloproteinases (MMP-1, -3, -9), which inhibit collagen synthesis.[25]

It is proposed that growth factors from PRP induce processes of inflammation and cell recruitment, angiogenesis, and matrix formation by delivering a large quantity of platelets to the site of injury; however, this is still the subject of ongoing research. It is important to note that PRP's effects through a complex sequence of growth factor

TABLE 7.1 Key Regenerative Growth Factors Stored in Platelet Alpha Granules and Their Functions.

Growth Factor	Function
PDGF	Stimulates cell proliferation, chemotaxis, and differentiation Stimulates angiogenesis
TGF-β	Stimulates production of collagen type I and type III, angiogenesis, re-epithelialization, and synthesis of protease inhibitors to inhibit collagen breakdown
VEGF	Stimulates angiogenesis by regulating endothelial cell proliferation and migration
EGF	Influences cell proliferation and cytoprotection Accelerates re-epithelialization Increases tensile strength in wounds Facilitates organization of granulation tissue
bFGF	Stimulates angiogenesis Promotes stem cell differentiation and cell proliferation Promotes collagen production and tissue repair
IGF-1	Regulates cell proliferation and differentiation Influences matrix secretion from osteoblasts and production of proteoglycan, collagen, and other noncollagen proteins

bFGF, Basic fibroblast growth factor; *EGF*, epidermal growth factor; *IGF-1*, insulin-like growth factor-1; *PDGF*, platelet-derived growth factor; *TGF-β*, transforming growth factor-β; *VEGF*, vascular endothelial growth factor.

Data from Refs.

Malanga GA, Goldin M. PRP: review of the current evidence for musculoskeletal conditions. *Curr Phys Med Rehabil Rep*. 2014;2:1–5.

Davis VL, Abukabda AB, Radio NM, et al. Platelet-rich preparations to improve healing. Part I: workable options for every size practice. *J Oral Implantol*. 2014;40(4):500–510.

Boswell SG, Cole BJ, Sundman EA, et al. Platelet-rich plasma: a milieu of bioactive factors. *Arthroscopy*. 2012;28(3):429–439.

Blair P, Flaumenhaft R. Platelet alpha-granules: basic biology and clinical correlates. *Blood Rev*. 2009:23(4):177–189.

communication within the tissue microenvironment facilitates healing of the remaining tissue and does not regenerate absent tissue.

Common clinical applications for PRP use include, but are not limited to: tendinopathies (patellar, rotator cuff, gluteal, lateral epicondylitis, plantar fasciitis), ligamentous tears (ulnar collateral ligament, anterior cruciate ligament [ACL]), muscular strains (hamstring, gastrocnemius, lumbar multifidus), peripheral mononeuropathies (carpal tunnel syndrome), spine pathology (sacroiliitis, facet arthropathy, degenerative disc disease, and radiculopathy), and peripheral joints (knee osteoarthritis, carpometacarpal joint pain, and temporomandibular joint syndrome).[26–30]

Data on Efficacy

The main limitation for clinical use of PRP is not a lack of data but rather heterogeneous data. There is a large variation in standardization in its preparation and delivery, making it difficult to discern potential beneficial effects of PRP. For instance, while PRP has demonstrated overall favorable outcomes in some systematic reviews, the studies had varying methods of PRP preparation, patient populations, and stages of disease.

Shen and colleagues conducted a systematic review that found that most patients had significantly improved pain relief and self-reported function after PRP injection for knee osteoarthritis compared to saline placebos, hyaluronic acid (HA), ozone, and corticosteroid injections. It was also reported that 10 of the 14 included studies had high risk of bias associated with them, mostly due to lack of investigator blinding.[27] Laver and colleagues published a recent systematic review of PRP in knee and hip osteoarthritis encompassing 29 studies, including 1 hip and 8 knee randomized controlled trials (RCTs) and 11 total studies controlled with HA. For the studies controlled with HA, 9 of 11 studies found that PRP was significantly superior to HA in terms of symptom improvement.[9] In general, beneficial effects of PRP therapy in osteoarthritis have been more effective in cohorts with milder disease and younger populations.[9,25]

A 2017 systematic review and meta-analysis comprised exclusively from Level 1 RCTs in rotator cuff injuries and lateral epicondylitis reports significantly less pain in PRP-treated groups compared to control in the long term.[31] This differs from prior meta-analysis, largely including low-powered studies and heterogenicity in comparator outcomes, which have published contrasting results.[32–34]

A double-blinded RCT by Dragoo and colleagues compared the clinical outcomes in patients with patellar tendinopathy after a single ultrasound-guided, leukocyte-rich PRP injection with dry needling compared to dry needling in 23 patients.[35] They reported that while the regimen of standardized eccentric exercise and PRP injection with dry needling appeared to help patients with patellar tendinopathy more than dry needling alone at 12 weeks ($P = .02$) as evaluated by the Victorian Institute of Sports Assessment (VISA), the benefits of PRP was not long lasting ≥26 weeks ($P = .66$).[35] An RCT of a single injection of LR-PRP or LP-PRP was not found to be more effective than saline for the improvement of patellar tendinopathy symptoms in a study by Scott and colleagues.[36] There was no significant difference in the VISA score, pain during activity, or global rating of change at 12 weeks, 6 months, and 12 months.[36] A systematic review and meta-analysis of nonsurgical treatments of patellar tendinopathy by Andriolo and colleagues noted that while eccentric exercises seem to be the most beneficial with short-term follow-ups less than 6 months ($P < .05$), multiple PRP injections may offer more satisfactory results at long-term follow-up (≥6 months, $P < .05$).[37]

Wu and colleagues conducted a single-blind RCT to assess the 6-month effect of PRP in patients with mild to moderate carpal tunnel syndrome (CTS). Sixty patients with unilateral CTS were randomized into two groups of 30, with one group receiving one dose of 3 mL of PRP using ultrasound guidance and the control group receiving a night splint.[38] The patients who received PRP exhibited a significant reduction in the visual analog scale (VAS), Boston Carpal Tunnel Syndrome Questionnaire score, and cross-sectional area of the median compared to those of the control group 6 months post-treatment ($P < .05$).[38]

A systematic review and meta-analysis by Sheth and colleagues comparing PRP to control therapies (such as physiotherapy or placebo injections) in acute muscle injuries (≤7 days) found that while the use of PRP did not significantly decrease the rate of injury at 6 months follow-up, there was significant decrease in return to play times except with a subgroup with grade 1 or 2 hamstring muscle strain.[39] A literature review by Setayesh and colleagues on the treatment of muscle injuries with PRP found that while there were numerous clinical case series demonstrating faster healing, less swelling, and quicker return to play times for patients with muscles strains who received PRP, most studies were retrospective and few RCTs demonstrate a clear clinical benefit.[40] They also observed variability in the injectant preparation, the platelet concentration, the presence of leukocytes, the volume of PRP injected, and the timing of treatments.[40]

Figueroa and colleagues conducted a systematic review of prospective cohort studies or RCTs on PRP compared to control in the treatment of ACL tears, assessing graft-to-bone healing, graft maturation, and/or clinical outcomes.[41] While they found that more studies had evidence of faster graft maturation, it appears there were mixed results, with overall findings leaning to no significant improvement in graft-to-bone healing or clinical outcomes.[41]

Overall, there is currently a need for systematic characterization of PRP therapy, which along with appropriately conducted prospective trials, could better understand PRP's efficacy and formulations.

Caveats/Side Effects

PRP has demonstrated an excellent safety profile with no reported major adverse events or reactions.[42] The side effects are similar to those for any intra- or extraarticular injection, such as infection, pain, bleeding, and injury to nearby blood vessels or nerves.

Drug interactions with PRP have not been well studied and documented in literature. Nonsteroidal antiinflammatory drugs (NSAIDs), such as aspirin and naproxen, have been shown to interfere with growth factor release given the direct inhibition of cyclooxygenase pathway.[7,43] Although there is no research correlating growth factor release and efficacy of PRP treatment in vivo, these studies suggest NSAIDs and aspirin should be held prior to PRP, and other analgesics, such as acetaminophen, should be prescribed for post-injection pain control.

US Food and Drug Administration (FDA) Regulations

PRP is regulated under the FDA Center for Biologics Evaluation and Research (CBER), which exempts it from the traditional regulatory pathway. The 510(k) application for "substantially equivalent" devices is used to bring PRP products to market. There are a myriad of FDA-approved devices ranging from traditional, injectable PRP to PRP-based biomaterials intended for enhancing bone graft healing. Most of the 33 systems on the market have FDA 510(k) clearance to enhance bone graft preparations with PRP. Although PRP injections are considered off-label use, physicians are allowed to administer them under CBER as long as they are "well informed about the product…base its use on firm scientific rationale and on sound medical evidence, and… maintain records of the product's use and effects."[44]

The World Anti-Doping Agency (WADA), an international independent agency that regulates doping-free sport, had prohibited PRP in 2010, but removed it from the list in 2011. The initial concern from the experts was that growth factors in PRP may stimulate muscle growth beyond the normal physiologic state and give individuals an unfair advantage; however, the prohibition was lifted as there was limited evidence for a systemic ergogenic effect of PRP.[42] PRP appears to trigger an increase in circulating growth factors systemically, including elevated serum insulin-like growth factor-1 (IGF-1), VEGF, and basic fibroblast growth factor (bFGF), which may be banned by governing agencies, and should be used with caution in athletes as this may cause false negatives in doping tests.[45]

Conclusion

PRP continues to be a promising therapy, especially in early osteoarthritis- and tendinopathy-related injuries. However, its use is currently limited by mechanistic understanding, cost burden, a lack of standardization in its formulation protocols, and calls for more robust blinded studies.

Platelet Lysate

PL is a cell- and platelet-free supernatant rich in growth factors and cytokines, created when the platelet membranes have been lysed, releasing intracellular proteins.[46] Anecdotally, this is thought to have inherent antiinflammatory properties.[47]

PL became of increasing interest in the 1980s as the growth-promoting effects of PL became studied in multiple clinical applications including wound and soft tissue injury, ocular disorders, and equine musculoskeletal injuries, and more recently in human musculoskeletal conditions.[48,49] Its main advantages include that it can be stored in a freezer and used for future or consecutive applications.[46] Studies with in vitro and animal models demonstrate PL promote the proliferation of various cell types, including equine mesenchymal stem cells (MSCs) and tenocytes, chondrocytes, keratinocytes, osteoblasts, and bone marrow mesenchymal cells.[50,51]

PL is derived from a platelet concentrate by mechanical disruption of PRP by freezing and thawing followed by centrifugation to separate platelet debris. There is no consensus protocol for preparation of PL. One reported protocol included freezing a PRP sample to −80°C for 30 minutes to lyse the platelets and release the growth factors. After thawing to 37°C in the water bath, the lysate is centrifuged at 1600× g for 10 minutes to separate the cell debris.[52] Other protocols call for repeating of the freeze-thaw cycle for higher yields.[53]

Mechanism of Action and Clinical Applications

The mechanism of action of PL is poorly understood; however, theoretically, the mechanism of action and clinical effectiveness should be similar to PRP.[54] There are no clear indications for the use of PL, but case reports and case series have reported the use of PL for knee osteoarthritis, lumbar radiculopathy, and lateral elbow tendinopathy.[47,55,56] It has been theorized that PL may be of more benefit around nerves as it is thought to be more antiinflammatory than PRP. However, this has not been studied in detail and there is no published literature on the effect of PL on nerve injuries outside of the Centeno and colleagues' lumbar radiculopathy study mentioned above.

Data on Efficacy

There are limited data regarding clinical efficacy of PL. In a prospective open-label study of 48 patients, Al-Ajlouni and colleagues suggests intra-articular (IA) injection of autologous PL in patients with osteoarthritis of the knee is effective in reducing pain and restoring function without provoking local or systemic adverse events.[55] This is consistent with the in vitro study in 2017 that suggested PL induces quiescent cartilage cell activation and proliferation leading to new cartilage formation.[51] In 2017 Centeno and colleagues suggested in a retrospective review of 470 patients that PL decreases pain in lumbar radiculopathy with a significantly improvement in pain scores up to 2 years post-injection.[47] Tan and colleagues observed in a prospective study of 56 patients significant improvement in VAS score and Mayo score for function following PL in chronic lateral epicondylitis who failed conservative therapy.[56] There are limited data regarding clinical efficacy of PL, or in vivo study of PL on human cells.

Caveats/Side Effects

Studies on clinical efficacy of PL are limited to small case series or case reports, and the study results have not been repeated. PL as an autologous therapy has similar complications and side effects to PRP. A more comprehensive review of drugs and their effects of PL remains to be conducted, but it is possible aspirin and NSAIDs can cause an inhibitory effect on growth factor release, and therefore should be withheld in the days prior and after injection.[7]

FDA Regulations

The use of PL is not FDA approved, however, its off-label use may be allowed by regulatory exemption per Title 21 United States Code of Federal Regulations Part 1271 (21 CFR 1271) and the 361-product exemption.[57] In the author's opinion, PL is exempt as it is derived from an autologous source, has a homologous use of tissue, and is processed with minimal manipulation.

Alpha-2 Macroglobulin

Alpha-2 macroglobulin protein (A2M) is a protease inhibitor, produced by the liver, and to a lesser extent by chondrocytes and synoviocytes. A2M can be found throughout the body but is greatest in the blood where it binds to and inactivates a wide variety of proteins and cytokines throughout the body. Its orthobiologic activity involves binding to proinflammatory and catabolic proteins to make a more favorable healing environment.

A2M can also be derived from autologous whole blood. Utilizing a centrifuge process similar to PRP, the platelet-poor concentrate is then used to create a concentrated volume of A2M. There are various commercial systems that can be used to purify A2M concentrate.

Mechanism of Action and Clinical Applications

In the IA environment, A2M inhibits endoproteases, particularly matrix metalloproteinases, responsible for catabolic activity.[58] Although A2M is found in the serum, A2M is a large molecule and does not cross into synovial fluid and joint spaces at large concentrations for significant IA effect. Injection of autologous A2M concentrate, such as Cytonics APIC System, into the joint allows for the in vivo delivery of high-volume A2M, which can bind and inhibit catabolic enzymes, inhibit the inflammatory cascade, and create a favorable healing environment in the joint or other area of tissue pathology.

Data on Efficacy

Although used clinically, A2M has not been extensively studied and to date there is minimal in vivo human studies. Of the available studies, most have involved assessing osteoarthritis of the knee in preclinical models. Elevated levels of catabolic proteases and cytokines in synovial fluid have been shown to induce chondrocyte death and cartilage matrix degeneration. In a rat model of osteoarthritis induced by ACL transection, IA A2M provided chondral protection and treated knees demonstrated less cartilage damage compared to controls.[59,60] There is also suggestion in a rabbit model that it may help in healing of a ruptured ACL.[61] Theoretically, since A2M is thought to be antiinflammatory, it is thought to potentially have utility in patients with increased joint inflammation or inflammatory arthropathies. An in vivo study by Cuellar suggests there may be efficacious use of A2M in discogenic pain in patients positive for the fibronectin-aggrecan complex (a protein biomarker of disc disease), as measured by VAS and Oswestry Disability Index (ODI) scores at 6 months following an intradiscal injection.[62]

Caveats/Side Effects

There are limited data on clinical efficacy and there are no known specific risks of A2M other than general adverse procedural risks.

FDA Regulations

A2M is not FDA approved; however, its off-label use may be allowed by regulatory exemption per 21 CFR 1271 and the 361-product exemption.[57] In the author's opinion, current products to concentrate A2M from whole blood undergo "minimal manipulation" and therefore would be exempt.

Interleukin-1 Receptor Antagonist Protein

IL-1 is a proinflammatory cytokine, produced in response to injury. IL-1 causes tissue degeneration and upregulates inflammatory mediators that can result in pain.[63] Elevated levels of IL-1 has long been associated with inflammation in rheumatologic disease and osteoarthritis, and IA levels of IL-1 correlates with osteoarthritis (OA) severity.[64] IL-1 action is mediated by the interleukin-1 receptor antagonist (IL-1Ra) protein, or IRAP, making IRAP an attractive therapy for mediating pain and potentially modifying disease.[65]

IL-1Ra can be obtained in two ways: (1) derived from autologous whole blood using commercial systems (Orthokine, Regenokine or Arthrex IRAP II System) or specific lab processing protocol; or (2) commercially available recombinant proteins. Recombinant forms of IL-1Ra have been FDA approved for the treatment of rheumatoid arthritis and are marketed as the drug anakinra (Kineret) and administered as daily subcutaneous injections. Autologous processing uses specialized equipment to process autologous whole blood. Glass beads bind monocytes, which then produce antiinflammatory cytokines, particularly IL-1Ra, and a milieu of regenerative growth factors as the solution is incubated typically for 6 to 24 hours. The process creates a cell-free solution, autologous conditioned serum (ACS), which is then recovered by centrifugation.[66]

Mechanism of Action and Clinical Applications

The proposed mechanism of action of IRAP is by competitive inhibition at the IL-1 receptor, blocking the proinflammatory IL-1 effect. There are no clear indications for the use of autologous IL-1Ra at this time. Some possible indications are in osteoarthritis of major joints. In osteoarthritis specifically, IL-1 directly contributes to cartilage loss through upregulation of extracellular proteolytic enzymes while simultaneously suppressing cartilage anabolism through downregulation of collagen and proteoglycan synthesis.[67,68]

Data on Efficacy

A 2019 systematic review of IL-1Ra products for knee osteoarthritis concluded that autologous IL-1Ra may improve pain and functionality for mild to moderate OA, and may be an effective adjunct for those unresponsive to traditional IA therapies.[69] In a randomized, double-blind, placebo-controlled clinical trial in knee OA patients a one-time injection of IL-1Ra significantly improved pain scores compared to placebo; however, there was no significant difference 4 weeks after the injection.[70] ACS with high-concentration IL-1Ra has also been studied for the treatment of lumbar and cervical radiculopathy with improvement in pain, function, and quality of life similar to that of corticosteroids with epidural injections, but with possibly a longer efficacy.[71] There is early preclinical work in a rat model of tendon disease, where IL1-Ra improved structural endpoints with histologic analysis.[72]

Current research is exploring long-term IL-1Ra delivery by gene therapy, or injecting the gene encoding the protein using a virus vector. This has been proposed to be a superior method of increasing IA IL-1Ra expression. Gene therapy IL-1Ra has been studied in animal models and found to be safe, symptomatically effective, and disease modifying; however, to date, there are no human trials.[73]

FDA Regulations

There is no FDA-approved system to produce autologous whole-blood–derived IL-1Ra proteins at this time. It is the opinion of the author that the Orthokine system (or Regenokine in the United States) to produce ACS is more than minimally manipulating the whole blood product, and thus would not categorize under regulatory exemption per 21 CFR 1271 and the 361-product exemption.[57]

Bone Marrow Aspirate Concentrate

Bone marrow aspirate concentrate (BMAC), also known as bone marrow concentrate (BMC), is a preparation of harvested autologous bone marrow. After harvesting, centrifugation is used to concentrate MSCs, hematopoietic cells (HCSs), platelets, and bioactive molecules such as cytokines.[74] Similar to PRP, BMAC utilizes cytokines to harness the body's ability for tissue healing. Unlike PRP, BMAC utilizes multipotent stem cells that can theoretically differentiate into damaged cell types, and also indirectly assist with healing by stimulating angiogenesis and recruiting local tissue-specific progenitor cells through paracrine effects.[75] It is important to note that there has been efforts to rename what is currently known as mesenchymal stem cells to medicinal signaling cells.[76] Dr. Caplan, one of the pioneers to first coin the term "mesenchymal stem cells" in the 1970s–80s, has suggested now using the new terminology to more accurately reflect that the cells migrate to the sites of injury or disease and then secrete bioactive factors.[76] It appears that the MSCs do not necessarily function in the body as progenitor cells for new tissues, and instead the bioactive factors secreted by the exogenously supplied MSC stimulate the patient's own site–specific and tissue–specific resident stem cells to construct the new tissue.[76] Currently, there is no clear consensus on the mechanism of action of these cells and how they ultimately influence the observed effects on the tissue microenvironment.

The International Society for Cellular Therapy (ISCT) proposed that MSCs must be plastic-adherent (such as to a tissue culture flask); must express the surface markers CD73, CD90, and CD105 and not express the hematopoietic markers CD14, CD34, CD45, CD11b, CD79a, CD19, or HLA class II; and should be able to undergo multilineage differentiation (osteogenic, adipogenic, and chondrogenic) in vitro.[77–79] MSC's low immunoreactivity and high immunosuppressive properties make it a promising stem cell source for therapy.

The two currently available bone marrow stem cell preparations are cultured bone marrow stem cell (referred to in the text as BMSCs) and noncultured BMAC that contains MSCs but also a variety of other cells (referred to in the text as BMACs). Cultured BMSCs require a two-step procedure for expansion of BMSCs in vitro to increase cell counts to 100- to 10,000-fold during several weeks in culture.[75,80] In this section, we will be focusing on non-cultured BMACs, with a subsequent section elaborating on cultured BMSCs.

BMAC is harvested from the patient's bone marrow, most commonly from the posterior iliac crest, due to higher yield, though other sites include tibia, femur, sternum, and humerus.[74,81] The physician inserts a needle percutaneously into the posterior iliac crest, past the cortical bone and into the medullary cavity to obtain bone marrow.[74] Detailed techniques, yield, and additional information on bone marrow harvest are described in Chapter 6 of this text.

BMAC is a concentrated milieu of MSCs, HCSs, pericytes, endothelial progenitor cells (EPCs), osteochondroreticular (OCRs) skeletal progenitor cells, stromal cells, multilineage-differentiating stress-enduring (Muse) cells, platelets, and various cytokines such as but not limited to IL-1RA, PDGF, and VEGF. Cell components include erythroblasts, neutrophils, eosinophils, basophils, monocytes, lymphocytes, macrophages, plasma cells, and megakaryocytes.[75,82] The end composition is reduced in RBCs and blood plasma. It is important to note that while there are multiple commercial BMAC devices available to the practitioner, the composition and consistency of the preparations vary.[83,84] Cassano and colleagues noted a significant difference in the IL-1B, TGF-β, and PDGF concentration between two commercial BMC systems.[83,84] Dragoo and Guzman compared three commercially available BMAC preparation systems in a controlled laboratory study with 10 patients.[84] While the authors noted a variation in the WBC concentration consistency between two systems, there was not a significant difference in consistently among the platelet, CD34+ cells concentration, and colony-forming unit (CFU) fibroblasts.[84] However, the composition of the concentrate products did differ across the systems.[84]

Mechanism of Action and Clinical Applications

While the exact mechanism of how BMAC functions is not known, the various components of BMAC have been shown to induce differentiation and proliferation of resident stem cells, and have chondrogenic and osteogenic potential, as well as antiinflammatory effects in vitro.[75] HCSs, also found in BMAC, can differentiate into red blood cells and muscle, are involved in muscle repair, and stimulate osteogenesis with direct contact with MSCs.[75,85] In addition to the platelet's ability to release growth factors to initiate stem cell migration to the injury site and provide adhesion sites for migrating stem cells, platelets can also decrease pain via a peripheral endocannabinoid related pathway.[75,86]

There is evidence that the dose of progenitor cells can affect clinical outcomes. Hernigou reported that for the treatment of nonunion tibia fractures with BMC, the total number and concentration of bone marrow progenitor cells had a significant effect on fracture healing.[87] Pettine reported that in the treatment of discogenic pain with BMC, higher MSC concentration was linked to pain reduction post procedure.[88] Centeno reported that in the treatment of knee arthritis with BMC, in patients with a total nucleated cell (TNC) count above 400 million there was significant improvement in all studied pain and functional metrics compared to the lower cell count group.[89] Both groups did report significant improvement from baseline.[89]

The addition of a supplementary PRP injection to the BMAC treatment protocol can potentially influence the results of an isolated BMAC injection for OA. A single, image-guided IA injection of BMAC followed by a supplementary IA injection with PRP at 8 weeks follow-up was well-tolerated and significantly improved pain at short-term follow-up among patients with moderate-to-severe OA.[90] An ongoing clinical trial called the CASCADE trial is examining the use of BMAC with and without HA for discogenic low back pain.[91,92]

Data on Efficacy

Few studies have compared the use of noncultured (nonexpanded) BMSCs with cultured (expanded) stem cell therapy, and it is unclear which method may be superior.[75] While there are no RCTs on the efficacy of noncultured BMAC for patients with cartilage disease, there have been many publications illustrating its safety profile and therapeutic potential.[75] Furthermore, the harvested stem cell quantity and quality can vary by patient, which makes research comparisons difficult.[74] Baseline pain and functional limitations, BMAC dose, PRP dose (if given at the same time), and individual biologic factors can all influence treatment efficacy.

Some of the current indications and uses for BMAC under evaluation include chondral defects of the knee,[93] full-thickness and moderate-to-large cartilage defects of the knee, osteoarthritis of the knee,[90] meniscal tears,[94] spine-mediated pain,[95] partial tear of the rotator cuff tendon,[96,97] shoulder arthritis,[98] osteochondral lesions of the talus,[81] ACL repair,[99] hip arthritis,[100] and hip osteonecrosis.[101] Autologous BMAC has also been used intraoperatively as an adjunct to debridement or microfracture surgery for cartilage defect[102] and has been shown to improve healing and reduce rotator cuff retears when augmenting RTC surgery.[103]

Studies of autologous BMC for the treatment of IA knee pathology are among the most numerous. Shapiro and colleagues performed a prospective, single-blind, placebo-controlled trial that compared BMAC and saline placebo injection for patients with bilateral knee osteoarthritis and found no serious adverse events from the BMAC procedures as well as a significant decrease in VAS pain scores at 1 week, 3 months, and 6 months.[104]

With respect to the spine, there is an increasing number of studies. Pettine and colleagues examined outcomes in 26 patients following intradiscal percutaneous injection of BMC for discogenic low back pain.[105] At 3-year follow-up, six patients went on to surgery. Of the remaining 20 patients, average ODI improved from baseline of 56.7 to 17.5 and average VAS improved from 82 to 22 at 36 months. At 1 year, 40% of patients had an improvement of one modified Pfirrmann grade on magnetic resonance imaging (MRI) and no patients had worsening of their imaging.

Caveats/Side Effects

Adverse reactions include general procedural risks, including but not limited to pain, swelling, bleeding, infection, damage to nearby structures, and potential detrimental effects of erythrocytes when used for IA joints.[74] Contraindications include bone marrow–derived cancer (lymphoma), active systemic infection, blood thinners, and non-bone marrow–derived cancers which is a relative contraindication.[75] However, a study by Hernigou and colleagues found no increased cancer risk in patients after application of autologous cell-based therapy using bone marrow–derived stromal progenitor cells either at the treatment site or elsewhere in the patients after an average follow-up period of 12.5 years.[101]

Centeno and colleagues performed a large prospective study on 339 patients who were treated for various orthopedic conditions with culture-expanded autologous, bone marrow–derived MSCs that were harvested from the posterior superior iliac crest between 2006 and 2010.[106] The mean patient age was 53 ± 13.85 years (214 males and 125 females) and follow up varied from 3 to 36 months.[106] Using high-field MRI tracking and complications surveillance, they noted that while there were two patients who reported the development of cancer, the cancers were not at the injection sites and the percentage of patients that developed cancer was not far from the annual rate of cancer in the general population.[106] The most common complaints were pain and swelling (2% of patients), with no reports of infections and procedure-related complications were self-limited or remediated with simple therapeutic measures.[106] Centeno and colleagues subsequently performed a larger prospective multicenter study investigating the safety of same day autologous BMC aspiration isolation, and injection (n = 1590 patients, 1949 injections), same day autologous BMC aspiration, isolation and injection with an addition of minimally processed lipoaspirate (n = 247 patients, 364 injections), and cultured expanded BMSCs re-implanted weeks or months after bone marrow aspiration (n = 535 patients, 699 injections), orthopedics procedures across 18 sites. The discrepancy in the number of procedures and patients can be explained by multiple joint procedures that occurred during the same session, and/or serial injections occurring at different treatment sessions for the same patient. 3012 procedures were performed over 9 years with 2372 patients reporting on adverse advents (AEs) with a mean follow up time of 2.2 years.[107] Follow-up ranged from 1 month to 8.8 years with an average of 2.2 years.[107]A total of 325 (12.1%) AEs were reported, with 38 adjudicated to be definitely related to the procedure (1.6% of the population).[107] The majority of the AEs were post-procedure pain or pain due to degenerative joint disease.[107] Thirty-six (1.5% of the population) reported a serious side effect, with 19 of those adjudicated to be not related to the procedure and 4 definitely related.[107] There were 7 neoplasms reported with none at the site of injections. The BMC only group was less likely to report AEs compared to the BMC with addition of minimally processed lipoaspirate and culture BMSC groups.[107]

Blood-thinning medications such as coumadin and aspirin may be discontinued and managed appropriately by the cardiologist or primary doctor prior to the procedure. Lastly, the financial costs associated with BMAC procedures may be prohibitive for some patients as they are often not covered by insurance for elective orthopedic procedures.

FDA Regulations

There are two currently available BMSC preparations: cultured BMSCs and noncultured (nonexpanded) BMACs. The culturing method is currently prohibited in the United States as current regulatory guidelines consider in vitro expansion of the BMA more than "minimally manipulated." In contrast, noncultured BMACs do not require laboratory cell expansion and culturing, and are available after centrifugation for same-day treatment.[75] Given that this is a single-step process with "minimal manipulation" of cells, this meets the criteria established by the US FDA for homologous use.[74,75] As defined in 21 CFR 1271.3(c), "homologous use means the repair, reconstruction, replacement, or supplementation of a recipient's cells or tissues with an HCT/P that performs the same basic function or functions in the recipient as in the donor."[57] Bone marrow meets this criterion for orthopedic uses as its constituents are involved in bone, cartilage, tendon, and muscle repair. Care should be taken when processing BMAC to not combine the BMAC with other agents, except for water, crystalloids, or a sterilizing, preserving, or storage agent to satisfy the minimally manipulated guidelines.

Minimally manipulated BMAC used for cartilage resurfacing therapies is not regulated by 21 CFR 1271 and therefore does not require premarket approval, preclinical research, or clinical trials to be marketed for treatment in the United States.[57,108] The FDA released a guidance document in November 2017 to explain the regulatory demands of manufacturers of human cells, tissue, and cellular and tissue-based products by specifically delineating the definition of "minimal manipulation."[57,108] BMAC preparation kits and concentration systems require only a 510(k) Premarket Notification to the FDA 90 days before marketing the product.[108] Thus, it highlights the importance of the clinician to counsel the patients effectively on the risks, benefits, and potential outcomes.[108]

Adipose Tissue

Since the first isolation and classification of adipose tissue stem cells (ASCs), human studies related to ASCs have increased, reaching up to 187 clinical trials in 2015 and more registered trials in 2019.[109] Subcutaneous adipose tissue is a common reservoir of progenitor cells, such as MSCs, and the clinical application of fat has been used in cosmetic, reconstructive, and corrective indications. MSCs have vast potential in regenerative medicine due to their ability to proliferate and differentiate into multiple lineages, including adipocytes, chondrocytes, myocytes, and osteoblasts.[77,110] MSCs can be obtained from different sources, including bone marrow, adipose tissue, dental pulp, synovium, muscle, and other tissues.[111] The evidence and proliferation of human use have vastly expanded since the first isolation and description of the progenitor cells in rodents in 1964 by Rodbell.[112–114]

Current applications have included knee osteoarthritis,[115–121] osteonecrosis of the femoral head,[116] hip osteoarthritis,[122] and shoulder osteoarthritis and rotator cuff pathologies.[123] Some studies have assessed ASCs in varying conditions in human and animal models,[109] such as multiple system atrophy,[124] Crohn disease,[110] cardiac disease,[125] ischemic heart disease,[126] amyotrophic lateral sclerosis,[127–129] Parkinson's disease,[130,131] spinal cord injury,[132] rheumatoid arthritis,[133–135] type 1 diabetes mellitus,[136] type 2 diabetes mellitus,[137] and Alzheimer disease.[138,139]

Methods for harvesting adipose tissue include resection, tumescent, conventional liposuction, and ultrasound-assisted liposuction (UAL; these are covered in more details in Chapter 5: Autologous Tissue Harvesting Techniques: Bone Marrow Aspirate and Adipose Tissue).[140,141] After harvesting, the raw lipoaspirate can be processed using various methods and protocols to produce an injectable MFAT, enzyme digested stromal vascular fraction (SVF), or cultured ASC product.[78,141] When the adipose tissues are further processed into the SVF or cultured ASC, they are considered more than minimally manipulated and do not meet the current regulations and criteria established by the FDA. Information regarding SVF and ASCs will be described in further detail in the subsequent section under cultured cellular injectates. There are FDA-compliant devices that can make MFAT with intact stromal vascular niche and MSCs that can then be injected back into the patients, such as Lipogems, PureGraft, and IntelliFat.[142–145]

MFAT preserves the stromal vascular architecture and stem cell niche; however, robust studies that have assessed its molecular profile are lacking. SVF has been better characterized, and is composed of a heterogeneous mixture of cells including pre-adipocytes, pericytes, mast cells, fibroblasts, smooth muscle cells, endothelial cells, hematopoietic stem cells, and adipose tissue–derived mesenchymal stem cells (AT-MSCs).[78,146] Adipose tissue can yield up to 500,000 to 2,000,000 cells per gram of tissue.[116]

The AT-MSC yield, proliferation, and differentiation capacity can be influenced by the location of adipose tissue harvested, the method of harvesting, the age of the patient, and other factors such as donor's body mass index.[114,147] Adipose has a high heterogeneity among individuals and within the same individuals with the various stem/precursor cells, different types of adipocytes (white, beige, brown), endothelial cells, and even pericytes.[114] The quality of AT-MSCs can also fluctuate based on the purifying method and storage conditions.[109]

The most common locations to extract adipose tissue include the abdomen and hip/thigh region, with the infrapatellar fat pad being a less commonly used location.[115,140,146] More studies illustrate that the abdomen is the optimal location to harvest adipose tissue.[146,148]

Depending on the methods of extracting adipose tissue, the yield, number of viable cells, and growth characteristics of AT-MSCs may differ. The viability of ADSCs may be affected by the stress applied to the adipose tissue during harvesting and processing. Oedayrajsingh-Varma and colleagues compared adipose tissue resection, tumescent, conventional liposuction, and UAL, and their effects on the ACS yields and growth characteristics.[140] The number of viable cells in SVF was similar regardless of the harvesting technique, but UAL contained fewer stem cells, and viable stem cells had a longer population doubling time.[140] Keck and colleagues compared power-assisted liposuction with manual aspiration in nine subjects undergoing abdominoplasty.[149] Both conditions had a comparable number of viable ASCs per mL of aspirated fat, similar proliferation rates, and ability to differentiate into mature adipocytes, though the cells harvested using power-assisted liposuction had significantly higher expression levels of differentiation markers adiponectin, GLUT4, and PPARg.[149] Duscher and colleagues compared an UAL device versus standard suction-assisted lipoaspiration in three patients with paired collection.[150] They reported that both methods had comparable ASC yield, viability, osteogenic and adipogenic differentiation capacity, and certain cytokine expressions such as VEGF, hepatocyte growth factor, stromal cell–derived factor 1, and bFGF, though the UAL method had more expression of the monocyte chemotactic protein 1.[150]

The effectiveness of AT-MSCs when obtained from and utilized in elderly patients must be considered. Choudhery and colleagues noted that aged AT-MSCs displayed senescent features when compared with cells isolated from young donors, and also exhibited reduced viability and proliferation.[151] The authors noticed a significant drop in the osteogenic potential of AT-MSCs with increased donor age; however, the adipogenic and the neurogenic potential of the AT-MSCs seemed to be maintained during aging.[151] Schipper and colleagues assessed the composition of cells harvested from 12 female patients within 3 age ranges (25 to 30, 40 to 45, and 55 to 60 years old) and from 5 different subcutaneous adipose depots.[152] They observed sensitivity to apoptosis was linked to the anatomic depot, with the superficial abdominal depot (above Scarpa layer) more resistant to apoptosis compared to the other sites (deep abdominal layer, arm, thigh, and trochanteric).[152] They also noted faster cell proliferation rates in younger patients than the older age groups, and that younger patients had increased peroxisome proliferator activated receptor (PPAR)-γ-2 expression, which is required for adipogenesis both in vivo and in vitro. The older patients only have elevated PPAR-γ-2 expression in the arm and thigh depots.[152]

In addition to age and harvest location influencing the composition and effectiveness of AT-MSCs, a systematic review by Varghese and colleagues noted decreased proliferation and differentiation potential of the AT-MSCs with increasing body mass index, diabetes mellitus, exposure to radiotherapy, and tamoxifen.[153] In one study, ASCs in adipose tissue of obese patients had lower capacity for repair than ASCs from nonobese patients, likely due to higher incidence of metabolic syndrome in obese patients.[154] Another study showed that ASCs from obese donors had shorter life spans, increased DNA damage, and more adipogenic differential potential than ASCs from normal-weight donors.[155] ASCs from type 2 diabetics showed higher levels of senescence and apoptosis, and reduced osteogenic and chondrogenic potential, while enhancing adipogenic potential.[156]

Furthermore, it appeared that there is not a significant impact of hypertension, renal disease, physical exercise, peripheral vascular disease, and total cholesterol on AT-MSC yield, though the authors noted it is very difficult to make conclusive recommendations due to the variability in studies.[153]

Mechanism of Action and Clinical Applications

MSCs are adult stem cells that can differentiate into a variety of cell types, including osteoblasts, chondrocytes, and adipocytes.[75,157] MSCs assist with tissue regeneration by differentiating into damaged cell types or indirectly by stimulating angiogenesis, limiting inflammation, and recruiting local tissue-specific progenitor cells. MSCs also secrete growth factors and cytokines, including but not limited to prostaglandins, TGF-B1, nitrous oxide, IL-4, IL-6, and IL-10, and IL-1 receptor antagonist.[75,157] HCSs can support the vascular system by differentiating into blood cells and stimulating osteogenesis with direct contact with MSCs.[75] A study by Ceserani and colleagues on MFAT harvested using Lipogems Systems reported that the MFAT has the capacity to induce vascular stabilization and even retain antiinflammatory effects.[142]

A study by Vezzani and colleagues noticed that the microanatomy of MFAT is similar to that of intact adipose tissue, with capillaries, microvessels, and pericytes wrapped around endothelial cells; however, they noted a higher frequency of pericytes in MFAT than in manual lipoaspirate and SVF.[158] It is notable that recent literature has suggested that in vivo the main functionality of MSCs may not be multipotency.[159] While pericytes have been widely believed to function as MSCs, others speculate that all MSCs could be pericytes due to the locations and cell marker signatures.[160] Crisan and colleagues observed the expression of MSC markers on the surface of perivascular cells, suggesting blood vessel walls may harbor a reserve of progenitor cells.[161] Guimarães-Camboa and colleagues' lineage-tracing experiments suggest that the plasticity observed in vitro, or following transplantation in vivo, may be due to the artificial cell culture environment.[159]

Microvascular fragments from adipose tissue exhibit a high angiogenic activity, representing a rich source of MSCs, and can rapidly develop into microvascular networks.[162] When the resulting MFAT is processed, such as with Lipogems, pericytes can be retained within the intact stromal vascular niche as well as retaining the MSCs.[143]

AT-MSCs isolated from younger donors are anticipated to be a more useful cell source for tissue engineering and regenerative medicine applications. There is theoretical potential for cell-based therapies for the elderly by banking adipose tissue at a younger age, preserving the stem and progenitor cells when biologic activity is at its greatest potential.[79]

Acknowledging a need for further high-quality research, the American Academy of Orthopaedic Surgeons in 2018 collaborated and called for establishing high-quality patient registries that can assist with continued surveillance and quality assessment.[163]

Caveats/Side Effects

Adverse reactions include general procedural risks including but not limited to pain, swelling, bleeding, infection, and damage to nearby structures. Kuah and colleagues evaluated the safety and tolerability of in vitro expanded MSCs derived from human donor adipose tissue combined with cell culture supernatant, and did not find any severe side effects when administered as a single IA injection to patients with symptomatic knee osteoarthritis.[116] Swelling of injected joints can be a common side effect, and is thought to be associated with the death of stem cells.[164] Other potential side effects, though less common, include tenosynovitis and tendonitis, arthralgia, joint stiffness, effusion, and paresthesia or malaise.[117,164,165]

Theoretically, MSCs can divide into unwanted oncologic cell lineages, and could contribute to tumor behavior by influencing the tumor microenvironment and promoting angiogenesis; however, this has not been seen with adult-derived MSCs.[166] No literature documenting neoplastic complications at ADSC implantation sites have been reported, and a longitudinal cohort study by Pak and colleagues on SVF with PRP into various joints found no evidence of neoplastic complications in any implantation site.[164]

The cost of the procedure is generally not covered by insurance, and can be prohibitive for some.

FDA Regulations

There are some FDA-compliant devices that can make MFAT with intact stromal vascular niche and MSCs such as Lipogems, PureGraft, and IntelliFat,[143–145] which can then be injected back into the patients through the use in orthopedic applications, and whether it counts as homologous use is debatable. The FDA defines the basic function of adipose tissue as providing cushioning and support. Some argue MFAT acts to cushion and/or support orthopedic tissue injuries, such as tendon and meniscal tears, and should be considered homologous.

Recently published guidelines that indicate enzymatically or mechanically processed lipoaspirate (PLA) alters these relevant characteristics and is not considered homologous use or minimal manipulation by the FDA.[57,167] SVF is adipose tissue that undergoes further processing (such as with enzymatic digestion) to break down and eliminate the adipocytes and surrounding structural components that provide cushioning and support, and thus is considered more than minimally manipulated.[57,167] Further laboratory cell sorting and culture expansion would also be considered more than minimally manipulated due to the steps involved in isolating and culturing of cells. Adipose tissue that is processed into SVF or cultured ASC is more than minimally manipulated and not FDA approved based on the current guidelines. Minimally manipulated ADSC used for cartilage resurfacing therapies is not regulated by 21 CFR 1271 and therefore does not require premarket approval, preclinical research, or clinical trials to be marketed for treatment in the United States. Consequently, some products are not FDA approved and may qualify instead for investigational new drug process.[167]

Bone Marrow–Derived Versus Adipose-Derived Stem Cells

MSCs can be obtained from different sources, including bone marrow, adipose tissue, dental pulp, synovium, muscle, and other tissues.[111] To date, bone marrow–derived MSCs are the best characterized and studied.[151] Recently, other MSC sources, particularly adipose tissue, have gained clinical interest for use in regenerative medicine.[168,169] Zuk and colleagues were one of the initial researchers to assess PLA cells obtained from liposuctioned adipose tissue, and found it represented a potential source of multilineage mesodermal stem cells.[170] Few studies have compared the efficacy of BMAC and MFAT.[171,172]

There are vast differences in the reported stem cell yields in adipose and bone marrow, with some studies reporting 100 to 500 times higher stem cell numbers found in adipose versus bone marrow.[109] However, based on donor-matched studies the differences volume per volume or gram for gram appear far less than that. In one study, patients undergoing ACL reconstruction donated samples of several tissues including bone marrow and adipose.[173] Bone marrow had about 93× more TNCs per volume compared to adipose (2045 vs 22).[173] Adipose had about 148.5× more CFUs per 1000 TNCs, but bone marrow had the most cells per colony.[173] Given that bone marrow had more TNCs, adipose contained about 1.6× as many MSCs per volume compared to bone marrow.[173] BMC was also found to contain 6x more nucleated cells compared to SVF.[174] SVF contained 4× more adherent cells.[174] Colony-forming frequency was 0.5% in SVF versus 0.01% in BMC. MSC population was 4.28% of the TNC in SVF versus 0.42% in BMC or about 10× more in SVF.[174] In summary, bone marrow has more nucleated cells than adipose but only a small percentage are MSCs. Adipose has less nucleated cells but a higher percentage of those are MSCs. Pending variability in harvesting techniques and patient characteristics, adipose per volume likely has 1.6 to 10× as many MSCs as bone marrow. It has been reported that the lipoaspirate harvesting, when compared to bone marrow harvesting, can yield more absolute MSCs, the MSCs have faster rapid in vitro expansion, and may yield more stem cells per gram of tissue.[169,175,176]

While there are similar and varying cell surface marker profiles between bone marrow–derived mesenchymal stem cells (BM-MSCs) and adipose tissue–derived mesenchymal stem cells (AT-MSCs), they both have the potential to differentiate into multiple lineages, including osteogenic, chondrogenic, adipogenic, cardiomyocytic, hepatic, and neurogenic differentiation.[109,177,178]

BM-MSCs and AT-MSCs have comparable immunophenotypes; however, AT-MSCs retain their phenotype more consistently over BM-MSCs across multiple culture passages, and also have higher proliferation capacities in part due to their lower senescence ratio.[179] A donor-matched study comparing culture-expanded AT-MSCs vs BT-MSCs showed that AT-MSCs underwent faster proliferation and doubling times.[180] They had longer life spans possibly due to the fact they had longer telomeres, which may suggest a smaller dose is required in vivo.[180] Both had similar differentiation capacity and decreased proliferation the longer the in vitro expansion was performed.[180] On the other hand, Mohamed-Ahmed and colleagues found BM-MSCs were superior to AT-MSCs in terms of osteogenic and chondrogenic differentiation, while AT-MSCs had higher proliferation and adipogenic potential.[77] Chondrogenesis was more efficient in human BM-MSCs versus AT-MSCs in vitro.[181] Human BM-MSCs showed more chondrogenic potential in vitro compared to AT-MSCs.[182] Xu and colleagues noted that BM-MSCs possessed stronger osteogenic and lower adipogenic differentiation potentials compared to AT-MSCs, but found no significant difference in the chondrogenic differentiation potential.[177] Xu and colleagues' results demonstrated that the DNA methylation status of the main transcription factors controlling MSC fate influenced their expression, and subsequently different differentiation capacities of AT-MSCs and BM-MSCs.[177]

Clinically, there are limited clinical data comparing BMAC to MFAT. Mautner and colleagues conducted a retrospective study of 110 patients comparing the pain and functional outcomes of patients with symptomatic knee osteoarthritis who received BMAC or MFAT or injections.[183] At a mean follow-up time for BMAC of 1.8 years and 1.0 years for MFAT, they noted both groups had significant improvement in Emory Quality of Life, VAS for pain, and Knee Injury and Osteoarthritis Outcome Score questionnaire ($P < .001$) without a significant difference between BMAC and MFAT.[183]

Cultured Cellular Injectates

Mesenchymal stem cells/stromal cells (MSCs) have a vast potential in regenerative medicine due to their ability to proliferate and differentiate into multiple lineages including adipocytes, chondrocytes, myocytes, and osteoblasts.[77] Cultured cells are in theory attractive, given their ability to potentially differentiate to the desired cell type of an injured tissue. MSCs can be obtained from different sources.

Mesenchymal Stem Cells/Stromal Cells From Bone Marrow

After harvesting BMA, the sample is processed in a centrifuge and subsequent buffy coat layer and platelet-poor plasma layers are removed. The cells are subsequently isolated, generally by their adherence to plastic, and then cultured.[75,184] Culturing methods can vary, though one method by DiGirolamo and colleagues includes diluting the aspirate marrow with Hank's balanced salt (HBS; Gibco), washing gently with inversion, adding a layer of Ficoll (Ficoll–Paque; Pharmacia) beneath the sample, and then spinning the sample at 2500 g for 30 minutes at room temperature.[184] The mononuclear cell layer was then washed again with HBS and the cells spun at 1500 g for 15 minutes and resuspended in complete medium (Minimum Essential Medium, alpha medium without deoxyribonucleotides or ribonucleotides, Gibco; 20% fetal calf serum lot–selected for rapid growth of human marrow stromal cells (hMSCs) FCS, Atlanta Biologicals; 100 units/mL penicillin, 100 μg/mL streptomycin, Gibco; and 2 mm L–glutamine, Gibco).[184] Cells were then plated in a 25 cm^2 tissue cultured flask (Nunc), incubated at 37°C with 5% humidified CO_2 for 1 day before the non-adherent cells were removed.[184] Adherent cells were then washed twice with PBS and shaken to remove adherent hematopoietic precursors, and fresh complete medium was added.[184] The medium was replaced every 3 to 4 days until the cells grew to 70% to 90% confluency, and harvested with trypsin and ethylenediaminetetraacetic acid (EDTA), with the entire process generally repeated to expand the cells through various passages.[184]

Mesenchymal Stem Cells/Stromal Cells From Adipose Tissue

After harvesting adipose tissue, the raw lipoaspirate can be processed using various methods and protocols to produce an injectable, including MFAT, enzyme-digested SVF, or cultured ASC.[78,141] After isolation from the raw lipoaspirate (refer to formulation section in Adipose Tissue section above), the SVF can either be used directly in clinical procedures or can be cultured to increase the number of cells before using them clinically. With cell culturing, only ASCs and their precursor cells (supra-adventitial cells and pericytes) are able to adhere and survive.[147,170] It is thought that the predominant benefit of SVF relies on the presence of ASCs.[147] The process of isolating and culturing ASCs is generally a long procedure that is not performed at the same time as surgery.[78,147]

When the adipose tissues are further processed into the SVF or cultured ASC, they are considered more than minimally manipulated and do not meet the criteria established by the FDA and do not comply with current regulations. To make SVF, the raw lipoaspirate is washed with PBS and subsequently undergoes enzymatic digestion with collagenase, dispase, trypsin, or other enzymes (ranging from 30 minutes to 1 to 2 hours).[78] After neutralization of the enzymes, the remaining elements are now called the stromal vascular fraction or SVF, and are separated from the mature adipocytes by centrifugation.[78] The SVF is composed of a heterogeneous mixture of cells, including pre-adipocytes, pericytes, mast cells, fibroblasts, smooth muscle cells, endothelial cells, hematopoietic stem cells, and AT-MSCs.[78,148]

When SVF cells are cultured, a subset of cells adheres to the tissue culture plasticware. After purification with washing and culture expansion with media, the HCSs (nonplastic adhesive cells) are separated from the SVF cells, leaving behind the adipose tissue–derived stromal cells which include the stem cells, which can be expanded in a culture medium.[78,109] The cells are then resuspended in a mixture of culture medium and cryoprotective medium and frozen and stored under good manufacturing practice. Cells can then be expanded in a culture medium for extended periods and utilized later.[77,140] Digesting the triple helix region of the peptide bonds in the collagen of adipose tissue with collagenase can be both time consuming and expensive.[141] In some cases, it may be possible to obtain ASCs without enzymatic digestion.[141,185] Baptista and colleagues isolated a population of MSC from lipoaspirate samples without tissue digestion and found that it is possible to store freshly isolated mechanically processed lipoaspirate adipose tissue (MPLA) cells by cryopreservation without a significant loss of MSCs.[185]

Jurgens and colleagues investigated whether the yield and functional characteristics of ASCs are affected by the adipose tissue-harvesting site and reported that the percentage of ASCs in the SVF of adipose tissue harvested from the abdomen was significantly greater than those harvested from the hip/thigh region ($P < .05$).[146] The authors noted that while there not was a significant difference in the ASC proliferation or differentiation capacity from cells harvested in the abdomen compared to cells harvested from the hip and thigh, there was a significantly increased yield of ASCs found in SVF of abdominal adipose tissue compared to SVF of adipose from hip/thigh regions.[146] Furthermore, Iyyanki and colleagues similarly found higher total SVF, but not tissue–derived stem cell yields in fat harvested from the abdomen compared to the flank or axilla.[148] Tsekouras and colleagues assessed 53 lipoaspirates in various locations (inner thigh, outer thigh, abdomen, waist, and inner knee) and found that the outer thigh exhibited significantly higher SVF cell count compared to other donor sites and both the inner and outer thigh showed a significantly higher number of ASCs.[186] No significant differences in the viability of SVF cells and ASCs were noted.[186] Fraser and colleagues evaluated the stem and progenitor cell content of subcutaneous adipose tissue in the hips and the abdomen of 10 subjects undergoing elective liposuction.[187] Using clonogenic culture assays and a paired analysis of tissue obtained from the different subcutaneous sites, the authors noted that tissue harvested from the hip yielded a statistically significant 2.3-fold more fibroblast CFU volume and a 7-fold higher frequency of alkaline phosphatase-positive colony-forming unit (CFU-AP, a widely used marker for osteogenesis) than that obtained from the abdomen.[187] One caveat is that the results could reflect the differences in ratio of deep and superficial subcutaneous adipose tissue collected from the two sites, as deep subcutaneous adipose tissue generally has a higher frequency of blood vessels, and thus more pericytes which may be detected by the CFU-AP assay[188] Pericytes, as mentioned before, have been shown to possess an adipogenic potential.[159]

FDA Regulations

Cultured MSCs are currently prohibited in the United States, as the methods for culture and isolation are currently considered more than minimal manipulation of the cells. The culturing method is performed outside of the United States; however, some institutions through special approval for research have been able to utilize culture-expanded cells.[75] The FDA released a guidance document in November 2017 to explain the regulatory demands of manufacturers of human cells, tissue, and cellular and tissue-based products by specifically delineating the definition of "minimal manipulation."[57]

Conclusion

Culture-expanded MSCs certainly have potential in clinical applications; however, more robust science is necessary to better understand their safety profile and efficacy in musculoskeletal applications.

References

1. Andia I, Martin JI, Maffulli N. Advances with platelet rich plasma therapies for tendon regeneration. *Expert Opin Biol Ther.* 2018;18(4):389–398. https://doi.org/10.1080/14712598.2018.1424626.
2. Dhurat R, Sukesh M. Principles and methods of preparation of platelet-rich plasma: a review and author's perspective. *J Cutan Aesthet Surg.* 2014;7(4):189. https://doi.org/10.4103/0974-2077.150734.
3. Fadadu PP, Mazzola AJ, Hunter CW, Davis TT. Review of concentration yields in commercially available platelet-rich plasma (PRP) systems: a call for PRP standardization. *Reg Anesth Pain Med.* 2019;44(6):652–659. https://doi.org/10.1136/rapm-2018-100356.
4. Hsu WK, Mishra A, Rodeo SR, et al. Platelet-rich plasma in orthopaedic applications: evidence-based recommendations for treatment. *J Am Acad Orthop Surg.* 2013;21(12):739–748. https://doi.org/10.5435/00124635-201312000-00004.
5. Oudelaar BW, Peerbooms JC, Huis in 't Veld R, Vochteloo AJH. Concentrations of blood components in commercial platelet-rich plasma separation systems: a review of the literature. *Am J Sports Med.* 2019;47(2):479–487. https://doi.org/10.1177/0363546517746112.
6. Fitzpatrick J, Bulsara MK, McCrory PR, Richardson MD, Zheng MH. Analysis of platelet-rich plasma extraction: variations in platelet and blood components between 4 common commercial kits. *Orthop J Sport Med.* 2017;5(1):2325967116675272-2325967116675272. https://doi.org/10.1177/2325967116675272.
7. Jayaram P, Yeh P, Patel SJ, et al. Effects of aspirin on growth factor release from freshly isolated leukocyte-rich platelet-rich plasma in healthy men: a prospective fixed-sequence controlled laboratory study. *Am J Sports Med.* 2019;47(5):1223–1229. https://doi.org/10.1177/0363546519827294.
8. Foster TE, Puskas BL, Mandelbaum BR, Gerhardt MB, Rodeo SA. Platelet-rich plasma. *Am J Sports Med.* 2009;37(11):2259–2272. https://doi.org/10.1177/0363546509349921.
9. Laver L, Marom N, Dnyanesh L, Mei-Dan O, Espregueira-Mendes J, Gobbi A. PRP for degenerative cartilage disease: a systematic review of clinical studies. *Cartilage.* 2017;8(4):341–364. https://doi.org/10.1177/1947603516670709.
10. Milants C, Bruyère O, Kaux J-F. Responders to platelet-rich plasma in osteoarthritis: a technical analysis. *Biomed Res Int.* 2017;2017:7538604. https://doi.org/10.1155/2017/7538604.
11. Toyoda T, Isobe K, Tsujino T, et al. Direct activation of platelets by addition of $CaCl_2$ leads coagulation of platelet-rich plasma. *Int J Implant Dent.* 2018;4(1). https://doi.org/10.1186/s40729-018-0134-6.
12. Cavallo C, Roffi A, Grigolo B, et al. Platelet-rich plasma: the Choice of activation method affects the release of bioactive molecules. *Biomed Res Int.* 2016;2016. https://doi.org/10.1155/2016/6591717.
13. Lana JFSD, Purita J, Paulus C, et al. Contributions for classification of platelet rich plasma—proposal of a new classification: MARSPILL. *Regen Med.* 2017;12(5):565–574. https://doi.org/10.2217/rme-2017-0042.
14. Rossi LA, Murray IR, Chu CR, Muschler GF, Rodeo SA, Piuzzi NS. Classification systems for platelet-rich plasma. *Bone Joint Lett J.* 2019;101-B(8):891–896. https://doi.org/10.1302/0301-620X.101B8.BJJ-2019-0037.R1.
15. Delong JM, Russell RP, Mazzocca AD. Platelet-rich plasma: the PAW classification system. *Arthrosc J Arthrosc Relat Surg.* 2012;28(7):998–1009. https://doi.org/10.1016/j.arthro.2012.04.148.
16. Mautner K, Malanga GA, Smith J, et al. A call for a standard classification system for future biologic research: the rationale for new PRP nomenclature. *Pharm Manag PM R.* 2015;7(4):S53–S59. https://doi.org/10.1016/j.pmrj.2015.02.005.
17. Zhou Y, Zhang J, Wu H, Hogan MCV, Wang JHC. The differential effects of leukocyte-containing and pure platelet-rich plasma (PRP) on tendon stem/progenitor cells—implications of PRP application for the clinical treatment of tendon injuries. *Stem Cell Res Ther.* 2015;6(1):1–13. https://doi.org/10.1186/s13287-015-0172-4.
18. Yamaguchi R, Terashima H, Yoneyama S, Tadano S, Ohkohchi N. Effects of platelet-rich plasma on intestinal anastomotic healing in rats: PRP concentration is a key factor. *J Surg Res.* 2012;173(2):258–266. https://doi.org/10.1016/j.jss.2010.10.001.
19. Berger DR, Centeno CJ, Steinmetz NJ. Platelet lysates from aged donors promote human tenocyte proliferation and migration in a concentration-dependent manner. *Bone Joint Res.* 2019;8(1):32–40. https://doi.org/10.1302/2046-3758.81.BJR-2018-0164.R1.
20. Toumi H, F'guyer S, Best TM. The role of neutrophils in injury and repair following muscle stretch. *J Anat.* 2006;208(4):459–470. https://doi.org/10.1111/j.1469-7580.2006.00543.x.
21. Wang J. Neutrophils in tissue injury and repair. *Cell Tissue Res.* 2018;371(3):531–539. https://doi.org/10.1007/s00441-017-2785-7.
22. Schäffer M, Barbul A. Lymphocyte function in wound healing and following injury. *Br J Surg.* 1998;85(4):444–460. https://doi.org/10.1046/j.1365-2168.1998.00734.x.
23. Braun HJ, Kim HJ, Chu CR, Dragoo JL. The effect of platelet-rich plasma formulations and blood products on human synoviocytes: implications for intra-articular injury and

therapy. *Am J Sports Med*. 2014;42(5):1204–1210. https://doi.org/10.1177/0363546514525593.

24. Kaux J-F. Reflections about the optimisation of the treatment of tendinopathies with PRP. *Muscles Ligaments Tendons J*. Published online. 2015. https://doi.org/10.11138/mltj/2015.5.1.001.
25. Barrientos S, Stojadinovic O, Golinko MS, Brem H, Tomic-Canic M. Growth factors and cytokines in wound healing. *Wound Repair Regen*. 2008;16(5):585–601. https://doi.org/10.1111/j.1524-475x.2008.00410.x.
26. Le ADK, Enweze L, DeBaun MR, Dragoo JL. Current clinical recommendations for use of platelet-rich plasma. *Curr Rev Musculoskelet Med*. 2018;11(4):624–634. https://doi.org/10.1007/s12178-018-9527-7.
27. Shen L, Yuan T, Chen S, Xie X, Zhang C. The temporal effect of platelet-rich plasma on pain and physical function in the treatment of knee osteoarthritis: systematic review and meta-analysis of randomized controlled trials. *J Orthop Surg Res*. 2017;12(1):16. https://doi.org/10.1186/s13018-017-0521-3.
28. Riboh JC, Saltzman BM, Yanke AB, Fortier L, Cole BJ. Effect of leukocyte concentration on the efficacy of platelet-rich plasma in the treatment of knee osteoarthritis. *Am J Sports Med*. 2015; 44(3):792–800. https://doi.org/10.1177/0363546515580787.
29. Nguyen RT, Borg-Stein J, McInnis K. Applications of platelet-rich plasma in musculoskeletal and sports medicine: an evidence-based approach. *Pharm Manag PM R*. 2011;3(3): 226–250. https://doi.org/10.1016/j.pmrj.2010.11.007.
30. Mautner K, Colberg RE, Malanga G, et al. Outcomes after ultrasound-guided platelet-rich plasma injections for chronic tendinopathy: a multicenter, retrospective review. *PM&R*. 2013;5(3):169–175. https://doi.org/10.1016/j.pmrj.2012.12.010.
31. Chen X, Jones IA, Park C, VangsnessJr CT. The efficacy of platelet-rich plasma on tendon and ligament healing: a systematic review and meta-analysis with bias assessment. *Am J Sports Med*. 2018;46(8): 2020–2032. https://doi.org/10.1177/0363546517743746.
32. Cai Y, Zhang C, Lin X. Efficacy of platelet-rich plasma in arthroscopic repair of full-thickness rotator cuff tears: a meta-analysis. *J Shoulder Elb Surg*. 2015;24(12):1852–1859. https://doi.org/10.1016/j.jse.2015.07.035.
33. Warth RJ, Dornan GJ, James EW, Horan MP, Millett PJ. Clinical and structural outcomes after arthroscopic repair of full-thickness rotator cuff tears with and without platelet-rich product supplementation: a meta-analysis and meta-regression. *Arthrosc J Arthrosc Relat Surg*. 2015;31(2):306–320. https://doi.org/10.1016/j.arthro.2014.09.007.
34. Andia I, Latorre PM, Gomez MC, Burgos-Alonso N, Abate M, Maffulli N. Platelet-rich plasma in the conservative treatment of painful tendinopathy: a systematic review and meta-analysis of controlled studies. *Br Med Bull*. 2014;110(1):99–115. https://doi.org/10.1093/bmb/ldu007.
35. Dragoo JL, Wasterlain AS, Braun HJ, Nead KT. Platelet-rich plasma as a treatment for patellar tendinopathy: a double-blind, randomized controlled trial. *Am J Sports Med*. 2014;42(3):610–618. https://doi.org/10.1177/0363546513518416.
36. Scott A, LaPrade RF, Harmon KG, et al. Platelet-rich plasma for patellar tendinopathy: a randomized controlled trial of leukocyte-rich PRP or leukocyte-poor PRP versus saline. *Am J Sports Med*. 2019;47(7):1654–1661. https://doi.org/10.1177/0363546519837954.
37. Andriolo L, Altamura SA, Reale D, Candrian C, Zaffagnini S, Filardo G. Nonsurgical treatments of patellar tendinopathy: multiple injections of platelet-rich plasma are a suitable option: a systematic review and meta-analysis. *Am J Sports Med*. 2019;47(4):1001–1018. https://doi.org/10.1177/0363546518759674.
38. Wu YT, Ho TY, Chou YC, et al. Six-month efficacy of platelet-rich plasma for carpal tunnel syndrome: a prospective randomized, single-blind controlled trial. *Sci Rep*. 2017;7(1):1–11. https://doi.org/10.1038/s41598-017-00224-6.
39. Sheth U, Dwyer T, Smith I, et al. Does platelet-rich plasma lead to earlier return to sport when compared with conservative treatment in acute muscle injuries? A systematic review and meta-analysis. *Arthrosc J Arthrosc Relat Surg*. 2018;34(1):281–288. e1. https://doi.org/10.1016/j.arthro.2017.06.039.
40. Setayesh K, Villarreal A, Gottschalk A, Tokish JM, Choate WS. Treatment of muscle injuries with platelet-rich plasma: a review of the literature. *Curr Rev Musculoskelet Med*. 2018;11(4):635–642. https://doi.org/10.1007/s12178-018-9526-8.
41. Figueroa D, Figueroa F, Calvo R, Vaisman A, Ahumada X, Arellano S. Platelet-rich plasma use in anterior cruciate ligament surgery: systematic review of the literature. *Arthrosc J Arthrosc Relat Surg*. 2015;31(5):981–988. https://doi.org/10.1016/j.arthro.2014.11.022.
42. Dhillon RS, Schwarz EM, Maloney MD. Platelet-rich plasma therapy—future or trend? *Arthritis Res Ther*. 2012;14(4):219. https://doi.org/10.1186/ar3914.
43. Mannava S, Whitney KE, Kennedy MI, et al. The influence of naproxen on biological factors in leukocyte-rich platelet-rich plasma: a prospective comparative study. *Arthrosc J Arthrosc Relat Surg*. 2019;35(1):201–210. https://doi.org/10.1016/j.arthro.2018.07.030.
44. Beitzel K, Allen D, Apostolakos J, et al. US definitions, current use, and FDA stance on use of platelet-rich plasma in sports medicine. *J Knee Surg*. 2015;28(1):29–34. https://doi.org/10.1055/s-0034-1390030.
45. Wasterlain AS, Braun HJ, Harris AHS, Kim H-J, Dragoo JL. The systemic effects of platelet-rich plasma injection. *Am J Sports Med*. 2012;41(1):186–193. https://doi.org/10.1177/0363546512466383.
46. Bieback K. Platelet lysate as replacement for fetal bovine serum in mesenchymal stromal cell cultures. *Transfus Med Hemother*. 2013;40(5):326–335. https://doi.org/10.1159/000354061.
47. Centeno C, Markle J, Dodson E, et al. The use of lumbar epidural injection of platelet lysate for treatment of radicular pain. *J Exp Orthop*. 2017;4(1):38. https://doi.org/10.1186/s40634-017-0113-5.
48. Dellera E, Bonferoni MC, Sandri G, et al. Development of chitosan oleate ionic micelles loaded with silver sulfadiazine to be associated with platelet lysate for application in wound healing. *Eur J Pharm Biopharm*. 2014;88(3):643–650. https://doi.org/10.1016/j.ejpb.2014.07.015.
49. Pezzotta S, Fante CD, Scudeller L, Cervio M, Antoniazzi ER, Perotti C. Autologous platelet lysate for treatment of refractory ocular GVHD. *Bone Marrow Transplant*. 2012;47(12):1558–1563. https://doi.org/10.1038/bmt.2012.64.
50. Del Bue M, Riccò S, Conti V, Merli E, Ramoni R, Grolli S. Platelet lysate promotes in vitro proliferation of equine mesenchymal stem cells and tenocytes. *Vet Res Commun*. 2007;31(S1):289–292. https://doi.org/10.1007/s11259-007-0099-z.
51. Nguyen VT, Cancedda R, Descalzi F. Platelet lysate activates quiescent cell proliferation and reprogramming in human articular cartilage: involvement of hypoxia inducible factor 1. *J Tissue Eng Regen Med*. 2017;12(3). https://doi.org/10.1002/term.2595.

52. Klatte-Schulz F, Schmidt T, Uckert M, et al. Comparative analysis of different platelet lysates and platelet rich preparations to stimulate tendon cell biology: an in vitro study. *Int J Mol Sci.* 2018;19(1):212. https://doi.org/10.3390/ijms19010212.
53. Yan L, Zhou L, Xie D, et al. Chondroprotective effects of platelet lysate towards monoiodoacetate-induced arthritis by suppression of TNF-α-induced activation of NF-κB pathway in chondrocytes. *Aging (Albany NY).* 2019;11(9):2797–2811. https://doi.org/10.18632/aging.101952.
54. Molloy T, Wang Y, Murrell GAC. The roles of growth factors in tendon and ligament healing. *Sport Med.* 2003;33(5):381–394. https://doi.org/10.2165/00007256-200333050-00004.
55. Al-Ajlouni J, Awidi A, Samara O, et al. Safety and efficacy of autologous intra-articular platelet lysates in early and intermediate knee osteoarthrosis in humans. *Clin J Sport Med.* Published online. 2014:1. https://doi.org/10.1097/jsm.0000000000000166.
56. Tan X, Ju H, Yan W, et al. Autologous platelet lysate local injections for the treatment of refractory lateral epicondylitis. *J Orthop Surg Res.* 2016;11:17. https://doi.org/10.1186/s13018-016-0349-2.
57. FDA/CBER. Regulatory considerations for human cell, tissues, and cellular and tissue-based products; minimal manipulation and homologous use guidance for industry and Food and Drug Administration staff. *Fda.* 2017: November, Accessed April 1, 2020. https://www.fda.gov/CombinationProducts/default.htm.
58. Tortorella MD, Arner EC, Hills R, et al. α2-Macroglobulin is a novel substrate for ADAMTS-4 and ADAMTS-5 and represents an endogenous inhibitor of these enzymes. *J Biol Chem.* 2004;279(17):17554–17561. https://doi.org/10.1074/jbc.m313041200.
59. Wang S, Wei X, Zhou J, et al. Identification of α2-macroglobulin as a master inhibitor of cartilage-degrading factors that attenuates the progression of posttraumatic osteoarthritis. *Arthritis Rheumatol (Hoboken, NJ).* 2014;66(7):1843–1853. https://doi.org/10.1002/art.38576.
60. Li S, Xiang C, Wei X, et al. Early supplemental α2-macroglobulin attenuates cartilage and bone damage by inhibiting inflammation in collagen II-induced arthritis model. *Int J Rheum Dis.* 2019;22(4):654–665. https://doi.org/10.1111/1756-185X.13457.
61. Demirag B, Sarisozen B, Durak K, Blgen ÖF, Ozturk C. The effect of alpha-2 macroglobulin on the healing of ruptured anterior cruciate ligament in rabbits. *Connect Tissue Res.* 2004;45(1):23–27. https://doi.org/10.1080/03008200490278115.
62. Cuellar JM. Intradiscal injection of an autologous alpha-2-macroglobulin (A2M) concentrate alleviates back pain in FAC-positive patients. *Orthop Rheumatol Open Access J.* 2017;4(2):4–8. https://doi.org/10.19080/oroaj.2017.04.555634.
63. Goldring MB. Osteoarthritis and cartilage: the role of cytokines. *Curr Rheumatol Rep.* 2000;2(6):459–465. https://doi.org/10.1007/s11926-000-0021-y.
64. Mabey T, Honsawek S. Cytokines as biochemical markers for knee osteoarthritis. *World J Orthop.* 2015;6(1):95–105. https://doi.org/10.5312/wjo.v6.i1.95.
65. Dinarello CA. The role of the interleukin-1–receptor antagonist in blocking inflammation mediated by interleukin-1. *N Engl J Med.* 2000;343(10):732–734. https://doi.org/10.1056/nejm200009073431011.
66. Meijer H, Reinecke J, Becker C, Tholen G, Wehling P. The production of anti-inflammatory cytokines in whole blood by physico-chemical induction. *Inflamm Res.* 2003;52(10):404–407. https://doi.org/10.1007/s00011-003-1197-1.
67. Chandrasekhar S, Harvey AK, Higginbotham JD, Horton WE. Interleukin-1-induced suppression of type II collagen gene transcription involves DNA regulatory elements. *Exp Cell Res.* 1990;191(1):105–114. https://doi.org/10.1016/0014-4827(90)90042-9.
68. van Beuningen HM, Arntz OJ, Van den Berg WB. In vivo effects of interleukin-1 on articular cartilage. Prolongation of proteoglycan metabolic disturbances in old mice. *Arthritis Rheum.* 1991;34(5):606–615. https://doi.org/10.1002/art.1780340513.
69. Ajrawat P, Dwyer T, Chahal J. Autologous interleukin 1 receptor antagonist blood-derived products for knee osteoarthritis: a systematic review. *Arthrosc J Arthrosc Relat Surg.* 2019;35(7):2211–2221. https://doi.org/10.1016/j.arthro.2018.12.035.
70. Chevalier X, Goupille P, Beaulieu AD, et al. Intraarticular injection of anakinra in osteoarthritis of the knee: a multicenter, randomized, double-blind, placebo-controlled study. *Arthritis Rheum.* 2009;61(3):344–352. https://doi.org/10.1002/art.24096.
71. H S RK, Goni VG, Y K B. Autologous conditioned serum as a novel alternative option in the treatment of unilateral lumbar radiculopathy: a prospective study. *Asian Spine J.* 2015;9(6):916–922. https://doi.org/10.4184/asj.2015.9.6.916.
72. Majewski M, Ochsner PE, Liu F, Flückiger R, Evans CH. Accelerated healing of the rat Achilles tendon in response to autologous conditioned serum. *Am J Sports Med.* 2009;37(11):2117–2125. https://doi.org/10.1177/0363546509348047.
73. Nixon AJ, Grol MW, Lang HM, et al. Disease-modifying osteoarthritis treatment with interleukin-1 receptor antagonist gene therapy in small and large animal models. *Arthritis Rheumatol.* 2018;70(11):1757–1768. https://doi.org/10.1002/art.40668.
74. Chahla J, Mannava S, Cinque ME, Geeslin AG, Codina D, LaPrade RF. Bone marrow aspirate concentrate harvesting and processing technique. *Arthrosc Tech.* 2017;6(2):e441–e445. https://doi.org/10.1016/j.eats.2016.10.024.
75. Sampson S, Bemden AB, Aufiero D. Autologous bone marrow concentrate: review and application of a novel intra-articular orthobiologic for cartilage disease. *Phys Sportsmed.* 2013;41(3):7–18. https://doi.org/10.3810/psm.2013.09.2022.
76. Caplan AI. Mesenchymal stem cells: time to change the name!. *Stem Cells Transl Med.* 2017;6(6):1445–1451. https://doi.org/10.1002/sctm.17-0051.
77. Mohamed-Ahmed S, Fristad I, Lie SA, et al. Adipose-derived and bone marrow mesenchymal stem cells: a donor-matched comparison. *Stem Cell Res Ther.* 2018;9(1):168. https://doi.org/10.1186/s13287-018-0914-1.
78. Bourin P, Bunnell BA, Casteilla L, et al. Stromal cells from the adipose tissue-derived stromal vascular fraction and culture expanded adipose tissue-derived stromal/stem cells: a joint statement of the International Federation for Adipose Therapeutics and Science (IFATS) and the International Society for Cellular Therapy (ISCT). *Cytotherapy.* 2013;15(6):641–648. https://doi.org/10.1016/j.jcyt.2013.02.006.
79. Dominici M, Le Blanc K, Mueller I, et al. Minimal criteria for defining multipotent mesenchymal stromal cells. The International Society for Cellular Therapy position statement. *Cytotherapy.* 2006;8(4):315–317. https://doi.org/10.1080/14653240600855905.
80. Xiang Y, Zheng Q, Jia B, et al. Ex vivo expansion and pluripotential differentiation of cryopreserved human bone marrow

mesenchymal stem cells. *J Zhejiang Univ Sci B*. 2007;8(2):136–146. https://doi.org/10.1631/jzus.2007.B0136.

81. Giannini S, Buda R, Vannini F, Cavallo M, Grigolo B. One-step bone marrow-derived cell transplantation in talar osteochondral lesions. *Clin Orthop Relat Res*. 2009;467(12):3307–3320. https://doi.org/10.1007/s11999-009-0885-8.
82. Ziegler CG, Van Sloun R, Gonzalez S, et al. Characterization of growth factors, cytokines, and chemokines in bone marrow concentrate and platelet-rich plasma: a prospective analysis. *Am J Sports Med*. 2019;47(9):2174–2187. https://doi.org/10.1177/0363546519832003.
83. Cassano JM, Kennedy JG, Ross KA, Fraser EJ, Goodale MB, Fortier LA. Bone marrow concentrate and platelet-rich plasma differ in cell distribution and interleukin 1 receptor antagonist protein concentration. *Knee Surg Sport Traumatol Arthrosc*. 2018; 26(1):333–342. https://doi.org/10.1007/s00167-016-3981-9.
84. Dragoo JL, Guzman RA. Evaluation of the consistency and composition of commercially available bone marrow aspirate concentrate systems. *Orthop J Sport Med*. 2020;8(1):2325967119893634. https://doi.org/10.1177/2325967119893634.
85. Corbel SY, Lee A, Yi L, et al. Contribution of hematopoietic stem cells to skeletal muscle. *Nat Med*. 2003;9(12):1528–1532. https://doi.org/10.1038/nm959.
86. Descalzi F, Ulivi V, Cancedda R, et al. Platelet-rich plasma exerts antinociceptive activity by a peripheral endocannabinoid-related mechanism. *Tissue Eng Part A*. 2013;19(19–20):2120–2129. https://doi.org/10.1089/ten.tea.2012.0557.
87. Hernigou P, Poignard A, Beaujean F, Rouard H. Percutaneous autologous bone-marrow grafting for nonunions: influence of the number and concentration of progenitor cells. *J Bone Jt Surg—Ser A*. 2005;87(7):1430–1437. https://doi.org/10.2106/JBJS.D.02215.
88. Pettine, K., Suzuki, R., Sand, T. et al. Treatment of discogenic back pain with autologous bone marrow concentrate injection with minimum two year follow-up. International Orthopaedics (SICOT) 40, 135–140 (2016). https://doi.org/10.1007/s00264-015-2886-4.
89. Centeno CJ, Al-Sayegh H, Bashir J, Goodyear S, Freeman MD. A dose response analysis of a specific bone marrow concentrate treatment protocol for knee osteoarthritis. *BMC Musculoskelet Disord*. 2015;16(1):1–8. https://doi.org/10.1186/s12891-015-0714-z.
90. Sampson S, Smith J, Vincent H, Aufiero D, Zall M, Botto-van-Bemden A. Intra-articular bone marrow concentrate injection protocol: short-term efficacy in osteoarthritis. *Regen Med*. 2016;11(6):511–520. https://doi.org/10.2217/rme-2016-0081.
91. Nct. Placebo-controlled study to evaluate rexlemestrocel-L alone or combined with hyaluronic acid in subjects with chronic low back pain. Https://clinicaltrials.gov/show/nct02412735 2015;(PG-). Accessed April 1, 2020. https://clinicaltrials.gov/ct2/show/NCT02412735.
92. Sampson S, Vincent H, Ambach MA, Amirianfar E. *Nov Tech Arthritis Bone Res Orthobiologics*. 2017;2(1). https://doi.org/10.19080/NTAB.2017.02.555576. Where are we Now?.
93. LaPrade RF, Geeslin AG, Murray IR, et al. Biologic treatments for sports injuries II think tank—current concepts, future research, and barriers to advancement, Part 1. *Am J Sports Med*. 2016;44(12):3270–3283. https://doi.org/10.1177/0363546516634674.
94. Centeno CJ, Busse D, Kisiday J, Keohan C, Freeman M, Karli D. Regeneration of meniscus cartilage in a knee treated with percutaneously implanted autologous mesenchymal stem cells. *Med Hypotheses*. 2008;71(6):900–908. https://doi.org/10.1016/j.mehy.2008.06.042.
95. Pettine KA, Murphy MB, Suzuki RK, Sand TT. Percutaneous injection of autologous bone marrow concentrate cells significantly reduces lumbar discogenic pain through 12 months. *Stem Cell*. 2014;33(1):146–156. https://doi.org/10.1002/stem.1845.
96. Centeno C, Fausel Z, Stemper I, Azuike U, Dodson E. A randomized controlled trial of the treatment of rotator cuff tears with bone marrow concentrate and platelet products compared to exercise therapy: a midterm analysis. *Stem Cells Int*. 2020;2020. https://doi.org/10.1155/2020/5962354.
97. Kim SJ, Kim EK, Kim SJ, Song DH. Effects of bone marrow aspirate concentrate and platelet-rich plasma on patients with partial tear of the rotator cuff tendon. *J Orthop Surg Res*. 2018;13(1):1. https://doi.org/10.1186/s13018-017-0693-x.
98. Centeno CJ, Al-Sayegh H, Bashir J, Goodyear SH, D Freeman M. A prospective multi-site registry study of a specific protocol of autologous bone marrow concentrate for the treatment of shoulder rotator cuff tears and osteoarthritis. *J Pain Res*. 2015;8:269–276. https://doi.org/10.2147/JPR.S80872.
99. Centeno C, Markle J, Dodson E, et al. Symptomatic anterior cruciate ligament tears treated with percutaneous injection of autologous bone marrow concentrate and platelet products: a non-controlled registry study. *J Transl Med*. 2018;16(1):246. https://doi.org/10.1186/s12967-018-1623-3.
100. J Centeno C. Efficacy and safety of bone marrow concentrate for osteoarthritis of the hip; treatment registry results for 196 patients. *J Stem Cell Res Ther*. 2014;04(10). https://doi.org/10.4172/2157-7633.1000242.
101. Hernigou P, Homma Y, Flouzat-Lachaniette C-H, Poignard A, Chevallier N, Rouard H. Cancer risk is not increased in patients treated for orthopaedic diseases with autologous bone marrow cell concentrate. *J Bone Jt Surg Am*. 2013;95(24):2215–2221. https://doi.org/10.2106/jbjs.m.00261.
102. Youn GM, Woodall BM, Elena N, et al. Arthroscopic bone marrow aspirate concentrate harvesting from the intercondylar notch of the knee. *Arthrosc Tech*. 2018;7(11):e1173–e1176. https://doi.org/10.1016/j.eats.2018.07.016.
103. Hernigou P, Flouzat Lachaniette CH, Delambre J, et al. Biologic augmentation of rotator cuff repair with mesenchymal stem cells during arthroscopy improves healing and prevents further tears: a case-controlled study. *Int Orthop*. 2014;38(9):1811–1818. https://doi.org/10.1007/s00264-014-2391-1.
104. Shapiro SA, Kazmerchak SE, Heckman MG, Zubair AC, O'Connor MI. A prospective, single-blind, placebo-controlled trial of bone marrow aspirate concentrate for knee osteoarthritis. *Am J Sports Med*. 2016;45(1):82–90. https://doi.org/10.1177/0363546516662455.
105. Pettine KA, Suzuki RK, Sand TT, Murphy MB. Autologous bone marrow concentrate intradiscal injection for the treatment of degenerative disc disease with three-year follow-up. *Int Orthop*. 2017;41(10):2097–2103. https://doi.org/10.1007/s00264-017-3560-9.
106. Centeno C, Schultz J, Cheever M, Robinson B, Freeman M, Marasco W. Safety and complications reporting on the re-implantation of culture-expanded mesenchymal stem cells using autologous platelet lysate technique. *Curr Stem Cell Res Ther*. 2010; 5(1):81–93. https://doi.org/10.2174/157488810790442796.
107. Centeno CJ, Al-Sayegh H, Freeman MD, Smith J, Murrell WD, Bubnov R. A multi-center analysis of adverse events among

two thousand, three hundred and seventy two adult patients undergoing adult autologous stem cell therapy for orthopaedic conditions. *Int Orthop*. 2016;40(8):1755–1765. https://doi.org/10.1007/s00264-016-3162-y.
108. Cavinatto L, Hinckel BB, Tomlinson RE, Gupta S, Farr J, Bartolozzi AR. The role of bone marrow aspirate concentrate for the treatment of focal chondral lesions of the knee: a systematic review and critical analysis of animal and clinical studies. *Arthrosc J Arthrosc Relat Surg*. 2019;35(6):1860–1877. https://doi.org/10.1016/j.arthro.2018.11.073.
109. Chu D-T, Nguyen Thi Phuong T, Tien NLB, et al. Adipose tissue stem cells for therapy: an update on the progress of isolation, culture, storage, and clinical application. *J Clin Med*. 2019;8(7):917. https://doi.org/10.3390/jcm8070917.
110. Fraser JK, Wulur I, Alfonso Z, Hedrick MH. Fat tissue: an underappreciated source of stem cells for biotechnology. *Trends Biotechnol*. 2006;24(4):150–154. https://doi.org/10.1016/j.tibtech.2006.01.010.
111. Beane OS, Darling EM. Isolation, characterization, and differentiation of stem cells for cartilage regeneration. *Ann Biomed Eng*. 2012;40(10):2079–2097.https://doi.org/10.1007/s10439-012-0639-8.
112. Rodbell M. Metabolism of isolated fat cells. II. The similar effects of phospholipase C (*Clostridium perfringens* alpha toxin) and of insulin on glucose and amino acid metabolism. *J Biol Chem*. 1966;241(1):130–139.
113. Yoshimura K, Suga H, Eto H. Adipose-derived stem/progenitor cells: roles in adipose tissue remodeling and potential use for soft tissue augmentation. *Regen Med*. 2009;4(2):265–273. https://doi.org/10.2217/17460751.4.2.265.
114. Argentati C, Morena F, Bazzucchi M, Armentano I, Emiliani C, Martino S. Adipose stem cell translational applications: from bench-to-bedside. *Int J Mol Sci*. 2018;19(11). https://doi.org/10.3390/ijms19113475.
115. Koh Y-G, Choi Y-J. Infrapatellar fat pad-derived mesenchymal stem cell therapy for knee osteoarthritis. *Knee*. 2012;19(6):902–907. https://doi.org/10.1016/j.knee.2012.04.001.
116. Pak J. Regeneration of human bones in hip osteonecrosis and human cartilage in knee osteoarthritis with autologous adipose-tissue-derived stem cells: a case series. *J Med Case Rep*. 2011;5:296. https://doi.org/10.1186/1752-1947-5-296.
117. Song Y, Du H, Dai C, et al. Human adipose-derived mesenchymal stem cells for osteoarthritis: a pilot study with long-term follow-up and repeated injections. *Regen Med*. 2018;13(3):295–307. https://doi.org/10.2217/rme-2017-0152.
118. Jo CH, Chai JW, Jeong EC, et al. Intra-articular injection of mesenchymal stem cells for the treatment of osteoarthritis of the knee: a 2-year follow-up study. *Am J Sports Med*. 2017;45(12):2774–2783. https://doi.org/10.1177/0363546517716641.
119. Lee WS, Kim HJ, Kim KI, Kim GB, Jin W. Intra-articular injection of autologous adipose tissue-derived mesenchymal stem cells for the treatment of knee osteoarthritis: a phase IIb, randomized, placebo-controlled clinical trial. *Stem Cells Transl Med*. 2019;8(6):504–511. https://doi.org/10.1002/sctm.18-0122.
120. Freitag J, Bates D, Wickham J, et al. Adipose-derived mesenchymal stem cell therapy in the treatment of knee osteoarthritis: a randomized controlled trial. *Regen Med*. 2019;14(3):213–230. https://doi.org/10.2217/rme-2018-0161.
121. Koh YG, Jo SB, Kwon OR, et al. Mesenchymal stem cell injections improve symptoms of knee osteoarthritis. *Arthrosc J Arthrosc Relat Surg*. 2013;29(4):748–755. https://doi.org/10.1016/j.arthro.2012.11.017.
122. Pak J, Lee JH, Park KS, Lee SH. Efficacy of autologous adipose tissue-derived stem cells with extracellular matrix and hyaluronic acid on human hip osteoarthritis. *Biomed Res*. 2017;28(4):1654–1658. Accessed April 1, 2020. www.biomedres.info.
123. Striano RD. *Refractory Shoulder Pain with Osteoarthritis, and Rotator Cuff Tear, Treated with Micro-fragmented Adipose Tissue*; 2018. Published online.
124. Singer W, Dietz AB, Zeller AD, et al. Intrathecal administration of autologous mesenchymal stem cells in multiple system atrophy. *Neurology*. 2019;93(1):e77–e87. https://doi.org/10.1212/WNL.0000000000007720.
125. Valina C, Pinkernell K, Song Y-H, et al. Intracoronary administration of autologous adipose tissue-derived stem cells improves left ventricular function, perfusion, and remodelling after acute myocardial infarction. *Eur Heart J*. 2007;28(21):2667–2677. https://doi.org/10.1093/eurheartj/ehm426.
126. Qayyum AA, Mathiasen AB, Mygind ND, et al. Adipose-derived stromal cells for treatment of patients with chronic ischemic heart disease (MyStromalCell trial): a randomized placebo-controlled study. *Stem Cells Int*. 2017;2017:5237063. https://doi.org/10.1155/2017/5237063.
127. Kim KS, Lee HJ, An J, et al. Transplantation of human adipose tissue-derived stem cells delays clinical onset and prolongs life span in ALS mouse model. *Cell Transplant*. 2014;23(12):1585–1597. https://doi.org/10.3727/096368913x673450.
128. Marconi S, Bonaconsa M, Scambi I, et al. Systemic treatment with adipose-derived mesenchymal stem cells ameliorates clinical and pathological features in the amyotrophic lateral sclerosis murine model. *Neuroscience*. 2013;248:333–343. https://doi.org/10.1016/j.neuroscience.2013.05.034.
129. Uccelli A, Milanese M, Principato MC, et al. Intravenous mesenchymal stem cells improve survival and motor function in experimental amyotrophic lateral sclerosis. *Mol Med*. 2012;18(1):794–804. https://doi.org/10.2119/molmed.2011.00498.
130. Schwerk A, Altschüler J, Roch M, et al. Human adipose-derived mesenchymal stromal cells increase endogenous neurogenesis in the rat subventricular zone acutely after 6-hydroxydopamine lesioning. *Cytotherapy*. 2015;17(2):199–214. https://doi.org/10.1016/j.jcyt.2014.09.005.
131. Berg J, Roch M, Altschüler J, et al. Human adipose-derived mesenchymal stem cells improve motor functions and are neuroprotective in the 6-hydroxydopamine-rat model for Parkinson's disease when cultured in monolayer cultures but suppress hippocampal neurogenesis and hippocampal memory function. *Stem Cell Rev Reports*. 2014;11(1):133–149. https://doi.org/10.1007/s12015-014-9551-y.
132. Hur JW, Cho T-H, Park D-H, Lee J-B, Park J-Y, Chung Y-G. Intrathecal transplantation of autologous adipose-derived mesenchymal stem cells for treating spinal cord injury: a human trial. *J Spinal Cord Med*. 2016;39(6):655–664. https://doi.org/10.1179/2045772315Y.0000000048.
133. Lopez-Santalla M, Mancheño-Corvo P, Menta R, et al. Human adipose-derived mesenchymal stem cells modulate experimental autoimmune arthritis by modifying early adaptive T cell responses. *Stem Cell*. 2015;33(12):3493–3503. https://doi.org/10.1002/stem.2113.
134. Baharlou R, Ahmadi-Vasmehjani A, Faraji F, et al. Human adipose tissue-derived mesenchymal stem cells in rheumatoid arthritis: regulatory effects on peripheral blood mononuclear cells activation. *Int Immunopharmacol*. 2017;47:59–69. https://doi.org/10.1016/j.intimp.2017.03.016.

135. Baharlou R, Rashidi N, Ahmadi-Vasmehjani A, Khoubyari M, Sheikh M, Erfanian S. Immunomodulatory effects of human adipose tissue-derived mesenchymal stem cells on T cell subsets in patients with rheumatoid arthritis. *Iran J Allergy Asthma Immunol*. Published online 2019. https://doi.org/10.18502/ijaai.v18i1.637.
136. Dang LT-T, Bui AN-T, Le-Thanh Nguyen C, et al. Intravenous infusion of human adipose tissue-derived mesenchymal stem cells to treat type 1 diabetic mellitus in mice: an evaluation of grafted cell doses. *Stem Cells Biol Eng*. Published online 2017:145–156. https://doi.org/10.1007/5584_2017_127.
137. Wang M, Song L, Strange C, Dong X, Wang H. Therapeutic effects of adipose stem cells from diabetic mice for the treatment of type 2 diabetes. *Mol Ther*. 2018;26(8):1921–1930. https://doi.org/10.1016/j.ymthe.2018.06.013.
138. Yan Y, Ma T, Gong K, Ao Q, Zhang X, Gong Y. Adipose-derived mesenchymal stem cell transplantation promotes adult neurogenesis in the brains of Alzheimer's disease mice. *Neural Regen Res*. 2014;9(8):798–805. https://doi.org/10.4103/1673-5374.131596.
139. Kim S, Chang K-A, Kim J a, et al. The preventive and therapeutic effects of intravenous human adipose-derived stem cells in Alzheimer's disease mice. *PloS One*. 2012;7(9):e45757-e45757. https://doi.org/10.1371/journal.pone.0045757.
140. Oedayrajsingh-Varma MJ, van Ham SM, Knippenberg M, et al. Adipose tissue-derived mesenchymal stem cell yield and growth characteristics are affected by the tissue-harvesting procedure. *Cytotherapy*. 2006;8(2):166–177. https://doi.org/10.1080/14653240600621125.
141. Shah FS, Wu X, Dietrich M, Rood J, Gimble JM. A non-enzymatic method for isolating human adipose tissue-derived stromal stem cells. *Cytotherapy*. 2013;15(8):979–985. https://doi.org/10.1016/j.jcyt.2013.04.001.
142. Ceserani V, Ferri A, Berenzi A, et al. Angiogenic and anti-inflammatory properties of micro-fragmented fat tissue and its derived mesenchymal stromal cells. *Vasc Cell*. 2016;8(1). https://doi.org/10.1186/s13221-016-0037-3.
143. Tremolada C, Colombo V, Ventura C. Adipose tissue and mesenchymal stem cells: state of the art and Lipogems® technology development. *Curr Stem Cell Reports*. 2016;2(3):304–312. https://doi.org/10.1007/s40778-016-0053-5.
144. Mestak O, Sukop A, Hsueh YS, et al. Centrifugation versus PureGraft for fat grafting to the breast after breast-conserving therapy. *World J Surg Oncol*. 2014;12(1):178. https://doi.org/10.1186/1477-7819-12-178.
145. About - Cellmyx. Accessed April 6, 2020. https://cellmyx.com/about/.
146. Jurgens WJFM, Oedayrajsingh-Varma MJ, Helder MN, et al. Effect of tissue-harvesting site on yield of stem cells derived from adipose tissue: implications for cell-based therapies. *Cell Tissue Res*. 2008;332(3):415–426. https://doi.org/10.1007/s00441-007-0555-7.
147. van Dongen JA, Tuin AJ, Spiekman M, Jansma J, van der Lei B, Harmsen MC. Comparison of intraoperative procedures for isolation of clinical grade stromal vascular fraction for regenerative purposes: a systematic review. *J Tissue Eng Regen Med*. 2017;12(1):e261–e274. https://doi.org/10.1002/term.2407.
148. Iyyanki T, Hubenak J, Liu J, Chang EI, Beahm EK, Zhang Q. Harvesting technique affects adipose-derived stem cell yield. *Aesthetic Surg J*. 2015;35(4):467. https://doi.org/10.1093/ASJ/SJU055.
149. Keck M, Kober J, Riedl O, et al. Power assisted liposuction to obtain adipose-derived stem cells: impact on viability and differentiation to adipocytes in comparison to manual aspiration. *J Plast Reconstr Aesthetic Surg*. 2014;67(1):e1. https://doi.org/10.1016/j.bjps.2013.08.019.
150. Duscher D, Atashroo D, Maan ZN, et al. Ultrasound-assisted liposuction does not compromise the regenerative potential of adipose-derived stem cells. *Stem Cells Transl Med*. 2016;5(2):248–257. https://doi.org/10.5966/sctm.2015-0064.
151. Choudhery MS, Badowski M, Muise A, Pierce J, Harris DT. Donor age negatively impacts adipose tissue-derived mesenchymal stem cell expansion and differentiation. *J Transl Med*. 2014;12:8. https://doi.org/10.1186/1479-5876-12-8.
152. Schipper BM, Marra KG, Zhang W, Donnenberg AD, Rubin JP. Regional anatomic and age effects on cell function of human adipose-derived stem cells. In: *Annals of Plastic Surgery*. Vol 60; 2008:538–544. https://doi.org/10.1097/SAP.0b013e3181723bbe.
153. Varghese J, Griffin M, Mosahebi A, Butler P. Systematic review of patient factors affecting adipose stem cell viability and function: implications for regenerative therapy. *Stem Cell Res Ther*. 2017;8(1):45. https://doi.org/10.1186/s13287-017-0483-8.
154. Oñate B, Vilahur G, Ferrer-Lorente R, et al. The subcutaneous adipose tissue reservoir of functionally active stem cells is reduced in obese patients. *FASEB J*. 2012;26(10):4327–4336. https://doi.org/10.1096/fj.12-207217.
155. Mitterberger MC, Mattesich M, Zwerschke W. Bariatric surgery and diet-induced long-term caloric restriction protect subcutaneous adipose-derived stromal/progenitor cells and prolong their life span in formerly obese humans. *Exp Gerontol*. 2014;56:106–113. https://doi.org/10.1016/j.exger.2014.03.030.
156. Cramer C, Freisinger E, Jones RK, et al. Persistent high glucose concentrations alter the regenerative potential of mesenchymal stem cells. *Stem Cells Dev*. 2010;19(12):1875–1884. https://doi.org/10.1089/scd.2010.0009.
157. Malanga G, Abdelshahed D, Jayaram P. Orthobiologic interventions using ultrasound guidance. *Phys Med Rehabil Clin N Am*. 2016;27(3):717–731. https://doi.org/10.1016/j.pmr.2016.04.007.
158. Vezzani B, Shaw I, Lesme H, et al. Higher pericyte content and secretory activity of microfragmented human adipose tissue compared to enzymatically derived stromal vascular fraction. *Stem Cells Transl Med*. 2018;7(12):876–886. https://doi.org/10.1002/sctm.18-0051.
159. Guimarães-Camboa N, Cattaneo P, Sun Y, et al. Pericytes of multiple organs do not behave as mesenchymal stem cells in vivo. *Cell Stem Cell*. 2017;20(3):345–359. e5. https://doi.org/10.1016/j.stem.2016.12.006.
160. Caplan AI. All MSCs are pericytes? *Cell Stem Cell*. 2008;3(3):229–230. https://doi.org/10.1016/j.stem.2008.08.008.
161. Crisan M, Yap S, Casteilla L, et al. A perivascular origin for mesenchymal stem cells in multiple human organs. *Cell Stem Cell*. 2008;3(3):301–313. https://doi.org/10.1016/j.stem.2008.07.003.
162. Laschke MW, Menger MD. Adipose tissue-derived microvascular fragments: natural vascularization units for regenerative medicine. *Trends Biotechnol*. 2015;33(8):442–448. https://doi.org/10.1016/j.tibtech.2015.06.001.
163. Chu CR, Rodeo S, Bhutani N, et al. Optimizing clinical use of biologics in orthopaedic surgery: consensus recommendations from the 2018 AAOS/NIH U-13 Conference. *J Am Acad Orthop Surg*. 2019;27(2):e50–e63. https://doi.org/10.5435/JAAOS-D-18-00305.
164. Pak J, Chang J-J, Lee JH, Lee SH. Safety reporting on implantation of autologous adipose tissue-derived stem cells with

platelet-rich plasma into human articular joints. *BMC Musculoskelet Disord.* 2013;14:337. https://doi.org/10.1186/1471-2474-14-337.
165. Kuah D, Sivell S, Longworth T, et al. Safety, tolerability and efficacy of intra-articular Progenza in knee osteoarthritis: a randomized double-blind placebo-controlled single ascending dose study. *J Transl Med.* 2018;16(1):49. https://doi.org/10.1186/s12967-018-1420-z.
166. Freese KE, Kokai L, Edwards RP, et al. Adipose-derived stems cells and their role in human cancer development, growth, progression, and metastasis: a systematic review. *Cancer Res.* 2015;75(7):1161–1168. https://doi.org/10.1158/0008-5472.can-14-2744.
167. Rodeo SA. Moving toward responsible use of biologics in sports medicine. *Am J Sports Med.* 2018;46(8):1797–1799. https://doi.org/10.1177/0363546518782182.
168. Zuk PA, Zhu M, Mizuno H, et al. Multilineage cells from human adipose tissue: implications for cell-based therapies. In: *Tissue Engineering.* Vol 7; 2001:211–228. https://doi.org/10.1089/107632701300062859.
169. Mizuno H, Tobita M, Uysal AC. Concise review: adipose-derived stem cells as a novel tool for future regenerative medicine. *Stem Cell.* 2012;30(5):804–810. https://doi.org/10.1002/stem.1076.
170. Zuk PA, Zhu M, Mizuno H, et al. Multilineage cells from human adipose tissue: implications for cell-based therapies. *Tissue Eng.* 2001;7(2):211–228. https://doi.org/10.1089/107632701300062859.
171. Alves H, van Ginkel J, Groen N, et al. A mesenchymal stromal cell gene signature for donor age. *PloS One.* 2012;7(8). https://doi.org/10.1371/journal.pone.0042908.
172. Mosna F, Sensebé L, Krampera M. Human bone marrow and adipose tissue mesenchymal stem cells: a user's guide. *Stem Cells Dev.* 2010;19(10):1449–1470. https://doi.org/10.1089/scd.2010.0140.
173. Sakaguchi Y, Sekiya I, Yagishita K, Muneta T. Comparison of human stem cells derived from various mesenchymal tissues: superiority of synovium as a cell source. *Arthritis Rheum.* 2005;52(8):2521–2529. https://doi.org/10.1002/art.21212.
174. Jang Y, Koh YG, Choi YJ, et al. Characterization of adipose tissue-derived stromal vascular fraction for clinical application to cartilage regeneration. *Vitr Cell Dev Biol—Anim.* 2014;51(2):142–150. https://doi.org/10.1007/s11626-014-9814-6.
175. Strem BM, Hicok KC, Zhu M, et al. Multipotential differentiation of adipose tissue-derived stem cells. *Keio J Med.* 2005;54(3):132–141. https://doi.org/10.2302/kjm.54.132.
176. Cowan CM, Shi Y-Y, Aalami OO, et al. Adipose-derived adult stromal cells heal critical-size mouse calvarial defects. *Nat Biotechnol.* 2004;22(5):560–567. https://doi.org/10.1038/nbt958.
177. Xu L, Liu Y, Sun Y, et al. Tissue source determines the differentiation potentials of mesenchymal stem cells: a comparative study of human mesenchymal stem cells from bone marrow and adipose tissue. *Stem Cell Res Ther.* 2017;8(1):275. https://doi.org/10.1186/s13287-017-0716-x.
178. Huang S-J, Fu R-H, Shyu W-C, et al. Adipose-derived stem cells: isolation, characterization, and differentiation potential. *Cell Transplant.* 2013;22(4):701–709. https://doi.org/10.3727/096368912x655127.
179. Kern S, Eichler H, Stoeve J, Klüter H, Bieback K. Comparative analysis of mesenchymal stem cells from bone marrow, umbilical cord blood, or adipose tissue. *Stem Cell.* 2006;24(5):1294–1301. https://doi.org/10.1634/stemcells.2005-0342.
180. Burrow KL, Hoyland JA, Richardson SM. Human adipose-derived stem cells exhibit enhanced proliferative capacity and retain multipotency longer than donor-matched bone marrow mesenchymal stem cells during expansion in vitro. *Stem Cells Int.* 2017;2017. https://doi.org/10.1155/2017/2541275.
181. Jakobsen RB, Shahdadfar A, Reinholt FP, Brinchmann JE. Chondrogenesis in a hyaluronic acid scaffold: comparison between chondrocytes and MSC from bone marrow and adipose tissue. *Knee Surg Sport Traumatol Arthrosc.* 2010;18(10):1407–1416. https://doi.org/10.1007/s00167-009-1017-4.
182. Danisovic L, Varga I, Polak S, et al. Comparison of in vitro chondrogenic potential of human mesenchymal stem cells derived from bone marrow and adipose tissue. *Gen Physiol Biophys.* 2009;28(1):56–62.
183. Mautner K, Bowers R, Easley K, Fausel Z, Robinson R. Functional outcomes following microfragmented adipose tissue versus bone marrow aspirate concentrate injections for symptomatic knee osteoarthritis. *Stem Cells Transl Med.* 2019;8(11):1149–1156. https://doi.org/10.1002/sctm.18-0285.
184. DiGirolamo CM, Stokes D, Colter D, Phinney DG, Class R, Prockop DJ. Propagation and senescence of human marrow stromal cells in culture: a simple colony-forming assay identifies samples with the greatest potential to propagate and differentiate. *Br J Haematol.* 1999;107(2):275–281. https://doi.org/10.1046/j.1365-2141.1999.01715.x.
185. Baptista LS, do Amaral RJFC, Carias RBV, Aniceto M, Claudio-da-Silva C, Borojevic R. An alternative method for the isolation of mesenchymal stromal cells derived from lipoaspirate samples. *Cytotherapy.* 2009;11(6):706–715. https://doi.org/10.3109/14653240902981144.
186. Tsekouras A, Mantas D, Tsilimigras DI, Moris D, Kontos M, Zografos GC. Comparison of the viability and yield of adipose-derived stem cells (ASCs) from different donor areas. *Vivo (Brooklyn).* 2017;31(6):1229–1234. https://doi.org/10.21873/invivo.11196.
187. Fraser JK, Wulur I, Alfonso Z, Zhu M, Wheeler ES. Differences in stem and progenitor cell yield in different subcutaneous adipose tissue depots. *Cytotherapy.* 2007;9(5):459–467. https://doi.org/10.1080/14653240701358460.
188. El-Mrakby HH, Milner RH. Bimodal distribution of the blood supply to lower abdominal fat: histological study of the microcirculation of the lower abdominal wall. *Ann Plast Surg.* 2003;50(2):165–170. https://doi.org/10.1097/01.SAP.0000032305.93832.9B.

8

Allograft Tissues

ALBERTO J. PANERO, ALAN M. HIRAHARA, LUGA PODESTA, AMIR A. JAMALI, WYATT ANDERSEN, AND ALYSSA A. SMITH

Introduction

Allograft tissues are obtained from a donor source and transplanted into a different recipient or host, while autologous tissues are obtained and redirected into the same individual. Allograft tissue has been used in interventional orthopedics to provide structural support, act as a scaffold for the growth of new tissue, or initiate and regulate the body's innate healing response. Allografts offer several advantages over autografts. Use of an autologous tissue requires harvesting of the blood, bone, bone marrow, or adipose tissue, which can be painful, require additional time to process the tissue, and carry procedural risks not associated with allografts. Moreover, allograft tissues can provide patients with access to orthobiologic treatments when autologous are not feasible, such as in the setting of systemic comorbidities or when pharmacologic interactions may not allow for autologous harvesting.

The potential therapeutic benefits of allogenic tissues are apparent; however, their true cellular composition and role in clinical practice is still debated. Furthermore, potential risks of cellular allografts include contamination with bacteria during tissue processing or graft rejection as a result of the allograft's donor cell population persisting. The greatest risk of cell-based treatments is graft versus host disease. In large-scale allograft transplantation, a chimeric cell population has been noted in soft tissue transplants[1] and osteochondral allograft transplantation.[2] Fortunately, in some applications, the cellular allograft elements may exert their beneficial effects and subsequently be cleared from the recipient. The risk of disease is always possible when transplanting tissue from one source to another, and although rare, this possibility must always be considered when evaluating potential allograft products for clinical use.[3]

The goal of this chapter is to review the basic science, clinical applications, and logistic considerations of several allograft tissues within the spectrum of interventional orthopedic procedures.

Cellular Versus Acellular Allografts

Allografts in interventional orthopedics should be categorized as either cellular or acellular. For musculoskeletal purposes, cellular allografts theoretically contain living nucleated cells, including leukocytes, hematopoietic stem cells, or mesenchymal stem cells (MSCs), in addition to platelets, growth factors, and other cytokines. These tissues are typically derived from blood, bone marrow, adipose, or placental tissues. The MSC has traditionally been the focus of cellular allografts for interventional orthopedics. Outside of the United States, clinicians are allowed to isolate and expand cells like MSCs in culture prior to transplantation into a patient. Culture-expanded products contain a greater concentration of MSCs than their nonexpanded counterparts; however, this practice is not currently allowed within the United States per Food and Drug Administration (FDA) regulations and is considered more than "minimal manipulation."[4] Per current FDA regulations, use of biologic tissues must fall under the Human Cells, Tissues, and Tissue Based-Products (HCT/Ps) guidance reports[4]:

1. The HCT/P is minimally manipulated;
2. The HCT/P is intended for homologous use only, as reflected by the labeling, advertising, or other indications of the manufacturer's objective intent;
3. The manufacture of the HCT/P does not involve the combination of the cells or tissues with another article, except for water, crystalloids, or a sterilizing, preserving, or storage agent, provided that the addition of water, crystalloids, or the sterilizing, preserving, or storage agent does not raise new clinical safety concerns with respect to the HCT/P; and
4. Either:
   i. The HCT/P does not have a systemic effect and is not dependent upon the metabolic activity of living cells for its primary function; or

ii. The HCT/P has a systemic effect or is dependent upon the metabolic activity of living cells for its primary function, and:
  a. Is for autologous use;
  b. Is for allogeneic use in a first-degree or second-degree blood relative; or
  c. Is for reproductive use.

Acellular allografts are those that have been irradiated or processed in such a manner where the product contains no nucleated cells or the cells that are present are no longer viable. These products rely on growth factor and cytokine content to mediate the healing processes. The presence of various growth factors and cytokines can be tested by performing enzyme-linked immunosorbent assay (ELISA) and further confirmed with tests such as a Western blot analysis. Acellular allografts, like demineralized bone matrix (DBM), also have the capability to provide structural support or act as a scaffold for the proliferation of cellular components.

Placental-derived products (amnion, cord blood, Wharton jelly) and exosome preparations characterize this subset of acellular allogenic products. While these tissues are known to have or be associated with MSCs in vivo, commercial processing techniques have been shown to negatively affect the viability of these cells.[5] Therefore, even though these products possess the potential to stimulate healing, they should not be considered "stem cell therapies."

Despite being acellular, there are many growth factors and cytokines that are relevant to interventional orthopedics.[6] Growth factor and cytokine concentrations present in the allograft tissue may vary by the host donor tissues utilized. Additionally, the concentrations of growth factors and cytokines may also be altered by the time between tissue acquisition and processing, and administration by the clinician. Highlighted below are just some examples of these biomolecules along with their respective roles and functions.

Bone morphogenetic protein-2 (BMP-2)
- Induces chondrogenic and osteogenic differentiation
- Vital in regulating cell interactions
- Role in cartilage restoration has been theorized, but not thoroughly proven (fully elucidated

Platelet derived growth factor-β (PDGF-β)
- Accelerates extracellular matrix deposition and collagen formation
- Upon injury, stimulates influx of inflammatory factors and fibroblasts

Transforming growth factor-β1 (TGF-β1)
- Important mediator of tissue repair
- Released by platelets during acute injury response
- Influx to a wound is critical for macrophage and fibroblast chemotaxis

Interleukin-8 (IL-8)
- Induces neutrophil chemotaxis
- Increases vascular endothelial growth factor expression
- Secreted by monocytes in response to inflammatory stimuli

Vascular endothelial growth factor
- Potent stimulator of angiogenic cascade
- Regulates endothelial migration and proliferation
- Induces vascular permeability for increased nutrient delivery
- Promotes epithelization

The Mesenchymal Stem Cell

The name "mesenchymal stem cell," first coined in 1991,[7] has undergone multiple iterations. This is due, in part, to the fact that upon transplantation in clinical practice the cell may differentiate into the target tissue, but it is unclear whether the cell retains its stem capabilities. Recently, terms like "connective tissue progenitor cell,"[8] "mesenchymal stromal cell,"[9] and "medicinal signaling cell"[10] have been offered as successors to the term "mesenchymal stem cell" in hopes of more accurately representing the true capabilities and biology of this type of cell. As the terminology and precise role of these cells in clinical practice remains a topic for debate, we will utilize the traditional name "mesenchymal stem cell" (MSC) for the purposes of this chapter. The specific name notwithstanding, the International Society of Cellular Therapy (ISCT) has offered explicit criteria that must be met in order to be considered an MSC (Table 8.1).[9]

A tissue sample can be evaluated for MSCs by identifying nucleated cells using a hemocytometer or cell counter. The mere presence of cells in a sample does not indicate viability; fluorescent dyes and various assays need to be used to properly determine a cell's viability. Even so, clinicians should pay specific attention to the type of test and fluorescent marker used, as some dyes only indicate a cell's presence without regard to whether the cell is alive or dead. If viable cells have been identified, additional testing must be performed to confirm the presence of MSCs based on the definition put forth by the ISCT (see Table 8.1).[9] Simply assuming MSCs are present based on the expression or lack of expression of a single or few of the cluster of differentiation (CD) surface molecules can lead to an improper determination of MSC content in a given product.

MSCs are derived from various sources, either autologously or allogenically, and have been employed in animal and human studies for a variety of conditions in the nonoperative setting and as a surgical adjunct.[11–18] MSCs are perivascular cells that, when activated in response to injury, migrate to the damaged site and serve as the main repair modulator of the musculoskeletal system. Upon arrival, they secrete various trophic and immunomodulatory factors that direct the body's healing response. Clinically, isolating and applying multipotent MSCs can assist, or even generate, a healing cascade.

Autologous MSCs derived from bone marrow and adipose have been used to treat osteoarthritic conditions, particularly knee osteoarthritis[19–26]; however, autologous MSCs used in the setting of tendinopathies, bone pathologies, and other soft tissue injuries have also garnered attention.[27–33] Application of allogenic MSCs and other

TABLE 8.1 International Society of Cellular Therapy Definition of Mesenchymal Stromal Cells.

1. Display plastic-adherence in standard culture conditions
2. Capacity for tri-lineage differentiation into osteoblasts, adipocytes, or chondroblasts in vitro
3. Expression of: CD105, CD73, and CD90; Lack expression of: CD45, CD34, CD14 or CD11b, CD79α or CD19, and HLA-DR surface molecules

International Society of Cellular Therapy Mesenchymal Stromal Cell Definition. *CD*, Cluster of differentiation; *HLA-DR*, human leukocyte antigen–DR isotype.
From Dominici M, Le Blanc K, Mueller I, et al. Minimal criteria for defining multipotent mesenchymal stromal cells. The International Society for Cellular Therapy position statement. *Cytotherapy*. 2006;8(4):315–317.

biologics mimic those described in autologous studies, but a paucity of human studies using these products are present in the literature. There are numerous studies using animal models for the treatment of various muscular and tendon pathologies[34–37]; however, degenerative joint disease is the most thoroughly studied.[38–44]

In the few human trials available, the focus has been on osteoarthritis and these studies have demonstrated good results.[45–52] Allogenic tissues have also been used as surgical adjuncts in spinal fusions and osteochondritis dissecans (OCD).[53–55] The current literature for other soft tissue pathologies, including lateral epicondylitis, plantar fasciitis, Achilles tendinopathy, and meniscal injury is limited, but the initial studies are promising.[56–58] There is still a great degree of research to be done to properly evaluate the true potential of allogenic biologic therapies and to identify whether each donor source carries the same therapeutic potential.

Culture-Expanded Allografts

Culture-expanded allografts are an attractive source of MSC, due to the ability to deliver a homogenized product with a high yield of MSCs. MSCs have classically been derived from autologous bone marrow or adipose tissue; however, patients are not always amenable to these types of harvests. Autologous aspirations may not be possible for patients with significant comorbidities and may yield a collection with a heterogeneous cell population with varying volumes of MSCs. Allogeneic sources offer numerous advantages. Cells can be derived from bone marrow and adipose, as well as placental tissues like the amnion, chorion, or umbilical cord. The opportunity to expand cells prior to administration and deliver a standardized, homogeneous product with low immunogenic properties makes MSCs isolated from allogeneic sources an attractive therapeutic option.

MSCs can be isolated from various portions of the umbilical cord: Wharton jelly, umbilical cord blood, or the umbilical cord as a whole.[59–64] Umbilical cord blood has been shown to yield fewer total MSCs than those isolated from bone marrow, adipose tissue, Wharton jelly, or umbilical cord matrix.[65–70] Furthermore, isolation efficiency is significantly lower when attempting to expand MSCs from umbilical cord blood compared to the other sources.[66,69,71] Umbilical cord matrix MSCs have demonstrated faster doubling times than bone marrow isolates,[72] as well as displaying minimal to no deterioration in division and growth power, or senescence, after multiple cell expansion passages.[73,74] Reports on the proliferative capacities of various tissue sources are conflicting and continue to be debated in the literature.[66,69,71,72,75–78]

As MSCs can be derived from different sources, it must be considered whether these various isolates carry the same biologic potential. It has been well established that MSCs expanded from adult and neonatal tissues have the capacity for chondrogenic differentiation; however, the capability for osteogenic and adipogenic differentiation is less consistent across cell sources. MSCs derived from adult bone marrow or adipose tissue have been thoroughly established to have tri-lineage differentiation,[66,79,80] and cells isolated from Wharton jelly have been shown to exhibit similar differentiation capacities to adult bone marrow.[78,81] Umbilical cord matrix MSCs have also proven capable of tri-lineage differentiation.[72] MSCs expanded from the amniotic membrane have displayed poor adipogenic and superior osteogenic differentiation capabilities compared to those derived from the chorionic plate, which have exhibited superior adipogenicity and poor osteogenicity.[78,82] Umbilical cord blood-derived MSCs represent the most conflicting source of cells. It has been confirmed these MSCs have the capability of adequate osteogenic and chondrogenic differentiation, with reports of reduced matrix formation,[67] but their capacity for adipogenicity is debated in the literature (Table 8.2).[66,67,69,83]

Neonatal tissues have been suggested to be the optimal sources of MSCs compared to adult tissues due to a theoretically greater capacity for expansion, differentiation, and engraftment.[60,84–86] Ultimately, Wharton jelly may be the most promising source of MSCs for musculoskeletal tissue engineering due to its cellular yield, immunocompatability, proliferative capacity, and noninvasive collection procedure.[78,87]

Cellular expansion has classically been completed in a two-dimensional (2D) monolayer characterized by repeated culturing of stem cells in plates or flasks. These methods ultimately lead to cell senescence and diminished multipotent capabilities. As such, three-dimensional (3D) culture systems have been developed, including perfusion cell systems,[88] rotatory culture systems,[89] stirred suspension systems,[90] and microcarrier systems.[91–94] These 3D expansion techniques are simple, reproducible, efficient, and offer advantages not observed in 2D systems. 3D cultures more favorably mimic the in vivo microenvironment of stem cells and ultimately increase their therapeutic potential.[95–97] These systems are not influenced by substrate attachments as heavily as 2D systems, which improves cellular fortitude

TABLE 8.2 **Tri-lineage Differentiation Capacity of Mesenchymal Stem Cells Isolated From Various Tissue Sources.**

Tissue Source	Chondrogenic	Adipogenic	Osteogenic
BM	+	+	+
AT	+	+	+
WJ	+	+	+
AM	+	–	+
CP	+	+	–
UCB	+	±	+

AM, Amniotic membrane; *AT*, adipose tissue; *BM*, bone marrow; *CP*, chorionic plate; *UCB*, umbilical cord blood; *WJ*, Wharton jelly. +, Significant capacity for differentiation; –, poor or absent capacity for differentiation; ±, inconclusive capacity for differentiation.

and differentiation capacity.[95,98] Additionally, they exhibit numerous advantages at the genomic level.[96,99] Expression of OCT4, SOX2, NANOG, and C-MYC is better maintained in 3D culturing systems than 2D.[96,99] These core transcription factors develop networks that preserve stem cells' pluripotent state and capacity for self-renewal, are found in various sources of MSCs, and gradually disappear as cells are continuously cultured.[96,99] MSCs isolated from bone marrow have been shown to demonstrate a greater expression of these transcription factors than Wharton jelly or umbilical cord blood.[69]

While there are studies that show that higher quantities of autologous MSCs yield better clinical results,[14] this premise has not yet been substantiated. It is theorized that allogenic cells may be immune evasive, but not immune privileged and after transplantation eventually get removed by the host immune system. The closer a donor is to a human leukocyte antigen (HLA) match the more likely cells are to survive. Their potential therapeutic effects may be reduced as they have less time to secrete their paracrine factors. It would be unlikely that these allogenic cells could differentiate successfully to target tissue, as they may be removed by the host prior to differentiation.[100,101] Furthermore, clinical evidence supporting the use of culture-expanded autologous or allogenic MSC grafts over nonculture-expanded MSC grafts for musculoskeletal disease is not currently available. It is worth again emphasizing that culture-expansion of MSCs is not currently allowed in clinical practice in the United States.

Placental-Derived Allografts

Amniotic Tissue

The placental membrane is composed of the outer chorion and the thin, innermost amniotic membrane (Fig. 8.1). The amniotic membrane, in conjunction with the amniotic fluid, envelop the developing fetus and provide nutritional, immunomodulatory, and structural benefits.[102–105] Stem cells present in the amniotic membrane contribute and interact with the developing innate and adaptive immune systems in part by hindering leukocyte differentiation into dendritic cells and diminishing T-cell proliferation.[102] The amniotic membrane and fluid also have numerous antimicrobial and antiviral effects.[102,106–113] The amniotic membrane and amniotic fluid have been identified in vivo as substantial sources of pluripotent and MSCs, and are considered advantageous due to minimal ethical concerns regarding the harvest of these tissues.[105,114–119] Cells derived from amniotic tissues have been used to treat human skin wounds,[120] induce corneal reepithelization,[121] and promote neochondrogenesis and peripheral nerve regeneration.[122,123] The pluri- and multipotent potential of these cells have made amniotic tissues attractive sources of MSCs in orthopedic tissue regeneration.[105,114–119]

While the amniotic membrane can be used intraoperatively in the form of tissue sheets, the membrane can also be lyophilized and pulverized to particulate matter and used as an injectable. These products are often a combination of amniotic membrane and umbilical cord tissue and have functioned as an anti-inflammatory, anti-scarring, and regenerative agent.[124–133] A primary therapeutic efficacy of amniotic membrane-umbilical cord tissue is due to its unique biochemical complex: heavy chain-hyaluronan-PTX3 (HC-HA/PTX3). This complex assists in the promotion of macrophage phagocytic activity,[126] neutrophil apoptosis,[124,126] and suppression of TGF-β activity.[130,134] The amniotic membrane-umbilical cord products are received in a solid state. These can be stored at room temperature in the office, have a longer shelf life, and are reconstituted with saline prior to transplantation.

Amniotic fluid is typically harvested at the time of birth or in the second trimester, and is known to contain a heterogeneous population of cells in vivo, including MSCs.[117,119,135,136] The composition of the amniotic fluid varies dependent on the gestational age at the time of harvest,[137] which likely affects the therapeutic potential of the tissue. Typically, the commercial fluid preparations are cryopreserved at −80°C and are shipped to the provider overnight in dry ice. Upon receipt, the product must be thawed out and transplanted into patient. Alternatively, the clinic may store the product in a freezer at −80°C until ready for use.

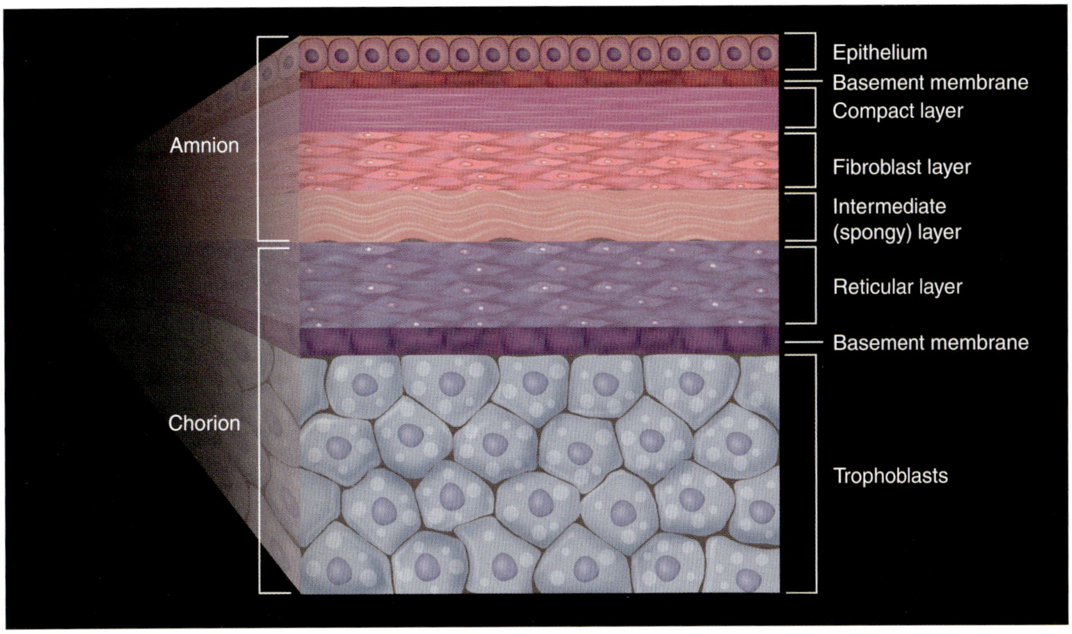

• **Fig. 8.1** Anatomy of Amniotic and Chorionic Tissue Layers of the Placenta.

Umbilical Cord Blood

Umbilical cord blood is a rich source of progenitor cells that has the potential to be used as a therapeutic.[138] Hematopoietic progenitor and stem cells from cord blood have a high recovery efficiency even after years of cryopreservation.[139] First used to treat hematologic malignancies,[140] umbilical cord blood is currently being explored for orthopedic applications. Cord blood has been employed in surgical cartilage repair with promising results when used in conjunction with a hyaluronate hydrogel,[141] allowing clinicians to theorize about its use in nonsurgical interventions. The main limitations of the use of cord blood are the current need for HLA matching as well as the risk of graft versus host disease.[142]

Wharton Jelly

Wharton jelly, the connective tissue of the umbilical cord, has also gained increasing interest as a potential source of stem and progenitor cells. Compositionally, Wharton jelly is agreed to have progenitor populations in the various tissue layers; however, there is no consensus on whether the cells in the regions are phenotypically identical.[143,144] It has been postulated that the MSCs derived from Wharton jelly originate as perivascular cells, but recent literature has brought this assertion into question.[143] Similar to umbilical cord blood, Wharton jelly as a source of MSCs is currently being examined in interventional orthopedics. There are currently registered clinical trials underway for its use for a variety of orthopedic conditions.

The true capacity for these tissues to deliver MSCs as commercial products have come into question as it is unclear whether commercial processing, including tissue preservation and storage, affects the viability of cells in the products.[5,145–147] In an analysis of commercial amniotic fluid products, it was found that those advertised as "stem cell" and cellular products either did not contain any cells, or if cells were present, were unable to be cultured to an appreciable level.[5] Known to be a potent source of growth factors and cytokines in vivo, the products were found to retain a number of these biomolecules—although the specific proteins present and volume of each varied across products. Such studies indicate that the therapeutic potential of allogenic amnion-derived products likely does not depend solely on cellular viability.[5,145–148] While the content of MSCs in commercial products is debatable,[5] both amniotic membrane and amniotic fluid-derived products offer the opportunity to deliver growth factors and cytokines that can be used to treat a variety of orthopedic injuries. While the legal aspects regarding the use of such products are largely outside of the scope of this section, the concepts of minimal manipulation and homologous use as laid out by the FDA still apply.[4] The processing and packaging methods of the amniotic membrane must be considered. Methods that compromise the original relevant characteristics of the tissue may change the product's consideration as an HCT/P. Furthermore, while cells derived from secreted body fluids like amniotic fluid are considered HCT/Ps, the body fluids themselves are generally not considered HCT/Ps.[4] Human clinical evidence on these commercial products for safety and efficacy for orthopedic issues is lacking as well.

Exosomes

Use of allogenic and autologous MSCs in interventional orthopedics has failed to completely fulfill clinical expectations due to concern over a lack of cell differentiation, loss of cells, and poor engraftment at target sites.[149,150] Research regarding the structure, makeup, physiologic, and pathologic function of the numerous substances secreted by MSCs (secretomes) has exponentially increased over the past several years. These unique MSC secretomes have anti-apoptotic and immunoregulatory properties and have been utilized for a wide variety of diagnostic and therapeutic applications.[151]

Secretomes have both a vesicular and soluble part. The vesicular components secreted by MSCs are categorized as extracellular vesicles, and further subcategorized based on cellular origin, size, and biologic function.[152,153] A variety of extracellular vesicle subtypes have been described, including exosome, microvesicles, membrane particles, peptides, and cytokines. Exosomes are small, spherical particles (70 to 150 nm) that are enclosed by a phospholipid bilayer and capable of passing through a 0.1-µm filter.[154] They were first described by Pan and Johnstone in 1983[155] and were initially believed to eliminate unwanted cellular components and waste during sheep reticulocyte maturation.[155,156] Recently, exosomes have received a great deal of interest due to their role in intracellular communication and immunomodulatory function, and their potential for use in identifying and treating a variety of disease states.[150,151]

Exosomes originate from the cell membrane by endocytic internalization (budding inward). The most well-established mechanism of exosome biogenesis has three stages: the endosomes stage, the multivesicular bodies (MVBs) stage, and the exosomes stage.[157] First, endocytic vessels are transferred to early endosomes—tube-like structures that are located near the outer edge of the cytoplasm. Early endosomes eventually mature into late endosomes, which are more spherical and located closer to the nucleus of the cell. Late endosomes, or MVBs, carry intraluminal vesicles that contain a variety of biomolecules, including proteins, lipids, and various types of RNAs. In the second stage, MVBs are either degraded by fusing with lysosomes or transported to the cell's plasma membrane. Upon fusion with the plasma membrane, the MVB releases its contents into the extracellular space as exosomes—completing the third stage.[153] In the extracellular space, recipient cells take up exosomes through paracrine or juxtracrine actions (exosomal fusion) or endocytosis (Fig. 8.2).[158]

The function and composition of exosomes are highly dependent on the physiologic state of the parent MSCs, where the MSCs are derived from, and the medium in which the MSCs are grown.[159,160] Exosomes act as cellular messengers conveying information to distant tissues through proteins and genetic material contained within that can ultimately alter the recipient cell's physiology and function. Exosomes can be released by most cell types, normal and pathologic, and are present in conditioned cell medium in vitro, especially when derived from MSCs.[161] They are stable in biologic fluids including blood, urine, saliva, breast milk, synovial fluid, and amniotic fluid.[158] The majority of exosomes express surface protein Alix; Tsg 101; and

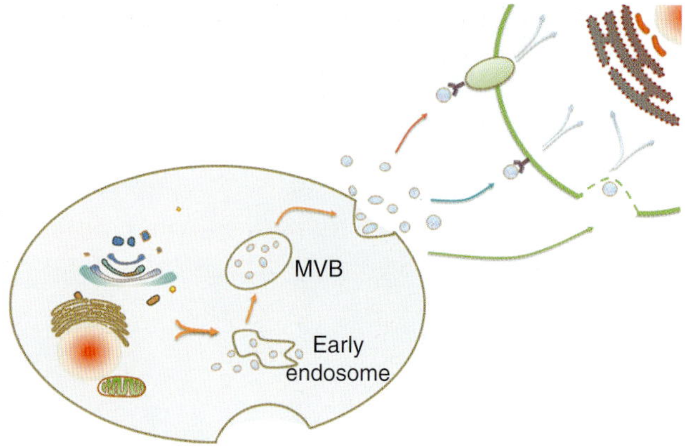

• **Fig. 8.2** The Formation and Mechanism of Exosomes. Exosomes originate through endocytic internalization and follow three stages: the endosomes stage, the multivesicular bodies *(MVBs)* stage, and the exosomes stage. When exosomes are released from the cell, they act as intercellular communication molecules that interact with cell receptors and elicit various actions. (Image retrieved from Ju C, Liu R, Zhang Y, et al. Exosomes may be the potential new direction of research in osteoarthritis management. *Biomed Res Int*. 2019. https://doi.org/10.1155/2019/7695768.)

transmembrane proteins CD9, CD63, and CD81, in addition to other proteins.[150,154]

To be able to utilize exosomes for diagnostic or therapeutic applications, it will become necessary to establish efficient and effective methods to isolate exosomes with minimal alteration to their structure and/or content.[150] Additionally, it is imperative to identify and only isolate exosomes with the desired trait. Several isolation methods have been developed and are currently in use.[150,162]

The currently accepted gold standard for isolation of exosomes involves differential ultracentrifugation. This is performed by applying sequentially increasing centrifugal forces to a solution with exosomes to separate them from cells, large debris, and organelles.[163] Ultracentrifugation is typically used in combination with sucrose density gradients or sucrose cushions to remove contaminants with densities different from exosomes. This method produces high-purity exosomal preparations,[164] but is limited to only generating exosome-enriched samples. Pure exosome isolates are difficult to obtain due to the large number of similar-sized nanoparticles in samples.

As research continues to expand our knowledge regarding these cellular secretions, exosomes have the potential to become a truly disease-modifying orthobiologic drug with a number of clinical benefits. As a therapeutic tool, exosomes could potentially be produced and available as an "off-the-shelf" product with a defined composition, potency, and dose. These products could provide immediate bioavailability of the active allogenic agents, with consistent content and quality independent of the patient's age and underlying health.[165]

Based on basic science research, exosomes exhibit a range of biologic capabilities including regulation of angiogenesis and apoptosis, antigen presentation, and endocytosis.[166] Through their miRNA contents, exosomes have the potential to regulate chondrocyte apoptosis and promote cartilage proliferation in the setting of osteoarthritis.[167–169] In tendinopathies, the therapeutic application of exosomes has been shown to promote tendon healing by establishing a balanced microenvironment and increasing the expression of tenogenic markers.[170] The ability of exosomes to play a crucial role in cell-to-cell signaling and mediate disease responses make them attractive options in regenerative medicine.

The legal considerations regarding these products remain out of the scope of this text; however, it should be noted that there are currently no FDA-approved exosome products. Given that these products require cell culture expansion, they are regulated as a drug as opposed to an HCT/P and are not approved for clinical use in the United States. Furthermore, to date there are no current human clinical trials evaluating the efficacy or safety of exosome treatments for any condition.

Of note, extracellular vesicles and exosomes have also been studied diagnostically. The presence of exosome-derived lncRNA has the potential to function as an indicator of osteoarthritis progression.[171] Disease-state biomarkers are often low in bodily fluids and can be masked by other proteins in the sample. Extracellular vesicles can reflect the biologic state of the host cell, and if isolated have the potential to prove information of various disease states. While exosomes have immense potential diagnostically and are an ideal choice for biomarker analysis, this field is also still in its infancy make them.[170]

Demineralized Bone Matrix

One of the most powerful tools in interventional orthopedics is in the percutaneous treatment of skeletal defects associated with fracture nonunion, osseous cysts, and avascular necrosis. In these conditions, the capacity for bone healing is diminished and, as a result, it is necessary to deliver bone grafts. Bone grafts are generally considered along two spectrums: osteoconductive and osteoinductive. Osteoconductivity refers to the ability of the material to act as a scaffold for the ingrowth of vessels and osteoprogenitor cells.[172,173] Osteoinductivity is the ability to promote the mitogenesis and differentiation of nearby cells into the osteogenic lineage.[173–176] Bone grafts employing these factors must be combined with an appropriate source of progenitor cells that are either found in vivo in the surrounding perivascular tissue or delivered concurrently with the graft.[172]

Autologous iliac crest bone graft is widely considered the gold standard in bone grafting of skeletal defects. It possesses all three characteristics of osteoconductivity, osteoinductivity, and osteogenic cells.[173] Unfortunately, donor site morbidity and the high costs of graft harvesting can be limiting. Furthermore, iliac crest bone grafts are not easily delivered percutaneously. A valuable alternative to autogenous bone is the use of DBM (Fig. 8.3). DBM is manufactured by acid digestion of bone, leading to a combination of collagens (predominantly type I), noncollagenous proteins, residual calcium phosphate, and residual cellular debris.[175] DBM has a long history of clinical use dating back more than a century.[177] The decalcification process used in the preparation of DBM causes the release of bone morphogenetic proteins into the surrounding tissue when it is implanted, leading to the osteoinductive properties of the material.[176]

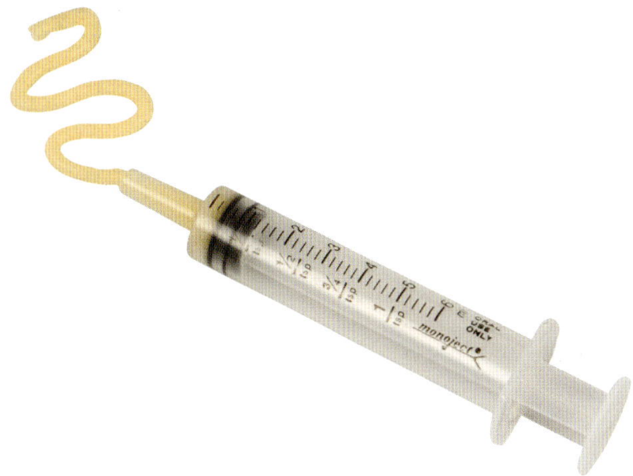

• **Fig. 8.3** StimuBlast (Arthrex, Inc., Naples, FL), a demineralized bone matrix allograft product, can be used in minimally invasive procedures with a wide range of clinical applications.

In its pure form, DBM exists as a powder. This form is difficult for the clinician to control and to conform to various skeletal defects. As a result, DBM is often combined with a number of carrier materials. These carrier materials are divided into two broad categories. The first category is composed of polymer materials such as collagen, chitosan, hyaluronic acid, or carboxymethylcellulose; the second category is characterized by low molecular weight carriers such as glycerol, calcium sulfate, and bioactive glass.[173] The carrier materials have specific advantages based on biocompatibility, viscosity, and rates of resorption. For most interventional orthopedic procedures, the selected DBM should strike the balance of viscosity, in order to be injectable, but also to be physically viscous enough to remain at the delivery site to exert its effect.

The clinical applications of the DBM were initially limited to open surgeries.[174,178–180] The percutaneous use of DBM was first reported in the treatment of simple bone cysts.[181–183] More recently, DBM has been explored in the augmentation of core decompression for the treatment of avascular necrosis of the femoral head.[184,185] The value of DBM in minimally invasive surgery has been expanded using both arthroscopic treatment of degenerative bone cysts[186] as well as the percutaneous treatment of degenerative bone cysts.[187,188]

In the future, we anticipate that DBM will remain an excellent option for the delivery of osteoinductive and osteoconductive bone grafts through minimally invasive techniques in combination with an extensive array of carriers and cell populations.

References

1. Starzl TE, Demetris AJ, Trucco M, et al. Systemic chimerism in human female recipients of male livers. *Lancet.* 1992;340(8824):876–877.
2. Jamali AA, Hatcher SL, You Z. Donor survival in a fresh osteochondral allograft at twenty-nine years. A case report. *J Bone Joint Surg Am.* 2007;89(1):166–169.
3. Hinsenkamp M, Muylle L, Eastlund T, Fehily D, Noel L, Strong DM. Adverse reactions and events related to musculoskeletal allografts: reviewed by the World Health Organisation Project NOTIFY. *Int Orthop.* 2012;36(3):633–641.
4. Food and Drug Administration. Regulatory Considerations for Human Cells, Tissues, and Cellular and Tissue-Based Products: Minimal Manipulation and Homologous Use. FDA-2017-D-6146. https://www.fda.gov/regulatory-information/search-fda-guidance-documents/regulatory-considerations-human-cells-tissues-and-cellular-and-tissue-based-products-minimal. Published December 2017. Accessed November 4, 2019.
5. Panero AJ, Hirahara AM, Andersen WJ, Rothenberg J, Fierro F. Are amniotic fluid products stem cell therapies? A study of amniotic fluid preparations for mesenchymal stem cells with bone marrow comparison. *Am J Sports Med.* 2019;47(5):1230–1235.
6. Bashir J, Panero AJ, Sherman AL. The emerging use of platelet-rich plasma in musculoskeletal medicine. *J Am Osteopath Assoc.* 2015;115(1):24–31.
7. Caplan AI. Mesenchymal stem cells. *J Orthop Res.* 1991;9(5):641–650.
8. Muschler GF, Midura RJ. Connective tissue progenitors: practical concepts for clinical applications. *Clin Orthop Relat Res.* 2002;395:66–80.
9. Dominici M, Le Blanc K, Mueller I, et al. Minimal criteria for defining multipotent mesenchymal stromal cells. The International Society for Cellular Therapy position statement. *Cytotherapy.* 2006;8(4):315–317.
10. Caplan AI. Mesenchymal stem cells: time to change the name! *Stem Cells Transl Med.* 2017;l6(6):1445–1451.
11. Ellera Gomes JL, da Silva RC, Silla LM, Abreu MR, Pellanda R. Conventional rotator cuff repair complemented by the aid of mononuclear autologous stem cells. *Knee Surg Sports Traumatol Arthrosc.* 2012;20(2):373–377.
12. Freitag J, Li D, Wickham J, Shah K, Tenen A. Effect of autologous adipose-derived mesenchymal stem cell therapy in the treatment of a post-traumatic chondral defect of the knee. *BMJ Case Rep.* 2017. https://doi.org/10.1136/bcr-2017-220852.
13. Freitag J, Ford J, Bates D, et al. Adipose derived mesenchymal stem cell therapy in the treatment of isolated knee chondral lesions: design of a randomized controlled pilot study comparing arthroscopic microfracture versus arthroscopic microfracture combined with postoperative mesenchymal stem cell injections. *BMJ Open.* 2015;5(12):e009332. https://doi.org/10.1136/bmjopen-2015-009332.
14. Hernigou P, Flouzat Lachaniette CH, Delambre J, et al. Biologic augmentation of rotator cuff repair with mesenchymal stem cells during arthroscopy improves healing and prevents further tears: a case-controlled study. *Int Orthop.* 2014;38(9):1811–1818.
15. Kim YS, Sung CH, Chung SH, Kwak SJ, Koh YG. Does an injection of adipose-derived mesenchymal stem cells loaded with fibrin glue influence rotator cuff repair outcomes? A clinical and magnetic resonance imaging study. *Am J Sports Med.* 2017;45(9):2010–2018.
16. Shapiro SA, Kazmerchak SE, Heckman MG, Zubair AC, O'Connor MI. A prospective, single-blind, placebo-controlled trial of bone marrow aspirate concentrate for knee osteoarthritis. *Am J Sports Med.* 2017;45(1):82–90.
17. Stein BE, Stroh DA, Schon LC. Outcomes of acute Achilles tendon rupture repair with bone marrow aspirate concentrate augmentation. *Int Orthop.* 2015;29(5):901–905.
18. Usuelli FG, Grassi M, Maccario C, et al. Intratendinous adipose-derived stromal vascular fraction (SVF) injection provides a safe, efficacious treatment for Achilles tendinopathy: results of a randomized controlled clinical trial at a 6-month follow-up. *Knee Surg Sports Traumatol Arthrosc.* 2018;26(7):2000–2010.
19. Centeno CJ, Al-Sayegh H, Bashir J, Goodyear S, Freeman MD. A prospective multi-site registry study of a specific protocol of autologous bone marrow concentrate for the treatment of shoulder rotator cuff tears and osteoarthritis. *J Pain Res.* 2015;8:269–276. https://doi.org/10.2147/JPR.S80872.
20. Chahla J, Dean CS, Moatshe G, Pascual-Garrido C, Serra Cruz R, LaPrade RF. Concentrated bone marrow aspirate for the treatment of chondral injuries and osteoarthritis of the knee: a systematic review of outcomes. *Orthop J Sports Med.* 2016;4(1):2325967115625481. https://doi.org/10.1177/2325967115625481.
21. Di Matteo B, Vandenbulcke F, Vitale ND, et al. Minimally manipulated mesenchymal stem cells for the treatment of knee osteoarthritis: a systematic review of clinical evidence. *Stem Cells Int.* 2019:1735242. https://doi.org/10.1155/2019/1735242.
22. Jo CH, Chai JW, Jeong EC, et al. Intra-articular injection of mesenchymal stem cells for the treatment of osteoarthritis of the knee: a 2-year follow-up study. *Am J Sports Med.* 2017;45(12):2774–2783.
23. Kim SH, Ha CW, Park YV, Nam E, Lee JE, Lee HJ. Intra-articular injection of mesenchymal stem cells for clinical outcomes and cartilage repair in osteoarthritis of the knee: a meta-analysis of randomized controlled trials. *Arch Orthop Trauma Surg.* 2019;139(7):971–980.
24. Lu L, Dai C, Zhang Z, et al. Treatment of knee osteoarthritis with intra-articular injection of autologous adipose-derived mesenchymal progenitor cells: a prospective, randomized, double-blind, active-controlled, phase IIb clinical trial. *Stem Cell Res Ther.* 2019;10(1):143. https://doi.org/10.1186/s13287-019-1248-3.
25. Mautner K, Bowers R, Easley K, Fausel Z, Robinson R. Functional outcomes following microfragmented adipose tissue versus bone marrow aspirate concentrate injections for symptomatic knee osteoarthritis. *Stem Cells Transl Med.* 2019;8(11):1149–1156.
26. Ozeki N, Muneta T, Koga H, et al. Not single but periodic injections of synovial mesenchymal stem cells maintain viable cells in knees and inhibit osteoarthritis progression in rats. *Osteoarthritis Cartilage.* 2016;24(6):1061–1070.
27. Campbell KJ, Boykin RE, Wijdicks CA, Erik Giphart J, LaPrade RF, Philippon MJ. Treatment of a hip capsular injury in a professional soccer player with platelet-rich plasma and bone marrow aspirate concentrate therapy. *Knee Surg Sports Traumatol Arthrosc.* 2013;21(7):1684–1688.
28. Pak J. Autologous adipose tissue-derived stem cells induce persistent bone-like tissue in osteonecrotic femoral heads. *Pain Physician.* 2012;15(1):75–85.
29. Pak J. Regeneration of human bones in hip osteonecrosis and human cartilage in knee osteoarthritis with autologous

adipose-tissue-derived stem cells: a case series. *J Med Case Rep.* 2011;5:296. https://doi.org/10.1186/1752-1947-5-296.
30. Pak J, Lee JH, Lee SH. Regenerative repair of damaged meniscus with autologous adipose tissue-derived stem cells. *Biomed Res Int.* 2014. https://doi.org/10.1155/2014/436029.
31. Pascual-Garrido C, Rolon A, Makino A. Treatment of chronic patellar tendinopathy with autologous bone marrow stem cells: a 5-year-followup. *Stem Cells Int.* 2012. https://doi.org/10.1155/2012/953510.
32. Singh A, Gangwar DS, Singh S. Bone marrow injection: a novel treatment for tennis elbow. *J Nat Sci Biol Med.* 2014;5(2):389–391.
33. Wyles CC, Houdek MT, Crespo-Diaz RJ, et al. Adipose-derived mesenchymal stem cells are phenotypically superior for regeneration in the setting of osteonecrosis of the femoral head. *Clin Orthop Relat Res.* 2015;473(10):3080–3090.
34. Gulecyuz MF, Macha K, Pietschmann MF, et al. Allogenic myocytes and mesenchymal stem cells partially improve fatty rotator cuff degeneration in a rat model. *Stem Cells Rev Rep.* 2018;14(6):847–859.
35. McDougall RA, Canapp SO, Canapp DA. Ultrasonographic findings in 41 dogs treated with bone marrow aspirate concentrate and platelet-rich plasma for a supraspinatus tendinopathy: a retrospective study. *Front Vet Sci.* 2018;5:98. https://doi.org/10.3389/fvets.2018.00098.
36. Muttini A, Russo V, Rossi E, et al. Pilot experimental study on amniotic epithelial mesenchymal cell transplantation in natural occurring tendinpathy in horses. Ultrasonographic and histological comparison. *Muscles Ligaments Tendons J.* 2015;5(1):5–11.
37. Ricco S, Renzi S, Del Bue M, et al. Allogeneic adipose tissue-derived mesenchymal stem cells in combination with platelet rich plasma are safe and effective in the therapy of superficial digital flexor tendonitis in the horse. *Int J Immunopathol Pharmacol.* 2013;26(suppl 1):61–68.
38. Broeckx SY, Seys B, Suls M, et al. Equine allogeneic chondrogenic induced mesenchymal stem cells are an effective treatment for degenerative joint disease in horses. *Stem Cells Dev.* 2019;28(6):410–422.
39. Chiang ER, Ma HL, Wang JP, Liu CL, Chen TH, Hung SC. Allogeneic mesenchymal stem cells in combination with hyaluronic acid for the treatment of osteoarthritis in rabbits. *PLoS One.* 2016;11(2):e0149835. https://doi.org/10.1371/journal.pone.0149835.
40. Feng C, Luo X, He N, et al. Efficacy and persistence of allogeneic adipose-derived mesenchymal stem cells combined with hyaluronic acid in osteoarthritis after intra-articular injection in a sheep model. *Tissue Eng Part A.* 2018;24(3-4):219–233.
41. Marinas-Pardo L, Garcia-Castro J, Rodriguez-Hurtado I, Rodriguez-Garcia MI, Nunez-Naveira L, Hermida-Prieto M. Allogeneic adipose-derived mesenchymal stem cells (Horse Allo 20) for the treatment of osteoarthritis-associated lameness in horses: characterization, safety, and efficacy of intra-articular treatment. *Stem Cells Dev.* 2018;27(17):1147–1160.
42. Marino-Martinez IA, Martinez-Castro AG, Pena-Martinez VM, et al. Human amniotic membrane intra-articular injection prevents cartilage damage in an osteoarthritis model. *Exp Ther Med.* 2019;17(1):11–16.
43. Xia T, Yu F, Zhang K, et al. The effectiveness of allogeneic mesenchymal stem cells therapy for knee osteoarthritis in pigs. *Ann Transl Med.* 2018;6(20):404. https://doi.org/10.21037/atm.2018.09.55.
44. Yang X, Zhu TY, Wen LC, et al. Intraarticular injection of allogenic mesenchymal stem cells has a protective role for the osteoarthritis. *Chin Med J (Engl).* 2015;128(18):2516–2523.
45. Bhattacharya N. *Clinical Use of Amniotic Fluid in Osteoarthritis: A Source of Cell Therapy. Regenerative Medicine Using Pregnancy-Specific Biological Substances.* London: Springer-Verlag; 2011. https://doi.org/10.1007/978-1-84882-718-9_38.
46. Castellanos R, Tighe S. Injectable amniotic membrane/umbilical cord particulate for knee osteoarthritis: a prospective, single-center pilot study. *Pain Med.* 2019. https://doi.org/10.1093/pm/pnz143.
47. Gupta PK, Chullikana A, Rengasamy M, et al. Efficacy and safety of adult human bone marrow-derived, cultured, pooled, allogeneic mesenchymal stromal cells (Stempeucel®): preclinical and clinical trial in osteoarthritis of the knee joint. *Arthritis Res Ther.* 2016;18(1):301.
48. O'Brien D, Kia C, Beebe R, et al. Evaluating the effects of platelet-rich plasma and amniotic viscous fluid on inflammatory markers in a human coculture model for osteoarthritis. *Arthroscopy.* 2019;35(8):2421–2433.
49. Preitschopf A, Zwicki H, Li K, et al. Chondrogenic differentiation of amniotic fluid stem cells and their potential for regenerative therapy. *Stem Cell Rev Rep.* 2012;8(4):1267–1274.
50. Raines AL, Shih MS, Chua L, Su CW, Tseng SC, O'Connell J. Efficacy of particulate amniotic membrane and umbilical cord tissues in attenuating cartilage destruction in an osteoarthritis model. *Tissue Eng Part A.* 2017;23(1-2):12–19.
51. Vega A, Martin-Perrero MA, Del Canto F, et al. Treatment of knee osteoarthritis with allogeneic bone marrow mesenchymal stem cells: a randomized controlled trial. *Transplantation.* 2015;99(8):1681–1690.
52. Willett NJ, Thote T, Lin AS, et al. Intra-articular injection of micronized dehydrated human amnion/chorion membrane attenuates osteoarthritis development. *Arthritis Res Ther.* 2014;16(1):R47. https://doi.org/10.1186/ar4476.
53. Anderson JJ, Swayzee Z. The use of human amniotic allograft on osteochondritis dissecans of the talar dome: a comparison with and without allografts in arthroscopically treated ankles. *Surgical Science.* 2015;6(9):412–417.
54. Nunley PD, Kerr 3rd EJ, Utter PA, et al. Preliminary results of bioactive amniotic suspension with allograft for achieving one and two-level lumbar interbody fusion. *Int J Spine Surg.* 2016;10:12. https://doi.org/10.14444/3012.
55. Sclafani JA, Liang K, Mosley D, Prevost M. A retrospective chart assessment of clinical outcomes after amniotic suspension allograft is used during spinal arthrodesis procedures. *Surgical Science.* 2016;7(7):150–156.
56. Lee SY, Kim W, Lim C, Chugn SG. Treatment of lateral epicondylosis by using allogeneic adipose-derived mesenchymal stem cells: a pilot study. *Stem Cells.* 2015;33(10):2995–3005.
57. Vangsness Jr CT, Farr 2nd J, Boyd J, Dellaero DT, Mills CR, LeRoux-Williams M. Adult human mesenchymal stem cells delivered via intra-articular injection to the knee following partial medial meniscectomy: a randomized, double-blind, controlled study. *J Bone Joint Surg Am.* 2014;96(2):90–98.
58. Werber B. Amniotic tissues for the treatment of chronic plantar fasciosis and Achilles tendinosis. *J Sports Med (Hindawi Publ Corp).* 2015:219896. https://doi.org/10.1155/2015/219896.

59. Can A, Karahuseyinoglu S. Concise review: human umbilical cord stroma with regard to the source of fetus-derived stem cells. *Stem Cells*. 2007;25(11):2886–2895.
60. Hass R, Kasper C, Bohm S, Jacobs R. Different populations and sources of human mesenchymal stem cells (MSC): a comparison of adult and neonatal tissue-derived MSC. *Cell Commun Signal*. 2011;9:12. https://doi.org/10.1186/1478-811X-9-12.
61. Karahuseyinoglu S, Cinar O, Kilic E, et al. Biology of stem cells in human umbilical cord stroma: in situ and in vitro surveys. *Stem Cells*. 2007;25(2):319–331.
62. Majore I, Moretti P, Stahl F, Hass R, Kasper C. Growth and differentiation properties of mesenchymal stromal cell populations derived from whole human umbilical cord. *Stem Cell Rev Rep*. 2011;7(1):17–31.
63. McNiece IK, Almeida-Porada G, Shpall EJ, Zanjani E. Ex vivo expanded cord blood cells provide rapid engraftment in fetal sheep but lack long-term engrafting potential. *Exp Hematol*. 2002;30(6):612–616.
64. Wang HS, Hung SC, Peng ST, et al. Mesenchymal stem cells in the Wharton's jelly of the human umbilical cord. *Stem Cells*. 2004;22(7):1330–1337.
65. Hatlapatka T, Moretti P, Lavrentieva A, et al. Optimization of culture conditions for the expansion of umbilical cord-derived mesenchymal stem or stromal cell-like cells using xeno-free culture conditions. *Tissue Eng Part C Methods*. 2011;17(4):485–493.
66. Kern S, Eichler H, Stoeve J, Kluter H, Bieback K. Comparative analysis of mesenchymal stem cells from bone marrow, umbilical cord blood, or adipose tissue. *Stem Cells*. 2006;24(5):1294–1301.
67. Montesinos JJ, Flores-Figueroa E, Castillo-Medina S, et al. Human mesenchymal stromal cells from adult and neonatal sources: comparative analysis of their morphology, immunophenotype, differentiation patterns and neural protein expression. *Cytotherapy*. 2009;11(2):163–176.
68. Moretti P, Hatlapatka T, Marten D, et al. Mesenchymal stromal cells derived from human umbilical cord tissues: primitive cells with potential for clinical and tissue engineering applications. *Adv Biochem Eng Biotechnol*. 2010;123:29–54. https://doi.org/10.1007/10_2009_15.
69. Secunda R, Vennila R, Mohanashankar AM, Rajasundari M, Jeswanth S, Surendran R. Isolation, expansion and characterization of mesenchymal stem cells from human bone marrow, adipose tissue, umbilical cord blood and matrix: a comparative study. *Cytotechnology*. 2015;67(5):793–807.
70. Zeddou M, Briquet A, Relic B, et al. The umbilical cord matrix is a better source of mesenchymal stem cells (MSC) than the umbilical cord blood. *Cell Biol Int*. 2010;34(7):693–701.
71. Rebelatto CK, Aguiar AM, Moretao MP, et al. Dissimilar differentiation of mesenchymal stem cells from bone marrow, umbilical cord blood, and adipose tissue. *Exp Biol Med (Maywood)*. 2008;233(7):901–913.
72. Lu LL, Liu YJ, Yang SG, et al. Isolation and characterization of human umbilical cord mesenchymal stem cells with hematopoiesis-supportive function and other potentials. *Haematologica*. 2006;91(8):1017–1026.
73. La Rocca G, Anzalone R, Corrao S, et al. Isolation and characterization of Oct-4+/HLA-G+ mesenchymal stem cells from human umbilical cord matrix: differentiation potential and detection of new markers. *Histochem Cell Biol*. 2009;131(2):267–282.
74. Weiss ML, Medicetty S, Bledsoe AR, et al. Human umbilical cord matrix stem cells: preliminary characterization and effect of transplantation in a rodent model of Parkinson's disease. *Stem Cells*. 2006;24(3):781–792.
75. Baksh D, Song L, Tuan RS. Adult mesenchymal stem cells: characterization, differentiation, and application in cell and gene therapy. *J Cell Mol Med*. 2004;8(3):301–316.
76. Baksh D, Yao R, Tuan RS. Comparison of proliferative and multilineage differentiation potential of human mesenchymal stem cells derived from umbilical cord and bone marrow. *Stem Cells*. 2007;25(6):1384–1392.
77. Chen MY, Lie PC, Li ZL, Wei X. Endothelial differentiation of Wharton's jelly-derived mesenchymal stem cells in comparison with bone marrow-derived mesenchymal stem cells. *Exp Hematol*. 2009;37(5):629–640.
78. Kim MJ, Shin KS, Jeon JH, et al. Human chorionic-plate-derived mesenchymal stem cells and Wharton's jelly-derived mesenchymal stem cells: a comparative analysis of their potential as placenta-derived stem cells. *Cell Tissue Res*. 2011;346(1):53–64.
79. Bieback K, Kern S, Kluter H, Eichler H. Critical parameters for the isolation of mesenchymal stem cells from umbilical cord blood. *Stem Cells*. 2004;22(4):625–634.
80. Wagner W, Wein F, Seckinger A, et al. Comparative characteristics of mesenchymal stem cells from human bone marrow, adipose tissue, and umbilical cord blood. *Exp Hematol*. 2005;33(11):1402–1416.
81. Hou T, Xu J, Wu X, et al. Umbilical cord Wharton's jelly: a new potential cell source of mesenchymal stromal cells for bone tissue engineering. *Tissue Eng Part A*. 2009;15(9):2325–2334.
82. Ma J, Wu J, Han L, et al. Comparative analysis of mesenchymal stem cells derived from amniotic membrane, umbilical cord, and chorionic plate under serum-free condition. *Stem Cell Res Ther*. 2019;10(1):19. https://doi.org/10.1186/s13287-018-1104-x.
83. Chang YJ, Shih DT, Tseng CP, Hsieh TB, Lee DC, Hwang SM. Disparate mesenchyme-lineage tendencies in mesenchymal stem cells from human bone marrow and umbilical cord blood. *Stem Cells*. 2006;24(3):679–685.
84. Barlow S, Brook G, Chatterjee K, et al. Comparison of human placenta- and bone marrow-derived multipotent mesenchymal stem cells. *Stem Cells Dev*. 2008;17(6):1095–1107.
85. Brooke G, Tong H, Levesque JP, Atkinson K. Molecular trafficking mechanisms of multipotent mesenchymal stem cells derived from human bone marrow and placenta. *Stem Cells Dev*. 2008;17(5):929–940.
86. 't Anker PS, Scherjon SA, Kleijburg-van der Keur C, et al., eds. Isolation of mesenchymal stem cells of fetal or maternal origin from human placenta. *Stem Cells*. 2004;22(7):1338–1345.
87. Wang L, Ott L, Seshareddy K, Weiss ML, Detamore MS. Musculoskeletal tissue engineering with human umbilical cord mesenchymal stromal cells. *Regen Med*. 2011;6(1):95–109.
88. Braccini A, Wendt D, Jaquiery C, et al. Three-dimensional perfusion culture of human bone marrow cells and generation of osteoinductive grafts. *Stem Cells*. 2005;23(8):1066–1072.
89. Tang Y, Xu Y, Xiao Z, et al. The combination of three-dimensional and rotary cell culture system promotes the proliferation and maintains the differentiation potential of rat BMSCs. *Sci Rep*. 2017;7(1):192. https://doi.org/10.1038/s41598-017-00087-x.

90. Kwok CK, Ueda Y, Kadari A, et al. Scalable stirred suspension culture for the generation of billions of human induced pluripotent stem cells using single-use bioreactors. *J Tissue Eng Regen Med.* 2018;12(2):e1076–e1087. https://doi.org/10.1002/term.2435.
91. Boo L, Selvaratnam L, Tai CC, Ahmad TS, Kamarul T. Expansion and preservation of multipotentiality of rabbit bone-marrow derived mesenchymal stem cells in dextran-based microcarrier spin culture. *J Mater Sci Mater Med.* 2011;22(5):1343–1356.
92. Liu JY, Hafner J, Dragieva G, Burg G. A novel bioreactor microcarrier cell culture system for high yields of proliferating autologous human keratinocytes. *Cell Transplant.* 2006;15(5):435–443.
93. Liu JY, Hafner J, Dragieva G, Burg G. Bioreactor microcarrier cell culture system (Bio-MCCS) for large-scale production of autologous melanocytes. *Cell Transplant.* 2004;13(7-8):809–816.
94. Liu JY, Hafner J, Dragieva G, Burg G. High yields of autologous living dermal equivalents using porcine gelatin microbeads as microcarriers for autologous fibroblasts. *Cell Transplant.* 2006;15(5):445–451.
95. Baraniak PR, McDevitt TC. Scaffold-free culture of mesenchymal stem cell spheroids in suspension preserves multilineage potential. *Cell Tissue Res.* 2012;347(3):701–711.
96. Miceli V, Pampalone M, Vella S, Carreca AP, Amico G, Conaldi PG. Comparison of immunosuppressive and angiogenic properties of human amnion-derived mesenchymal stem cells between 2D and 3D culture systems. *Stem Cells Int.* 2019. https://doi.org/10.1155/2019/7486279.
97. Saleh FA, Frith JE, Lee JA, Genever PG. Three-dimensional in vitro culture techniques for mesenchymal stem cells. *Methods Mol Biol.* 2012;916:31–45. https://doi.org/10.1007/978-1-61779-980-8_4.
98. Sart S, Tsai AC, Li Y, Ma T. Three-dimensional aggregates of mesenchymal stem cells: cellular mechanisms, biological properties, and applications. *Tissue Eng Part B Rev.* 2014;20(5):365–380.
99. Zhao G, Liu F, Lan S, et al. Large-scale expansion of Wharton's jelly-derived mesenchymal stem cells on gelatin microbeads, with retention of self-renewal and multipotency characteristics and the capacity for enhancing skin wound healing. *Stem Cell Res Ther.* 2015;6:38. https://doi.org/10.1186/s13287-015-0031-3.
100. Ankrum JA, Ong JF, Karp JM. Mesenchymal stem cells: immune evasive, not immune privileged. *Nature.* 2014;32:252–260.
101. Rowland AL, Xu JJ, Joswig AJ, et al. In vitro MSC function is related to clinical reaction in vivo. *Stem Cell Res Ther.* 2018;9(1):295. https://doi.org/10.1186/s13287-018-1037-4.
102. Insauti CL, Blanquer M, Garcia-Hernandez AM, Castellanos G, Moraleda JM. Amniotic membrane-derived stem cells: immunomodulatory properties and potential clinical application. *Stem Cells Cloning.* 2014;7:53–63. https://doi.org/10.2147/SCCAA.S58696.
103. Mamede AC, Carvalho MJ, Abrantes AM, Laranjo M, Maia CJ, Botelho MF. Amniotic membrane: from structure and functions to clinical applications. *Cell Tissue Res.* 2012;349(2):447–458.
104. McIntyre JA, Jones IA, Danilkovich A, Vangsness Jr CT. The placenta: applications in orthopaedic sports medicine. *Am J Sports Med.* 2018;46(1):234–247.
105. Riboh JC, Saltzman BM, Yanke AB, Cole BJ. Human amniotic membrane-derived products in sports medicine: basic science, early results, and potential clinical applications. *Am J Sports Med.* 2016;44(9):2425–2434.
106. Akinbi HT, Narendran V, Pass AK, Markart P, Hoath SB. Host defense proteins in vernix caseosa and amniotic fluid. *Am J Obstet Gynecol.* 2004;191(6):2090–2096.
107. Galask RP, Snyder IS. Antimicrobial factors in amniotic fluid. *Am J Obstet Gynecol.* 1970;106(1):59–65.
108. Ismail MA, Salti GI, Moawad AH. Effect of amniotic fluid on bacterial recovery and growth: clinical implications. *Obstet Gynecol Surv.* 1989;44(8):571–577.
109. Kjaegaard N, Hein M, Hyttel L, et al. Antibacterial properties of human amnion and chorion in vitro. *Eur J Obstet Gynecol Reprod Biol.* 2001;94(2):224–229.
110. Mao Y, Pierce J, Singh-Varma A, Boyer M, Kohn J, Reems JA. Processed human amniotic fluid retains its antibacterial activity. *J Transl Med.* 2019;17(1):68. https://doi.org/10.1186/s12967-019-1812-8.
111. Niknejad H, Peirovi H, Jorjani M, Ahmadiani A, Ghanavi J, Seifalian AM. Properties of the amniotic membrane for potential use in tissue engineering. *Eur Cell Mater.* 2008;15:88–99.
112. Yoshio H, Tollin M, Gudmundsson GH, et al. Antimicrobial polypeptides of human vernix caseosa and amniotic fluid: implications for newborn innate defense. *Pediatr Res.* 2003;53(2):211–216.
113. Yung SC, Murphy PM. Antimicrobial chemokines. *Front Immunol.* 2012;3:276. https://doi.org/10.3389/fimmu.2012.00276.
114. Kmiecik G, Niklinska W, Kuc P, et al. Fetal membranes as a source of stem cells. *Adv Med Sci.* 2013;58(2):185–195.
115. Loukogeorgakis SP, De Coppi P. Concise review: amniotic fluid stem cells: the known, the unknown, and potential regenerative medicine applications. *Stem Cells.* 2017;35(7):1663–1673.
116. Loukogeorgakis SP, De Coppi P. Stem cells from amniotic fluid — potential for regenerative medicine. *Best Pract Res Clin Obstet Gynaecol.* 2016;31:45–57. https://doi.org/10.1016/j.bpobgyn.2015.08.009.
117. Pierce J, Jacobson P, Benedetti E, et al. Collection and characterization of amniotic fluid from scheduled C-section deliveries. *Cell Tissue Bank.* 2016;17(3):413–425.
118. Toda A, Okabe M, Yoshida T, Nikaido T. The potential of amniotic membrane/amnion-derived cells for regeneration of various tissues. *J Pharmacol Sci.* 2007;105(3):215–228.
119. Zia S, Toelen J, Mori da Cunha M, Dekoninck P, de Coopi P, Deprest J. Routine clonal expansion of mesenchymal stem cells derived from amniotic fluid for perinatal applications. *Prenat Diagn.* 2013;33(10):921–928.
120. Nyman E, Huss F, Nyman T, Junker J, Kratz G. Hyaluronic acid, an important factor in the wound healing properties of amniotic fluid: in vitro studies of re-epithelialisation in human skin wounds. *J Plast Surg Hand Surg.* 2013;47(2):89–92.
121. Castro-Combs J, Noguera G, Cano M, et al. Corneal wound healing is modulated by topical application of amniotic fluid in an ex vivo organ culture model. *Exp Eye Res.* 2008;87(1):56–63.
122. Ozgenel GY, Filiz G. Effects of human amniotic fluid on peripheral nerve scarring and regeneration in rats. *J Neurosurg.* 2003;98(2):371–377.
123. Ozgenel GY, Filiz G, Ozcan M. Effects of human amniotic fluid on cartilage regeneration from free perichondrial grafts in rabbits. *Br J Plast Surg.* 2004;57(5):423–428.
124. He H, Li W, Chen SY, et al. Suppression of activation and induction of apoptosis in RAW264.7 cells by amniotic membrane extract. *Invest Ophthalmol Vis Sci.* 2008;49(10):4468–4475.

125. He H, Li W, Tseng DY, et al. Biochemical characterization and function of complexes formed by hyaluronan and the heavy chains of inter-alpha-inhibitor (HC*HA) purified from extracts of human amniotic membrane. *J Biol Chem.* 2009;284(30):20136–20146.
126. He H, Zhang S, Tighe S, Son J, Tseng SC. Immobilized heavy chain-hyaluronic acid polarizes lipopolysaccharide-activated macrophages toward M2 phenotype. *J Biol Chem.* 2013;288(36):25792–25803.
127. Li W, He H, Chen YT, Hayashida Y, Tseng SC. Reversal of myofibroblasts by amniotic membrane stromal extract. *J Cell Physiol.* 2008;215(3):657–664.
128. Shimmura S, Shimazaki J, Ohashi Y, Tsubota K. Antiinflammatory effects of amniotic membrane transplantation in ocular surface disorders. *Cornea.* 2001;20(4):408–413.
129. Tseng SC. HC-HA/PTX3 purified from amniotic membrane as novel regenerative matrix: insight into relationship between inflammation and regeneration. *Invest Ophthalmol Vis Sci.* 2016;57(5):ORSFh1–ORSFh8. https://doi.org/10.1167/iovs.15-17637.
130. Tseng SC, Li DQ, Ma X. Suppression of transforming growth factor-beta isoforms, TGF-beta receptor type II, and myofibroblast differentiation in cultured human corneal and limbal fibroblasts by amniotic membrane matrix. *J Cell Physiol.* 1999;179(3):325–335.
131. Wang MX, Gray TB, Park WC, et al. Reduction in corneal haze and apoptosis by amniotic membrane matrix in excimer laser photoablation in rabbits. *J Cataract Refract Surg.* 2001;27(2):310–319.
132. Zhang S, He H, Day AJ, Tseng SC. Constitutive expression of inter-α-inhibitor (IαI) family proteins and tumor necrosis factor-stimulated gene-6 (TSG-6) by human amniotic membrane epithelial and stromal cells supporting formation of the heavy chain-hyaluronan (HC-HA) complex. *J Biol Chem.* 2012;287(15):12433–12444.
133. Zhang S, Zhu YT, Chen SY, He H, Tseng SC. Constitutive expression of pentraxin 3 (PTX3) protein by human amniotic membrane cells leads to formation of the heavy chain (HC)-hyaluronan (HA)-PTX3 complex. *J Biol Chem.* 2014;289(19):13531–13542.
134. Lee SB, Li DQ, Tan DT, Meller DC, Tseng SC. Suppression of TGF-beta signaling in both normal conjunctival fibroblasts and pterygial body fibroblasts by amniotic membrane. *Curr Eye Res.* 2000;20(4):325–334.
135. Bottai D, Cigognini D, Nicora E, et al. Third trimester amniotic fluid cells with the capacity to develop neural phenotypes and with heterogeneity among sub-populations. *Restor Neurol Neurosci.* 2012;30(1):55–68.
136. 't Anker PS, Scherjon SA, Kleijburg-van der Keur C, et al. Amniotic fluid as a novel source of mesenchymal stem cells for therapeutic transplantation. *Blood.* 2003;102(4):1548–1549.
137. Da Sacco S, Sedrakyan S, Boldrin F, et al. Human amniotic fluid as a potential new source of organ specific precursor cells for future regenerative medicine applications. *J Urol.* 2010;183(3):1193–1200.
138. Broxmeyer HE, Douglas GW, Hangoc G, et al. Human umbilical cord blood as a potential source of transplantable hematopoietic stem/progenitor cells. *Proc Natl Acad Sci U S A.* 1989;86(10):3828–3832.
139. Broxmeyer HE, Srour EF, Hangoc G, Cooper S, Anderson SA, Bodine DM. High-efficiency recovery of functional hematopoietic progenitor and stem cells from human cord blood cryopreserved for 15 years. *Proc Natl Acad Sci U S A.* 2003;100(2):645–650.
140. Munoz J, Shah N, Rezvani K, et al. Concise review: umbilical cord blood transplantation: past, present, and future. *Stem Cells Transl Med.* 2014;3(12):1435–1443.
141. Park YB, Ha CW, Lee CH, Yoon YC, Park YG. Cartilage regeneration in osteoarthritic patients by a composite of allogeneic umbilical cord blood-derived mesenchymal stem cells and hyaluronate hydrogel: results from a clinical trial for safety and proof-of-concept with 7 years of extended follow-up. *Stem Cells Transl Med.* 2017;6(2):613–621.
142. Shpall EJ, Quinones R, Giller R, et al. Transplantation of ex vivo expanded cord blood. *Biol Blood Marrow Transplant.* 2002;8(7):368–376.
143. Davies JE, Walker JT, Keating A. Concise review: Wharton's jelly: the rich, but enigmatic, source of mesenchymal stromal cells. *Stem Cells Transl Med.* 2017;6(7):1620–1630.
144. Subramanian A, Fong CY, Biswas A, Bongso A. Comparative characterization of cells from the various compartments of the human umbilical cord shows that Wharton's jelly compartment provides the best source of clinically utilizable mesenchymal stem cells. *PLoS One.* 2015;10(6):e0127992. https://doi.org/10.1371/journal.pone.0127992.
145. Fujisato T, Tomihata K, Tabata Y, Iwamoto Y, Burczak K, Ikada Y. Cross-linking of amniotic membranes. *J Biomater Sci Polym Ed.* 1999;10(11):1171–1181.
146. Kruse FE, Joussen AM, Rohrschneider K, et al. Cryopreserved human amniotic membrane for ocular surface reconstruction. *Graefe's Arch Clin Exp Ophthalmol.* 2000;238(1):68–75.
147. Kubo M, Sonoda Y, Muramatsu R, Usui M. Immunogenicity of human amniotic membrane in experimental xenotransplantation. *Invest Ophthalmol Vis Sci.* 2001;42(7):1539–1546.
148. Parolini O, Soncini M, Evangelista M, Schmidt D. Amniotic membrane and amniotic fluid-derived cells: potential tools for regenerative medicine? *Regen Med.* 2009;4(2):275–291.
149. Ankrum J, Karp JM. Mesenchymal stem cell therapy: two steps forward, one step back. *Trends Mol Med.* 2010;16:203–209.
150. Vitha AE, Kollefrath AW, Huang CC, Garcia-Godoy F. Characterization and therapeutic uses of exosomes: a new potential tool in orthopedics. *Stem Cells and Development.* 2019;28(2):141–146.
151. Privoraite U, Jarmalaviciute A, Tunaitis V, Ramanauskaite G, Vaitkuviene A, Kaseta V, et al. Exosomes from human dental pulp stem cells suppress carrageenan-induced acute inflammation in mice. *Inflammation.* 2015;38:1933–1941.
152. Burke J, Kolhe R, Hunter M, Isales C, Hamrick M, Fulzele S. Stem cell-derived exosomes: a potential alternative therapeutic agent in orthopedics. *Stem Cell Int.* 2016:5802529.
153. Hessvik NP, Lloorente A. Current knowledge on exosome biogenesis and release. *Cell Mol Life Sci.* 2016;164:1226–1232.
154. Zhao T, Sun F, Liu J, Ding T, She J, et al. Emerging role of mesenchymal stem cell-derived exosomes in regenerative medicine. *Curr Stem Cell Res Ther.* 2019;14:482–494.
155. Pan BT, Johnstone RM. Fate of the transferrin receptor during maturation of sheep reticulocytes in vitro: selective externalization of the receptor. *Cell.* 1983;33:967–978.
156. Li Z, Wang Y, Xiao K, Xiang S, Li Z, Weng X. Emerging role of exosomes in the joint diseases. *Cell Physio Biochem.* 2018;47:2008–2017.
157. Conde-Vancells J, Rodriguez-Suarez J, Embade N, et al. Characterization and comprehensive proteome profiling of exosomes secreted by hematocytes. *J Proteome Res.* 2008;7:5157–5166.

158. Thery C, Zitvogel L, Amigorena S. Exosomes. Composition, biogenesis and function. *Nat Rev Immunol.* 2002;2:569–579.
159. Jarmalaviciute A, Pivoriunas A. Exosomes as a potential novel therapeutic tools against neurodegenerative diseases. *Pharmacol Res.* 2016;113:816–822.
160. Vlassov AV, Magdaleno S, Setterquist R, Conrad R. Exosomes: current knowledge of their composition, biological functions and diagnostic and therapeutic potentials. *Biochem Biophys Acta.* 2012;1820:940–948.
161. Tkach M, Thery C. Communication by extracellular vesicles: where we are and where we need to go. *Cell.* 2016;164:1226–1232.
162. Huang F, Wan J, Hu W, Hao S. Enhancement of anti-leukemia immunity by leukemia-derived exosomes via downregulation of TGF-beta1 expression. *Cell Physiol Biochem.* 2017;44:240–254.
163. Colombo M, Raposo G, Thery C. Biogenesis, secretion, and intercellular interactions of exosomes and other extracellular veicles. *Annu Rev Cell Dev Biol.* 2014;30:255–2899.
164. Skotland T, Sandvig K, Llorente A. Lipids in exosomes: current knowledge and the way forward. *Prog Lipid Res.* 2017;66:30–41.
165. Thery C, Amigorena S, Raposo G, Clayton A. Isolation and characteristics of exosomes from cell culture supernatants and biological fluids. *Curr Protoc Cell Biol.* 2006. Chapter 3:Unit 3.22.
166. Ju C, Liu R, Zhang Y, et al. Exosomes may be the potential new direction of research in osteoarthritis management. *Biomed Res Int.* 2019. https://doi.org/10.1155/2019/7695768.
167. Mao G, Zhang Z, Hu S, et al. Exosomes derived from miR-92a-3p-overexpressing human mesenchymal stem cells enhance chondrogenesis and suppress cartilage degradation via targeting WNT5A. *Stem Cell Res Ther.* 2018;9:247. https://doi.org/10.1186/s13287-018-1004-0.
168. Tao SC, Yuan T, Zhang YL, Yin WJ, Guo SC, Zhang CQ. Exosomes derived from miR-140-5p-overexpressing human synovial mesenchymal stem cells enhance cartilage tissue regeneration and prevent osteoarthritis of the knee in a rat model. *Theranostics.* 2017;7(1):180–195.
169. Wang R, Xu B, Xu H. TGF-β1 promoted chondrocyte proliferation by regulating Sp1 through MSC-exosomes derived miR-135b. *Cell Cycle.* 2018;17(24). https://doi.org/10.1080/15384101.2018.1556063.
170. Wang Y, He G, Guo Y, et al. Exosomes from tendon stem cells promote injury tendon healing through balancing synthesis and degradation of the tendon extracellular matrix. *J Cell Mol Med.* 2019;23(8):5475–5485.
171. Zhao Y, Xu J. Synovial fluid-derived exosomal lncRNA PCGEM1 as a biomarker for the different stages of osteoarthritis.
172. Finkemeier CG. Bone-grafting and bone-graft substitutes. *J Bone Joint Surg Am.* 2002;84(3):454–464.
173. Zhang H, Yang L, Yang XG, et al. Demineralized bone matrix carriers and their clinical applications: an overview. *Orthop Surg.* 2019;11(5):725–737.
174. Campana V, Milano G, Pagano E, et al. Bone substitutes in orthopaedic surgery: from basic science to clinical practice. *J Mater Sci Mater Med.* 2014;25(10):2445–2461.
175. Gruskin E, Doll BA, Futrell FW, Schmitz JP, Hollinger JO. Demineralized bone matrix in bone repair: history and use. *Adv Drug Deliv Rev.* 2012;64(12):1063–1077.
176. Urist MR, Dowell TA. Inductive substratum for osteogenesis in pellets of particulate bone matrix. *Clin Orthop Relat Res.* 1968;61:61–78.
177. Senn on the healing of aseptic bone cavities by implantation of antiseptic decalcified bone. *Ann Surg.* 1889;10(5):352–368.
178. Connolly JF. Injectable bone marrow preparations to stimulate osteogenic repair. *Clin Orthop Relat Res.* 1995;(313):8–18.
179. Connolly JF, Guse R, Tiedeman J, Dehne R. Autologous marrow injection as a substitute for operative grafting of tibial nonunions. *Clin Orthop Relat Res.* 1991;(266):259–270.
180. Wilkins RM, Kelly CM. The effect of allomatrix injectable putty on the outcome of long bone applications. *Orthopedics.* 2003;26(suppl 5):s567–s570.
181. Kanellopoulos AD, Yiannakopoulos CK, Soucacos PN. Percutaneous reaming of simple bone cysts in children followed by injection of demineralized bone matrix and autologous bone marrow. *J Pediatr Orthop.* 2005;25(5):671–675.
182. Killian JT, Wilkinson L, White S, Brassard M. Treatment of unicameral bone cyst with demineralized bone matrix. *J Pediatr Orthop.* 1998;18(5):621–624.
183. Rougraff BT, Kling TJ. Treatment of active unicameral bone cysts with percutaneous injection of demineralized bone matrix and autogenous bone marrow. *J Bone Joint Surg Am.* 2002;84(6):921–929.
184. Noth U, Rackwitz L, Steinert AF, Tuan RS. Cell delivery therapeutics for musculoskeletal regeneration. *Adv Drug Deliv Rev.* 2010;62(7-8):765–783.
185. Petrigliano FA, Lieberman JR. Osteonecrosis of the hip: novel approaches to evaluation and treatment. *Clin Orthop Relat Res.* 2007;465:53–62.
186. Jamali AA, Fritz AT, Reddy D, Meehan JP. Minimally invasive bone grafting of cysts of the femoral head and acetabulum in femoroacetabular impingement: arthroscopic technique and case presentation. *Arthroscopy.* 2010;26(2):279–285.
187. Elena N, Woodall BM, Lee K, et al. Intraosseous bioplasty for a chondral cyst in the lateral tibial plateau. *Arthrosc Tech.* 2018;7(11):e1149–e1156.
188. Hinsekamp M, Muylle L, Eastlund D, et al. Adverse reactions and events related to musculoskeletal allografts: reviewed by the World Health Organization Project NOTIFY. *Int Orthop.* 2011;36:633–641.

9

Therapeutic Dextrose Injection: Prolotherapy, Perineural Injection Therapy, and Hydrodissection

KENNETH D. REEVES, STANLEY K.H. LAM AND DAVID RABAGO

KEY POINTS

- Dextrose prolotherapy has level B strength of recommendation for chronic pain in eight areas based on a growing number of RCTs and meta-analyses.
- Dextrose, when used in perineural and hydrodissection procedures, often has a prompt analgesic effect and is an alternative to anesthetic injection for treatment of neuropathic pain.
- The evidence base supporting dextrose prolotherapy, perineural injection therapy, and hydrodissection of nerves is growing.
- Treatment of individual regions of the body should consider nociceptive sources in joints, connective tissue, and their related nerves due to shared neural origins (Hilton's law).
- Image guidance is often crucial in the performance of dextrose prolotherapy, and ultrasound guidance is required to visualize nerves for hydrodissection.

Introduction

Therapeutic injection of dextrose is a potentially disease-modifying treatment for chronic pain. Three related but discreet approaches have emerged using dextrose injectates, comprising dextrose prolotherapy (DPT), perineural injection therapy (PIT), and hydrodissection (HD). These approaches have significant overlap but are distinct enough to merit individual consideration. This chapter addresses the evidence associated with each, and the contribution of ultrasound guidance.

Prolotherapy

Prolotherapy is the oldest regenerative injection technique for chronic musculoskeletal pain conditions, emerging as a modality to treat chronic pain in the early 20th century.[1] Initially called "sclerotherapy" due to the scarring produced by early caustic injectants, clinicians treated the same conditions as today, but also chronic, repetitive joint subluxations and inguinal hernias.[2] George Hackett, MD, a general surgeon in the United States, formalized these injection techniques in the 1950s based on clinical experience and research.[3] Considering proliferation of injected tissue to be an essential aspect of prolotherapy's effects, he renamed the procedure: "To the treatment of proliferating new cells I have applied the name prolotherapy."[4]

One of the most common agents used for prolotherapy is hypertonic dextrose[5] but several other injectates can be utilized as well.[6] Hackett's early injection protocols and comprehensive textbook informed the field's procedural work for the rest of the 20th century.[4] His central diagnostic principle was that ligament laxity led to pain and disability. The location of laxity was understood to be the entheses of ligaments and tendons. This was prescient, as we now understand that degenerative change[7] and laxity[8] are core features of overuse tendinopathies. Injections at tender entheses and adjacent joint spaces defined the core procedure and could be done at any joint. Out of necessity, identification of bony anatomy for localization was based on palpation, and a cadre of clinicians with advanced skills in superficial anatomy comprised the early clinical and research endeavors, and published clinically based research reports.[9] While palpation guidance was the previous gold standard, teaching organizations are in the process of developing protocols including high-resolution ultrasound (HRUS) and fluoroscopy to augment palpation guidance, particularly for difficult-to-identify and higher-risk anatomic targets.

Mechanism/Animal Model Research

The in vitro mechanism of action of DPT has received little attention, and it is unclear how cellular changes associated with dextrose affect pain. Small concentrations of dextrose (15 mM, 0.27%) have been shown to alter the expression of various cytokines in multiple cell lines with less than 20 minutes of exposure,[10,11] while exposure to 0.6% dextrose in culture for 24 hours results in significant cellular death and dysfunction.[12,13] However, in vitro studies have not attempted to simulate the declining concentrations and limited exposure time seen in vivo.

Research using an in vivo rabbit model reported a proliferative effect of 10% dextrose in ligament tissue in the absence of an inflammatory response or cellular death.[14] The same researchers confirmed organized connective tissue proliferation with 10% dextrose injections in three randomized controlled trials (RCTs) using the same rabbit model.[15-17] All three studies demonstrated nearly a doubling of the ligament's thickness after the dextrose injection, greater force was required to rupture the ligament, and histologic findings were normal.[17] Studies have not compared the relative proliferative effect of differing dextrose concentrations in vivo. Although a proliferative effect of hypertonic dextrose injection has been documented,[17] the therapeutic effects of hypertonic dextrose injection are likely multifactorial and a combination of proliferative and other biologic effects.

Clinical Research and Strength of Recommendations

Clinical research has been limited to relatively small studies. Despite modest sample sizes, numerous rigorous RCTs have reported a clinically meaningful effect of DPT in knee osteoarthritis (OA),[18-21] temporomandibular dysfunction,[22-24] rotator cuff tendinopathy,[25,26] lateral epicondylosis,[27,28] wrist pain,[29] finger/thumb OA,[30,31] sacroiliac pain,[32] hip OA due to hip dysplasia,[33] Osgood-Schlatter disease,[34,35] Achilles tendinosis,[36] and plantar fasciosis.[37,38]

Strength of recommendation (SOR) criteria[39] are commonly used to summarize the cumulative status of evidence in a given area with level A or B SOR indicating likely benefit. DPT for knee OA has level A evidence.[5,40-48] In a clinical model of grade IV knee OA, exposure to intra-articular 12.5% dextrose injection was followed by the appearance of new, metabolically active, type I and II cartilage in post-treatment arthroscopies.[49] While patients in this small case series improved clinically, the relationship between such improvement and apparent cartilage growth is not clear. Assessment of prolotherapy for several conditions meet B SOR criteria including temporomandibular dysfunction,[50] rotator cuff tendinopathy,[5,46,47,51-53] lateral epicondylosis,[5,28,45-47,51,54,55] wrist pain,[29] painful finger or thumb OA,[5,42,46,47,51] sacroiliac pain,[32] Osgood-Schlatter disease,[5,45-47,56] and Achilles tendinopathy.[5,45-47,56-59] Treatment of plantar fasciosis has level B-C evidence.[37,56]

Training and Protocols

Over time, individual clinicians have refined the injection protocols and developed consensus-based guidelines.[60,61] Professional medical societies with a focus on prolotherapy, including the Hackett Hemwall Patterson Foundation (HHPF) and American Association of Orthopedic Medicine (AAOM), offer conferences and training worldwide. (Table 9.1). HHPF has recently released "The Prolotherapy Procedural and Study Guides," using an iterative consensus model.[62]

TABLE 9.1 Organizations Offering Training With a Focus on Prolotherapy.

Organization	Website
Australia	
Australian Association of Musculoskeletal Medicine	aamm.org.au
Asia	
Hong Kong Institute of Musculoskeletal Medicine	hkimm.hk
Taiwan Association of Prolotherapy and Regenerative Medicine	taprm.org
Europe	
European School of Prolotherapy	proloterapia.it/en
North America	
American Association of Orthopaedic Medicine	aaomed.org
The American Osteopathic Association of Prolotherapy Regenerative Medicine	prolotherapycollege.org/
Canadian Association of Orthopaedic Medicine	caom.ca
Hackett Hemwall Patterson Foundation /International Association of Regenerative Therapy	hhpfoundation.org/ iart.org
South America	
Latin American Association of Orthopaedic Medicine	www.laomed.org

Perineural Injection Therapy

The injection of dextrose around painful peripheral nerves emerged from the prolotherapy tradition, and was first introduced in 2006[63] as "neural prolotherapy." The more descriptive term "perineural injection therapy" was soon adopted, since the proposed goal of treatment was restoration of nerve function, and not proliferation.

Mechanism/Clinical Research

Neurogenic inflammation is characterized by an absence of leukocytes,[64] and is due to peptidergic nerve fibers releasing pain-producing and degenerative neuropeptides.[64] These neuropeptides, including calcitonin gene–related peptide (CGRP) and substance P, are primarily released by type C peptidergic nerve fibers.[64] Clinical findings of allodynia and hyperalgesia are common due to alteration of C nerve fiber firing rates and thresholds. The rapid analgesic (not anesthetic) effect after subcutaneous 5% dextrose (D5W) injection over painful peripheral nerves suggests a neurogenic effect of dextrose.[65]

In an RCT assessing caudal epidural injection of D5W versus normal saline in participants with back and buttock or leg pain, dextrose provided a significant analgesic effect within 15 minutes, lasting 48 hours or more,[66] and this pattern was repeated after each of the 4 consecutive biweekly treatments.[67] Proposed mechanisms for an apparent calming effect of dextrose in the presence of neurogenic pain include alteration of key cation channels[68] or restoration of the normal cation-pump-maintained transmembrane potential by correction of relative neural hypoglycemia.[69]

Multiple case series report pain reduction from subcutaneous dextrose injections over painful superficial cutaneous nerves in the knee, shoulder, elbow,[70] Achilles tendon,[71] and lumbar region,[72] though assignment of causality is not possible in the absence of control.[72] One randomized controlled trial has been reported using PIT in chronic Achilles tendinopathy, with injections about the Achilles tendon showing results comparable with eccentric lengthening exercises (ELE).[36]

Training and Protocols

Neurogenic inflammation is common with dysfunction of superficial sensory or mixed motor and sensory nerves,[65,73] which can be located by palpation with training and injected with minimal risk using small-gauge needles. Training in PIT is largely outside of conventional medical education and is often taught without ultrasound guidance. Conference-based training was introduced by and remains available from content experts John Lyftogt and HHPF/IART.[70-72,74]

Hydrodissection

HD is the process of injecting fluid around a nerve to release the nerve from potentially constricting fascia. Symptomatic nerve compression or entrapment can result in fusiform swelling or flattening of the nerve,[75] and ultrasound-guided injection of fluid between the nerve and surrounding fascia can release adherent fascial tissue. With the constriction removed, the nerve is free to resume a normal, more circular cross-section appearance.[76]

Mechanism/Clinical Research

A hypothesized mechanism of action for dextrose HD follows Bennett's sciatic ligature model,[77] where even mild constriction of a nerve caused neurogenic inflammation with sciatic nerve swelling, loss of axons distal to the ligatures, and neuroma formation at the level of the ligatures. A variety of injectates have been used, and saline, dextrose, corticosteroid, and platelet-rich plasma (PRP) HD injectates have been compared in the treatment of carpal tunnel syndrome (CTS). A favorable effect of HD using saline was reported in a study of CTS participants.[78] Wu et al. reported that D5W outperformed saline[79] and triamcinolone[80] in treatment of CTS. PRP and D5W injection resulted in similar symptomatic benefit in a treatment-comparison trial in CTS.[81]

Dextrose may offer advantages compared with other injectants. The risk of potential lidocaine toxicity is avoided with use of D5W or PRP without lidocaine.[76] In addition, D5W HD without lidocaine does not result in nerve depolarization. In contrast, lidocaine depolarizes the nerve and renders distal fibers non-functional, limiting precise localization of the primary nociceptive source.

Training and Protocols

HD procedures will be discussed in this chapter and throughout this Atlas.

Regional Injection Approaches Utilizing Dextrose and Current Clinical Evidence

The goal of this section is to briefly review relevant research for each of the three modalities and identify key nociceptors. Detailed injection methods are covered in later chapters.

Head/Facial Region

Publications regarding the head/facial region have focused on DPT in or about the temporomandibular joint (TMJ). Three small RCTs with moderate to high bias compared the effect of dextrose to anesthetic injection in participants with painfully subluxing TMJs.[22,23,82] The protocols included injections of the TMJ capsule on multiple occasions in addition to an intra-articular injection. In all three studies, there was significant improvement in TMJ pain in both the dextrose and control injection groups, favoring dextrose upon meta-analysis.[50] Despite a consistent reduction in frequency of perceived subluxation, a single-arm prospective study showed no change in measurable subluxation upon comparison of pre- and post-injection tomography of joint motion.[83] The one complication observed in both the RCTs[22,23,82] and open-label studies[83-87] was a significant reduction in mouth opening.[50]

Louw et al., in a larger, low-bias, RCT, injected the TMJ intra-articular space and avoided capsular injection.[24] They reported similar clinical benefit favoring dextrose over lidocaine injection in all types of TMJ dysfunction (myofascial, disc dysfunction, and arthritic), but the dextrose group showed improved mouth opening at the 3- and 12-month follow-up. The results argue for avoidance of capsular injection clinically and in future study protocols.[24,50]

Key Nociceptors

Nociceptive sources that are implicated in difficult pain presentations involving the head and/or face include:

1. Superficial nerves: Auriculotemporal, zygomaticotemporal, lacrimal, supraorbital, supratrochlear, zygomaticofacial, infraorbital, external nasal, buccal, mental, greater auricular, greater occipital, lesser occipital, third occipital, and suboccipital.

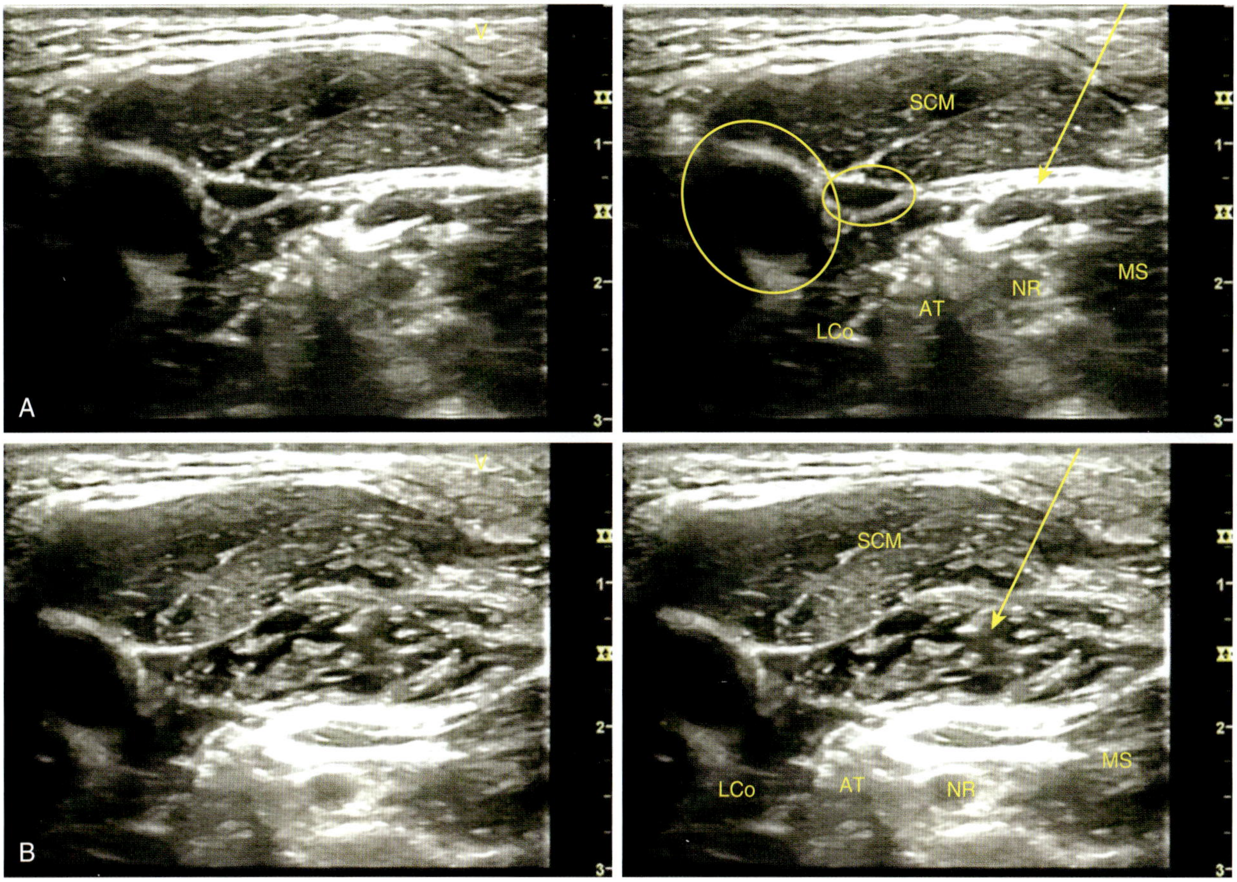

• **Fig. 9.1** (A) Cervical plexus location: The lesser occipital and greater auricular nerves are branches of the cervical plexus. Pandit et al. demonstrated through cadaveric dye study that fluid injected about the cervical plexus travels through the deep cervical fascia and is found about the cervical nerve roots.[97] The cervical plexus can be accessed through the posterior investing fascia of the sternocleidomastoid (*arrow* indicates needle placement location). Injection of the cervical plexus should avoid the carotid artery and internal jugular vein (*large and small circles,* respectively). The external jugular may also need to be avoided by adjusting needle entry slightly cephalad or caudal. Because the vagus nerve is located within the nearby vascular sheath, and the phrenic nerve has partial supply from the cervical plexus, lidocaine should not be included in this injection to avoid a vagal and phrenic nerve block. (B) Hydrodissection of the cervical plexus: The arrow tip (representing the 30-gauge needle tip which is not visible in this image) is in the same location as in image A. Shown here is the area of expansion of the space under the investing fascia of the sternocleidomastoid. *AT,* Anterior tubercle of transverse process; *LCo*, longus coli; *MS*, middle scalene; *NR*, nerve root; *SCM*, sternocleidomastoid.

2. Deeper nerves/ganglion/plexi: Cervical plexus (Fig. 9.1A and B).
3. Entheses: Capiti and trapezius.
4. Joints: Temporomandibular.

Cervical Spine/Neck

DPT was studied in a small group of participants (n = 6) with cervical laxity with greater than 2.7 mm of cervical translation on flexion-extension x-rays and referred shoulder pain.[88] Using fluoroscopic guidance, subjects underwent injections with 12.5% dextrose into the involved posterior elements, lamina, and spinous processes. Reduced cervical translation in flexion-extension x-rays, along with a significant reduction in pain, was observed. For facet-mediated pain, Hooper et al., in a small case series (n = 18) involving 20% dextrose injection into the zygapophysial joint at 2 to 4 levels using fluoroscopic guidance in post whiplash patients, found DPT improved pain and function.[89]

Key Nociceptors

Nociceptive sources that are commonly important in difficult pain presentations involving the neck include:

1. Superficial nerves: Posterior supraclavicular and superficial cervical rami.
2. Deeper nerves/ganglion/plexi: Cervical dorsal rami and cervical plexus.
3. Entheses: Cervical multifidi and facet ligaments 3 to 7 (Fig. 9.2A), levator scapulae origin (Fig. 9.2B), and C2 facet ligament (Fig. 9.3A and B).

Thoracic Spine/Upper to Mid Back

In a study of 70 subjects with chronic axial spine pain treated with 20% DPT targeting the ligaments and facet joint capsules at symptomatic levels, Hooper et al. reported clinically significant improvement as measured by the patient-specific functional scale (PSFS).[90] Of interest is that 50 of the 70

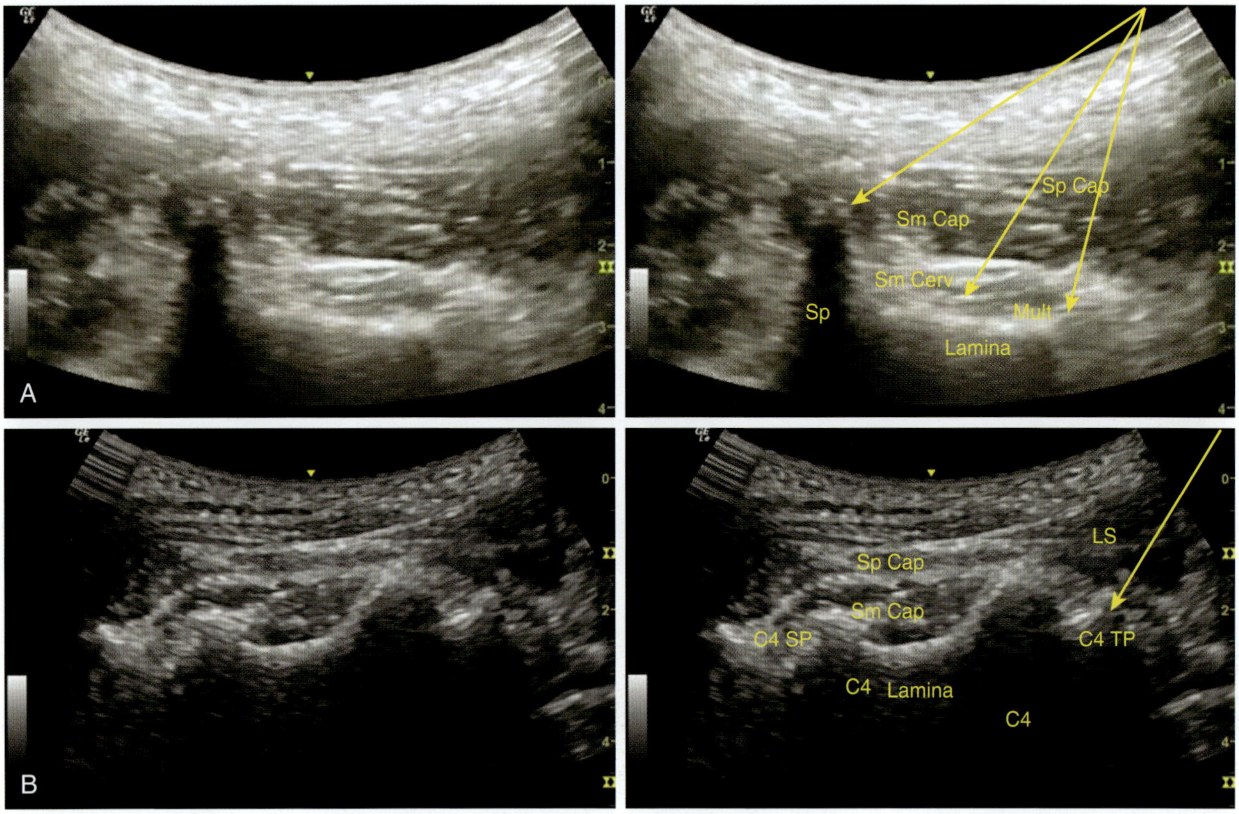

• **Fig. 9.2** (A) Injection of posterior cervical structures: The posterior cervical elements, including the posterior capsular ligaments and enthesis along the lamina and spinous process, can be accessed with a single entry and needle redirection, illustrated by the three arrows on the right. The interspinous ligament between posterior spinous processes (not depicted) can be targeted using a similar approach. (B) Injection of levator scapulae origin: Ultrasound visualization is important to inject the levator scapulae origin from the C2 to C4 posterior tubercles, either by advancing a few millimeters anterior to the cervical facets to avoid nerve root contact using an axial view to visualize the posterior tubercle (arrow) or using a sagittal view showing multiple tubercles (not depicted). *LS*, Levator scapulae; *Mult*, multifidus; *Sm Cap*, semispinalis capitis; *Sm Cerv*, semispinalis cervicis; *Sp Cap*, splenius capitis; *SP*, spinous process; *TP*, transverse process.

participants were litigants, with outcomes comparable to non-litigants.

Key Nociceptors

For the thoracic spine region, nociceptive sources that are commonly important include:

1. Superficial nerves/penetrators: Posterior supraclavicular and medial and lateral penetrators of the posterior thoracic rami.
2. Deeper nerves/ganglion/plexi: Dorsal scapular nerve (Fig. 9.4A), thoracic dorsal rami, and the paravertebral ganglia/space (Fig. 9.4B).
3. Entheses: Thoracic multifidi and facet ligaments (Fig. 9.5).
4. Joints: Costotransverse (Fig. 9.6A and B).

Shoulder Girdle

DPT for rotator cuff tendinopathy has been the object of considerable research. Bertrand et al. conducted a three-arm blinded RCT (n = 73) comparing landmark-guided injection with dextrose into the painful enthesis to lidocaine at the enthesis and superficially.[25] Seven et al., in an open label RCT (n = 101), compared ultrasound-guided dextrose injections into the subacromial bursa and tender entheses to extensive physiotherapy.[26] While both groups had significant improvement from baseline measures, the dextrose group significantly outperformed the control at 6 and 12 weeks in pain score reductions, Western Ontario Rotator Cuff (WORC) index, and Shoulder Pain and Disability Index (SPADI).

In a pairwise and network meta-analysis by Lin et al. comparing all injection therapies in the treatment of rotator cuff tendinopathy,[53] platelet-rich plasma and prolotherapy injections yielded better outcomes than control injections in the long term (>24 weeks). Study heterogenicity limited conclusions to level B confidence. A systematic review by Catapano et al. of DPT for symptomatic rotator cuff tendinopathy[52] concluded that dextrose demonstrated at least short-term improvements in pain and function compared to physical therapy alone. There was a high risk of bias and variable efficacy within the studies, but repeated multisite injections showed more consistent improvements.

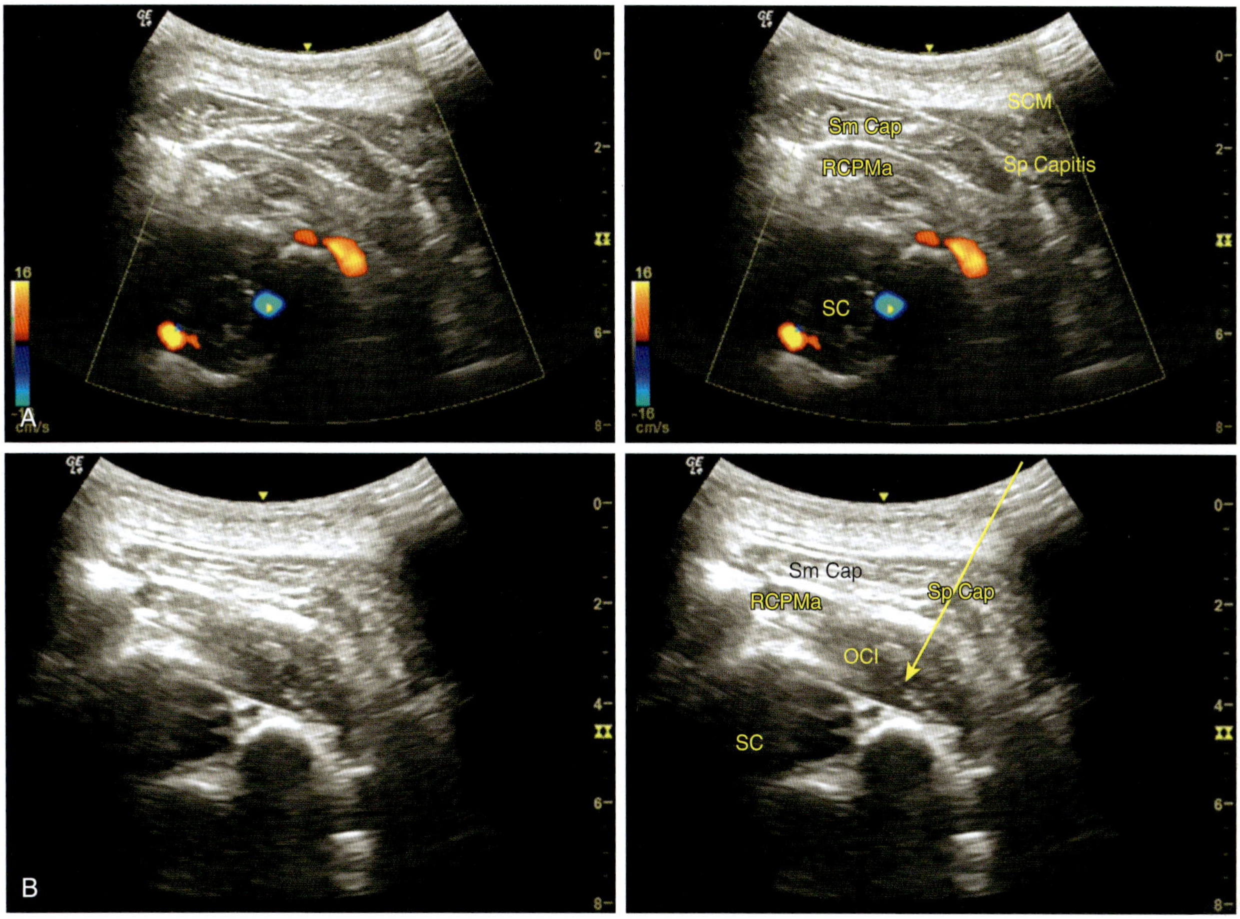

• **Fig. 9.3** (A) Visualization of the vertebral artery by Doppler: This is critical when targeting the C1 to C2 capsular ligaments and the lateral occipitoatlantal capsular ligament (latter not depicted). (B) Injection of C2 superior articular facet: Injections in this region should utilize hydrodissection technique when advancing the needle to push away the vertebral artery until bone contact. Lidocaine concentions of 0.1% or less and aspiration at the point of bone contact is advised to minimize the risk of complications from inadvertent vertebral artery injection. *OCI*, Obliquus capitis inferior; *RCPMa*, rectus capitis posterior major; *SC*, spinal cord; *SCM*, sternocleidomastoid; *Sm Cap*, semispinalis capitis; *Sp Capitis*, splenius capitis; *VA*, vertebral artery.

Key Nociceptors

Nociceptive sources of particular importance for this region include:

1. Superficial nerves/penetrators: Posterior and intermediate supraclavicular, suprascapular, axillary, subscapular, and musculocutaneous nerves.
2. Deeper nerves/ganglion/plexi: Suprascapular, interscalene, supraclavicular, and axillary brachial plexus.
3. Entheses: Supraspinatus insertion, infraspinatus insertion, subscapularis insertion, inferior and anteroinferior glenohumeral ligament, and origins of the infraspinatus, teres major, and teres minor.
4. Joints: acromiocalvular (AC) joint, sternoclavicular (SC) joint, and glenohumeral (GH) joint.
5. Other: Subscapular bursa, subdeltoid bursa, and biceps long head.

Elbow

Rabago et al., in a three-arm RCT, compared prolotherapy with dextrose and dextrose-morrhuate injections to watchful waiting for lateral epicondylosis.[27] Patient-Rated Tennis Elbow Evaluation scores at 16 weeks in both prolotherapy injection groups were significantly better than in the watchful waiting group, and there was no difference between the dextrose and dextrose-morrhuate injection groups. Bayat et al. compared DPT to methylprednisolone. While both injections resulted in significant clinical improvements at 3-month follow-up, dextrose was superior in Quick DASH (Disabilities of Arm, Shoulder and Hand) and pain improvements.[28] In the most rigorous study of dextrose injection therapy for lateral epicondylosis, Yelland et al. conducted a single-blind RCT (n = 120) comparing 20% DPT, physiotherapy, and combined treatment with prolotherapy and physiotherapy.[54] At 1 year, all groups showed significant improvement with no significant differences between groups.[55] Dong et al., in a systematic review and Bayesian network meta-analysis of all injection therapies for lateral epicondylalgia,[54] concluded that botulinum toxin, platelet-rich plasma, autologous blood injection, hyaluronate injection, and prolotherapy can be considered for lateral epicondylitis, but cortisone was not recommended.

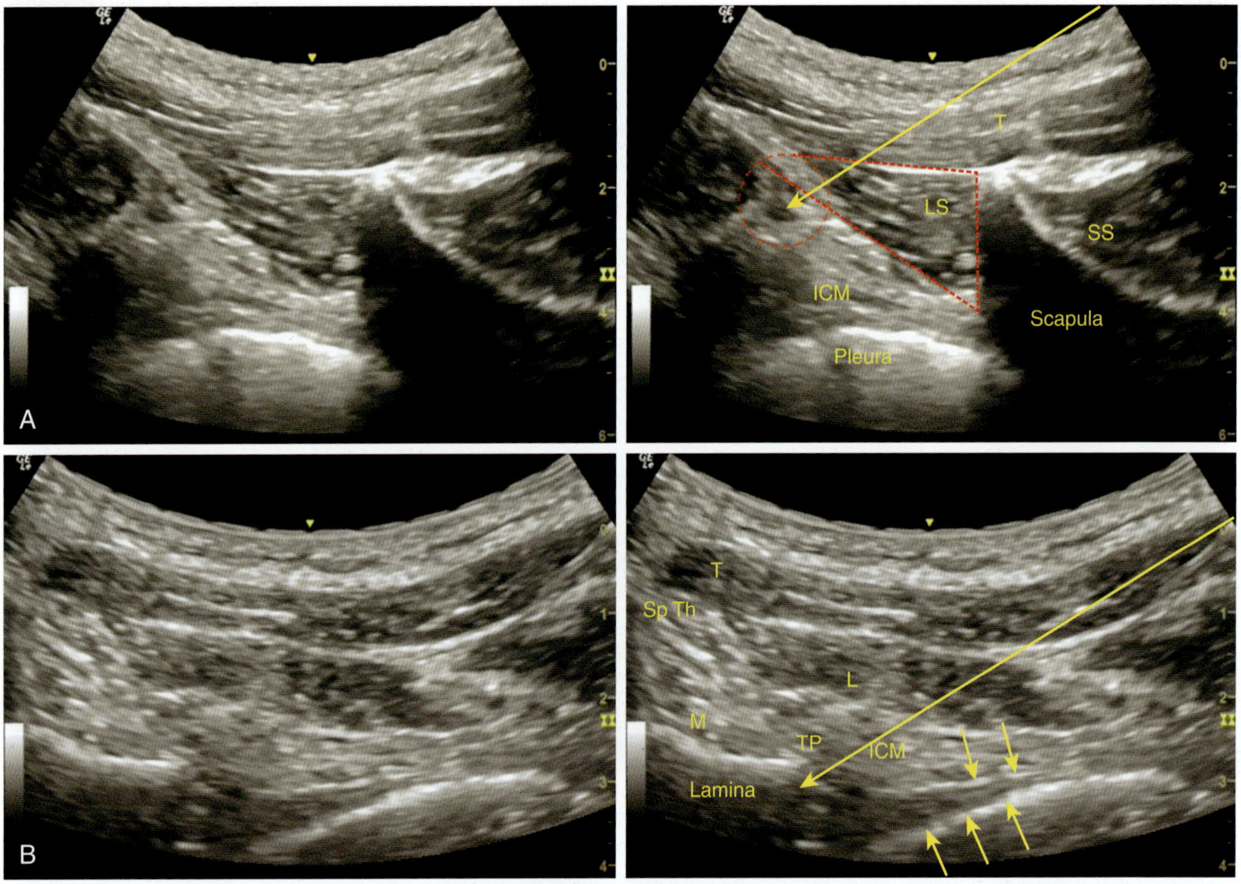

• **Fig. 9.4** (A) Hydrodissection (HD) of dorsal scapular nerve: The dorsal scapular nerve branches off the brachial plexus and can be involved in a whiplash injury. The dorsal scapular nerve travels with the dorsal scapular artery (both nerve and artery are within the *dashed circle*), lateral and inferior to the levator scapulae (*dotted red triangle*). The needle is represented by the *arrow*. (B) HD of the paravertebral space: This can be helpful in severe neuropathic pain such as in post-herpetic neuralgia. HD into the paravertebral space surrounds the spinal nerves as they emerge from the intervertebral foramen and surrounds the sympathetic ganglion. The needle passes just lateral to the transverse process. As the needle approaches the target (path shown by the long arrow), the bevel of the needle is down to avoid contacting the parietal pleura with a sharp needle tip. The paravertebral space is seen opening between the intercostal muscle and the parietal pleura (area between small arrows). *ICM*, Intercostal muscles and membrane; *L*, longissimus: *LS*, levator scapulae; *M*, multifidus; *Sp Th*, splenius thoracis; *SS*, supraspinatus; *T*, trapezius; *TP*, transverse process.

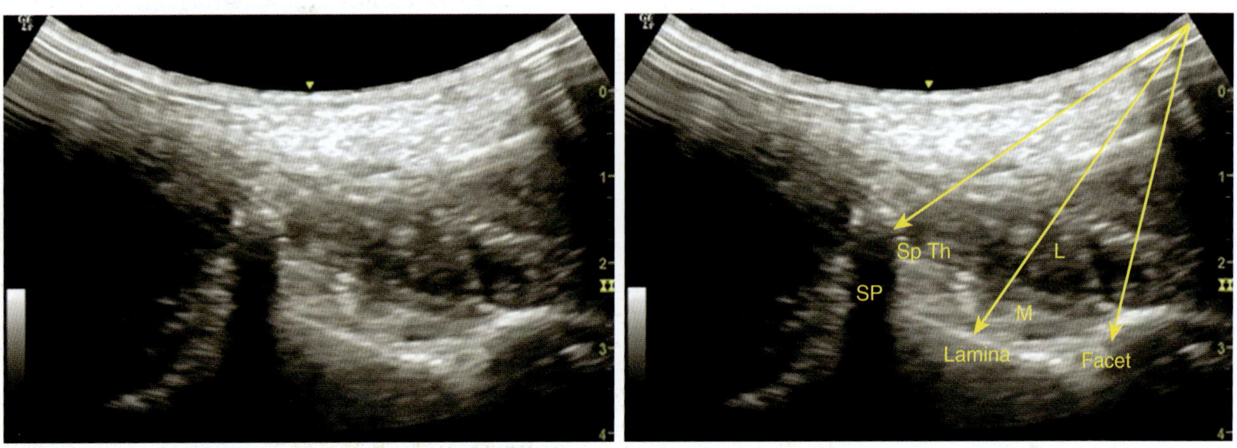

• **Fig. 9.5** Injection of posterior elements of thoracic spine: The posterior elements, including the facet ligaments, entheses along the lamina, and spinous process can be accessed with a single entry and multiple needle redirections (arrows in image). *L*, longissimus; *M*, multifidus; *SP*, spinous process; *Sp Th*, splenius thoracis.

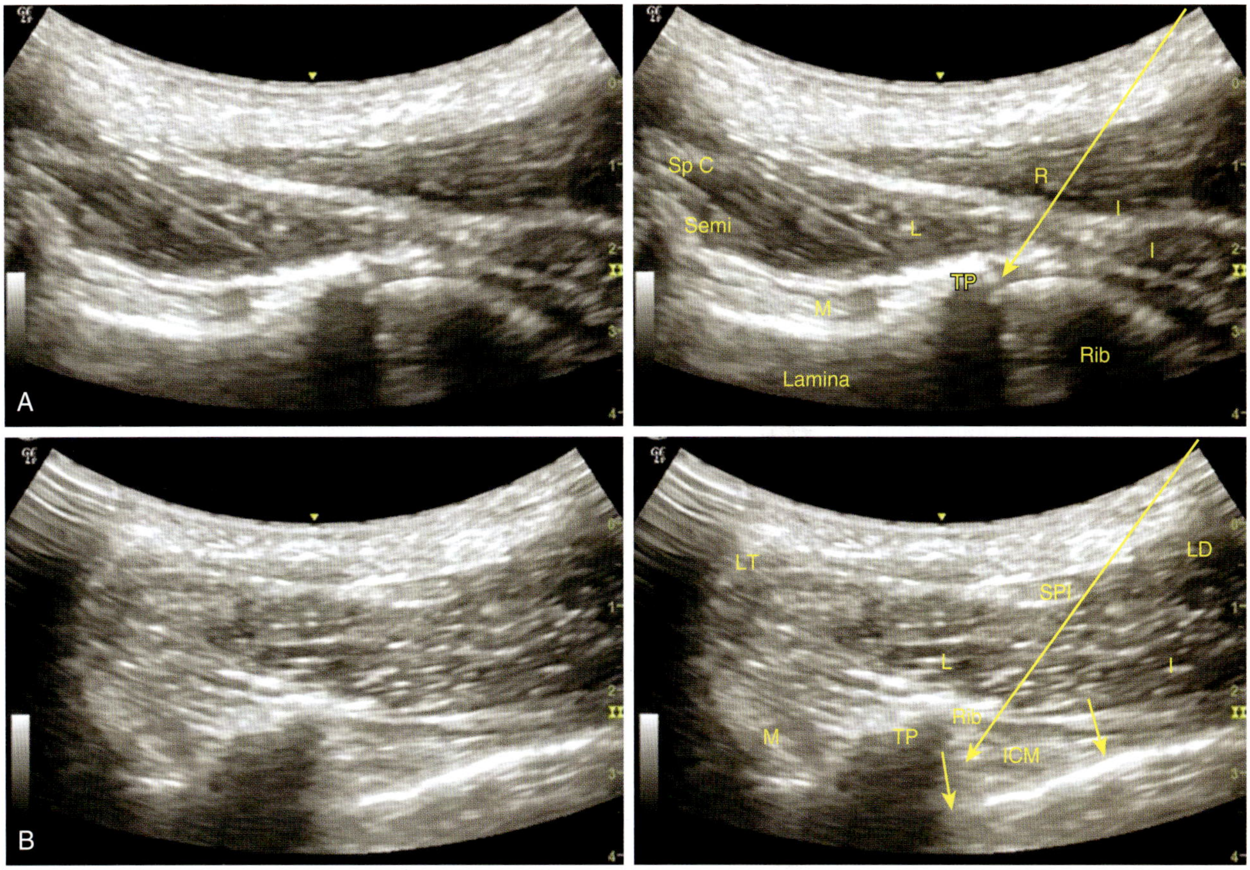

• **Fig. 9.6** (A) Injections of T1 to T2 costotransverse junctions: The costotransverse junctions of the upper rib levels can be injected by visualizing the rib blocking the lung and injecting the joint between rib and transverse process. (B) Option for injecting lower (T3 to T12) costotransverse junctions: At lower rib levels (3 to 12) an easier approach with good visualization involves altering the angle of the probe parallel with the rib but below the rib so the rib is not seen in ultrasound. All that is seen then is the transverse progress with intercostal muscle to its right. This allows for a clear view of the pleura *(arrows)* with injection maximizing safety by visualizing the needle while infiltrating against or close to the transverse process. This injection appears to be a reasonable substitute for intra-articular injection at each level. *ICM*, Intercostal muscles and membrane; *I*, iliocostalis; *L*, longissimus; *LD*, latissimus dorsi; *LT*, lower trapezius, *M*, multifidus; *R*, rhomboid; *Sp C*, splenius cervicis; *SPI*, serratus posterior inferior; *TP*, transverse process.

Hyaluronic acid injection and prolotherapy might be superior, but Dong and colleagues suggested additional research is needed.

Key Nociceptors

Nociceptive sources/targets for dextrose proliferant or perineural injection are grouped below according to lateral or medial elbow:

Lateral elbow:

1. Superficial nerves/penetrators: Posterior and lateral antebrachial cutaneous nerves.
2. Deeper nerves/ganglion/plexi: Median nerve under pronator teres, and ulnar nerve across elbow.
3. Entheses: Common extensor origin, and radial head ligament.

Medial elbow:

1. Superficial nerves/penetrators: Medial antebrachial cutaneous nerve.
2. Deeper nerves/ganglion/plexi: Radial nerve in spiral groove, at elbow, and within the supinator.
3. Entheses: Common flexor origin.

Wrist/Hand

Reeves et al. compared hypertonic dextrose (10%) solution to lidocaine alone injection for proximal interphalangeal (PIP), distal interphalangeal (DIP), and trapeziometacarpal (TMC) OA at 0, 2, and 4 months.[30] There was no significant difference at rest, but a significant improvement in pain with finger function and finger flexion range of motion in the dextrose group was reported at 6-month follow-up. Jahangiri et al.[31] in an RCT (n = 60) compared 3 monthly dextrose injections for TMC OA to a group with saline (at 0 and 1 months) and methylprednisolone (at 2 months). At 6-month follow-up, pain and pinch improvements were significantly more in the dextrose group. The above studies were included in two systematic analysis of RCTs for the treatment of knee and hand OA.[42,44] Krsticevic et al. in a narrative review[44] concluded that there was limited evidence indicating a beneficial effect of prolotherapy for finger/thumb OA management, and Hung et al. in a systematic review and meta-analysis[42] concluded that dextrose injection reduced pain in patients with hand OA.

At the wrist, Hooper et al. in an RCT (*n* = 39) compared periscaphoid and perilunate injections with hypertonic dextrose to lidocaine in participants with dorsal wrist pain and normal x-rays.[29] At 3 months there was no difference in outcomes, but at 12 months the Patient Rated Wrist Evaluation (PRWE) scores were significantly improved in the DPT group compared to the lidocaine group. Both groups improved more than the minimal clinically important difference (MCII) for PRWE, indicating a clinical benefit from lidocaine needling as well.

Wu et al. have reported three RCTs on HD for CTS. One trial (*n* = 34) compared saline HD (5 mL) into the intracarpal region to superficial injection of saline outside the carpal tunnel, and found a therapeutic benefit to HD in mild-to-moderate CTS.[78] A second study (*n* = 49) compared a single HD with 5 mL of D5W to HD with saline around the median nerve, and showed the D5W group had a significant reduction in pain and disability, improvement on electrophysiologic response measures, and decreased cross-sectional area of the median nerve compared to the saline HD control group.[79] A third study (*n* = 54) compared a single HD with 5 mL of D5W to triamcinolone injection 3 mL, and showed a significant reduction in pain and disability compared to triamcinolone.[80] Shen et al., in an RCT (*n* = 52) comparing HD with dextrose to HD with PRP for the treatment of mild to moderate CTS, reported significant and comparable improvements in pain and functional status in both groups.[81]

Studies by Wu et al. are among the most rigorous RCTs for any dextrose-related therapy and strongly support an independent biologic action for dextrose D5W HD compared to saline or corticosteroid injection.

Key Nociceptors

Nociceptive sources about the hand include:

1. Superficial nerves/penetrators: Superficial ulnar, median, and radial cutaneous nerves.
2. Deeper nerves/ganglion/plexi: Radial, median, and ulnar nerves at the elbow, median nerve at the wrist, and interdigital nerves.
3. Entheses: Radiocarpal, ulnocarpal, and intercarpal ligaments, triangular fibrocartilage complex, 1st dorsal interosseous, adductor pollicis, and abductor pollicis brevis.
4. Joints: Trapeziometacarpal joint/capsule, wrist joint, metacarpophalangeal (MCP), PIP, or DIP joints.

Lumbosacral Area

Yelland et al. assessed the efficacy of needling the entheses of symptomatic lumbo-pelvic ligaments and sacroiliac joints with dextrose versus lidocaine (*n* = 110).[91] Both groups reported a clinically significant improvement in pain and disability at the 2-year follow-up irrespective of the solution injected, suggesting that needling of entheses has a therapeutic effect. These findings are consistent with other DPT studies with a needling control,[25,29] and imply that needling controls should not be considered as a control in future research design. Instead, inclusion of a non-injection control should be considered.

Maniquis-Smigel et al. in a prospective uncontrolled cohort study (*n* = 32) evaluated the effect of caudal epidural injection of D5W (without an anesthetic or corticosteroid component) in participants with chronic low back pain radiating to the gluteal area or lower extremities.[67] Participants received 10 mL D5W caudally biweekly (x4) and then as needed. At the 1-year follow-up, 66% of participants reported a 50% or more reduction in chronic pain, and improved disability ratings on Oswestry Disability Index.[66]

Kim et al. in a single-blind RCT (*n* = 48) compared 25% dextrose to triamcinolone injections into the sacroiliac joint using fluoroscopic guidance with up to three biweekly injections.[32] At 15-month follow-up, dextrose injection showed a significant improvement in pain compared to cortisone, with more subjects reporting a ≥50% reduction in back pain (58.7% vs. 10.2%). For coccygodynia, Khan et al. published the largest case series with 37 consecutive patients with > 6 months of pain treated with 25% DPT at the area of maximum pain.[92] There was a reduction in VAS pain score in excess of 70% after 2 injections, but only 2-month follow-up was reported. Thirty patients had good relief and seven had minimal or no relief.

Key Nociceptors

For this area important nociceptive sources to consider in treatment of the complex pain patient using therapeutic dextrose injection include:

1. Superficial nerves/penetrators: Superficial dorsal rami medial and lateral branches, superficial superior, middle, and inferior cluneal nerves, and superficial iliohypogastric and ilioinguinal nerves.
2. Deeper nerves/ganglion/plexi: Dorsal rami, superior cluneal (Fig. 9.7A), and middle cluneal nerves, iliohypogastric and ilioinguinal nerves, and lumbar plexus (see Fig. 9.7B).
3. Entheses: Lumbar multifidi, facet ligaments and intertransversarii (Fig. 9.8A), sacroiliac (SI) ligament (see Fig. 9.8B), and iliolumbar (IL) ligaments.
4. Other: Sacrococcygeal joint, and caudal epidural injection.

Hip/Pelvic Area

There are no randomized trials of DPT for primary hip OA. Gul et al. in an open-label RCT[33] treated 41 patients (46 hips) with hip OA secondary to developmental dysplasia with hypertonic dextrose injections to tender periarticular tendons at 21-day intervals for a maximum of 6 injections versus 30 sessions of supervised progressive resistance

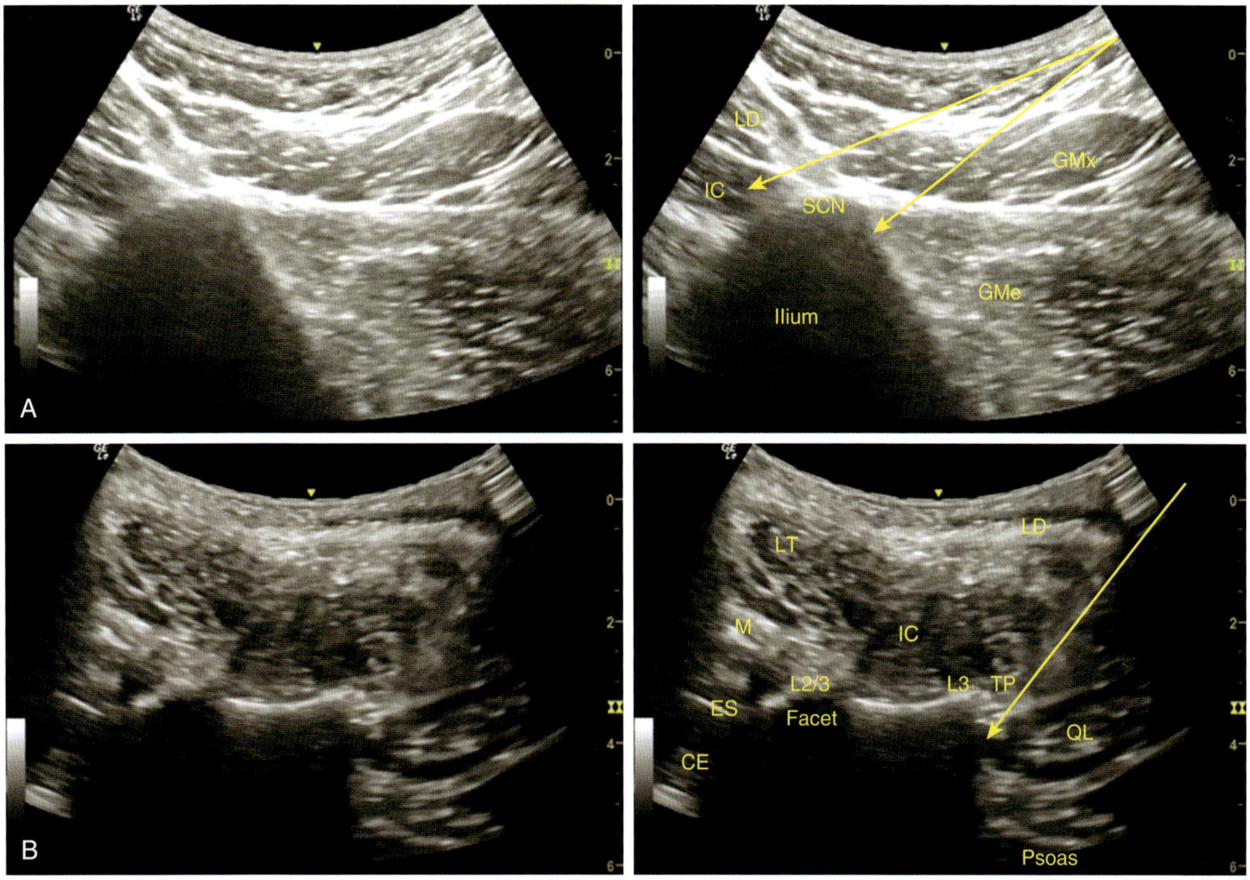

• **Fig. 9.7** (A) Superior cluneal nerve hydrodissection (HD): superior cluneal nerve *(SCN)* entrapment can be a source of low back and leg pain. The SCN can be localized as it crosses the iliac crest by finding the accompanying vessel. If the vessel is difficult to localize, HD under the fascia both above and below the iliac crest at the maximal area of tenderness is likely to release the entrapment of the SCN in its osteofibrous tunnel (two arrows in figure A showing injection under fascia above *[left]* and below *[right]* the iliac crest and under the fascial layer). (B) Lumbar plexus HD: HD of the lumbar plexus can downregulate neurogenic pain originating at mid to lower lumbar levels. If the needle passes lateral to the transverse process, and infiltration occurs bevel down for optimum safety, fluid will be observed filling the space posterior to the psoas. That space (located at the arrow tip) communicates with the lumbar plexus. *CE*, Cauda equina; *ES*, epidural space; *GMe*, gluteus medius muscle; *GMx*, gluteus maximus muscle; *IC*, iliocostalis lumborum muscle; *LD*, latissimus dorsi muscle; *LT*, longissimus thoracis muscle; *M*, multifidus muscle; *TP*, transverse process; *QL*, quadratus lumborum.

training. DPT outperformed the exercise control for improvements in Harris Hip Score (HHS) and pain scores at the 6-month and 1-year follow-ups.[9] These improvements were clinically significant, exceeding twice the minimal clinically important difference (MCID) for VAS pain improvement and above the MCID for HHS.

DPT has been reported as a treatment for athletic pubalgia. Topol et al. reported on a case series of 72 consecutive elite soccer or rugby athletes with chronic adductor origin or pubic symphysis pain. Subjects received 3 monthly treatments of palpation-guided 12.5% DPT, and 66 of 72 (92%) returned to full sport within 3 months.[93]

Key Nociceptors

Primary nociceptive sources to consider in therapeutic dextrose injection in this area include the following:

1. Superficial nerves/penetrators: Ventral rami medical branches, superior cluneal, middle and inferior cluneal, gluteal, iliohypogastric, ilioinguinal, femoral component of genitofemoral, inferior cluneal gluteal branches, perineal branches of inferior cluneal and pudendal nerves, lateral femoral cutaneous, and common fibular nerves.
2. Deeper nerves/ganglion/plexi: Ilioinguinal nerve at its quadratus lumborum penetration point, sacral and potentially lumbar ganglia via caudal epidural injection, and femoral nerve proximal just distal to the inguinal ligament, inferior cluneal nerve at ischial tuberosity level, pudendal medial to ischial spine, pudendal nerve in Alcock canal, and along ischiopubic ramus.
3. Entheses: Inferior gemellar origin (Fig. 9.9A), superior gemellar origin, gemellar and obturator externus insertions at base of trochanter and piriformis on top edge of trochanter (see Fig. 9.9B), ischiofemoral and iliofemoral ligaments (Fig. 9.10A) proximal gluteal origins, gluteal insertions onto the greater trochanter, gluteus maximus junction with the iliotibial band (see Fig. 9.10B), mid to distal iliotibial band,

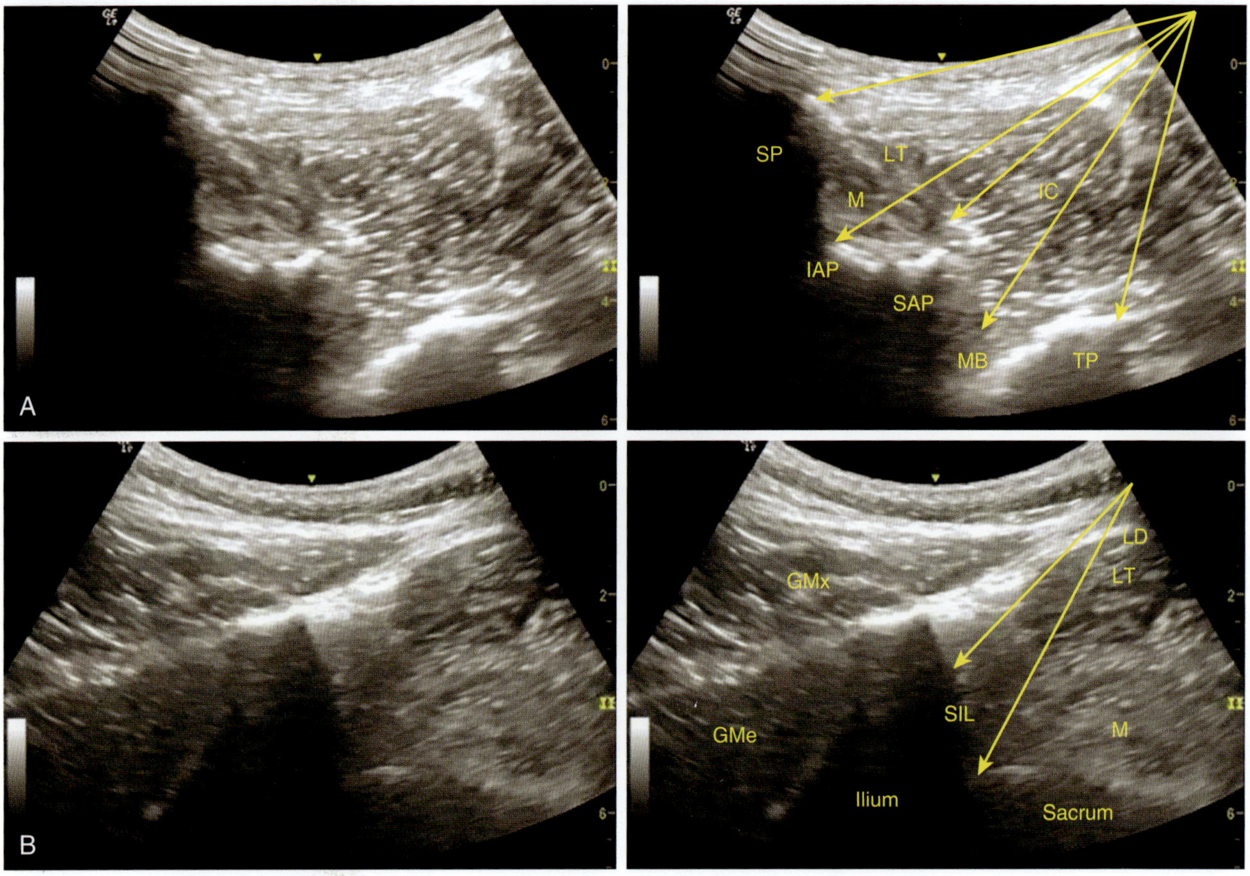

• **Fig. 9.8** (A) Injection of posterior elements of lumbar spine: The intertransverse ligament, facet ligaments, and multifidi/posterior lumbar rami can be treated from the same needle insertion. Targeting transverse processes requires the use of ultrasound for accuracy, and for avoidance of pleural contact at L1 and L2. (B) Sacroiliac ligament injection: The sacroiliac ligament can be targeted at both deep and superficial levels. The deeper injection is below the ligament and may be intra-articular. *GMe*, Gluteus medius muscle; *GMx*, gluteus maximus muscle; *IAP*, inferior articular pillar; *IC*, iliocostalis lumborum muscle; *LD*, latissimus dorsi muscle; *LT*, longissimus thoracis muscle; *M*, multifidus muscle; *MB*, medial branch; *SAP*, superior articular pillar; *SIL*, sacroiliac ligament; *SP*, spinous process *TP*, transverse process.

pectineus origin, pyramidalis insertion, rectus abdominus insertion, adductor origins, posterior insertions on ischiopubic ramus, and rectus femoris origin.

4. Joints: Sacrococcygeal joint, symphysis pubis, and iliofemoral joint.

Knee

For knee OA, Rabago et al. in an RCT (n = 90) of landmark guided intra-articular (25% dextrose) and extra-articular (15% dextrose) injections at 1, 5, and 9 weeks reported that DPT outperformed both the saline control and exercise groups at 1 year.[18] All groups reported improved composite Western Ontario and McMaster Universities Index (WOMAC) scores compared to baseline, but the DPT group exceeded the MCID for WOMAC scores. Dumais et al., using a randomized open-label crossover trial (n = 36), compared landmark guided intra-articular (20% dextrose) and collateral ligaments (15% dextrose) DPT to exercise.[19] At the 36-week follow-up, hypertonic dextrose was significantly better than exercise alone, accounting for a 29.5% improvement and 11.9 point decrease in WOMAC scores beyond that of exercise alone. Sert et al. in an RCT of participants with Kellgren-Lawrence grade II or III OA (n = 66) randomized into DPT, saline, or control home exercise treatment groups,[20] found a significant decrease in WOMAC pain and VAS activity scores at 18 weeks in the DPT group treated with intra- and extra-articular prolotherapy at 0, 3, and 6 weeks. Multiple meta-analyses and systematic reviews evaluating DPT for knee OA have shown favorable results.[40,42-44]

In cases of Osgood-Schlatter disease, Topol et al. in an RCT (n = 54; 65 knees) compared physical therapy to double-blind injection of lidocaine with or without 12.5% dextrose monthly for 3 months. Asymptomatic return to sport was significantly more common in the DPT cohort than the lidocaine-only or usual care group at 1 year. Nakase et al. compared 3 monthly injections of 20% dextrose or lidocaine into the deep infrapatellar bursa.[35] Neither treatment was reported as superior, with both showing a decrease in VISA score. However, the dextrose cohort had a greater change in pain scores than the lidocaine group (27 vs. 19.8

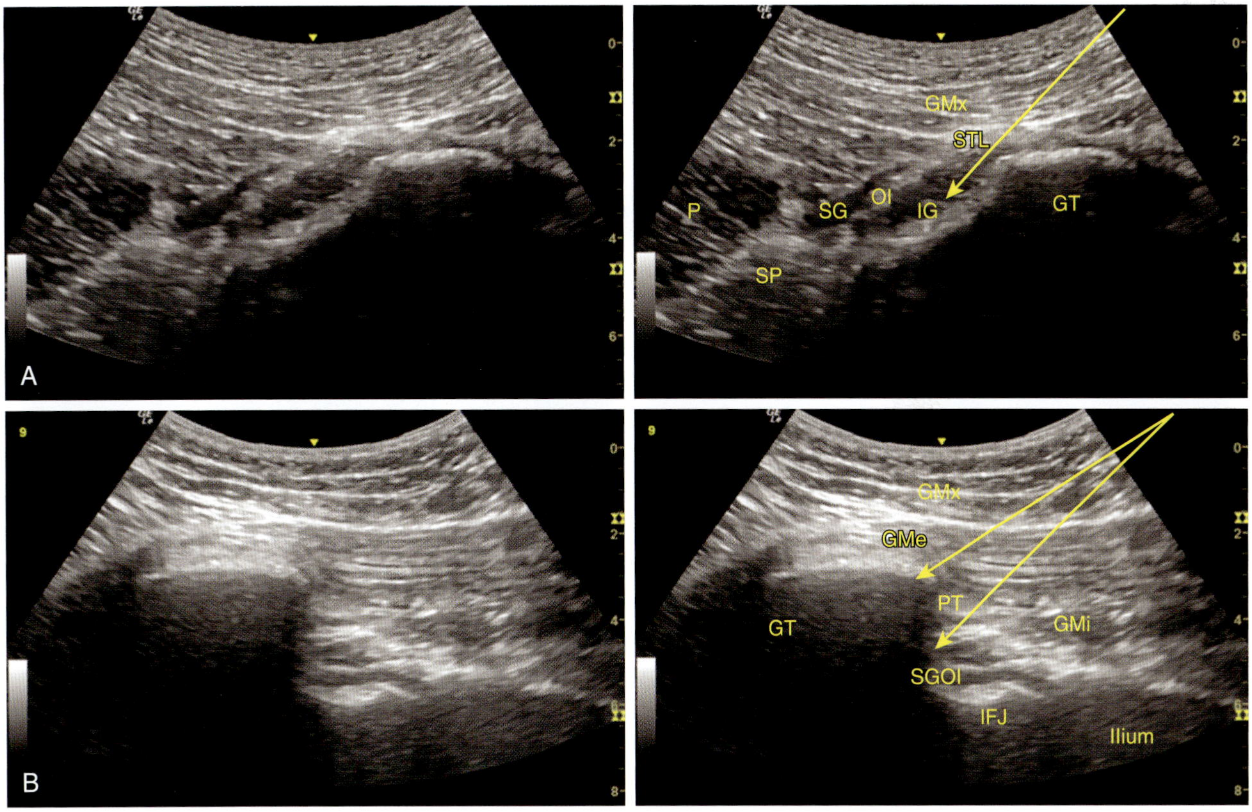

• **Fig. 9.9** (A) External rotator origins. Ultrasound offers the ability to accurately target the origin of several external rotators of the hip, including the inferior gemellus (at arrow tip) and superior gemellus. (B) External rotator insertions. Ultrasound also allows for targeting of insertions of the gemelli and obturator externus at the base of the greater trochanter (right arrow), and the piriformis insertion (left arrow) at the top edge of the greater trochanter laterally. *GMe*, Gluteus medius muscle; *GMi*, gluteus minimus muscle; *GMx*, gluteus maximus muscle; *GT*, greater trochanter; *IFJ*, iliofemoral joint; *IG*, inferior gemellus muscle; *P*, piriformis muscle; *PT*, piriformis tendon; *SG*, superior gemellus muscle; *SGOI*, tendons of superior gemellus, obturator internus and inferior gemellus; *SP*, sacral plexus.

points), and statistical results may have favored dextrose if the study was appropriately powered or used change scores rather than raw scores.[94] In addition, unlike Topol et al., Nakase et al.'s method did not target entheses, which may be important for successful management of Osgood-Schlatter disease.

Key Nociceptors

Nociception about the knee in the difficult-pain patient, as with other regions, is heavily influenced by multiple neurogenic sources, including:

1. Superficial nerves/penetrators: Saphenous, anterior femoral cutaneous, and common fibular.
2. Deeper nerves/ganglion/plexi: Femoral at inguinal canal, saphenous in Hunter canal, common fibular at knee, obturator nerve to the medial joint line, and the tibial nerve at the knee.
3. Entheses: Lateral and medial coronary and collateral ligaments, anterior cruciate ligament (ACL), medial and lateral retinaculum, quads insertion, and patellar tendon origin.
4. Other/Joints: Infrapatellar (Hoffa) fat pad, tibiofemoral joint, and large Baker cysts.

Ankle/Foot

Pilot studies and case series have examined prolotherapy for Achilles tendinosis[95,96] and subcutaneous PIT.[71] Yelland et al. in an RCT (n = 43) compared dextrose injection along the midsubstance Achilles tendon to eccentric lengthening exercises (ELE) or dextrose plus exercise.[36] Forty patients completed the study and at 12 months' dextrose and the combined dextrose and ELE treatment had a higher percentage of participants reaching the MCID for VISA-A. The combined dextrose and ELE group had more rapid improvement than ELE alone. Morath et al. in a meta-analysis on sclerotherapy and prolotherapy included four RCTs with a low risk of selection bias and concluded sclerotherapy and prolotherapy are safe and possibly effective treatments for Achilles tendinosis.[57]

For plantar fasciosis, Ersen et al. in an RCT (n = 50) compared three sonographically guided 15% DPT injections every 21 days to an exercise control.[37] The VAS pain, Foot and Ankle Outcome Score (FAOS), and Foot Function Index (FFI) were significantly improved in both groups. The prolotherapy group did have higher VAS and FAOS scores than the control group at 42, 90, and 360 days, but both

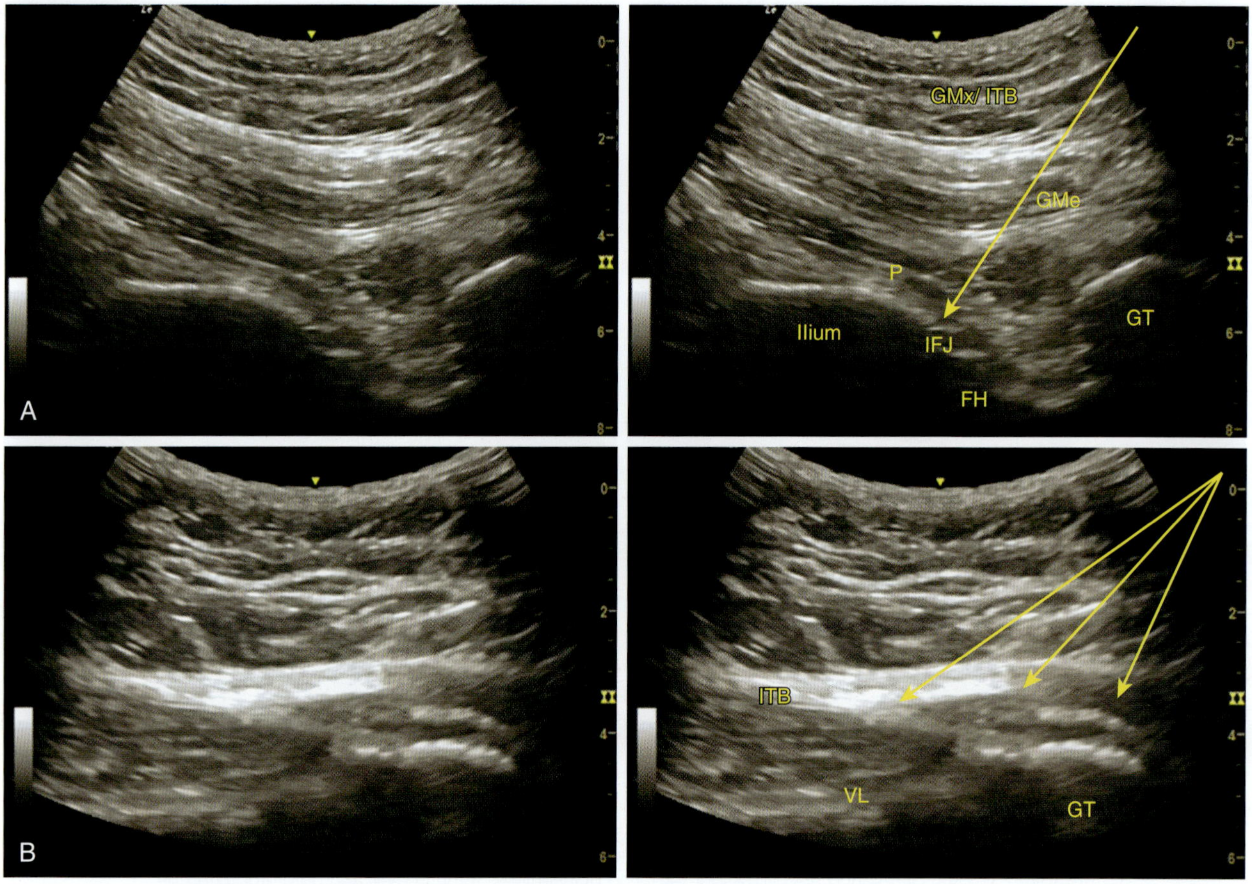

• **Fig. 9.10** High-resolution ultrasound (HRUS) application examples about the mid and lateral gluteus, posterolateral hip, and iliotibial band. (A) Hip capsular injection posterolaterally: For the patient with hip laxity, the origins of ischiofemoral and iliofemoral ligaments can be targeted at the iliac edge just proximal to the iliofemoral joint (arrow indicates needle direction and injection site). (B) Proximal iliotibial band injection. The junction of the gluteus maximus muscle *(GMx)* with the iliotibial band *(ITB)* can be a source of pain and requires ultrasound localization to treat the appropriate layers. This shows needling within the iliotibial band (multiple arrow tip) as it condenses over the greater trochanter. *FH*, Femoral head; *GMe*, gluteus medius muscle; *GT*, greater trochanter; *IFJ*, iliofemoral joint; *P*, piriformis muscle; *VL*, vastus lateralis.

groups had similar FFI scores at 360 days. Kim and Lee, in an RCT comparing sonographically guided PRP and 15% dextrose injection for plantar fasciosis,[38] reported significant improvement in mean FFI and found no statistically significant difference between PRP and prolotherapy at 6 months.

Key Nociceptors

Common sources of nociception within/affecting the ankle and/or foot include:

1. Superficial nerves/penetrators: Saphenous, superficial fibular, and lateral sural cutaneous.
2. Deeper nerves/ganglion/plexi: Tibial nerve at knee, posterior tibial in tarsal tunnel, fibular nerve at knee, fibular nerve about the fibular head, interdigital nerves, and nerves dorsal to the plantar fascia.
3. Entheses: Talofibular ligament origin and insertion, calcaneofibular ligament origin and insertion, talocalcaneal ligament origin and insertion, plantar fascia origin, short plantar ligament insertion, bifurcate ligament origin and insertion, tibiofibular ligament origin and insertion, spring ligament origin and insertion, and naviculocuboidal ligament origin and insertion.
4. Joints/other: Subtalar and tibiotalar joints, cubometatarsal, cuneometatarsal, cuneonavicular, and metatarsophalangeal (MTP) joints, posterior tibial synovium, and Kager fat pad/injection about the Achilles tendon.

Summary

Dextrose injection has been reported in numerous RCTs to be clinically effective in a variety of pain conditions. While its mechanism of action is not well understood, dextrose is hypothesized to be biologically active in the treatment of connective tissue: for example, ligament, tendon, cartilage, and nerve. It is used in three related but distinct modalities: prolotherapy, perineural injection therapy (PIT), and HD. The use of ultrasound is increasingly used to guide or confirm needle placement in many prolotherapy procedures that have historically been palpation-guided, and is essential in performing safe HD and some prolotherapy techniques.

References

1. Schultz LW. A treatment for subluxation of the temporomandibular joint. *J Am Med Assoc.* 1937;109(13):1032–1035.
2. Rice CO, Mattson H. Histologic changes in the tissues of man and animals following the injection of irritating solutions intended for the cure of hernia. *Ill Med J.* 1936:271–278.
3. Hackett GS. Prolotherapy in whiplash and low back pain. *Postgrad Med.* 1960;27:214–219.
4. Hackett GS, Hemwall GA, Montgomery GA. *Ligament and Tendon Relaxation Treated by Prolotherapy.* 5th ed. Madison, WI: Hackett Hemwall Patterson Foundation; 1993. http://hhpfoundation.org/.
5. Reeves KD, Sit RWS, Rabago D. Dextrose prolotherapy: a narrative review of basic science and clinical research, and best treatment recommendations. *Phys Med Rehabil Clin N Am.* 2016;27(4):783–823.
6. Scarpone M, Rabago DP, Zgierska A, Arbogast G, Snell E. The efficacy of prolotherapy for lateral epicondylosis: a pilot study. *Clin J Sport Med.* 2008;18(3):248–254.
7. Cook JL, Rio E, Purdam CR, Docking SI. Revisiting the continuum model of tendon pathology: what is its merit in clinical practice and research? *Brit Jnl Sports Med.* 2016;50:1187–1191.
8. Churgay CA. Diagnosis and treatment of biceps tendinitis and tendinosis. *Am Fam Physician.* 2009;80(5):470–476.
9. Rabago D, Best TM, Beamsley M, Patterson JJ. A systematic review of prolotherapy for chronic musculoskeletal pain. *Clin J Sport Med.* 2005;15(5):376–380.
10. Murphy M, Godson C, Cannon S, et al. Suppression subtractive hybridization identifies high glucose levels as a stimulus for expression of connective tissue growth factor and other genes in human mesangial cells. *J Biol Chem.* 1999;274(9):5830–3834.
11. Grosick R, Alvarado-Vazquez PA, Messersmith AR, Romero-Sandoval EA. High glucose induces a priming effect in macrophages and exacerbates the production of pro-inflammatory cytokines after a challenge. *J Pain Res.* 2018;11:1769–1778.
12. Ekwueme EC, Mohiuddin M, Yarborough JA, et al. Prolotherapy induces an inflammatory response in human tenocytes in vitro. *Clin Orthop Relat Res.* 2017;475:2117–2127.
13. Freeman JW, Empson YM, Ekwueme EC, Paynter DM, Brolinson PG. Effect of prolotherapy on cellular proliferation and collagen deposition in MC3T3-E1 and patellar tendon fibroblast populations. *Transl Res.* 2011;158:132–139.
14. Oh S, Ettema AM, Zhao C, et al. Dextrose-induced subsynovial connective tissue fibrosis in the rabbit carpal tunnel: a potential model to study carpal tunnel syndrome? *Hand (N Y).* 2008;3(1):34–40.
15. Yoshii Y, Zhao C, Schmelzer JD, Low PA, An KN, Amadio PC. Effects of hypertonic dextrose injections in the rabbit carpal tunnel. *J Orthop Res.* 2011;29(7):1022–1027.
16. Yoshii Y, Zhao C, Schmelzer JD, Low PA, An KN, Amadio PC. The effects of hypertonic dextrose injection on connective tissue and nerve conduction through the rabbit carpal tunnel. *Arch Phys Med Rehabil.* 2009;90(2):333–339.
17. Yoshii Y, Zhao C, Schmelzer JD, Low PA, An KN, Amadio PC. Effects of multiple injections of hypertonic dextrose in the rabbit carpal tunnel: a potential model of carpal tunnel syndrome development. *Hand (N Y).* 2014;9(1):52–57.
18. Rabago D, Patterson JJ, Mundt M, et al. Dextrose prolotherapy for knee osteoarthritis: a randomized controlled trial. *Ann Fam Med.* 2013;11:229–237.
19. Dumais R, Benoit C, Dumais A, et al. Effect of regenerative injection therapy on function and pain in patients with knee osteoarthritis: a randomized crossover study. *Pain Med.* 2012;13(8):990–999.
20. Sert AT, Sen EI, Esmaeilzadeh S, Ozcan E. The effects of dextrose prolotherapy in symptomatic knee osteoarthritis: a randomized controlled study. *J Altern Complement Med. Pain Med.* 2020;26(5):409–417.
21. Sit RWS, Wu RWK, Rabago D, et al. Efficacy of intra-articular hypertonic dextrose (prolotherapy) for knee osteoarthritis: a randomized controlled trial. *Ann Fam Med.* 2020;18(3):235–242.
22. Refai H, Altahhan O, Elsharkawy R. The efficacy of dextrose prolotherapy for temporomandibular joint hypermobility: a preliminary prospective, randomized, double-blind, placebo-controlled clinical trial. *J Oral Maxilofac Surg.* 2011;69(12):2962–2970.
23. Kilic SC, Güngörmüş M. Is dextrose prolotherapy superior to placebo for the treatment of temporomandibular joint hypermobility? A randomized clinical trial. *Int J Oral Maxillofacial Surg.* 2016;43(7):813–819.
24. Louw WF, Burrils F, Reeves KD, Cheng AL, Rabago D. Treatment of temporomandibular dysfunction with dextrose prolotherapy: a randomized controlled trial with long term follow-up. *Mayo Clinic Proc.* 2019;94(5):820–832.
25. Bertrand H, Reeves KD, Bennett CJ, Bicknell S, Cheng AL. Dextrose prolotherapy versus control injections in painful rotator cuff tendinopathy. *Arch Phys Med Rehabil.* 2016;97(1):17–25.
26. Seven MM, Ersen O, Akpancar S, et al. Effectiveness of prolotherapy in the treatment of chronic rotator cuff lesions. *Orthop Traumatol Surg Res.* 2017;103(3):427–433.
27. Rabago D, Lee KS, Ryan M, et al. Hypertonic dextrose and morrhuate sodium injections (prolotherapy) for lateral epicondylosis (tennis elbow): results of a single-blind, pilot-level, randomized controlled trial. *Am J Phys Med Rehabil.* 2013;92(7):587–596.
28. Bayat M, Raeissadat SA, Mortazavian Babiki M, Rahimi-Dehgolan S. Is dextrose prolotherapy superior to corticosteroid injection in patients with chronic lateral epicondylitis?: a randomized clinical trial. *Orthop Res Rev.* 2019;11:167–175.
29. Hooper RA, Hildebrand K, Faris P, Westaway M, Freiheit E. Randomized controlled trial for the treatment of chronic dorsal wrist pain with dextrose prolotherapy. *Int Musculoskeletal Med.* 2011;33(3):100–106.
30. Reeves KD, Hassanein K. Randomized prospective placebo-controlled double-blind study of dextrose prolotherapy for osteoarthritic thumbs and fingers (DIP, PIP and trapeziometacarpal joints): evidence of clinical efficacy. *Jnl Alt Compl Med.* 2000;6(4):311–320.
31. Jahangiri A, Moghaddam FR, Najafi S. Hypertonic dextrose versus corticosteroid local injection for the treatment of osteoarthritis in the first carpometacarpal joint: a double-blind randomized clinical trial. *J Orthop Sci.* 2014;19(5):737–743.
32. Kim WM, Lee HG, Jeong CW, Kim CM, Yoon MH. A randomized controlled trial of intra-articular prolotherapy versus steroid injection for sacroiliac joint pain. *J Altern Complement Med.* 2010;16(12):1284–1290.
33. Gul D, Orselik A, Akpancar S. Treatment of osteoarthritis secondary to developmental dysplasia of the hip with prolotherapy injection versus a supervised progressive exercise control. *Med Sci Monit.* 2020;26:e919166.
34. Topol GA, Podesta LA, Reeves KD, Raya MF, Fullerton BD, Yeh HW. Hyperosmolar dextrose injection for recalcitrant Osgood-Schlatter disease. *Pediatrics.* 2011;128(5):e1121–1128.

35. Nakase J, Oshima T, Takata Y, Shimozaki K, Asai K, Tsuchiya H. No superiority of dextrose injections over placebo injections for Osgood-Schlatter disease: a prospective randomized double-blind study. *Arch Orthop Trauma Surg*. 2020;140(2):197–202.
36. Yelland MJ, Sweeting KR, Lyftogt JA, Ng SK, Scuffham PA, Evans KA. Prolotherapy injections and eccentric loading exercises for painful Achilles tendinosis: a randomised trial. *Br J Sports Med*. 2009;45(5):421–428.
37. Ersen O, Akpancar S, Seven MM, Akyildiz F, Yildiz Y, Ozkan H. A randomized-controlled trial of prolotherapy injections in the treatment of plantar fasciitis. *Turk J Phys Med Rehab*. 2018;64(1):59–65.
38. Kim E, Lee JH. Autologous platelet-rich plasma versus dextrose prolotherapy for the treatment of chronic recalcitrant plantar fasciitis. *PMR*. 2014;6(2):152–158.
39. Ebell MH, Siwek J, Weiss BDW,SH, Susman J, Ewigman BB,M. Strength of recommendation taxonomy (SORT): a patient-centered approach to grading evidence in the medical literature. *Am Fam Physician*. 2004;69(3):549–556.
40. Sit RWS, Chung VCH, Reeves KD, et al. Hypertonic dextrose injections (prolotherapy) in the treatment of symptomatic knee osteoarthritis: a systematic review and meta-analysis. *Sci Rep*. 2016;6:25247.
41. Nourani B, Rabago D. Prolotherapy for knee osteoarthritis: a descriptive review. *Curr Phys Med Rehab Rep*. 2016;4:42–49.
42. Hung CY, Hsiao MY, K.V. C, Han DS, Wang TG. Comparative effectiveness of dextrose prolotherapy versus control injections and exercise in the management of osteoarthritis pain: a systematic review and meta-analysis. *J Pain Res*. 2016;9:847–857.
43. Hassan F, Trebinjac S, Murrell WD, Maffulli N. The effectiveness of prolotherapy in treating knee osteoarthritis in adults: a systematic review. *Br Med Bull*. 2017;4(1–18).
44. Krsticevic M, Jeric M, Dosenovic S, Jelicic KA, Puljak L. Proliferative injection therapy for osteoarthritis: a systematic review. *Int Orthop*. 2017;41(4):671–679.
45. Covey CJ, Sineath MHJ, Penta JF, Leggit JC. Prolotherapy: can it help your patient? *J Fam Pract*. 2015;64(12):763–768.
46. Hauser RA, Lackner JB, Steilen-Matias D, Harris DK. A systematic review of dextrose prolotherapy for chronic musculoskeletal pain. *Clin Med Insights Arthritis Musculoskelet Disord*. 2016;9:139–159.
47. Borg-Stein J, Osoaria HL, Hayano T. Regenerative sports medicine: past, present, and future (adapted from the PASSOR legacy award presentation; AAPMR; October 2016). *Pharm Manag PM R*. 2018;10(10):1083–1005.
48. Billesberger LM, Fisher KM, Qadri YJ, Boortz-Marx RL. Procedural treatments for knee osteoarthritis: a review of current injectable therapies. *Pain Res Manag*. 2020:3873098. https://doi.org/10.1155/2020/3873098.
49. Topol GA, Podestá L, Reeves KD, et al. Hypertonic-dextrose intra-articular injections in severe knee osteoarthritis: a pilot study suggesting disease modification through chondrogenesis (Abs). *Arch Phys Med Rehabil*. 2015;96(10):e104.
50. Nagori SA, Jose A, Gopalakrishnan V, Roy ID, Chattopadhyay PK, Roychoudhury A. The efficacy of dextrose prolotherapy over placebo for temporomandibular joint hypermobility: a systematic review and meta-analysis. *J Oral Rehabil*. 2018;45(12):998–1006.
51. Dwivedi S, Sobel AD, DaSilva MF, Akelman E. Utility of prolotherapy for upper extremity pathology. *J Hand Surg Am*. 2019;44(3):236–239.
52. Catapano M, Zhang K, Mittal N, Sangha H, Onishi K, de Sa D. Effectiveness of dextrose prolotherapy for rotator cuff tendinopathy: a systematic review. *PM R*. 2020;12(3):288–300.
53. Lin MT, Chiang CF, Wu CH, Huang YT, Tu YK, Wang TG. Comparative effectiveness of injection therapies in rotator cuff tendinopathy: a systematic review, pairwise and network meta-analysis of randomized controlled trials. *Arch Phys Med Rehabil*. 2019;100(2):336–349.
54. Dong W, Goost H, Lin XB, et al. Injection therapies for lateral epicondylalgia: a systematic review and Bayesian network meta-analysis. *Br J Sports Med*. 2015;50(15):900–908.
55. Yelland M, Rabago D, Ryan M, et al. Prolotherapy injections and physiotherapy used singly and in combination for lateral-epicondylalgia: a single-blinded randomised clinical trial. *BMC Musculoskelet Disord*. 2019;20(509). https://doi.org/10.1186/s12891-019-2905-5.
56. Sanderson LM, Bryant A. Effectiveness and safety of prolotherapy injections for management of lower limb tendinopathy and fasciopathy: a systematic review. *J Foot Ankle Res*. 2015;(8):57.
57. Morath O, Kubocsh EJ, Taeymans J, et al. The effect of sclerotherapy and prolotherapy on chronic painful Achilles tendinopathy—a systematic review including meta-analysis. *Scand J Med Sci Sports*. 2018;28(1):4–15.
58. Pavone V, Vescio A, Mobilia G, et al. Conservative treatment of chronic Achilles tendinopathy: a systematic review. *J Funct Morphol Kinesiol*. 2019;4:46.
59. Smith WB, Melton W, Davies J. Midsubstance tendinopathy, percutaneous techniques (platelet-rich plasma, extracorporeal shock wave therapy, prolotherapy, radiofrequency ablation). *C Podiatr Med Surg*. 2017;34(2):161–174.
60. Ravin TH, Cantieri MS, Pasquarello GJ. *Principles of Prolotherapy.* Friesens, Altona, Manitoba, Canada: American Academy of Musculoskeletal Medicine; 2008.
61. Baumgartner JJ. *Prolotherapy; the Art of Healing. Complete Injection Manual.* St. Cloud, Minnesota: Baumgartner, J.J.; 2011.
62. Hackett Hemwall Patterson Foundation. *Basic Prolotherapy Study Guide*. Madison, Wisconsin; 2010. https://hhpfoundation.org.
63. Lyftogt J. Chronic exertional compartment syndrome and prolotherapy. *Aust M Med*. 2006;11:83–85.
64. Ji R, Nackley A, Huh Y, Terrando N, Maixner W. Neuroinflammation and central sensitization in chronic and widespread pain. *Anesthesiology*. 2018;192(2):343–366.
65. Lyftogt J. Pain conundrums: which hypothesis? Central nervous system sensitization versus peripheral nervous system autonomy. *Aust M Med*. 2008;13(11):72–74.
66. Maniquis-Smigel L, Reeves KD, Rosen JH, et al. Short term analgesic effects of 5% dextrose epidural injection for chronic low back pain. A randomized controlled trial. *Anesth Pain Med*. 2017;7(1):e42550.
67. Maniquis-Smigel L, Reeves KD, Rosen JH, et al. Analgesic effect and potential cumulative benefit from caudal epidural D5W in consecutive participants with chronic low back and buttock/leg pain. *Jnl Alt Compl Med*. 2018;12(12):1189–1196.
68. Bertrand H, Kyriazis M, Reeves KD, Lyftogt J, Rabago D. Topical mannitol reduces capsaicin-induced pain: results of a pilot level, double-blind randomized controlled trial. *PM R*. 2015;7(11):1111–1117.
69. MacIver MB, Tanelian DL. Activation of C fibers by metabolic perturbations associated with tourniquet ischemia. *Anesthesiology*. 1992;76(4):617–623.

70. Lyftogt J. Subcutaneous prolotherapy treatment of refractory knee, shoulder and lateral elbow pain. *Aust M Med.* 2007;12(2):110–112.
71. Lyftogt J. Subcutaneous prolotherapy for Achilles tendinopathy. *Aust M Med.* 2007;12(11):107–109.
72. Lyftogt J. Prolotherapy for recalcitrant lumbago. *Aust M Med.* 2008;13(5):18–20.
73. Jancsó N, Jancsó-Gábor A, Szolcsányi J. Direct evidence for neurogenic inflammation and its prevention by denervation and by pretreatment with capsaicin. *Br J Pharmacol Chemother.* 1967;31(1):138–151.
74. Lyftogt J. Neuopathic pain therapies. 2020. *lyftogtmed.com.* 2020. Accessed April 21.
75. Klauser AS, Halpern EJ, De Zordo T, et al. Carpal tunnel syndrome assessment with US: value of additional cross-sectional area measurements of the median nerve in patients versus healthy volunteers. *Radiology.* 2009;250(1):171–177.
76. Lam SKH, Reeves KD, Cheng AL. Transition from deep regional blocks toward deep nerve hydrodissection in the upper body and torso. Method description and results from a retrospective chart review of the analgesic effect of 5% dextrose water as the primary hydrodissection injectate. *Biomed Res Int.* 2017:7920438. (Available at https://www.hindawi.com/journals/bmri/2017/7920438/).
77. Bennett GJ, Xie YK. A peripheral mononeuropathy in rat that produces disorders of pain sensation like those seen in man. *Pain.* 1988;33:87–107.
78. Wu YT, Chen SR, Li TY, et al. Nerve hydrodissection for carpal tunnel syndrome: a prospective, randomized, double-blind, controlled trial. *Muscle Nerve.* 2019;59(2):174–180.
79. Wu YT, Ho TY, Chou YC, et al. Six-month efficacy of perineural dextrose for carpal tunnel syndrome: a prospective, randomized, double-blind, controlled trial. *Mayo Clin Proc.* 2017;92(8):1179–1189.
80. Wu YT, Ke MJ, Ho TY, Li TY, Shen YP, Chen LC. Randomized double-blinded clinical trial of 5% dextrose versus triamcinolone injection for carpal tunnel syndrome patients. *Ann Neurol.* 2018;84(4):601–610.
81. Shen YP, Li TY, Chou YC, et al. Comparison of perineural platelet-rich plasma and dextrose injections for moderate carpal tunnel syndrome: a prospective randomized, single-blind, head-to-head comparative trial. *J Tissue Eng Regn Med.* 2019;13(11):2009–2017.
82. Mustafa R, Güngörmüş M, Mollaoğlu N. Evaluation of the efficacy of different concentrations of dextrose prolotherapy in temporomandibular joint hypermobility treatment. 2018;29(5): e461–e465.
83. Refai H. Long-term therapeutic effects of dextrose prolotherapy in patients with hypermobility of the temporomandibular joint: a single-arm study with 1-4 years' follow up. *Br J Oral Maxillofac Surg.* 2017;55(5):465–470.
84. Ungor C, Atasoy KT, Taskesen F, et al. Short-term results of prolotherapy in the management of temporomandibular joint dislocation. *J Craniofac Surg.* 2013;24(2):411–415.
85. Zhou H, Hu K, Ding Y. Modified dextrose prolotherapy for recurrent temporomandibular joint dislocation. *Br J Oral Maxillofac Surg.* 2014;52(1):63–66.
86. Fouda AA. Change of site of intra-articular injection of hypertonic dextrose resulted in different effects of treatment. *Br J Oral Maxillofac Surg.* 2018;56(8):715–718.
87. Majumdar SK, Krishna S, Chatterjee A, Chakraborty R, Ansari N. Single injection technique prolotherapy for hypermobility disorders of TMJ using 25% dextrose: a clinical study. *J Maxillofac Oral Surg.* 2016;16(2):226–230.
88. Centeno CJ, Elliott J, Elkins WL, Freeman M. Fluoroscopically guided cervical prolotherapy for instability with blinded pre and post radiographic reading. *Pain Physician.* 2005;1:67–72.
89. Hooper RA, Frizzell JB, Faris P. Case series on chronic whiplash related neck pain treated with intraarticular zygapophysial joint regeneration injection therapy. *Pain Physician.* 2007;10(2):313–318.
90. Hooper RA, Yelland MJ, Fonstad P, Southern D. Prospective case series of litigants and non-litigants with chronic spinal pain treated with dextrose prolotherapy. *Int Musculoskelet Med.* 2011;33(1):15–20.
91. Yelland MJ, Glasziou PP, Bogduk N, Schluter PJ, McKernon M. Prolotherapy injections, saline injections, and exercises for chronic low-back pain: a randomized trial. *Spine (Phila Pa 1976).* 2004;29(1):9–16.
92. Khan SA, Kumar A, Varshney MK, Trikha V, Yadav CS. Dextrose prolotherapy for recalcitrant coccygodynia. *J Orthop Surg.* 2008;16(1):27–29.
93. Topol GA, Reeves KD. Regenerative injection of elite athletes with career-altering chronic groin pain who fail conservative treatment: a consecutive case series. *Am J Phys Med Rehabil.* 2008;87(11):890–902.
94. Rabago D, Reeves KD, Topol GA, Podesta LA, Cheng AL, Fullerton BD. Infrapatellar bursal injection with dextrose and saline are both effective treatments for Osgood-Schlatter disease. Letter to editor for: no superiority of dextrose injections over placebo injections for Osgood-Schlatter disease: a prospective randomized double blind study. *Arch Orthop Trauma Surg.* 2020;140(4):591–592.
95. Maxwell NJ, Ryan MB, Taunton JE, Gillies JH, Wong AD. Sonographically guided intratendinous injection of hyperosmolar dextrose to treat chronic tendinosis of the Achilles tendon: a pilot study. *Am J Roentgenol.* 2007;189(4):W215–W220.
96. Ryan M, Wong A, Taunton J. Favorable outcomes after sonographically guided intratendinous injection of hyperosmolar dextrose for chronic insertional and midportion Achilles tendinosis. *Am J Roentgenol.* 2010;194(4):1047–1053.
97. Pandit JJ, Dutta D, Morris JF. Spread of injectate with superficial cervical plexus block in humans: an anatomical study. *Br J Anaesth.* 2003;91(5):733–735.

10
Sclerosing Agents

COLTON L. WOOD, DAVID J. BERKOFF, AND JUSTIN R. LOCKREM

Introduction

Sclerotherapy is the process of injecting a proinflammatory agent into an enlarged potential space (e.g., bursa, Morel-Lavallee lesion, tendon sheath) with the goal of alleviating pain, restoring function, and achieving cosmetic normalcy. Published literature to date details the sclerosing effects of an array of agents, including fibrin glue, doxycycline, other tetracycline derivatives, ethyl alcohol, polidocanol, and sodium morrhuate. Case reports, case series, and a limited number of randomized controlled trials (RCTs) report how these agents can serve as therapeutic options for numerous orthopedic conditions, including aseptic olecranon bursitis, aseptic prepatellar bursitis, subacromial bursitis, malleolar bursitis, Morel-Lavallee lesions, chronic idiopathic finger flexor tenosynovitis, chronic Achilles tendinosis, intraosseous low-flow vascular lesions, and chronic shoulder impingement syndrome.

This chapter reviews the current body of evidence and sets forth evidence-based treatment guidelines regarding sclerotherapy for orthopedic conditions. Prolotherapy is discussed within a separate chapter.

Indications for Use

Sclerotherapy in Bursitis: Theory and Clinical Evidence

Initial reports of using injectable caustic agents to accomplish sclerodesis in refractory bursitis date back to the 1930s.[1] Sclerodesis for recalcitrant bursitis fell out of favor with the increased popularity of surgical resection, percutaneous drain placement, or autologous blood injection ("blood patch").[2–5] However, surgical resection is not without significant complications, including recurrent bursitis, iatrogenic infection, chronic sinus tract formation, nerve damage, scar formation, increased pain, reduced range of motion (ROM), and delayed return to sport.[6,7] In the past 10 years, there has been a reemergence of interest in percutaneous sclerotherapy as a treatment for refractory bursitis.

In 2009, Ike detailed a case series of two patients (one with systemic lupus erythematosus, the other healthy) with chronic post-traumatic prepatellar bursitis refractory to rest, nonsteroidal antiinflammatory drugs (NSAIDs), compression bandage, and bursa aspiration in conjunction with a corticosteroid injection. Both patients had resolution of prepatellar swelling after blind aspiration and injection of the sclerosing agent sodium morrhuate. The agent was combined with methylprednisone and lidocaine to prevent previously described post-injection flares. At a 17-month follow-up, there was no recurrence of prepatellar swelling or pain.[12,13]

In 2016, Hong et al. completed a case series of two patients with aseptic olecranon bursitis and 22 patients with aseptic malleolar bursitis at the ankle with over 4 months of symptoms refractory to NSAIDs, bandaging, and aspiration with corticosteroid injection. All patients were treated with ultrasound (US)-guided bursa aspiration followed by irrigation with 50% dehydrated ethyl alcohol. After 1 minute the alcohol was aspirated and a compressive bandaging applied. This was repeated weekly if the bursa was not smaller on follow-up. In 13 of 24 study participants (54%), decreased bursal size was noted after one injection and patients went on to have complete resolution of the bursitis. The remaining 11 patients began to show clinical response after the second injection and these patients went on to a partial resolution of their bursitis. The mean follow-up period was 16 months, with no recurrence of bursa fluid or pain after initial resolution, with "local heat with tolerable pain" the only side effect reported in 4 of 24 patients. Patients with >3 months of symptoms required fewer injections (2.4 ± 1.7 injections) compared to those with <3 months of symptoms (4.7 ± 5.5 injections), suggesting ethyl alcohol sclerotherapy be reserved for patients who have failed >3 months of conservative therapy.[11]

In 2016, Berkoff et al. published a case report on the novel use of fibrin glue for persistent aseptic olecranon bursitis for patients who failed four prior aspirations and one steroid injection with compressive wrapping. In this case report, after aspiration of the olecranon bursa 2 mL of TISSEEL fibrin glue was injected using US guidance and compression wrap was applied. Follow-up evaluation at 3 weeks, 2 months, and 6 months showed no recurrence of the bursitis or pain.[14]

In 2018, Parker and Leggit authored a case report of a soldier with an 8-month history of refractory prepatellar bursitis treated successfully with two rounds of US-guided aspiration, injection with the sclerosing agent polidocanol (based on hospital formulary), and compression bandage. Improved function was reported at the 2-week follow-up visit, and at the 10-month follow-up no bursal fluid had reaccumulated and the patient had returned to prior level of function with no adverse effects.[8]

Concomitantly in 2018, Close and Hill published a case series of three patients with aseptic olecranon bursitis, including one with recurrent bursitis after a surgical bursectomy, refractory to over 1 month of conservative treatment. All patients had a single-blind injection with doxycycline 100 mg diluted in 10 mL sterile saline and compressive wrap for 2 weeks, and had improvement in bursal swelling and pain within 3 weeks. One patient reported mild burning at the injection site, controlled with over-the-counter analgesics. At the 6-month follow-up, no patient had recurrence of pain or swelling.[9]

Sclerotherapy in Morel-Lavallee Lesions and Seromas: Theory and Clinical Evidence

Morel-Lavallee lesions (MLLs) result from traumatic shearing forces to the tissue plane between subcutaneous fat and underlying muscle. The closed degloving-type injury disrupts the vessels that penetrate the fascia, leading to rapid accumulation of blood within the potential space between the subcutaneous fat and fascia. Complications include risk of secondary infection, fat necrosis and resultant deformity, or persistent pseudocyst formation.[15–18] Although MLL has historically been treated with open debridement and healing by secondary intention or drain placement, there is an emerging push toward minimally invasive treatments to avoid disturbing the subdermal arterial plexus. This plexus is the only remaining vascular supply to the overlying cutaneous flap, and its disruption can result in tissue flap necrosis.[15,17,19,20] Drainage and sclerotherapy is one proposed alternative to surgery for MLL, and includes sclerodesis with talc, bleomycin, and doxycycline. Talc can lead to severe pain as well as increased infection risk and bleomycin is very costly, making doxycycline is an appealing sclerosing agent for treating MLL.[15,20–32]

In 2007, Tejwani et al. reported a case series of 24 National Football League players who sustained a MLL to their knee(s) after a shearing blow from field impact or a tackle. Players presented an average of 3 days from the date of injury, and a total of 27 knees were included in this study. All 27 lesions were initially treated with ice, compression wrapping of the knee and thigh, and immediate passive/active ROM exercises; 13 lesions ultimately required aspiration. Three lesions (11%) persisted after three aspirations, but all subsequently resolved with one intralesional injection with 20 mg/mL doxycycline and compression wrapping. The doxycycline sclerodesis group had a successful full return to play within 1 day post-injection, but no extended follow-up was reported.[27]

In 2013, Bansal et al. focused on chronic MLL in a case series of 16 patients with MLL persisting for greater than 6 months. Patients had lesions located at the thigh, greater trochanter, gluteus, lower back, or abdominal wall. Most patients had undergone conservative therapy and multiple aspirations, and all patients underwent a blind MLL aspiration and sclerotherapy with 25 mL of doxycycline. The doxycycline was left in the lesion for 60 minutes with position changes every 10 minutes to ensure distribution, followed by aspiration of the sclerosing agent and compression wrapping for 4 weeks. At 4-week follow-up, 11 of the 16 patients (69%) had complete resolution of MLL. Four of the five remaining patients had MLL located on the anterior abdominal wall and were instructed to continue continuous compression wrapping. At 8-week follow-up, 15 of the 16 patients (94%) had complete resolution of MLL. The remaining patient was found to be noncompliant with compression therapy, and 13 of the 16 patients had no recurrent swelling or pain at the 3-year follow-up. The remaining three patients were lost to follow-up. Side effects included mild to moderate post-procedural pain and low-to-high grade fever for the first day post-procedure in the first 3 subjects. The remaining patients were treated with 1 day of Tylenol (acetaminophen) prophylaxis and reported no adverse effects.[33]

Fibrin agents have also been used over the years in various surgeries and procedures.[34–36] Berkoff et al. reported successfully using US-guided fibrin glue sclerodesis for a chronic post-arthroscopic knee seroma. In a 2013 case report, a persistent 7.5 × 7 cm seroma over the posterolateral knee that did not resolve with three US-guided aspirations and a corticosteroid injection was treated with aspiration and fibrin glue injection across the fascial defect and adjacent stalk. There was complete resolution at 2 weeks, with no re-accumulation at the 1-year follow-up.[37] In 2017, Koc et al. described the use of fibrin glue injection following endoscopic debridement of a suprapatellar MLL in a professional soccer player following failed conservative management, including doxycycline sclerodesis. The patient returned to sport at 6 weeks following treatment. US at 6 weeks showed complete resolution of MLL, with no recurrence at the 1-year follow-up.[38]

Sclerotherapy in Tendinosis and Tenosynovitis: Theory and Clinical Evidence

Sclerosing agents have also been investigated for treatment of chronic, refractory tendinopathy. Neonerves usually travel with neovessels inside the tendon. These sensory nerves have been implicated as possible pain generators, and it has been hypothesized that destroying the local neonerves adjacent to neovessels can decrease pain. Polidocanol is an analgesic and vascular irritant with established tolerability and efficacy in the treatment of varicose veins at various sites such as lower extremity varicosities, esophageal varices, telangiectasias, and hemorrhoids.[39–41]

In 2002 and 2003, two case series by Öhberg and Alfredson reported the effects of polidocanol injections at sites of neovascularization in chronic Achilles tendinosis with a symptom duration greater than 4 months. The polidocanol was injected under US-guided and Doppler imaging into the area adjacent to the neovessels as they entered the Achilles tendon until all vessels were sclerosed and no further Doppler flow was visualized. These pilot studies both revealed clinically and statistically significant improvements in visual analog scale (VAS) pain levels, patient satisfaction ratings, and Achilles tendon neovascularization for the first 6 months after polidocanol sclerotherapy.[42,43] Unpublished follow-up data for the 2002 case series revealed all eight patients had no recurrence of pain or neovascularization at 2 years, with normalization of tendon diameter and fibrillar structure on US.[44]

Öhberg and Alfredson also conducted a double-blind randomized controlled trial that randomized 20 consecutive patients with chronic mid-portion Achilles tendinopathy to US-guided polidocanol injections versus US-guided lidocaine injections into sites of tendon neovascularization. At 3 to 6 weeks post-injection, VAS pain scores with Achilles-loading activity, patient satisfaction ratings, and neovascularization were significantly improved ($P < .005$) in 5 of the 10 patients (50%) randomized to polidocanol compared to 0% of patients in the control group ($P < .878$). Neovascularization was fully resolved in all polidocanol subjects who reported no pain but remained present in all patients with persistent pain. At the trial's completion, subjects were allowed to cross over to the polidocanol group; 14 of the 15 crossover subjects (93%) noted statistically significant ($P < .04$) improvement in pain, satisfaction, and neovascularization on US. No adverse effects were reported by any patients.[44] Similar improvements in pain and return to preinjury level of activity have been reported after US-guided polidocanol sclerotherapy in seven elite and eight recreational-level athletes with chronic patellar tendinosis refractory to more than 3 months of rest and NSAIDs.[45]

Polidocanol also showed promising results in a 2006 case series as a treatment for chronic shoulder impingement syndrome. Alfredson et al. reported the results of US-guided polidocanol injections at sites of supraspinatus or subacromial bursa neovascularization in 15 patients who had failed rest, NSAIDs, physical rehab, and/or multiple subacromial corticosteroid injections. After a median of two polidocanol injections and gentle ROM exercises over at least 4 months, 14 of 15 patients (93%) reported clinically and statistically significant ($P < .05$) improvement in VAS shoulder pain scores with daily movements. No adverse outcomes were reported.[46]

There is one case report of a 56-year-old male with chronic idiopathic finger flexor tenosynovitis successfully treated with two injections of 50% ethyl alcohol. Injections were 10 months apart with initial improvement in pain after first injection and gradual resolution of swelling after two injections. Follow-up at 22 months revealed no adverse effects, pain-free normal ROM, and complete resolution of symptoms.[47]

Few studies have examined the association between neovascularization and pain, and results have been conflicting.[48–50] Due to the conflicting results and limited high-quality evidence, it is difficult to make a recommendation for sclerosing injection.[51] In addition, while fibrin products and fibrin carriers have been extensively studied in animal models for promotion of postsurgical healing of tendons, tendinopathy, and tendon ruptures,[52–57] no research has been published with human subjects for tendonitis or tendinosis.

Sclerotherapy in Intraosseous Lesions: Theory and Clinical Evidence

Although limited evidence exists, doxycycline has been used for treatment of postoperative lymphoceles, head and neck lymphatic malformations, and intramuscular and intraosseous vascular lesions with good results.[58–61] In 2009, Wible and Mitchell published a case report of a 19-year-old male with a chronic, severely painful intraosseous lymphatic malformation. Following two sequential injections with doxycycline under US guidance, the patient's pain decreased from a pre-injection rating of 9 on a 10-point pain scale to 2/10 at rest 9 months after injection and 3/10 after running 1 mile at the same time point; his lymphatic lesion filling dimensions on magnetic resonance imaging (MRI) were also slightly reduced as well. No adverse effects were found or reported after 9 months of follow-up.[62]

Suggested Sclerosing Agents and Dosing

See Table 10.1.

Patient Selection, Management, and Rationale

Olecranon and Patellar Bursitis

Based on the current limited evidence, a treatment guideline for *aseptic* superficial bursitis should include the following patient-oriented, resource-conscientious steps:

1. Trial period of conservative therapy for 2 weeks including rest from aggravating activities, elbow or patellar padding, ice twice daily for 20 minutes, NSAID (i.e., naproxen 500 mg by mouth twice daily), and compression bandage.
2. Aspiration of bursa contents (preferably with US guidance) followed by compression bandage for 12 to 24 hours.
3. US-guided aspiration of bursa followed by injection of a corticosteroid injection with concomitant conservative therapies as listed in step 1.
4. US-guided aspiration of bursa followed by injection of a sclerosing agent (preferably doxycycline given current safety, cost, efficacy, and tolerability data) with concomitant conservative measures and scheduled follow-up in 2 to 4 weeks.
5. If no improvement by 12-week follow-up, repeat step 4 or discuss role of US-guided fibrin glue injection.
6. If suboptimal or no response, offer surgical referral for bursal resection.

TABLE 10.1 Recommended Sclerosing Agents and Dosing for Various Pathologies

Sclerosing Agent	Bursitis	Tendinosis/ Tenosynovitis	Morel-Lavallee Lesions/Seromas	Intraosseous Lesions
Doxycycline	100 mg of doxycycline powder in 10 mL of sterile saline (10 mg/mL).[9,a]	No prior studies.	100 mg of doxycycline powder in 5 mL of sterile saline (20 mg/mL).[27,a]	100 mg of doxycycline powder in 10 mL of sterile saline (10 mg/mL).[62,a]
Fibrin glue	Off-label use.	No prior human trials.	Off-label use.	No prior studies.
Polidocanol	4–6 mL of polidocanol (unspecified concentration).[8,a]	1–4 mL of 5 mg/mL polidocanol.[42–45,a]	No prior studies.	No prior studies.
Ethyl alcohol	Anesthesia with 3 mL of 2% lidocaine aspirated to the bursa sac. After lidocaine aspiration, inject a mixture of 2.5 mL of 50% dehydrated ethyl alcohol and 2.5 mL normal saline into the bursa sac.[11,a]	1 mL of 50% ethanol injected (tendon sheath of finger).[47,a]	No prior studies.	No prior studies.
Sodium morrhuate	Aspirate bursa, then instill 2 mL of 50 mg/mL sodium morrhuate (NDC 0517-3065-01), 40 mg of methylprednisolone, and 1 mL of 1% lidocaine.[13,a]	No prior studies.	No prior studies.	No prior studies.

[a]Adjust injectate volume to size of lesion.
This table compiles the recommended doses of sclerosing agents for the pathologies of bursitis, tendinosis, tendinitis, Morel-Lavallee lesions, seromas, and intraosseus lesions as discussed in this chapter.

Morel-Lavallee Lesions

Based on the current limited evidence, a treatment guideline for MLLs should include the following patient-oriented, resource-conscientious steps:

- For acute MLL characterized by small fluid collections and full ROM: compressive wrapping, ice for 20 minutes twice daily, and immediate physical therapy targeting active/passive joint ROM.
- For acute MLL with large fluid collections or limited ROM: compression wrapping, ice, and lesion aspiration. Attempt three series of aspirations prior to doxycycline sclerodesis.
- For chronic MLL: aspiration followed by doxycycline sclerodesis and compression wrapping for at least 4 weeks; may reattempt sclerodesis if not optimally resolved at follow-up.
- For resistant MLL: consideration of US-guided fibrin sealant following aspiration.

Techniques for Administration

Bursal (olecranon, prepatellar, etc.), Morel-Lavallee, and seroma injections

- Identify lesion and para-lesion structures with US
  - Note any neurovascular structures and alter procedural approach to avoid them
- Mark site of lesion
- Sterilize field
  - Take care to avoid contamination of sterile field with US probe/gel
  - Alternatively, consider sterile draping over US probe
- Anesthetize aspiration/injection tract

- 1% lidocaine w/o epinephrine drawn up in 5 to 10 mL syringe
- Use higher-gauge needle with appropriate needle length for anesthetizing (i.e., 25- or 27-guage, 1.5-inch needle)
- Consider use of anesthetizing cold (i.e., ethyl chloride) spray over the site of needle entry
- Introduce needle into skin and raise small wheal within subcutaneous tissue
- Under US guidance, advance needle along the planned aspiration-needle trajectory and gradually inject anesthetic along the entire tract
- Continue advancing needle into lesion as well and inject a small bolus of anesthetic within lesion
- Retract needle slowly along entry trajectory, slowly injecting the remaining anesthetic along the tract

- Aspirate
  - Use lower-gauge needle with appropriate needle length (i.e., 18- or 20-gauge needle)
  - Under US guidance, introduce aspiration needle into skin and retrace the trajectory of previously anesthetized tract and advance tip of needle to the lesion and aspirate contents
  - Leave needle in place and exchange syringe for sclerosant-containing syringe
  - Make use of a hemostat to facilitate maintaining needle position during syringe exchange.
- Use US to confirm needle position after syringe exchange and inject sclerosant
  - Fibrin use is off label
  - Doxycycline or tetracycline derivative
- Apply compression wrap (i.e., Coban wrap)
  - Confirm neurovascular status post-application, taking care to avoid high pressure that may lead to limb ischemia
- Review post-procedure instructions
  - Leave or reapply Coban to complete compressive wrapping for 24 hours post-procedure
  - Patient should be instructed on how to take down and reapply Coban wrapping if paresthesia or discomfort develops
  - Post-procedure rehab
  - Minimal movement for initial 72 hours

    Gentle passive ROM at 72 hours with gradual progression to full active ROM and subsequent strengthening exercises,

References

1. Kaplan L, Ferguson LK. Bursitis. *Am J Surg.* 1937;37:455–465.
2. Nontraumatic soft tissue disorders. Knee. Prepatellar bursitis. In: Canale ST, ed. *Campbell's Operative Orthopedics.* 10th ed. Philadelphia: Mosby; 2003:894–895.
3. Nardella FA. Blood-patch treatment for prepatellar bursitis (housemaid's knee). *New Engl J Med.* 1982;306:1553.
4. Stimson H. Bursitis. *Am J Surg.* 1940;50:527–533.
5. Fisher RH. Conservative treatment of distended patellar and olecranon bursae. *Clin Orthop.* 1979;123:98.
6. Baumbach SF, Lobo CM, Badyine I, Mutschler W, Kanz KG. Prepatellar and olecranon bursitis: literature review and development of a treatment algorithm. *Arch Orthop Trauma Surg.* 2014;134(3):359–370.
7. Quayle JB, Robinson MP. An operation for chronic prepatellar bursitis. *J Bone Joint Surg Am.* 1976;58-B(4):504.
8. Parker CH, Leggit JC. Novel treatment of prepatellar bursitis. *Military Med.* 2018;183(11-12):e768–e770.
9. Close E, Hill G. Doxycycline as sclerotherapy for recurrent aseptic olecranon bursitis, a new application of an existing therapy. *EC Orthopaedics.* 2018;9(4):211–217.
10. Hassell AB, Fowler PD, Dawes PT. Intra-bursal tetracycline in the treatment of olecranon bursitis in patients with rheumatoid arthritis. *Br J Rheumatol.* 1994;33(9):859–860.
11. Hong JS, Kim HS, Lee JH. Ultrasound-guided 50% ethyl alcohol injection for patients with malleolar and olecranon bursitis: a prospective pilot study. *Ann Rehabil Med.* 2016;40(2):310–317.
12. Menninger H, Reinhardt S, Söndgen W. Intra-articular treatment of rheumatoid knee-joint effusion with triamcinolone hexacetonide versus sodium morrhuate. A prospective study. *Scand J Rheumatol.* 1994;23:249–254.
13. Ike RW. Chemical ablation as an alternative to surgery for treatment of persistent prepatellar bursitis. *J Rheumatol.* 2009;36(7):1560.
14. Berkoff DJ, Sandbulte ZW, Stafford HC, Berkowitz JN. Fibrin glue for olecranon bursitis: a case report. *Ther Adv Musculoskelet Dis.* 2016;8(1):28–30.
15. Hak DJ, Olson SA, Matta JM. Diagnosis and management of closed internal degloving injuries associated with pelvic and acetabular fractures: the Morel-Lavallée lesion. *J Trauma.* 1997;42(6):1046–1051.
16. Hudson DA. Missed closed degloving injuries: late presentation as a contour deformity. *Plast Reconstr Surg.* 1996;98(2):334–337.
17. Kottmeier SA, Wilson SC, Born CT, Hanks GA, Iannacone WM, DeLong WG. Surgical management of soft tissue lesions associated with pelvic ring injury. *Clin Orthop Relat Res.* 1996;(329):46–53.
18. Kudsk KA, Sheldon GF, Walton RL. Degloving injuries of the extremities and torso. *J Trauma.* 1981;21(10):835–839.
19. Helfet DL, Schmeling GJ. Complications. In: Tile M, ed. *Fractures of the Pelvis and Acetabulum.* 2nd ed. Baltimore, Md: Williams & Wilkins; 1995:451–467.
20. Routt Jr ML, Kregor PJ, Simonian PT, Mayo KA. Early results of percutaneous iliosacral screws placed with the patient in the supine position. *J Orthop Trauma.* 1995;9(3):207–214.
21. Hudson DA, Knottenbelt JD, Krige JE. Closed degloving injuries: results following conservative surgery. *Plast Reconstr Surg.* 1992;89:853–855.
22. Mir Y, Mir L, Novell AM. Repair of necrotic cutaneous lesions, secondary to tangential traumatism over detachable zones. *Plast Reconstr Surg.* 1950;6:264–274.
23. Luria S, Applbaum Y, Weil Y, Liebergall M, Peyser A. Talc sclerodhesis of persistent Morel-Lavalle´e lesions (posttraumatic pseudocysts): case report of 4 patients. *J Orthop Trauma.* 2006;20(6):435–438.
24. Gericke KR. Doxycycline as a sclerosing agent. *Ann Pharmacother.* 1992;26(5):648–649.
25. Caliendo MV, Lee DE, Queiroz R, Waldman DL. Sclerotherapy with use of doxycycline after percutaneous drainage of postoperative lymphoceles. *J Vasc Interv Radiol.* 2001;12:73–77.

26. Robinson LA, Fleming WH, Galbrainth TA. Intrapleural doxycycline control of malignant pleural effusions. *Ann Thorac Surg.* 1993;55:1115–1121.
27. Tejwani SG, Cohen SB, Bradley JP. Management of Morel-Lavallee lesion of the knee: twenty-seven cases in the National Football League. *Am J Sports Med.* 2007;35(7):1162–1167.
28. Harma A, Inan M, Ertem K. The Morel-Lavallee lesion: a conservative approach to closed degloving injuries. *Acta Orthop Traumatol Turc.* 2004;38:270–273.
29. Kothe M, Lein T, Weber AT, Bonnaire F. Morel-Lavallee lesion: a grave soft tissue injury. *Unfallchirurg.* 2006;109:82–86.
30. Luria S, Yaakov A, Yoram A, Meir L, Peyser A. Talc sclerodhesis of persistent Morel-Lavallee lesions (posttraumatic pseudocysts): case report of 4 patients. *J Orthop Trauma.* 2006;20:435–438.
31. Tseng S, Tornetta P. Percutaneous management of Morel-Lavallee lesions. *J Bone Joint Surg Am.* 2006;88:92–96.
32. Tsur A, Galin A, Kogan L, Loberant N. Morel-Lavallee syndrome after crush injury. *Harefuah.* 2006;145:111–113. 166.
33. Bansal A, Bhatia N, Singh A, Singh AK. Doxycycline sclerodesis as a treatment option for persistent Morel-Lavallée lesions. *Injury.* 2013;44(1):66–69.
34. Kulber DA, Bacilious N, Peters ED, Gayle LB, Hoffman L. The use of fibrin sealant in the prevention of seromas. *Plast Reconstr Surg.* 1997;99:842–849.
35. Schwabegger AH, Ninkovic MM, Anderl H. Fibrin glue to prevent seroma formation. *Plast Reconstr Surg.* 1998;101(6):1744–1745.
36. Shigeno Y, Harada I, Katayama S. Treatment of cystic lesions of soft tissue using fibrin sealant. *Clin Orthop Relat Res.* 1995;321:239–244.
37. Berkoff DJ, Kanaan M, Kamath G. Fibrin glue as a non-invasive outpatient treatment for post-arthroscopic knee seromas. *Knee Surg Sports Traumatol Arthrosc.* 2013;21:1922.
38. Koc BB, Somorjai N, Kiesouw PM, Egid, et al. Endoscopic debridement and fibrin glue injection of a chronic Morel-Lavallée lesion of the knee in a professional soccer player: a case report and literature review. *The Knee.* 2017;24(1):144–148.
39. Conrad P, Malouf GM, Stacey MC. The Australian polidocanol (aethoxysklerol) study. Results at 2 years. *Dermatol Surg.* 1995;21:334–336.
40. Guex JJ. Indications for the sclerosing agent polidocanol. *J Dermatol Surg Oncol.* 1993;19:959–961.
41. Winter H, Drager E, Sterry W. Sclerotherapy for treatment of hemangiomas. *Dermatol Surg.* 2000;26:105–108.
42. Ohberg L, Alfredson H. Ultrasound guided sclerosis of neovessels in painful chronic Achilles tendinosis: pilot study of a new treatment. *Br J Sports Med.* 2002;36(3):173–175; discussion 176–177.
43. Ohberg L, Alfredson H. Sclerosing therapy in chronic Achilles tendon insertional pain—results of a pilot study. *Knee Surg Sports Traumatol Arthrosc.* 2003;11(5):339–343.
44. Alfredson H, Ohberg L. Sclerosing injections to areas of neovascularisation reduce pain in chronic Achilles tendinopathy: a double-blind randomized controlled trial. *Knee Surg Sports Traumatol Arthrosc.* 2005;13(4):338–344.
45. Alfredson H, Ohberg L. Neovascularisation in chronic painful patellar tendinosis—promising results after sclerosing neovessels outside the tendon challenge the need for surgery. *Knee Surg Sports Traumatol Arthrosc.* 2005;13(2):74–80.
46. Alfredson H, Harstad H, Haugen S, Ohberg L. Sclerosing polidocanol injections to treat chronic painful shoulder impingement syndrome—results of a two-centre collaborative pilot study. *Knee Surg Sports Traumatol Arthrosc.* 2006;14(12):1321–1326.
47. Shin JE, Park JH, Yi HS, Ye BK, Kim HS. Treatment of chronic isolated finger flexor tenosynovitis through 50% dehydrated alcohol installation. *Ann Rehabil Med.* 2013;37(4):586–590.
48. de Vos RJ, Weir A, Cobben LP, Tol JL. The value of power Doppler ultrasonography in Achilles tendinopathy: a prospective study. *Am Journal Sports Med.* 2007;35(10):1696–1701.
49. Tol J, de Jonge S, Weir A, de Vos RJ, Verhaar J. Relationship between neovascularization and clinical severity in Achilles tendinopathy: a prospective analysis of 556 paired measurements. *Knee Surg Sports Traumatol Arthrosc.* 2012;20(suppl 1):S63.
50. van Sterkenburg MN, de Jonge MC, Sierevelt IN, van Dijk CN. Less promising results with sclerosing ethoxysclerol injections for midportion Achilles tendinopathy: a retrospective study. *Am J Sports Med.* 2010;38(11):2226–2232.
51. Tol JL, Spiezia F, Maffulli N. Neovascularization in Achilles tendinopathy: have we been chasing a red herring? *Knee Surg Sports Traumatol Arthrosc.* 2012;20:1891–1894.
52. Chong AK, Ang AD, Goh JC, et al. Bone marrow-derived mesenchymal stem cells influence early tendon-healing in a rabbit Achilles tendon model. *J Bone Joint Surg Am.* 2007;89:74–81.
53. Andres BM, Murrell GA. Treatment of tendinopathy: what works, what does not, and what is on the horizon. *Clin Orthop Relat Res.* 2008;466(7):1539–1554.
54. Hohendorff B, Siepen W, Staub L. Treatment of acute Achilles tendon rupture: fibrin glue versus fibrin glue augmented with the plantaris longus tendon. *J Foot Ankle Surg.* 2009;48(4):439–446.
55. Kim HJ, Park JH, Lim HC, et al. The healing effect of bone morphogenic protein with fibrin glue on an injury of the tendon-bone junction. *J Korean Orthop Assoc.* 2007;42(1):115–124.
56. He M, Gan AWT, Lim AYT, et al. The effect of fibrin glue on tendon healing and adhesion formation in a rabbit model of flexor tendon injury and repair. *J Plast Surg Hand Surg.* 2013;47(6):509–512.
57. Kuskucu M, Mahirogullari M, Solakoglu C, et al. Treatment of rupture of the Achilles tendon with fibrin sealant. *Foot & Ankle International.* 2005;26(10):826–831.
58. Nehra D, Jacobson L, Barnes P, Mallory B, Albanese C, Sylvester K. Doxycycline sclerotherapy as primary treatment of head and neck lymphatic malformations in children. *J Pediatr Surg.* 2008;43:451–460.
59. Cordes B, Seidel F, Sulek M, Giannoni C, Friedman E. Doxycycline sclerotherapy as the primary treatment for head and neck lymphatic malformations. *Otolaryngol Head Neck Surg.* 2007;137:962–964.
60. Caliendo MV, Lee DE, Queiroz R, et al. Sclerotherapy with use of doxycycline after percutaneous drainage of postoperative lymphoceles. *J Vasc Interv Radiol.* 2001;12:73–77.
61. Mautner KR, Sussman WI. Intramuscular vascular malformations: a rare cause of exertional leg pain and a novel treatment approach with ultrasound-guided doxycycline sclerotherapy. *Am J Sports Med.* 2015;43(3):729–733.
62. Wible BC, Mitchell S. Doxycycline sclerotherapy of an intraosseous femoral lymphatic malformation: case report and literature review. *J Vasc Interv Radiol.* 2009;20(5):660–663.

11

Toxins for Orthopedics

ZACH BOHART, WALTER I. SUSSMAN, JACOB SELLON, AND NATALIE SAJKOWICZ

Introduction

Botulinum toxin (BTX) is produced by the bacteria *Clostridium botulinum* as a complex of proteins containing neurotoxin and various non-toxic proteins. There are seven immunologically distinct serotypes of the botulinum neurotoxin, named A to G.[1,2] Botulinum toxin A (BTX-A) is the most commonly used in clinical practice. Commercially available in the United States as onabotulinumtoxin A (Botox), abobotulinumtoxin A (Dysport), incobotulinumtoxin A (Xeomin). BTX-B is also used in clinical practice and is available as rimabotulinumtoxinB (Myobloc). There are no clear differences in effectiveness between the commercial formulations.[2]

Mechanism of Action

Botulinum toxin prevents the release of the neurotransmitter acetylcholine into the neuromuscular junction. The toxins bind to cholinergic neurons and prevent acetylcholine-containing vesicles from fusing with the synaptic membrane, inhibiting muscular activity. Traditionally, pain relief has been attributed to a reduction in muscle hyperactivity. Recent studies have suggested that there is a direct analgesic effect based on BTX action on neurotransmitters other than acetylcholine, including substance P and glutamate.[1]

Clinically, muscle weakness occurs after 2 to 5 days and lasts for about 2 to 3 months before starting to wear off. The duration of effect varies among patients, and subjective effects may be seen up to 6 months. There is a correlation between the amount of BTX used and duration of action, though even with higher doses the duration appears to plateau at about 3 months.[1]

Dosing of Botulinum Toxin

The potency of commercially available BTX is determined by in vivo mouse assays. One unit of BTX is defined as the intraperitoneal amount of toxin lethal to 50% (LD_{50}) of Swiss Webster mice.[1,3] Units are not comparable or interchangeable between different commercial formulations. For example, 20 units of onabotulinumtoxin A (ONA) (Botox) does not have the same potency as 20 units of abobotulinumtoxin A (ABO) (Dysport) or rimabotulinumtoxinB (RIMA) (Myobloc). The dose required to effectively weaken a muscle varies with the density of neuromuscular junction in any given muscle and the pathology being treated. Toxicity can occur, and recommendations for a safe total body dose are 12 units/kg for ONA and 30 units/kg for ABO.[3a]

Reconstitution of Botulinum Toxin

Botulinum toxin typically is available in a vacuum-dried crystalline form. The toxin appears as a barely visible thin crystalline complex at the bottom of the vial (Figs. 11.1 and 11.2) and must be reconstituted with sterile preservative-free normal saline (0.9% sodium chloride injection). RimabotulinumtoxinB (Myobloc) does not require reconstitution. These authors routinely use a dilution of 2 mL preservative-free saline per 100 units of onabotulinumtoxin A, though for small muscles concentration of 1 mL normal saline per 100 units has been used. For ABO, 1.5 mL normal saline per 300 units or 2.5 mL per 500 units is used.

For reconstitution, saline should be slowly injected into the BTX vial, checking that vacuum is present in the vial to ensure sterility; the vacuum can then be released by disconnecting the syringe from the needle. The botulinum toxin is gently mixed with the saline by moving vial side to side prior to drawing up the botulinum toxin solution. Reconstituted BTX should be refrigerated, but there is some concern that BTX may lose potency if stored.

Techniques for Administration

To maximize clinical effectiveness of BTX, the toxin must be injected into the fascial compartment of the muscle, and the dose must be sufficient to neutralize the neuromuscular junction. Localization of the target muscle can be aided using electrical stimulation. Ultrasound (US), fluoroscopy, and computed tomography (CT) can also ensure accurate

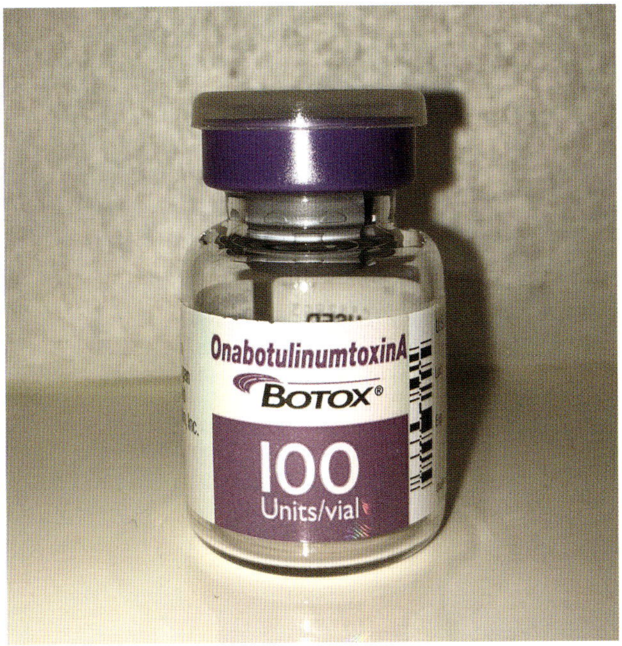

• **Fig. 11.1** Vial Containing Onabotulinumtoxin A. (© 2020 Allergan. Used with permission. All rights reserved.)

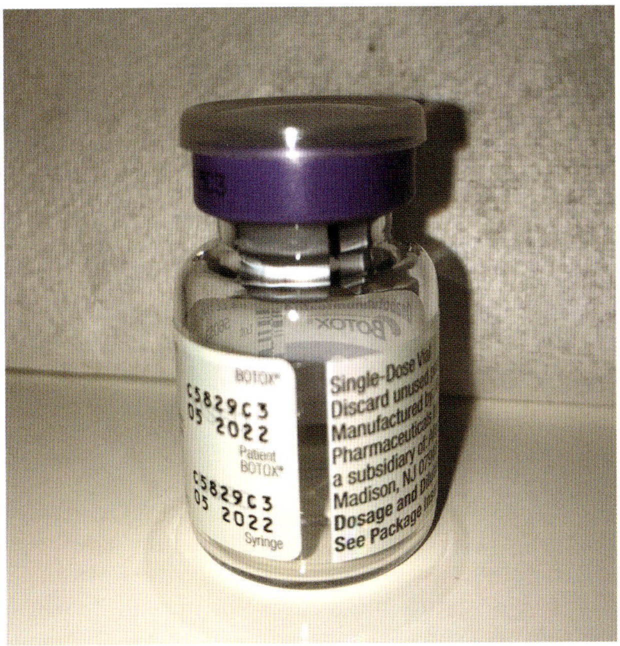

• **Fig. 11.2** Posterior view of a vial of onabotulinumtoxin A illustrating that the toxin is in dried crystalline form which is a barely visible thin complex at the bottom of the vial. (© 2020 Allergan. Used with permission. All rights reserved.)

placement of the BTX (Table 11.1). The number of injection sites should take into account the spread of medication, with animal studies showing that the toxin diffuses 30 to 45 mm from the injection site.[4]

Indications for Use

The use of BTX has evolved since its discovery in the 19th century.[1] BTX was first applied therapeutically as a treatment

TABLE 11.1 Supplies utilized for botulinum toxin injection

Supplies
• 3-mL syringe • 21-gauge 2-inch needle for reconstitution • Sterile, preservative-free normal saline (0.9% sodium chloride) • 2-inch needle for injection (EMG needle if EMG guidance being used) • Alcohol to prepare skin • EMG machine if being used with sticker electrodes (Fig. 11.3) • Ultrasound

EMG, Electromyography.

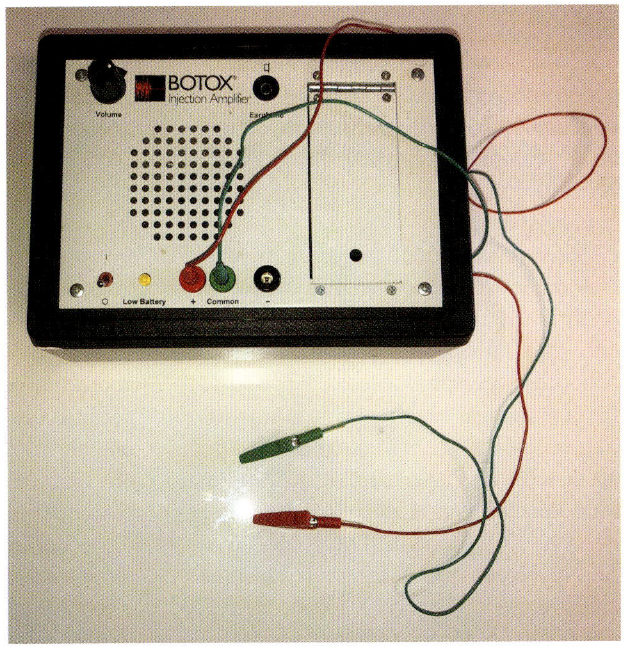

• **Fig. 11.3** Electromyography Amplifier With Electrodes Attached. (© 2020 Allergan. Used with permission. All rights reserved.)

for strabismus in the 1980s,[5] but its role in musculoskeletal medicine has continued to expand. Food and Drug Administration (FDA)-approved indications for BTX are limited, and there has been a growing interest in exploring the broader role of BTX in musculoskeletal medicine. The literature has explored the value of BTX in different musculoskeletal disorders. The following clinical indications are considered off-label uses of BTX, and many of these emerging applications require further validation.

Muscle

Researchers have utilized BTX-A for various muscle pathologies, primarily to treat muscle spasm or hypertrophy.

Myofascial Pain Syndrome (Trigger Points)

The exact pathogenesis of myofascial pain is unknown, and diagnostic criteria have varied across the literature.

Myofascial pain is characterized by "trigger points," defined as "a hyperirritable spot in skeletal muscle that is associated with a hypersensitive palpable nodule in a taut band. The spot is tender when pressed and can give rise to characteristic referred pain, motor dysfunction, and autonomic phenomena."[6] While the mechanism of BTX on myofascial pain is unclear, one theory is that BTX interrupts the pathologic muscle contraction allowing the muscle to relax.[7] BTX may be an alternative treatment for recalcitrant trigger points that have not responded to dry needling or anesthetic injections. Despite not clearly understanding the pathology, multiple studies have reported improved pain following BTX-A injections, including three randomized controlled trials (RCTS) comparing BTX-A injection to injection of saline and one RCT comparing BTX-A injection to dry needling.[8–15] Five RCTs found no significant difference between a single BTX injection and placebo.[16–21] In one study, some subjects were asymptomatic after a second injection,[17] and an additional RCT has shown significant improvement with a second dose,[22] suggesting possible benefit with sequential injections. Studies comparing BTX to local anesthetic or methylprednisolone have had heterogeneous results, some suggesting the injectates are equally beneficial.[8,14,23]

Most studies used palpation for localization, injecting into the most tender area. A local twitch response can help confirm the trigger point. Electromyography (EMG) guidance and fluoroscopic guidance have also been used.[18,24–26] All studies except one used BTX-A, with onabotulinumtoxin A dosages ranging from 10 to 100 units per injection site, up to 300 units total, and ABO dosages ranging from 40 to 120 units per site, 480 units total (Table 11.2). A randomized open-label prospective study comparing ABO doses of 60, 80, and 120 units for lower back trigger points found no dose–response relationship.[27] A retrospective chart review compared BTX-A and BTX-B for myofascial pain and found BTX-A had a significantly greater mean reduction in pain scores and longer duration of relief.[28]

The current body of literature provides no strong evidence to recommend or reject this treatment modality.[29–31] RCTs comparing BTX to saline placebo injection are complicated by the fact that the saline is an active control.[32] Further investigation is needed to determine the most efficacious BTX dosing and injection techniques.

TABLE 11.2 Botulinum Toxin Dosing for Muscle Applications

Toxin (Total Dose)	Area Targeted (Dose per Injection Site)
Myofascial Pain (Trigger Points)	
BTX-A NOS (20–600 U) BTX-B NOS (2500–20,000 U) ONA (50–150 U) ABO (240–480 U)	Trapezius (5–20 U ONA; 40 U ABO; 25–50 U BTX-A NOS) Splenius capitis (20 U ONA; 5–40 U ABO, 50 U BTX-A NOS) Cervical and thoracic paraspinal muscles (25–100 U NOS) Sternocleidomastoid (25 U BTXA-NOS) Infraspinatus (5–50 U ONA) Scalene (80 U ONA) Levator scapulae (5 U ONA; 50 U BTX-A NOS) Piriformis (100 U ONA) Iliopsoas (150 U ONA)
Chronic Exertional Compartment Syndrome	
ABO (76–108 U) BTX-A NOS (20–65 U) INCO (20 U)	Anterior compartment (tibialis anterior, extensor hallucis longus, extensor digitorum longus) (25–108 U ABO) Lateral compartment (peroneus brevis and longus) (25–108 U ABO) First dorsal interossei (10 U INCO) Adductor pollicis (10 U INCO)

ABO, abobotulinumtoxin A (Dysport); *INCO*, incobotulinumtoxin A (Xeomin); *NOS*, not otherwise specified; *ONA*, onabotulinumtoxin A (Botox); *RIMA*, rimabotulinumtoxinB (Myobloc); *U*, units.

Chronic Exertional Compartment Syndrome

Chronic exertional compartment syndrome (CECS) is caused by a reversible increase in the pressure within a fascial compartment. CECS most often involves the anterior and lateral compartments of the leg, leading to decreased tissue perfusion during periods of exertion. The symptoms quickly resolve with rest. The diagnosis is confirmed by checking the compartment pressures at rest and after exercise with needle manometry.

Initial treatment is typically nonoperative, and chemodenervation with BTX has been reported. Robust research including RCTs is still lacking. In one case series with 16 patients, BTX-A was used to treat CECS involving the anterior compartments (targeting tibialis anterior, extensor hallucis longs, extensor digitorum longs) and lateral compartments (targeting peroneus brevis and longus muscles).[33] Subjects showed a significant decrease in intra-compartmental pressures for up to 9 months.[33] Three other case reports, including a case of CECS involving the forearm, have shown sustained benefit at end of follow-up period at 10 to 15 months post treatment.[34,35] Some loss of muscle strength was noted as a potential side effect, though in all cases, posttreatment weakness resolved over the course of months.[34–36]

Tendon and Fascia

Plantar Fasciitis

Plantar fasciitis has been associated with hyperpronation and mechanical overload resulting in excessive tension on the fascia.[37] Nonoperative management of plantar fasciitis includes nonsteroidal antiinflammatory drugs (NSAIDs), corticosteroid injections, and physical therapy.[38] Corticosteroids have been a mainstay of treatment, but studies have shown similar or superior results with BTX injections. The plantar fascia is not composed of muscle, but palpation- or EMG-guided botulinum toxin injections have targeted the adjacent abductor hallucis and flexor digitorum brevis (FDB) muscles[39–42] or the gastrocnemius and soleus[43] with significant pain relief. Ultrasound (US)- and landmark-guided injections directly into the plantar fascia have also been used,[44–46] resulting in significant pain relief.

BTX-A to treat plantar fasciitis has been studied in multiple RCTs comparing BTX-A to placebo,[39,46–48] three of which showed significant improvement in pain compared to placebo, one finding no difference in treatment groups. Studies have also compared BTX to steroids[40] (concluding no difference in pain relief between treatment groups) and extracorporeal shock wave (ECSW)[42] therapy (suggesting the ECSW group had greater pain relief). Studies showed benefit from single BTX-A injection lasting from follow-up at 8 weeks[39] up to 12 months.[41,48] The dose of BTX-A has ranged from 50 units up to 250 units, with the most common dose being 70 units divided between the FDB muscle and abductor hallucis muscle.[39–42,49]

Lateral Epicondylitis

Lateral epicondylitis is often an overuse injury leading to degenerative changes of the common extensor tendon.[50] Standard treatment involves antiinflammatories, physical therapy, bracing, and corticosteroid injections. Corticosteroid injections have shown a short-term improvement in pain, but one study showed worse clinical outcomes with cortisone compared to placebo at the 1-year follow-up.[51,52] Botulinum toxin for lateral epicondylitis was initially reported in case studies and an early prospective study.[53,54] Since then, four randomized placebo-controlled trials have been performed which support BTX-A injection as beneficial treatment for lateral epicondylitis,[55–58] though three studies have not shown significant superiority in pain relief in the BTX treatment group compared to placebo[59] or steroids.[61,56]

BTX is thought to ease the tension on the enthesis site, allowing the tendon to heal.[60] BTX-A doses have ranged from 20 to 50 units onabotulinumtoxin A[59,61–63] and 40 to 60 units ABO[55–58,64] with the extensor carpi radialis brevis most commonly targeted using EMG guidance,[58,64,65] palpation guidance,[57] or electric stimulation (Table 11.3).[61] EMG and palpation guidance have been used to target the extensor digitorum communis.[54,57] Other studies have injected the most tender spot using landmark guidance,[55,56,59] with one recent study using US to inject 10 to 30 units incobotulinumtoxin A to specific symptomatic forearm extensor muscles. Sustained benefit after a single injection has been seen up to 18 months in one study.[56]

The most significant adverse effect is weakness of finger and wrist extensors, with studies showing mild paresis lasting from 2 to 16 weeks.[55–57] This weakness may not be tolerated by patients whose work requires intricate hand movements.

TABLE 11.3 Botulinum Toxin Dosing for Tendon and Fascia Applications.

Toxin (Total Dose)	Area Targeted (Dose per Injection Site)
Plantar Fasciitis	
BTX-A NOS (70–250 U)	Origin of plantar fascia (50–200 U BTX-A NOS) Tender area of heel medial to base of plantar fascia insertion (40–50 U BTX-A NOS) Tender area between 1 inch anterior to heel and midpoint of the plantar arch (30–50 U BTX-A NOS) Gastrocnemius (200 U BTX-A NOS) Soleus (50 U BTX-A NOS) Point of maximal tenderness along plantar arch (100 U BTX-A NOS)
Lateral Epicondylitis	
BTX-A NOS (20–40 U) ONA (50–100 U) ABO (60 U) INCO (10–30 U)	ECRB (30–40 U BTX-A NOS; 50–100 U ONA; 40 U ABO; 20 U INCO) EDC (20–40 U BTX-A NOS); Distance 1/3 length of forearm from lateral epicondyle on course of PIN (60 U ABO) Extensor carpi ulnaris (20 U INCO) Extensor digiti minimi (10 U INCO) Extensor digitorum longus (30 U INCO) 5 cm distal to maximum point of tenderness at lateral epicondyle (50 U ONA) Tender point 1 cm from lateral epicondyle (60 U ABO, 20 U ONA) 3–4 cm distal to tender lateral epicondyle (60 U ABO)

ABO, Abobotulinumtoxin A (Dysport); *ECRB*, extensor carpi radialis brevis; *EDC*, extensor digitorum communis; *INCO*, incobotulinumtoxin A (Xeomin); *NOS*, not otherwise specified; *ONA*, onabotulinumtoxin A (Botox); *RIMA*, rimabotulinumtoxinB (Myobloc); *U*, units.

Intra-Articular Applications

Most clinical applications of BTX are based on blocking the release of acetylcholine and causing muscle paralysis. Intra-articular (IA) BTX for painful joint conditions likely works through a different mechanism. BTX has been shown to suppress the release of various neuropeptides and inflammatory mediators, and inhibiting the release of these neurotransmitters is thought to reduce neurogenic inflammation and pain.[66] While the exact mechanism of pain relief is still unsertain, there is a growing interest in intra-articular applications for BTX.

BTX was first described for intra-articular pain in 11 patients with refractory joint pain from osteoarthritis (OA), rheumatoid arthritis, and psoriatic arthritis by Mahowald et al. in 2006.[67] In this case series, 15 joints (ankle, knee, and shoulder) were treated with BTX, and patients reported decreased pain and improved quality of life lasting for

3 to 13 months. The majority of studies have examined the role of IA BTX for OA, but BTX also been used for rheumatoid or psoriatic arthritis,[67–69] persistent pain after total joint replacement,[70–72] adhesive capsulitis,[73] sacroiliac joint pain,[74,75] and patellofemoral pain syndrome.[30,76–78]

Osteoarthritis

OA is the most common type of arthritis.[79] There are no treatments to cure or reverse the disease process, and various therapeutic and lifestyle interventions have been proposed for the management of symptomatic OA. In recent years, there has been a growing interest in new applications of BTX. A 2018 meta-analysis showed IA BTX has beneficial and significant short-term effects in decreasing refractory joint pain, but a nonsignificant improvement at 6 months.[80] BTX has been studied in ankle, knee, hip, and shoulder OA, with the majority of studies examining the impact of BTX on knee OA. RCTs have compared BTX to a 0.9% normal saline control,[67,81–84] hyaluronate injection,[83] corticosteroid injection,[85] and education.[86] Most studies showed that pain and quality-of-life parameters improved with IA BTX, but not all studies found IA BTX to be superior to placebo,[81,87] steroids,[87] or hyaluronic acid.[83]

The evidence for IA BTX is limited, and the clinical value is unclear. The severity of OA, type and dose of BTX, location of injection, and number of injections may impact results. One study showed benefit of BTX in Kellgren-Lawrence stage III OA, but no improvement in stage IV OA.[88] For the knee, shoulder, and ankle OA, ONA (100 units) was the most common botulinum toxin and dose used (Table 11.4), with doses ranging from as low as 25 units for ankle and knee OA[67,68,72] to 300 units for knee OA.[72] Higher doses of BTX may be less effective, with one study showing benefit with 100 units, but that 200 units of IA BTX had no effect.[70,81]

The IA application of BTX is novel, but the evidence is still limited. Most studies have been uncontrolled, single center, and with a small sample size and short-term follow-up. Studies have varied in BTX brand and dosing, number of injections, and protocols (i.e., multiple injections, co-administration with other injectates). In addition, not all IA pathology has been treated with IA BTX. Hip OA has been treated with BTX injected into the adductor longus and magnus muscle to reduce pressure on the femoral head and acetabulum[84,89] and patellofemoral pain syndrome treated with BTX injection into the vastus lateralis muscle.[76–78,90] More studies are needed to better define BTX's role in managing IA pathology.

TABLE 11.4 Botulinum Toxin Dosing for Intra-Articular Applications.

Toxin (Total Dose)	Area Targeted (Dose per Injection Site)
Knee	
ONA (25–300 U) ABO (300–700 U)	Intra-articular (25–300 ONA; 250 U ABO) Vastus lateralis (120–500 U ONA; 500–700 U ABO)
Hip	
ABO 400 U	Adductor longus (250 U) Adductor magnus (150 U)
Sacroiliac Joint	
ONA (50–100 U) ABO (100 U) RIMA (5000 U)	
Ankle	
ONA (25–100 U)	Intra-articular ankle (25–100 U) MTP joint (25 U)
Intra-Articular Shoulder	
ONA (50–300 U) ABO (200 U) INCO (100 U	

ABO, Abobotulinumtoxin A (Dysport); *INCO*, incobotulinumtoxin A (Xeomin); *NOS*, not otherwise specified; *ONA*, onabotulinumtoxin A (Botox); *RIMA*, rimabotulinumtoxinB (Myobloc); *U*, units.

Entrapment Syndromes

Botulinum toxin has been studied for a number of entrapment syndromes. The proposed mechanism is chemodenervation of the muscles decreasing neural or vascular compression. BTX treatments have been successful in treating thoracic outlet syndrome (TOS), piriformis syndrome (PS), and functional popliteal artery entrapment syndrome (PAES). While the literature is limited, clinical applications are promising.

BTX has been reported for the treatment of carpal tunnel syndrome (CTS), but literature is limited.[91,92] Only one randomized, double-blind, placebo-controlled study has explored BTX for CTS and showed BTX was not superior to placebo.[91]

Thoracic Outlet Syndrome

TOS is due to compression of the neurovascular bundle in the neck. Compression can occur at the interscalene triangle, costoclavicular space, or retropectoralis minor space. Patients can present with neurogenic or vascular symptoms. Neurogenic TOS resulting in irritation of the brachial plexus trunk or cords accounts for the majority of all TOS cases.[93] Botulinum toxin has been used for the management of TOS, weakening the muscles that impinge the brachial plexus. Successful treatment of neurogenic[94–96] and arterial TOS[97,98] has been reported. BTX was superior to corticosteroid in a prospective longitudinal study,[99] but the majority of studies are case reports[97,98,100] or retrospective.[94,96,101] Only one randomized double-blind controlled trial exists, which found no clinically or statistically significant difference between BTX and the normal saline control at 6 months.[95] The use of imaging can help minimize complications from the inadvertent spread of toxin. There is

TABLE 11.5 Botulinum Toxin Dosing for Entrapment Syndromes.

Toxin (Total Dose)	Muscle Targeted (Dose per Injection Site)
Thoracic Outlet Syndrome	
ONA (100–150 U)	Anterior scalene (12–30 U) Middle scalene (12–30 U) Trapezius and levator scapula (75–100 U) Subclavius (12–20 U) Pectoralis minor (15–35 U)
Piriformis Syndrome	
ONA (50–103 U) ABO (150 U) INCO (40–130 U) RIMA (5–12,000 U)	Piriformis Obturator internus
Popliteal Artery Entrapment Syndrome	
ONA (100–200 U) ABO (400 U)	Medial gastrocnemius (50–100 U) Lateral gastrocnemius (50–100 U) plantaris (50 U)

ABO, Abobotulinumtoxin A (Dysport); *INCO*, incobotulinumtoxin A (Xeomin); *NOS*, not otherwise specified; *ONA*, onabotulinumtoxin A (Botox); *RIMA*, rimabotulinumtoxinB (Myobloc); *U*, units.

no statistically significant difference in complication rate or outcomes with a combination of US and EMG versus fluoroscopy with EMG.[101] Studies have targeted the anterior scalene,[94,95,97–99,101,102] middle scalene,[95,99–101] trapezius,[101] subclavius,[94,101] and pectoralis minor[94,101] muscles. The majority of studies used onabotulinumtoxin A, with doses ranging from 15 to 100 units depending on the number of muscles being targeted (Table 11.5).[a] One study suggested improved outcomes when targeting the scalenes, subclavius, and pectoralis minor, compared to the anterior and middle scalene alone.[101] Long-term outcomes are limited, with the majority of studies providing outcomes at 3 months or less and only 1 study showing benefit at 6 months.[101] It is unclear from the literature if repeat injections provide any additive benefit.

Piriformis Syndrome

PS is a compression neuropathy of the sciatic nerve as it passes between the piriformis and obturator internus muscle. Various etiologies may account for PS, but the diagnosis is complicated as PS lacks a well-established laboratory or imaging study.

US-guided injections for PS have been validated, with an accuracy of 90% to 95%.[103,104] Fluoroscopy-assisted contrast injections have a reported accuracy of only 30%, with the majority of missed injections into the gluteus maximus muscle in a cadaveric study.[104] In the majority of studies of BTX for PS, the piriformis muscle was targeted alone. In one retrospective study, the piriformis and obturator internus muscle were targeted.[105] The majority of studies used onabotulinumtoxin 100 units,[103,105–109] but doses as low as 50 units have also been used.[108] Myobloc (5000 to 12,000 units),[110,111] Dysport (150 units),[112] and Xeomin (40 to 130 units)[113–115] have also been used. Chronic PS treated with botulinum toxin has been shown to cause atrophy[106,107,112] and fatty infiltration of the piriformis muscle.[105] Sustained clinical benefits have been reported up to 9 months after the treatment.[107]

[a] References 94, 95, 97, 99, 101, 102.

Popliteal Artery Entrapment Syndrome

PAES is a compression of the neurovascular structures in the popliteal fossa resulting in exercise-induced claudication. There are two types of PAES: anatomic and functional. Anatomic PAES is caused by an anatomic lesion directly causing entrapment and occlusion of the artery. Functional popliteal artery entrapment syndrome (FPAES) is more common,[116] and involves overcrowding of the popliteal fossa and compression of the artery. Bilateral presentation is common, and can occur in 25% to 76% of cases.[117]

Dynamic duplex US can confirm the diagnosis if there is a 75% or more reduction in the diameter of the popliteal artery at the two heads of the gastrocnemii with the ankle in plantar flexion.[118] Stress-position magnetic resonance imaging (MRI) with the ankle at rest and in plantar flexion can confirm vascular occlusion, and rule out anatomic anomalies of the popliteal fossa or artery. A patient may not be able to hold active plantarflexion during US and MRI due to discomfort and fatigue, making diagnosis challenging. BTX has been described as both a diagnostic tool and therapeutic alternative to surgery, and post-BTX imaging has demonstrated resolution of arterial occlusion.[119,120] The majority of studies targeted the medial gastrocnemius[118–122] with 50 units of onabotulinumtoxin A,[118–120,122] with some studies also injecting the lateral gastrocnemius[121,122] or plantaris muscle.[118,119] The injection can be repeated if recurrent symptoms present.[119] No major complications have been reported, but denervation atrophy of the medial gastrocnemius has been reported in one study.[120]

Adverse Effects

Botulinum toxin is generally considered safe for therapeutic indications, though adverse effects should be discussed during the consent process. BTX is not recommended in pregnant or lactating women. BTX-A and BTX-B have been associated with systemic adverse reactions including dysphagia, muscle weakness and atrophy, allergic reaction, injection-site trauma, myocardial infarction, respiratory failure, and death. In the majority of these cases with serious adverse events, significant comorbidities existed and may have had a causal role.[4,123] These adverse events are rare, and in one review the most common adverse event was dysphagia and was reported in only 26 of 1437 patients.[123]

Patients with neuromuscular disorders are at increased risk of a serious adverse event.

There have been reports of antibody formation to the toxin, considered a long-term adverse event, though newer formulations of BTX-A appear to be associated with reduced antibody formation.[124] In general, BTX is contraindicated in patients with disorders of the neuromuscular junction. The authors also would recommend avoiding botulinum toxin in patients with joint instability, especially in the cervical region. Patients with genetic hypermobility, such as Ehlers-Danlos syndrome or other diseases that affect collagen synthesis, rely more on muscular strength to compensate for ligamentous laxity, and therefore weakening of muscle strength by BTX injection may worsen symptoms caused by joint hypermobility.

References

1. Dressler D, Adib Saberi F. Botulinum toxin: mechanisms of action. *Eur Neurol.* 2005;53(1):3–9.
2. Scaglione F. Conversion Ratio between Botox(R), Dysport(R), and Xeomin(R) in clinical practice. *Toxins (Basel).* 2016;8(3).
3. Godoy IR, Donahue DM, Torriani M. Botulinum toxin injections in musculoskeletal disorders. *Semin Musculoskelet Radiol.* 2016;20(5):441–452.

3a. Ramachandran M, Eastwood D. Botulinum toxin and its orthopaedic applications. *J Bone Joint Surg.* 2006;88-B:981-7.

4. Yiannakopoulou E. Serious and long-term adverse events associated with the therapeutic and cosmetic use of botulinum toxin. *Pharmacology.* 2015;95(1-2):65–69.
5. Scott AB. Botulinum toxin injection of eye muscles to correct strabismus. *Trans Am Ophthalmol Soc.* 1981;79:734–770.
6. Simons DG. *Travell & Simons' Myofascial Pain and Dysfunction : The Trigger Point Manual.* 2nd ed. Baltimore: Williams & Wilkins; 1999.
7. Kamanli A, Kaya A, Ardicoglu O, Ozgocmen S, Zengin FO, Bayik Y. Comparison of lidocaine injection, botulinum toxin injection, and dry needling to trigger points in myofascial pain syndrome. *Rheumatol Int.* 2005;25(8):604–611.
8. Benecke R, Heinze A, Reichel G, Hefter H, Gobel H. Botulinum type A toxin complex for the relief of upper back myofascial pain syndrome: how do fixed-location injections compare with trigger point-focused injections? *Pain Med.* 2011;12(11):1607–1614.
9. Gobel H, Heinze A, Reichel G, Hefter H, Benecke R. Efficacy and safety of a single botulinum type A toxin complex treatment (Dysport) for the relief of upper back myofascial pain syndrome: results from a randomized double-blind placebo-controlled multicentre study. *Pain.* 2006;125(1-2):82–88.
10. Cheshire WP, Abashian SW, Mann JD. Botulinum toxin in the treatment of myofascial pain syndrome. *Pain.* 1994;59(1):65–69.
11. Acquadro MA, Borodic GE. Treatment of myofascial pain with botulinum A toxin. *Anesthesiology.* 1994;80(3):705–706.
12. Miller D, Richardson D, Eisa M, Bajwa RJ, Jabbari B. Botulinum neurotoxin-A for treatment of refractory neck pain: a randomized, double-blind study. *Pain Med.* 2009;10(6):1012–1017.
13. Porta M. A comparative trial of botulinum toxin type A and methylprednisolone for the treatment of myofascial pain syndrome and pain from chronic muscle spasm. *Pain.* 2000;85(1-2):101–105.
14. Kim DY, Kim JM. Safety and efficacy of prabotulinumtoxinA (Nabota((R))) injection for cervical and shoulder girdle myofascial pain syndrome: a pilot study. *Toxins (Basel).* 2018;10(9).
15. Ferrante FM, Bearn L, Rothrock R, King L. Evidence against trigger point injection technique for the treatment of cervicothoracic myofascial pain with botulinum toxin type A. *Anesthesiology.* 2005;103(2):377–383.
16. Wheeler AH, Goolkasian P, Gretz SS. A randomized, double-blind, prospective pilot study of botulinum toxin injection for refractory, unilateral, cervicothoracic, paraspinal, myofascial pain syndrome. *Spine (Phila Pa 1976).* 1998;23(15):1662–1666; discussion 1667.
17. Qerama E, Fuglsang-Frederiksen A, Kasch H, Bach FW, Jensen TS. A double-blind, controlled study of botulinum toxin A in chronic myofascial pain. *Neurology.* 2006;67(2):241–245.
18. Ojala T, Arokoski JP, Partanen J. The effect of small doses of botulinum toxin A on neck-shoulder myofascial pain syndrome: a double-blind, randomized, and controlled crossover trial. *Clin J Pain.* 2006;22(1):90–96.
19. Wheeler AH, Goolkasian P, Gretz SS. Botulinum toxin A for the treatment of chronic neck pain. *Pain.* 2001;94(3):255–260.
20. Lew HL, Lee EH, Castaneda A, Klima R, Date E. Therapeutic use of botulinum toxin type A in treating neck and upper-back pain of myofascial origin: a pilot study. *Arch Phys Med Rehabil.* 2008;89(1):75–80.
21. Nicol AL, Wu, II, Ferrante FM. Botulinum toxin type A injections for cervical and shoulder girdle myofascial pain using an enriched protocol design. *Anesth Analg.* 2014;118(6):1326–1335.
22. Graboski CL, Gray DS, Burnham RS. Botulinum toxin A versus bupivacaine trigger point injections for the treatment of myofascial pain syndrome: a randomised double blind crossover study. *Pain.* 2005;118(1-2):170–175.
23. De Andres J, Cerda-Olmedo G, Valia JC, Monsalve V, Lopez A, Minguez A. Use of botulinum toxin in the treatment of chronic myofascial pain. *Clin J Pain.* 2003;19(4):269–275.
24. Lang AM. Botulinum toxin type A therapy in chronic pain disorders. *Arch Phys Med Rehabil.* 2003;84(3 suppl 1):S69–S73; quiz S74-65.
25. Braker C, Yariv S, Adler R, Badarny S, Eisenberg E. The analgesic effect of botulinum-toxin A on postwhiplash neck pain. *Clin J Pain.* 2008;24(1):5–10.
26. Hubbard DR, Berkoff GM. Myofascial trigger points show spontaneous needle EMG activity. *Spine (Phila Pa 1976).* 1993;18(13):1803–1807.
27. Muller-Schwefe GHH, Uberall MA. Dysport(R) for the treatment of myofascial back pain: results from an open-label, phase II, randomized, multicenter, dose-ranging study. *Scand J Pain.* 2011;2(1):25–33.
28. Lang AM. A preliminary comparison of the efficacy and tolerability of botulinum toxin serotypes A and B in the treatment of myofascial pain syndrome: a retrospective, open-label chart review. *Clin Ther.* 2003;25(8):2268–2278.
29. Ahmed S, Subramaniam S, Sidhu K, et al. Effect of local anesthetic versus botulinum Toxin-A injections for myofascial pain disorders: a systematic review and meta-analysis. *Clin J Pain.* 2019;35(4):353–367.
30. Chen YW, Chiu YW, Chen CY, Chuang SK. Botulinum toxin therapy for temporomandibular joint disorders: a systematic review of randomized controlled trials. *Int J Oral Maxillofac Surg.* 2015;44(8):1018–1026.

31. Climent JM, Kuan TS, Fenollosa P, Martin-Del-Rosario F. Botulinum toxin for the treatment of myofascial pain syndromes involving the neck and back: a review from a clinical perspective. *Evid Based Complement Alternat Med.* 2013;2013:381459.
32. Hsieh RL, Lee WC. Are the effects of botulinum toxin injection on myofascial trigger points placebo effects or needling effects? *Arch Phys Med Rehabil.* 2008;89. United States.
33. Isner-Horobeti ME, Dufour SP, Blaes C, Lecocq J. Intramuscular pressure before and after botulinum toxin in chronic exertional compartment syndrome of the leg: a preliminary study. *Am J Sports Med.* 2013;41(11):2558–2566.
34. Orta C, Petit J, Gremeaux V. Chronic exertional compartment syndrome in hands successfully treated with botulinum toxin-A: a case. *Ann Phys Rehabil Med.* 2018;61(3):183–185.
35. Hutto WM, Schroeder PB, Leggit JC. Botulinum toxin as a novel treatment for chronic exertional compartment syndrome in the U.S. military. *Mil Med.* 2019;184(5-6):e458–e461.
36. Baria MR, Sellon JL. Botulinum toxin for chronic exertional compartment syndrome: a case report with 14 month follow-up. *Clin J Sport Med.* 2016;26(6):e111–e113.
37. Cornwall MW, McPoil TG. Plantar fasciitis: etiology and treatment. *J Orthop Sports Phys Ther.* 1999;29(12):756–760.
38. Thomas JL, Christensen JC, Kravitz SR, et al. The diagnosis and treatment of heel pain: a clinical practice guideline-revision 2010. *J Foot Ankle Surg.* 2010;49(3 suppl):S1–S19.
39. Babcock MS, Foster L, Pasquina P, Jabbari B. Treatment of pain attributed to plantar fasciitis with botulinum toxin A: a short-term, randomized, placebo-controlled, double-blind study. *Am J Phys Med Rehabil.* 2005;84(9):649–654.
40. Diaz-Llopis IV, Rodriguez-Ruiz CM, Mulet-Perry S, Mondejar-Gomez FJ, Climent-Barbera JM, Cholbi-Llobel F. Randomized controlled study of the efficacy of the injection of botulinum toxin type A versus corticosteroids in chronic plantar fasciitis: results at one and six months. *Clin Rehabil.* 2012;26(7):594–606.
41. Diaz-Llopis IV, Gomez-Gallego D, Mondejar-Gomez FJ, Lopez-Garcia A, Climent-Barbera JM, Rodriguez-Ruiz CM. Botulinum toxin type A in chronic plantar fasciitis: clinical effects one year after injection. *Clin Rehabil.* 2013;27(8):681–685.
42. Roca B, Mendoza MA, Roca M. Comparison of extracorporeal shock wave therapy with botulinum toxin type A in the treatment of plantar fasciitis. *Disabil Rehabil.* 2016;38(21):2114–2121.
43. Elizondo-Rodriguez J, Araujo-Lopez Y, Moreno-Gonzalez JA, Cardenas-Estrada E, Mendoza-Lemus O, Acosta-Olivo C. A comparison of botulinum toxin A and intralesional steroids for the treatment of plantar fasciitis: a randomized, double-blinded study. *Foot Ankle Int.* 2013;34(1):8–14.
44. Placzek R, Deuretzbacher G, Buttgereit F, Meiss AL. Treatment of chronic plantar fasciitis with botulinum toxin A: an open case series with a 1 year follow up. *Ann Rheum Dis.* 2005;64.
45. Placzek R, Deuretzbacher G, Meiss AL. Treatment of chronic plantar fasciitis with botulinum toxin A: preliminary clinical results. *Clin J Pain.* 2006;22(2):190–192.
46. Huang YC, Wei SH, Wang HK, Lieu FK. Ultrasonographic guided botulinum toxin type A treatment for plantar fasciitis: an outcome-based investigation for treating pain and gait changes. *J Rehabil Med.* 2010;42(2):136–140.
47. Peterlein CD, Funk JF, Holscher A, Schuh A, Placzek R. Is botulinum toxin A effective for the treatment of plantar fasciitis? *Clin J Pain.* 2012;28(6):527–533.
48. Ahmad J, Ahmad SH, Jones K. Treatment of plantar fasciitis with botulinum toxin. *Foot Ankle Int.* 2017;38(1):1–7.
49. Chou LW, Hong CZ, Wu ES, Hsueh WH, Kao MJ. Serial ultrasonographic findings of plantar fasciitis after treatment with botulinum toxin A: a case study. *Arch Phys Med Rehabil.* 2011;92(2):316–319.
50. Kraushaar BS, Nirschl RP. Tendinosis of the elbow (tennis elbow). Clinical features and findings of histological, immunohistochemical, and electron microscopy studies. *J Bone Joint Surg Am.* 1999;81(2):259–278.
51. Olaussen M, Holmedal O, Lindbaek M, Brage S, Solvang H. Treating lateral epicondylitis with corticosteroid injections or non-electrotherapeutical physiotherapy: a systematic review. *BMJ Open.* 2013;3(10):e003564.
52. Coombes BK, Bisset L, Brooks P, Khan A, Vicenzino B. Effect of corticosteroid injection, physiotherapy, or both on clinical outcomes in patients with unilateral lateral epicondylalgia: a randomized controlled trial. *Jama.* 2013;309(5):461–469.
53. Keizer SB, Rutten HP, Pilot P, Morre HH, v Os JJ, Verburg AD. Botulinum toxin injection versus surgical treatment for tennis elbow: a randomized pilot study. *Clin Orthop Relat Res.* 2002(401):125–131.
54. Morre HH, Keizer SB, van Os JJ. Treatment of chronic tennis elbow with botulinum toxin. *Lancet.* 1997;349. England.
55. Wong SM, Hui AC, Tong PY, Poon DW, Yu E, Wong LK. Treatment of lateral epicondylitis with botulinum toxin: a randomized, double-blind, placebo-controlled trial. *Ann Intern Med.* 2005;143(11):793–797.
56. Placzek R, Drescher W, Deuretzbacher G, Hempfing A, Meiss AL. Treatment of chronic radial epicondylitis with botulinum toxin A. A double-blind, placebo-controlled, randomized multicenter study. *J Bone Joint Surg Am.* 2007;89(2):255–260. doi: 210.2106/JBJS.F.00401.
57. Espandar R, Heidari P, Rasouli MR, et al. Use of anatomic measurement to guide injection of botulinum toxin for the management of chronic lateral epicondylitis: a randomized controlled trial. *Cmaj.* 2010;182(8):768–773.
58. Creuze A, Petit H, de Seze M. Short-term effect of low-dose, electromyography-guided botulinum toxin A injection in the treatment of chronic lateral epicondylar tendinopathy: a randomized, double-blinded study. *J Bone Joint Surg Am.* 2018;100(10):818–826. doi: 810.2106/JBJS.2117.00777.
59. Hayton MJ, Santini AJ, Hughes PJ, Frostick SP, Trail IA, Stanley JK. Botulinum toxin injection in the treatment of tennis elbow. A double-blind, randomized, controlled, pilot study. *J Bone Joint Surg Am.* 2005;87(3):503–507. doi: 510.2106/JBJS.D.01896.
60. Kalichman L, Bannuru RR, Severin M, Harvey W. Injection of botulinum toxin for treatment of chronic lateral epicondylitis: systematic review and meta-analysis. *Semin Arthritis Rheum.* 2011;40(6):532–538.
61. Oskarsson E, Piehl Aulin K, Gustafsson BE, Pettersson K. Improved intramuscular blood flow and normalized metabolism in lateral epicondylitis after botulinum toxin treatment. *Scand J Med Sci Sports.* 2009;19(3):323–328.
62. Lin YC, Tu YK, Chen SS, Lin IL, Chen SC, Guo HR. Comparison between botulinum toxin and corticosteroid injection in the treatment of acute and subacute tennis elbow: a prospective, randomized, double-blind, active drug-controlled pilot study. *Am J Phys Med Rehabil.* 2010;89(8):653–659.
63. Guo YH, Kuan TS, Chen KL, et al. Comparison between steroid and 2 different sites of botulinum toxin injection in the

treatment of lateral epicondylalgia: a randomized, double-blind, active drug-controlled pilot study. *Arch Phys Med Rehabil.* 2017;98(1):36–42.

64. Cogne M, Creuze A, Petit H, Delleci C, Dehail P, de Seze M. Number of botulinum toxin injections needed to stop requests for treatment for chronic lateral epicondylar tendinopathy. A 1-year follow-up study. *Ann Phys Rehabil Med.* 2019.
65. Lim EC, Seet RC, Cheah AE, Lim AY. Injection of botulinum toxin to the extensor carpi radialis brevis for tennis elbow. *J Hand Surg Eur.* 2010;35. England.
66. Singh JA. Botulinum toxin therapy for osteoarticular pain: an evidence-based review. *Ther Adv Musculoskelet Dis.* 2010;2(2):105–118.
67. Mahowald ML, Singh JA, Dykstra D. Long term effects of intra-articular botulinum toxin A for refractory joint pain. *Neurotox Res.* 2006;9(2-3):179–188.
68. Singh JA, Mahowald ML, Kushnaryov A, Goelz E, Dykstra D. Repeat injections of intra-articular botulinum toxin A for the treatment of chronic arthritis joint pain. *J Clin Rheumatol.* 2009;15(1):35–38. doi: 10.1097/RHU.1090b1013e31819 53b3181914.
69. Singh JA, Mahowald ML, Kushnaryov A, Goelz E, Dykstra D. Repeat injections of intra-articular botulinum toxin A for the treatment of chronic arthritis joint pain. *J Clin Rheumatol.* 2009;15(1):35–38.
70. Boon AJ, Smith J, Dahm DL, et al. Efficacy of intra-articular botulinum toxin type A in painful knee osteoarthritis: a pilot study. PM R. 2010;2(4):268–276.
71. Singh JA, Fitzgerald PM. Botulinum toxin for shoulder pain. *Cochrane Database Syst Rev.* 2010(9):CD008271.
72. Singh JA. Efficacy of long-term effect and repeat intraarticular botulinum toxin in patients with painful total joint arthroplasty: a retrospective study. *Br J Med Med Res.* 2014;4(1).(doi):10.9734/BJMMR/2014/4897.
73. Joo YJ, Yoon SJ, Kim CW, et al. A comparison of the short-term effects of a botulinum toxin type A and triamcinolone acetate injection on adhesive capsulitis of the shoulder. *Ann Rehabil Med.* 2013;37(2):208–214.
74. Lee JH, Lee SH, Song SH. Clinical effectiveness of botulinum toxin A compared to a mixture of steroid and local anesthetics as a treatment for sacroiliac joint pain. *Pain Med.* 2010;11(5):692–700. doi: 610.1111/j.1526-4637.2010.00838.x.
75. Dykstra DD, Stuckey MW, Schimpff SN, Singh JA, Mahowald ML. The effects of intra-articular botulinum toxin on sacroiliac, cervical/lumbar facet and sterno-clavicular joint pain and C-2 root and lumbar disc pain: a case series of 11 patients. *The Pain Clinic.* 2007;19(1):27–32.
76. Singer BJ, Silbert PL, Dunne JW, Song S, Singer KP. An open label pilot investigation of the efficacy of botulinum toxin type A [Dysport] injection in the rehabilitation of chronic anterior knee pain. *Disabil Rehabil.* 2006;28(11):707–713.
77. Singer BJ, Silbert PL, Song S, Dunne JW, Singer KP. Treatment of refractory anterior knee pain using botulinum toxin type A (Dysport) injection to the distal vastus lateralis muscle: a randomised placebo controlled crossover trial. *Br J Sports Med.* 2011;45(8):640–645. doi: 610.1136/bjsm.2009.069781. Epub 062010 Apr 069723.
78. Silbert BI, Singer BJ, Silbert PL, Gibbons JT, Singer KP. Enduring efficacy of botulinum toxin type A injection for refractory anterior knee pain. *Disabil Rehabil.* 2012;34(1):62–68.
79. Lawrence RC, Felson DT, Helmick CG, et al. Estimates of the prevalence of arthritis and other rheumatic conditions in the United States. Part II. *Arthritis Rheum.* 2008;58(1):26–35.
80. Courseau M, Salle PV, Ranoux D, de Pouilly Lachatre A. Efficacy of intra-articular botulinum toxin in osteoarticular joint pain: a meta-analysis of randomized controlled trials. *Clin J Pain.* 2018;34(4):383–389. doi: 310.1097/AJP.0000000000000538.
81. Kalunian KC, Arendt-Nielsen L, Turkel CC, et al. Results from a single center, double-blind, randomized, placebo-controlled, parallel-group study of the efficacy and safety of intra-articular onabotulinumtoxin A for osteoarthritis knee pain. *Osteoarthritis and Cartilage.* 2014;22:S192.
82. Arendt-Nielsen L, Jiang GL, DeGryse R, Turkel CC. Intra-articular onabotulinumtoxinA in osteoarthritis knee pain: effect on human mechanistic pain biomarkers and clinical pain. *Scand J Rheumatol.* 2017;46(4):303–316. doi: 310.1080/03009742.0 3002016.01203988. Epub 03002016 Oct 03009713.
83. Bao X, Tan JW, Flyzik M, Ma XC, Liu H, Liu HY. Effect of therapeutic exercise on knee osteoarthritis after intra-articular injection of botulinum toxin type A, hyaluronate or saline: a randomized controlled trial. *J Rehabil Med.* 2018;50(6):534–541.
84. Eleopra R, Rinaldo S, Lettieri C, et al. AbobotulinumtoxinA: a new therapy for hip osteoarthritis. a prospective randomized double-blind multicenter study. *Toxins (Basel).* 2018;10(11).
85. Shukla D, Sreedhar SK, Rastogi V. A Comparative study of botulinum toxin A with triamcinolone compared to triamcinolone alone in the treatment of osteoarthritis of knee. *Anesth Essays Res.* 2018;12(1):47–49. doi: 10.4103/aer.AER_4210_4117.
86. Hsieh LF, Wu CW, Chou CC, et al. Effects of botulinum toxin landmark-guided intra-articular injection in subjects with knee osteoarthritis. *Pm r.* 2016;8(12):1127–1135.
87. Mendes JG, Natour J, Nunes-Tamashiro JC, Toffolo SR, Rosenfeld A, Furtado RNV. Comparison between intra-articular botulinum toxin type A, corticosteroid, and saline in knee osteoarthritis: a randomized controlled trial. *Clin Rehabil.* 2019;33(6):1015–1026.
88. Chou CL, Lee SH, Lu SY, Tsai KL, Ho CY, Lai HC. Therapeutic effects of intra-articular botulinum neurotoxin in advanced knee osteoarthritis. *J Chin Med Assoc.* 2010;73(11):573–580. doi: 510.1016/S1726-4901(1010)70126-X.
89. Marchini C, Acler M, Bolognari MA, et al. Efficacy of botulinum toxin type A treatment of functional impairment of degenerative hip joint: preliminary results. *J Rehabil Med.* 2010;42(7):691–693. doi: 610.2340/16501977-16500546.
90. Chen JT, Tang AC, Lin SC, Tang SF. Anterior knee pain caused by patellofemoral pain syndrome can be relieved by botulinum toxin type A injection. *Clin Neurol Neurosurg.* 2015;129(suppl 1):S27–S29. doi: 10.1016/S0303-8467(1015)30008-30001.
91. Breuer B, Sperber K, Wallenstein S, et al. Clinically significant placebo analgesic response in a pilot trial of botulinum B in patients with hand pain and carpal tunnel syndrome. *Pain Med.* 2006;7(1):16–24.
92. Tsai CP, Liu CY, Lin KP, Wang KC. Efficacy of botulinum toxin type A in the relief of carpal tunnel syndrome: a preliminary experience. *Clin Drug Investig.* 2006;26(9):511–515.
93. Sanders RJ, Hammond SL, Rao NM. Thoracic outlet syndrome: a review. *Neurologist.* 2008;14(6):365–373.
94. Torriani M, Gupta R, Donahue DM. Botulinum toxin injection in neurogenic thoracic outlet syndrome: results and experience using a ultrasound-guided approach. *Skeletal Radiol.* 2010;39(10):973–980.

95. Finlayson HC, O'Connor RJ, Brasher PM, Travlos A. Botulinum toxin injection for management of thoracic outlet syndrome: a double-blind, randomized, controlled trial. *Pain.* 2011;152(9):2023–2028.
96. Lum YW, Brooke BS, Likes K, et al. Impact of anterior scalene lidocaine blocks on predicting surgical success in older patients with neurogenic thoracic outlet syndrome. *J Vasc Surg.* 2012;55(5):1370–1375.
97. Danielson K, Odderson IR. Botulinum toxin type A improves blood flow in vascular thoracic outlet syndrome. *Am J Phys Med Rehabil.* 2008;87(11):956–959.
98. Le EN, Freischlag JA, Christo PJ, Chhabra A, Wigley FM. Thoracic outlet syndrome secondary to localized scleroderma treated with botulinum toxin injection. *Arthritis Care Res (Hoboken).* 2010;62(3):430–433.
99. Jordan SE, Ahn SS, Freischlag JA, Gelabert HA, Machleder HI. Selective botulinum chemodenervation of the scalene muscles for treatment of neurogenic thoracic outlet syndrome. *Ann Vasc Surg.* 2000;14(4):365–369.
100. Rahman A, Hamid A, Inozemtsev K, Nam A. Thoracic outlet syndrome treated with injecting botulinum toxin into middle scalene muscle and pectoral muscle interfascial planes: a case report. *A A Pract.* 2019;12(7):235–237.
101. Jordan SE, Ahn SS, Gelabert HA. Combining ultrasonography and electromyography for botulinum chemodenervation treatment of thoracic outlet syndrome: comparison with fluoroscopy and electromyography guidance. *Pain Physician.* 2007;10(4):541–546.
102. Christo PJ, Christo DK, Carinci AJ, Freischlag JA. Single CT-guided chemodenervation of the anterior scalene muscle with botulinum toxin for neurogenic thoracic outlet syndrome. *Pain Med.* 2010;11(4):504–511.
103. Fabregat G, Rosello M, Asensio-Samper JM, et al. Computer-tomographic verification of ultrasound-guided piriformis muscle injection: a feasibility study. *Pain Physician.* 2014;17(6):507–513.
104. Finnoff JT, Hurdle MF, Smith J. Accuracy of ultrasound-guided versus fluoroscopically guided contrast-controlled piriformis injections: a cadaveric study. *J Ultrasound Med.* 2008; 27(8):1157–1163.
105. Al-Al-Shaikh M, Michel F, Parratte B, Kastler B, Vidal C, Aubry S. An MRI evaluation of changes in piriformis muscle morphology induced by botulinum toxin injections in the treatment of piriformis syndrome. *Diagn Interv Imaging.* 2015;96(1):37–43.
106. Fanucci E, Masala S, Sodani G, et al. CT-guided injection of botulinic toxin for percutaneous therapy of piriformis muscle syndrome with preliminary MRI results about denervative process. *Eur Radiol.* 2001;11(12):2543–2548.
107. Yang HE, Park JH, Kim S. Usefulness of magnetic resonance neurography for diagnosis of piriformis muscle syndrome and verification of the effect after botulinum toxin type A injection: two cases. *Medicine (Baltimore).* 2015;94(38):e1504.
108. Michel F, Decavel P, Toussirot E, et al. Piriformis muscle syndrome: diagnostic criteria and treatment of a monocentric series of 250 patients. *Ann Phys Rehabil Med.* 2013; 56(5):371–383.
109. Childers MK, Wilson DJ, Gnatz SM, Conway RR, Sherman AK. Botulinum toxin type A use in piriformis muscle syndrome: a pilot study. *Am J Phys Med Rehabil.* 2002;81(10):751–759.
110. Lang AM. Botulinum toxin type B in piriformis syndrome. *Am J Phys Med Rehabil.* 2004;83(3):198–202.
111. Fishman LM, Konnoth C, Rozner B. Botulinum neurotoxin type B and physical therapy in the treatment of piriformis syndrome: a dose-finding study. *Am J Phys Med Rehabil.* 2004;83(1):42–50; quiz 51-43.
112. Yoon SJ, Ho J, Kang HY, et al. Low-dose botulinum toxin type A for the treatment of refractory piriformis syndrome. *Pharmacotherapy.* 2007;27(5):657–665.
113. Santamato A, Micello MF, Valeno G, et al. Ultrasound-guided injection of botulinum toxintype A for piriformis muscle syndrome: a case report and review of the literature. *Toxins (Basel).* 2015;7(8):3045–3056.
114. Rodriguez-Pinero M, Vidal Vargas V, Jimenez Sarmiento AS. Longterm efficacy of ultrasound-guided injection of incobotulinumtoxinA in piriformis syndrome. *Pain Med.* 2018;19. England.
115. Fishman LM, Wilkins AN, Rosner B. Electrophysiologically identified piriformis syndrome is successfully treated with incobotulinum toxin A and physical therapy. *Muscle Nerve.* 2017;56(2):258–263.
116. Turnipseed WD. Popliteal entrapment in runners. *Clin Sports Med.* 2012;31(2):321–328.
117. Baltopoulos P, Filippou DK, Sigala F. Popliteal artery entrapment syndrome: anatomic or functional syndrome? *Clin J Sport Med.* 2004;14(1):8–12.
118. Gandor F, Tisch S, Grabs AJ, Delaney AJ, Bester L, Darveniza P. Botulinum toxin A in functional popliteal entrapment syndrome: a new approach to a difficult diagnosis. *J Neural Transm (Vienna).* 2014;121(10):1297–1301.
119. Hislop M, Brideaux A, Dhupelia S. Functional popliteal artery entrapment syndrome: use of ultrasound guided Botox injection as a non-surgical treatment option. *Skeletal Radiol.* 2017;46(9):1241–1248.
120. Murphy M, Charlesworth J, Koh E. The effects of botulinum toxin injection in an elite sportsman with functional popliteal artery entrapment syndrome: a case report. *Phys Ther Sport.* 2017;27:7–11.
121. Isner-Horobeti ME, Muff G, Masat J, Daussin JL, Dufour SP, Lecocq J. Botulinum toxin as a treatment for functional popliteal artery entrapment syndrome. *Med Sci Sports Exerc.* 2015;47(6):1124–1127.
122. Wadhwani A, Nutley M, Bakshi D, Mirakhur A. Treatment of functional popliteal artery entrapment syndrome with ultrasound-guided Botox injection. *J Vasc Interv Radiol.* 2018;29(12):1780–1782.
123. Coté TR, Mohan AK, Polder JA, Walton MK, Braun MM. Botulinum toxin type A injections: adverse events reported to the US Food and Drug Administration in therapeutic and cosmetic cases. *J Am Acad Dermatol.* 2005;53(3):407–415
124. Fabbri M, Leodori G, Fernandes RM, et al. Neutralizing antibody and botulinum toxin therapy: a systematic review and meta-analysis. *Neurotox Res.* 2016;29(1):105-117.

12 Cervical Injection Techniques

MARKO BODOR, STEPHEN DERRINGTON, JOHN PITTS, JASON MARKLE, SAIRAM ATLURI, NAVNEET BODDU, AND VIVEK MANOCHA

Ultrasound Guided Techniques

Posterior Muscles

Cervical

Cervical multifidus
Rectus capitis posterior major
Rectus capitis posterior minor
Obliquus capitus superior
Obliquus capitus inferior

KEY POINTS

These paraspinal muscles are important in postural control of the head on the neck and assist with rotation and extension of the head and upper neck. The suboccipital muscles can become overworked following ligament injuries with resulting instability in the upper cervical spine.

Pertinent Anatomy

Obliquus capitis inferior runs from the spinous process of the axis (C2) to the transverse process of the atlas (C1).

Obliquus capitis superior runs from the transverse process of the atlas (C1) to the occiput, below the superior nuchal line.

Rectus capitis posterior major runs from the posterior tubercle of the axis (C2) to the lateral occiput, inferior to the nuchal line.

Rectus capitis posterior minor runs from the posterior tubercle of the atlas (C1) to the medial occiput, inferior to the nuchal line.

The cervical multifidus muscles originate from the facet joint capsules in the lower cervical and transverse processes of the upper thoracic spine, span 2 to 5 segments, and insert on the spinous processes and laminae of the vertebrae above.[1]

Common Pathology

Atrophy of the multifidus can occur with cervical pathology, including radiculopathy and myelopathy.[2,3] Suboccipital muscles can become atrophied after whiplash[4] and have been shown to be associated with cervicogenic headaches.[5]

The rectus capitis posterior minor has been noted to be hypertrophied following trauma, possibly leading to headaches related to its myodural connection.[6]

All of these muscles can become tight and painful from compensatory overactivity in the setting of segmental instability.

Equipment

An ultrasound with high-frequency linear or curvilinear transducers. Transducer choice is dependent on body habitus and clinician preference.

27 to 25 gauge 1.25 to 2 inch needle

Common Injectates

Orthobiologics (PRP, PPP, etc.)

Injectate Volume

0.25 to 1 mL

Technique

Patient Position. Prone

Clinician Position. At the side of the patient, contralateral to the side of the muscle being treated, with the ultrasound monitor next to or on the opposite side of the patient.

Transducer Position. Short axis to the target muscle (Figs. 12.1 to 12.3)

Rectus capitis posterior minor visualization and injection can be performed in the long axis to the muscle belly (Fig. 12.4)

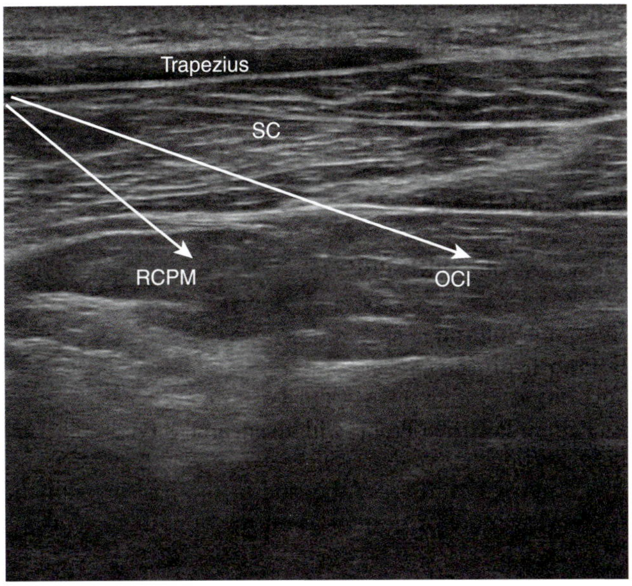

• **Fig 12.1** Transverse view of rectus capitis posterior major *(RCPM)* and obliquus capitis inferior *(OCI)* muscles. Arrow demonstrating needle trajectory from medial to lateral into muscle bellies. *SC,* Semispinalis cervicis.

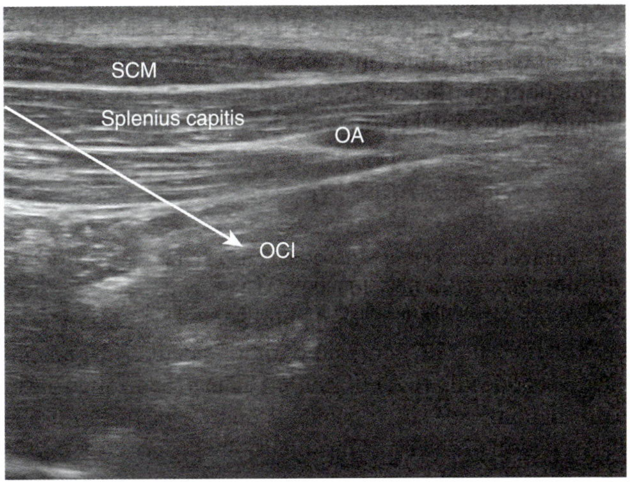

• **Fig 12.2** Obliquus capitis superior (OCS) transverse view. Occipital artery (OA) located lateral and superficial to OCS. Arrow demonstrating needle trajectory from medial to lateral into muscle belly. *SCM*: Sternocleidomastoid muscle cervical facet figure: Cervical facet. Inferior articular process (IAP) from cephalad vertebra and superior articular process (SAP) from caudal vertebra are identified. Needle can be visualized from anterior approach (*right* of image) with needle tip in the joint. *OCI,* Obliquus capitis inferior.

The obliquus capitis inferior can be visualized, and the injection can be performed in the long axis with the same positioning as for a GON injection (Fig. 12.5)

Needle Position. In-plane needle visualization, lateral to medial approach

Target. Muscle belly

PEARLS AND PITFALLS

Care should be taken when performing these injections, with ultrasound visualization of the needle tip at all times for in-plane injections and starting shallow and doing a careful walk-down for out-of-plane injections to avoid going too deep.

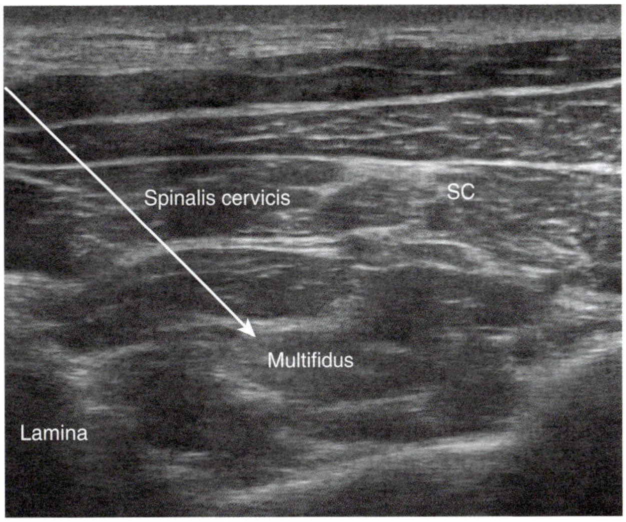

• **Fig 12.3** Transverse view of multifidus muscle, immediately superficial to the cervical lamina. Arrow demonstrating needle trajectory from medial to lateral into muscle belly. *SC*: Semispinalis cervicis and upper trapezius.

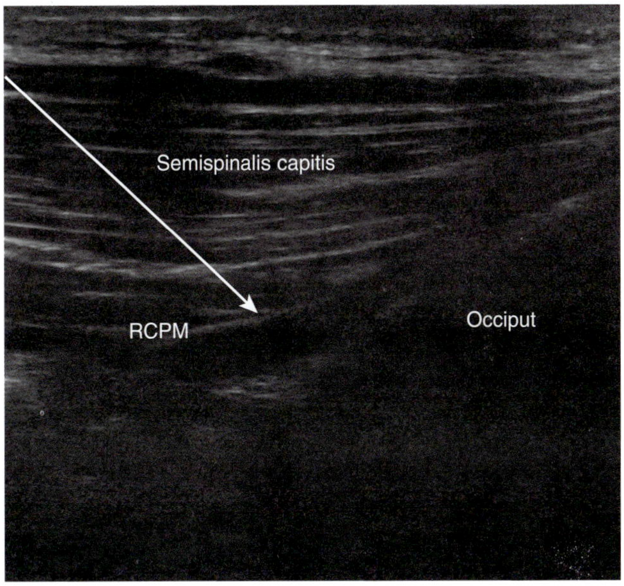

• **Fig 12.4** Longitudinal view of rectus capitis posterior minor, with semispinalis capitis running superficially. Arrow demonstrating needle trajectory from caudal to cephalad into muscle belly. *RCPM,* Rectus capitis posterior major.

Cervical Supraspinous and Interspinous Ligaments

KEY POINTS

These ligaments can be targeted in isolation for specific injuries, but more commonly are targeted in combination with other components of the functional spinal unit,[7,8] including the spinal nerves in the epidural space, facet joints, paraspinal muscles, and sometimes the intervertebral discs.

Treatment with prolotherapy has demonstrated a reduction in translation with cervical spine flexion and extension associated with pain reduction.[9]

Pertinent Anatomy

The interspinous ligament is a thin membranous ligament that traverses adjacent spinous processes. The ligament runs from the root to the apex of each spinous process and connects anteriorly with the ligamentum flavum and posteriorly with the nuchal ligament.

The nuchal ligament is a large midline ligament lying superficial (posterior) to the spinous processes of the cervical spine spanning from the inion to C7, where it becomes continuous with the supraspinous ligament. The nuchal ligament connects anteriorly with the interspinous ligament (Fig. 12.6).

Common Pathology

Ligament strain, partial tear,[10,11] relative laxity related to disc and facet pathology

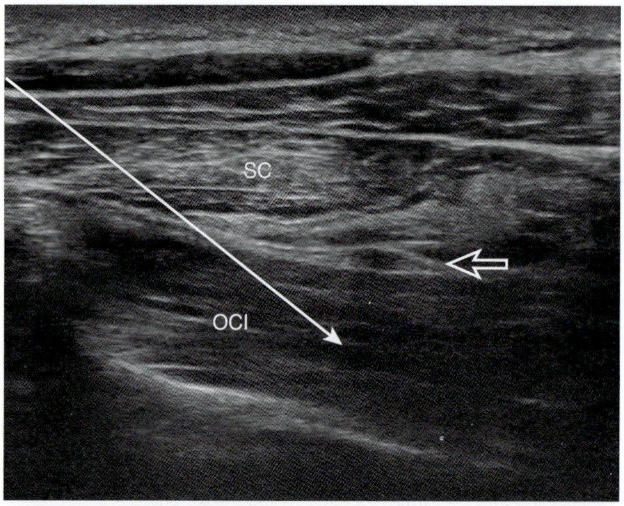

• **Fig 12.5** OCI figure labeled. *OCI*, Obliquus capitis inferior; *SC*, semispinalis cervicis.

Equipment

Ultrasound machine with linear or curvilinear transducer. Transducer choice is dependent on patient body habitus and clinician preference.

27 to 25 gauge 1.25 to 2 inch needle

Common Injectates

Prolotherapy
Orthobiologics (PRP, PPP, etc.)

Injectate Volume

0.25 to 1 mL

Technique

Patient Position. Prone, with the neutral cervical spine and head position.

Clinician Position. At the side of the patient with the ultrasound monitor next to or on the opposite side of the patient.

Transducer Position. Long axis to the ligaments, with visualization of both the ligament and spinous processes (Fig. 12.7)

Needle Position. In-plane needle visualization, caudal to cephalad approach

Target. Direct injection into the ligaments at the desired spinal level, injecting into areas of hypoechogenicity and throughout the ligaments, including the bony insertion. Filling of interstitial injuries can be seen with injectate

PEARLS AND PITFALLS

- Fluoroscopic contrast-dye confirmation may be used to ensure accurate placement of injectate
- These ligaments are difficult to visualize entirely, so adjacent and adjoining anatomy needs to be visualized

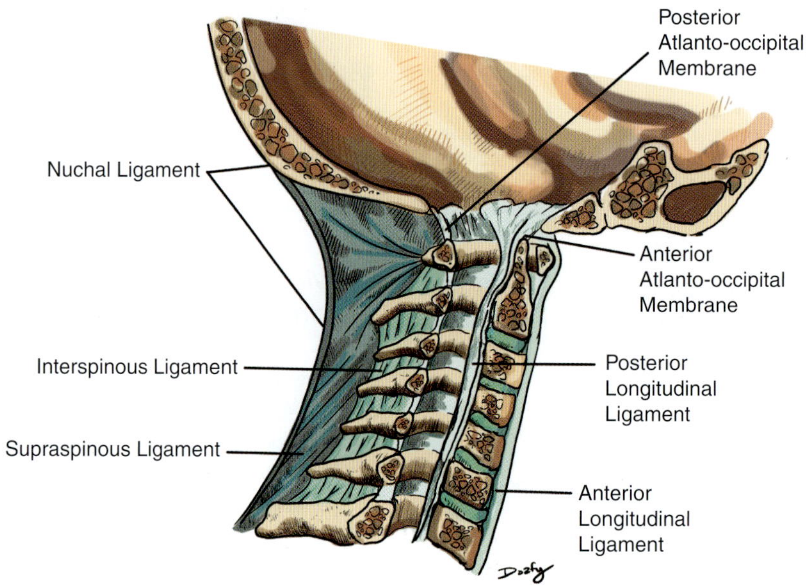

• **Fig 12.6** Cervical spine ligamentous anatomy. The posterior ligament are relatively easily to inject under image guidance.

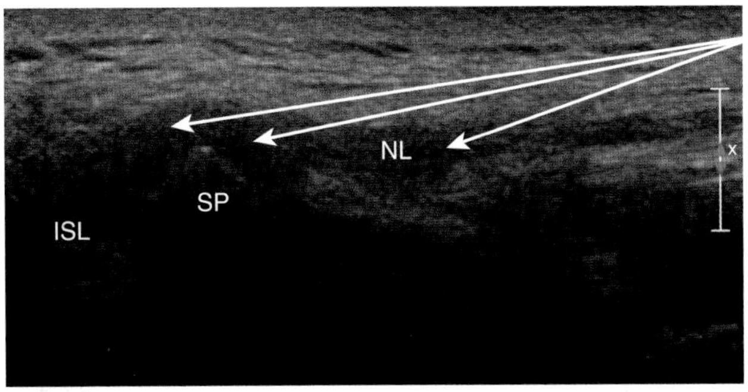

• **Fig 12.7** Nuchal ligament/interspinous figure: Long-axis view of the Nuchal ligament *(NL)*, spinous process *(SP)*, and interspinous ligament *(ISL)*. Arrow demonstrating multiple targets for injection throughout the nuchal and interspinous ligaments.

Greater and Lesser Occipital Nerve Block

KEY POINTS

Occipital neuralgia can come from compression or irritation of the greater or lesser occipital nerves, with greater occipital nerve (GON) irritation being much more common.[12]

Pertinent Anatomy

The greater occipital nerve originates from the dorsal ramus of the C2 spinal nerve, loops around the obliquus capitis inferior (OCI), then courses medially and superiorly through the semispinalis capitis to reach the skin of the occiput, where it provides sensory innervation.

The lesser occipital nerve (LON) originates from the ventral ramus of the C2 and C3 spinal nerves, emerging from under the posterior margin of the sternocleidomastoid muscle to provide sensory innervation to the lateral occiput and posterior ear.[13,14]

Common Pathology

Compression between muscles, acute or repetitive trauma, or other irritation resulting in pain between the posterior occiput and temporal region (GON) or posterior auricle (LON).[12]

Equipment

Ultrasound with a high-frequency linear transducer.
27 to 25 gauge 1.25 to 2 inch needle

Common Injectates

Local anesthetics for blocks +/− corticosteroids
Neuroprolotherapy (5% dextrose solution)
Orthobiologics: (preferably platelet lysate, PRP, etc.)

Injectate Volume

1 to 3 mL

Technique

Patient Position. Prone, or seated, arms crossed, leaning with head on hands.

Clinician Position. At the side of the patient, contralateral to the nerve being treated for prone position, or standing behind the patient for a seated position.

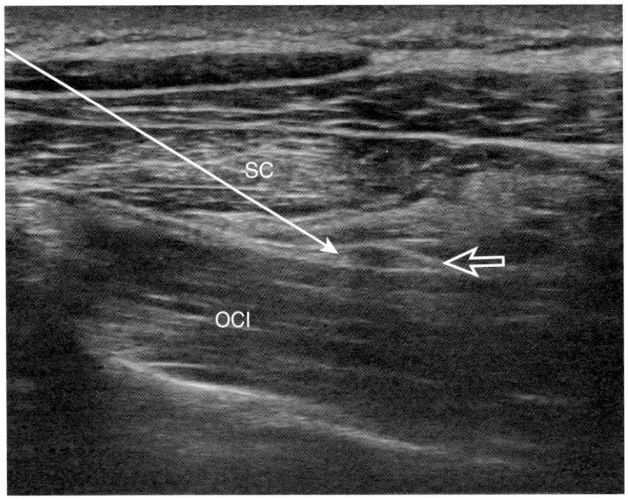

• **Fig 12.8** GON figure: GON (open *arrow*) visualized between the obliquus capitis inferior *(OCI)* and semispinalis cervicis *(SC)* muscles. Arrow demonstrating needle trajectory from medial to lateral immediately adjacent to the nerve.

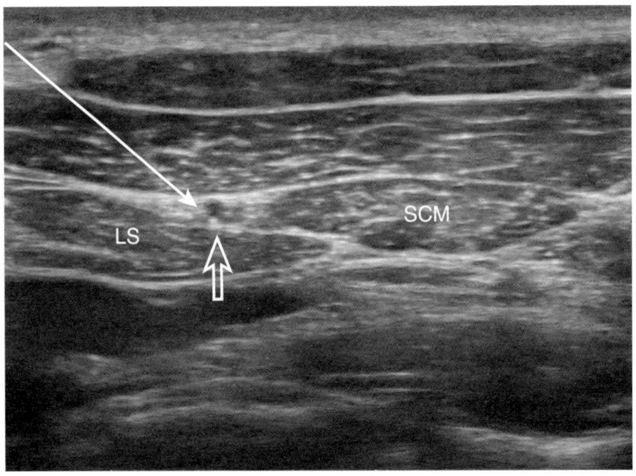

• **Fig 12.9** LON figure: The LON (open *arrow*) is visualized posterior to the sternocleidomastoid *(SCM)* muscle. Arrow demonstrating needle trajectory from medial to lateral immediately adjacent to the nerve. *LS,* Levator scapulae muscle.

Transducer Position. GON: The bifid C2 spinous process is located, then the ultrasound transducer is translated laterally and superiorly in the direction of the transverse process of the C1 vertebra. The obliquus capitis inferior muscle is identified along its long axis. The GON can be visualized in its short axis between the obliquus capitis inferior and the overlying semispinalis capitis (Fig. 12.8)

LON. Scan the sternocleidomastoid (SCM) transversely, inferior to the mastoid. The LON will be visualized at the posterior margin of the SCM, traversing superiorly towards the lateral occiput. (Fig. 12.9)

Needle Position

GON: In-plane needle visualization, posteromedial to anterolateral.

LON: In-plane needle visualization, medial to lateral

Target

GON: Perineural injection, in the fascial layer between obliquus capitis inferior and semispinalis capitis muscles

LON: perineural injection, superficial to the levator scapulae muscle and posterior to the SCM

PEARLS AND PITFALLS

Visual assessment of pulsations and Doppler imaging should be performed prior to needle insertion to help identify and avoid the vertebral artery. The needle tip must be kept in view at all times as it is advanced and during injection to ensure safety.

Cervical Facets

KEY POINTS

The cervical facet joints are the most common cause of chronic neck pain, most often secondary to osteoarthritis or trauma.[15] Ultrasound can be used for the precise identification of painful facets and treatment but requires advanced skills, capability, and equipment.

Pertinent Anatomy

Cervical facet joints are diarthrodial joints formed by the articular pillars of adjacent vertebrae. Each joint is stabilized by a tough collagen capsule enclosing a fine synovial membrane, with joint fluid and hyaline-cartilage-covered articular surfaces inside. The joints are gradually inclined 40° to 60° posteriorly and 20° to 0° medially from C2-3 to C6-7. The medial branches of the dorsal rami of the respective spinal nerves innervate the joints, with the exception of the third occipital nerve (TON), which innervates the top half of C2-3.

Pain from the facet joints is experienced in the neck, radiating to the trapezius and typically exacerbated by neck rotation (Fig. 12.10). Pain from the C2-3 facet joint can cause occipital headaches.[16] X) [7 (link from fluoro cervical facet anatomy section)].?

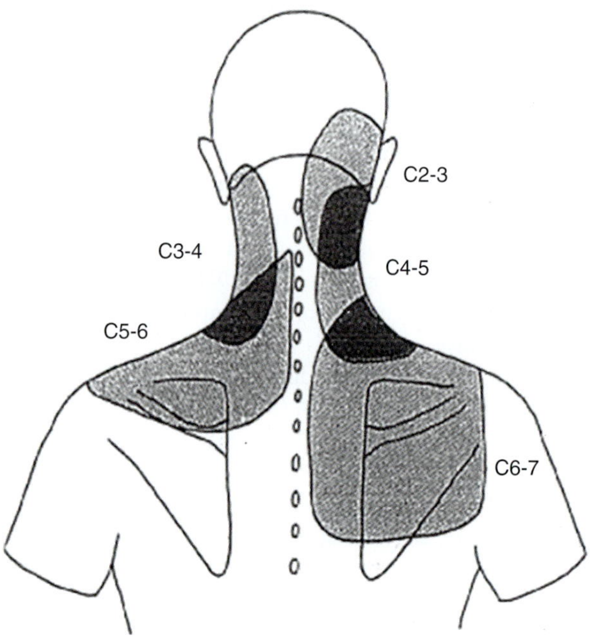

• **Fig 12.10** Cervical facet joint pain provocation patterns, composite map from 5 subjects. (From Dwyer et al.)

Common Pathology

Osteoarthritis, post-traumatic microfractures, and capsular ruptures. Capsular ruptures may be present when the capsule does not distend or distends then collapses during injection.

Indications

Neck Pain
Trapezius Pain
Occipital Headache
Impaired Neck Rotation
Facet Joint Tenderness

Equipment

High-performance ultrasound machine with high-frequency (5-12 MHz) linear transducer

27-gauge 1.25 inch needle.

Common Injectates

Local anesthetics for diagnostics, corticosteroids, Orthobiologics (PRP).

Technique

Patient Position. Side-lying with the head on a pillow, slightly tilted and rotated away from the side being injected, the neck relaxed.

Clinician Position. Standing next to the patient's head and neck, looking at and over the transducer and needle (aerial view) as the needle is advanced in-plane to ensure correct angle and alignment.

Transducer Position. The initial position is with the long axis of the transducer placed along the lateral aspect of the neck (Figs. 12.11 to 12.14). The cervical facet joints appear as undulations. The C2-3 facet joint is the most superior and a bit posterior, beyond which the pulsations of the vertebral artery can be seen (see Fig. 12.13B). Younger joints have smooth undulations with small joint openings, whereas older ones have a rough appearance, larger gaps,

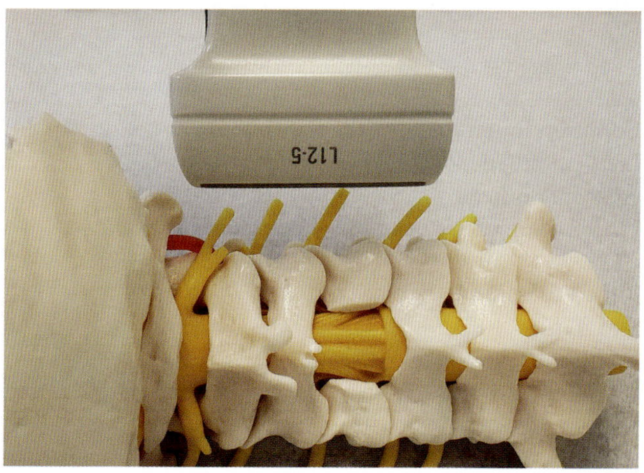

• **Fig 12.11** Right side cervical facet joint scan depicted with an anatomical model.

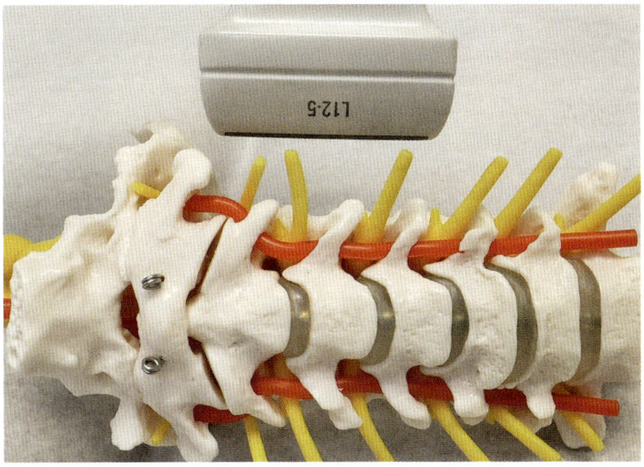

• **Fig 12.12** Left side cervical facet joint scan depicted with an anatomical model.

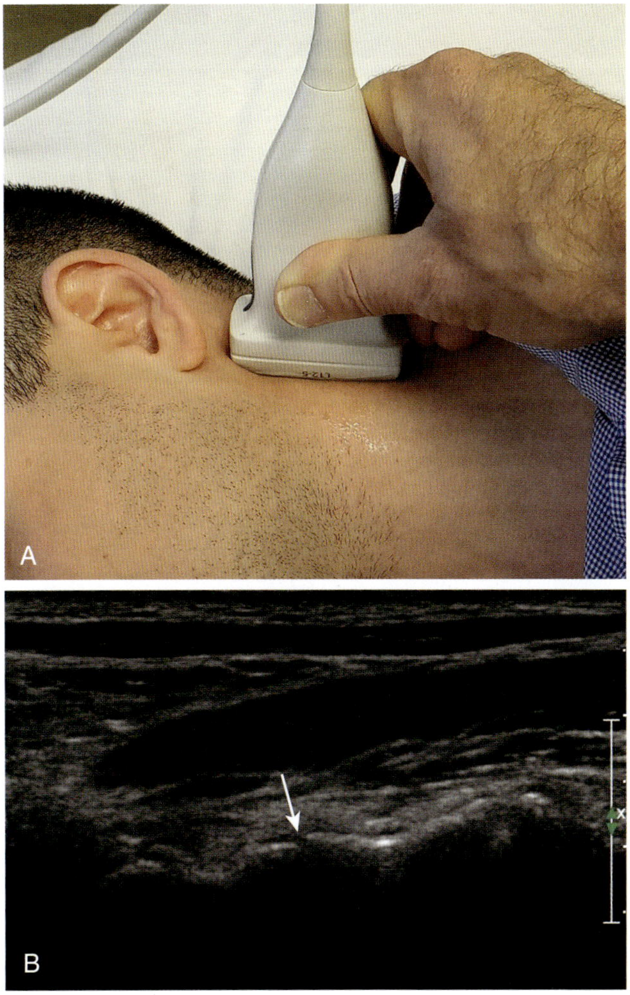

• **Fig 12.13** Left side cervical facet joint scan in a young subject with a muscular neck: (A) Photo; (B) ultrasound image, optimized for the C3-4 facet joint. The tip of the arrow is touching the capsule and pointing to the joint opening. The C2-3 joint is on the left, beyond which no further joints are seen. Scale on the right is in centimeters.

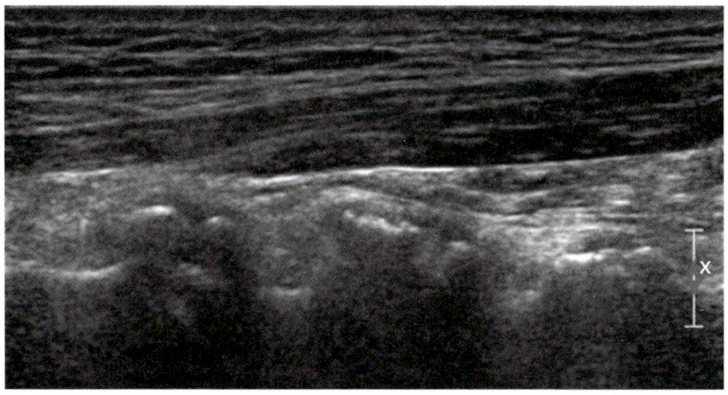

• **Fig 12.14** Cervical facet joints in an older individual. The joints have a rough appearance with osteophytes, enlarged joint spaces, and effusions.

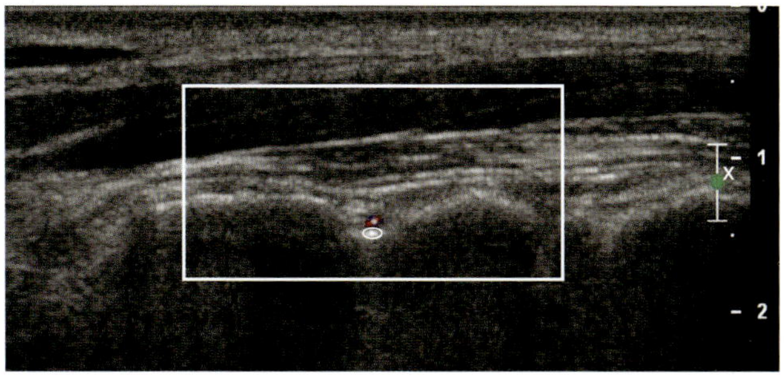

• **Fig 12.15** Cervical facet joint Doppler ultrasound showing normal location of a medial branch nerve (*white circle*) next to an artery *(red)*.

osteophytes, and effusions (Fig. 12.15; see also Fig. 12.13B). The transducer is rotated carefully over the opening of the C2-3 facet joint to obtain a transverse view (Fig. 12.16). Sonopalpation is then performed, one joint at a time. Once the desired joint is selected for injection, the transducer is aligned with the ramus of the mandible and adjusted to optimize the joint opening. The needle is inserted typically using an anterior or posterior approach, typically anterior for a right hand dominant physician injecting the patient's right side, but also depending on the orientation of the joint opening (Figs. 12.17 and 12.18).

Needle Position. In-plane.

Target. Joint opening, effusion, or capsule.

Injectate Volume

0.25 to 1 mL

PEARLS AND PITFALLS

The transducer is kept immobile over the target during the injection. This is done via the two-tripod technique, with the first consisting of the thumb, index, and middle finger holding the transducer, and the second consisting of the ring and little finger and transducer maintaining a stable position on the neck. Cervical facet joint openings are very small, so a slight slip of the transducer means that the target disappears from view. Successful performance of this procedure requires steady alignment of the transducer, needle, and the joint opening, requiring superior equipment, experience, skill, and hand-eye coordination. Patients with thick necks and difficult to see anatomy are not candidates for this procedure. Once the needle enters the joint, it should not be advanced more than a few millimeters because of the unlikely possibility of passing through the joint. Particulate injectates should not be used because of the remote possibility of an intra-arterial injection.

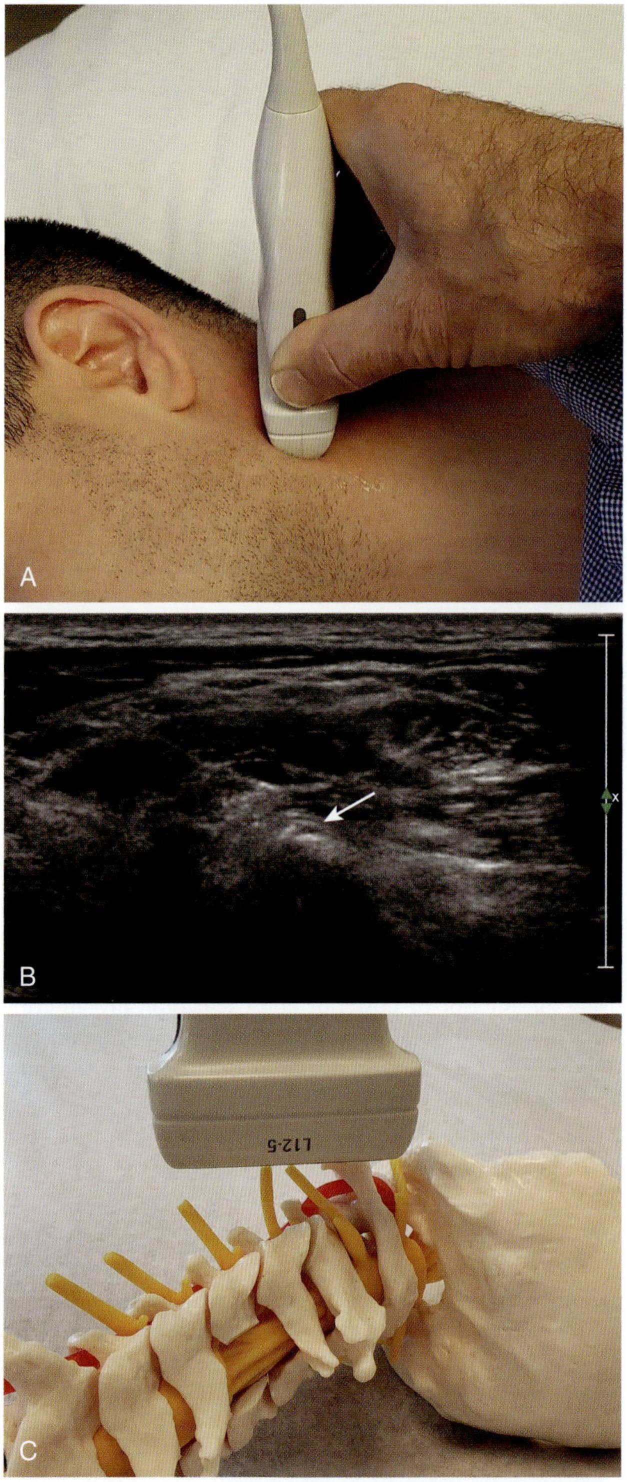

• **Fig 12.16** C2-3 facet joint scan following transducer rotation: (A) Photo, (B) ultrasound image with arrow pointing to joint opening, and (C) depiction with an anatomical model, seen from a posterior-inferior view.

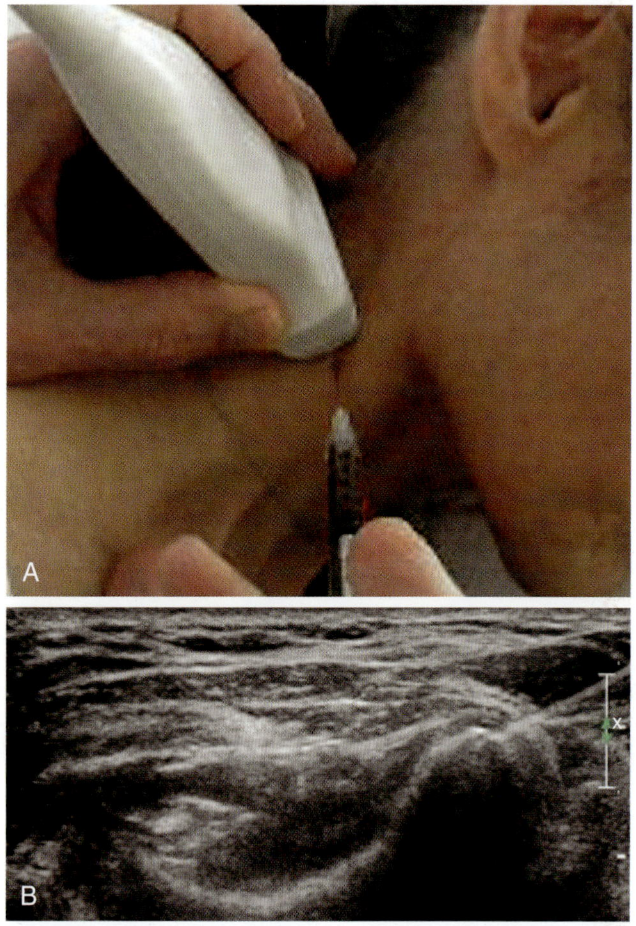

• **Fig 12.17** Cervical facet injection. (A) Non-dominant hand keeps the transducer immobile while the dominant hand advances the needle to the target; (B) ultrasound image of needle in the joint.

Interscalene Brachial Plexus Block

KEY POINTS

- The Interscalene brachial plexus block is performed at the interscalene groove where the roots of the plexus pass between anterior scalene and middle scalene muscles, at the level of C6 tubercle or Chassaignac's tubercle.
- The block can be performed by paresthesia technique, neuromuscular stimulation, or by using ultrasound.
- It can be used as an anesthetic or adjunct to general anesthesia or postoperative pain control.
- Ultrasound is used for defining anatomic landmarks, identification of blood vessels, and identification of nerves. The use of ultrasound has increased the safety and accuracy of the block.

Pertinent Anatomy

- The brachial plexus is a network of nerves formed by the ventral rami of the lower four cervical nerves (C5-C8) and 1st Thoracic nerve.
- The plexus is responsible for sensory innervations of the upper extremity with the exception of the axilla and motor innervations of all the upper extremity muscle groups with the exception of trapezius and levator scapulae.

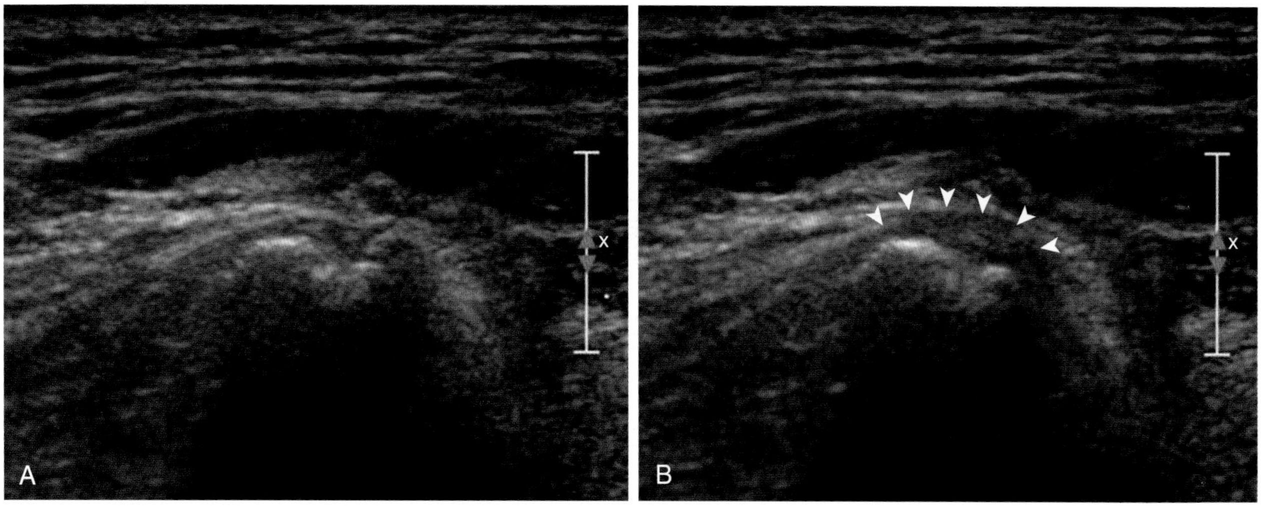

• **Fig 12.18** Ultrasound images taken (A) before and (B) after a cervical facet injection, showing normal distention of the joint capsule (*arrowheads*).

- The plexus communicates with the sympathetic chain.
- The brachial plexus can be divided into roots, trunks, divisions, and cords which can be further divided into peripheral nerves.
- Interscalene block is performed at the posterior border of sternocleidomastoid muscle at the level of C6 anterior tubercle known as Chassaignac or carotid tubercle.
- This is most prominent among the anterior tubercle of the transverse process of the cervical vertebra, and it corresponds with the level of Cricoid cartilage.
- Chassaignac's tubercle separates the carotid artery and vertebral artery.
- Internal Jugular vein and anterior scalene muscles are located lateral to the carotid artery (Fig. 12.20).

Common Pathology

- Interscalene block is used in surgeries or procedures of the shoulder joint, upper arm, and clavicle.

Equipment

- High frequency (9 to 18 MHz) linear ultrasound probe
- 25 to 22 gauge 2-inch short bevel needle

Common Injectates

- Local anesthetic

Injectate Volume

- 5 to 20 mL

Technique

Patient Position

- The patient can be placed supine or in the lateral decubitus position.
- Instruct the patient to rotate his neck at an angle of 45 degrees and raise his head off the bed keeping the head rotated. This contracts the scalene muscles, and one can palpate the interscalene groove between the muscles running in craniocaudal direction.

Clinician Position

- Ipsilateral side of the patient if supine or standing behind the patient if in the lateral decubitus position.

Transducer Position

- The probe is placed transversely over the anterolateral part of the neck at the level of Chassaignac's tubercle
- The ultrasound view shows a pulsating anechoic structure, which is the Carotid artery, then the ultrasound probe is moved posterior-laterally, maintaining the same level at C6 to view the Internal Jugular vein and anterior scalene muscle (ASM).
- The roots of the brachial plexus can be visualized laterally to ASM in the interscalene groove between the anterior scalene and middle scalene muscles.
- The ultrasound probe can be rotated or tilted slightly to obtain a clearer view. The probe can be moved craniocaudal directions to see the formation of the brachial plexus trunks and divisions from the cervical roots and to obtain an optimal site for injection where 2 or 3 roots are visualized.
- Sternocleidomastoid (SCM) muscle lies superficial to the plexus and is seen as a triangle structure on ultrasound. The plexus lies 1 to 3 cm deep from the skin level.

Needle Position

- In-plane technique going from lateral to medial.
- Avoiding the external jugular vein.
- Needle travels through interscalene groove, crossing the middle scalene muscle
- Injectionists may feel the pop entering the prevertebral fascia.

Target

- Needle tip should end just adjacent to the plexus
- Aspirate to check for blood or CSF, then inject, visualizing the spread of the injectate as it infiltrates the vicinity of nerve roots keeping the roots intact.

PEARLS AND PITFALLS

- Intravascular injection:
    - Brachial plexus lies lateral to carotid artery, external and Internal jugular vein and vertebral artery; therefore, there is a high risk for intravascular injection.
    - Visualize the needle tip at all times with ultrasound during the procedure.
    - Confirm the tip of the needle seen under ultrasound is the real tip and not the needle falling off the ultrasound beam by injecting small amounts of local anesthetic and watch it exiting the needle tip.
- Phrenic nerve block:
    - Performing the interscalene block higher than the C6 level or injection of high volumes of local anesthetics can cause ipsilateral phrenic nerve block.
    - Healthy patients may not be symptomatic, but patients with compromised pulmonary function may have shortness of breath or difficulty maintaining oxygen saturation.
    - Using a lower concentration of local anesthetic and keeping local anesthetic injection to lower volumes may avoid phrenic nerve block.
- Horner's syndrome:
    - Horner's syndrome is due to sympathetic block caused by an accidental spill of local anesthetic into the stellate ganglion.
    - A patient complains of ptosis, anhydrosis, mydriasis, redness of the eye on the ipsilateral side.
- Pneumothorax:
    - It can rarely occur with lower cervical injection site, though patients with obstructive lung disease can be prone because of the higher pleural dome, and it should be suspected if the patient complains of shortness of breath or is unable to maintain normal saturation.
    - Pneumothorax may share the same clinical picture as phrenic nerve paralysis; however, there are reduced or absent breath sounds in patients with pneumothorax.
    - An upright chest x-ray will help diagnose both conditions.
- Subarachnoid injection:
    - Although rare, injection into dural sleeves of cranial nerves or spread of local anesthetic injection into cervical epidural space can cause a high spinal block, resulting in hypotension, difficulty breathing, numbness and muscle weakness of upper extremities, and loss of consciousness.[17-21]

Supraclavicular Brachial Plexus Block

KEY POINTS

- Supraclavicular block can be used as an alternative or adjunct to general anesthesia or used for postoperative pain control for the upper extremity from the upper part of the arm to the hand.
- The brachial plexus above the clavicle area forms trunks and divisions as they pass under the clavicle in very close proximity to the chest cavity.
- Brachial plexus trunks and divisions are arranged very close, so the local anesthetic spreads easier, and a superior block can be obtained.
- The plexus passes over above the 1st rib between the insertions of middle scalene and anterior scalene muscles roughly at the midpoint of the clavicle.
- The plexus is in very close proximity to the pleura and lung, increasing the risk of pneumothorax.

Pertinent Anatomy

- Surface Anatomy
- Supraclavicular block can be performed in the supraclavicular fossa at the midpoint of the superior border of the clavicle.
- The plexus forms three trunks, upper (C5 & C6), middle (C7), and lower (C8 &T1).
- Both the brachial plexus and subclavian artery lie on top of the 1st rib between the insertions of the anterior scalene muscle and the middle scalene muscle.
- The brachial plexus is located posterior and lateral to the subclavian artery, and in very close proximity to the pleura.
- You can palpate pulsations of the subclavian artery and the 1st rib in the midclavicular area above the clavicle.
- Ultrasound Anatomy:
    - The ultrasound probe is placed horizontally above the clavicle in the midclavicular area. The subclavian artery is seen as a round anechoic pulsating structure.
    - Located underneath the subclavian artery, you can see the hyperechoic 1st rib. Since the ultrasound waves are completely reflected back, it casts a dark shadow underneath the rib.
    - On either side of the first rib, you can see a hyperechoic pleural shadow.
    - Some of the ultrasound waves pass through the pleura into lung tissue filled with air, so it gives the characteristic appearance of cosmic dust under the pleura.
    - Make a mental note of the location and depth of the 1st rib and pleura since you have to make sure the needle does not pass beyond this depth.
    - Now focus your attention on the subclavian artery, where the brachial plexus can be seen as hypoechoic fascicles both superficial and deep to the artery.
    - The ultrasound probe can be moved proximally and distally along the brachial plexus to visualize its trunks and divisions.
    - The brachial plexus lies at 1 to 2 cm depth below the skin at this location.

Common Pathology

- Used for anesthesia for upper extremity procedures
- Also, consider for brachial plexus neuritis or plexopathy

Equipment

- Linear ultrasound transducer
- 25 gauge 2-inch spinal needle

Common Injectates

- Local Anesthetic

Injectate Volume

- 10 to 25 mL

Technique

Patient Position

- Supine position with neck in the midline position. Turn the patient's chin to 45 degrees in the opposite direction to open up the supraclavicular fossa

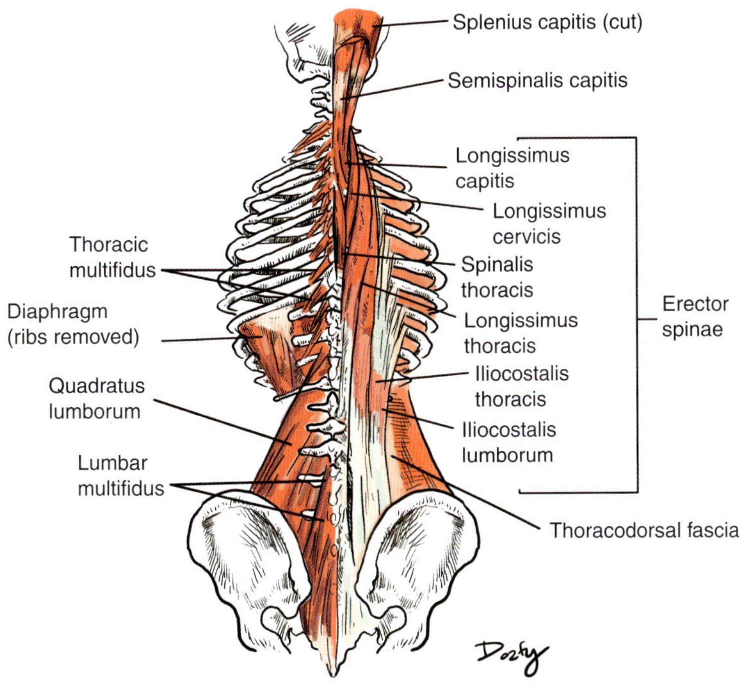

• **Fig 12.19** Spinal muscular anatomy. Note Splenius capitis is more superficial that semispinalis capitus and suboccipital muscles and cervical multifidus are deep to these.

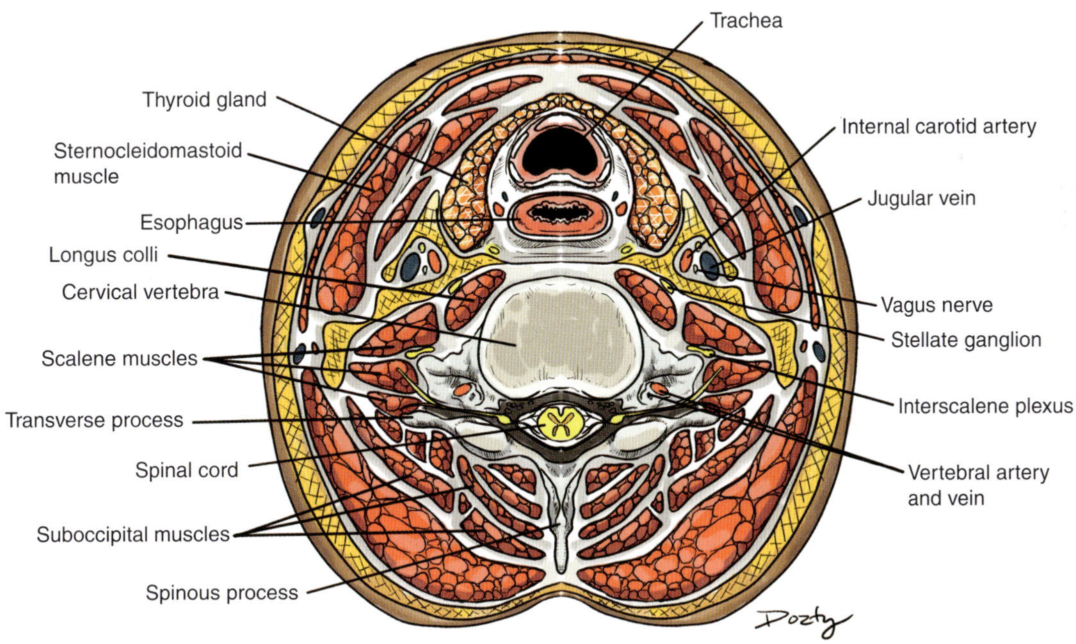

• **Fig 12.20** Cervical spine cross-sectional anatomy. Note the relationship between the interscalene plexus and scalene muscles and the longus colli muscle and the stellate ganglion.

- Lateral decubitus with 1 pillow under the head so that the neck is tilted slightly away from the targeted side.
- It can be done in a sitting position but is not preferred.

Clinician Position

- Ipsilateral side of the patient.

Transducer Position

- The transducer is placed transversely above the clavicle in the midclavicular area.
- Identify the hyperechoic line that the 1st rib casts and the pleura on either side of the rib. It is mandatory to stay superficial to 1st rib and pleura

Needle Position

- Introduce the needle in-plane from the lateral side of the probe using ultrasound guidance.
- Visualize the needle tip and direct it towards the brachial plexus, which is seen as hypoechoic fascicles. It is

mandatory that the needle tip stays superficial to 1st rib and pleura.

Target

- Enter the fascia that covers the brachial plexus; a pop may be felt
- Target injection inside the fascia sheath in between the brachial plexus trunks

PEARLS AND PITFALLS

- Vascular Injection: The brachial plexus is close to the subclavian artery and lies superficial and deep to the artery.
- Intra-arterial injection can be minimized by aspirating the needle prior to injection, watching the spread of local anesthetic live as the injection is performed, and using incremental doses during the injection.
- Pneumothorax: Brachial plexus block has the highest incidence of pneumothorax. It is mandatory to identify the 1st rib and pleura prior to insertion of the needle and keep needle tip superficial to those structures.

Nerve injury: The use of ultrasound has reduced the risk of nerve injury. Nerve injury can be avoided by performing the block in-plane technique, making sure the nerve bundle maintains its integrity during the injection, and performing it on an awake or minimally sedated patient so that the patient can alert the practitioner to nerve pain.[22-26]

Cervical Plexus Block

KEY POINTS

- Cervical plexus blocks were first performed by Halsted in 1884.
- The cervical plexus can be done by the posterior or lateral approach.
- Currently, the most commonly performed is the lateral approach of cervical plexus block.
- Superficial cervical plexus block is used for superficial surgeries of the neck and shoulder.
- Deep cervical plexus block is used for surgeries on deeper structures of the anterior and lateral neck, like surgeries of the carotid artery, thyroid, neck lymph nodes, etc.

Pertinent Anatomy

- The cervical plexus is formed by anterior divisions of upper cervical nerve nerves C2 to C4.
- The cervical nerves emerge for their respective foramina and divide into anterior and posterior divisions. The anterior divisions exit behind the vertebral artery in a gutter formed by the anterior and posterior tubercle of the transverse process at corresponding cervical vertebrae.
- The anterior rami divide into ascending and descending branches forming series of loops known as the cervical plexus.
- The plexus divides into superficial and deep branches giving rise to a series of nerves.
- The branches of the superficial cervical plexus pierce the deep fascia of the neck at the midpoint of the posterior margin of sternocleidomastoid muscle to emerge, forming the lesser occipital nerve, greater auricular nerve, transverse cervical nerve, and supraclavicular nerve.
- It supplies the skin area of the anterior neck and shoulder area.
- The deep cervical plexus supplies the deep structures of the anterior and lateral neck and also gives branches to the phrenic nerve.
- To locate the deep cervical plexus, a straight line is drawn from the tip of the mastoid process to Chassaignac's (C6) tubercle; the line will indicate the positions of cervical transverse processes.
- On this line, the transverse process of C2 is located 2 cm below the tip of the mastoid process corresponding to the level of the hyoid bone; the transverse processes of C3 and C4 are located 1.5 and 3 cm below the mark for the C2 transverse process.
- C4 transverse process corresponds to the level of the superior border of the thyroid cartilage.

Common Pathology

- The cervical plexus can be used as an anesthetic or adjunct to general anesthesia or postoperative pain relief for surgeries of the neck and shoulders.

Equipment

- High frequency (9 to 18 MHz) linear ultrasound probe

Common Injectates

- Local anesthetics

Injectate Volume

- 5 to 10 mL

Technique

Patient Position

- The patient is positioned in a supine position
- The head is rotated 45 degrees away to slide the SCM muscle away from the site of injection.

Clinician Position

- Ipsilateral to targeted side

Transducer Position

- The superficial cervical plexus block is performed by placing the probe transversely over the posterior border of SCM at the midpoint of the muscle.
- Visualize hypoechoic fascicles under the posterior border or emerging out through the fascia posterior to the SCM muscle.
- The deep cervical plexus block is performed by placing the high-frequency linear ultrasound probe over the posterior border of the SCM muscle; therefore, SCM is seen as a triangle.
- The transverse process of the C4 vertebra can be seen as a hyperechoic structure.
- By tilting the probe in the craniocaudal direction, you can visualize the C4 nerve root exiting the foramen

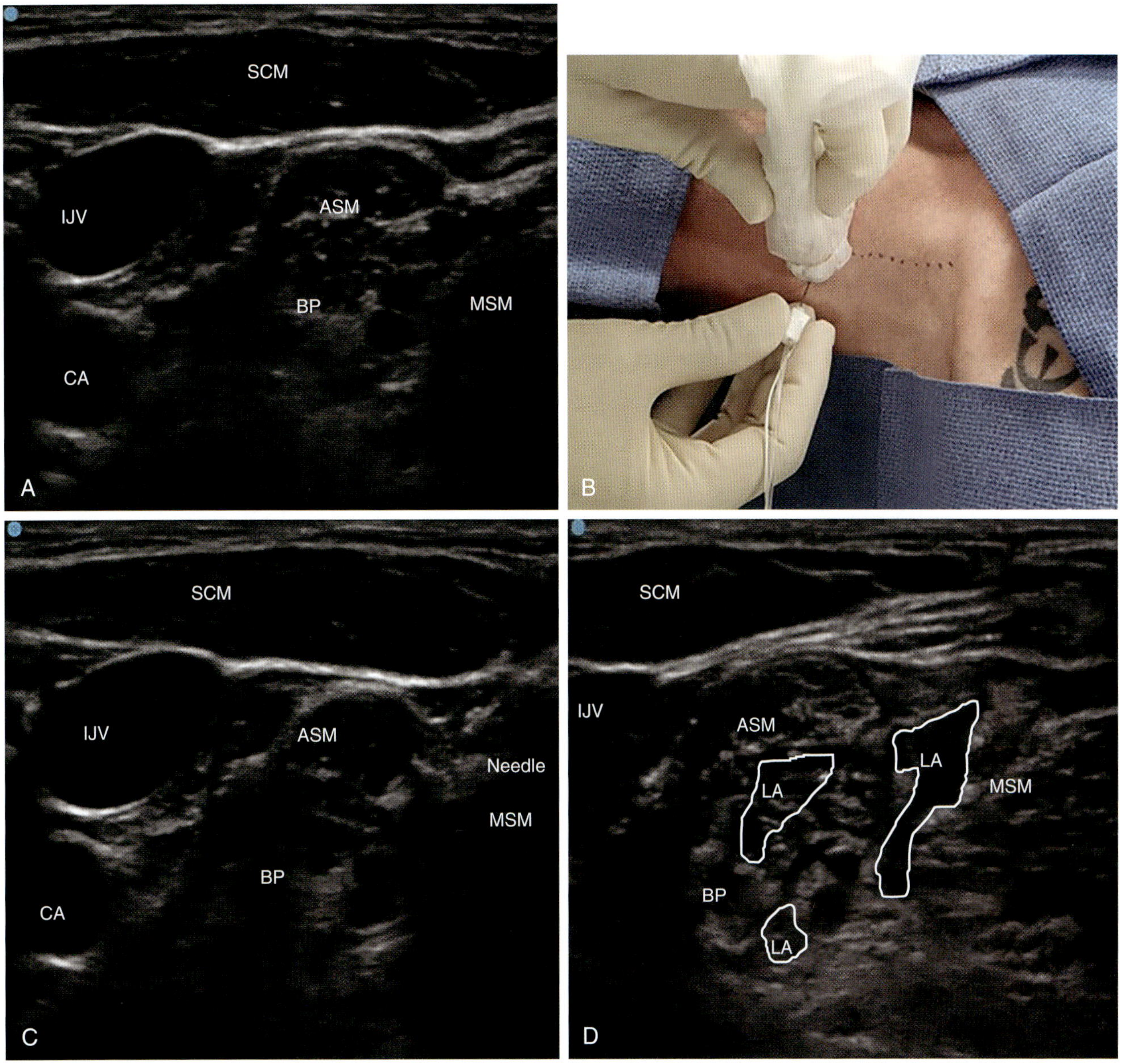

• **Fig 12.21** *ASM,* Anterior scalene muscle; *BP,* brachial plexus; *CA,* carotid artery; *IJV,* internal jugular vein; *LA,* local anesthetic; *MSM,* middle scalene muscle; *SCM,* sternocleidomastoid muscle.

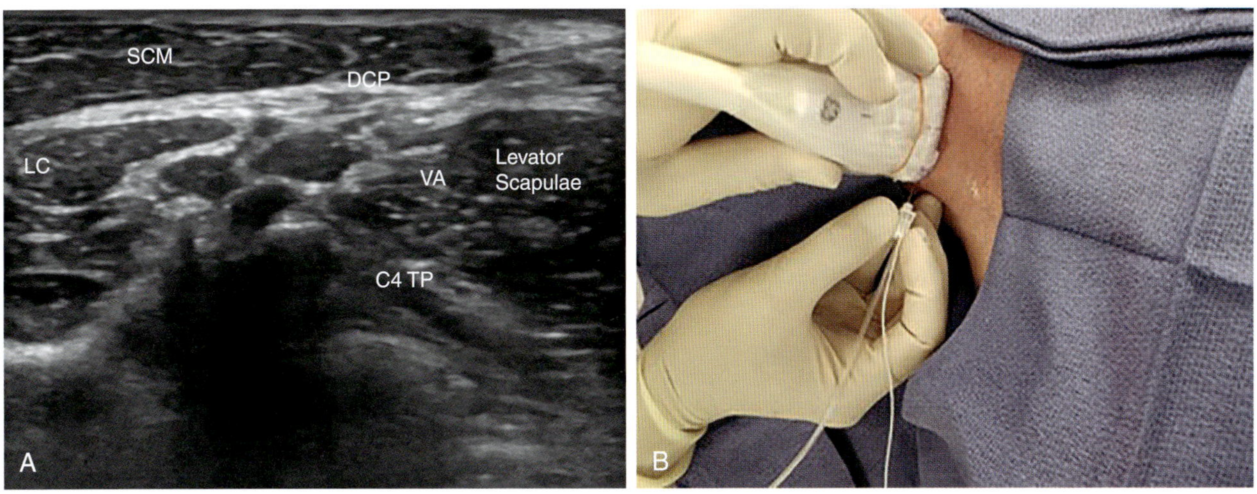

• **Fig 12.22** *C4 TP,* transverse process of 4th cervical vertebra; *DCP,* deep cervical plexus; *LC,* Longus Coli; *VA,* vertebral artery; *SCM,* Sternocleidomastoid muscle.

and going in between the anterior and middle scalene muscles.

Needle Position

- For a superficial cervical plexus block, enter the skin over the midpoint of the posterior border of SCM muscle.
- Guide the needle through the long axis to pass through the superficial part of the deep cervical fascia.
- For the deep cervical plexus block, the needle is inserted and directed towards the C4 nerve root in the groove between the anterior and middle scalene muscles

Target

- For a superficial cervical plexus injection, under the superficial layer of deep cervical fascia near the superficial cervical plexus
- Aspirate first to ensure no vascular uptake and make sure there is an adequate spread of injectate near the nerve branches
- For the deep cervical plexus, the needle should contact the anterior tubercle of the C4 transverse process
- Aspirate to make sure there is no blood or cerebrospinal fluid, then inject
- Apply gentle pressure over the C5 tubercle to prevent the local anesthetic spread in the caudal direction

PEARLS AND PITFALLS

- Intravascular injection: The neck is highly vascular; accidental intravascular injection of local anesthetic can occur into external and internal jugular veins, external and internal carotid arteries, or vertebral artery. A very small amount of local anesthetic injected into the carotid artery, or vertebral artery can cause seizures or loss of consciousness.
- High spinal block: Local anesthetic injection into epidural and subdural spaces can occur due to penetration of the dural sleeve. Careful aspiration prior to injection can avoid intravascular or subarachnoid injection.
- Phrenic nerve block: Transient phrenic nerve block occurs in 100% of the patients as the phrenic nerve mainly arises from the C4 nerve root with minor branches from C3 and C5 nerve roots. Cervical plexus block should be avoided in patients who have severe respiratory illnesses.
- Horner's syndrome: Upper and middle cervical sympathetic ganglion can be blocked during this procedure if the local anesthetic spreads anteriorly to the prevertebral fascia.[27-31]

Fluoroscopy Guided Techniques

Transforaminal Cervical Epidural Injections

KEY POINTS

- A transforaminal cervical epidural injection can be used for both diagnostic and therapeutic purposes.
- Since the injection is done at a specific level, it has a higher diagnostic value as long as the injectate volume is kept low.
- Radiculitis at the cervical region can be secondary to disc, uncovertebral joint, or cervical facet pathology.
- Transforaminal epidural steroid injection is done to suppress the inflammation of the cervical nerve root and treat radicular pain.
- Under fluoroscopy, the cervical facets joints look like pillars on both sides of the vertebral column and therefore are called lateral masses or articular pillars.
- The location of the needle tip in relation to the articular pillar during the cervical injections is crucial to avoid complications.
- In the cervical region, the dural sleeve around the cranial nerve can extend up to the midpoint of the articular pillar.

Anatomic Consideration

- The roof of the intervertebral foramen is formed by the corresponding vertebral pedicle, and the floor of the foramen is formed by the pedicle of the vertebra below. The anterior part foramen is formed by the uncovertebral joint, and the posterolateral part is formed by the facet joints.
- The facet joints are formed by the inferior articular process of the corresponding vertebra and the superior articular process of the vertebral below.
- The transverse process of the cervical vertebra has a foramen called the transverse foreman.
- The vertebral artery (VA) runs through the transverse foramen of C1 to C6 vertebra and lies medial to the midline of the lateral masses or articular pillar; however, there is significant variation of the position of VA along the lateral masses.
- The cervical intervertebral foramina are positioned anterolaterally at 45 degrees and directed slightly inferior.
- The cervical spinal nerves from C3 to C7 exit in the groove for the spinal nerve. The groove has an inferior bony floor and anterior and posterior tubercle formed by the transverse process of the vertebra (see Figs 12.23 and 12.24).

Equipment

- C-arm fluoroscopy
- Needle: 25 gauge 2 to 3.5 inch spinal needle depending on neck girth
- non-ionic contrast material (Omnipaque or Isovue)

Common Injectates

- local anesthetics for diagnostics, nonparticulate corticosteroids
- Orthobiologics (platelet lysate)
- Do not use particulate steroids epidurally

Injectate Volume

- 1 to 3 mL

Technique

Patient Position

- The patient is in the supine position, and the head should be turned away from the side of the procedure. This will

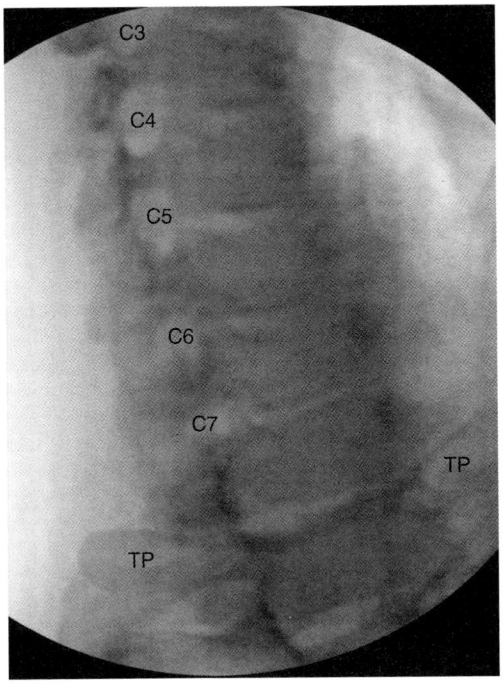

• **Fig 12.23** C3 to C7 Neural foramen openings seen in the initial scout oblique view. *TP,* Large transverse process of TI.

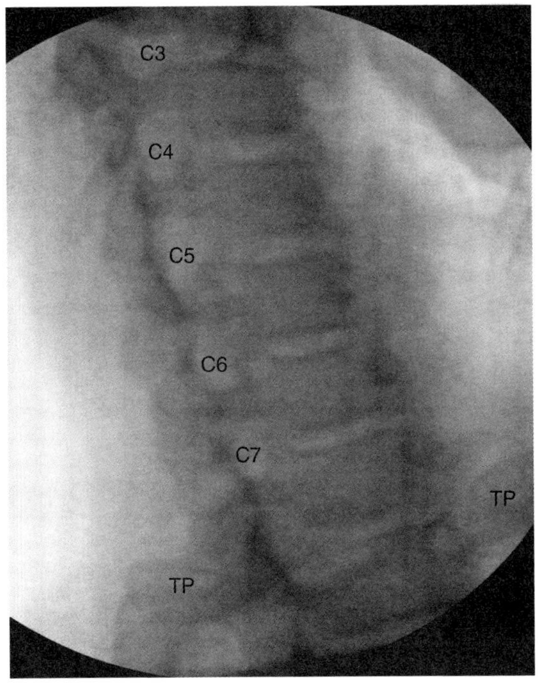

• **Fig 12.24** Openings of the neural foramen especially at C5, C6, C7 levels when compared to the image in Figure 12.23. Sometimes caudal angulation may be additionally required to maximize the foraminal opening.

prevent the overlap of the jaw and facial bones and optimizes the visualization of the foramen.

Clinician Position

- Ipsilateral side of the injection

C-Arm Position

- The C-arm is turned into oblique position significantly, usually 30 degrees or more, to maximize the opening of the neural foramen (Fig. 12.23).
- Caudal angulation [image intensifier angled to the feet] is usually required to additionally maximize the opening of the neural foramen.
- Sometimes cranial angulation may be needed. The goal is to optimally visualize the opening of the neural foramen at the level of the injection being performed (Fig. 12.24).
- The most superior neural foramen seen is the C3 level. This is used as a landmark to count the level of the neural foramen of interest.
- Alternatively, the large transverse process of T1 can also be used to count (see Fig. 12.24).

Needle Position

- Skin is marked over the posterior and inferior part of the foramen (Fig. 12.25).
- The needle is introduced under fluoroscopic guidance using the hub shot technique.
- As soon as the needle is stabilized in the tissues, further advancement is stopped in the oblique view to avoid entering the spinal canal. It is absolutely critical for the needle to remain in the posterior part of the foramen.
- The author prefers to have the needle touch the posterior boney wall of the foramen (anterior lateral border of the inferior articular pillar IAP) to ascertain the depth and for safety. Then, the needle can be "walked off" just anterior to the IAP but remaining in the posterior foramen.

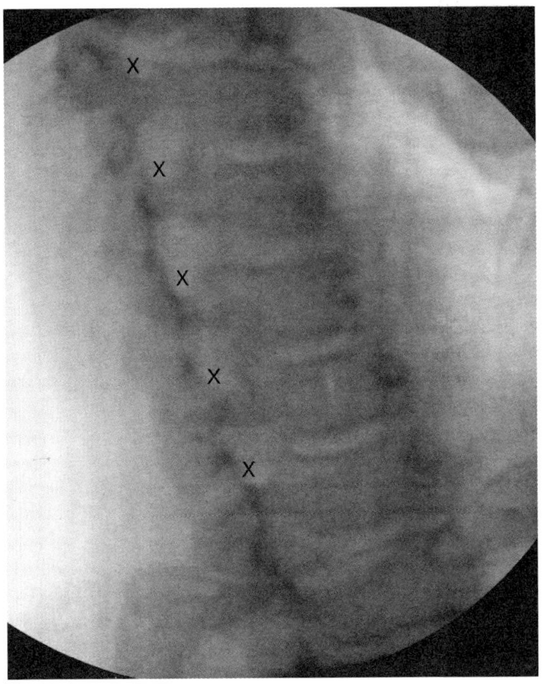

• **Fig 12.25** X: Site of needle entry in the posterior and inferior part of the foramen.

- Anterior deviation of the needle would bring it near the vertebral artery, which can lead to dangerous consequences.
- True AP view [spinous process in the middle of the vertebral body] is now obtained.
- The needle can be advanced here and can begin to direct the needle slightly superior as the nerve root exits anterior and inferiorly into the foramen.

Target

- Target the tip of the needle at the middle of the lateral masses (articular pillars). Needle position beyond the middle of the articular pillar risks entry into the spinal canal (Fig. 12.26).
- A small extension tube (K 50) can be used to minimize the mobilization of the needle during the procedure.
- Aspiration should be negative for blood or CSF.
- Under real-time fluoroscopy, inject 0.5 to 1 mL of contrast dye to confirm the correct position of the needle. The dye should be seen entering the epidural space and tracking the nerve exiting the foramen. A second still image can be taken a few seconds later to confirm there is no change in the dye pattern.

PEARL AND PITFALLS

Complications

- Penetration of great vessels:
  - Carotid artery and Internal Jugular vein are present anterior lateral to the intervertebral foramen. The artery and vein lie over the body of the cervical vertebra in an oblique view.
  - The vertebral artery lies over the anterior border of the intervertebral foramen in the oblique fluoroscopic view. One can avoid injury to the vertebral artery by targeting the posterior part of the intervertebral foramen.
  - Staying lateral to the midline of lateral masses in AP view does not guarantee avoiding vertebral artery injection.
  - There have been case reports of injection into the radicular artery at the corresponding level causing spinal cord injury.[32]
- Intrathecal injection:
  - Cervical spinal nerves have dural sleeves that extend up to the midline of the lateral masses or articular pillars.
  - Make sure the needle tip is lateral to the midline of the articular pillar.
  - Intrathecal injection causes high spinal block where the patient may have numbness and weakness of upper extremities, difficulty breathing, and hypotension.
  - The symptoms should be managed accordingly.
- Nerve Injury:
  - The exiting nerve lies in the anterior and inferior part of the intervertebral foramen. One can avoid nerve injury by targeting the posterior part of the foramen.[33-38]

Cervical Interlaminar Epidural

KEY POINTS

- Cervical epidural injections are done to treat neck and radicular pain.
- The proposed mechanism of action of steroids in the epidural space includes anti-inflammatory effect, direct membrane stabilization, and perhaps modulating the input of peripheral nociceptors.

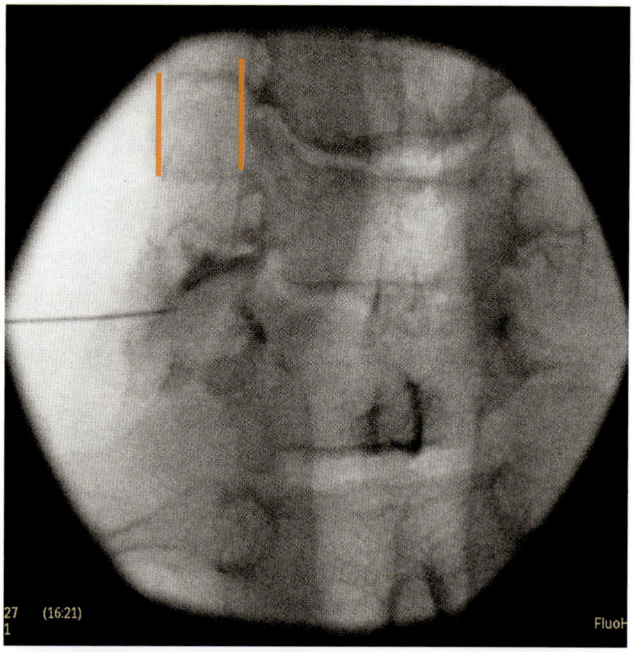

• **Fig 12.26** Needle tip in the center of the facet column. The needle should not be advanced more medial. Dye spread along the nerve root. Orange lines depict the medial and lateral margins of the facet column.

Pertinent Anatomy

- Epidural space lies between the dura mater and osteoligamentous structure lining the vertebral canal.
- The epidural space starts at the foramen magnum and terminates at the sacral hiatus at S4 and S5 levels.
- Epidural space is subdivided into anterior and posterior compartments.[39,40]
- The anterior epidural space is bordered anteriorly by the vertebral body, discs, and the posterior longitudinal ligament.
- The posterior epidural space is bordered anteriorly by the thecal sac and posteriorly by ligamentum flavum and lamina.[41]
- The epidural space contains fat, areolar tissue, and the internal vertebral venous plexus.[42]
- Posterior epidural space varies throughout the length of the spine.
- It is widest at the upper thoracic levels, where the posterior space measures 7.5 mm. The dimensions at C7-T1 are 0.4 mm.[43]

Equipment

- C-arm fluoroscopy
- Needle: Tuohy 18 gauge 3.5 inch if using a catheter OR 20 gauge if not using a catheter.
- Option to use an 18 gauge Tuohy for patients with higher BMI for better maneuverability.
- Radiopaque catheter
- non-ionic contrast material (Omnipaque or Isovue)

Common Injectates

- Corticosteroids
- Orthobiologics (platelet lysate)

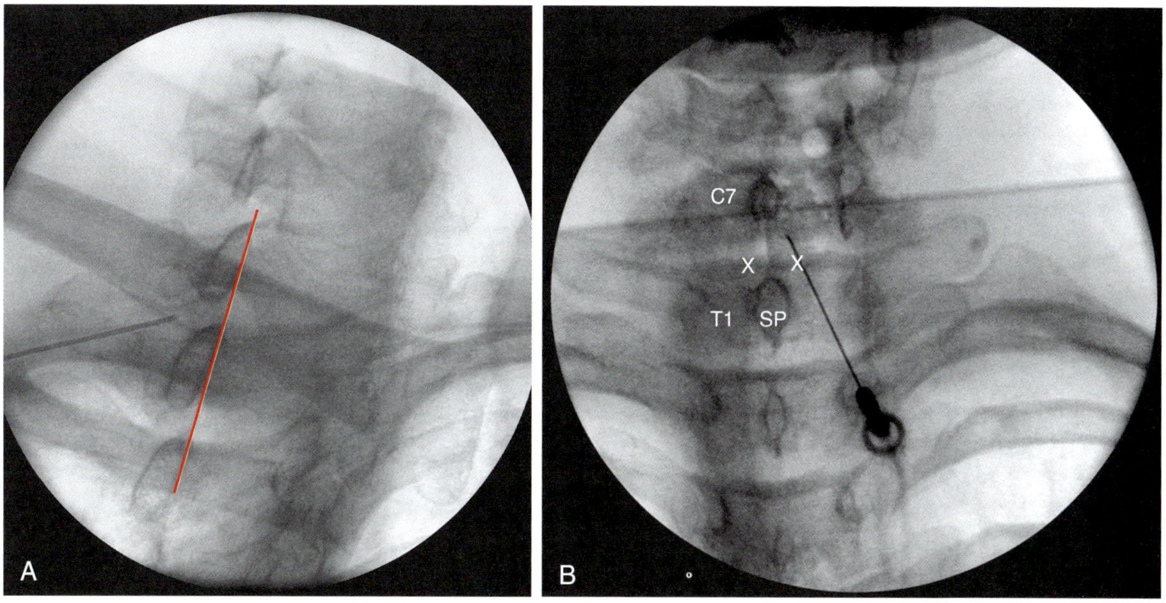

• **Fig. 12.27** C7-T1 Paramedian cervical interlaminar needle placement. A. Contralateral oblique view of Touhy needle posterior to ligamentum flavum. B. AP view of contrast showing epidural flow.

- Avoid local anesthetics in the epidural space as the upper cervical nerve block could arrest breathing

Injectate Volume

- 1 to 3 mL

Technique

Patient Position

- Place the patient in a prone position with a pillow or two under the chest.
- The neck should be slightly flexed (to increase the intralaminar space).
- The head could be turned to the contralateral side to injection to improve visualization of the interlaminar space.

Clinician Position

- Opposite of the C-arm base

Transducer Position or C-Arm Position Fluoro Technique

- The C-arm is placed in a position to get an AP view.
- Then the image-intensifier is tilted caudally or cranially to maximize the interlaminar space.
- The edges of the inferior and superior lamina should be sharp and well seen.
- Although epidural injections can be done at C5-6 and C6-7, C7-T1 has the most space and is the preferred site.

Needle Position

- One side of the T1 lamina [T1 is identified with a large spinous process] is marked on the skin (Fig. 12.27B).
- The entry point is anesthetized with a local anesthetic
- The Touhy needle is advanced using a paramedian approach, preferably on the side where the patient is experiencing radicular pain.
- The needle is aimed at the upper border of the T1 lamina.
- Touch the lamina for safety.
- Once the needle touches the lamina, the C-arm is rotated in the contralateral oblique position.
- At this point, the needle should be behind the "interlaminar line" (ligamentum flavum) (see Fig. 12.27A, shown in *red*).
- Generally, a loss of resistance syringe is attached to the needle after removing the stylet. The author also prefers to fill the needle all the way to the hub with contrast material.
- Following this, the LOR syringe is attached, and the needle is directed upward using the loss of resistance technique.
- Attention should be kept at the hub as the contrast material is seen getting sucked in as the loss is achieved.

Target

- The needle should be just past the interlaminar line, when the loss of resistance occurs. Loss of resistance can occur further posterior as well.
- Attach a syringe connected to a small volume extension tubing containing the contrast to the needle.
- Gently aspirate for the presence of any blood or CSF.
- Once negative aspiration is confirmed, slowly inject contrast under live fluoroscopy to assess its spread within the epidural space in contralateral oblique and AP views (Figs 12.28 and 12.29).

Needle and Catheter technique:

- If the target pathology is at a higher level, use an epidural catheter.
- Use an 18 gauge Tuohy needle to access the epidural space.
- After confirming the needle tip in the epidural space using the above technique, a radiopaque 20 gauge catheter can be threaded cephalad within the epidural space to the specific target level.

PEARLS AND PITFALLS

- Interlaminar epidural injections in the levels above C5-6 are not recommended even for experienced clinicians as the ligamentum flavum is very thin.
- MRI or CT scan should be reviewed to assess the spinal anatomy prior to doing the injection.
- Should not attempt the procedure if stenosis or large disc herniation is present at the target entry point.
- Use a catheter to deliver the medication if the pathology is higher up, at C3-4, C4-5, C5-6.
- IV access should be obtained in the patient prior to doing the procedure.
- Potential complications are rare and are usually attributable to the needle placement and include the following:
  - Spinal cord injury (if the needle is advanced too far)
  - Epidural hematoma (anticoagulation medications should be held per ASRA guidelines prior to doing the procedure)
  - Infection (procedure should be done with full sterile protocol)
  - Postdural puncture headaches
  - Allergic reaction to the contrast material

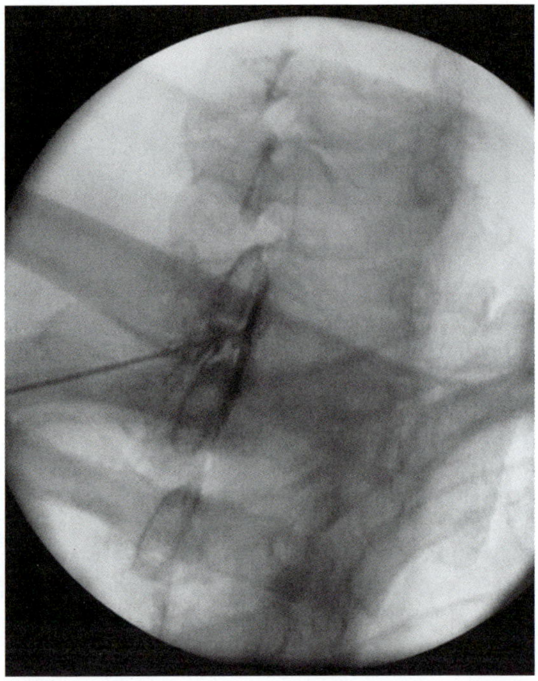

• **Fig. 12.28** Contralateral Oblique view on interlaminar injection with epidural contrast flow.

Facet Joints

Atlanto-Occipital and Atlanto-Axial Interventions

KEY POINTS

- The atlanto-occipital (AO) joint is an ellipsoid (bean-like) joint with its lateral edges sloping upwards. It allows passive flexion, an extension of 10 degrees, as well as 10 degrees of rotation.[44]
- The atlanto-axial (AA) joint is not a true facet joint. It is an anterior structure rather than a posterior one. It lies ventral to the vertebral artery, spinal cord, and C2 dorsal root ganglion and is innervated by the C2 root.

Pertinent Anatomy

- The atlanto-occipital (AO) joint is the articulation of the superior articular facet of C1 (Atlas) and the occiput.
- The atlanto-axial (AA) joint is the articulation of the Atlas and C2 (Axis).
- AO and AA joints have a high degree of mobility and are primarily supported by ligaments, whose function is to transmit information to the Central Nervous System concerning head and neck position. No discs or uncinate processes are present.
- The vertebral artery runs on the lateral aspect of the AA joint, however, variations could be present, including bypass of the transverse foramen of C1, close relation to the C1-2 facet joints, and variable course along the posterior arch of C1.[45]
- The normal AA joint allows for 5 degrees of flexion and 10 degrees of extension. The axial rotation is 70 degrees which allows for over 40% of total cervical spine rotation.
- The C2 dorsal ramus innervates both the AO and AA joints.

Common Pathology

- The AO joint and the AA joint are implicated in approximately 9% of cervicogenic headaches. Dreyfuss et al. showed that noxious stimulation of these joints in normal volunteers with injections of contrast medium produces pain in the suboccipital region and the occiput.[46]
- Typical pain patterns:
  - Deep pain in the suboccipital region, often unilateral
  - Pain with rotation, flexion, and extension of the neck
  - Crepitus/pain associated with movement
  - Cervicogenic headaches impairing function

Equipment

- Emergency equipment (crash cart)
- C-arm fluoroscopy
- 25 to 22 gauge, 3 to 3.5 inch spinal needle
- Non-ionic contrast (omnipaque or Isovue)

Common Injectates

- Local anesthetics for diagnostics, corticosteroids, orthobiologics (Dextrose prolotherapy, PRP)

Injectate Volume

- 0.5 to 1 mL

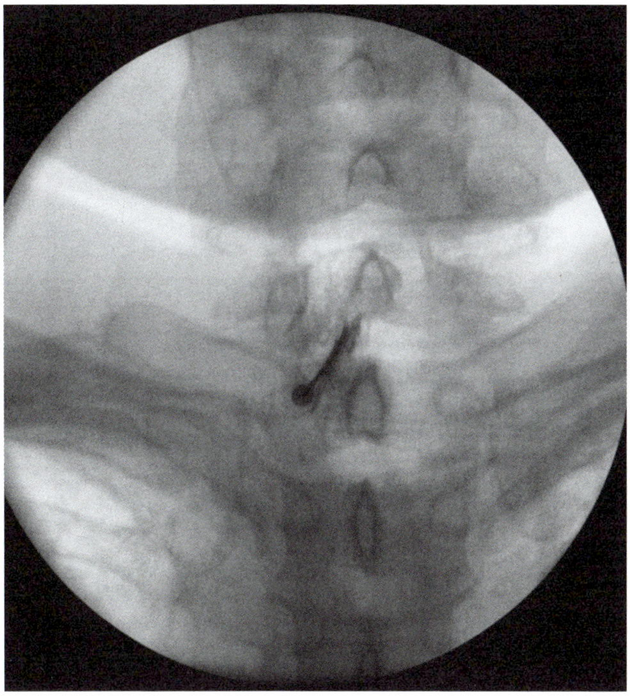

• **Fig. 12.29** AP view C7-T1left paramedian interlaminar injection with contrast showing epidural flow.

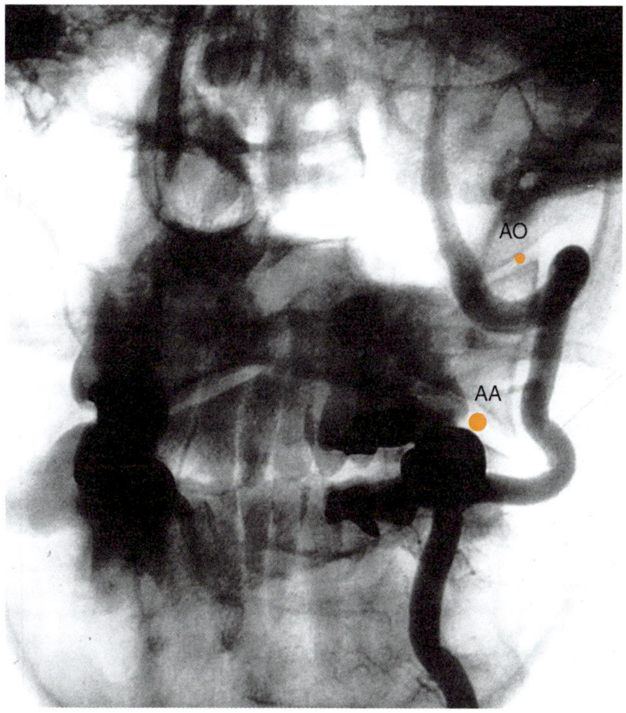

• **Fig. 12.30** Target entry points for AO and AA joint with relation to the vertebral artery. *AA,* Atlanto-axial; *AO,* Atlanto-occipital. (Photo Courtesy: Dr. Paul Dreyfuss.)

Technique: AO (C0-1) joint

Patient Position

- The patient is placed in a prone position with the neck slightly flexed. The head and neck should be supported, and the mouth should be unobstructed as the patient may need to open it during the procedure.
- Another technique described by Centeno et al.[47] suggests placing the patient in a prone position with the head slightly flexed and rotated to the ipsilateral side (approximately 30 degrees). Ipsilateral rotation of the head displaces the vertebral artery medially.

Clinician Position

- The opposite side of the base of the C-arm

C-Arm Position Fluoro Technique

- Caudal tilt to move occiput from needle trajectory
- Slight C-arm rotation along the long axis of the joint to visualize the joint in the nasal cavity.

Needle Position

- The needle is placed in the palpable groove between the mastoid process and the occipital rim.
- A reliable entry point is the posterolateral aspect of the joint capsule, which is drawn upwards, above the edge of the cup, over the posterolateral edge of the occipital condyle.[47]
- The "gun barrel" approach should be used.

Target

- Target is the most superior and posterior aspect of the joint just inside its lateral edge (Fig. 12.30).
- After negative aspiration, inject a small amount of non-ionic contrast
- Confirm proper needle placement and contrast flow in the AP and lateral views.

PEARLS AND PITFALLS

- Care should be taken not to advance the needle too far in.
- NOTE: if venous runoff is seen, you are not in the joint as there is a rich venous plexus present. If arterial runoff is seen or the contrast material is seen in the epidural space, the injection should be terminated.
- The joint volume is around 1 mL.
- BMAC and lipoaspirates should be considered particulate injections with potential to occlude vessels if injected intravascularly.

Technique: AA (C1-2) joint

Patient Position

- The patient is placed in a prone position with the neck slightly flexed. The head and neck should be supported, and the mouth should be unobstructed as the patient may need to open it during the procedure.

Clinician Position

- The opposite side of the base of the C-arm

C-Arm Position Fluoro Technique

- Direct AP view with cephalad tilt to "open" the AA joint.

Needle Position

- In AP view, the start point is over the lateral third of the lower end of the posterior surface of the lateral mass of the Atlas (see Fig. 12.30).
- Make sure that the needle does not stray from this path.

Target

- Target is the lateral third of the joint. After the needle touches bone, redirect intraarticularly
- Confirm depth in the lateral view.
- Inject contrast and confirm intra-articular flow in the AP and lateral views.

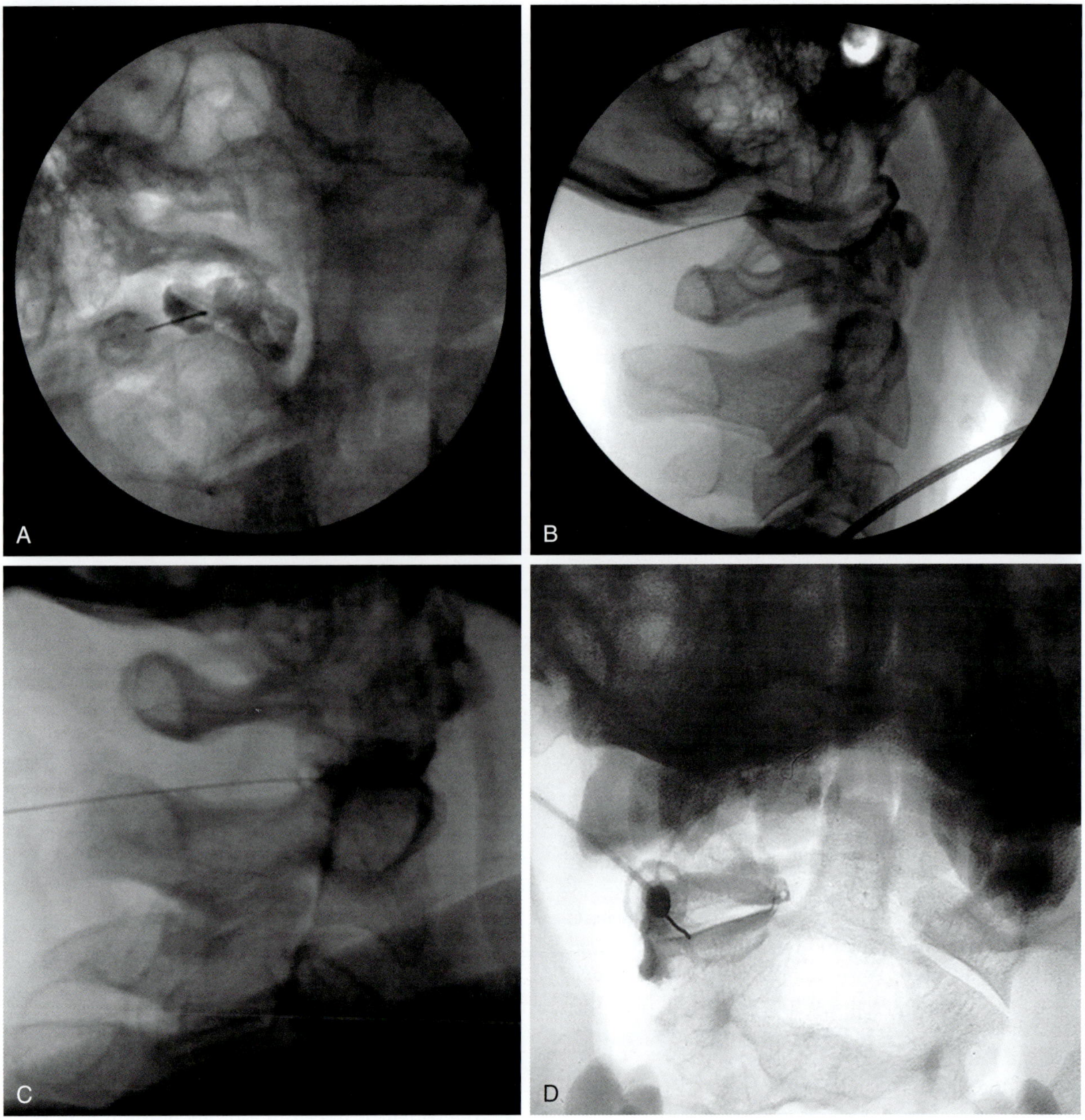

• **Fig. 12.31** (A) Contrast filling the AO joint oblique. (B) Lateral view. (C) Lateral view of AA joint (D) AP view of the AA joint. (Courtesy Dr. Paul Dreyfuss.)

PEARLS AND PITFALLS

- Keep the needle in lateral 1/3 area of the joint/lateral mass. If the needle strays laterally, it could enter the vertebral artery and if it strays medially the C2 ganglion or spinal cord.

C2-3 to C7-T1 Facet Joints

Pertinent Anatomy

- The cervical facet joint or zygapophysial joint (Z-joint) is a diarthrodial, synovial joint formed by the superior articular pillar of the inferior vertebral segment and the inferior articular pillar of the superior vertebral segment. There is a 45 degree joint inclination with increased angulation inferiorly. It is a relatively flat joint.
- The articular facets are covered by articular cartilage, and a synovial membrane bridges the margins of the articular cartilage of the two facets in each joint.
- Z-Joints are innervated by the medial branches of the dorsal rami.
- The C2-3 joint is innervated by the third occipital nerve (TON), while the joints below C2-3 are innervated by the medial branches of the cervical dorsal rami of above and below the joint.

Common Pathology

- Based on multiple studies, the prevalence of cervical facet joint pain has been shown to be 36% to 67% in

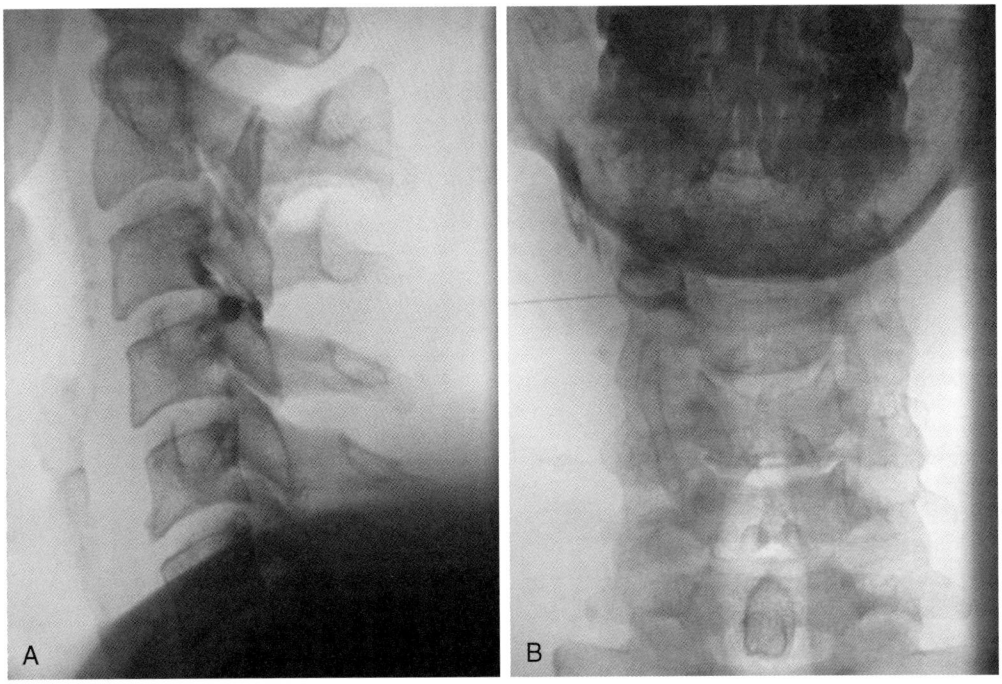

• **Fig. 12.32** (A and B) Lateral approach. AP and lateral views: needle in the C3-4 facet joint along with the contrast seen in the superior and inferior recesses. (Courtesy Vivek Manocha.)

patients with chronic neck pain suspected of facet joint pain.[48]

- Typical pain patterns: Dwyer et al. mapped out referred pain patterns by performing facet joint injections in normal volunteers.[49]
  - Axial neck pain, upper back pain
  - Crepitus/pain associated with movement
  - Cervicogenic headaches
  - No radicular pattern
  - No evidence of discogenic pain

Equipment

- Emergency equipment (crash cart)
- C-arm fluoroscopy
- 25 to 22 gauge, 3 to 3.5 inch spinal needle
- Non-ionic contrast (omnipaque or Isovue)

Common Injectates

- Local anesthetics for diagnostics, corticosteroids, orthobiologics (Prolotherapy, PRP, bone marrow concentrate, etc.)

Injectate Volume

- 0.5 to 1 mL

Technique

This procedure can be done in a posterior or lateral approach. The prone position is preferred for joints C5-6 and below as these are easily accessible from a posterior approach. For C2-3, C3-4, and C4-5 facet joints, the lateral approach is preferable.

Technique for lateral approach

Patient Position

- Lateral Decubitus or supine position. The key element to successfully performing this block is to obtain a near-perfect, true lateral view.
- In a lateral decubitus position, this can be achieved by putting a folded towel under the head to keep the head and neck parallel to the table.
- In most patients, C2-3, C3-4, and C4-5 facets can be blocked in supine and/or lateral decubitus positions. However, C5-6, C6-7, and C7-T1 will require access using the posterior approach while the patient is in the prone position.

Clinician Position

- Physician preference when the procedure is performed in a lateral decubitus position as long as the fluoroscope base is on the opposite side of the physician.
- For a supine position, the physician should stand on the side of the neck being injected.

Fluoroscope Position

- Position the C-arm to obtain a true lateral view. This minimizes the risk that the needle will be aimed toward the contralateral side.
- The silhouettes of the articular pillars at each segmental level should be superimposed.
- The joint line should be clear and visible.

Needle Position

- Start over the inferior or superior articular process just below or above the joint line.
- The needle should be advanced in small increments, and the directional adjustments should be made in a subtle manner (Fig. 12.32A and B).
- Touch needle down on bone for depth safety.
- A lateral view is obtained at this time.

Target

- The needle is then walked off into the joint capsule.
- A small dose (0.2 mL) of contrast material is injected, which can be seen filling the superior and inferior recesses (Fig. 12.32A).

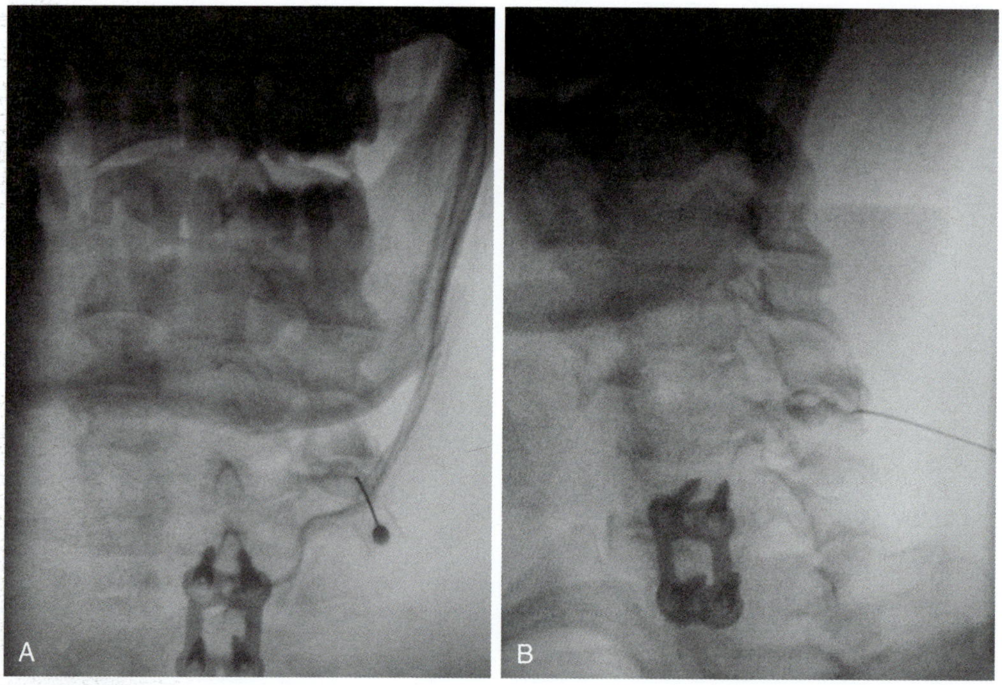

• **Fig. 12.33** (A and B) Posterior approach. AP and contralateral oblique view with contrast within the joint. (Courtesy Vivek Manocha.)

PEARLS AND PITFALLS

- Must have a true lateral view to see an accurate target
- Use lateral view to ensure needle not advancing too deep through the joint, which can risk puncturing the dura or spinal cord.

Technique for the Posterior Approach

Patient Position

- The patient is placed in a prone position with a pillow under the chest and the neck in a slight flexion.
- The head should be turned to the contralateral side to get the molars out of the way.

Clinician Position

- Opposite the fluoroscope base.

Fluoroscope Position

- The C-arm is brought in the AP position, and a caudal tilt is given to the image intensifier to obtain a pillar view (Fig. 12.33A).
- Align the spinous processes in the center of the pillars.

Needle Position

- The needle entry point is selected half to a full segment below the target joint.
- The needle is passed upwards and ventrally through the posterior neck muscles until it makes contact with the posterior surface of the articular pillar just below the joint line
- At this point, the contralateral oblique view is obtained, and the needle is "walked off" into the joint.

Target

- The lateral third of the joint should be the target entry point.
- Inject a small amount of contrast to confirm intraarticular spread in the AP view (Fig. 12.33A and B).
- Most patients have a communicating pathway between the facet joints and the extradural, interlaminar, and even the contralateral facet joint space (Okada[50]).

PEARLS AND PITFALLS

- A curved needle tip helps to navigate the needle more precisely with this approach

Cervical Medial Branch Block

KEY POINTS

- The main purpose of cervical medial branch blocks is to test if the patient's pain stems from a particular facet joint.
- Cervical medial branch blocks have diagnostic utility, in that if positive, they identify the source of pain
- A positive response predicts a good chance of obtaining complete relief of pain from radiofrequency ablation.
- A good history and physical exam and imaging review should be conducted to exclude serious possible causes of neck pain, such as infections, tumors, or vascular disease.
- Pain maps are used to select which nerves to target.

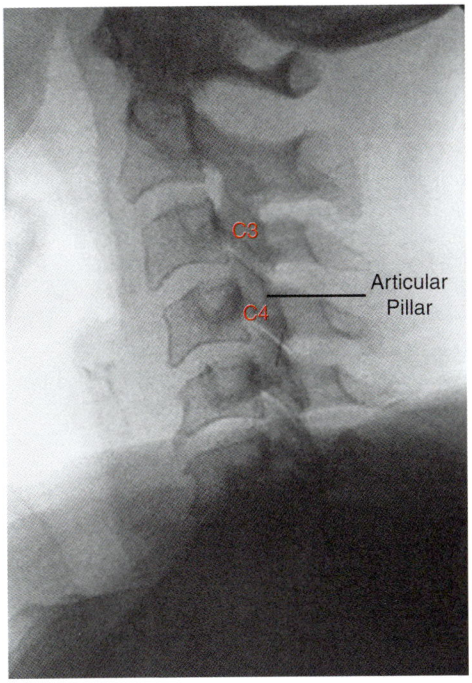

• **Fig. 12.34** A lateral view of the cervical spine showing the articular pillar (C3 and C4 marked in *red*). Needle shown at the middle of the C5 articular pillar over the C5 medial branch. (Courtesy Vivek Manocha.)

Pertinent Anatomy

- Medial branches arise from the dorsal rami of the spinal nerves, and innervate the facet joints.
- Each joint receives articular branches from the nerve above and the nerve below the joint.
- Those nerves have the same segmental numbers as the joint.
- Each nerve (except C7) crosses the middle of the articular pillar, which is the suitable target point for the block (Fig. 12.34).
- Lord et al. described the variation in the location of the medial branches. At C5, the medial branches are located over the middle of the C5 articular pillar; but are located higher on the pillars at levels above.[48]
- The third occipital nerve and C3 medial branch provides innervation to the C2-3 facet joint. It also innervates the semispinalis capitis muscle.

Common Pathology

- Unilateral or bilateral neck pain.
- Decreased range of motion of the neck.
- Local tenderness over the affected facet joint(s)
- Upper neck pain with associated headaches
- Pain referring to the shoulder girdle. It should not radiate distally to the elbow. The pain should follow a non-dermatomal (non-radicular) pattern.
- Referred pain from the C2-3 facet joint leads to headaches.

Equipment

- Emergency equipment (crash cart)
- C-arm fluoroscopy
- 25 to 22 gauge, 1.5 to 2 inch needle for lateral approach
- 25 to 22 gauge 3 to 3.5 inch spinal needle
- Non-ionic contrast (omnipaque or Isovue)

Common Injectates

- Local anesthetics for diagnostics, corticosteroids
- Typically 2% lidocaine or 0.5% bupivacaine (preservative free). Comparative blocks using a short-acting anesthetic and a long-acting anesthetic are recommended to decrease the false-positive response.

Injectate Volume

- 0.25 to 1 mL

Technique—Lateral Approach

Patient Position

- Lateral Decubitus or supine position. The key element to successfully performing this block is to obtain a near-perfect, true lateral view.
- In a lateral decubitus position, this can be achieved by putting a folded towel under the head to keep the head and neck parallel to the table.
- In most patients, the third occipital nerve and C3-5 medial branches can be blocked in supine and/or lateral decubitus position. However, C6 and C7 will require access using the posterior approach while the patient is in the prone position.

Clinician Position

- The physician's preference while the procedure is performed in a lateral decubitus position as long as the fluoroscope is on the opposite side of the physician.
- For a supine position, the physician should stand on the side of the neck being injected.

Fluoroscope Position

- Position the fluoroscope in such a fashion that a true lateral view is obtained.
- The silhouettes of the articular pillars at each segmental level should be superimposed.

Needle Position

- The needle should start directly over the targeted MBB and use the "gun barrel" approach.

Target

- For medial branches C3-6:
  - The target point is the centroid of the articular pillar with the same segmental number as the target nerve.
  - This centroid is found at the intersection of the two diagonals of the articular pillar (Fig. 12.34).
- For medial branch C7:
  - The target point lies high on the apex of the superior articular process of C7.
  - Keep in mind that the transverse process of the C7, which is often not visible in the lateral view, can obstruct the needle placement.
- For third occipital nerve block:
  - The target area is a rectangular area bounded by the anterior edge of the superior articular process of C3; upper and lower lines perpendicular to this edge

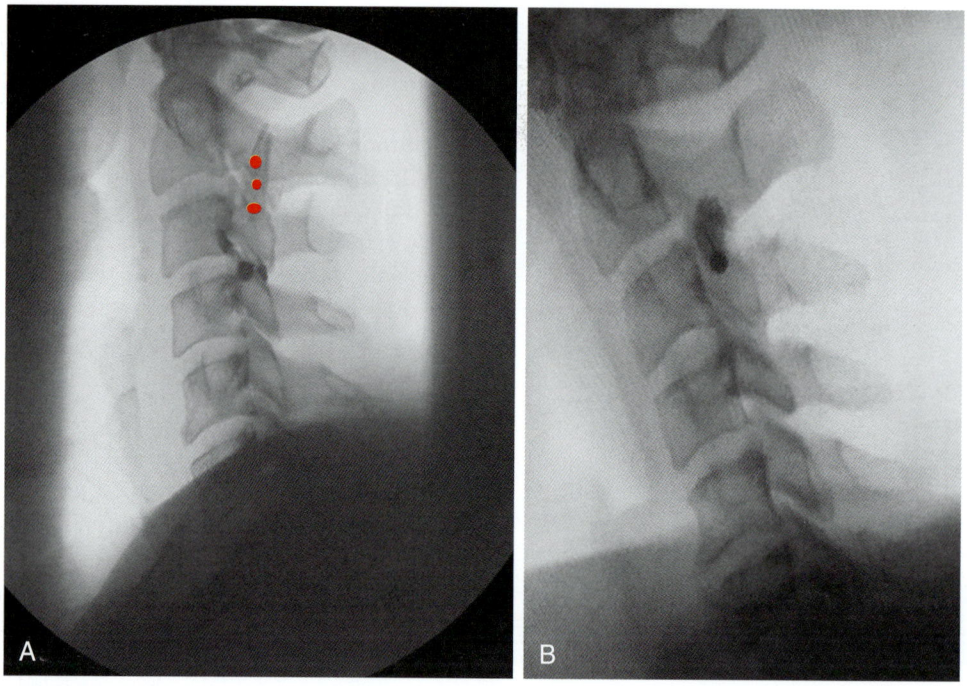

• **Fig. 12.35** (A) The three red dots represent the target area for the Third occipital nerve block. (B) shows contrast over the location of the third occipital nerve. (Courtesy Vivek Manocha).

passing posteriorly from the apex of the superior articular process and from the bottom of the C2-3 intervertebral foramen, and a posterior line approximately through the posterior edge of the inferior articular process of C2 (Fig. 12.35).

- The needle is inserted in the middle of the three target points.
- When the bone is contacted, the needle should be slightly withdrawn prior to injecting the contrast.

Technique—Posterior Approach

Patient Position

- Place the patient in the prone position.
- Patient positioning is the same as described above for the cervical facet injection.

Clinician Position

- Same as described above for cervical facet injections

Fluoroscope Position

- The C-arm is positioned to get the pillar view of the cervical spine which is obtained by tilting the C-arm caudally. (Fig. 12.36A).
- A pillar view is obtained by reorienting the plane of the fluoroscope so that it passes parallel to the plane of the z-joint at the target level.

Needle Position

- The needle should be inserted starting directly over and at the lateral margin of the target pillar.
- It is advisable to directly contact the bone immediately medial to the target pillar.
- The C-arm should then be rotated to a contralateral oblique position.
- In this view, the needle can be rotated 180 degrees and advanced to the target

Target

- Target is the lateral concavity of the articular pillar.

PEARLS AND PITFALLS

- In the posterior approach, a curved needle tip is required to navigate the needle safely and more accurately to the target
- The patient may not experience 100% pain relief as it is possible that the patient may have other sources of pain.
- Diagnostic medial branch blocks should be performed only if the clinician is trained to proceed with performing the RFA.

Cervical Radiofrequency Neurotomy of the Medial Branches

KEY POINTS

- Indication: A diagnostic block of the target medial branches has provided 80% or better relief for the duration of the anesthetic.
- A radiofrequency lesion is created with a temperature over 80 degrees. However, the higher the temperature, the bigger the lesion.

Equipment

- Emergency equipment (crash cart)
- C-arm fluoroscopy
- A 100 mm or 140 mm RF needle with a curved tip
- Radiofrequency generator that displays impedance, voltage, current, and temperature

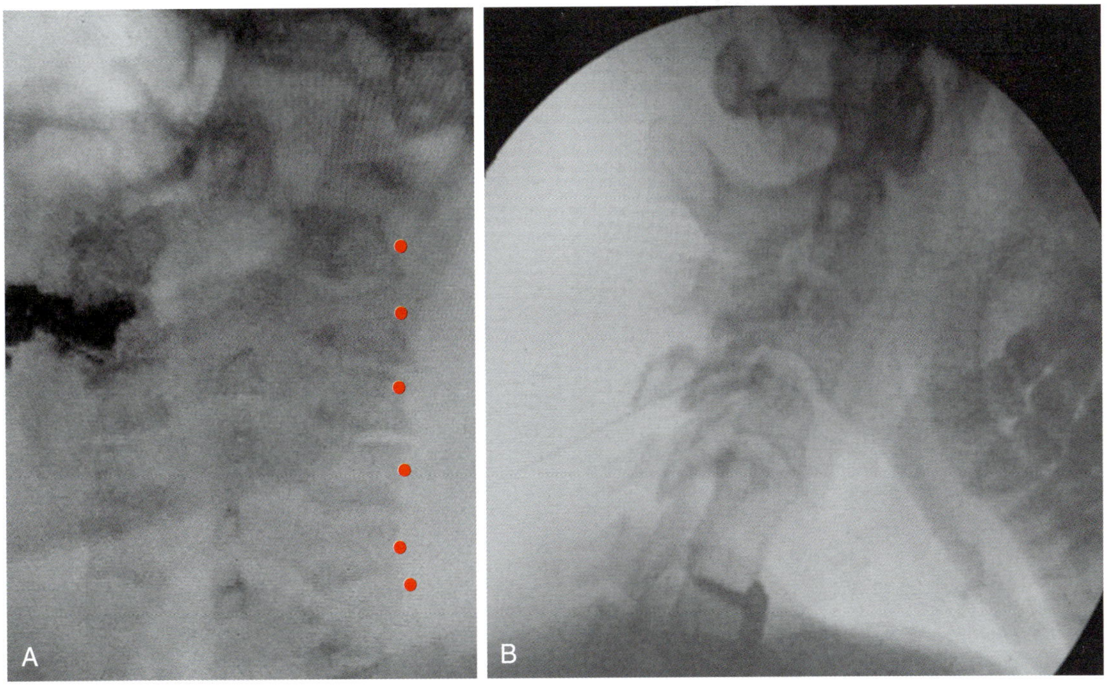

• **Fig. 12.36** (A) Waist of the articular pillars. Site for the placement of the needle *(red dots)*. (B) Contralateral oblique view. (Courtesy Vivek Manocha.)

- Grounding pad
- Local anesthetic

Technique—C3-6 Medial Branch

Patient Position

- Place the patient in the prone position. Patient positioning is the same as described above for the cervical facet injection.

Clinician Position

- Same as described above for cervical facet injections

Fluoroscope Position

- The C-arm is positioned to get the pillar view of the cervical spine which can be obtained by tilting the image intensifier in a caudate position (see Fig. 12.36A).
- A pillar view is obtained by reorienting the plane of the fluoroscope so that it passes parallel to the plane of the z-joint at the target level.

Needle Position

- A 100 mm 20 gauge with a 10 mm curved active tip is inserted starting directly over and at the lateral margin of the target pillar.
- It is advisable to directly contact the bone immediately medial to the target pillar.
- The C-arm can be rotated in a contralateral oblique position (Fig. 12.37B).
- In this view, the needle can be rotated 180 degrees and advanced to enter the lateral concavity of the articular pillar (see Fig. 12.37A).

Target

- For the C5 medial branch, this will be the center of the articular pillar, whereas, for C3, C4, and C6, the target region is more cephalad on the pillar.[51]
- Once the correct placement has been achieved and confirmed, sensory and motor stimulation is done.
- It is recommended that the patient report sensation during stimulation at 50 Hz at less than 0.5 volts and have no motor stimulation to the affected myotome at 2 Hz at no less than 3 times the sensory threshold or 3 volts.
- A twitching response is seen, which is due to the stimulation of the multifidus muscle.
- Then the level is anesthetized with 0.5 mL of local anesthetic, and the lesions are carried out at 80 degrees for 90 seconds.
- The cannula can be retracted and repositioned for a second lesion for 60 seconds.

Technique—C7 Medial Branch Neurotomy

- Setup is the same as C3-6 Medial Branch Neurotomy
- The C7 medial branch neurotomy follows the same principles and precautions as the other nerves. However, there are some differences, given that the C7 nerve exhibits significant variation in location.
- It can lie on the lateral aspect of the superior articular process, as high as the apex of this process, or it may be found on the superior aspect of the proximal end of the C7 transverse process.[52]

Moreover, the C7 medial branch crosses the superior articular process rather than the waist of the articular pillar.

Needle Position

- A 100 mm 20 gauge with a 10 mm curved active tip is inserted starting directly over and at the lateral margin of the superior articular pillar of C7.
- It is advisable to directly contact the bone immediately medial to the target pillar.

Target

- Once the bone has been contacted, the needle is redirected so as to pass into the lateral surface of the superior

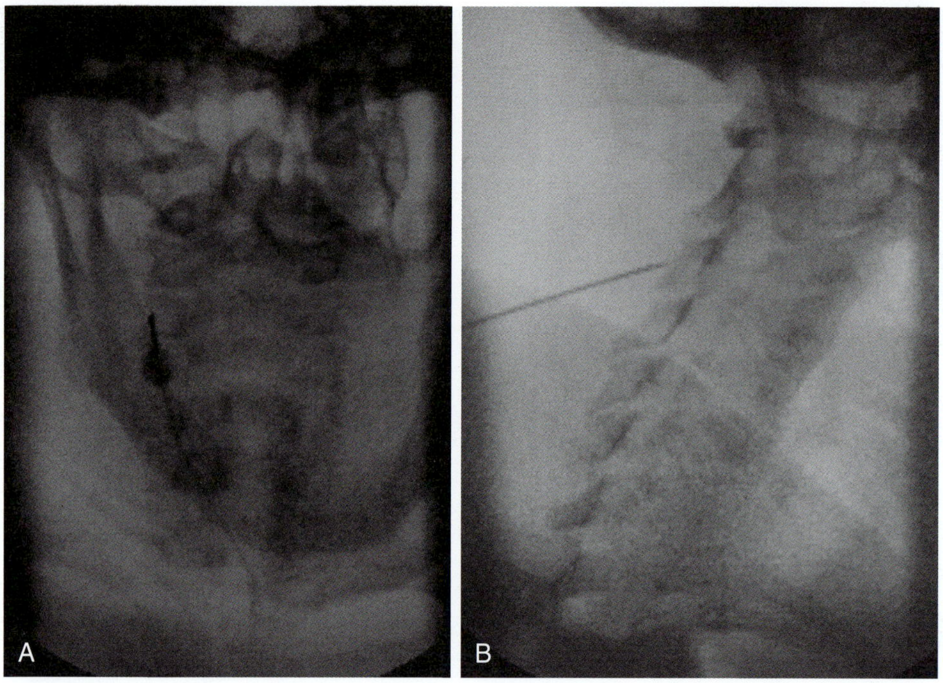

• **Fig 12.37** (A) RF needle position in an AP view. (B) Needle position in the contralateral oblique view. (Courtesy Vivek Manocha.)

articular process. Care should be taken not to advance more than 3 mm.

- Once the placement is confirmed, the lesion is created as previously described.

Technique—Third Occipital Nerve Neurotomy

- Setup is the same as C3-6 Medial Branch Neurotomy
- Third occipital radiofrequency neurotomy follows the same principles and precautions as the other nerves.
- Two separate lesions are typically performed to adequately ablate the third occipital nerve. The neurotomies are performed with both an oblique and sagittal pass.[51,52]

Target

- For the oblique pass
  - The target area is the entire anterolateral surface of the superior articular process of the C3, from its apex to its base opposite to the base of the C2-3 foramen.
  - On lateral views, the uninsulated portion of the electrode should lie over the anterior third of the SAP of C3, and its tip should coincide with the anterior margin of the process but should not project beyond this margin.
  - On AP view, the tip of the electrode should project just medial to the lateral silhouette of the C2-3 Z-joint.
- For the sagittal pass:
  - A direct posterior-anterior approach is used, and the pillar view is not required.
  - In lateral views, the uninsulated portion of the electrode should lie over the middle third of the C2-3 joint.
  - In AP views, it should abut directly against the lateral convexity of the joint.

PEARLS AND PITFALLS

- Complications from intra-articular facet joints, medial branch blocks, and radiofrequency ablation are exceedingly rare. However, serious complications can occur from incorrect placement of needles or administration of various drugs.[51]
- The proximity of the needle to the vertebral artery, spinal cord, and nerve root creates risk for injury, and so it is extremely important to place the needle in a precise and accurate location.
- Complications may include dural puncture, spinal cord trauma, subdural injections, neural trauma, intravascular injections.
- Complications from RFA lesion include worsening of the usual pain, burning or dysesthesias, decreased sensation and/or allodynia in the skin in the region of the facets denervated.

Cervical Intradiscal Technique

KEY POINTS

- The technique for cervical discography was first described in 1957 by Smith and Nichols.[53]
- The utility of cervical provocative or analgesic discography as a diagnostic tool has been controversial[54] and hence infrequently used.
- However, with the evolution of intradiscal biologics to successfully treat lumbar discogenic pain,[55,56] there has been a resurgence of interest in cervical disc needle placement and injection.
- IV access is recommended for emergent complications
- Surgical prep and drape are strongly encouraged. The proceduralist should also wear a surgical cap, mask,

KEY POINTS—CONT'D

and gown. C-arm should have a sterile cover. Every possible sterile precaution should be undertaken to reduce the risk of discitis.
- Prophylactic antibiotics can be given even though there is no strong evidence to support this reduces infection rates. The author prefers 1 to 2 g of cefazolin or 600 to 900 mg of clindamycin infused half an hour before the start of the procedure.

Pertinent Anatomy

- The cervical disc annulus does not consist of concentric ring-shaped laminae of collagen fibers as found in lumbar discs.
- Rather, a crescent-shaped mass of collagen fibers thicker anteriorly and tapered laterally toward the uncinate process characterizes the annulus fibrosus.
- Healthy cervical discs accept small amounts of contrast media, usually on the order of 0.25 mL to 0.5 mL, due to the very small nucleus and small size of the disc.
- Injection of greater volumes usually means extravasation of contrast from the posterolateral or uncovertebral portions of the annulus, with little resistance upon injection being appreciated.[57,58]
- Intervertebral disc innervation in the cervical spine is analogous to that in the lumbar spine, with cervical discs receiving innervation posteriorly from the sinuvertebral nerves, laterally from the vertebral nerve, and anteriorly from the sympathetic trunks.[54]
- Cervical sinuvertebral nerves have an upward course in the vertebral canal and supply the disc at their level of entry as well as the more cranial disc.[57]
- Both nerve fibers and proprioceptive receptors are found in the outer third of the annulus fibrosus.

Common Pathology

- After facet joints, the cervical discs are the second most common cause of neck pain.[59] Symptoms solely due to disc herniation are less common in the cervical region than in the lumbar region because of three reasons.[57]
  - Herniation laterally is first prevented by cervical facet joints, which form a bony barrier between the disc and the nerve root.
  - The dense posterior longitudinal ligament limits the posterior herniations
  - The nucleus also lies much more anteriorly in the cervical disc than in the lumbar disc, and its movement posteriorly is correspondingly much more difficult and less likely.
- Inflammation in the disc, usually from injury or degeneration, can fire up the nociceptors in the annulus.
- Inflammatory cytokines leaking from the disc can irritate or sensitize the annulus, adjacent spinal nerves, ligaments, and muscles.

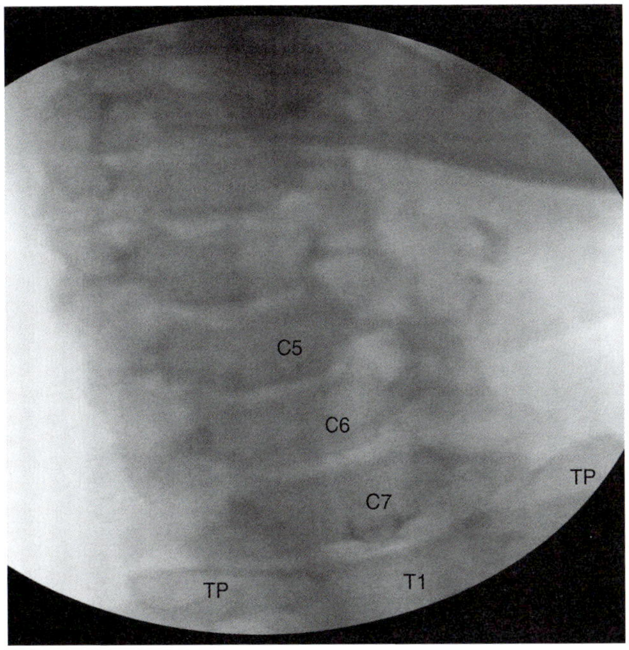

• **Fig 12.38** *TP,* The large transverse process of T1.

- Mesenchymal stem cells with known secretory and paracrine abilities have the potential to modify inflammation and provide pain relief by producing potent anti-inflammatory proteins like interleukin receptor antagonist protein [IRAP], transforming growth factor [TGF], interleukin 10, prostaglandin E2 [PGE2], etc. (Chapter 7).

Equipment

- C-arm fluoroscopy
- 25 gauge 2 to 3.5 inch spinal needle

Common Injectates

- Contrast for a provocative discogram
- Orthobiologics (PRP, bone marrow concentrate, etc.)

Injectate Volume

- 0.25 to 0.5 mL

Technique

Patient Position

- The patient is in the supine position.
- The head should be tilted to the patient's left.
- A pillow can be placed under the shoulder blades to extend the cervical spine.
- The patient's face is turned to the left so that the jaw does not obscure the visualization of the cervical spine(see Fig. 12.38).

Clinician Position

- The interventionist should be on the patient's right side, with the C-arm on the left side.

C-Arm Position

- AP view will identify the cervical disc levels. T1 level can be distinguished by the large transverse process (see Fig. 12.38). This is a useful landmark to count the disc levels.

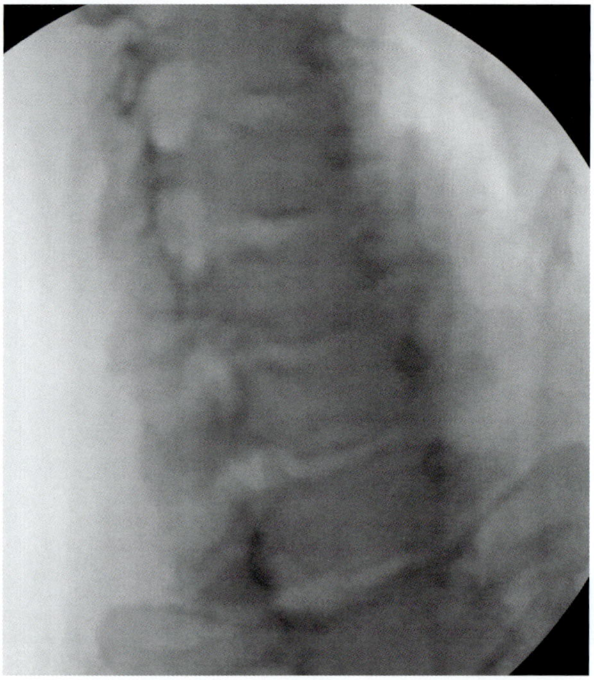

• **Fig 12.39** Ipsilateral oblique view of cervical foramen.

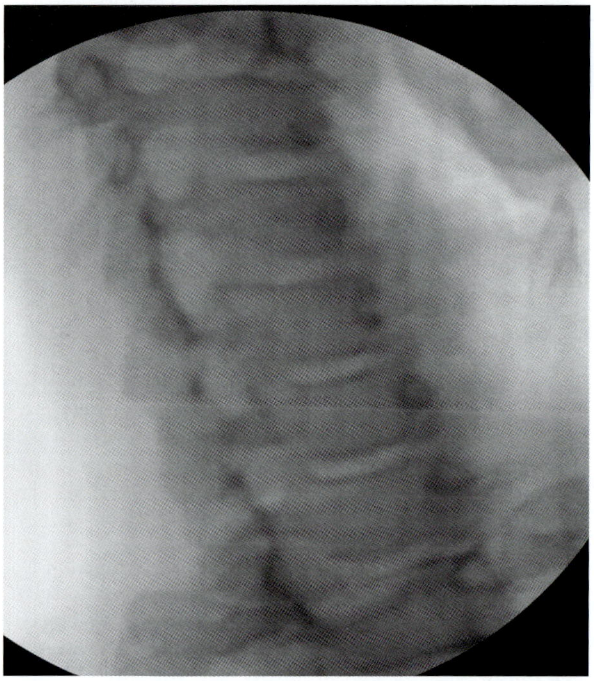

• **Fig 12.40** Squaring the endplates is a vital step. Usually, the caudal angulation helps. Notice that the discs are much better visualized in this figure compared to Fig. 12.37.

- Oblique the C-arm towards the right side of the patient until the neural foramen at the level of disc entry is maximized and the uncinate process is well seen (see Fig. 12.39).
- Next, craniocaudal angulation of the C-arm is done until the disc endplates are maximally squared off (see Fig. 12.40). Usually, caudal angulation [image intensifier angled towards the feet of the patient] is required. Most

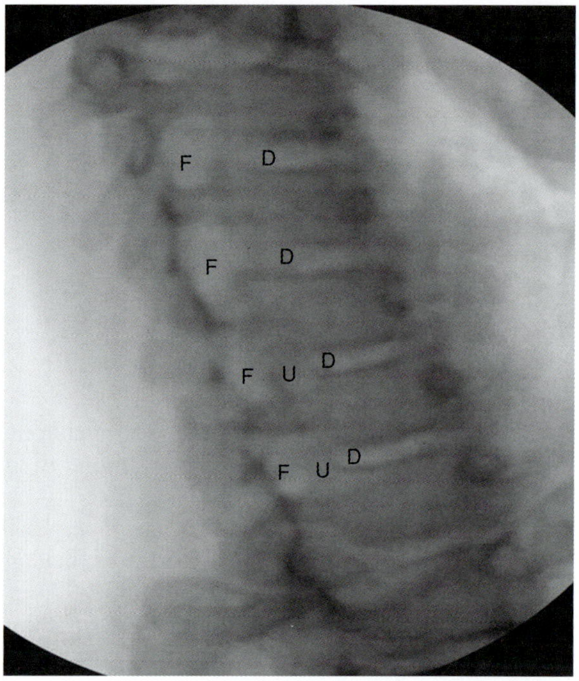

• **Fig 12.41** *D,* Entry site into disc; *F,* neural foramen maximized; *U,* uncincate process.

of the procedure is done in this oblique view, and it is important to do the following.
  - Maximize the neural foramen
  - The uncinate process should be clearly seen. This is an important landmark as most of the procedure revolves around it.
  - Disc endplates are maximally squared. If this step is not done, it is very difficult to enter the disc.

Needle Position

- Cervical disc entry should always be from the right side in order to avoid the esophagus. This is mandatory.
- A curved needle is highly encouraged.
- Skin entry after local anesthetic infiltration is done just anterior to the uncinate process, after palpating to ensure that the carotid artery is not in the way.
- The needle should be advanced parallel to the x-ray beam using the "gun barrel" approach.
- The goal is to contact the anterior border of the uncinate process (see Fig. 12.41).
  - It is imperative that the needle does not stray anterior to the uncinate on its way.
  - Anterior diversion increases the risk of encountering the carotid artery/jugular vein and the esophagus.
  - Posterior deviation of the needle risks the vertebral artery and the spinal nerve (see Fig. 12.42).
  - The carotid sheath should be palpated and manually moved to the left during needle placement.
- Once the anterior border of the uncinate process is contacted, the needle is advanced a few millimeters slightly anteriorly and medially into the disc, again with the needle as close as possible to the uncinate process (Fig. 12.43).

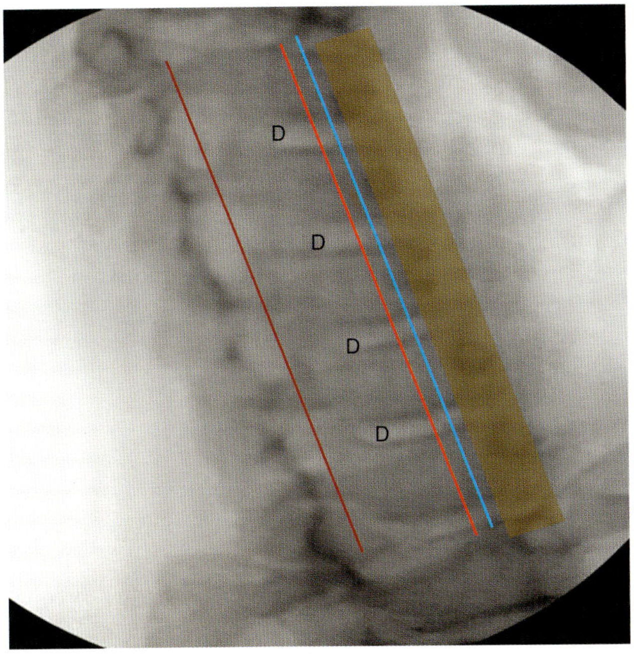

• **Fig 12.42** Ipsilateral Oblique view for cervical intradiscal access. *Blue,* Internal jugular vein; *bright red*: carotid artery; *brown,* esophagus; *D,* disc entry point; *dark red,* vertebral artery.

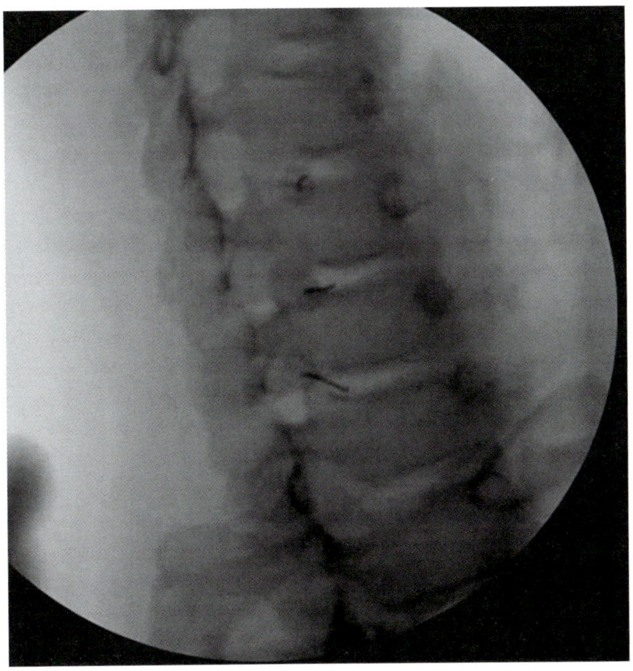

• **Fig 12.43** Needles very close to the uncinate process.

Target

- As soon as the disc is entered, further advancement should be stopped immediately.
- A true lateral view is obtained where the vertebral bodies are seen as squares and the discs seen clearly.
  - Occasionally, the shoulders impair the view at the C6-7 and C7-T1 levels.
  - An assistant should pull the arms down, then imaging is repeated.
  - This maneuver usually enhances the visualization of the lower cervical discs.

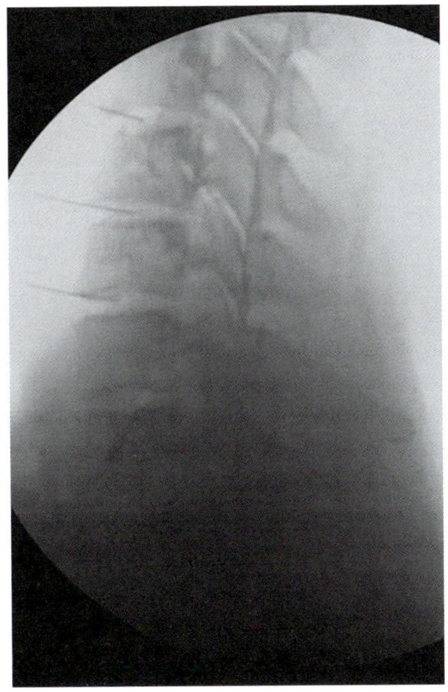

• **Fig 12.44** Lateral view of intradiscal placement.

- Only in the lateral view, further needle advancement is done to prevent the needle from violating the spinal canal and cord.
- In this view, the needle should not be advanced beyond the midpoint of the disc (Fig. 12.44).
- Since the nucleus is anterior to the midline compared to the lumbar spine, the needle will be in the nucleus.
- Option to use dye confirmation to ensure the needle is within the nucleus pulposus and for diagnostic discography.
  - The injectionist may choose to avoid dye also as the volume of the nucleus is usually 0.5 mL or less and want to use that volume for the orthobiologic. Contrast dye has been observed to have a dose-dependent effect on MSC in regard to cytotoxicity.
- Injection should be done slowly with as minimal pressure as possible to prevent disc rupture. After injection, remove the needle slowly.

PEARLS AND PITFALLS

- Discitis: Although rare, discitis is a devastating complication. Unfortunately, it is also a very painful condition.
  - If not recognized early, it can spread to the vertebral bodies resulting in their collapse and possible serious neurological sequelae.
  - Increasing pain 1 to 2 weeks after the procedure should alert the suspicion of discitis.
  - MRI with contrast is the best diagnostic tool to detect discitis.
  - Usually, the erythrocyte sedimentation rate (ESR) and C-reactive protein [CRP] are elevated. The WBC count may or may not be elevated.
  - Fever is not a consistent finding.
  - If the diagnosis of discitis is made, the patient should be admitted, and an infectious disease consult should be obtained. Neurosurgical consultation is also recommended, especially if any neural deficits are noted.

PEARLS AND PITFALLS—CONT'D

- Discitis requires aggressive intravenous antibiotics. It is imperative to get blood cultures and disc cultures prior to the initiation of antibiotics. In most cases, the cultures are negative. However, if they are positive, it will help in selecting the right antibiotics.
- Needle transgression through the esophagus on its way into the disc increases the chances of discitis.
- Penetration of the great vessels:
  - The location of the vertebral artery is highly variable. If the needle is anterior to the uncinate process in the oblique view, the risk of encountering the vertebral artery is low.
- Violating the spinal canal:
  - As soon as the needle is in the annulus, it is mandatory to check the lateral view before advancing the needle further. The needle should be advanced very cautiously in the lateral view. The final needle position should never be beyond the middle of the disc in the lateral view.
- Avoiding the Spinal Nerve:
  - Avoid the spinal nerve by staying anterior to the neural foramen.
- Risk of Pneumothorax:
  - This complication is possible at the C7-T1 level.

Clinical Studies

Stellate Ganglion Block

KEY POINTS

- Stellate ganglion block (SGB) is one of the oldest and a very common sympathetic block that is applied today.
- SGB can be done, under fluoroscopy or with ultrasound.
- The authors feel that ultrasound guidance is preferred for the following reasons:
  - SG lies in the fascial plane between the carotid artery and longus colli muscle which can be easily appreciated with ultrasound. This increases the accuracy of the block.
  - Moreover, only bony landmarks are seen under fluoroscopy, and they are only surrogate markers for the SG.
  - The location of the carotid artery, vertebral artery, and the recurrent laryngeal nerve can be assessed under ultrasound, making it a safer procedure.
- If available, confirm with fluoroscopy and contrast after ultrasound-guided procedure.

Pertinent Anatomy

- The cervical sympathetic chain is composed of superior, middle, and inferior cervical ganglia.
- In about 80 % of the cases, the inferior cervical ganglion is fused with the first thoracic ganglion, forming the cervicothoracic ganglion, also known as the stellate ganglion [SG].
- If the inferior cervical ganglion and the first thoracic ganglion are not fused, the inferior cervical ganglion lies in front of the C7 transverse process, and the first thoracic ganglion lies in front of the neck of the first rib.
- The stellate ganglion measures approximately 2.5 cm in length, 1 cm in width, and 0.5 cm in thickness (see Fig. 12.20A).[60]

Common Pathology

- There is increasing evidence for SB effectiveness in
  - CRPS types 1 and 2
  - postherpetic neuralgia (PHN)
  - intractable angina
  - hyperhidrosis
  - trigeminal neuralgia
  - arrhythmias.[61]
  - post-traumatic stress disorder (PTSD)

Equipment

- Linear transducer ultrasound and/or C-arm fluoroscopy
- 25 gauge 2.0 to 3.5 inch spinal needle
- Contrast agent (omnipaque or isovue) if using fluoroscopy

Common Injectates

- Local anesthetics

Injectate Volume

- 2 to 5 mL if using ultrasound, 10 mL if using fluoroscopy

Ultrasound Technique

Patient Position

- The patient is in a supine position.
- The head is turned away from the side of the procedure.

Clinician Position

- Ipsilateral side of the patient

Transducer Position

- The transducer is placed at the base of the neck in the midline around the C6-7 level.
- After the trachea and thyroid are visualized, it is then moved laterally until the carotid artery is seen.
- Posterolateral to the carotid artery, the longus colli muscle should be identified (Fig. 12.45).
- Identification of the carotid artery and longus colli muscle is key to the performance of this block.
- The SG lies in the plane between these two structures.

Needle Position

- Using an "in-plane" approach, the needle is advanced from the lateral side towards the medial structures.

Target

- The needle should be targeted posterolateral to the carotid artery and anterior to the longus colli muscle.
- Do not inject if the needle if the needle tip is not visualized. This is mandatory as there is a risk of injecting into the carotid resulting in seizures, immediate loss of consciousness, and respiratory arrest.
- Separation of the carotid artery from the longus colli by the local anesthetic should be seen.
- 2 to 10 cc of local anesthetic is injected.

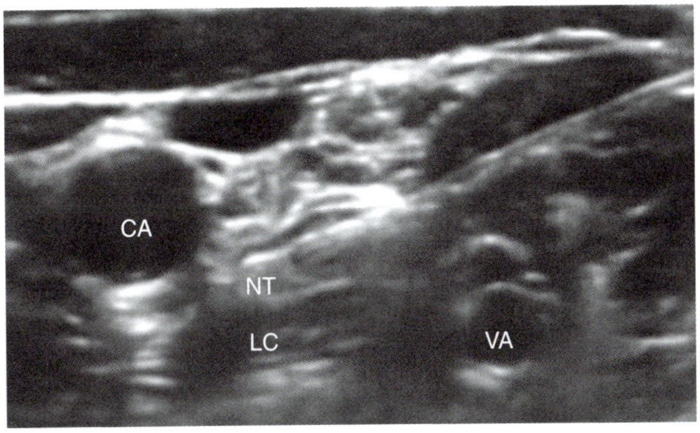

• **Fig 12.45** Needle seen in between the carotid artery and the longus colli muscle. *CA,* Carotid artery; *LC,* longus colli; *NT,* needle tip; *VA,* vertebral artery.

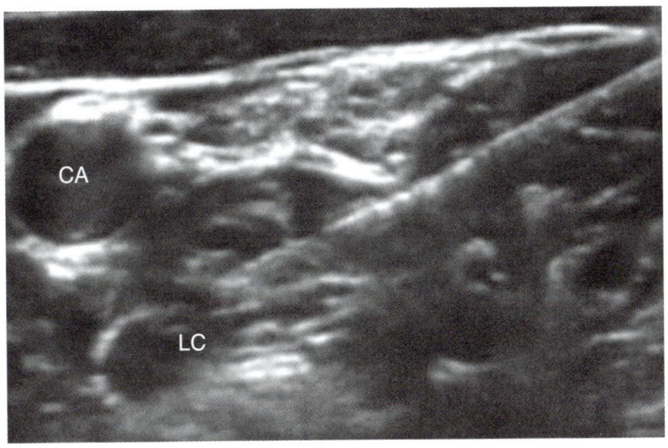

• **Fig 12.46** Separation of carotid artery from longus colli with local anesthetic. Needle is away from the carotid artery. *CA,* Carotid artery; *LC,* longus colli.

- The presence of Horner's syndrome [ptosis, myosis, and redness of the ipsilateral eye] within 5 minutes and increased temperature of the arm within 10 minutes indicates a successful block.

PEARLS AND PITFALLS

- The most dreaded complication is seizures, loss of consciousness and respiratory arrest from injecting the local anesthetic into the carotid or vertebral artery.
- The airway should be supported, and if needed the patient should be intubated.
- If seizures do not abate, intravenous valium or sodium pentothal should be administered.
- If arrhythmias are noted, ACLS protocol should be followed.
- If this procedure is done in an office setting, 911 should be called immediately.
- The risk of injecting the vertebral artery is extremely low with the technique described above, as it is further away from the injection site (see Fig. 12.45).
- Since the vagus nerve lies in the carotid sheath, care must be taken to avoid injecting the carotid sheath.
- The recurrent laryngeal nerve can be blocked and will lead to temporary hoarseness.
- Injecting the spinal canal and the spinal nerves is rare with this procedure if done as described above.

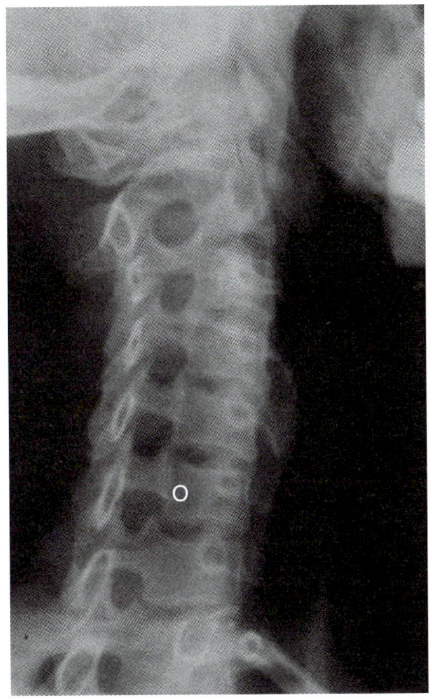

• **Fig 12.47** Right oblique view of the cervical spine showing the site for stellate ganglion block. This is marked by "O", which is the junction of the uncinate process and the vertebral body (C6 or C7).

Fluoroscopic Technique

Patient Position

- Place the patient in a supine position with the new slightly extended (roll under the neck and shoulders), and the head rotated slightly to the contralateral side to be blocked.[62]

Clinician Position

- The opposite side of the base of the C-arm

Transducer Position or C-Arm Position Fluoroscopy Technique

- In the AP view, caudocranial angulation of the C-arm is done to maximize the disc space of the C5-6 disc.
- Subsequently, the fluoroscope is rotated obliquely, ipsilateral to the side where the blockade is desired.
- Rotate until the C5-6 neural foramen is maximized.

Needle Position

- Start the needle at the junction of the uncinate process and the vertebral body.
- Palpate for the carotid artery, which should be medial to the entry point using this technique.
- Under real-time fluoroscopy, a single pass is made with a spinal needle to contact the bone.

Target

- The needle tip should be contacting and resting at the junction between the uncinate process and the vertebral body (Fig. 12.47).
- Withdraw the needle 2 to 3 mm
- Inject a small amount of contrast material, ideally using digital subtraction angiography, to confirm no intravascular uptake and dye spread along the longus colli muscle (Fig. 12.48A and B).
- Inject local anesthetic after negative aspiration of blood.

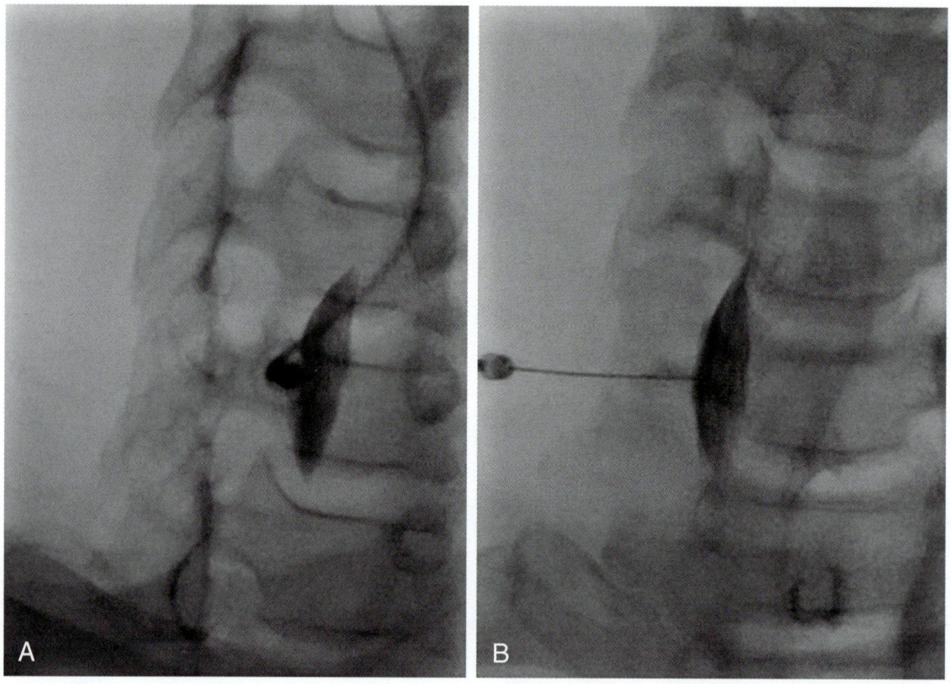

• **Fig 12.48** (A) Right oblique view showing the spread of the contrast material. (B) AP view showing the contrast spread from C5 to C7 (Courtesy Vivek Manocha.)

PEARLS AND PITFALLS

- Avoid directing the needle toward the neural foramina, thecal sac, and vertebral artery present posteriorly, the disc superiorly, and the esophagus, medially.

References

1. Anderson JS, Hsu AW, Vasavada AN. Morphology, architecture, and biomechanics of human cervical multifidus. *Spine (Phila Pa 1976)*. 2005;30(4):E86–E91.
2. Yeocheon Yun MD, Eun Jeong Lee MD, Yong Kim MD, et al. Asymmetric atrophy of cervical multifidus muscles in patients with chronic unilateral cervical radiculopathy. *Medicine (Baltim)*. 2019;98(32):e16041.
3. Cloney M, Smith AC, Coffey T, Paliwal M, Dhaher Y, Parrish T, Elliott J, Smith ZA. Fatty infiltration of the cervical multifidus musculature and their clinical correlates in spondylotic myelopathy. *J Clin Neurosci*. 2018;57:208–213.
4. Elliott JM, Pedler AR, Jull GA. Differential changes in muscle composition exist in traumatic and nontraumatic neck pain. *Spine (Phila Pa 1976)*. 2014;39(1):39–47.
5. Uthaikhup S, Assapun J, Kothan S, Watcharasaksilp K, Elliott JM. Structural changes of the cervical muscles in elder women with cervicogenic headache. *Musculoskelet Sci Pract*. 2017;29:1–6.
6. Hack GD, Hallgren RC. Chronic headache relief after section of suboccipital muscle dural connections: a case report. *Headache*. 2004;44:84–89.
7. Oxland TR. Fundamental biomechanics of the spine--What we have learned in the past 25 years and future directions. *J Biomech*. 2016;49(6):817–832.
8. Panjabi MM, White 3rd AA. Basic biomechanics of the spine. *Neurosurgery*. 1980;7(1):76–93.
9. Centeno C, Elliot J, Elkins WL, Freeman M. *Pain Physician*. 2005;81:67–72.
10. Panjabi MM, Pearson AM, Ito S, et al. Cervical spine ligament injury during simulated frontal impact. *Spine (Phila Pa 1976)*. 2004;29(21):2395–2403.
11. Benedetti PF, Fahr LM, Kuhns LR, Anne Hayman L. MR imaging findings in spinal ligamentous injury. *AJR Am J Roentgenol*. 2000;175.
12. Choi I, Jeon SR. Neuralgias of the head: occipital neuralgia. *J Korean Med Sci*. 2016;31(4):479–488.
13. Kim H-S, Shin K-J, Jehoon O, Kwon H-J, Lee M, Yang H-M. Stereotactic topography of the greater and third occipital nerves and its clinical implication. *Sci Rep*. 2018;8:870.
14. Platzgummer H, Moritz T, Gruber GM, Pivec C, Wöber C, Bodner G, Lieba-Samal D. The lesser occipital nerve visualized by high-resolution sonography—normal and initial suspect findings. *Cephalalgia*. 2015:35(9):816–24.
15. Yin W, Bogduk N. The nature of neck pain in a private pain clinic in the United States. *Pain Med*. 2008;92:196–203.
16. Dwyer A, Aprill C, Bogduk N. Cervical zygapophyseal joint pain patterns. [A study in normal volunteers]. *Spine (Phila Pa 1976)*. 1990;156:453–457.
17. Winnie AP. Interscalene brachial plexus block. *Anesth Analg*. 1970;49:455–466.
18. Kapral S, Greher M, Huber G, et al. Ultrasonograhic guidance improves the success rate of interscalene brachial plexus blockade. *Reg Anesth Pain Med*. 2008;33:253–258.
19. Bonica JJ (ed). Postoperative pain. *The Management of Pain*. 2nd ed. Philadelphia.
20. Ross S, Scarborough CD. Toltal spinal anesthesia following brachial plexus block. *Anesthesiology*. 1973;39:458.
21. Urmey WF, Talts KH, Shrarock NE. One hundred percent incidence of hemi-diaphragmatic paresis associated with interscelene brachial plexus anesthesia as diagnosed by ultrasonography. *Anesth Analg*. 1991;72:498–503.

22. Kapral S, Krafft P, Eibenberger K, et al. Ultrasound-guided supraclavicular approach for regional anesthesia of the brachial plexus. *Anesth Analg*. 1994;78:507–513.
23. William SR, Chouinard P, Arcand G, et al. Ultrasound guidance speeds execution and improves the quality of supraclavicular block. *Anesth Analg*. 2003;97:1518–1523.
24. Chan VW, Perlas A, Rawson R, Odukoya O. Ultrasound-guided supraclavicular brachial plexus block. Anesth Analg 203; 97:1514–1517.
25. Liu SS, Gordon MA, Shaw PM, et al. A prospective clinical registry of ultrasound-guided regional anesthesia for ambulatory shoulder surgery. *Anesth Analg*. 2010;111:617–623.
26. Guirguis M, Karroum R, Abd-Elsayed AA, Mounir-Soliman L. Acute respiratory distress following ultrasound-guided supraclavicular block. *Ochsner J*. 2012:159–162.
27. Aunac S, Cariter M, Singelyn F. The analgesic efficacy of bilateral combined superficial and deep cervical plexus block administered before thyroid surgery under general anesthesia. *Anesth Analg*. 2002;95:746–750.
28. Flaherty J, Horn JL, Derby R. Regional anesthesia for vascular surgery. *Anesthesiol Clin*. 2014;32:639–659.
29. Tran DQ, Dugani S, Finlayson RJ. A randomized comparison between ultrasound-guided and landmark based superficial cervical plexus block. *Reg Anesth Pain Med*. 2010;35:539–543.
30. Dhonneur G, Saidi NE, Merie JC, et al. Demonstration of the spread of the injectate with deep cervical plexus block: a case series. *Reg Anesth Pain Med*. 2007;32:16–119.
31. Sandeman DJ, Griffiths MJ, Lennox AF. Ultrasound guided deep cervical plexus block. *Anaesth Intensive Care*. 2006;34:240–244.
32. Verrills P, Nowesenitz G, Barnard A. Penetration of a cervical radicular artery during a transforaminal epidural injection. *Pain Med*. 2010;11(2):229–231. https://doi.org/10.1111/j.1526-4637.2009.00776.x.
33. Radhakrishnan K, Litchy WJ, O'Fallon WM, Kurland LT. Epidemiology of cervical radiculopathy: a population-based study of Rochester, Minnesota, 1976 through 1990. *Brain*. 1994;117:325–335.
34. Saal JS, Saal JA, Yurth EF. Nonoperative management of herniated cervical intervertebral disc with radiculopathy. *Spine (Phila Pa 1976)*. 1996;21:1877–1883.
35. Martin GM, Cobrin KB. An evaluation of conservative treatment for patients with cervical disk syndrome. *Arch Phys Med Rehabil*. 1954;35:87–92.
36. Bogduk N. *Medical Management of Acute Cervical Radicular Pain: An Evidence-Based Approach*. Newcastle, Australia: Newcastle Bone and Joint Institute; 1999.
37. Ali D, El Khousmi M, Gorur Y, Benoit C, Noel Lorenzo Villalba. Rare case of ischemic stroke following cervical transforiminal injection. *Eur J Case Rep Intern Med*. 2019;6(3):001082.
38. Ziai WC, Ardelta AA, Llinas RH. Brainstem stroke following uncomplicated cervical epidural steroid injection. *Arch Neurol*. 2006;63(11):1643–1646.
39. Bogduk N. In: *Clinical Anatomy of the Lumbar Spine and Sacrum*. 3rd ed. New York: Churchill Livingstone; 1997.
40. Hogan QH. Epidural anatomy examined by cryomicrotome section: influence of age, vertebral level and disease. *Reg Anesth*. 1996;21:295–306.
41. Fenton DS, Czervionke LF. *Image-guided Spine Intervention*. Saunders; 2003:101.
42. Parkin IG, Harrison GR. The Topographical anatomy of the lumbar spine. *J Anat*. 1985;141:211–217.
43. Nickalls RW, Kokri MS. The width of the posterior epidural space in obstetric patients. *Anaesthesia*. 1986;41(4):432–433.
44. Clark C, Goel V, Galles K. Kinematics of the occipito-atlanto-axial complex. *Transaction*. 1986. Cervical Spine Research Society; 1986.
45. Jagetia A, Mewda T, Bishnoi I, et al. Understanding the course of vertebral artery at craniovertebral junction in occipital assimilation of atlas: made simplified using conventional angiography. *J Neurol Surg B Skull Base*. 2017;78(2):173–178.
46. Dreyfuss P, Michaelsen M, Fletcher D. Atlanto-occipital and lateral atlanto-axial joint pain patterns. *Spine (Phila Pa 1976)*. 1994;19:1125–1131.
47. Centeno C, Williams C, Markle J, Dodson E. A new atlanto-occipital (C0-C1) joint injection technique. *Pain Med*. 2018;19:1499–1500.
48. Lord SM, McDonald GJ, Bogduk N. Percutaneous radiofrequency neurotomy of the cervical medial branches; a validated treatment for cervical zygapophyseal joint pain. *Neurosurg Q*. 1998;8:288–308.
49. Dwyer A, Aprill C, Bogduk N. Cervical zygapophysial joint patterns I: a study in normal volunteers. *Spine (Phila Pa 1976)*. 1990;6:453–457.
50. Okada K. Studies on the cervical facet joints using arthrography of the cervical facet joint. *J Jpn Orthop Assoc*. 1981;55(6):563–580.
51. Manchikanti L, Singh V. *Interventional Techniques in Chronic Spinal Pain*. Paducah, KY: ASIPP publishing; 2007.
52. Bogduk N. Cervical radiofrequency neurotomy. *Practice Guidelines for Spinal Diagnostic and Treatment Procedures*. ISIS; 2004: 249–284.
53. Smith GW, Nichols Jr P. Technique for cervical discography. *Radiology*. 1957;68:718–720.
54. Manchikanti L, Dunbar EE, Wargo BW, et al. Systematic review of cervical discography as a diagnostic test for chronic spinal pain. *Pain Physician*. 2009;12(2):305–321.
55. Pettine KA, Suzuki RK, Sand TT. Murphy MBAutologous bone marrow concentrate intradiscal injection for the treatment of degenerative disc disease with three-year follow-up. *Int Orthop*. 2017;41(10):2097–2103.
56. Tuakli-Wosornu YA, Terry A, Boachie-Adjei K, et al. Lumbar intradiskal Platelet-Rich Plasma (PRP) injections: a prospective, double-blind, randomized controlled study. *Pharm Manag PM R*. 2016;8(1):1–10.
57. Singh V. The role of cervical discography in interventional pain management. *Pain Physician*. 2004;7:249–255.
58. Saternus KS, Bornscheuer HH. Comparative radiologic and pathologic-anatomic studies on the value of discography in the diagnosis of acute intravertebral disc injuries in the cervical spine. *ROFO Fortschr Geb Roentgenstr Neuen Bildgeb Verfahr*. 1983;139:651–657.
59. Yin W, Bogduk N. The nature of neck pain in a private pain clinic in the United States. *Pain Med*. 2008;9(2):196–203.
60. Narouze S, et al. Ultrasound-guided stellate ganglion block: safety and efficacy. *Curr Pain Headache Rep*. 2014.
61. Gunduz OH, Kenis-Coskun O. Ganglion blocks as a treatment of pain: current perspectives. *J Pain Res*. 2017;10:2815–2826.
62. Abdi S, Zhou Y, Patel N, Saini B, Nelson J. A new and easy technique to block the stellate ganglion. *Pain Physician*. 2004;7(3):327–331.

13

Thoracic Injection Techniques

MARKO BODOR, STEPHEN DERRINGTON, JOHN PITTS, JASON MARKLE, AND ORLANDO LANDRUM

KEY POINTS

- The thoracic spine is a common source of mid-back pain and is frequently overlooked despite it having the greatest number of levels and the greatest diversity between vertebral levels.
- For injections, it is important to confirm the correct level. Identify the appropriate level by starting at either the first or twelfth rib and counting from there.

Pertinent Anatomy[1–6]

- The thoracic spine contains 12 levels, compared to 7 in the cervical and 5 in the lumbar spine.
- See Figs. 13.1–13.3.
- The T2-T9 thoracic vertebrae have costovertebral and costotransverse articulations of the rib with the vertebral body and the rib with the transverse process. The wedge shape of these vertebrae results in the kyphotic curve of the thoracic spine.
- The other vertebrae of the thoracic spine are similar to either the cervical vertebrae (T1) or lumbar spine (T10-T12).
- Typical ligamentous anatomy includes anterior longitudinal ligament (ALL), posterior longitudinal ligament (PLL), ligamentum flavum, interspinous ligament, supraspinous ligament (SSL), and intertransverse ligaments.
- Qualities unique to the thoracic spine include:
  - Radial and intraarticular ligaments (costovertebral articulation—connection of the head of the rib with the vertebral body)
  - Superior and lateral costotransverse ligaments (costotransverse articulation—connection of the neck/tubercle with the vertebral body)
  - Thoracic facet joints have a different orientation than cervical or lumbar facets, approximately 60 degrees superiorly and 20 degrees anteriorly.
- The thoracic spine has a major impact on alignment of the entire spine. These changes in alignment can have both clinical and subclinical effects on a person's biomechanical health.
- Three important measurements affecting biomechanics and pain are:
  - Coronal balance
  - Sagittal vertical axis
  - Pelvic incidence.
- The artery of Adamkiewicz may originate from a segmental artery between T7 and L4, typically on the left side.
- Concerns with thoracic injections include adjacent vascular structures (bleeding from non-compressible arteries and/or veins), lung puncture (resulting in pneumothorax), cardiac (direct cardiac injury or secondary tamponade), sympathetic chain side effects (hypotension) spinal cord or intrathecal injection (see Fig. 13.3).

Ultrasound Guided

Supraspinous and Interspinous Ligaments

KEY POINTS

These ligaments can be targeted in isolation for specific injuries but are more commonly treated in combination with other components of the functional spinal unit,[7,8] including the spinal nerves in the epidural space, facet joints, paraspinal muscles, and occasionally the intervertebral discs.

Pertinent Anatomy

The interspinous ligament (ISL) is a thin membranous ligament that connects adjacent spinous processes. The ligament spans from the root to the apex of each spinous process, anteriorly to the ligamentum flavum and posteriorly to the nuchal ligament.

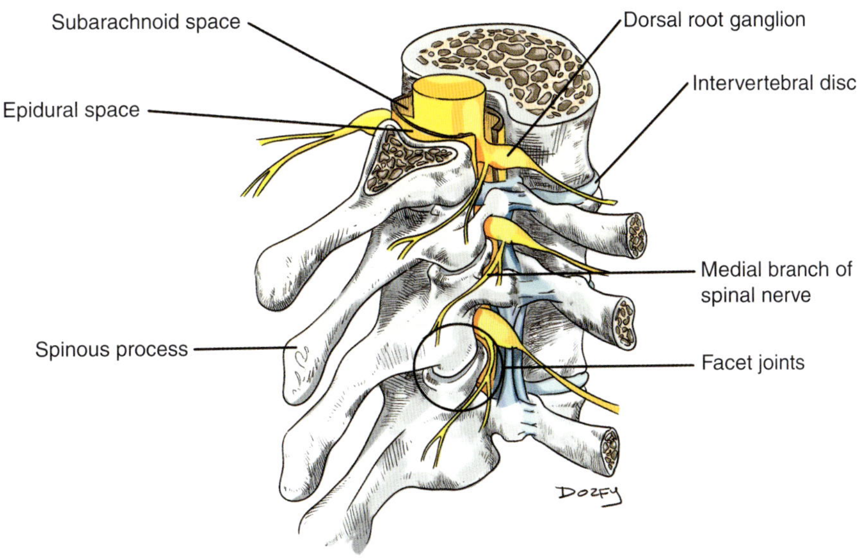

• **Fig. 13.1** Thoracic Spine Anatomy. Note the relationship of the medial branch nerve as it innervates the joint.

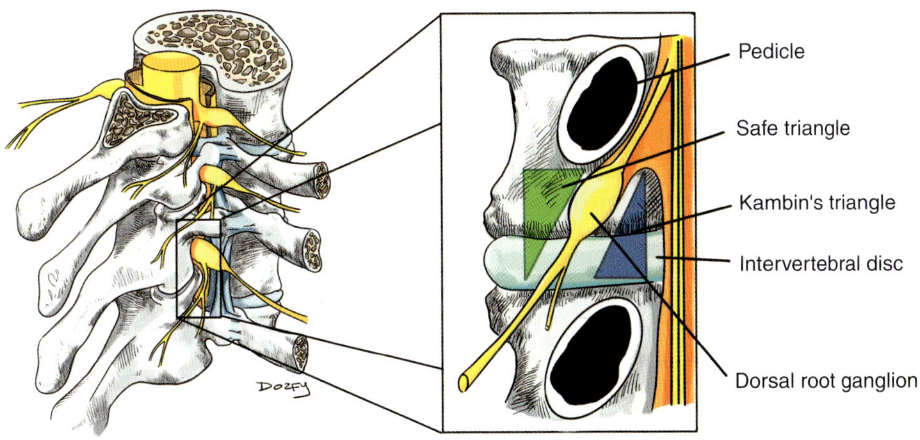

• **Fig. 13.2** Thoracic Spine Anatomy of the Neural Foramen.

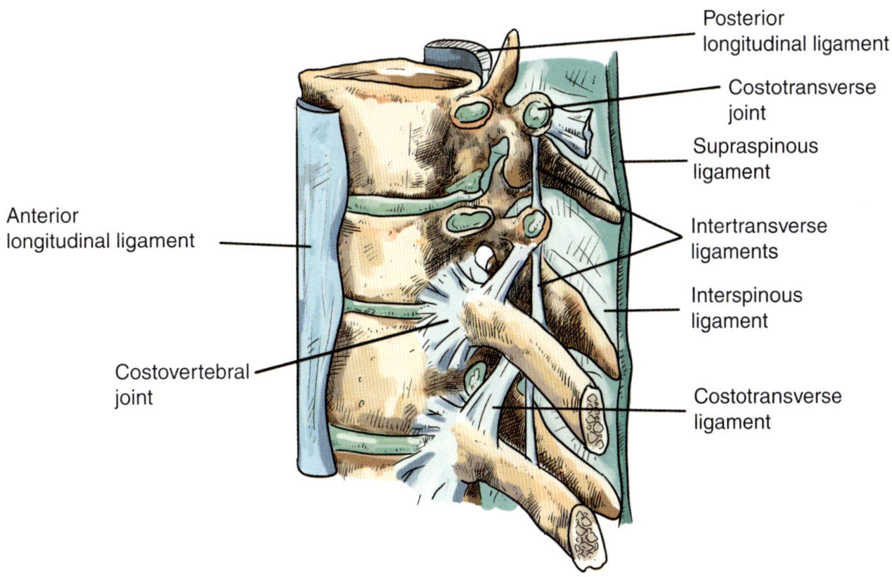

• **Fig. 13.3** Thoracic Spine Ligamentous Anatomy.

The supraspinous ligament (SSL) is a thin membranous ligament and lies superficial to the spinous processes of the thoracic spine overlying the interspinous ligament.

Common Pathology

Ligament strain, partial tear,[9] relative laxity related to disc, and facet pathology.[10]

Equipment

Ultrasound machine with high-frequency linear transducer.

Technique

Patient Position

Prone

Clinician Position

At the side of the patient, with the ultrasound monitor next to or on their opposite side.

Transducer Position

Long axis to the ISL and SSL with visualization of ligaments and spinous processes (Fig. 13.4).

Needle Position

In plane (author preference) or out of plane

Target

Direct injection into the ligaments at the desired spinal level, injecting into areas of hypoechogenicity and throughout the ligament, including the bony attachments. Filling of interstitial injuries can be seen with injectate.

- In plane:
  - With ligaments in long axis, introduce the needle in plane to the transducer with or without a gel stand-off to minimize anisotropy. Needle tip should be advanced to the spinous process to inject at the SSL, then walked and advanced into the interspinous space for the ISL.

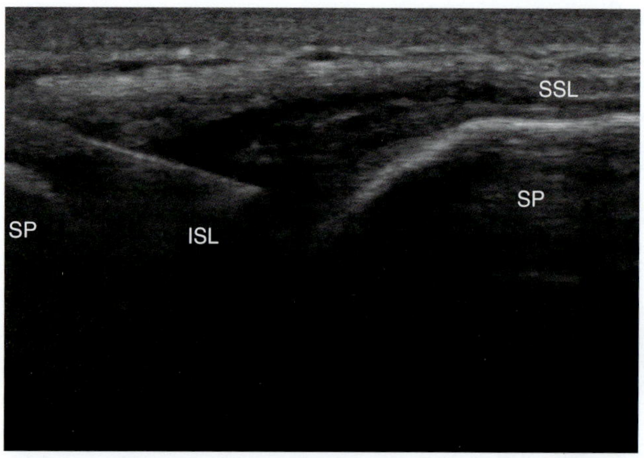

• **Fig. 13.4** Supraspinous and Interspinous Ligaments. Longitudinal view of supraspinous ligament *(SSL)* and interspinous ligament *(ISL)* with adjacent spinous processes *(SP)*. Needle visualized in plane, passing through the SSL into the ISL. Needle will be repositioned to cover the entire ISL and SSL of the target spinal segment.

Injectate Volume

0.25 to 1 mL at each spinal level

Prolotherapy, orthobiologics

Needle: 25- to 27-gauge 1.5- to 2-inch needle

> **PEARLS AND PITFALLS**
>
> - These ligaments are difficult to visualize entirely, so adjacent and adjoining anatomy needs to be visualized.

Thoracic Facet Joints

> **KEY POINTS**
>
> Whereas the fluoroscopic approach to the lumbar facet joints is typically at 0 to 45 degree rotation, the thoracic facet joint is oriented at 90 to 110 degrees, which needs to be taken into consideration when assessing the joints with ultrasound.

Pertinent Anatomy

Facet joint

Common Pathology

Osteoarthritis, rotational scoliosis

Equipment

Ultrasound machine with low-frequency linear or a curvilinear transducer, which provides better visualization of deeper structures and a wider field of view.

Technique

Patient Position

Prone

Clinician Position

Clinician preference for optimal needle guidance and ultrasound transducer control, typically at the patient's side with ultrasound monitor next to or on their opposite side.

Transducer Position

Midline along the long-axis, initially flat on the skin, but then angled 10 to 20 degrees medially to be perpendicular to the articular processes, which slope down from the midline to laterally.

Needle Position

Caudad-cephalad needle direction, in-plane visualization (Fig. 13.5).

Target

Facet joint opening

Injectate Volume

0.25 to 1 mL

Dextrose prolotherapy, orthobiologics

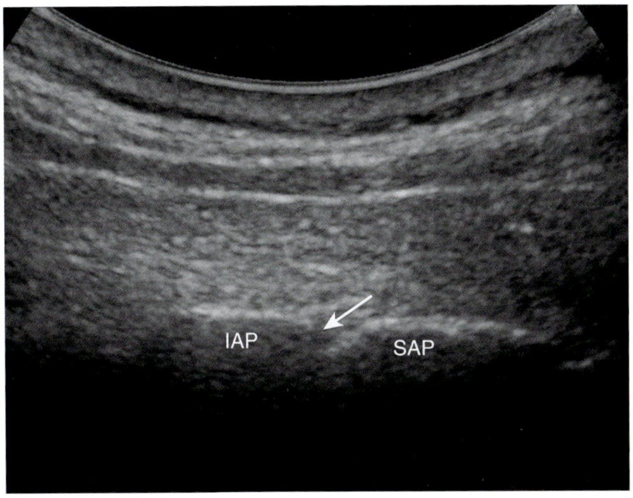

• **Fig. 13.5** Thoracic Facet. Inferior articular process *(IAP)* from cephalad vertebra and superior articular process *(SAP)* from caudal vertebra. *Arrow* demonstrates needle trajectory into joint.

PEARLS AND PITFALLS

Advanced ultrasound skills are required. Keep the needle and target in view at all times. Missing the target and going too deep laterally risks penetration into the lung, while going too medially risks penetrating the thecal sac. An echogenic or large-caliber can be helpful to optimize visualization, which can otherwise be difficult because of multiple overlying fascial planes.

Thoracic Costotransverse Joints

KEY POINTS

Important structure to consider in patients with chest and abdominal pain, difficulty breathing, or paresthesia in this area.

Pertinent Anatomy

Rib head, transverse process (TP) of thoracic vertebra

Common Pathology

Damaged or stretched ligaments from trauma[11,12] or hypermobility syndromes, osteoarthritis

Equipment

Ultrasound machine with high-frequency linear transducer

Technique

Patient Position

Prone

Clinician Position

At the side of the patient, with the ultrasound monitor next to or on the opposite side

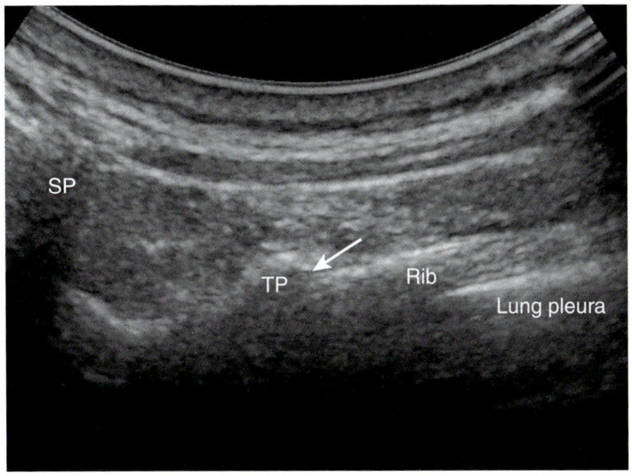

• **Fig 13.6** Thoracic Costal Facet. Target is articulation of the rib to the transverse process *(TP)*. Lung pleura can be seen deep to the rib if the rib is not parallel to the cartilage throughout the length of the transducer. *Arrow* demonstrates needle trajectory into joint. *SP,* Spinous process.

Transducer Position

Transverse, with ultrasound transducer overlying the head of the rib and transverse process (Fig. 13.6).

Needle Position

In-plane needle visualization, lateral to medial approach

Target

Posterior costal facet, costotransverse ligaments

Injectate Volume

0.25 to 0.75 mL

Dextrose prolotherapy, orthobiologics

PEARLS AND PITFALLS

Keep the needle and target in view at all times. Missing the target risks going into the pleura or thecal sac.

Costochondral Joints

KEY POINTS

Important structure to consider in patients with chest pain, abdominal pain, difficulty breathing, or paresthesia in this area. It is important to visualize the sternum, adjacent costal cartilage (typically hypoechoic), and rib (hyperechoic with typical bony acoustic shadowing).

Identify rib, costal cartilage, articulation at desired level, and lung pleura.

Pertinent Anatomy

Sternum, rib cartilage, lung pleura

Common Pathology

Damaged or stretched ligaments from trauma[11,12] or hypermobility syndromes, osteoarthritis

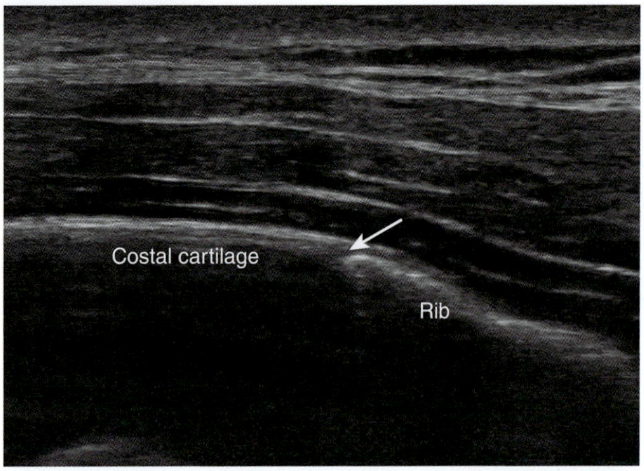

• **Fig. 13.7** Costochondral Joint. The articulation of costal cartilage and rib can be visualized. *Arrow* demonstrates needle trajectory into joint from lateral to medial.

Equipment

Ultrasound machine with high-frequency linear transducer

Technique

Patient Position
Supine

Clinician Position
At the side of the patient, with the ultrasound monitor next to or on the opposite side

Transducer Position
In plane, with costochondral joint (Fig. 13.7).

Needle Position
In plane: lateral to medial approach

Target
Costochondral joint

Injectate Volume

0.5 to 1.0 mL
Prolotherapy, orthobiologics

PEARLS AND PITFALLS

Keep the needle and target in view at all times. If the needle deviates away from view, it can easily bypass the target, go into the pleura, and cause a pneumothorax.

Sternocostal Joints

KEY POINTS

Important structure to consider in patients with chest pain, abdominal pain, difficulty breathing, or paresthesia in this area. It is important to visualize the sternum, adjacent costal cartilage (typically hypoechoic), and rib (hyperechoic with typical bony acoustic shadowing).

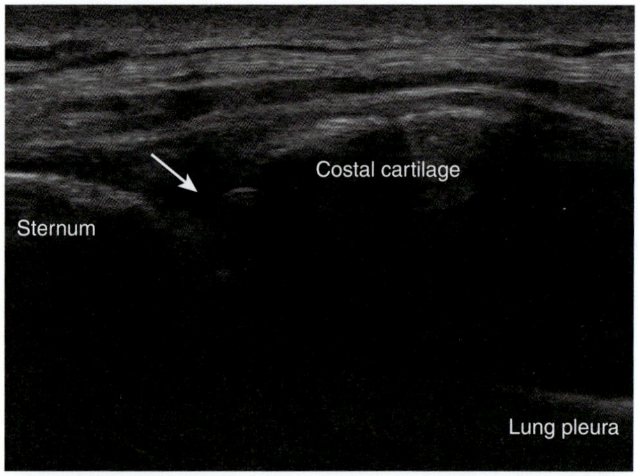

• **Fig. 13.8** Sternocostal Joint. Lung pleura can be visualized deep to the costal cartilage if the transducer is not parallel to the cartilage throughout the length of the transducer. *Arrow* demonstrates needle trajectory into joint.

Pertinent Anatomy

Sternum, costal cartilage, sternocostal joint, pleura of the lung.

Common Pathology

Damaged or stretched ligaments from trauma[11,12] or hypermobility syndromes, osteoarthritis

Equipment

Ultrasound machine with high-frequency linear transducer

Technique

Patient Position
Supine

Clinician Position
At the side of the patient, with the ultrasound monitor next to or on the opposite side

Transducer Position
Axial to the patient, in line with the sternocostal joint (Fig. 13.8).

Needle Position
Medial to lateral or vice-a-versa depending on the side

Target
Sternocostal joint

Injectate Volume

0.5 to 1 mL
Dextrose prolotherapy, orthobiologics

PEARLS AND PITFALLS

Keep the tip of the needle in view at all times to avoid going too deep and causing pneumothorax. Avoid vascular structures and aspirate prior to injection to avoid intravascular injection.

Sternoclavicular Joints

KEY POINTS

Clarify anatomy of sternum and clavicle; use real-time ultrasound visualization to maintain safe depth.

Pertinent Anatomy

Clavicle, sternum, sternoclavicular (SC) joint

Common Pathology

Damaged or stretched ligaments from trauma, osteoarthritis, capsular strain

Equipment

Ultrasound machine with high-frequency linear transducer.

Technique

Patient Position

Supine

Clinician Position

For in-plane needle visualization, at the side of the patient with the ultrasound monitor next to or on the opposite side of the patient.

For out-of-plane visualization, at the patient's side and ipsilateral to the joint being treated, with the ultrasound screen at or near the patient's head.

Transducer Position

Overlying the clavicle and sternum, spanning the SC joint

Needle Position

Author's preference: in-plane needle visualization. Slide the ultrasound transducer so that the SC joint lies close to its edge, reducing the distance from needle to target (Fig. 13.9).

Alternative: out of plane. Ensure the transducer is centered and perpendicular to the joint; use the scale on the monitor to determine target depth, then insert needle, erring on the side of being shallow at first.

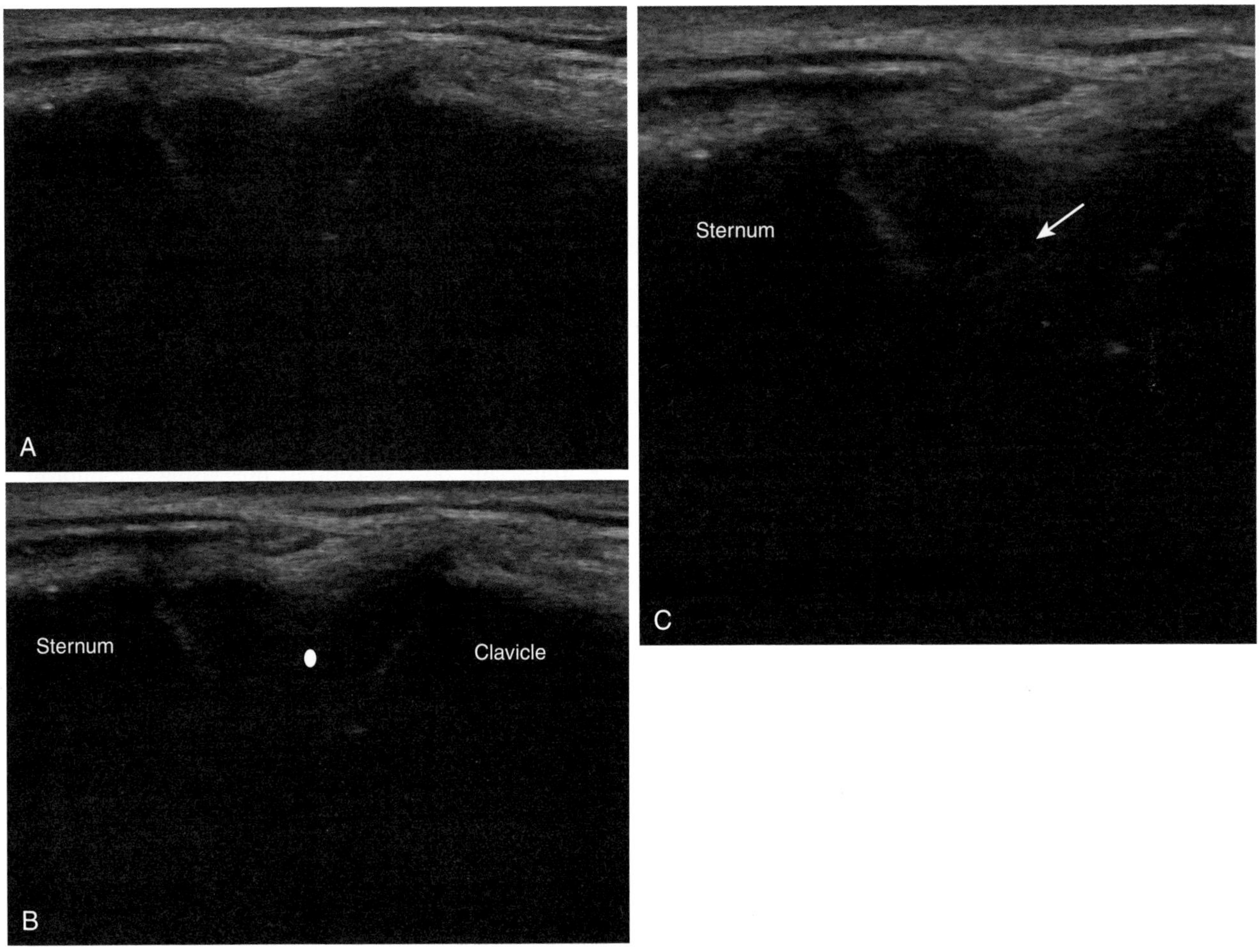

• **Fig. 13.9** (A to C) Sternoclavicular (SC) joint. Transducer parallel to the clavicle and spanning the SC joint. Out of plane: needle insertion midline to the transducer. *White* dot demonstrates target location. In plane: needle insertion lateral to medial (arrow), with joint offset near edge of transducer to reduce the distance the needle will travel to get to the target.

Target

Sternoclavicular joint

Injectate Volume

0.5 to 1 mL

Prolotherapy, orthobiologics

PEARLS AND PITFALLS

Use three fingers to hold the transducer and the remaining two to stabilize the transducer on the joint. Keep the needle in view at all times for an in-plane approach, and err on the side of going shallow for an out-of-plane approach. Missing the joint risks penetration into the pleura or great vessels.

Fluoroscopy Guided

Thoracic epidurals

KEY POINTS

- To appropriately identify level, "square off" endplates to adjust for parallax error.
- Epidural approach is similar to intradiscal approach.

Pertinent Anatomy

- Kambin's
- spinal nerve
- rib head
- vertebral body (Fig. 13.2).
- intervertebral disc

Common Pathology

- Radiculitis
- Disc herniation
- Endplate modic changes
- Intervertebral narrowing

Equipment

- C-arm fluoroscopy
- 25- to 22-gauge 3- to 3.5-inch spinal needle for transforaminals
- 20- to 21-gauge 3.5-inch Tuoy needle for interlaminar

Common Injectates

- Local anesthetics
- Corticosteroids
- Orthobiologics (platelet lysate, dextrose neuroprolotherapy)

Injectate Volume

- 1 to 5 mL

Technique for Transforaminal Infraneural Approach

Patient Position

- Prone

Clinician Position

- To the side of the patient contralateral to fluoroscopy unit base

C-Arm Position Fluoroscopy

- Angulate the C-arm to "square off" the level to be injected.
- Rotate 25 to 45 degrees to optimize foraminal view between superior articular process (SAP) of the lower vertebral bone and rib. Keep the lung field line lateral to the vertebral body.
- Use lateral view to check depth as needle nears target.
- Use anteroposterior (AP) view to check needle position and confirm epidural contrast flow.

Needle Position

- Aim for the posterior lateral disc space passing between the rib head laterally and the SAP medially (Fig. 13.10A and B).
- Visualize the lung field and keep the needle medial to the lung.
- Guide the needle with "tunnel" view orientation, periodically checking the AP view to ensure the needle does not go spinal medial to the pedicles.
- Once the needle is advanced deeper, the tip can be positioned over the vertebra to avoid entering the disc.
- If the needle touches the periosteal surface, it should be pulled back 1 to 2 mm.

Target

- Inferior aspect of intervertebral foramen at level of disc
- Once the needle is close to the foramen, check the lateral view. Needle should be in the central to anterior aspect of the foramen posterior to the inferior endplate.
- Check the AP view; the needle should not be beyond the 6 o'clock position of the inferior aspect of the pedicle.
- Inject and observe contrast flow using live fluoroscopy, ideally digital subtraction angiography. There should be anterior epidural flow in the lateral view and flow medial to the pedicle and around the nerve in the AP view (see Fig. 13.10C and D).

PEARLS AND PITFALLS

- The rib and SAP position can vary, so observe the spaces between the bones before starting the injection but maintain trajectory in Kambin's triangle.

Technique: interlaminar

Patient Position

- Prone

Clinician Position

- To the side of the patient, opposite the C-arm

C-Arm Position Fluoroscopy

Angulate the C-arm to "square off" the vertebrae at level to be injected; make sure the laminae are clearly visualized.

- Obtain a true AP view at the desired level.
- Use the contralateral oblique view to assess depth once the needle is near the target.

Needle Position

- The authors prefer paramedian approach, so start needle slightly off from midline on the more symptomatic side.
- The needle should be started in the interlaminar space (Fig. 13.11A and B).
- Advance the needle in the AP view, periodically checking depth in the contralateral oblique view. Stop at the ligamentum flavum behind the spinolaminar line in the contralateral oblique view.

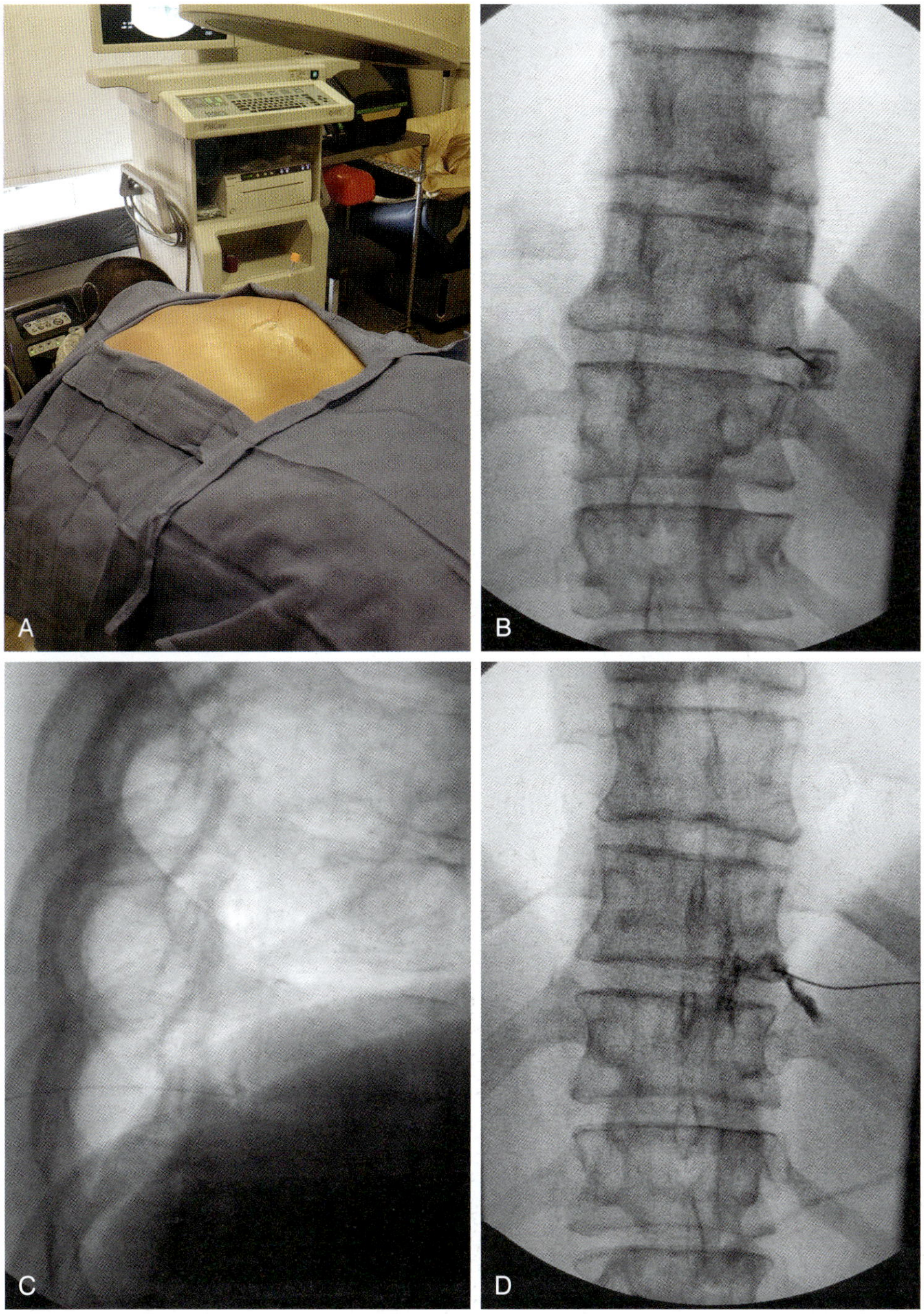

• **Fig. 13.10** (A) Thoracic transforaminal epidural fluoroscopy setup. (B) Thoracic transforaminal epidural oblique view of needle trajectory. (C) Thoracic transforaminal epidural lateral view with contrast. (D) Thoracic transforaminal epidural AP view with contrast.

- Alternatively, the needle can be advanced towards the superior border of the caudal lamina to touch the periosteal surface and ascertain depth in the AP view. Once the needle touches the lamina, "walk" the needle superior to the ligamentum flavum and confirm in the contralateral oblique view.
- Once the needle is at the ligamentum flavum, attach a loss of resistance syringe filled with normal saline.
- Advance the needle in the contralateral oblique view, obtaining an image after each advancement (see Fig. 13.11C).

Target

- Once loss of resistance is met, the needle should be in the posterior epidural space.
- Aspirate first to ensure no cerebrovascular fluid (CSF) or vascular flow, then slowly inject contrast.
- Confirm epidural flow in both contralateral oblique and AP views.
- In the contralateral oblique view, the contrast should be just anterior to the spinolaminar line (see Fig. 13.11D).

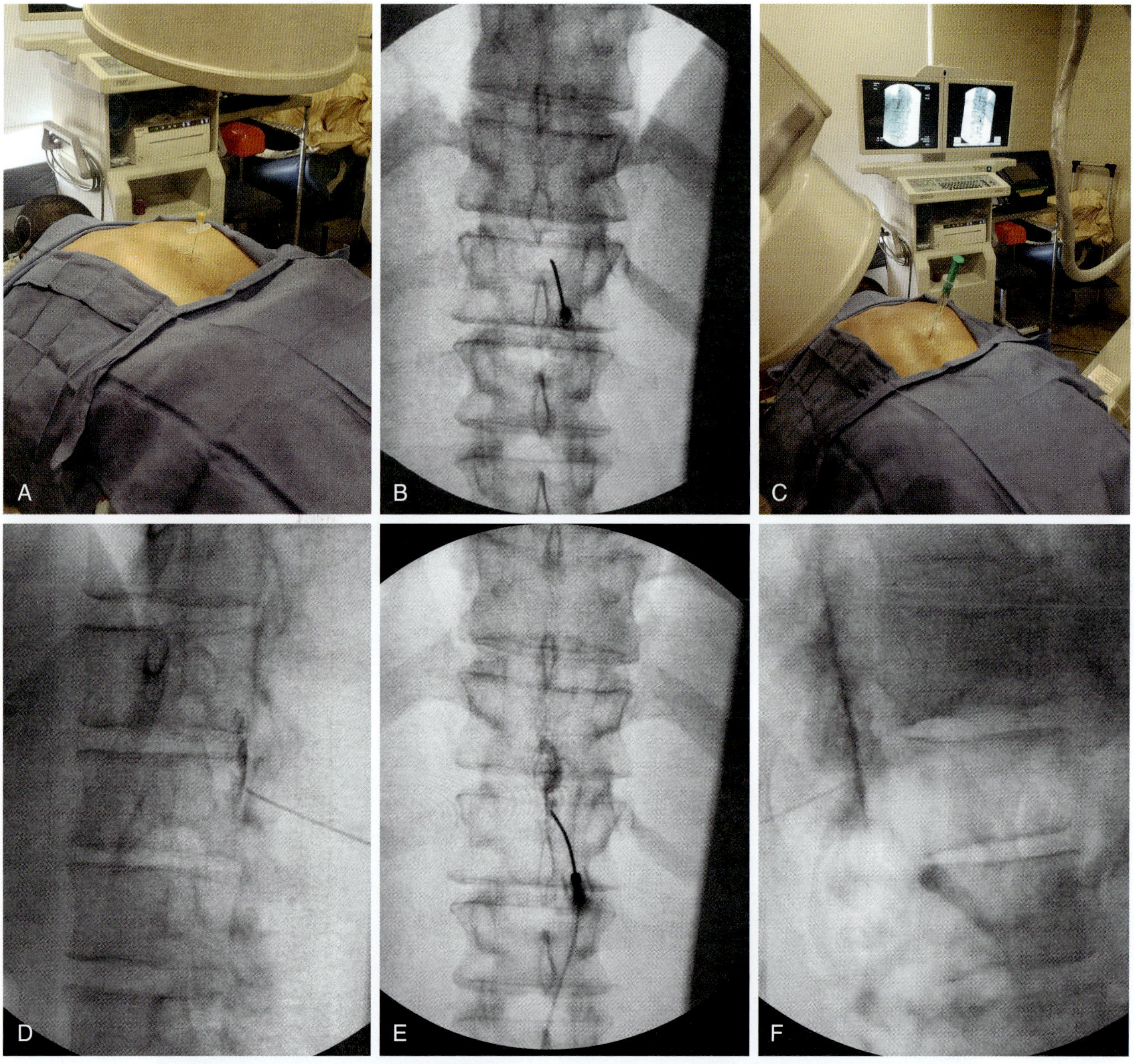

• **Fig. 13.11** (A) Thoracic interlaminal epidural (ILE) paramedial approach setup. (B) Thoracic ILE anteroposterior (AP) needle trajectory. (C) Thoracic ILE contralateral oblique view setup with loss of resistance syringe. (D) Thoracic IL contralateral oblique view with contrast. (E) Thoracic IL AP view with contrast. (F) Thoracic ILE lateral view with contrast.

- In the AP view, it should look irregular due to epidural fat and mostly on the side of the needle (see Fig. 13.11E).
- Option to view in the lateral view as well (see Fig. 13.11F).

PEARLS AND PITFALLS

- In the contralateral oblique view, the needle can appear more anterior than it actually is.
- If the needle is advanced where it appears too far anterior, but loss of resistance is not met, check the AP view to ensure the needle did not travel too far laterally.
- Possible complications include CSF leak or epidural hematoma.

Sternoclavicular and Sternocostal Joints

KEY POINTS

- Identify and clarify anatomy of sternum and clavicle prior to injection.
- Palpate tender joint(s) prior to the injection.

Pertinent Anatomy

- The sternoclavicular joint is a diarthrodial saddle joint with an intraarticular disc.[14]
- The sternocostal joints are formed between the sternum and medial end of the costal cartilage from ribs one to seven. The first rib joint is cartilaginous, and the remainder are synovial joints surrounded by a capsule.[15]

Common Pathology

- Traumatic, degenerative, or inflammatory arthritis[16]
- Osteitis condensans of the clavicle[17]
- Costochondritis
- Tietze's syndrome: rare inflammation, swelling, and pain at sternocostal joints[18]

Equipment

- C-arm fluoroscopy
- 25-gauge 2-inch needle

Common Injectates

- Anesthetic for diagnostics
- Corticosteroids
- Prolotherapy
- Orthobiologics (platelet-rich plasma [PRP], bone marrow concentrate)

Injectate Volume

- 0.5 to 1 mL

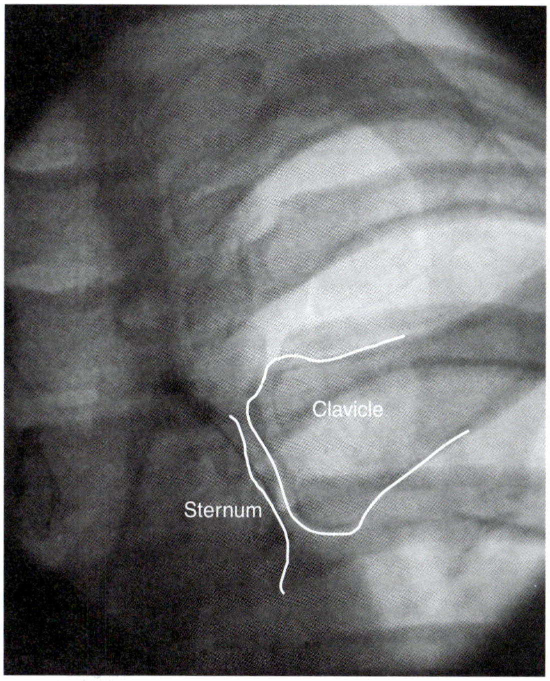

• **Fig. 13.12** Sternoclavicular joint injection with contrast.

Technique

Patient Position

- Supine

Clinician Position

- Standing on the side of patient opposite the C-arm

Fluoroscopy Position

- Direct AP view, optimizing view of desired joint
- Cephalad tilt is often required to best visualize joint space best.

Needle Position

- "Tunnel" view orientation in anterior to posterior approach, starting over the desired joint (Fig. 13.12A).

Target

- Sternoclavicular joint or costochondral joint
- Inject a small amount of contrast to confirm intraarticular placement and no vascular uptake (see Fig. 13.12B)
- Can also inject joint capsules while using orthobiologics if there is instability

PEARLS & PITFALLS

- Avoid going too deep to avoid pneumothorax.

Thoracic Rib Facets (Costotransverse Joints)

KEY POINTS

- Pain coming from the costotransverse joints is often underdiagnosed.

Pertinent Anatomy

- The joints form from the tubercle of the rib and the transverse process.
- The articular surface is curved in the cephalad 5 to 6 joints and flattened in the caudal joints.
- The joint openings are at 45 to 60 degrees rotation; thus for straight needle path the C-arm needs to be rotated.
- The joints are surrounded by a thin capsule.
- Costotransverse ligament and the superior and lateral costotransverse ligaments[19] (see Fig. 13.1)

Common Pathology

- Joint degeneration is most likely due to trauma or inflammation[20]
- Joint instability due to trauma.[21]
- The pain pattern is superficial and adjacent to the joint.[22]

Equipment

- C-arm fluoroscopy machine
- 25-gauge 2- to 3-inch needle

Common Injectates

- Anesthetic for diagnostics
- Corticosteroids
- Dextrose prolotherapy
- Orthobiologics (PRP, bone marrow concentrate)

Injectate Volume

- 0.5 to 1 mL

Technique

Patient Position

- Prone

Clinician Position

- Standing on the side of patient opposite the C-arm

Fluoroscopy Position

- "Square off" endplates with cephalad angulation for upper levels; possible caudal angulation for lower levels.
- Ipsilateral oblique 15 to 45 degrees rotation to optimize joint visualization.

Needle Position

- "Tunnel" view posterior-lateral to anterior-medial approach.
- Can start needle just over the lateral border of the transverse process to touch down on the periosteal surface, then slightly redirect into the joint.

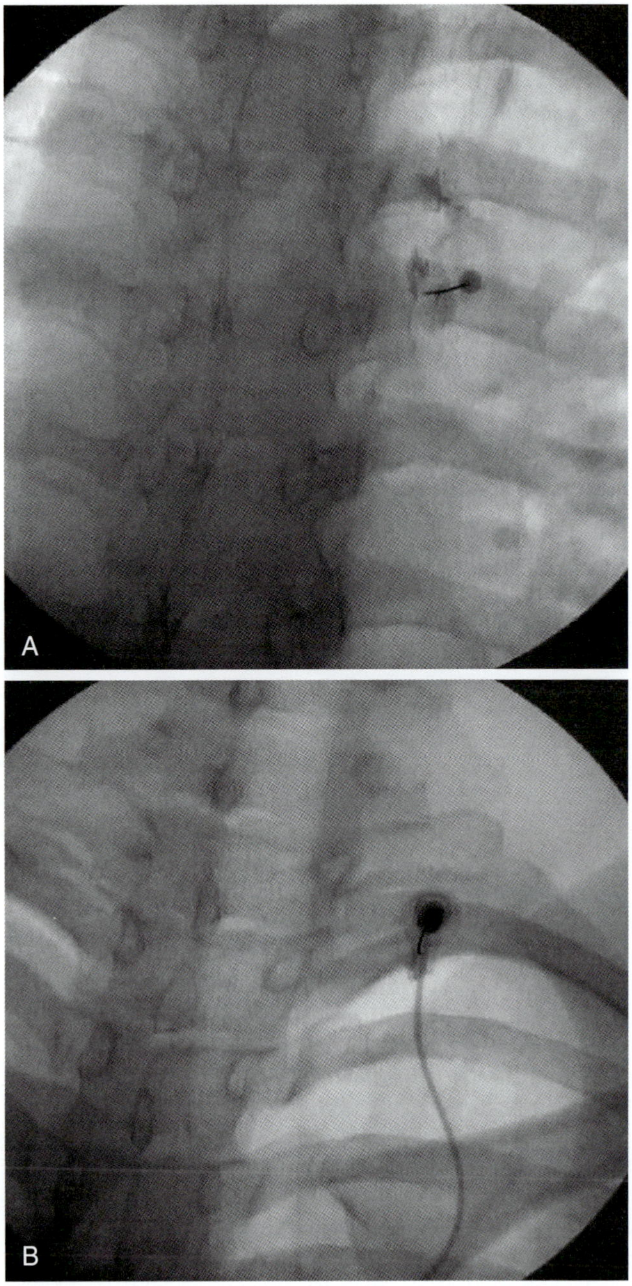

• **Fig. 13.13** (A) Costotransverse joint injection with contrast. (B). Upper costotransverse injection with contrast.

Target

- Rib joint connection to the TP
- Inject a small amount of contrast to confirm intraarticular placement (Fig. 13.13A and B).
- Can also inject joint capsule if instability is present and using prolotherapy or orthobiologics.

PEARLS AND PITFALLS

- Be sure the needle stays over the boney structures to avoid going too deep and risking pneumothorax.
- Avoid injury to the subcostal neurovascular structure just below the ribs.

Thoracic Intraarticular Facet Joint Injection

KEY POINTS

- Thoracic facet joints have different angulation than lumbar and cervical facets.

Pertinent Anatomy

- Thoracic facets are oriented much more coronal than cervical and lumbar facets.
- The medial border of the thoracic facets is about 9 to 10 mm from the posterior midline of the spine.
- The superior articular process (SAP) emanates from the upper part of the pedicle and lies caudal with the articular surface facing dorsal.
- The inferior articular process emanates from the lower part of the pedicle and lies cephalad with the articular surface facing ventral[23] (see Fig. 13.1).

Common Pathology

- Facet arthropathy; 34% to 48% of patients' pain with upper and mid-back pain comes from the thoracic facets.[24]
- Scoliosis can lead to facet arthropathy.[25]

Equipment

- C-arm fluoroscopy
- 25- to 22-gauge 3- to 3.5-inch needle

Common Injectates

- Local anesthetic
- Corticosteroids
- Dextrose prolotherapy
- Orthobiologics (PRP, bone marrow concentrate)

Injectate Volume

- 0.5 to 1 mL

Technique

Patient Position

- Prone

Clinician Position

- Standing on the side of patient opposite the C-arm

Fluoroscopy Position

- AP view and identify target level. Use this view to start needle trajectory, particularly for medial and lateral alignment.
- Contralateral oblique view to make final needle adjustments and ascertain depth safety.

Needle Position

- In the AP view start the needle over the pedicle 2 levels below the targeted facet. For example, if injecting the T7-8 facet, start the needle over the T10 pedicle (Fig. 13.14A and B).
- The needle will be angled close to about 60 degrees, aiming towards the targeted pedicle/inferior aspect of the SAP.
- The needle should be about 1cm from the middle; be sure not to advance more lateral to avoid the lung field.
- Once the needle touches the inferior SAP, switch to the contralateral oblique view. Advance the needle superior and anterior into the joint.

Target

- Mid portion of the facet joint in the AP view.
- Inject contrast to confirm intraarticular flow in the contralateral oblique and AP views (see Fig. 13.14C and D).

PEARLS AND PITFALLS

- Having a curve on the needle helps navigation.
- On AP view keep needle in line with the pedicles to avoid migrating medially into the spinal canal or laterally into the lung.
- Use the contralateral oblique view to ensure the needle does not travel too far anterior into the epidural space/intradural.
- Use a shallow angle to enter the joints due to the coronal orientation of the joints.

Medial Branch Blocks and Radiofrequency Ablation for Facet Joint Pain

KEY POINTS

- Be mindful of medial branch block (MBB) numbering and varying position of the nerves at the lowest 2 thoracic levels.
- For radiofrequency ablation (RFA), a successful diagnostic blockage must first be performed to confirm facetogenic pain.
- To denervate one joint, two medial branch nerves must be targeted.

Pertinent Anatomy

- The medial branch arises from the dorsal ramus and travels in the intertransverse space before curving dorsally over the superior lateral aspect of the transverse process (target for block) for the T1-T10 medial branches.
- After crossing the transverse process, the nerve travels dorsally, inferior, and medially along the TP. It then branches to the inferior aspect of the joint at the level and the superior aspect of the joint below the level.
- The thoracic facets are innervated by two median branches: one from the somatic nerve at the level of the joint and one from above.
- The medial branches are named by the somatic nerve they originate from, which in the thoracic spine are

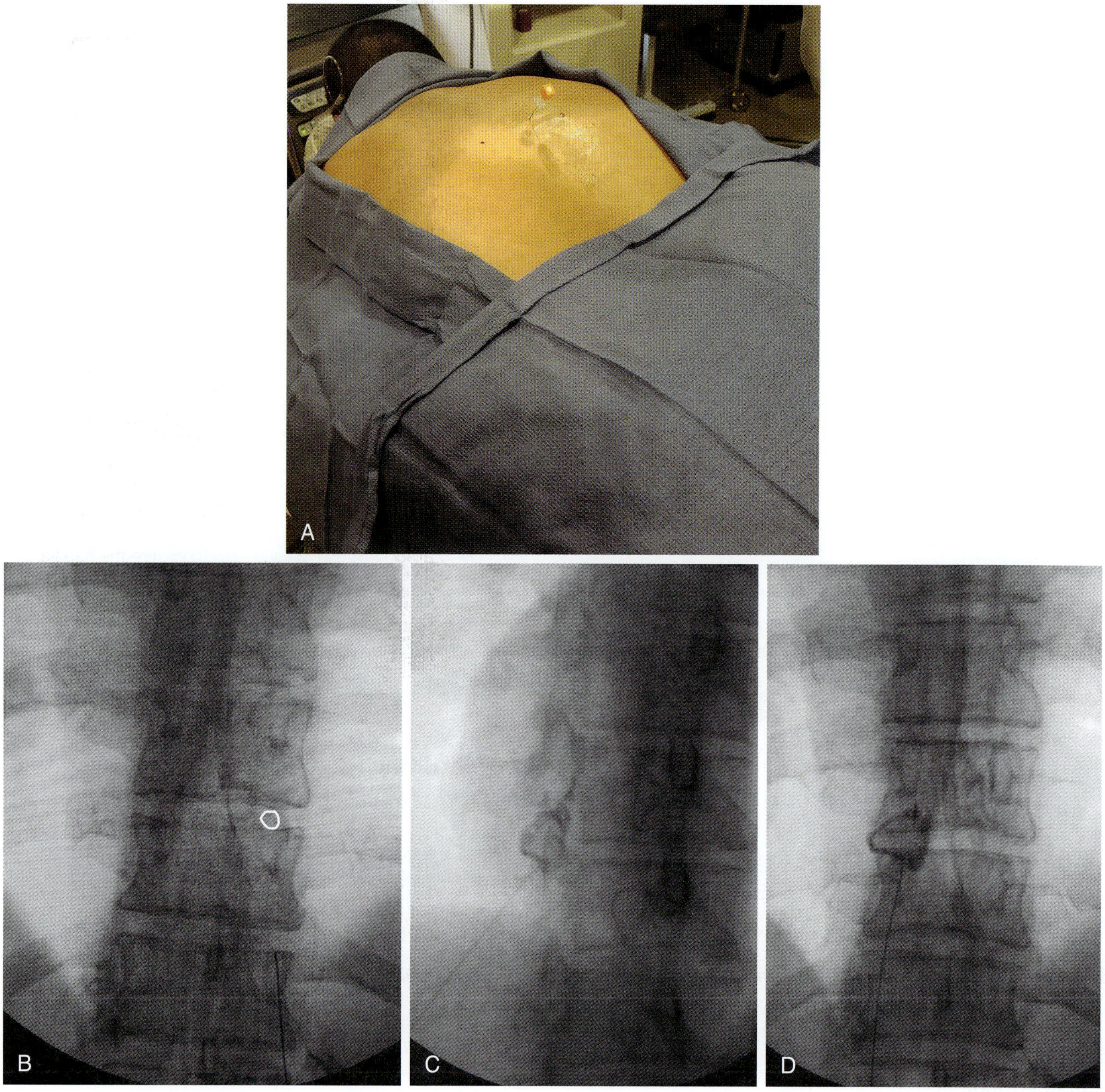

• **Fig. 13.14** (A) Thoracic facet setup. (B) Thoracic facet needle start point over T10 pedicle for injection of T8-9 facet. (C) Thoracic facet injection with contrast contralateral oblique view. (D) Thoracic facet injection with contrast contralateral AP view.

from one level above the transverse process they traverse over. For example, the T8-9 thoracic facet joint is innervated by the T7 and T8 medial branches. The T7 medial branch innervates the inferior aspect of the T7-8 facet and superior aspect of the T8-9 facet, whereas the T8 medial branch innervates the inferior aspect of the T8-9 facet and superior aspect of the T9-10 facet.

- The T11-T12 medial branches travel over the SAP and transverse process junction at T12 and L1, similar to the lumbar medial branches[26] (see Fig. 13.1).

Common Pathology

- Thoracic facet–mediated pain secondary to trauma, deformity, osteoarthritis.

Equipment

- C-arm fluoroscopy
- 25- to 22-gauge 3- to 3.5-inch needle

Common Injectates

- Local anesthetic
- Corticosteroids

Injectate Volume

- 1 to 2 mL

Technique for Medial Branch Block

Patient Position

- Prone

Clinician Position

- Standing on the side of patient opposite the C-arm

Fluoroscopy Position

- AP view and "square off" vertebrae of the targeted area, then rotate 10 degrees contralateral oblique.

Needle Position

- "Tunnel" view with needle tip starting over the superior lateral aspect of the transverse process for T1-T10 medial branches, and over SAP TP junction for T11-T12 medial branches.

Target

- For the T1-T10 medial branches, target over T2-T11 transverse processes (Fig. 13.15).
- For the T11-T12 medial branches, target over junction of SAP and transverse process of T12-L1.
- To denervate the joint, block the 2 corresponding medial branches. For example, to block T9-10, block the T8 and T9 medial branches over the T9 and T10 transverse process, respectively.
- Option to confirm no vascular uptake with contrast injection.

PEARLS AND PITFALLS

- Keep the needle tip over the bone at all times to avoid advancing too anterior or causing a pneumothorax.
- Collimating the image to exclude most of the vertebrae and rotating the C-arm 10 degrees contralateral oblique can enhance visualization of the TPs.

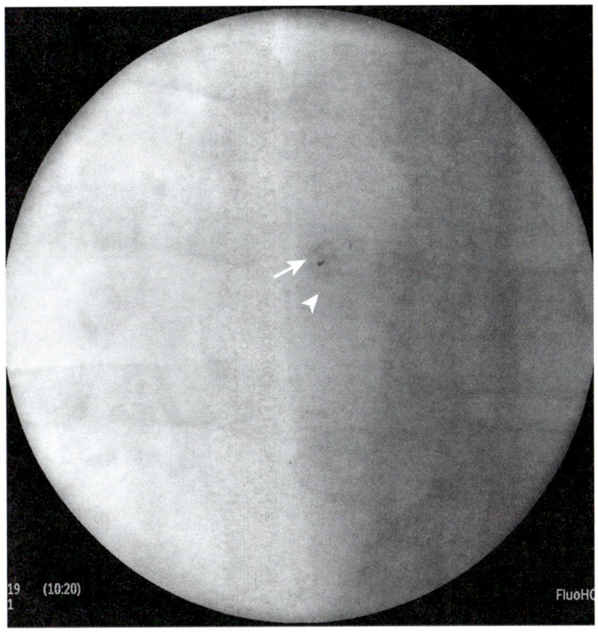

• **Fig. 13.15** Thoracic medial branch block using a 10 degree contralateral oblique view to optimize visualization of the transverse processes. A needle is seen targeting the left T7 medial branch (arrow) on the left T8 transverse process (arrowhead). The image is centered away from the vertebral bodies to reduce beam intensity via the auto-adjust feature.

Technique for Medial Branch Radiofrequency Ablation

Patient Position

- Prone

Clinician Position

- Standing on the side of the patient opposite the C-arm

Fluoroscopy Position

- For the T1-T10 medial branches:
    - AP view and "square off" endplates of the targeted area
    - Lateral view to advance the needle after touching the TP
- For the T11-T12 medial branches
    - "Square off" endplates of the desired level, then oblique about 10 degrees contralaterally
    - Use lateral view to track depth

Needle Position

For the T1-T10 medial branches:

- For RFA, the needle tip starts inferior and medial to the target so that the final position will cover more area of the nerve.
- Start over the medial aspect of the rib below the target level.
- Advance the needle superior lateral and touch down on the superior lateral transverse process; then obtain a lateral view.

For the T11-T12 medial branches, the approach will be similar to the lumbar medial branch RFA:

- Start inferior one level to the targeted level and guide the needle to the SAP TP junction from caudal to cephalad.
- Use contralateral oblique or lateral view to ascertain depth.

Target

- For the T1-T10 medial branches: target is just superior and lateral to the T2-T11 transverse processes (Fig. 13.16A). Depth in the lateral should be at the level of the transverse process (see Fig. 13.16B).
- For T11-T12 medial branches: target is over junction of SAP and transverse process of T12-L1.

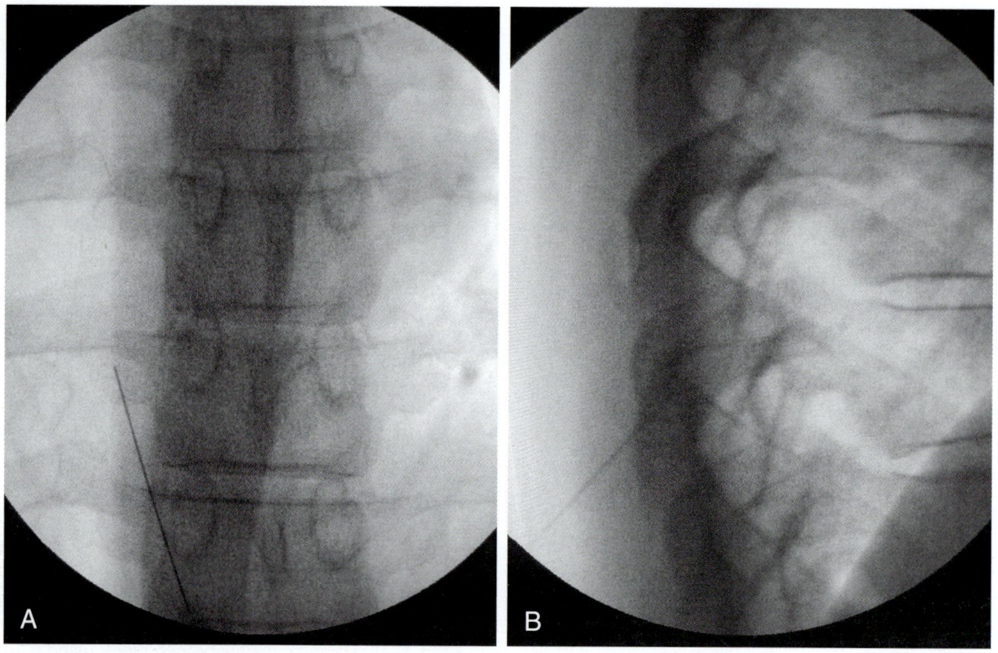

• **Fig. 13.16** (A) Radiofrequency ablation (RFA) at target in AP view. (B) RFA at target in lateral view.

- To denervate, the joint must block the two corresponding medial branches. For example, block T9-10, block the T8 and T9 medial branches over the T9 and T10 transverse process.
- Option to confirm no vascular uptake with contrast injection.

PEARLS AND PITFALLS

- Use lateral or contralateral oblique views to ensure the needle is not advanced too anteriorly.
- Ensure that the needle is placed at an angle so that there is parallel placement of the tip along the nerve.
- Before the ablation, motor and sensory stimulation should be performed to ensure there are no radicular symptoms or signs of muscle movement.
- 0.5 mL to 1 mL of local anesthetic is typically injected after stimulation and before the ablation to improve the patient's comfort.
- Practitioners vary in their ablation settings; it can be 80 to 85 degrees for 60-90 seconds. Some may do 2 or 3 rounds of the ablation, adjusting the RF cannula each time by a few millimeters to widen the ablation zone.

Thoracic Intradiscal

KEY POINTS

- Symptomatic thoracic disc herniation is rare. Greater incident occurs in patients between 40 and 60 years old with a slight male predominance.
- At the time of writing, there is no published literature for the role of orthobiologics in thoracic disc disease.
- Intradiscal approach is similar to epidural approach.

Pertinent Anatomy

- The thoracic spinal cord accounts for 40% of the canal size and the spinal cord lies just posterior to the PLL and disc. Small disc herniation can cause significant ventral cord compression.[27]
  - spinal nerve
  - rib head
  - vertebral body (Fig. 13.2)
  - intervertebral disc

Common Pathology

- Disc annular tear
- Disc bulge/protrusion
- Endplate modic changes
- Thoracic discs are most at risk for injury with combined bending and torsion, but less so than lumbar discs due to the stability of the ribcage.[27]

Equipment

- C-arm fluoroscopy
- 25- to 22-gauge 3- to 5-inch spinal needle

Common Injectates

- Contrast for provocative discography
- Orthobiologics (PRP, bone marrow concentrate)

Injectate Volume

- 1 to 2 mL

Technique

Patient Position

- Prone

Clinician Position

- To the side of the patient contralateral to the C-arm

C-Arm Position Fluoroscopy

- "Square off" the disc space at the level to be injected.
- Align 25 to 45 degrees oblique view, optimize foraminal view between SAP of the lower vertebral bone and the rib. Keep the lung field line lateral to the vertebral body.
- Use the lateral view to confirm depth once the needle is at the target.

Needle Position

- Start the needle over the posterior lateral disc space
- The needle should be directed between the rib laterally and the SAP medially (Fig. 13.17A).
- Visualize the lung field and keep the needle medial to the lung.
- Guide the needle in the "tunnel" view orientation.
- Advance the needle into the disc.
- Once the needle enters the disc, adjust using the lateral and AP views.

Target

- Middle of the disc space in the AP and lateral views (see Fig. 13.17B and C)
- Inject a small amount of contrast to show nucleogram if doing a discogram

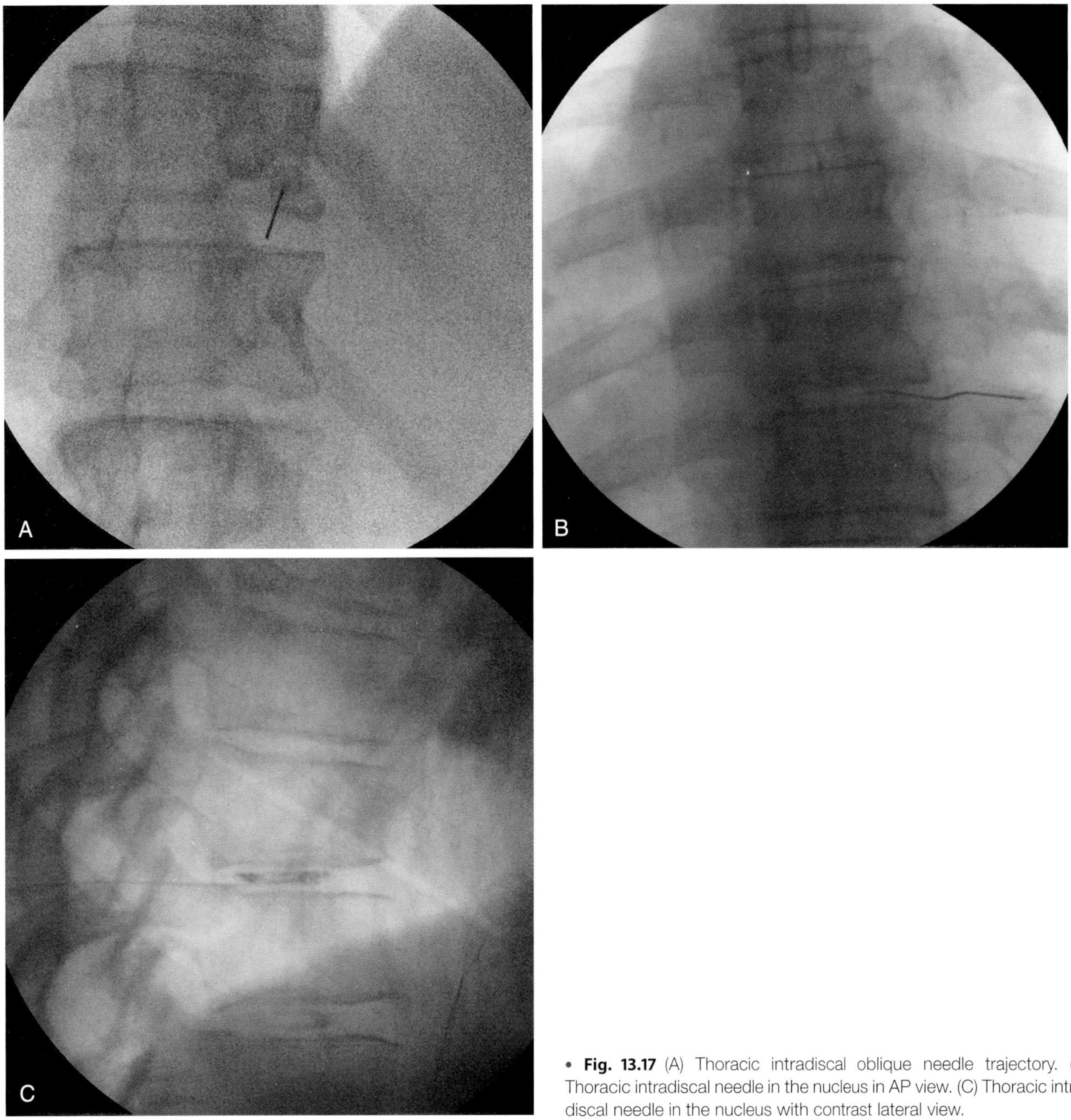

• **Fig. 13.17** (A) Thoracic intradiscal oblique needle trajectory. (B) Thoracic intradiscal needle in the nucleus in AP view. (C) Thoracic intradiscal needle in the nucleus with contrast lateral view.

PEARLS AND PITFALLS

- Visualize and stay medial to the lung line.
- Stay lateral to the dura to avoid intrathecal or spinal cord injury.
- Don't advance too ventral into the disc.

Superspinous and Interspinous Ligament Injection

KEY POINTS

- The thoracic supraspinous and interspinous ligaments are important structures to consider when patients have thoracic pain with excess kyphosis, hypermobility, or traumatic injury.
- The thoracic intertransverse ligaments are important to consider in patients with thoracic pain and scoliosis, traumatic injury, or side bending pain.

Pertinent Anatomy

- The supraspinous (SS) ligaments course between and just over the spinous processes[28]
- The interspinous (IS) ligaments course between the spinous processes[28]
- The intertransverse (IT) ligaments course between and just anterior to the transverse processes[28] (see Fig. 13.3)

Common Pathology

- Traumatic injury
- Thoracic spondylosis, degenerative disease, and wedge fractures can cause thoracic ligament laxity (and vice versa).
- Scoliosis: for a lateral curve, the intertransverse ligaments are over stretched with potential increased laxity at the convexity of the segmental curve and are possible targets for injection.

Equipment

- C-arm fluoroscopy
- 25- to 22-gauge 3- to 3.5-inch spinal needle

Common Injectates

- Prolotherapy, orthobiologics (PRP, bone marrow concentrate, etc.)
- Avoid intraligamentous corticosteroids.

Injectate Volume

- 0.5 to 1 mL per area/ligament

Technique for Supraspinous and Interspinous Ligaments

Patient Position

- Prone
- Arms above the head to remove the arms from view on the lateral projection

Clinician Position

- Standing on the side of the patient opposite of the C-arm

C-Arm Position Fluoroscopy

- True lateral view
- The upper levels can be difficult to have a clear lateral view due to the rib cage and organs.

Needle Position

- Palpate the spinous processes to ascertain midline; consider marking the skin prior to or at the time of the injection with a marker.
- Insert needle aiming for spinous process at the desired level to ensure midline placement.

Target

- Gently touch down on the spinous process and inject the SSL (Fig. 13.18A).
- Redirect the needle superior between the spinous processes to inject the interspinous ligaments (see Fig. 13.18B).

PEARLS AND PITFALLS

- Use smallest-length needle possible.
- Use two hands when injecting the deeper ligaments to ensure adequate control of the needle and also to limit accidental advancement of the needle too deep.
- If unable to obtain a clear lateral picture, only advance about 1 cm deep so as to not place the needle too anterior into the thecal sac or spinal cord.

Technique for Intertransverse

Patient Position

- Prone

Clinician Position

- Standing on the side of the patient opposite of the C-arm

C-Arm Position Fluoroscopy

- True AP view, so the spinous process of the desired level is centered between the vertebral bodies.
- "Square off" vertebral endplate of the desired level
- Center the transverse process

Needle Position

- The needle starts over the lateral border of the targeted transverse process. (For instance, if targeting the T7-8 IT ligament, start one needle over the T7 TP and redirect inferiorly. A second needle will start over the T8 transverse process and redirect superiorly.)

Target

- Transverse ligaments:
  - Either just superior and deep/anterior or inferior and deep/anterior to the transverse process to target the desired superior or inferior band.

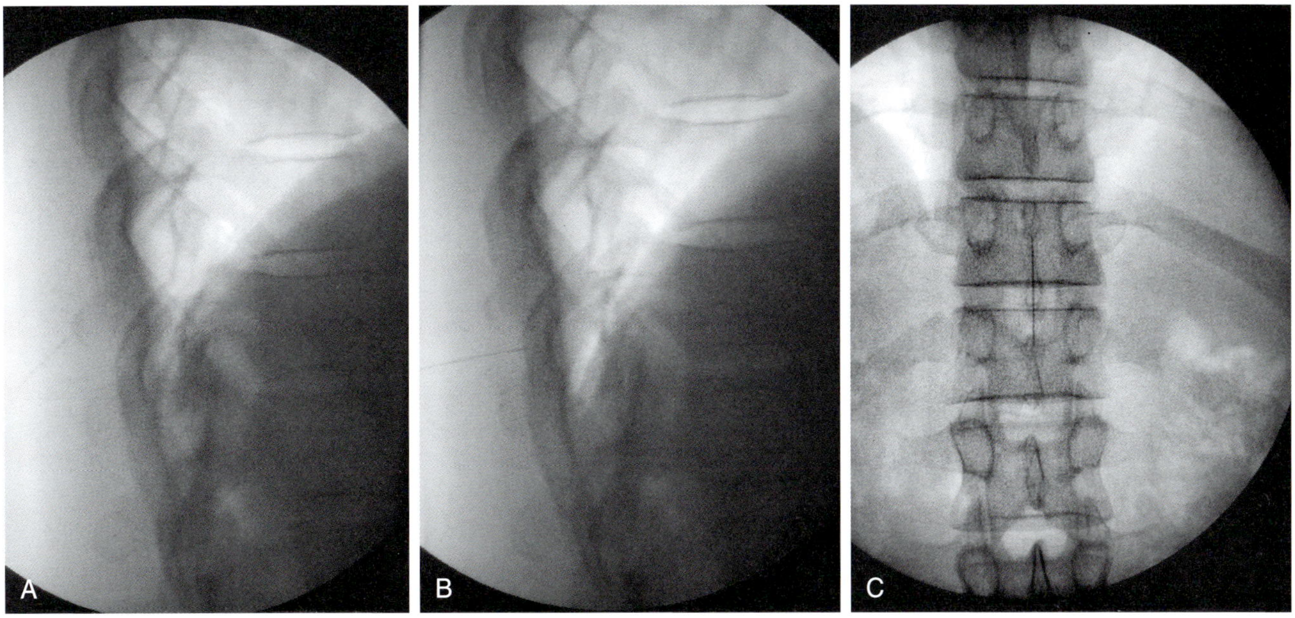

• **Fig. 13.18** (A) Supraspinous ligament in lateral view. (B) Interspinous ligament in lateral view. (C) Interspinous ligament in AP view.

- Inject a small amount of contrast that should show vertical flow along the ligament superiorly or inferiorly, depending on the target.
- Inject both the superior and inferior aspects of the ligament (Fig. 13.19).

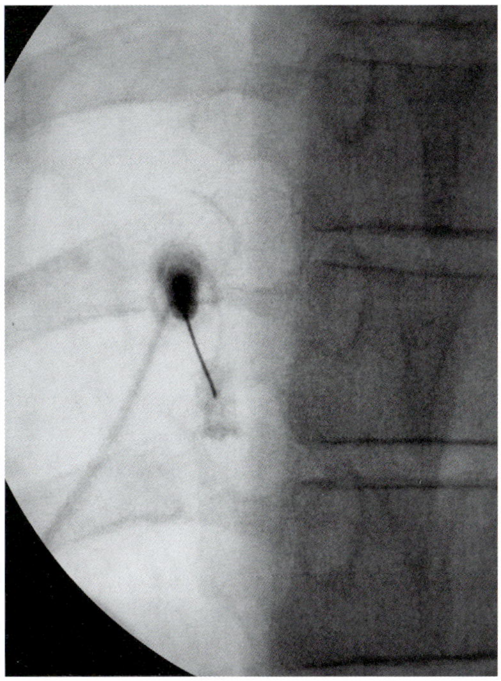

• **Fig. 13.19** Thoracic Intertransverse Ligament with Contrast in AP View.

PEARLS AND PITFALLS

- Always start over and touch down on the periosteal surface of the transverse process to ascertain depth and for safety.
- Only advance 1 to 2 mm deep/anterior to the TP to avoid going too anterior or causing a pneumothorax.
- Medial branches are in close proximity.
- The authors recommend using contrast to confirm ligamentous spread. This can serve as a diagnostic injection using an anesthetic agent.

Intercostal Nerve Block

KEY POINTS

- Used for short- or long-term pain relief for thoracic dermatomal and abdominal pain.[29]
- Can be done with either fluoroscopy or ultrasonography.[30]

Pertinent Anatomy

- The intercostal nerves are the anterior branches of the thoracic nerves. They provide sensory input from the chest and abdominal walls, and motor innervation to the intercostal and abdominal muscles.
- The intercostal neurovascular structures travel through the intercostal space between the pleura and intercostal membrane.
- They travel below the rib margin with the vein, artery, and nerve, from cranial to caudal, respectively.[31]

Common Pathology

- Painful rib fractures
- Intercostal neuropathy
- Herpes zoster[32]
- Pain related to thoracotomies, cardiothoracic, and breast surgeries[33-35]

Equipment

- C-arm fluoroscopy
- 25-gauge 2- to 3-inch needle

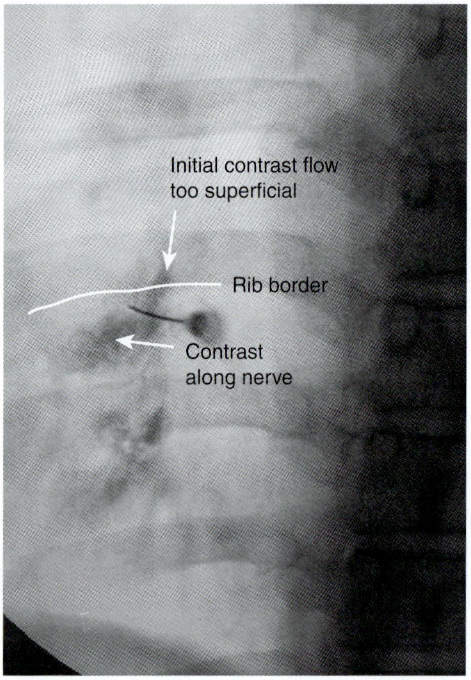

• **Fig. 13.20** Intercostal Nerve Block with Contrast in AP View.

Common Injectates

- Local anesthetic
- Corticosteroids

Injectate Volume

- 2 to 5 mL

Technique

Patient Position

- Prone

Clinician Position

- Stand on the side of the patient

Fluoroscopy Position

- AP view and clearly visualize the rib
- Can use the lateral view to confirm depth

Needle Position

- Start about 3 inches lateral to the costotransverse joint or anywhere along the rib, proximal to the patient's pain generator.
- Start a few millimeters below the rib margin and aim slightly superior to touch down on the rib, then walk off rib inferiorly.

Target

- Intercostal space 1 to 2 mm inferior to rib and 1 to 2 mm deep to posterior rib border (Fig. 13.20).
- Inject contrast to confirm flow along the nerve parallel to the rib with no vascular uptake.

PEARLS AND PITFALLS

- Due to the close proximity of the vasculature, there is a higher risk of anesthetic uptake, and care that should be given to the amount of anesthetic used.
- The needle should not be advanced more than 1 to 2 mm past the dorsal rib margin due to risk of going too anterior and pneumothorax.
- Avoid bilateral intercostal nerve blocks due to risk of pneumothorax.

References

1. Bogduk N. Functional anatomy of the spine. *Handb Clin Neurol.* 2016;136:675–688. https://doi.org/10.1016/B978-0-444-53486-6.00032-6.
2. Chiou-Tan FY, Miller JS, Goktepe AS, Zhang H, Taber KH. Sectional neuroanatomy of the upper thoracic spine and chest [published correction appears in *J Comput Assist Tomogr.* 2005;29(4):569]. *J Comput Assist Tomogr.* 2005;29(2):281–285. https://doi.org/10.1097/01.rct.0000159509.75575.8e.
3. Miller JS, Chiou-Tan F, Zhang H, Taber KH. Sectional neuroanatomy of the lower thoracic spine and chest. *J Comput Assist Tomogr.* 2007;31(1):160–164. https://doi.org/10.1097/01.rct.0000237813.26301.73.
4. Miller JS, Goktepe AS, Chiou-Tan F, Zhang H, Taber KH. Sectional neuroanatomy of the middle thoracic spine (t5-t8) and chest. *J Comput Assist Tomogr.* 2006;30(1):161–164. https://doi.org/10.1097/01.rct.0000187415.07698.56.
5. Vollmer DG, Banister WM. Thoracolumbar spinal anatomy. *Neurosurg Clin N Am.* 1997;8(4):443–453.
6. Maiman DJ, Pintar FA. Anatomy and clinical biomechanics of the thoracic spine. *Clin Neurosurg.* 1992;38:296–324.
7. Oxland TR. Fundamental biomechanics of the spin—What we have learned in the past 25 years and future directions. *J Biomech.* 2016;49(6):817–832.
8. Panjabi MM, White AA 3rd. Basic biomechanics of the spine. *Neurosurgery* 1980;7(1):76–93.
9. Panjabi MM, Pearson AM, Ito S, et al. Cervical spine ligament injury during simulated frontal impact. *Spine.* 2004;29(21):2395–2403.
10. Benedetti PF, Fahr LM, Kuhns LR, Hayman LA. MR. imaging findings in spinal ligamentous injury. *Am J Roentgenol.* 2000;175:661–665.
11. Turcios NL. Slipping rib syndrome: an elusive diagnosis. *Paediatr Respir Rev.* 2017;22:44–46.
12. Laurie L, Peterson, Cavanaugh DG, Two years of debilitating pain in a football spearing victim: slipping rib syndrome. *Med Sci Sports Exerc.* 2003;35(10):1634–1637.
13. Fanous AA, Tumialán LM, Wang MY. Kambin's triangle: definition and new classification schema [published online ahead of print, 2019 Nov 29]. *J Neurosurg Spine.* 2019:1–9. https://doi.org/10.3171/2019.8.SPINE181475.
14. Brossmann J, Stäbler A, Preidler KW, Trudell D, Resnick D, Sternoclavicular joint: MR imaging—anatomic correlation. *Radiology.* 1996;198(1):193–198.
15. Norris CM. *Managing Sports Injuries.* 4th ed. 2011:292–309.
16. Edwin J, Ahmed S, Verma S, Tytherleigh-Strong G, Karuppaiah K, Sinha J. Swellings of the sternoclavicular joint: review of traumatic and non-traumatic pathologies. *EFORT Open Rev.* 2018;3(8):471–484. https://doi.org/10.1302/2058-5241.3.170078.

17. Galla R, Basava V, Conermann T, Kabazie AJ. Sternoclavicular steroid injection for treatment of pain in a patient with osteitis condensans of the clavicle. *Pain Physician*. 2009;12(6):987–990.
18. Jurik AG, Graudal H. Sternocostal joint swelling—clinical Tietze's syndrome. Report of sixteen cases and review of the literature. *Scand J Rheumatol*. 1988;17(1):33–42. https://doi.org/10.3109/03009748809098757.
19. Lau LSW, Littlejohn GO. Costotransverse joint injection description of technique. *Australas Radiol*. 1987;31(1):47–49. https://doi.org/10.1111/j.1440-1673.1987.tb01781.x.
20. Sanzhang C, Rothschild BM. Zygapophyseal and costovertebral/costotransverse joints: an anatomic assessment of arthritis impact. *Br J Rheumatol*. 1993;32(12):1066–1071. https://doi.org/10.1093/rheumatology/32.12.1066.
21. Christensen EE, Dietz GW. Injuries of the first costovertebral articulation. *Radiology*. 1980;134(1):41–43. https://doi.org/10.1148/radiology.134.1.7350632.
22. Young BA, Gill HE, Wainner RS, Flynn TW. Thoracic costotransverse joint pain patterns: a study in normal volunteers. *BMC Musculoskelet Disord*. 2008;9:140. https://doi.org/10.1186/1471-2474-9-140.
23. Ebraheim NA, Xu R, Ahmad M, Yeasting RA. The quantitative anatomy of the thoracic facet and the posterior projection of its inferior facet. *Spine (Phila Pa 1976)*. 1997;22(16):1811–1818. https://doi.org/10.1097/00007632-199708150-00002.
24. Lee DG, Ahn SH, Cho YW, Do KH, Kwak SG, Chang MC. Comparison of intra-articular thoracic facet joint steroid injection and thoracic medial branch block for the management of thoracic facet joint pain. *Spine (Phila Pa 1976)*. 2018;43(2):76–80. https://doi.org/10.1097/BRS.0000000000002269.
25. Aebi M. The adult scoliosis. *Eur Spine J*. 2005;14(10):925–948. https://doi.org/10.1007/s00586-005-1053-9.
26. Chua WH, Bogduk N. The surgical anatomy of thoracic facet denervation. *Acta Neurochir*. 1995;136(3–4):140–144. https://doi.org/10.1007/bf01410616.
27. Vanichkachorn JS, Vaccaro AR. Thoracic disc disease: diagnosis and treatment. *J Am Acad Orthop Surg*. 2000;8(3):159–169. https://doi.org/10.5435/00124635-200005000-00003.
28. Behrsin JF, Briggs CA. Ligaments of the lumbar spine: a review. *Surg Radiol Anat*. 1988;10(3):211–219. https://doi.org/10.1007/BF02115239.
29. Niesel HC, Klimpel L, Kaiser H, al-Rafai S. Die einzeitige Interkostalblockade—operative und therapeutische Indikationen [The single intercostal block—surgical and therapeutic indications]. *Reg Anaesth*. 1989;12(1):1–12.
30. Shankar H, Eastwood D. Retrospective comparison of ultrasound and fluoroscopic image guidance for intercostal steroid injections. *Pain Pract*. 2010;10(4):312–317. https://doi.org/10.1111/j.1533-2500.2009.00345.x.
31. Court C, Vialle R, Lepeintre JF, Tadié M. The thoracoabdominal intercostal nerves: an anatomical study for their use in neurotization. *Surg Radiol Anat*. 2005;27(1):8–14. https://doi.org/10.1007/s00276-004-0281-8.
32. Cui JZ, Zhang JW, Yan F, et al. Effect of single intra-cutaneous injection for acute thoracic herpes zoster and incidence of postherpetic neuralgia. *Pain Manag Nurs*. 2018;19(2):186–194. https://doi.org/10.1016/j.pmn.2017.09.002.
33. Kristek J, Kvolik S, Sakić K, Has B, Prlić L. Intercostal catheter analgesia is more efficient vs. intercostal nerve blockade for post-thoracotomy pain relief. *Coll Antropol*. 2007;31(2):561–566.
34. Zinboonyahgoon N, Luksanapruksa P, Piyaselakul S, et al. The ultrasound-guided proximal intercostal block: anatomical study and clinical correlation to analgesia for breast surgery. *BMC Anesthesiol*. 2019;19(1):94. https://doi.org/10.1186/s12871-019-0762-2.
35. Thompson C, French DG, Costache I. Pain management within an enhanced recovery program after thoracic surgery. *J Thorac Dis*. 2018;10(suppl 32):S3773–S3780. https://doi.org/10.21037/jtd.2018.09.112.

14 Lumbar Injection Techniques

DI CUI, LISA FOSTER, BRIAN HART KEOGH JR., JASON MARKLE, HASSAN MONFARED, JAYMIN PATEL, SHOUNUCK I. PATEL, JOHN PITTS, AND DIYA SANDHU

Ultrasound-Guided Techniques

Facet Joints

KEY POINTS

- The facet joints (zygapophyseal or Z joints) can be targeted individually for isolated pathology or targeted in combination with treating other components of the functional spinal unit,[1,2] along with ligaments (supraspinous/interspinous, intertransverse, iliolumbar, ligamentum flavum), paraspinal multifidus muscles, the thoracodorsal fascia, nerve roots in the epidural space, and the intervertebral discs.
- Injections can be accomplished using a low-frequency curvilinear transducer with similar accuracy as fluoroscopy- or CT-or computed tomography (CT)-guided techniques.[3,4]
- Fluoroscopic contrast-dye confirmation may be used to ensure accurate placement of the injectate.

Pertinent Anatomy

- The facet joints or zygapophyseal Z joints are the synovial interface between the inferior and superior articular processes (SAPs) of adjacent vertebral bodies (Figs. 14.1–14.4).
- The orientation of facet joints may cause[5] or be otherwise associated with degenerative processes such as spondylosis,[6] spondylolisthesis, and/or disc degeneration.[7]

Common Pathology

- Facet arthropathy, facet capsule sprain, tropism.

Equipment

- Ultrasound machine with low-frequency curvilinear probe
- 22 to 25 gauge, 2- to 3-inch needle

Common Injectate

- Local anesthetics with or without corticosteroid[8]
- Prolotherapy
- Orthobiologics[9] (platelet-rich plasma [PRP], bone marrow concentrate, etc.)

Injectate Volume

- 0.25 to 0.5 mL into the joint, +/– peppering the capsule outside of the joint

Technique

Patient Position

- Prone with a pillow under the lower abdomen/pelvis to allow lumbar spine to be in a flattened or rounded kyphotic position. This allows the spinous processes to be gapped and the ligaments to be taut.

Clinician Position

- Standing at the side of the patient with the ultrasound screen on the opposite side.

Transducer Position

- Short axis with visualization of spinous process, lamina, and facet joint. Identification of levels should be done by starting in the region of the sacrum. The L5 spinous process and lamina are much steeper, and together with the bilateral facets and transverse processes further laterally form the appearance of a "crown." This is just cephalad to the S1 spinous process which comes off of a relatively flat sacral base that has more of a "tiara" appearance. After identifying your target level, scan so that the lateral aspect of the lamina is midline to the probe, then scan cephalad/caudad incrementally to visualize the facet joint which is lateral to the lamina but medial to the deeper transverse process—with the appearance of two small teeth (the superior and inferior articular processes). You may or may not be able to visualize a thin hyperechoic joint capsule overlying the facets (Figs. 14.5–14.7).
- Identification of levels can also be done with long-axis view; visualizing spinous processes from a midline axial position helps identify levels, starting caudally with the

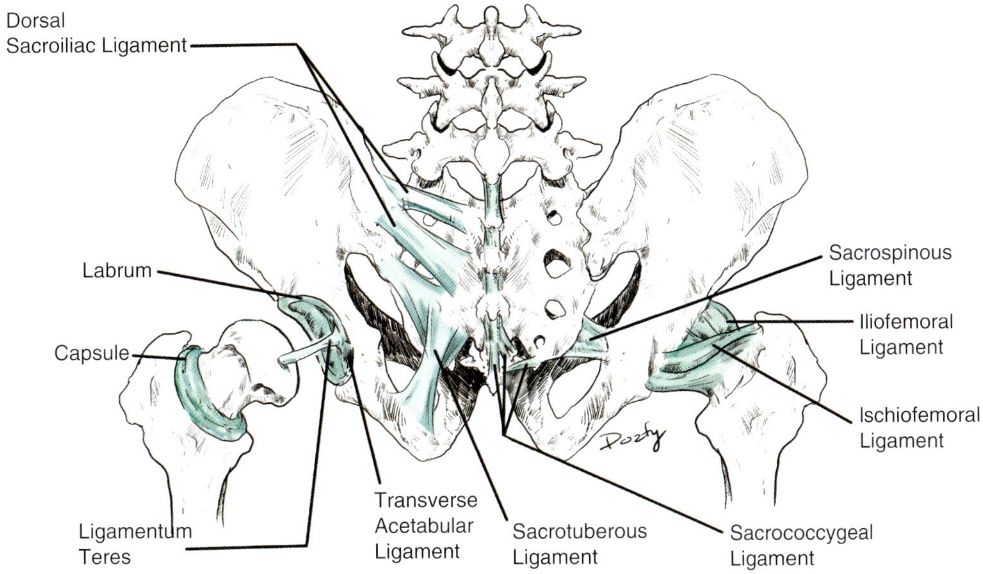

• **Fig. 14.1** Lumbosacral Pelvis Ligamentous Anatomy.

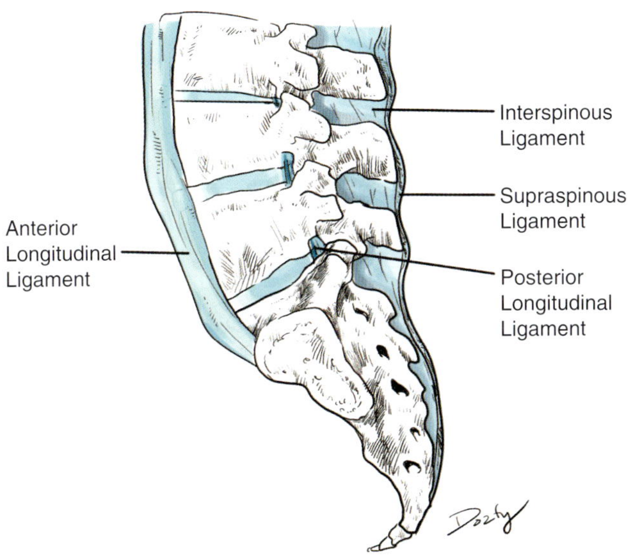

• **Fig. 14.2** Lower Lumbar Sagittal Key Ligamentous Anatomy.

shallow relatively flat sacral spinous processes, cephalad to the steeper lumbar spinous processes. With target level in mid-screen, turn the probe 90 degrees.

- Switching back and forth may optimize targeting of needle tip.

Needle Position

- In-plane[10]
  - With spine in short axis, introduce the needle lateral to medial at a steep angle with or without gel stand-off, directed into the gap between the superior and inferior articular processes (Fig. 14.6).
- Out-of-plane
  - With spine in short axis, introduce the needle out-of-plane just caudad to the mid-point of the transducer which is placed just lateral to the facet joint. Needle tip should be advanced superficially at first, withdrawn back from the plane of the transducer, and walked down to the gap between the superior and inferior articular processes (Fig. 14.8).

Target

- Direct placement into the desired facet joint and or capsule.

PEARLS AND PITFALLS

- The facet joint may be difficult to visualize in situations with significant facet hypertrophy.
- For in-plane injections, a gel stand-off may be beneficial at reducing anisotropy.
- Care must be taken to stay midline when doing an out-of-plane injection with a curvilinear probe because straying to one direction or the other can be skewed drastically due to the convex nature of the ultrasound beam.

Supraspinous and Interspinous Ligaments

KEY POINTS

- The supraspinous and interspinous ligaments can be targeted in isolation for specific injuries, but more commonly are targeted in combination with treating other components of the functional spinal unit,[11,2] along with other ligaments (intertransverse, iliolumbar, ligamentum flavum), paraspinal multifidus muscles, the thoracodorsal fascia, zygapophysial (Z joints or facet) joints, nerve roots in the epidural space, and the intervertebral discs.
- Injections can be accomplished using a high-frequency linear transducer; however, a low-frequency curvilinear transducer is preferred to have a wider visualization of the region and allow for steeper in-plane injections with minimized anisotropy.

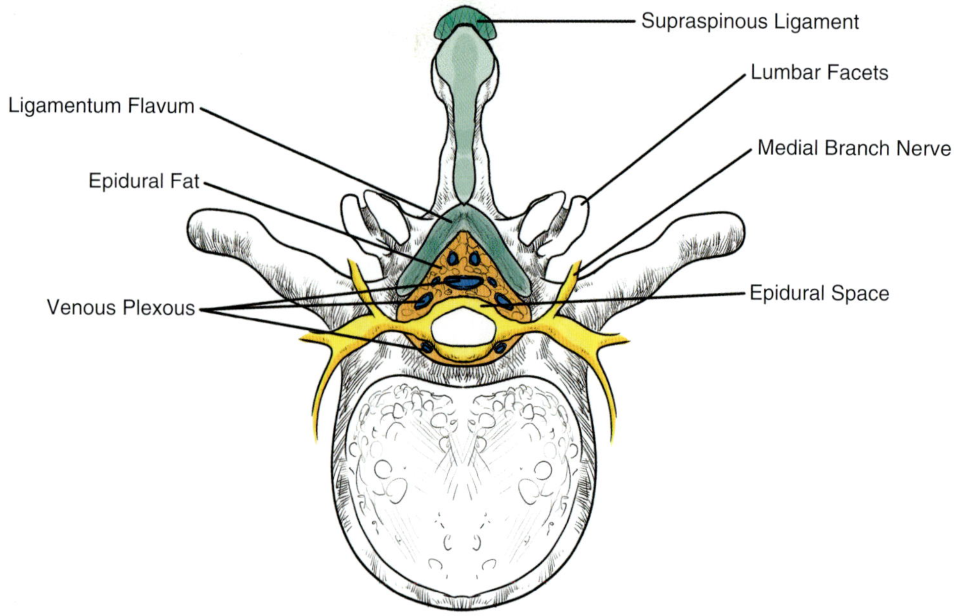

• **Fig. 14.3** Lumbar Axial Anatomy with Key Relationship Between the Supraspinous, Infraspinous, and Ligamentum Flavum.

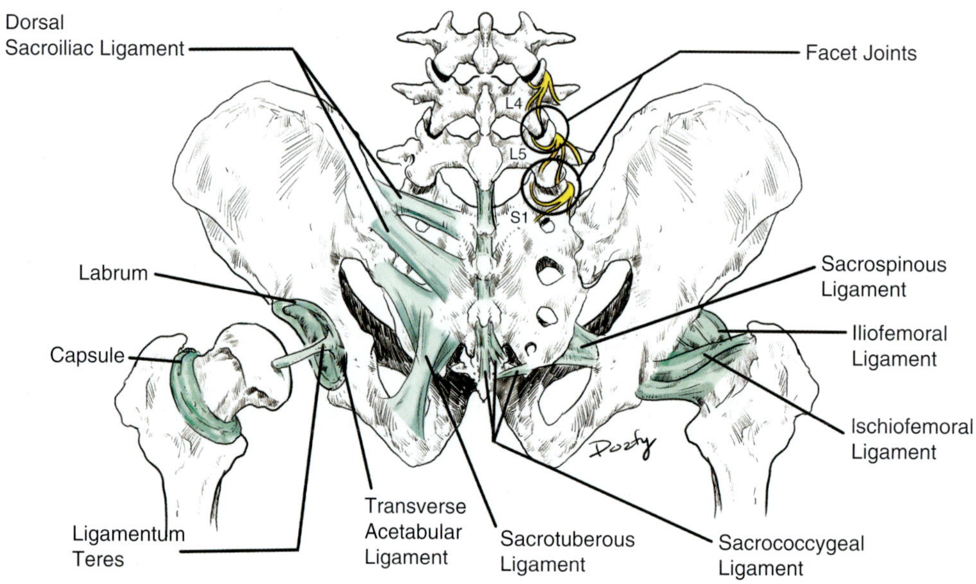

• **Fig. 14.4** Lumbosacral anatomy demonstrating facet joint innervation and pertinent ligaments.

Pertinent Anatomy

- The supraspinous ligament (SSL) is a strong fibrous cord-like structure that adjoins and overlies adjacent spinous processes.[12] The SSL is contiguous dorsally with the thoracodorsal fascia and ventrally with the interspinous ligament (ISL).
- The ISL is a thin membranous structure that traverses adjacent spinous processes from the root to the apex. The ISL connects dorsally with the SSL and ventrally with the ligamentum flavum (see Figs 14.2 and 14.3).

Common Pathology

- Ligament strain, partial tear,[13] relative laxity secondary to or underlying disc, and facet pathology.[14]

Equipment

- Ultrasound machine with low-frequency curvilinear probe. Alternatively, a high-frequency linear probe can be utilized in individuals with low body fat and minimal subcutaneous tissue.
- 22 to 25 gauge, 2- to 3-inch needle.

Common Injectate

- Prolotherapy
- Orthobiologics (PRP, bone marrow concentrate, etc.)

Injectate Volume

- 0.25 to 1 mL at each site

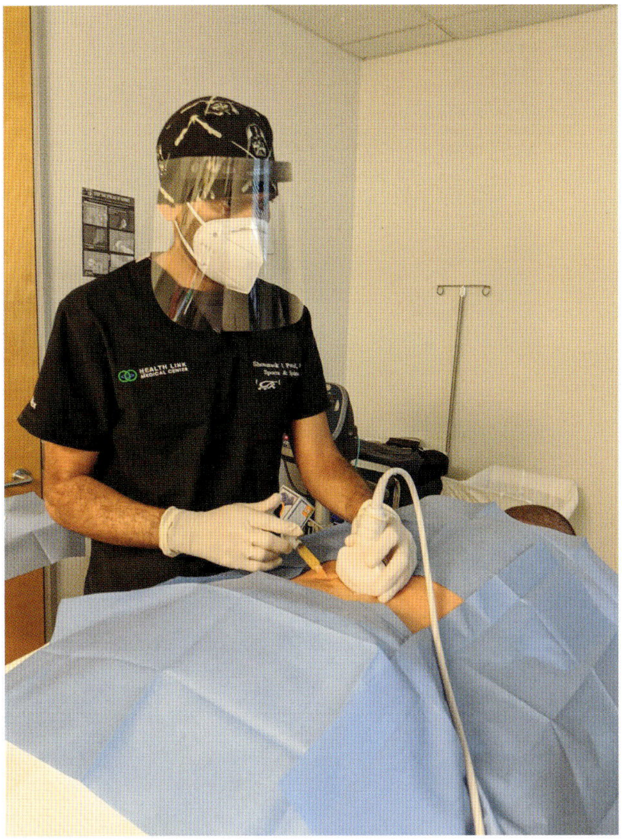

• **Fig. 14.5** Ultrasound-Guided Lumbar Facet Short-Axis In-Plane Setup.

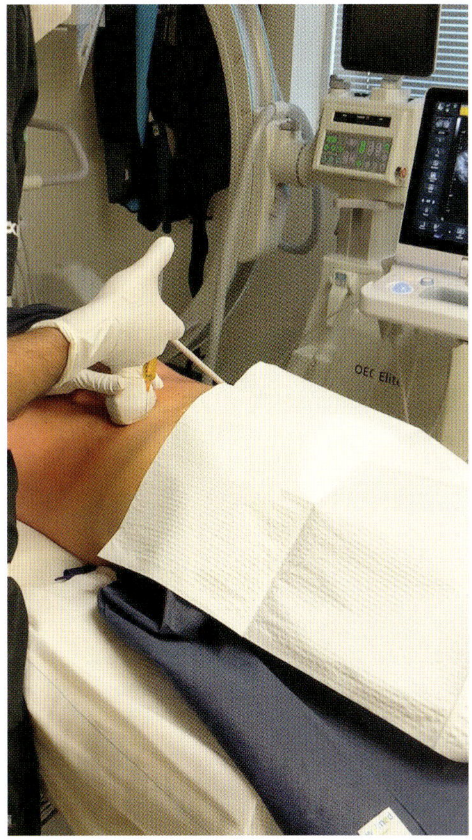

• **Fig. 14.7** Ultrasound-Guided Lumbar Facet Out-of-Plane Setup.

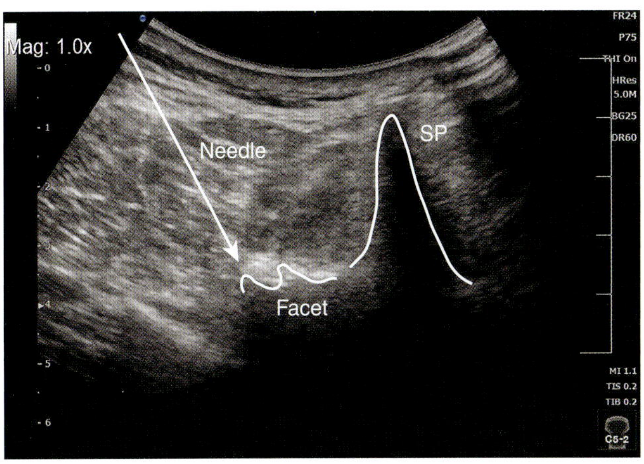

• **Fig. 14.6** Ultrasound Lumbar Facet Short-Axis In-Plane Injection. *SP*, Spinous process.

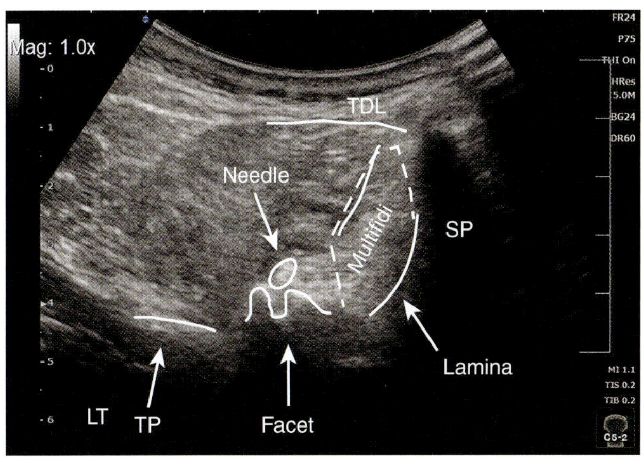

• **Fig. 14.8** Ultrasound-Guided Facet Short-Axis Out-of-Plane Injection. *SP*, Spinous process; *TP*, transverse process; *TDL*, thoracodorsal fascia; *LT*, left.

Technique

Patient Position

- Prone with a pillow under the lower abdomen/pelvis to allow lumbar spine to be in a flattened or rounded kyphotic position. This allows the spinous processes to be gapped and the ligaments to be taut.

Clinician Position

- Standing at the side of the patient with the ultrasound screen on the opposite side.

Transducer Position

- Short and/or long axis to the ligaments, with visualization of spinous processes (Figs 14.9 and 14.16).
- Switching back and forth may optimize targeting of needle tip.
- In short-axis view, identification of levels should be done by starting in the region of the sacrum. The L5 spinous process and lamina are much steeper and together with the bilateral facets and transverse processes further laterally form the appearance of a "crown." This is just

cephalad to the S1 spinous process, which comes off of a relatively flat sacral base that has more of a "tiara" appearance (Figs 14.9 and 14.13).

- Identification of levels can also be done with long-axis view; visualizing spinous processes from a midline axial position helps identify levels, starting caudally with the shallow relatively flat sacral spinous processes, cephalad to the steeper lumbar spinous processes (Figs 14.11 and 14.15).

Needle Position

- In-plane
    - With ligaments in short axis, introduce the needle in-plane lateral to medial to SSL superficial to the spinous process. Needle tip is walked cephalad or caudad and anteriorly into the interspinous gap. This is done while pivoting or fanning the ultrasound transducer to maintain the needle length in-plane (Fig. 14.10).
    - With ligaments in long axis, introduce the needle in-plane with the transducer from caudad to cephalad, with or without a gel stand-off to minimize anisotropy. Needle tip should be advanced to the spinous process to inject at the SSL, then walked cranially into the interspinous space for the ISL (Fig. 14.12).
- Out-of-plane
    - With ligaments in short axis, introduce the needle out-of-plane just caudad to the mid-point of the transducer. Needle tip should be advanced to the spinous process to inject at the SSL, then walked cranially into the interspinous space for the ISL. This is done while the transducer glides cephalad to follow the needle tip (Fig. 14.14).
    - With ligaments in long axis, introduce the needle out-of-plane just lateral to the mid-point of the transducer. Advance needle tip to the SSL superficial to or between the dorsal aspect of the spinous processes, then walk anteriorly into the interspinous space for the ISL (Fig. 14.16).

Target

- Diffusely through the SSL and ISL as deep as can safely be visualized.

PEARLS AND PITFALLS

- These ligaments may be difficult to visualize entirely, so adjacent and adjoining anatomy need to be visualized.
- For in-plane injections, needle angle and anisotropy need to be considered. With the ligaments in short axis, the needle can be obscured in the thoracodorsal fascia while approaching the SSL. With the ligaments in long axis, a gel stand-off may be required to limit anisotropy.
- For out-of-plane injections, the needle tip could inadvertently be advanced beyond the plane of the transducer Use doppler to see injectate flow can help (see Fig. 14.17).

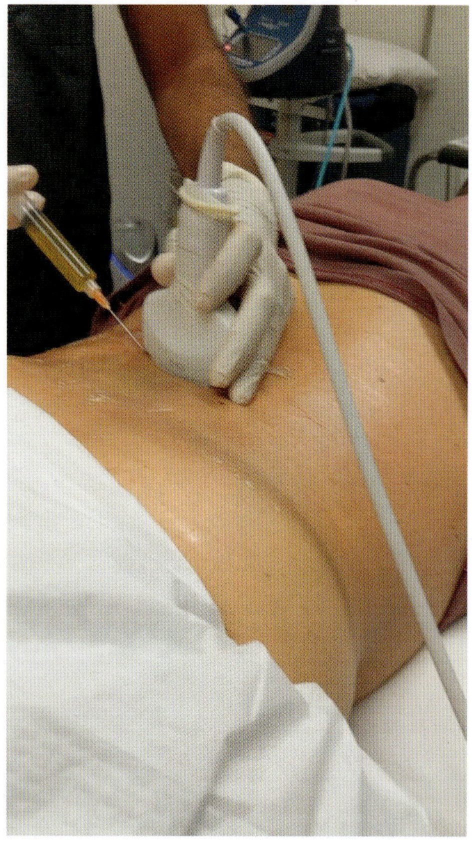

• **Fig. 14.9** Ultrasound-Guided Supraspinous and Interspinous Ligament Short-Axis In-Plane Injection Setup.

Multifidus Muscles

KEY POINTS

- The multifidus muscles can be targeted in isolation for specific injuries, but more commonly are targeted in combination with treating other components of the functional spinal unit, including ligaments (supraspinous/interspinous, intertransverse, iliolumbar, ligamentum flavum), the thoracodorsal fascia, zygapophysial (Z joints or facet) joints, nerve roots in the epidural space, and the intervertebral discs.
- Injections can be accomplished using a low-frequency curvilinear transducer.

Pertinent Anatomy

- The multifidus muscles are the most medial column of the three main lumbar paraspinal muscles, which are all enclosed between the thoracodorsal fascia posteriorly, the lamina, facet joints, transverse processes, and intertransverse (IT) ligaments anteriorly, and the spinous processes and ISLs medially. Unlike the erector spinae (the other two columns of the paraspinal muscles that run the length of the spine), the multifidus muscles consist of several fascicles that traverse three to six vertebral segments, attaching the spinous processes to the vertebral bodies, sacrum, posterior superior iliac spine (PSIS). and posterior sacroiliac ligaments.[15,16]

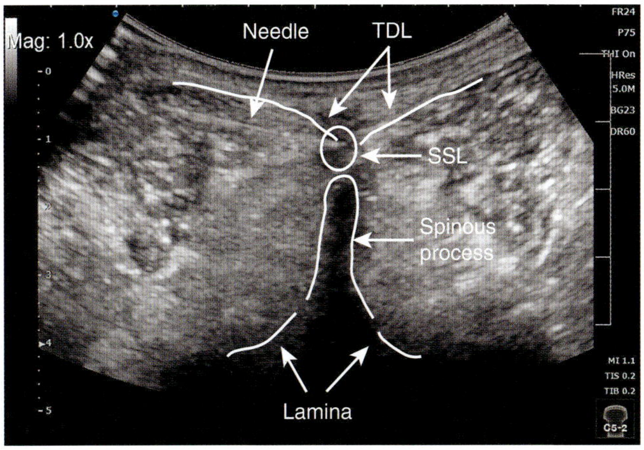

• **Fig. 14.10** Ultrasound-Guided Supraspinous and Interspinous Ligament Short-Axis In-Plane Injection. *SSL*, Supraspinous ligament.

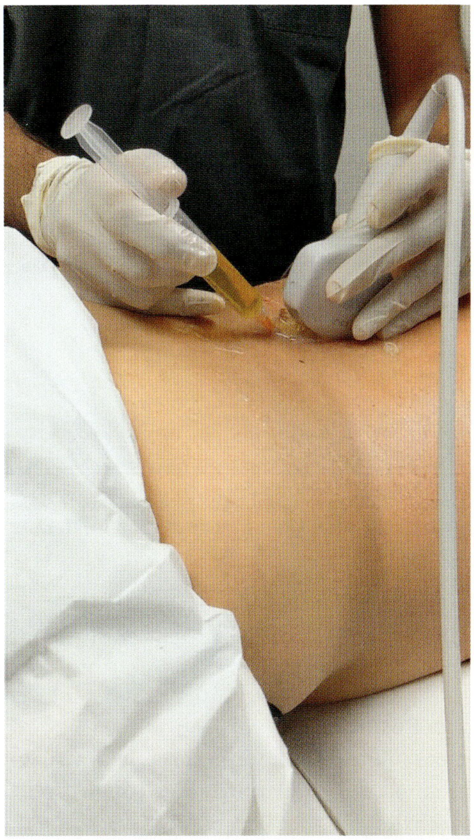

• **Fig. 14.11** Ultrasound-Guided Lumbar Supraspinous and Interspinous Ligament Long-Axis In-Plane Setup.

- The multifidus muscles provide functional stabilization, with deep and superficial fibers playing different roles in segmental motion.[17]

Common Pathology

- The multifidus muscles have been controversially linked to various low back conditions,[18,19] but ultimately they are involved as a part of the functional spinal unit. Pathology includes multifidus muscle atrophy associated with chronic degenerative spine pathology,[20,21] chronic low back pain,[22,23] chronic radiculopathy,[24] or iatrogenically from radiofrequency denervation,[25,5] or prior surgery.[26]

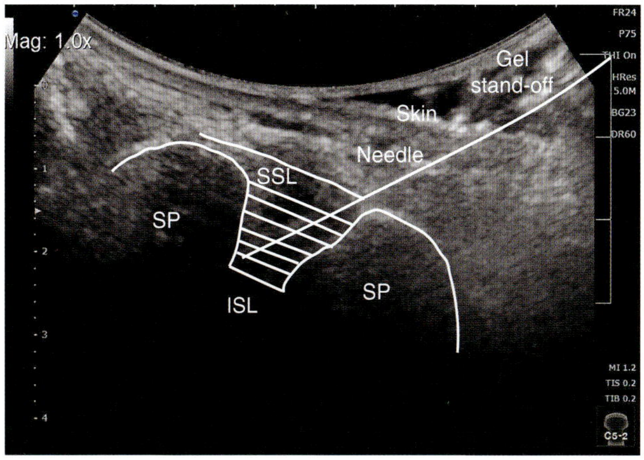

• **Fig. 14.12** Ultrasound-Guided Lumbar Supraspinous and Interspinous Ligament Long-Axis In-Plane Injection. *ISL*, Interspinous ligament; *SP*, spinous process; *SSL*, supraspinous ligament.

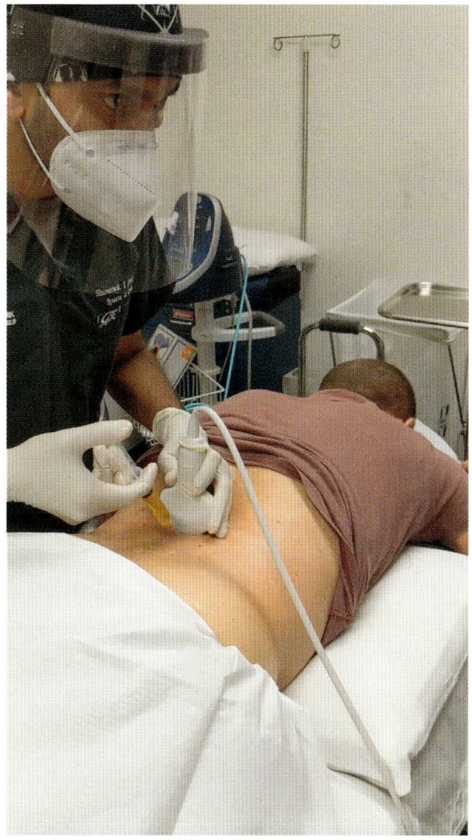

• **Fig. 14.13** Ultrasound-Guided Supraspinous and Interspinous Ligament Short-Axis Out-of-Plane Injection Setup.

- While often not mentioned in magnetic resonance imaging (MRI) radiology reports, pathology of the multifidus muscles is readily visible.[27]

Equipment

- Ultrasound machine with low-frequency curvilinear probe. Alternatively, a high-frequency linear probe can be utilized in individuals with low body fat and minimal subcutaneous tissue
- 22 to 27 gauge, 1.5- to 3-inch needle

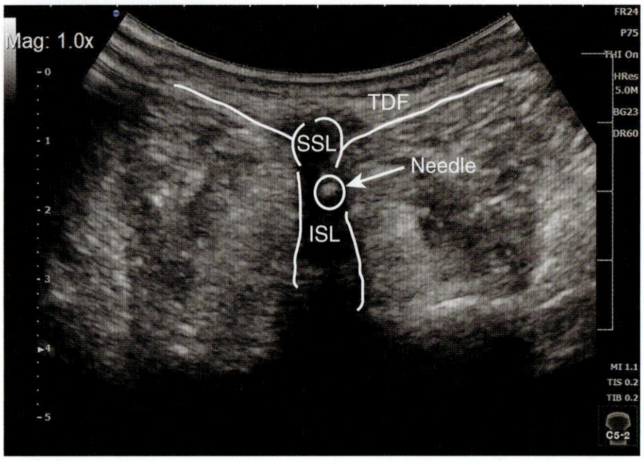

• **Fig. 14.14** Ultrasound-Guided Lumbar Supraspinous and Interspinous Ligament Short-Axis Out-of-Plane Injection. *ISL*, Interspinous ligament; *SSL*, supraspinous ligament.

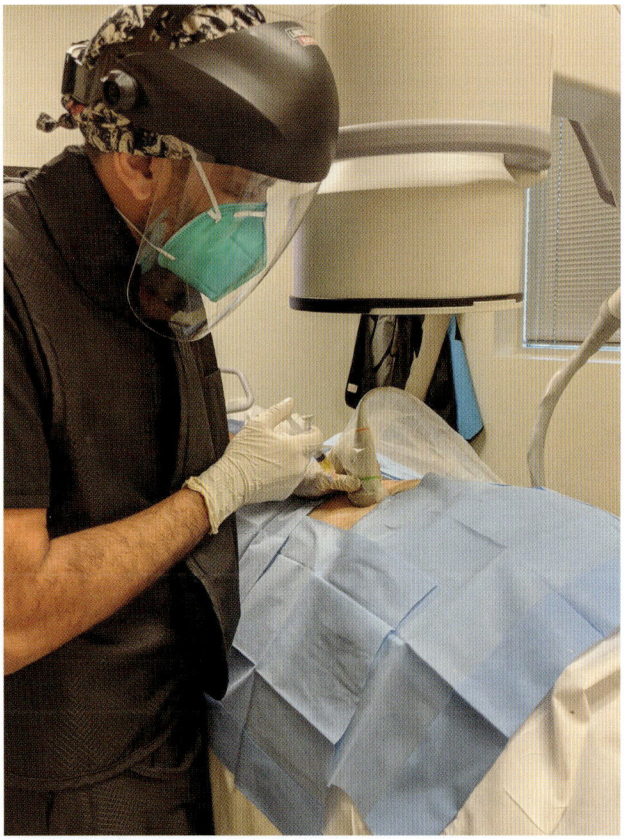

• **Fig. 14.15** Ultrasound-Guided Supraspinous and Interspinous Ligament Long-Axis Out-of-Plane Setup.

Common Injectate

- Local anesthetic for trigger point injection
- Orthobiologics (PRP, platelet-poor plasma [PPP])

Injectate Volume

- 0.25 to 2 mL at each site

Technique

Patient Position

- Prone with a pillow under the lower abdomen/pelvis to allow lumbar spine to be in a flattened or rounded kyphotic position.

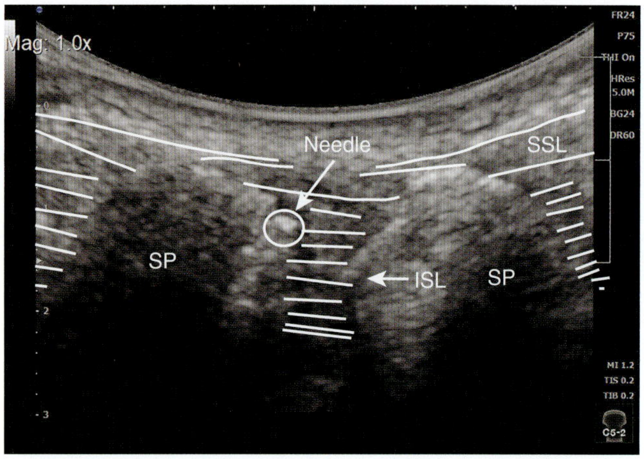

• **Fig. 14.16** Ultrasound-Guided Lumbar Supraspinous and Interspinous Ligament Long-Axis Out-of-Plane Injection. *ISL*, Interspinous ligament; *SP*, spinous process; *SSL*, supraspinous ligament.

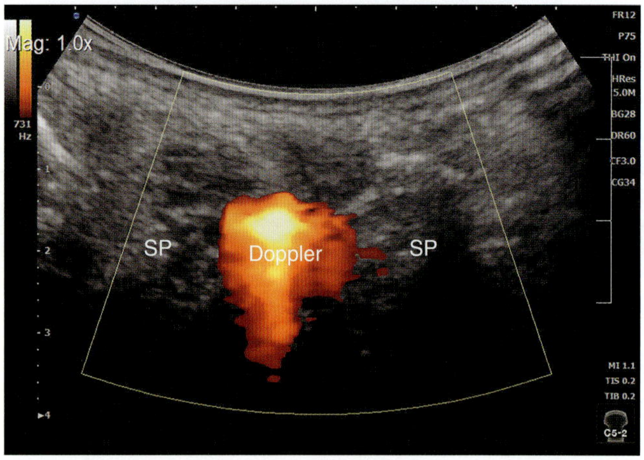

• **Fig. 14.17** Ultrasound-Guided Lumbar Supraspinous and Interspinous Ligament Long-Axis Out-of-Plane Injection with Doppler Flow. *SP*, Spinous process.

Clinician Position

- Standing at the side of the patient with the ultrasound screen on the opposite side.

Transducer Position

- Short axis to the multifidus muscles, with visualization of spinous processes and lamina (Figs 14.18A and 14.19A).
- In short-axis view, identification of levels should be done by starting in the region of the sacrum. The L5 spinous process and lamina are much steeper and together with the bilateral facets and transverse processes further laterally form the appearance of a "crown." This is just cephalad to the S1 spinous process, which comes off of a relatively flat sacral base that has more of a "tiara" appearance.
- Identification of levels can also be done with long-axis view, visualizing spinous processes from a midline axial position helps identify levels, starting caudally with the shallow relatively flat sacral spinous processes, cephalad to the steeper lumbar spinous processes. Turn 90 degrees at desired level.

Needle Position

- In-plane
  - Introduce the needle in-plane lateral to medial directed to lamina. Needle tip is walked anterior/

posterior and cephalad/caudad while injectate is administered (Fig 14.18B).
- Out-of-plane
  - Introduce the needle out-of-plane just caudad to the mid-point of the transducer, which is centered over the spinous process. Needle tip should be advanced to the spinous process, then walked off laterally into the multifidus muscle (Fig. 14.19B).

Target
- Multifidus lying just lateral to the spinous process and just superficial to the laminae.

PEARLS AND PITFALLS

- Take care to keep track of the needle tip. If a longer needle is used, the tip could be advanced into the interlaminar epidural space.
- For out-of-plane injections, the needle tip could inadvertently be advanced beyond the plane of the transducer. As the needle tip is advanced deeper, it can be tracked by tilting the probe in the direction of advancement.

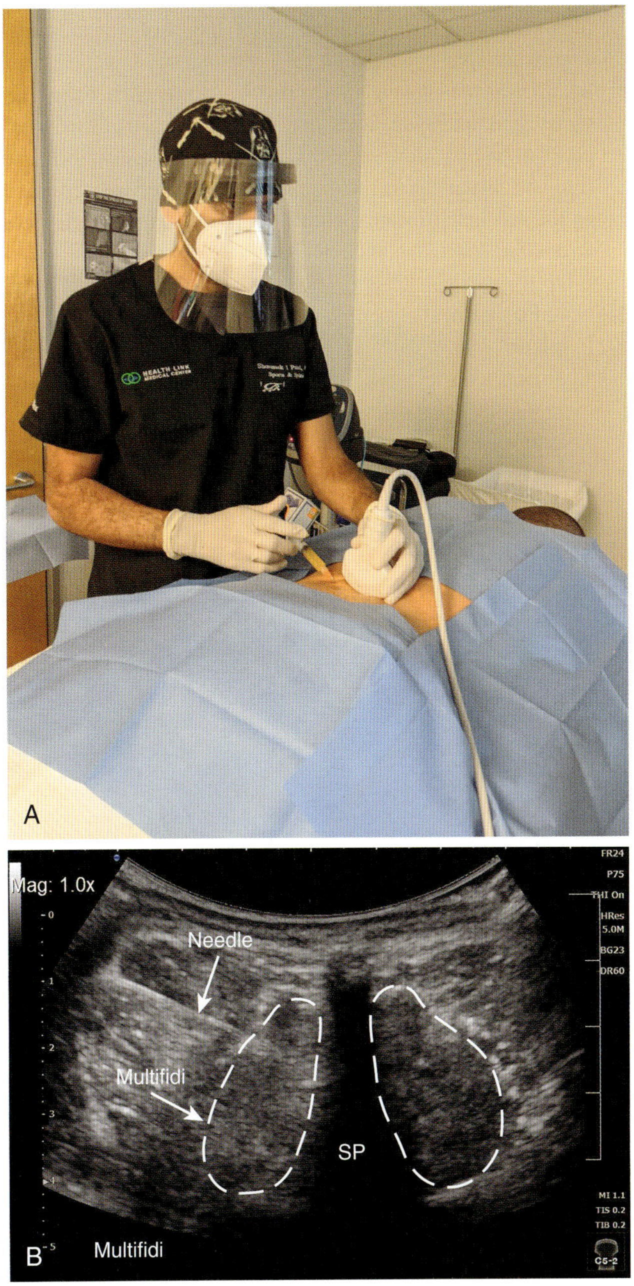

• **Fig. 14.18** Ultrasound-Guided Lumbar Multifidis Short Axis In-Plane (A) Setup; (B) Injection. *SP*, Spinous process.

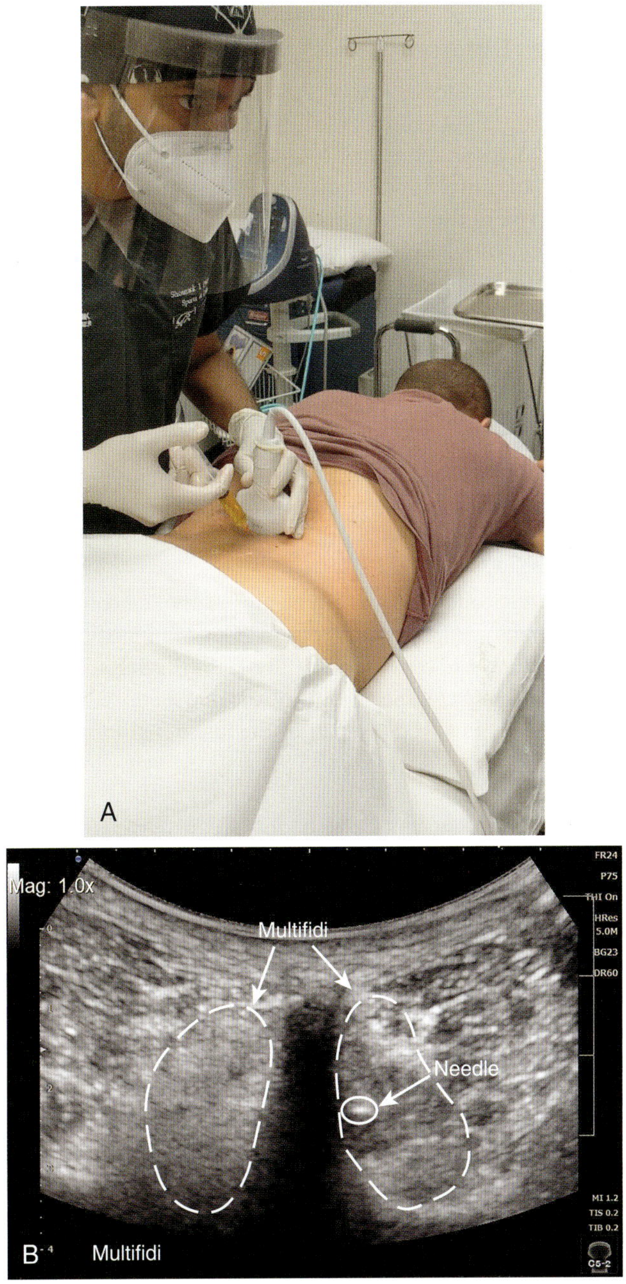

• **Fig. 14.19** (A) Ultrasound-Guided Lumbar Multifidis Short-Axis Out-of-Plane (A) Setup; (B) Injection.

Thoracodorsal Fascia

KEY POINTS

- The thoracodorsal fascia (also called the thoracolumbar fascia) can be targeted in isolation for focal injuries, but more commonly is targeted in combination with treating other components of the functional spinal unit,[28,29] along with ligaments (supraspinous/interspinous, intertransverse, iliolumbar, ligamentum flavum), paraspinal multifidus muscles, zygapophysial (Z joints or facet) joints, nerve roots in the epidural space, and the intervertebral discs.
- Injections can be accomplished using a low-frequency curvilinear transducer.

Pertinent Anatomy

- The thoracodorsal fascia is a thick retinaculum around the paraspinal muscles of the lumbar and sacral regions, composed of aponeurotic fascial tissue continuous with the paraspinal fascia throughout the spine from the cranial base to the sacrum.[30]
- Several muscles of the trunk and extremities insert into the thoracodorsal fascia.
- Laterally, the thoracodorsal fascia is in continuity with the fascia of all of the abdominal muscles, ultimately providing synchronization throughout the core muscles between the rectus abdominis and paraspinals.[31]
- Medially, the bilateral thoracodorsal fascia converges into the midline SSL, which in turn is contiguous ventrally with the ISLs into the ligamentum flavum (see Fig. 14.3).

Common Pathology

- The thoracodorsal fascia can be injured spontaneously with a hernia[32] or iatrogenically from even minimally invasive procedures like vertebroplasty[33] or LASER spine surgery.[34]
- In the absence of specific injury, the thoracodorsal fascia is ultimately involved as a part of the functional spinal unit.

Equipment

- Ultrasound machine with low-frequency curvilinear probe. Alternatively, a high-frequency linear probe can be utilized in individuals with low body fat and minimal subcutaneous tissue.
- 22 to 25 gauge, 2- to 3-inch needle.

Common Injectate

- Prolotherapy solution[35]
- Orthobiologics (PRP, etc.)

Injectate Volume

- 0.25 to 10 mL at each site

Technique

Patient Position

- Prone with a pillow under the lower abdomen/pelvis to allow lumbar spine to be in a flattened or rounded kyphotic position.

Clinician Position

- Standing at the side of the patient with the ultrasound screen on the opposite side.

Transducer Position

- Short axis to the SSL, ISL, and multifidus muscles, with the thoracodorsal fascia arching laterally off the midline spinous processes and SSL (Figs 14.20 and 14.22).
- In short-axis view, identification of levels should be done by starting in the region of the sacrum. The L5 spinous process and lamina are much steeper and together with the bilateral facets and transverse processes further laterally form the appearance of a "crown." This is just cephalad to the S1 spinous process, which comes off of a relatively flat sacral base that has more of a "tiara" appearance.
- Identification of levels can also be done with long-axis view; visualizing spinous processes from a midline axial position helps identify levels, starting caudally with the shallow relatively flat sacral spinous processes, cephalad to the steeper lumbar spinous processes. Turn 90 degrees at desired level.

Needle Position

- In-plane
  - Introduce the needle in-plane lateral to medial directed along the thoracodorsal fascia. Can redirect superior and inferior to get broader coverage (Fig. 14.21).
- Out-of-plane

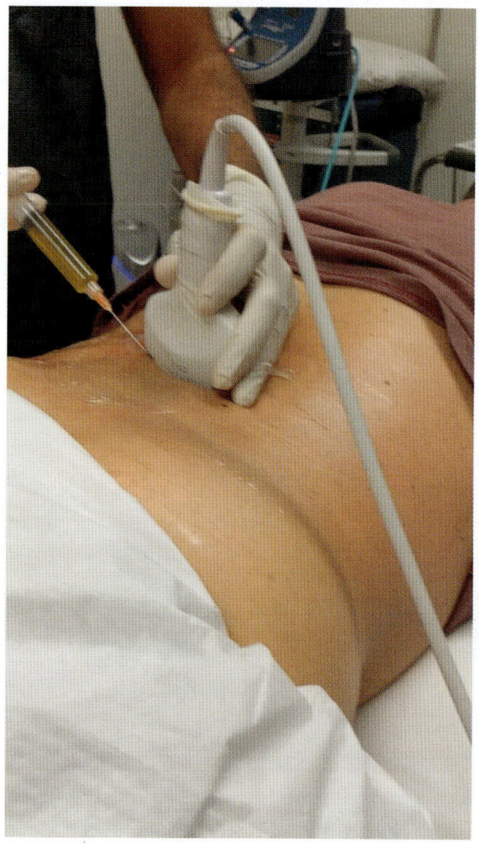

• **Fig. 14.20** Ultrasound-Guided Superficial TDF In-Plane Setup.

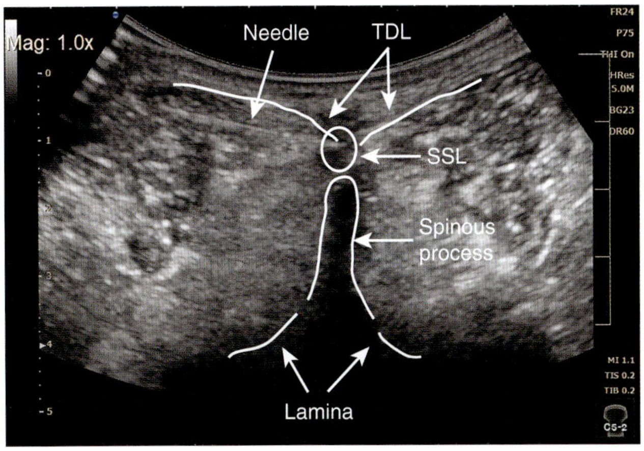

• **Fig. 14.21** Ultrasound-Guided Superficial TDF In-Plane Injection. *SSL*, Supraspinous ligament.

- Introduce the needle out-of-plane just caudad to the mid-point of the transducer, which is centered over the spinous process. Needle tip should be advanced to the spinous process, then walked off laterally and superficially into the thoracodorsal fascia (Fig. 14.23).

Target

- TDF fibers overlying the erector spinae muscles from the spinous process out as lateral as desired.

PEARLS AND PITFALLS

- For in-plane injections, needle angle and anisotropy need to be considered. With the ligaments in short axis, the needle can be obscured in the thoracodorsal fascia while approaching the SSL. With the ligaments in long axis, a gel stand-off may be required to limit anisotropy.
- For out-of-plane injections, the needle tip could inadvertently be advanced beyond the plane of the transducer.

Iliolumbar, Intertransverse Ligaments

KEY POINTS

- Injured iliolumbar intertransverse ligaments may or may not be primary pain generators but should be considered as part of the spinal functional unit (adjacent vertebrae, intervertebral disc, ligaments, and facet joints) in which injury to any part can cause biomechanical alterations leading to degeneration and pain.[36]
- These ligaments can get stressed with scoliosis.

Pertinent Anatomy

- The IT ligaments course between and just anterior to the transverse processes.
- The iliolumbar (IL) ligament can have several anatomic variations but mostly courses between the transverse processes of the lowest lumbar vertebra (typically L5) and the iliac crest.[12]

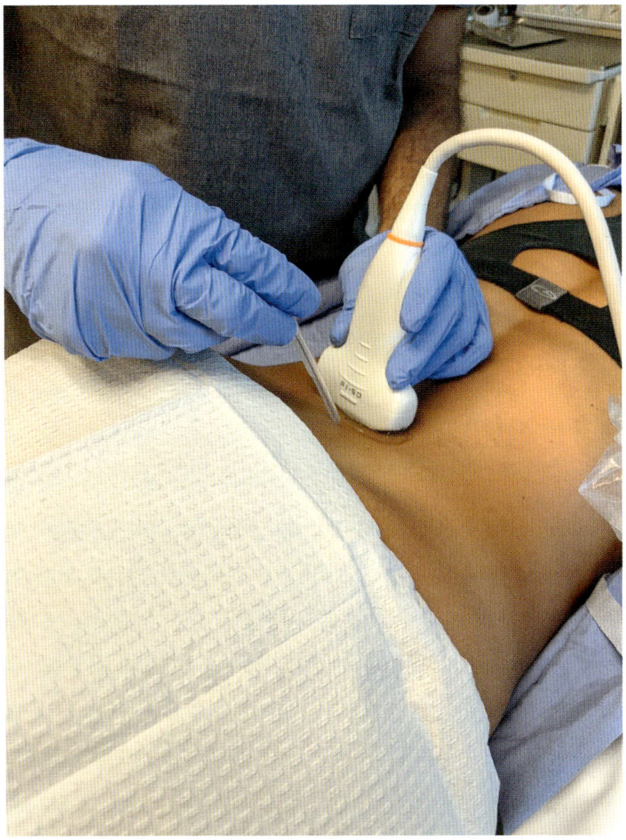

• **Fig. 14.22** Ultrasound-Guided Superficial TDF Out-of-Plane Setup.

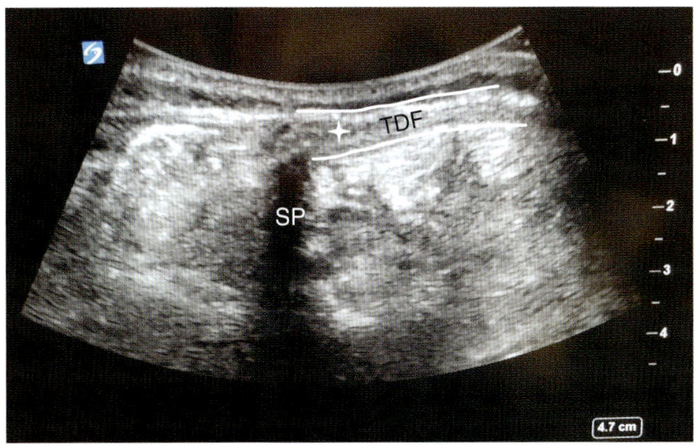

• **Fig. 14.23** Ultrasound-Guided Superficial TDF Out-of-Plane Injection. *SP*, spinous process; *TDF*; thoracodorsal fascia; *Star*, needle tip in TDF.

Common Pathology

- Traumatic injury.
- Lumbar ligament injuries are common after motor vehicle accidents (MVAs) or traumas.
- Lumbar spondylosis, degenerative disease, and loss of lordosis can cause lumbar ligament laxity and vice versa.
- Scoliosis: for a lateral curve the IT ligaments are stretched/lax at the convexity of the curve at that segment and are the targets for injection.

- Buckling and hypertrophy of the ligamentum flavum associated with degenerative disk disease, segmental motion abnormalities, spondylosis, and contributes to spinal stenosis.[36]
- Iliolumbar syndrome has been described as unilateral low back pain at the posterior iliac crest, reproduced by hip flexion and the Patrick test. One small study showed that 25% dextrose solution helped pain in 6/7 patients.[37]

Equipment

- Ultrasound machine with low-frequency curvilinear probe
- 22 to 25 gauge, 2- to 3-inch needle

Common Injectates

- Prolotherapy, orthobiologics (PRP, bone marrow concentrate, etc.)
- Avoid intraligamentous corticosteroids

Injectate Volume

- 0.5 to 1 mL per area/ligament

Technique

Patient Position

- Prone with a pillow under the lower abdomen/pelvis to allow lumbar spine to be in a flattened or rounded kyphotic position.

Clinician Position

- Standing at the side of the patient with the ultrasound screen on the opposite side.

Transducer Position

- Long axis to spine, short axis to the transverse processes (Fig. 14.24).
- Start scanning at the sacrum and count L5 up to targeted region.
- Scan laterally until the most lateral aspect of the transverse process are visualized.

Needle Position

- In-plane, distal to proximal or proximal to distal approach (Fig. 14.25).
- Alternatively, can inject out-of-plane medial to lateral (Figs 14.26 and 14.27).

Target

- IL ligament distal to the L5 spinous process.
- IT ligaments at levels above L5.
- Target the fibers traversing between the spinous processes just deep to bony tip.

PEARLS AND PITFALLS

- Heel toe maneuver with gel stand-off can be helpful to visualize the needle better.
- Always visualize needle tip and be careful not to go deep into the retroperitoneal space (higher risk with out-of-plane injections).

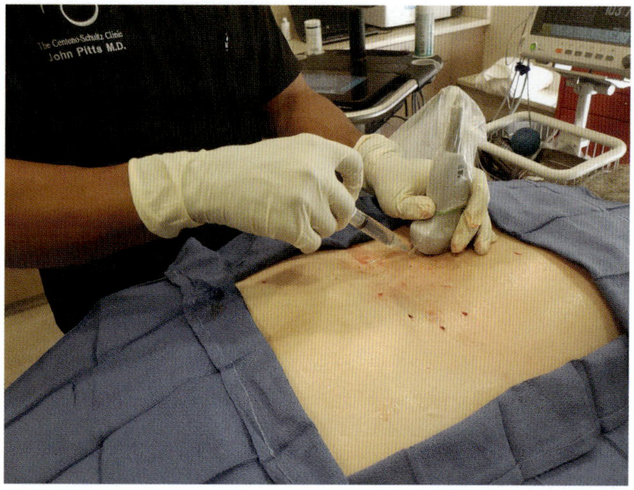

• **Fig. 14.24** Ultrasound-Guided Long-Axis Interspinous Ligament In-Plane Setup.

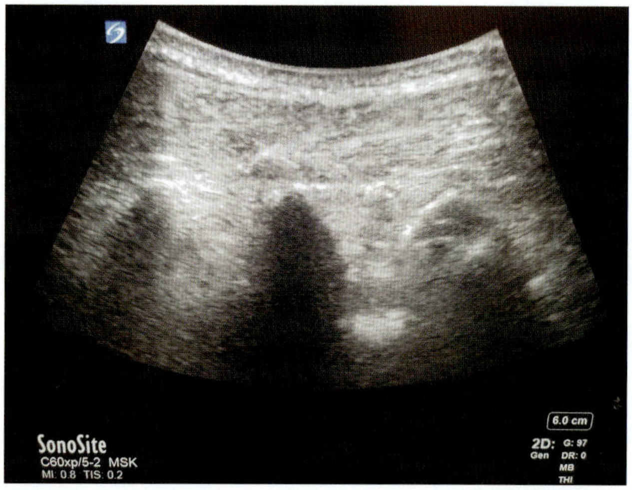

• **Fig. 14.25** Ultrasound-Guided Long Axis Interspinous Ligament In-Plane Injection.

Quadratus Lumborum Origins Off the Iliac Crest

KEY POINTS

- The quadratus lumborum (QL) has great anatomic variability; thus, ultrasound to visualize it is the best modality
- QL injury or pain syndromes are likely an underdiagnosed problem but typically result in myofascial pain.[38]
- The injection describes the tendon injections if typical myofascial treatments for QL pain fail or there is suspected tendon injury form trauma.

Pertinent Anatomy

- Originates on the superior wing of the posterior iliac crest (extends up to 5 to 7 cm laterally) and IL ligament
- Inserts on the anterior inferior border of the 12th rib (extending 4.5 to 7 cm laterally) and off the lateral borders of the L1-4 transverse processes

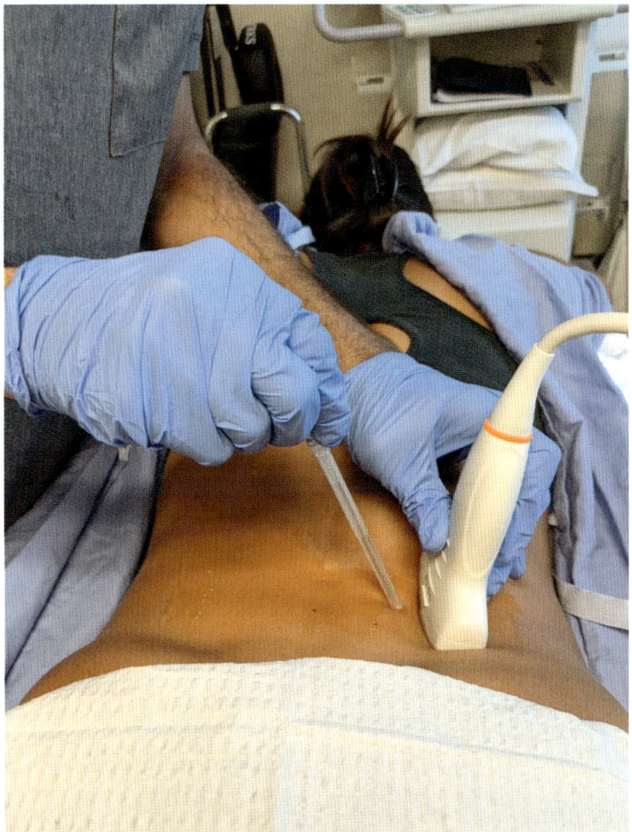

• **Fig. 14.26** Ultrasound-Guided Long-Axis Interspinous Ligament Out-of-Plane Setup.

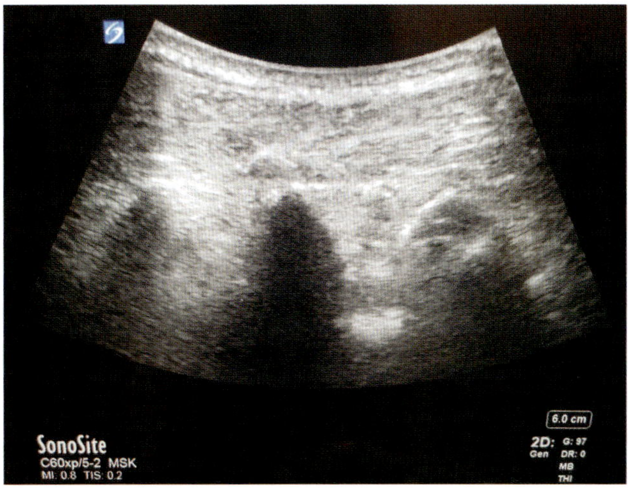

• **Fig. 14.27** Ultrasound-Guided Interspinous Ligament Out-of-Plane Injection.

- There is great variability to its locations and can have interwoven fibers of the different intrinsic spinal muscles
- The iliohypogastric and ilioinguinal nerves course along the ventral muscle fibers
- The QL lies posterior to the colon, kidneys, and diaphragm and deep to the spinal erectors
- The anterior primary ramus of the 12th thoracic spinal nerve runs in the abdominal wall inferior to the 12th rib, known as the subcostal nerve
- Unilateral contraction causes ipsilateral trunk flexion; bilateral contraction extends the trunk and flexes the 12th rib during inspiration
- These muscle actions are small and so may play more of a role in lumbar stability.[39]

Common Pathology

- Muscle and tendon injury after traumatic event via hyper-flexion or hyper-contralateral flexion mechanisms.

Equipment

- Ultrasound machine with low-frequency curvilinear probe
- 22 to 25 gauge, 2- to 3-inch needle

Common Injectates

- Local anesthetics for diagnostics or for muscle trigger point or QL blocks
- Orthobiologics (PRP, platelet poor plasma, bone marrow concentrate, etc.)

Injectate Volume

- 0.5 to 1 mL per tendon area

Technique

Patient Position

- Prone with a pillow under the lower abdomen/pelvis to allow lumbar spine to be in a flattened or rounded kyphotic position.

Clinician Position

- Standing at the side of the patient with the ultrasound screen on the opposite side.

Transducer Position

- Long axis to spine and QL (Fig. 14.28).
- Can rotate to visualize more medial or lateral fibers.
- Identify the posterior medial superior border of the iliac crest.
- Scan up to 5 to 7 cm laterally from the medial border.

Needle Position

- In-plane, proximal to distal approach (Fig. 14.29).
- May use two to four different needle entry sites to target multiple areas of the tendons.

Target

- Tendon fibers at and proximal to the iliac crest.
- Hypoechoic fibers and the enthesopathy points.

PEARLS AND PITFALLS

- Heel toe maneuver with gel stand-off can be helpful to visualize the needle better.

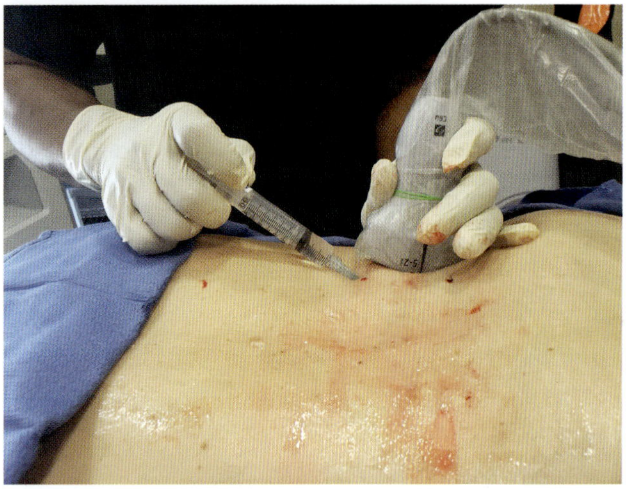

• **Fig. 14.28** Ultrasound-Guided Long-Axis Quadratus Lumborum In-Plane Setup.

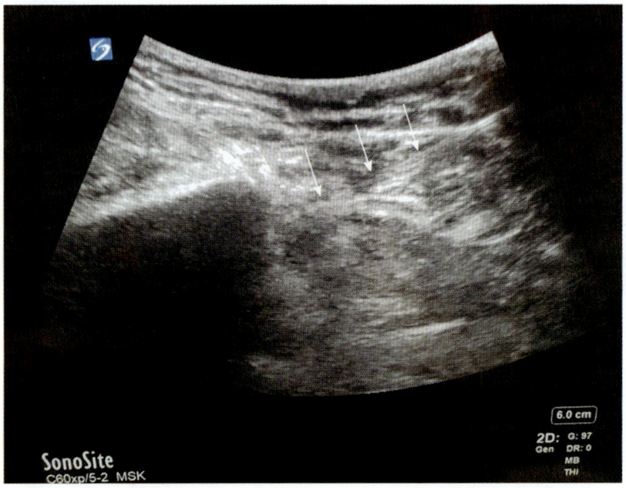

• **Fig. 14.29** Ultrasound-Guided Long Axis Quadratus Lumbar In-Plane Injection. *Arrows*, needle.

Fluoroscopy-Guided Techniques

Lumbar Transforaminal Epidurals

KEY POINTS

- Real-time live fluoroscopy is key for visualizing intravascular injection. Inject contrast slowly and carefully and assess the flow pattern. Do not rely on aspiration.
- Digital subtraction can be considered if there is a question of aberrant flow pattern or difficulty with visualization due to other factors such as contrast or hardware obscuring the view with live fluoroscopy.
- Particulate steroids are not recommended due the risk of catastrophic consequences thought to be from particulate steroid embolization via the arterial supply to the brain and spinal cord.[40–43]
- Particulate steroids have not been found to be consistently superior to soluble steroids (dexamethasone or betamethasone) in efficacy.[43]
- Platelet lysate epidural injections for lumbar radicular pain have evidence that they can help pain and function.[44]

Pertinent Anatomy

- The intervertebral foramen is bordered by:
  - Posterior: the inferior and superior articular processes
  - Superior/Inferior: The pedicles superiorly and inferiorly
  - Anterior: Vertebral body and intervertebral disc anteriorly from a lateral view
- The spinal canal (dural sac) lies medial from an anterior-posterior perspective
- Would add anatomy of vascularization of the spinal cord (Fig. 14.30)
  - Pedicle (P)—Eye
  - Pars interarticularis (PI)—Neck
  - Superior articulating process (SAP)—Ear
  - Transverse process—Nose
  - Spinous process (SP)—Tail
  - Lamina (L)—Body
  - Inferior articulating process (IAP)—Legs

Common Pathology

- Lumbar disc herniation
- Facet arthrosis or synovial cyst with nerve root impingement
- Disc osteophyte, resulting in subarticular narrowing
- Spinal stenosis with symptomatic neurogenic claudication

Equipment

- C-arm fluoroscope
- Extension tubing
- 22 to 25 gauge, 3.5- to 7-inch needle depending on body habitus
- Contrast

Common Injectates

- Local anesthetic and non-particulate corticosteroids
- Orthobiologics (platelet lysate)
- Avoid particulate steroids

Injectate Volume

- 2 to 5 mL, pending the degree of stenosis and patient tolerance
- Prior studies have shown that with an injectate volume of 2.8 mL, 95% of the lumbar transforaminal epidurals will spread to the superior aspect of the superior intervertebral disc and with 3.6 mL total volume, 95% with reach to the inferior aspect of the inferior intervertebral disc.[45]

Technique: Subpedicular Approach

Patient Position

- Prone with abdomen on a pillow to reduce lumbar lordosis.

C-Arm Position

- Confirm the level using the anteroposterior (AP) view and counting down from the 12th rib.
- Line up the superior endplate corresponding to the correct vertebrae by tilting the C-arm cephalad or caudal. This should "square off" the target segment.

- Oblique the C-arm ipsilateral to visualize the "Scotty Dog."
- The SAP of the level below will be below the 6 o'clock position of the pedicle above.
- Obtain a non-obstructed view of the chin of the "Scotty Dog" or 6 o'clock position of the pedicle.
- If the iliac crest obstructs the trajectory to the L5-S1 foramen, a more cephalad tilt and a less oblique angle may be required.
- It is recommended to have a more lateral rather than medial bias to decrease the risk of neural injury (6:30 if procedure is on the right side, or 5:30 if procedure is on the left side).[46]
- Will use the AP view to triangulate the needle position. Optimal position in the AP view requires:
  - "Squaring" of superior and inferior endplate of the target level using a cephalad or caudal tilt.
  - The spinous process should be midline using an oblique tilt.
- Optional to use "true" lateral view to ascertain depth. Optimal position in the lateral view requires:
  - "Squaring" the superior and inferior endplate of the target level using a wigwag.

Needle Position

- Slight bend in the needle can help with navigation.
- Start slightly inferior lateral to the final target as this starting point will make it easier to navigate around potential osteophytes off the SAP or transverse process.
- Place the needle coaxial to the fluoroscopic beam using intermittent fluoroscopic guidance in the oblique view, guiding the needle towards the 6 o'clock position of the pedicle.
- Do not advance too deep in the oblique view without checking an AP view.
- Authors recommend in the oblique view to gently touch os at the inferior aspect of the pedicle to ascertain depth.
- Withdraw the needle slightly; then redirect just inferior to the pedicle.
- Obtain an AP view to ascertain depth and medial trajectory. The needle tip should not pass the midpedicular line (6 o' clock of the pedicle) in the AP to avoid dural puncture.
- Optional to obtain lateral view to ascertain depth.

Target

- The target point is also known as the "safe triangle" formed by the pedicle superiorly and the spinal nerve that passes in a tangent inferomedially.[47]
- By staying in the superior one-sixth of the "safe triangle" there is less risk of neural injury; however, vascular penetration can still occur.[48]
- In the AP view the needle should not pass the 6 o'clock position of the pedicle.
- In the lateral view the needle should land close to the facet joint silhouette within the superior aspect of the foramen.

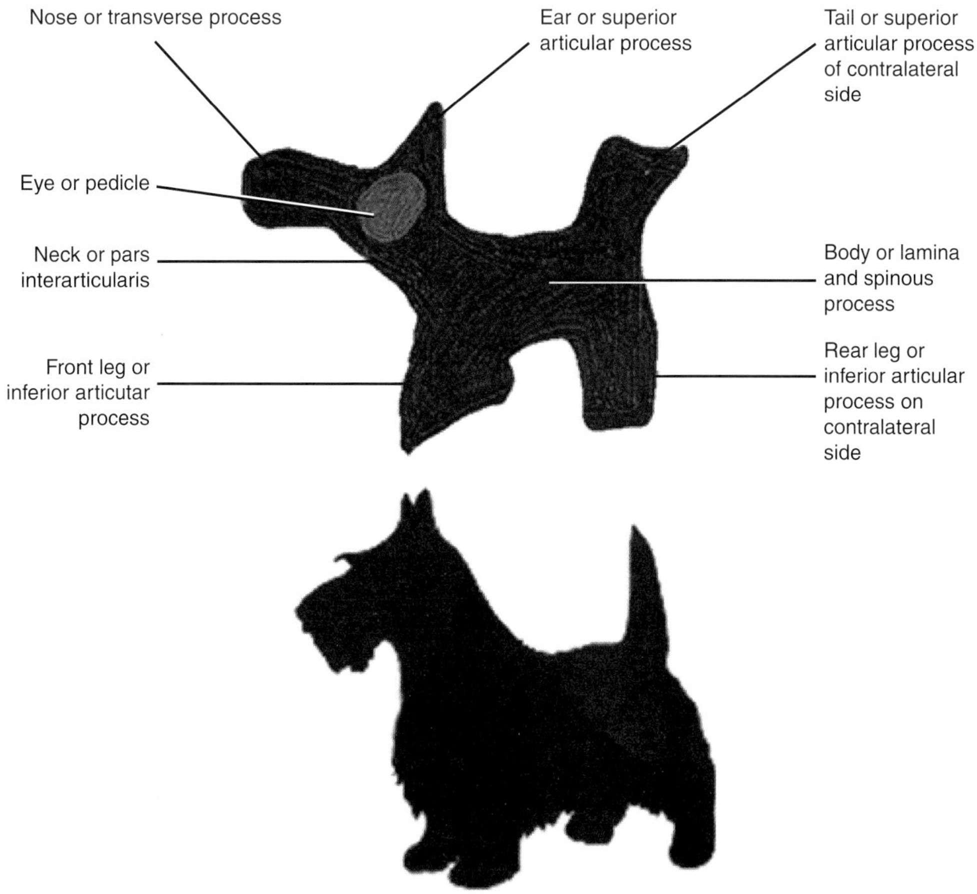

• **Fig. 14.30** Scotty dog fluoro image and anatomic sketch.

- The anterior or ventral aspect of the foramen should be avoided due to increased risk of vascular injury or vascular injection as the radicular arteries and intervertebral veins typically lie dorsal to the vertebral body.
- Attach extension tubing, keeping the needle still.
- Aspirate to ensure no vascular uptake; then inject a small amount of contrast under live fluoroscopy.
- In the AP view, contrast should flow epidurally along the medial pedicle border with or without peripheral extension around the spinal nerve.
- In the lateral view, contrast should flow against the posterior margin of the vertebral body.

PEARLS AND PITFALLS

- If the needle is adjusted in the lateral view, the AP view should also be checked to confirm that the needle has not advanced past the mid-pedicular line (6 o'clock of the pedicle).
- If at any point, neuropathic pain is elicited, the needle should be withdrawn and repositioned. If the pain does not resolve, the procedure should be aborted. Pain should not be used as an indicator of needle placement.
- The injection of contrast should be done under live fluoroscopy.
- Extension tubing should be used for stability to avoid inadvertent movements.
- Ideal flow should outline the desired spinal nerve and then flow medially into the epidural under the pedicle.
- Avoid intrathecal or subdural flow patterns.
- Avoid all vascular flow patterns.
- Be aware of the characteristic downward "hairpin" turn of the artery of Adamkiewicz (arteria radicularis magnus). This vessel supplies the spinal cord from T8 to the conus medullaris. It has a high degree of anatomic variation but typically enters the canal between T12-L3 and is more commonly found on the left side (Figs. 14.31–14.34).[49–52]

Technique: Infraneural Transforaminal Epidural

Patient Position

- Prone with abdomen on a pillow to reduce lumbar lordosis.

C-Arm Position

- Square off of vertebrae at injection level.
- Identify the pedicle, pars interarticularis, transverse process, spinous process.
- Ipsilateral oblique to rotate the SAP to approximately one-half to one-third of the width of disc space.

Needle Position

- The initial target is the lateral aspect of the SAP of the inferior vertebral level.
- For example, when targeting the L4-5 foramen, one should target the SAP of the L5 vertebrae.
- The needle is inserted just lateral to the SAP and advanced in a coaxial position.
- Once the needle contacts the SAP or is felt to be at the depth of the SAP, a lateral view should be obtained.
- Intermittent AP and lateral multiplanar views should be utilized to assess depth in relation to the foramen.
- The needle can slowly be advanced past the SAP with care to note any changes in "feel" consistent with inadvertent disc access.

Target

- In the AP view, the needle should not be advanced past the 6 o' clock position of the superior pedicle to avoid intrathecal or subdural needle placement.
- In a true lateral view, the needle should be just anterior to the SAP in its final position.

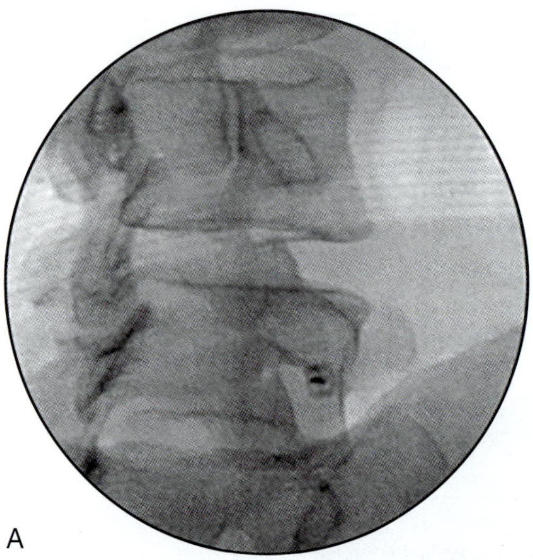

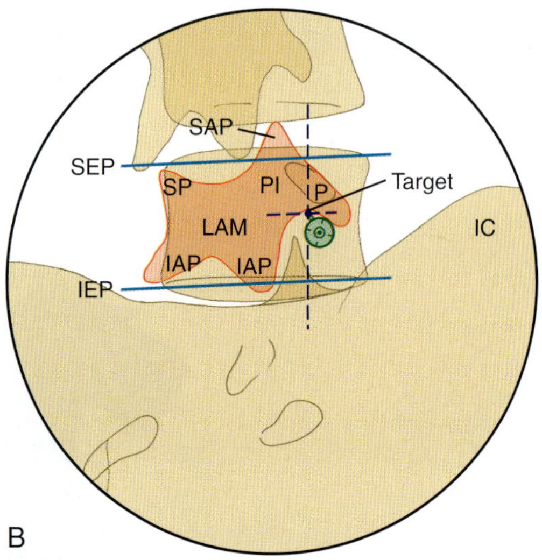

• **Fig. 14.31** (A) Fluoroscopic image of oblique "scotty dog" view with target below the chin of the Scotty dog with pertinent anatomy labeled. (B) Artist's rendition of the fluoroscopic image with pertinent anatomy labeled similar to shown. *IAP*, Inferior articular process; *IC*, iliac crest; *L*, lamina; *P*, pedicle; *SAP*, superior articular process; *SP*, spinal process; *TP*, transverse process. (From Furman MB. *Atlas of Image-Guided Spinal Procedures*. 2nd ed. Elsevier; 2018.[71])

- Attach extension tubing, keeping the needle still.
- Aspirate to ensure no vascular uptake; then inject a small amount of contrast under live fluoroscopy. Confirm epidural flow in both AP and lateral views.

PEARLS AND PITFALLS

- Multiplanar imaging is essential.
- If the needle is found too ventral on lateral view, the initially set up was likely not oblique enough. A less oblique trajectory results in a more ventral position on lateral view and a less medial needle position on AP.
- If the needle is found too medial on AP but has not reached the foramen on lateral, the initial trajectory was likely too oblique, and readjustment is required to make the trajectory less medial and more ventral. A more oblique trajectory results in a more medial needle position on AP and a less ventral position on lateral view.
- Do not advance too deep in the oblique or lateral view without checking an AP view.
- The needle tip should not pass the mid-pedicular line (6 o' clock of the pedicle) in the AP to avoid dural puncture.
- Be aware of the characteristic downward "hairpin" turn of the artery of Adamkiewicz.
- Beware of placing the needle too inferior and ventral to avoid intradiscal puncture. This is more common with an infraneural approach.
- Caution with needle advancement past the SAP given proximity of the intervertebral disc. With proper technique, Levi et al. reported intradiscal needle placement 4.7% occurrence.[53]
- Pre-procedure MRI review is imperative to confirm adequate epidural space for needle placement. Dural ectasia or Tarlov cysts should be noted prior to injection.
- Be aware of intrathecal, subdural, and vascular flow patterns (Figs 14.35 and 14.36).

Lumbar Interlaminar Epidural Injection

KEY POINTS

- Aseptic technique should be followed during the performance of any epidural injection.
- A fluoroscope should be used for routine performance of interlaminar epidural injections for the management of painful conditions.
- A loss of resistance technique is commonly performed to access the epidural space from an interlaminar approach.
- Contrast spread should cover the target of interest to ensure appropriate injectate delivery.

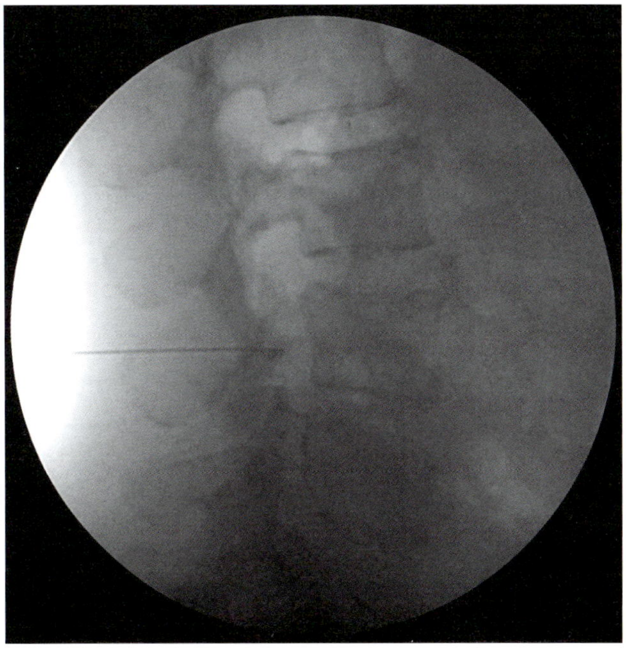

• **Fig. 14.33** Lateral View with the Needle in Superior and Dorsal Aspect of the Foramen Epidural Space.

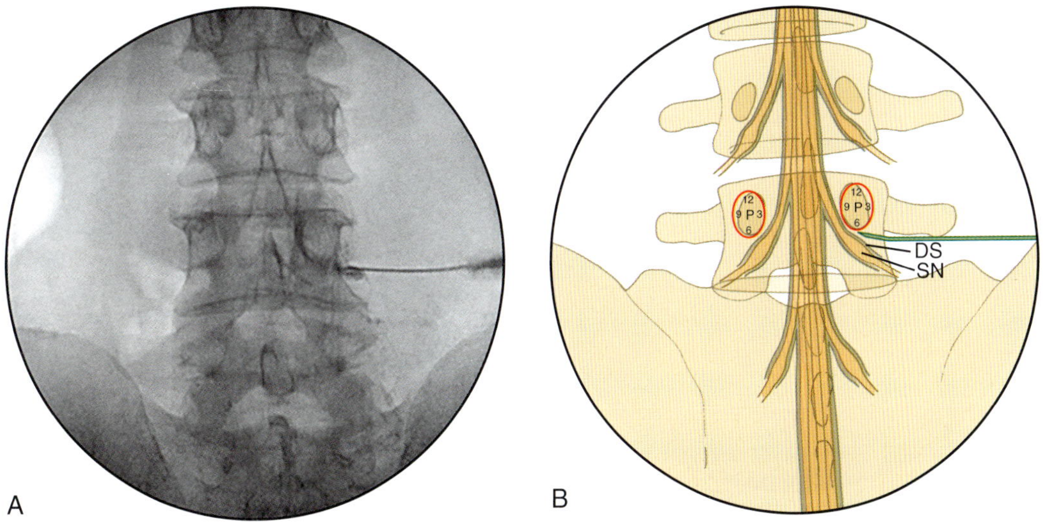

• **Fig. 14.32** (A) Anteroposterior view of a right L4-5 transforaminal epidural using the subpedicular approach. Contrast flow shows nerve root medial flow to the pedicle into the epidural space. (B) Artist rendition of the fluoroscopic image with pertinent anatomy labeled similar to shown. (From Furman MB. *Atlas of Image-Guided Spinal Procedures*. 2nd ed. Elsevier; 2018.)

Pertinent Anatomy

- The lumbar interlaminar space is a semicircular or ellipsoid space, with the laminar convexity at the superior aspect of the lamina. The lumbar interlaminar space is named by the lamina of the level above and below (e.g., the L4-5 interlaminar space is bound by the L4 lamina superiorly and the L5 lamina inferiorly). The epidural space proper is just deep to the spinolaminar line and bound by the ligamentum flavum posteriorly and the dura anteriorly (Figs. 14.37 and 14.38).
- The lumbar epidural space contains fat, vasculature including Batson's valveless venous plexus, and exiting nerve roots (see Fig. 14.3).

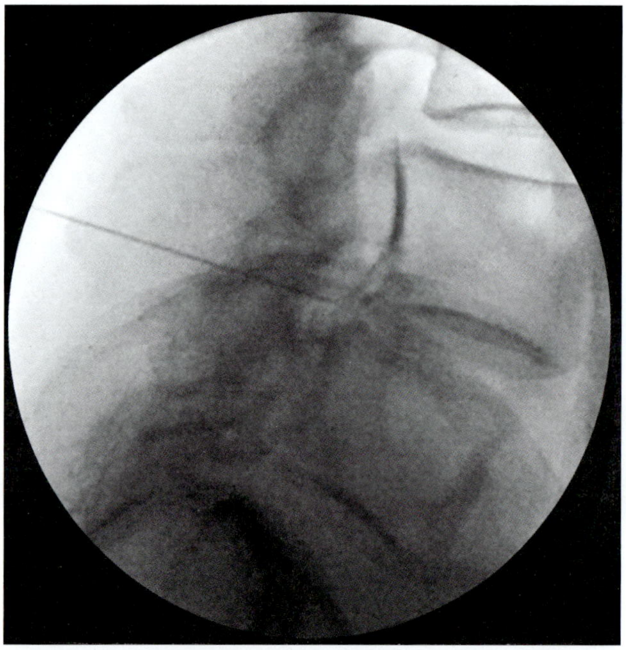

• **Fig. 14.34** Lateral View with Contrast Showing Flow Along the L4 Nerve Root and Epidural Space.

Common Pathology

- Neural impingement can occur in a number of regions, including the subarticular zone (lateral recess), neural foramina, extraforaminal zone (far lateral), and central canal.
- Impingement of the neural tissue may result from any combination of disc herniation, ligamentum flavum hypertrophy, facet arthropathy, disc-osteophyte complex development, spondylolisthesis, or facet synovial cyst formation.
- Epidural scarring postoperatively, can restrict neural mobility and lead to chronic radiculopathy.

Equipment

- Performed under sterile procedural conditions.
- Standard procedural kit, including sterile skin preparatory materials, hypodermic needle for skin anesthesia, syringes, small-bore extension tubing, and sterile gloves.
- Needles: Epidural loss of resistance needle (e.g., Tuohy, Weiss, Hustead needles). Some clinicians prefer to perform without loss of resistance and place anatomically with a standard spinal needle.
- Special equipment: Loss of resistance syringe, glass or plastic, slip tip or luer lock, typically 8 mL volume.
- Fluoroscope.
- Radiation protection equipment, including lead apron, leaded glasses (optional), and leaded gloves (optional).
- Radiolucent x-ray table.

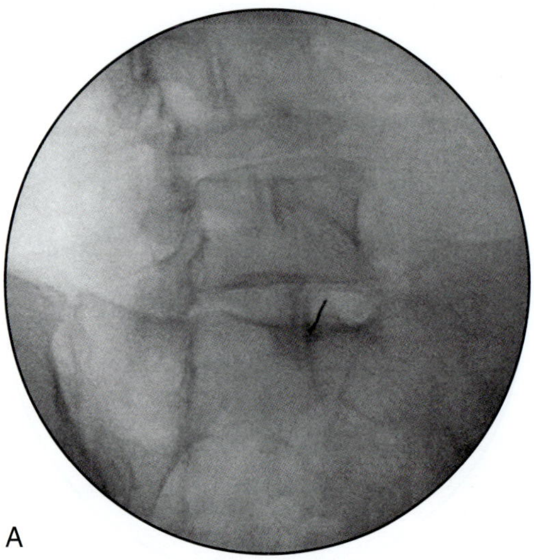

A

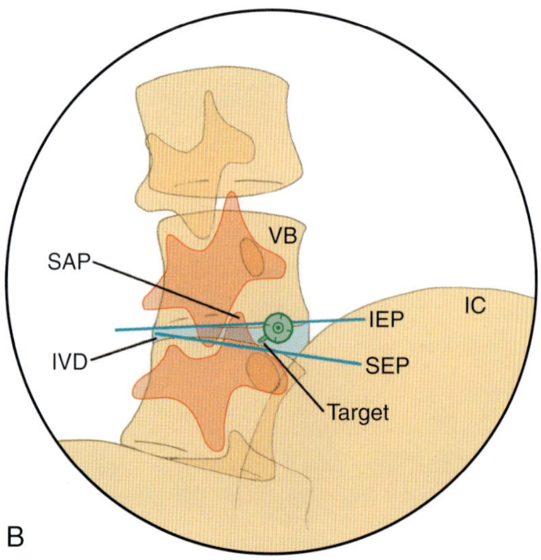

B

• **Fig. 14.35** (A) Fluoroscopic image of oblique "scotty dog" view with target at the superior articular process with pertinent anatomy labeled. (B) Artists rendition of the fluoroscopic image with pertinent anatomy labeled similar to shown. *IAP*, Inferior articular process; *IC*, iliac crest; *L*, lamina; *P*, pedicle; *SAP*, superior articular process; *SP*, spinal process; *TP*, transverse process. (From Furman MB. *Atlas of Image-Guided Spinal Procedures*. 2nd ed. Elsevier; 2018.)

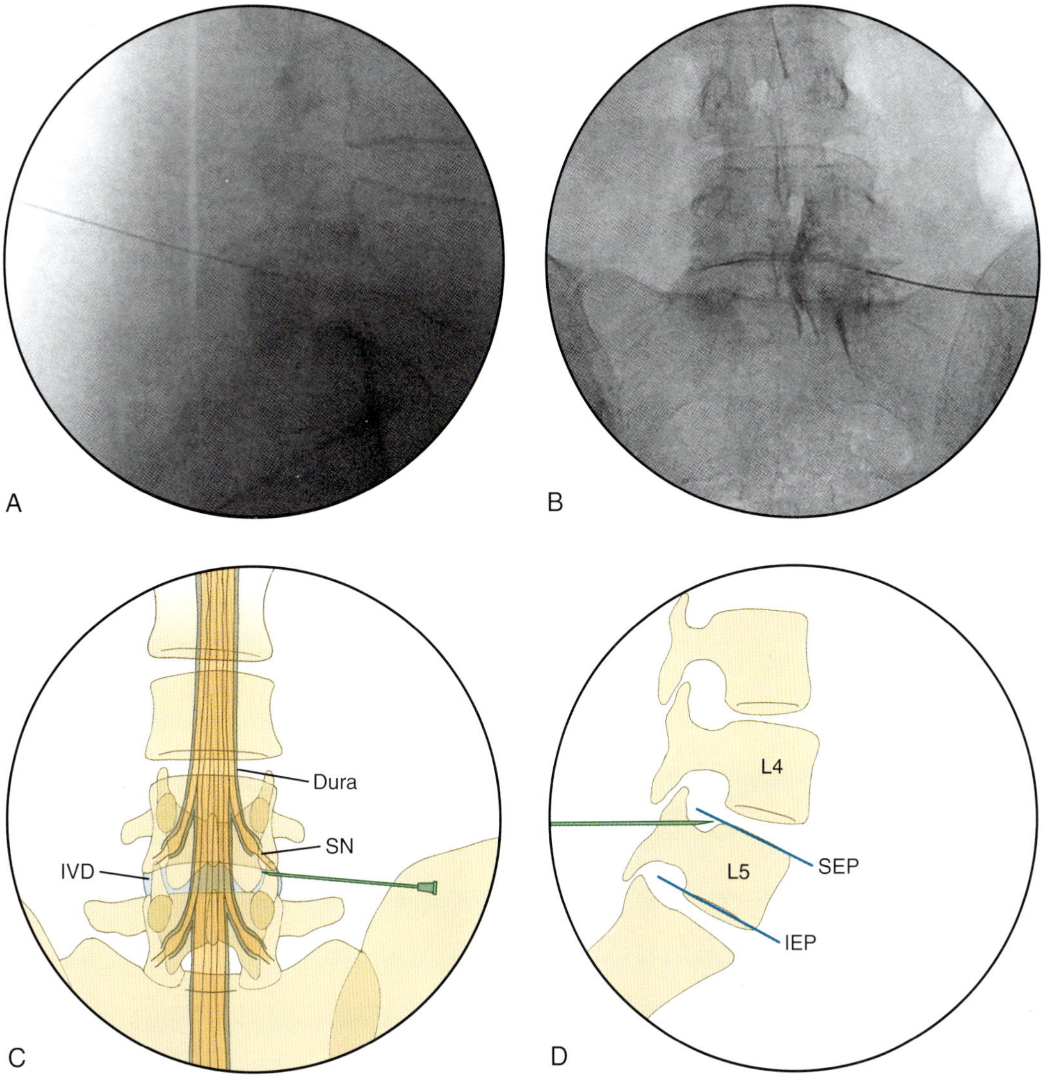

• **Fig. 14.36** (A) Lateral fluoroscopic image of needle placement with infraneural approach. Note needle is advanced just anterior to the superior articular process. (B) Anteroposterior (AP) view of final needle placement and contrast administration demonstrating epidural flow medial to pedicle and lobular flow pattern. (C) Artist rendering of lateral view identifying vertebral body (VB), Superior and articular processes at level of injection (SAP & IAP) and sacrum (S) with needle drawn in just past the SAP as in the fluoroscopic image. (D) Artist rendering of AP view with final needle placement just under inferolateral to the pedicle (labeled P) at the level of the disc space at l5-S1 past the lateral margin of the SAP as in the fluoroscopic image. *IAP*, Inferior articular process; *IEP*, Inferior Endplate; *IVD*, intervertebral disc; *SAP*, superior articular process; *SEP*, superior Endplate; *SN*, spinal nerve. (A–D, From Furman MB. *Atlas of Image-Guided Spinal Procedures*. 2nd ed. Elsevier; 2018.)

Common Injectates

- Preservative-free saline, preservative-free local anesthetic, single-dose steroid, including betamethasone sodium phosphate/sodium acetate mixture, methylprednisolone acetate, and dexamethasone sodium phosphate.
- Triamcinolone acetonide was a common steroid used in epidural injections until the Food and Drug Administration (FDA) placed a black box warning stating "not for epidural administration" in 2011. There is contention over the safety of injecting particulate steroids in the epidural space. There have been a few case reports of adhesive arachnoiditis reported after interlaminar and transforaminal particulate epidural steroid injection. Multiple cases of paraplegia and stroke have been reported after transforaminal injection of particulate steroids, though the interlaminar route has not been implicated in these side effects. It is recommended that the proceduralist become familiar with the risks and benefits of using a particulate versus a non-particulate steroid for epidural injections.
- Orthobiologics include 5% dextrose prolotherapy, platelet lysate, and PRP.

Volume

- Sufficient non-ionic contrast to visualize coverage of the desired structure, and ensure no vascular uptake, typically 0.5 to 2 mL (Figs. 14.39–14.41).

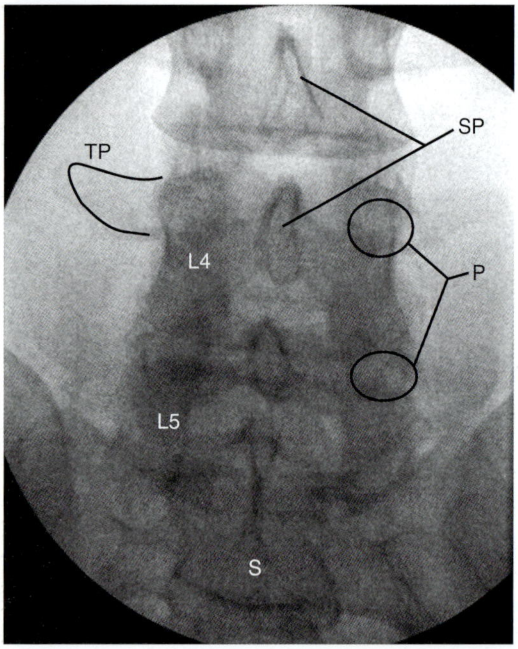

• **Fig. 14.37** Anteroposterior Fluoroscopic Image of the Lumbar Spine. *IL*, Interlaminar space; *L4*, fourth lumbar lamina; *L5*, fifth lumbar lamina; *P*, pedicle; *S*, sacrum; *SP*, spinous process; *TP*, transverse process.

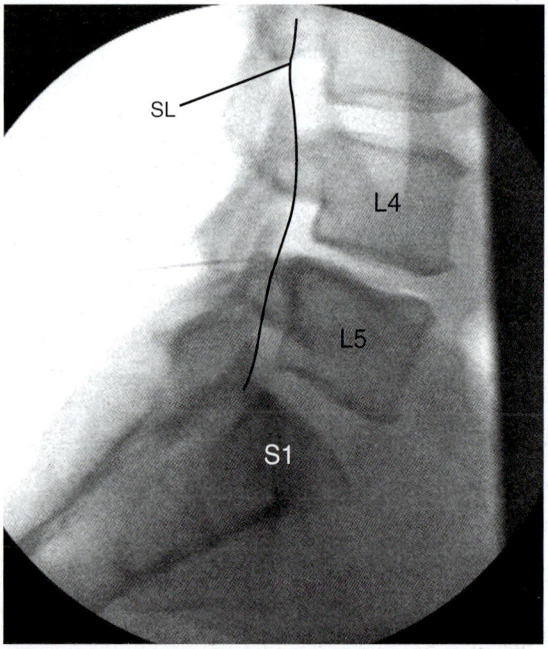

• **Fig. 14.38** Lateral Fluoroscopic Image of the Lumbar Spine. *L4 VB*, fourth lumbar vertebral body; *L5 VB*, fifth lumbar vertebral body; *S1*, S1 vertebral body; *SL*, spinolaminar line.

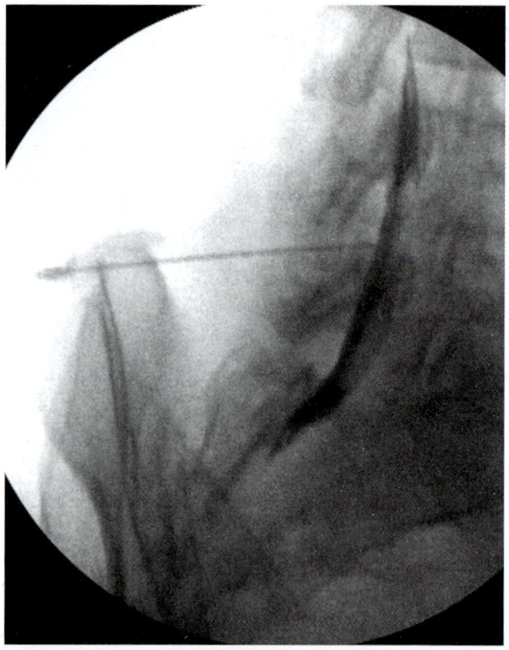

• **Fig. 14.39** Fluoroscopic Image of Final Needle Position with Contrast Flow Pattern in the Contralateral Oblique View for a Left Paramedian L4-5 Lumbar Interlaminar Epidural Steroid Injection.

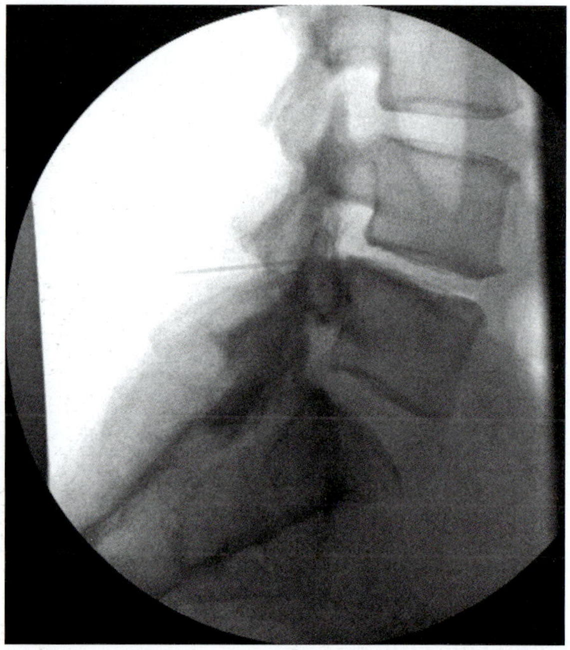

• **Fig. 14.40** Fluoroscopic Image of Final Needle Position with Contrast Flow Pattern in the Lateral View for a Left Paramedian L4-5 Lumbar Interlaminar Epidural Steroid Injection.

- Injectate volume varies depending upon contrast flow pattern and degree of patient stenosis. At least the volume required to cover the target of interest should be used: 5 mL of injectate is common but varies from 2 mL to over 8 mL.

Technique

Patient Position

- Prone with pillow under the abdomen to decrease lumbar lordosis and accentuate the interlaminar space.

Clinician Position

- Standing to the side of the patient, most commonly opposite the side of the fluoroscope controls.

Fluoroscope Position

- The fluoroscope most commonly will enter from the side of the patient opposite the physician, with the level of interest centered in the beam (Fig. 14.42).

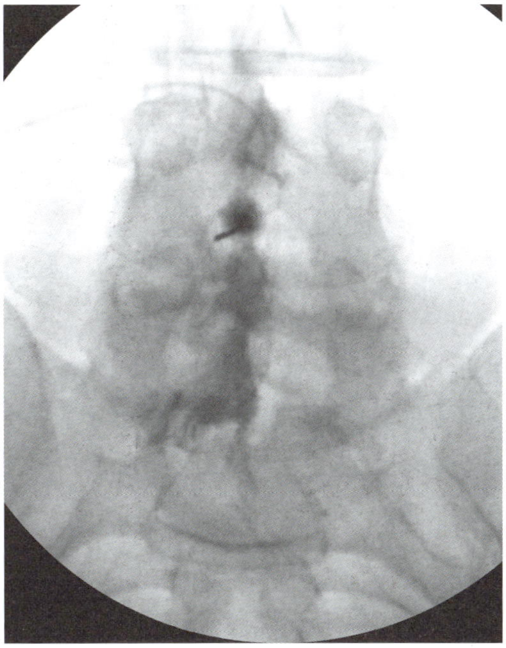

• **Fig. 14.41** Fluoroscopic Image of Final Needle Position with Contrast Flow Pattern in the Anteroposterior View for a Left Paramedian L4-5 Lumbar Interlaminar Epidural Steroid Injection.

Target

- Various aspects of the epidural space can be targeted, depending upon the site of pathology.
- Starting in the AP approach with the spinous process centered between the pedicles, obtain a trajectory view by caudally tilting until the interlaminar space appears sufficiently wide (Fig. 14.43).
- Placing the needle in a paramedian approach in the AP view, toward the side of pathology, will preferentially cover that side unilaterally (Fig. 14.44).
- Midline approach can result in bilateral spread, though contrast flow may be contained to the dorsal epidural space.

Final Approach and Needle Position

- The safety view is either lateral or contralateral oblique (CLO) to ensure needle placement is not too ventral into the thecal sac.
- The CLO view will vary from 45 to 55 degrees, depending upon the laminar shape and distance the needle is from midline.
- Upon engaging the ligamentum flavum at the ventral edge of the lamina, the loss of resistance syringe is attached

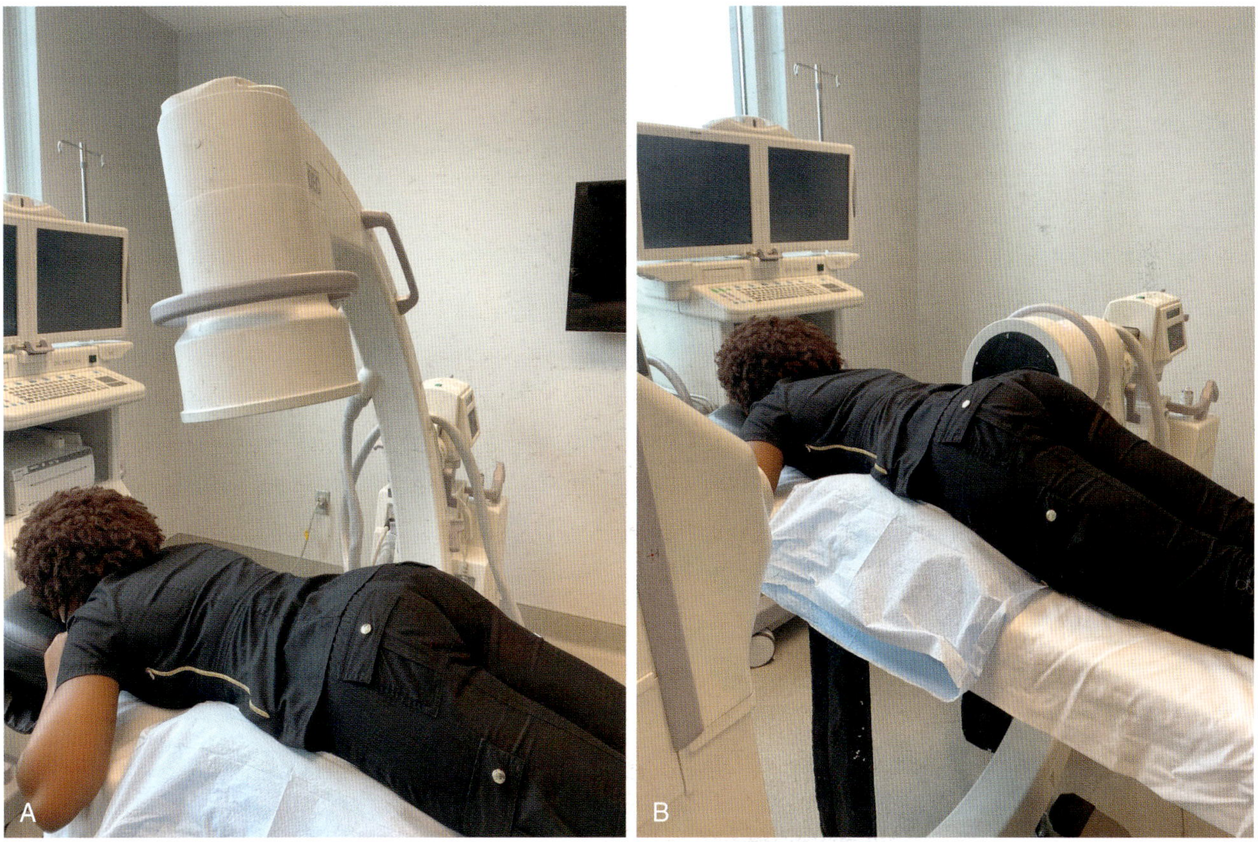

• **Fig. 14.42** Patient Positioned on Fluoroscopy Table with C-arm in Position and Clinician Standing on the Left Side of the Patient. (A) anteroposterior view; (B) lateral view.

to the needle hub and cautiously advanced slowly with either intermittent or continuous gentle pressure on the syringe plunger, until loss of resistance is obtained, which is a sudden acceptance of the material in the loss of resistance syringe. Physician preference dictates which material is used in the loss of resistance syringe: typically used options are air, saline, or an air/saline mixture.

- Final needle position is within the dorsal epidural space, which appears just deep to the spinolaminar line in a view lateral to the laminar edge (Fig. 14.45).

PEARLS AND PITFALLS

- The more laterally placed the needle, the more likely to have injectate spread over the dorsal root ganglion.
- A very narrow interlaminar space can be made wider by placing more pillows under the abdomen to give a higher degree of lumbar flexion.
- If the interlaminar space is narrow, caudal tilt and ipsilateral oblique rotation of the C-arm can help present an opening for access.
- Do not perform an interlaminar epidural injection through a laminectomy defect. The epidural space is obliterated during laminectomy, and a dural puncture is highly likely to occur.
- The epidural space is a low-pressure system; thus there are no compressive forces to abate bleeding and hemostasis in the epidural space; we rely purely upon the intrinsic clotting function of the patient. The risk of epidural hematoma, while low, is of greater theoretical risk in this approach compared to a transforaminal approach (apart from an S1 transforaminal), due to the needle tip violating the epidural space during interlaminar placement. Ensure that the physician has noted and held for an appropriate duration any medications that substantially affect hemostasis, such as aspirin and warfarin.
- The injectate will follow the path of least resistance. If attempting to target pathology above a level with high resistance or no epidural space, such as above a level of severe central stenosis, the injectate may not reach the desired target and an alternate approach may need to be considered.
- Reviewing the patient's MRI or computed tomography (CT) scans before the procedure can give the physician insight into the size and shape of the epidural space to plan the approach appropriately.
- Parallax occurs when the needle is not near the center of the fluoroscope beam. It results in the angle and position of the needle appearing different than it truly is anatomically. The physician must accommodate for this if working toward the edges of the field of view and obtain a final view with the needle in the center of the fluoroscope image.
- Caution should be exercised if advancing more than a short distance in the lateral or CLO views to avoid inadvertently straying too far medially or laterally off trajectory. This can result in needle placement in an unanticipated location, such as on the lamina or crossing over midline.

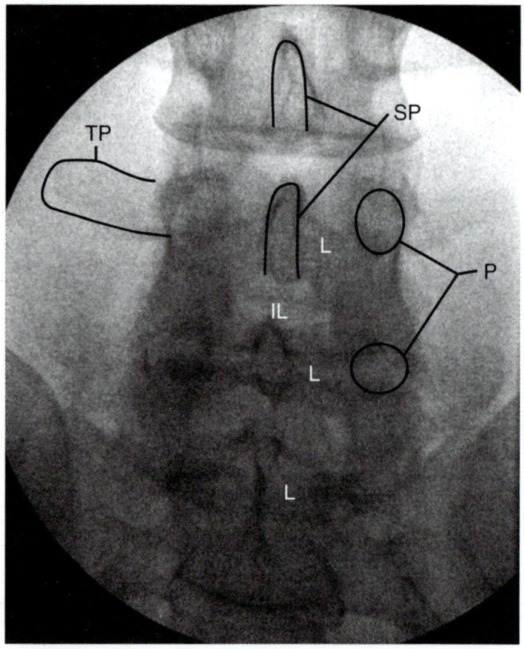

• **Fig. 14.43** **Trajectory View Anteroposterior Fluoroscopic Image for an L4-5 Lumbar Interlaminar Epidural Steroid Injection.** Note the wide appearance of the interlaminar space at the level of interest. *IL*, Interlaminar space; *L*, lamina; *P*, pedicle; *SP*, spinous process; *TP*, transverse process.

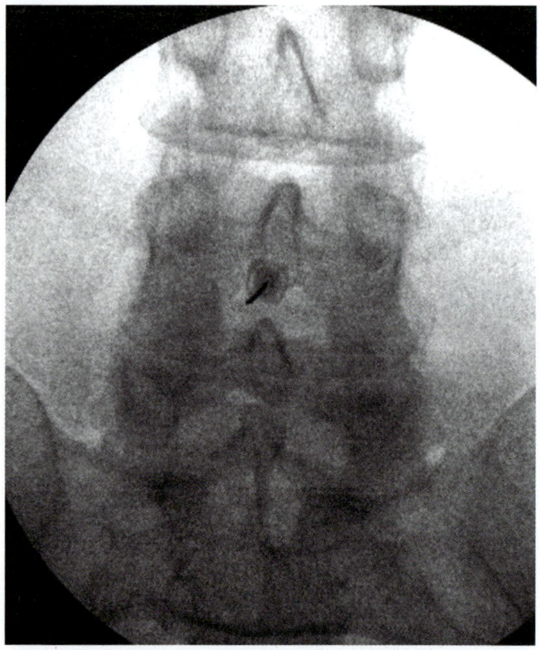

• **Fig. 14.44** **Fluoroscopic Image of Needle Position in the Anteroposterior Trajectory View for a Left Paramedian L4-5 Lumbar Interlaminar Epidural Steroid Injection.**

Suboptimal Flow Patterns

Retrodural Space of Okada (Figs. 14.46–14.50)

- The retrodural space of Okada is a potential space deep to the lamina and superficial to the ligamentum flavum.

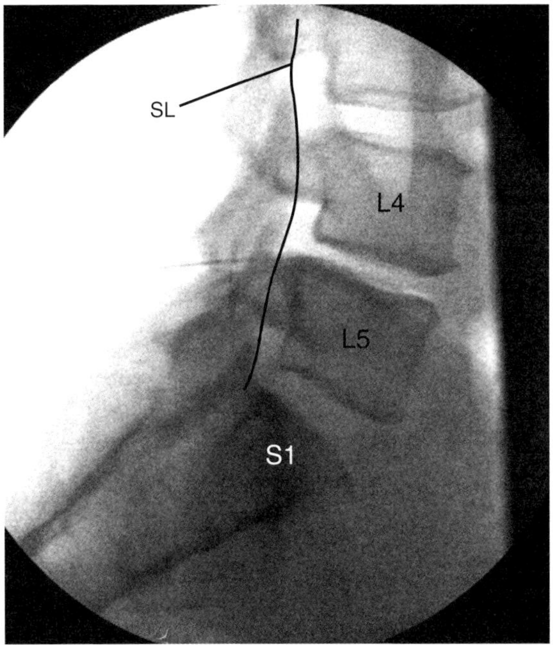

• **Fig. 14.45** Fluoroscopic Image of Final Needle Position in the Lateral View for a Left Paramedian L4-5 Lumbar Interlaminar Epidural Steroid Injection. *L4 VB*, Fourth lumbar vertebral body; *L5 VB*, fifth lumbar vertebral body; *LF*, ligamentum flavum; *S1*, S1 vertebral body; *SL*, spinolaminar line; *TS*, thecal sac.

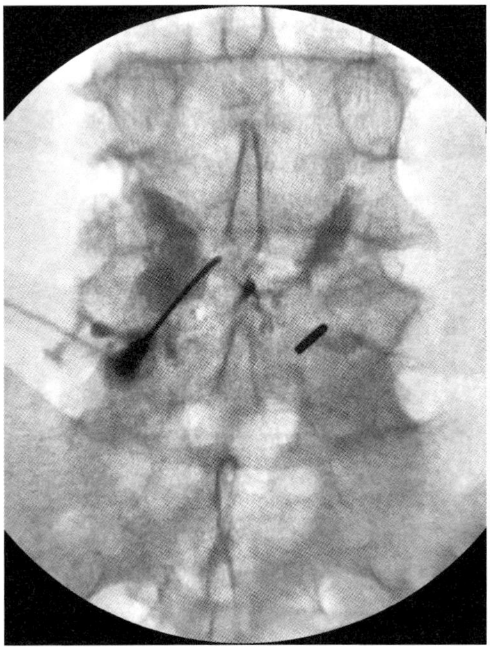

• **Fig. 14.46** Fluoroscopic image of contrast flow pattern demonstrating filling of the retrodural space of Okada during performance of a lumbar epidural steroid injection. Note the contrast flow into the bilateral facet joints.

It can communicate with the facet joints and the interspinous space to form an interspinous bursa. A false loss of resistance can occur, resulting in non-epidural placement of injectate. Careful attention to contrast spread can clue the clinician to an aberrant flow pattern and the need for correction prior to injectate delivery.

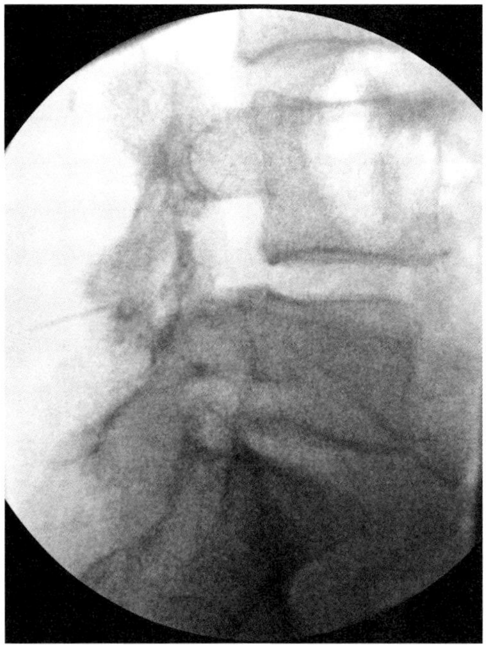

• **Fig. 14.47** Fluoroscopic Image of Contrast Flow Pattern Demonstrating Filling of the Retrodural Space of Okada in the Lateral View During Performance of a Lumbar Interlaminar Epidural Steroid Injection.

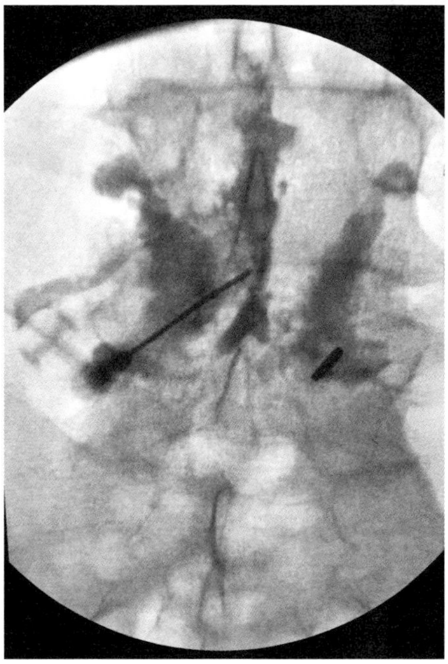

• **Fig. 14.48** Fluoroscopic Image of Contrast Flow Pattern Demonstrating Filling of the Retrodural Space of Okada in the Anteroposterior View, with Further Advancement of the Needle to Obtain Epidural Flow During Performance of a Lumbar Epidural Steroid Injection.

Intrathecal (Fig. 14.51)

- If there is insufficient epidural space to accommodate the needle, or the needle is placed deep to the epidural space, intrathecal injection can occur. The contrast should layer ventrally, and a hazy fluid–fluid interface may be appreciated, as opposed to the crisp delineation expected with epidural spread.

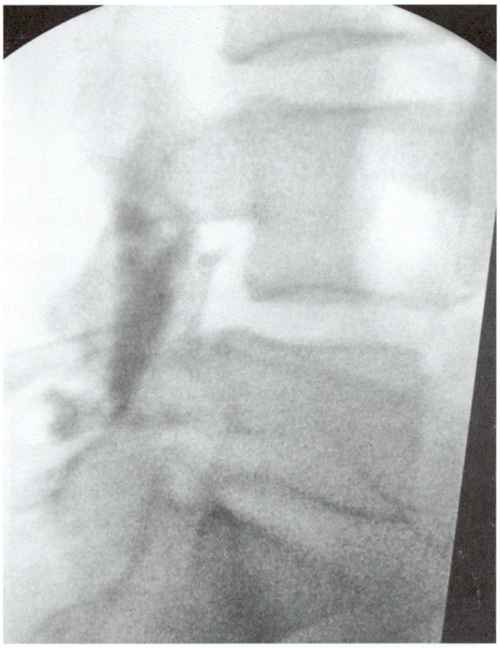

• **Fig. 14.49** Fluoroscopic Image of Contrast Flow Pattern Demonstrating Filling of the Retrodural Space of Okada in the Lateral View, with Further Advancement of the Needle to Obtain Epidural Flow During Performance of a Lumbar Interlaminar Epidural Steroid Injection.

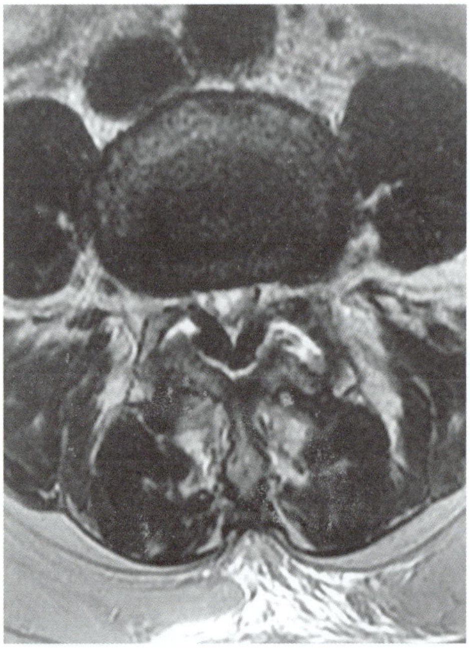

• **Fig. 14.50** Axial T2-Weighted Magnetic Resonance Imaging Demonstrating the Retrodural Space of Okada from the Preceding Figures During Attempted Lumbar Interlaminar Epidural Steroid Injection.

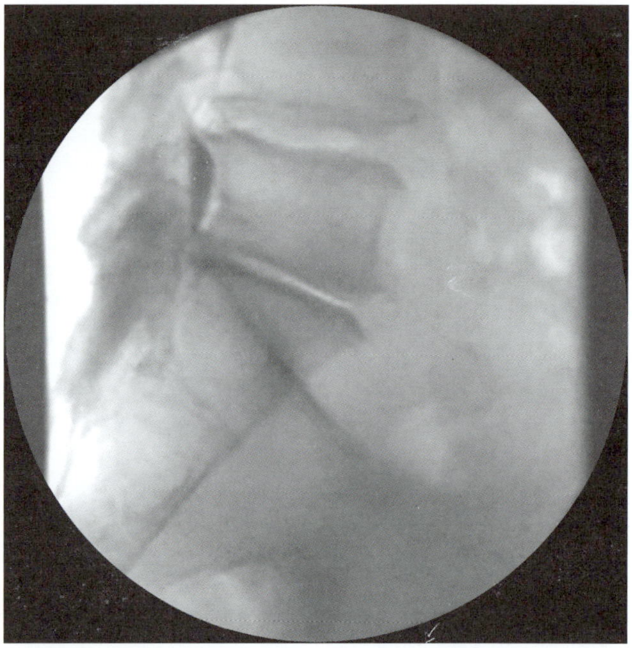

• **Fig. 14.51** Fluoroscopic Image of Contrast Flow Pattern Demonstrating Intrathecal Spread of Contrast During an Attempted Interlaminar Epidural Steroid Injection. Note the hazy fluid–fluid interface of the contrast with the cerebrospinal fluid, and the ventral layering of the contrast.

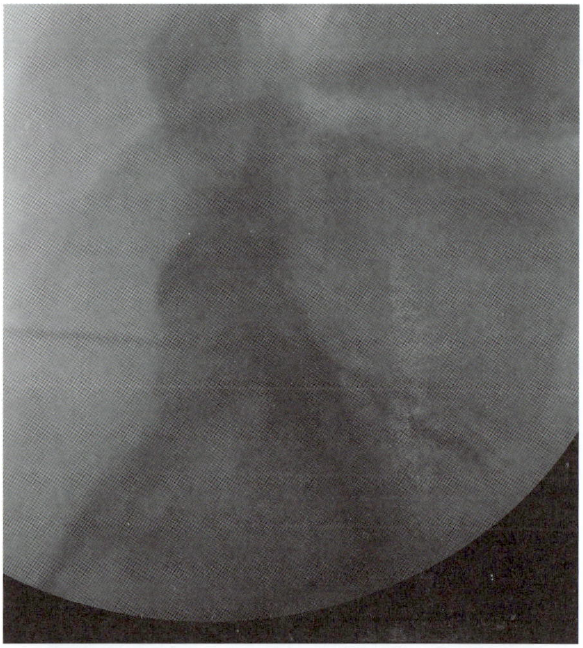

• **Fig. 14.52** Fluoroscopic Image of Contrast Flow Pattern Demonstrating Intradiscal Contrast Flow During an Attempted Right Paramedian Interlaminar Epidural Injection. The patient had a large disc herniation that had extruded to the ventral aspect of the ligamentum flavum.

Intradiscal (Fig. 14.52)

- It should be extraordinarily rare during an interlaminar epidural steroid injection to obtain intradiscal needle placement, as the needle is relatively posterior in the epidural space. A large enough disc extrusion that has migrated posteriorly and is contiguous with the parent disc could be encountered. Placement of the needle ventrally into the disc would not be expected to occur with careful attention to technique and utilizing appropriate lateral or CLO views.

Subdural

- The subdural space is just deep to the epidural space before piercing the arachnoid matter of the thecal sac. Subdural contrast spread will commonly demonstrate a railroad track pattern, showing circumferential spread of the subdural space. Aspiration will often remove nearly all of the injected contrast material.

Vascular

- Venous injection can occur in a posteriorly placed lumbar interlaminar epidural steroid injection, though it is uncommon.
- A far laterally placed paramedian lumbar interlaminar epidural steroid injection could theoretically encounter a radiculomedullary artery if placed ventrally into the periforaminal region.

Medial Branch Block

KEY POINTS

- The lumbar medial branch block is solely diagnostic. It is used to determine whether axial back pain is facet-mediated.
- Lumbar medial branch radiofrequency ablation is performed if patients receive substantial benefit from medial branch bocks.

Pertinent Anatomy

- Facet joints have dual innervation from a pair of medial branches from the dorsal primary rami. The joint is innervated by the branch at the same level and the above. For example, the L5-S1 joint is innervated by the L4 and L5 medial branch.
- The medial branch branches off of the dorsal primary ramus, run across the neck of the SAP, and then wraps around the transverse process one level below at the junction of the SAP; for example, the L4 medial branch lies on the transverse process of L5.
- L1-L4 medial branch pass under the mamillo-accessory ligament, which some time can be an obstacle; the medial branch is most accessible as it crosses the neck of the SAP.
- At the level of L5, the practitioner will target the primary dorsal ramus itself. The L5 dorsal ramus is located at the junction of the base of the S1 superior articulating process and the sacral ala (see Fig. 14.4).

Technique

Patient Position

- Prone with abdomen on a pillow to reduce lumbar lordosis.

C-Arm Position

- Confirm the appropriate level with an AP view.
- Tilt the C-arm cephalad or caudad to square off the superior endplate at the targeted level.

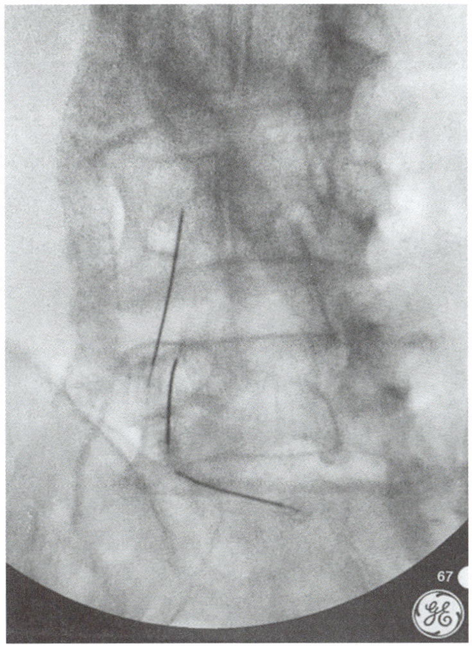

• **Fig. 14.53** Left contralateral oblique view demonstrating needle placement for medial branch block at L3-4, L4-5, and L5-S1 with optimal placement at the junction of the superior articulating process and transverse process (i.e. the eye of the scotty dog).

- Oblique the C-arm to the ipsilateral side until the "Scotty dog" is clearly visualized.

Needle Position

- Insert the needle coaxially, targeting the "eye" of the Scotty dog.

Target

- The "eye" of the Scotty dog, which is at the articulation of the SAP and the transverse process (Fig. 14.53).

Injectate Volume

- Use of contrast is optional. If the practitioner elects to use contrast, 0.2 to 0.5 mL should be injected per level, and contrast should spread along the lateral aspect of the SAP. It can be useful to ensure there is no vascular or epidural spread.
- Injectate should consist of 0.5 mL volume of lidocaine (1% or 2%), or bupivacaine (0.25%, 0.5%, or 0.75%).

PEARLS AND PITFALLS

- Lumbar tilt may need to be adjusted at each level to optimize the needle trajectory to the target due to lumbar lordosis and in patients with scoliosis.
- The L5 dorsal ramus maybe access coaxial in AP view; all other medial branches cannot be readily accessed if the needle is coaxial in AP views.

Radiofrequency Ablation

KEY POINTS

- Radiofrequency (RF) ablation uses a radiofrequency current through an electrode tip needle to create a thermal lesion.
- Neurodestructive temperatures range from 65°C to 90°C.
- The RF electrode tip should be placed parallel to the target medial branch.

Pertinent Anatomy

- Medial branch anatomy is described in the medial branch section (see Figs. 14.1–13).

Technique

Patient Position

- Prone with abdomen on a pillow to reduce lumbar lordosis.

C-Arm Position

- Confirm the appropriate level with an AP view.
- Tilt the C-arm cephalad or caudad to square off the superior endplate at the targeted level.
- Oblique the C-arm to 20 degrees to the ipsilateral side.
- Tilt the C-arm 45 degrees caudally.

Needle Position

- Insert the needle coaxially, targeting the "eye" of the Scotty dog.

Target

- The "eye" of the Scotty dog, which is at the articulation of the SAP and the transverse process (Fig. 14.54).

Injectate Volume

- 0.5 to 1 mL of local anesthetic is typically injected after stimulation and before the ablation to improve the patient's comfort. Practitioners may use lidocaine (1% or 2%), or bupivacaine (0.25%, 0.5%, or 0.75%).

PEARLS AND PITFALLS

- Ensure that the needle is placed at an angle so that there is parallel placement of the tip along the nerve; hence, the suggestion to oblique the C-arm 20 degrees and tilt 45 degrees.
- Before the ablation, motor and sensory stimulation should be performed to ensure there are no radicular symptoms or signs of muscle movement.
- 0.5 to 1 mL of local anesthetic is typically injected after stimulation and before the ablation to improve the patient's comfort.
- Practitioners vary in their ablation settings; it can be 70 to 85 degrees for up to 90 seconds. Some practitioners may do two or three rounds of the ablation.
- For monopolar RF, the temperature reading will not stay exactly at the preset temperature but will go over and under, typically within half a degree. This is due to the probe itself causing the surrounding tissue to oscillate to create heat. The probe then reads the tissue temperature and adjusts to keep the temperature constant.
- This also limits the size of the "zone of coagulation."

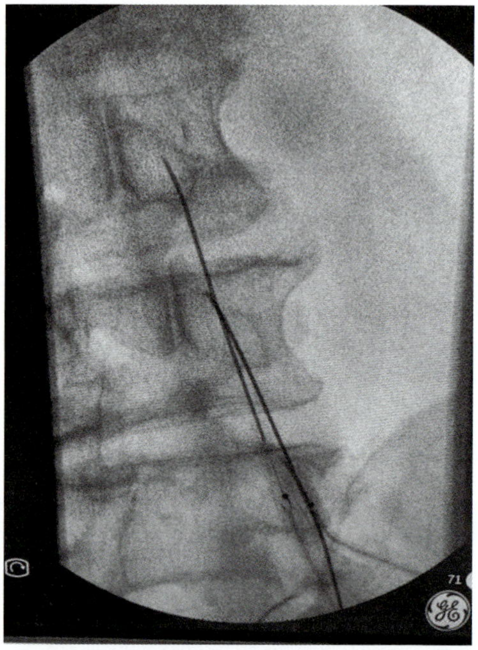

• **Fig. 14.54** Right contralateral oblique view demonstrating lead placement for radiofrequency ablation at L2-3, L3-4, and L4-5 with optimal placement at the junction of the superior articulating process and transverse process (i.e. the eye of the scotty dog).

Zygapophyseal or Facet Joint Injections

KEY POINTS

- The volume capacity of the facet joint is 1 to 1.5 mL.

Pertinent Anatomy

- Facet joints are J-shaped joints that are composed of the IAP and SAP of adjacent vertebral bodies.
- The joint is lined by articular cartilage and encapsulated by synovial lining.
- The obliquity of the joint increases as we go down from L1 to L5.
- The capsule of the lumbar facet joint attaches tight to the articulating cartilage, but at superior and inferior ends of the joint, the capsule relaxes, creating the superior and inferior subarticular recess when the joint is in neutral position.
- There are also small foramen at either end of the capsule that may allow contrast material to leak out during the injection.
- Subfascial channel communicates between the joint on one side and the opposite side; contrast material may flow to the opposite side.

Technique

Patient Position

- Prone with abdomen on a pillow to reduce lumbar lordosis.

C-Arm Position

- Confirm the appropriate level with an AP view.
- Square up the top endplate of the lower vertebrae (for example, square up L5 superior endplate for an L4-L5 facet injection).

- Oblique the fluoroscope ipsilaterally until the joint can be clearly identified.
- Due to the J-shape, the ventromedial segment may be mistaken for the dorsal opening.
- Next, it may be useful to decrease the tilt by 5 degrees from that position to facilitate entry into the joint from a medial to lateral trajectory.
- IAP and SAP should be clearly identified.
- Lateral images should be obtained to verify needle depth; the needle should land close to the facet joint silhouette.

Needle Position

- The needle should be inserted coaxially.
- Advance needle until the joint capsule is penetrated.
- "Purchase" should be achieved.
- Needle entry may be difficult due to most injections being on advanced arthritic joints.

Target

- Facet joint.

Injectate Volume

- 0.2 to 0.5 of contrast should be injected to confirm intra-articular positioning.
- Common injectates: Depo-Medrol (methylprednisolone) or dexamethasone with lidocaine or bupivacaine: 1 mL total volume.

PEARLS AND PITFALLS

- Cephalad or caudad tilt may be required to optimize entry into the joint, especially in scoliotic patients.
- When performing a facet injection at L5-S1, cephalad tilt can be used to create a clear needle trajectory if the iliac crest is superimposed.
- When there is significant facet arthropathy and overgrowth, it will be easier to enter the joint if the medial border of the joint is targeted. This is because overgrowth tends to occur on the SAP, which corresponds with the lateral aspect of the joint.
- Optimal contrast spread can be seen encircling the joint capsule and filling the joint line. Try to minimize volume of contrast used as the total volume capacity of the joint is only 1 to 1.5 mL.
- An ideal intra-articular spread may be shaped like an apple core or dumbbell.
- Needle placement superior to the joint in AP and oblique views or too ventral to the facet joint silhouette on lateral views can increase risk of injuring the exiting spinal nerve (Figs 14.55 and 14.56).

Pars Interarticularis Defect

KEY POINTS

- The pars can be injected for diagnostic purposes.
- Orthobiologics may play a role in treating symptomatic non-union pars fractures that have failed conservative management, but at the time of writing there are no studies published on this technique.

Pertinent Anatomy

- The "Scotty dog" sign represents the normal appearance of the posterior elements of the lumbar vertebra on the oblique radiograph.[54] The transverse process is the nose, the superior facet is the ear, the inferior facet is the front leg, the pars interarticularis reflects the neck or collar, and the pedicle forms the eye.[54]
- A gap through the dog's neck/collar indicates spondylolysis, a fractured pars interarticularis or a congenital pars defect, originally described by LaChapelle (Fig. 14.58).[54]

Common Pathology

- Congenital pars defect.
- Traumatic pars fracture can lead to non-union fracture. If an acute pars fracture is suspected, then MRI or a CT scan.[54a] and the initial x-ray is equivocal.[55]
- An x-ray is usually the imaging modality of choice and may assist in the confirmation of the diagnosis in 80% of cases. In cases with a high clinical suspicion and a negative x-ray, a CT-scan or MRI may be recommended.[54a]
- Trauma fracture: usually occurs with loaded hyperextension such that occurs in sports like soccer, basketball, football, gymnastics, wrestling, etc.[56]
  - Conservative management includes a thoracic lumbar sacral orthotic (TLSO) brace, activity modification, physical therapy, and bone growth stimulation. A review article showed the average time to return to sports was 3.7 months, and good clinical outcomes were achieved in 84% to 91% of patients and were not dependent on resolution or healing of the fracture.[56]
  - If conservative measures fail or the resulting non-union is symptomatic despite conservative care, surgery may be an option.[56]
  - A non-surgical alternative may include the injection of mesenchymal stem cells from bone marrow. There is some published literature on utilizing bone marrow aspirate concentrate (BMAC) for the treatment of non-union fractures; however, there is no literature published on treating non-union of pars interarticularis fractures.[57]
  - PRP, BMAC, and demineralized bone matrix (DBM) all have evidence for osteoinductivity.[58]
- Degenerative spondylolysis.

Equipment

- C-arm fluoroscopy.
- 22 to 25 gauge, 3- to 5-inch spinal needle used for diagnostics, degenerative spondylosis, and for injury with no callus.
- or 15 gauge, 3.5-inch trochar for defect with callus formation.
- Contrast medium.

Common Injectates

- Local anesthetic for diagnostics
- Orthobiologics (PRP, bone marrow concentrate, etc.)
- Demineralized bone matrix

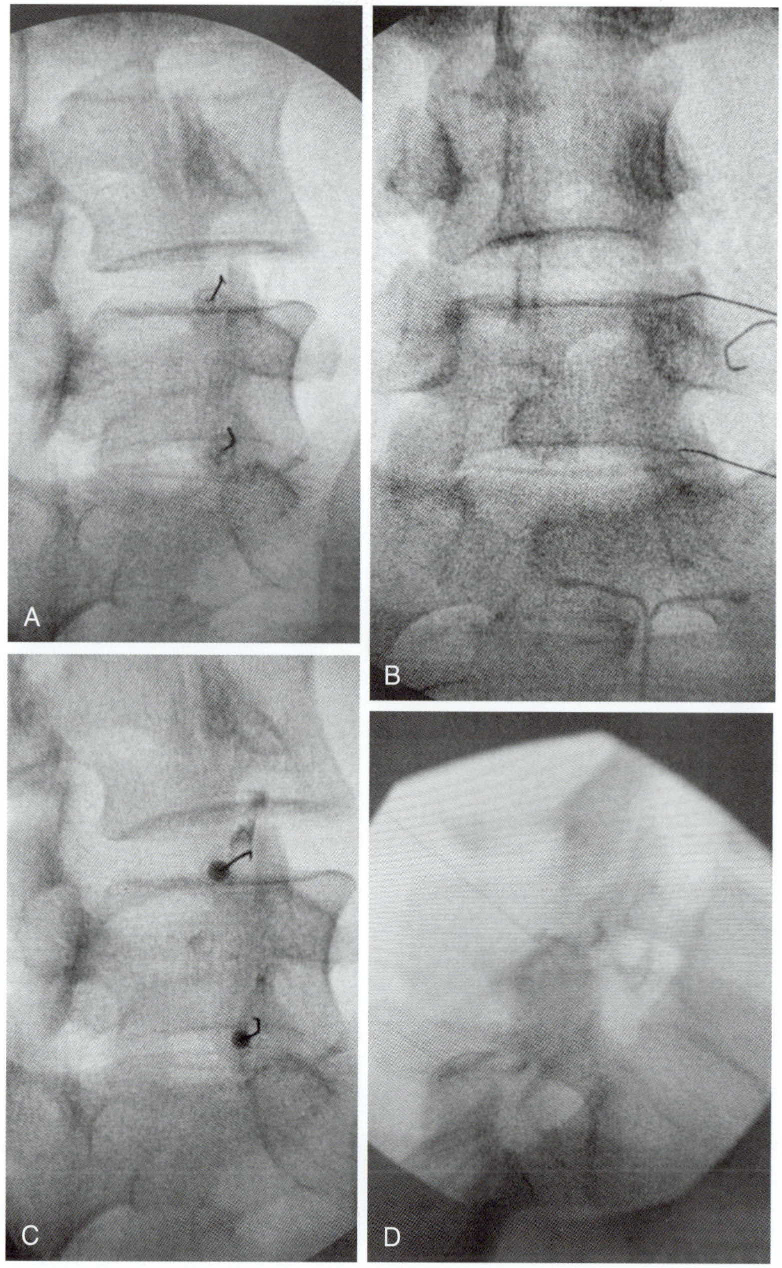

• **Fig. 14.55** Intra-articular facet needle position without contrast in the oblique view (A) and anteroposterior view (B). With contrast in the oblique view (C) and lateral view (D).

Injectate Volume

- 0..5 to 2 mL

Technique

Patient Position

- Prone with abdomen on a pillow to reduce lumbar lordosis.

C-Arm Position

- Confirm the appropriate level with an AP view.
- Square off the top endplate of the lower vertebrae (for example, square off L5 superior endplate for an L4-L5 injection).
- Oblique the C-arm to the ipsilateral side until the "Scotty dog" is clearly visualized.
- Lateral images should be obtained to verify needle depth.
- Use the AP view to confirm needle position and to inject contrast.

Needle Position

- The needle should start directly over the pars or neck of the "Scotty dog".
- The needle should be inserted coaxially.

Target

- Touch down on os right at the neck of the scotty dog/pars area.
- Confirm needle placement in the AP view, where it should be just inferior and medial to the pedicle 5 o'clock position on the left side, 7 o'clock position on the right side.

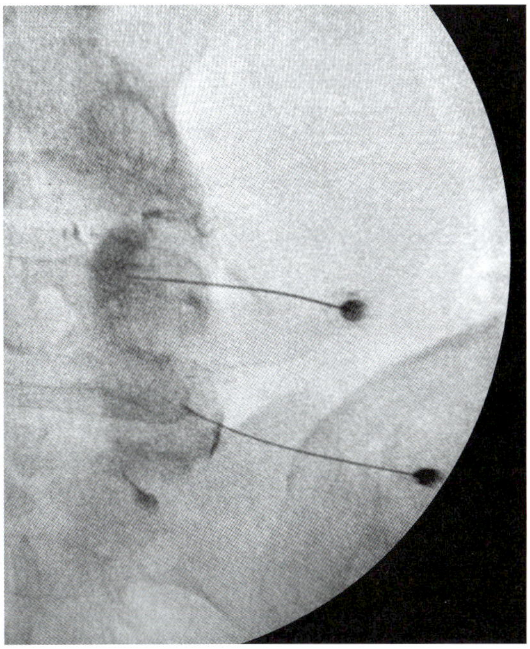

• **Fig. 14.56** Optimal Contrast Spread.

- Confirm depth in the lateral to ensure it is not in the foramen. It should be below the facet joint (for example, if injecting the L4 pars, the needle will be below the L3-4 facet joint).
- Inject a small amount of contrast to confirm contrast spread in the pars defect in both views.

PEARLS AND PITFALLS

- If there is a symptomatic non-union with bony callus, a 15 gauge, 3.5-inch trocar will be needed to get into the defect.
- Manually drill the trocar if possible. If not, and a power drill is utilized, then advance the trocar in the lateral view and proceed slowly and cautiously to prevent advancing the trocar into the foramen.
- If there is a large defect, there may be less bony resistance, and there is a chance the needle can go through the defect into the foramen. Also, if using a trocar, it is easier to advance too deep. Observe the needle in the lateral view to confirm trocar and needle depth.
- In the AP view, do not travel too far medially past the lamina into the central canal.

Intradiscal Injection

KEY POINTS

- All lumbar intradiscal injections should be done utilizing fluoroscopy or CT guidance.
- Intradiscal injections can be done for diagnostic and therapeutic purposes.

Introduction

- The prevalence of pain due to internal disc disruption, in patients with chronic low back pain, is 39%.[59]
- Intervertebral disc (IVD)-related pain can be caused by structural abnormalities, such as disc degeneration or disc herniation.
- Biochemical effects, such as inflammation, and neurobiologic processes may play a role.
- Nerve growth factor (NGF) may play an important role in discogenic back pain.[60,61]

Pertinent Anatomy

- Intervertebral disks constitute 25% of the height of the spine, which decrease with aging.[59,62]
- Disc nutrition is supported through lymphatics and extracellular fluid osmosis.
- Discs have three major components: nucleus pulposus, annulus fibrosus, and cartilaginous endplates.
- Nucleus pulposus: ovoid, yellowish, gelatinous paracentrally located and made of mucoprotein.
- Annulus fibrosus: firm concentric, meshwork of collagenous fibers called the annulus fibrosus.
- Disc innervation: receive innervation to outer third of annulus anteriorly, posteriorly, and laterally.
- Posteriorly, the annulus receives innervation from the sinovertebral nerves; laterally from the exiting spinal nerve roots; and anteriorly, fibers from the sympathetic chain (see Fig. 14.2).[59,62,63]

Indication

- Provocative discography for diagnostic purposes
- Intradiscal placement of device or therapeutic medication

Contraindication

- Absolute
  - Unable or unwilling to consent
  - Untreated localized infection in the procedural field
  - Systemic or local infection
  - Pregnancy
  - Known bleeding diathesis
  - Anticoagulants
- Relative contraindication
  - Anatomic derangements; congenital and acquired
  - Allergy to contrast medium, local anesthetic or antibiotics

Equipment

- A 22 or 25 gauge, 3.5- or 5-inch spinal needle
- An 18 or 20 gauge, 3.5- or 5-inch spinal needle as an outer needle for two-needle technique
- Local anesthetic
- Connecting tubing
- Prophylactic intravenous antibiotics
  - Consider diluted gentamicin
- Water-soluble, nonionic contrast dye
- Manometer for diagnostic discography

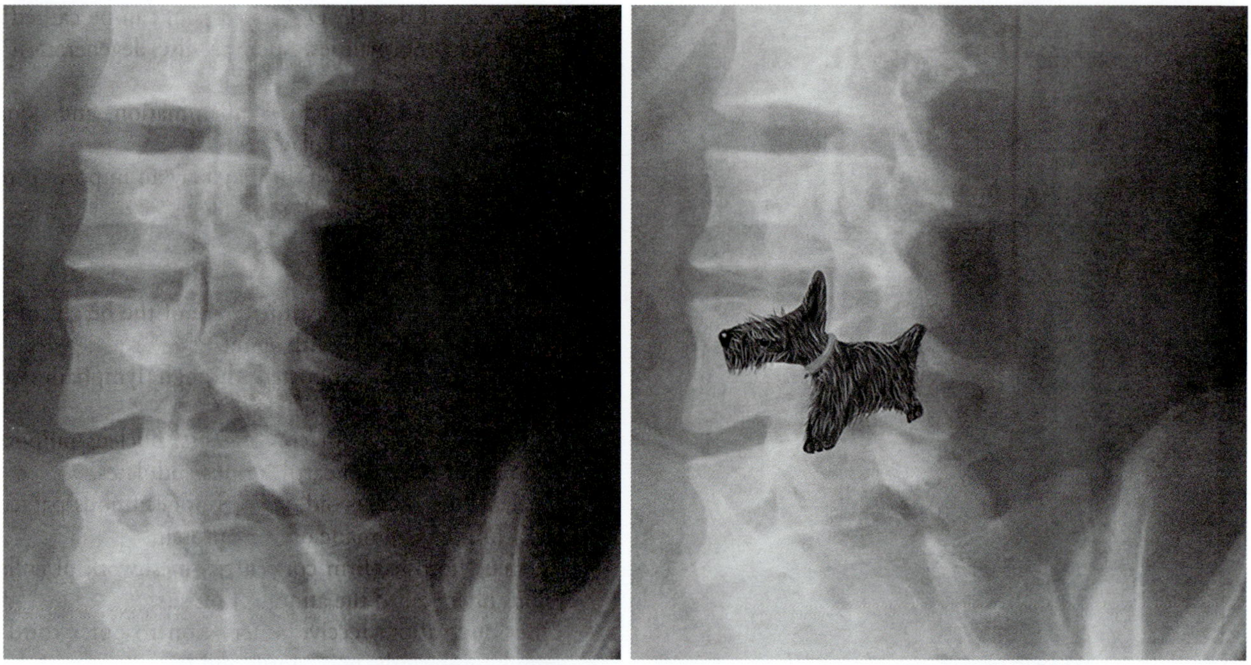

• **Fig 14.57** X-ray oblique view with scotty dog correlate. (From Ridley LJ, Han J, Ridley WE, Xiang H. Scotty dog: normal anatomy—pars interarticularis. *J Med Imaging Radiat Oncol*. 2018;62[Suppl 1]:152. https://doi.org/10.1111/1754-9485.26_12786.)

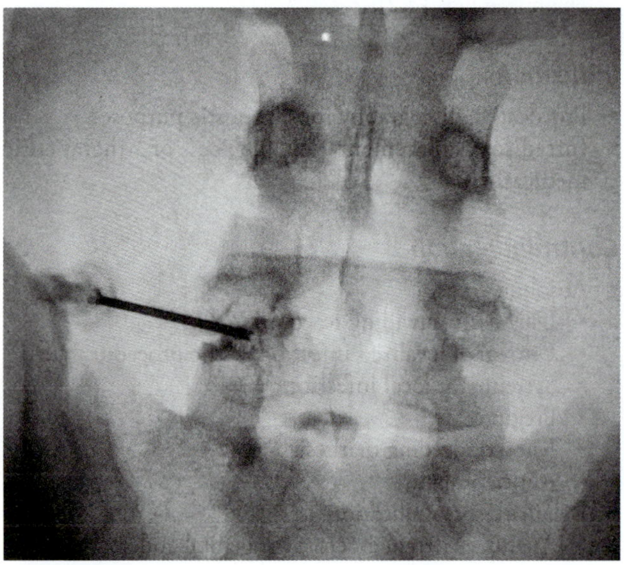

• **Fig. 14.58** L5 Injection in Anteroposterior with Contrast.

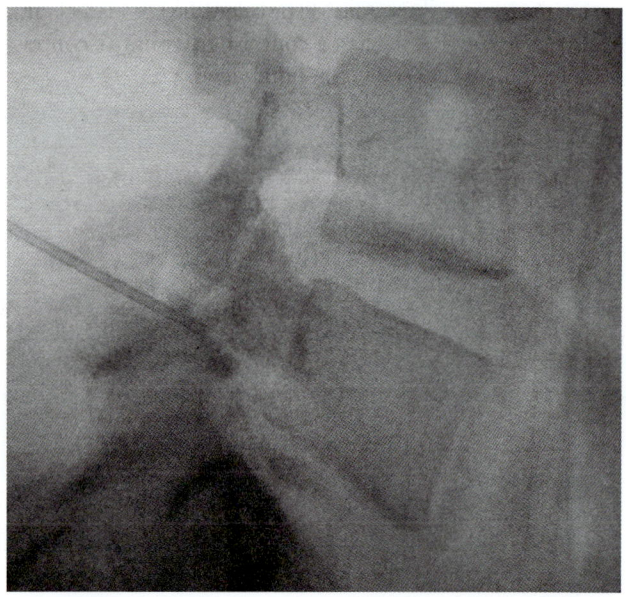

• **Fig. 14.59** L5 Defect Injection Lateral View with Contrast.

Technique

Patient Position

- Prone position on the fluoroscopy table with the pillow under the abdomen to reduce lumbar lordosis.

C-Arm Position

- Confirm the appropriate level with an AP view.
- Tilt: cephalic enough to open disc space at affected level; substantially tilt at L5-S1.
- Rotate toward affected side to create an acute oblique image. At L5-S1 you will visualize the entry point as a small triangle created by the iliac crest, the L5 vertebral body, and the body of S1.
- "Square off" the target disc by squaring off the vertebral endplate above or below the disc (Fig. 14.60).

Needle Position

- The needle should be inserted coaxially.
- Target the SAP at the midpoint of width of the disc.
- On a longitudinal plane navigate the needle lateral to the SAP of the same segment as the target disc; stay sufficiently lateral to SAP to avoid snagging the periosteum of SAP.

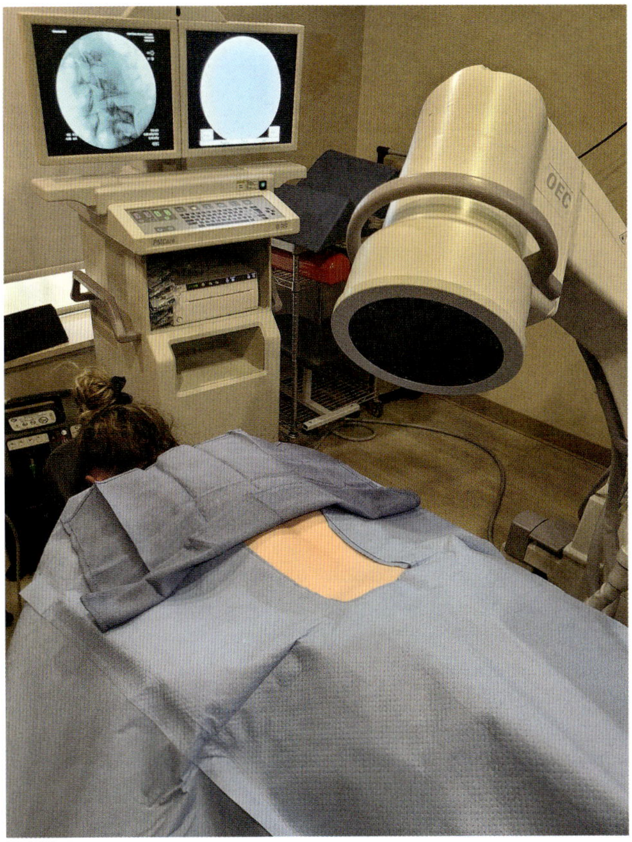

• **Fig. 14.60** Patient Positioning for Lumbar Discography.

- A two-needle technique can be used for an added precaution against infection and to facilitate the passage of a very fine needle through the back muscles.
- The depth of insertion should be checked periodically by briefly reverting to an AP and lateral view (Figs 14.61 and 14.62).

Complications

- Discitis; most common severe complication after discography
- Subdural abscess
- Epidural and prevertebral abscess
- Spinal cord injury
- Vascular injury
- Direct trauma to nerve roots

PEARLS AND PITFALLS

- Any needle tip should not be touched or handled by the glove hands. Always use sterile gauze or instrument.
- Obtain CT of lumbar spine following diagnostic discography within 2 to 4 hours.
- Consider a post-injection MRI if any worsening or prolonged lower back pain to rule out discitis.

Lumbar Ligaments: Supraspinous, Interspinous, Ligamentum Flavum, Iliolumbar, Intertransverse

KEY POINTS

- The lumbar ligaments are important structures to consider when patients have low back or lumbar radicular pain, especially in the presence of scoliosis, spondylolisthesis, loss of disc height, after trauma, or in patients with a hypermobility syndrome.
- Spine ligament injuries are often not seen or diagnosed on x-rays or MRI.[64]
- Flexion extension x-rays can show subtle movements in the vertebral bodies in different positions.
- Damaged ligaments may or may not be primary pain generators but should be considered as part of the spinal functional unit (adjacent vertebrae, intervertebral disc, ligaments, and facet joints) in which injury to any part can cause biomechanical alterations leading to degeneration and pain.[64,65]

Pertinent Anatomy

- The supraspinous (SS) ligaments course between and just over the spinous processes.[66]
- The interspinous (IS) ligaments course between the spinous processes.[66]
- The ligamentum flavum extends from the second cervical vertebra to the first sacral vertebra connecting the adjacent laminae.[65]
- The intertransverse (IT) ligaments course between and just anterior to the transverse processes.[66]
- The iliolumbar ligament can have several anatomic variations but mostly courses between the transverse processes of the lowest lumbar vertebra (typically L5) and the iliac crest.
- The iliolumbar ligament restricts lateral, rotational, and flexion movement of the lumbosacral junction and helps to stabilize the superior SI joint.
- There are two inferior bands off of the lowest (typically L5 transverse process):
  - The transverse (transverse process to the superior posterior medial aspect of the posterior iliac crest).
  - The inferior (which connects lower and medially on the posterior iliac crest and can have some connections to the superior SI joint capsule). This can have both ventral and dorsal components.
  - Sometimes a third band, the superior band can connect from the superior medial aspect of the posterior iliac crest to the lateral aspect of the second lowest transverse process (typically L4) and have some connections to the L5 spinous process, blending with the L4-5 IT ligament).

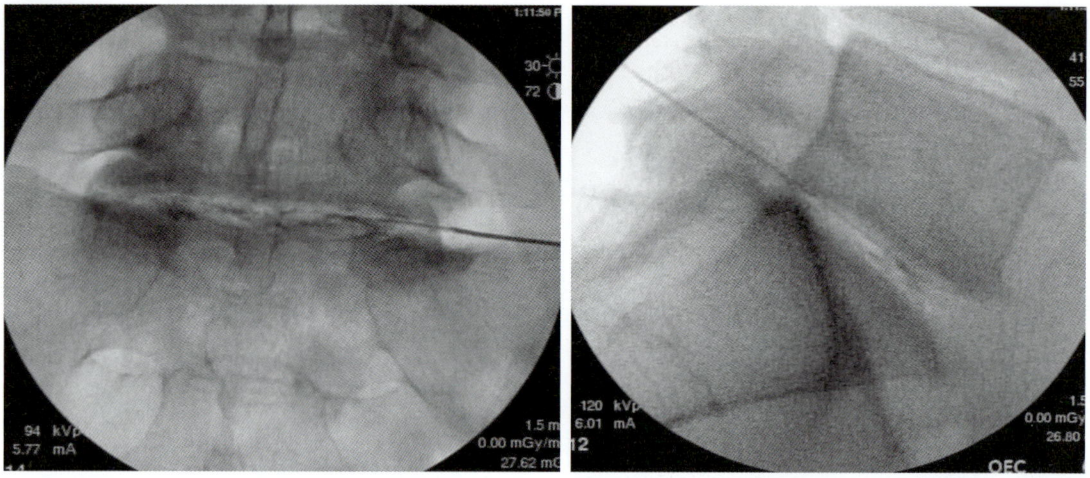

• **Fig. 14.61** Needle positioning at L5-S1 in the anteroposterior and lateral views.

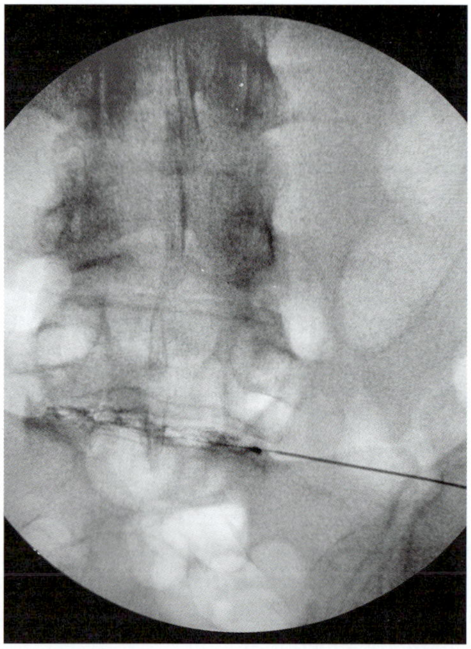

• **Fig. 14.62** Anteroposterior Contrast View Shows Normal Disc Appearance at L3-L4, L4-L5. and "Degenerative Appearing Disc at L5-S1."

- Muscle fibers of the erector spinae, iliacus quadratus lumborum, and the thoracodorsal fascia attach to different parts of the IL ligament.[67,68]

Common Pathology

- Traumatic injury.
- Lumbar ligament injuries are common after MVAs or traumas.
- Lumbar spondylosis, degenerative disease, and loss of lordosis can cause lumbar ligament laxity and vice versa.
- Scoliosis: for a lateral curve, the intertransverse ligaments are stretched. with increased laxity at the convexity of the segmental curve, and are the targets for injection.
- Buckling and hypertrophy of the ligamentum flavum has been associated with degenerative disc disease segmental motion abnormalities, spondylosis, and contributes to spinal stenosis.[67]
- Iliolumbar syndrome has been described as unilateral low back pain at the posterior iliac crest, reproduced by hip flexion and the Patrick test. One small study showed that 25% dextrose solution helped pain in six of seven patients.[69]

Equipment

- C-arm fluoroscopy
- 22 to 25 gauge, 3- to 3.5-inch spinal needle
- Optional: contrast

Common Injectates

- Prolotherapy, orthobiologics (PRP, bone marrow concentrate, etc.)
- Avoid intraligamentous corticosteroids

Injectate Volume

- 0.5 to 1 mL per area/ligament

Technique: SS/IS Mid Ligamentum Flavum

Patient Position

- Same as for other lumbar procedures.
- Prone with pillow under the waist to decrease lordosis.

Clinician Position

- Standing opposite of the C-arm.

C-Arm Position Fluoroscopy

- True lateral view.

Needle Position

- Palpate the spinous processes to ascertain midline; option to mark the skin.
- Insert needle aiming for spinous process at desired level to ensure midline placement.

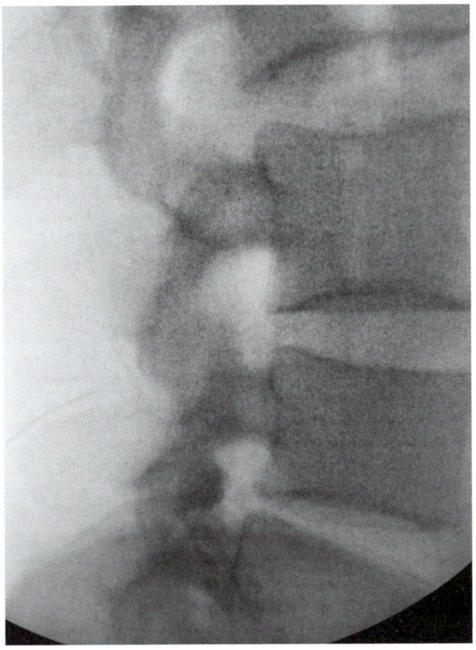

• **Fig. 14.63** Supraspinous (SS) Injection and Interspinous (IS) Injection Lateral Fluoroscopy Needle in Mid IS Ligament.

Target

- Gently touch down on the spinous process and inject the SSL.
- Redirect the needle superior between the spinous processes to inject the ISLs.
- Cautiously advance the needle towards the mid-portion of the ligamentum flavum. Stay posterior to the spinal laminar line.
- Option to inject contrast for the deeper structure to ensure no epidural flow.

PEARLS AND PITFALLS

- Use smallest needle possible.
- Use two hands when injecting the deeper ligaments to ensure adequate control of the needle, which will also limit accidental advancement of the needle too deep (Figs 14.63 and 14.64).

Technique for Iliolumbar, Intertransverse Ligaments

Patient Position

- Same as for other lumbar procedures.
- Prone with pillow under the waist to decrease lordosis.

Clinician Position

- Standing opposite of the C-arm.

C-Arm Position Fluoroscopy

- True AP view, so the spinous process of the desired level is centered between the vertebral bodies.
- "Square off" endplate of the desired level.
- Center the transverse process.

Needle Position

- For the iliolumbar ligament:
  - The needle starts over the inferior lateral border of the lowest lumbar transverse process.
  - Guide the needle coaxially to touch down on the periosteum of the lateral aspect of the transverse process.
- For the intertransverse ligaments:
  - The needle starts over the lateral border of the targeted transverse process.
  - For instance, if targeting the L3-4 IT ligament, start one needle over the L3 TP and redirect inferiorly. A second needle will start over the L4 transverse process and redirect superiorly.

Target

- Iliolumbar ligament:
  - To target the iliolumbar inferior band, redirect the needle inferiorly off of the periosteum and deep/ventral no more than 1 to 2 mm.
  - Inject a small amount of contrast to show vertical flow extending inferiorly to the posterior iliac crest and superior sacroiliac joint.
  - To target the transverse band, redirect the needle slightly laterally off of the periosteum and deep/ventral no more than 1 to 2mm.
  - Inject a small amount of contrast to show linear flow horizontally going toward the posterior iliac crest.
  - To target the superior band, redirect the needle superiorly and lateral to the lowest transverse process and go slightly deep/ventral no more than 1 to 2 mm
  - Inject a small amount of contrast to show flow going toward the L4 spinous process and toward the posterior iliac crest.
- Transverse ligaments:
  - The needle should be advanced to the lateral aspect of the transverse process until touching down on the periosteum. Redirect the needle either superior and deep/anterior or inferior and deep/anterior to target the desired superior or inferior band no more than 1 to 2 mm.
  - Inject a small amount of contrast that should show vertical flow along the ligament superiorly or inferiorly, depending on the target.
  - Inject both the superior and inferior aspects of the ligament.

PEARLS AND PITFALLS

- The iliolumbar ligament is an important stabilizer for the L5-S1 segment and for the superior sacroiliac (SI) joint.[70]
- Always start over and touch down on is to ascertain depth and for safety.
- If the patient is awake, injecting the iliolumbar ligament can reproduce some typical pain and may provide diagnostic information on if the IL ligament is a pain generator.
- The authors recommend using contrast to confirm ligamentous spread. Also, it can serve as a diagnostic injection using an anesthetic agent (Figs 14.65-14.67).

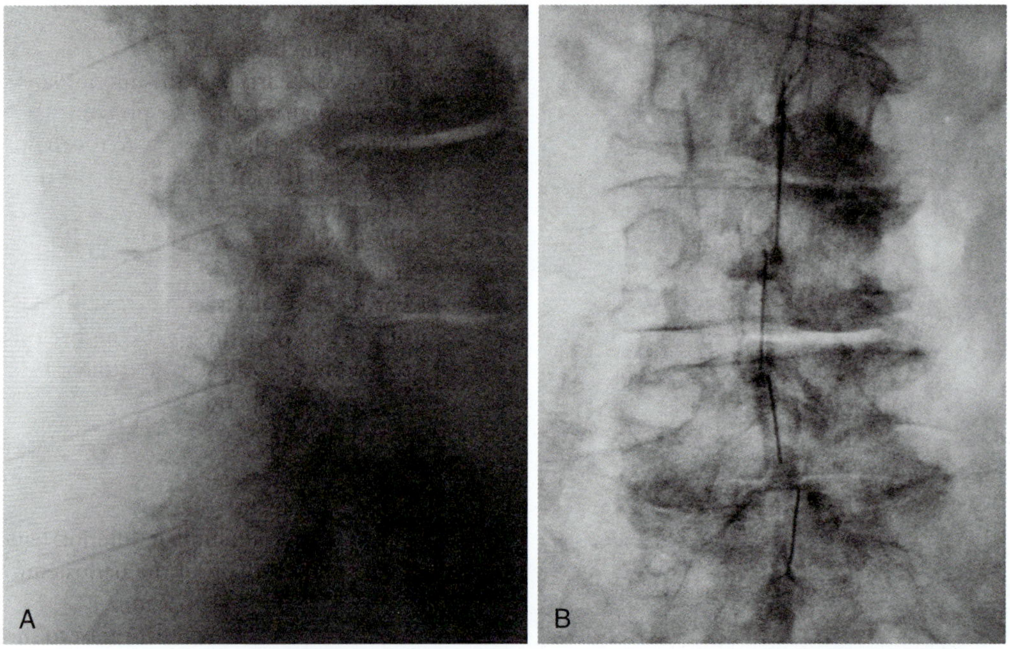

• **Fig. 14.64** (A) Mid-portion ligamentum flavum (LF) injection lateral fluoroscopy with contrast showing supraspinous injection and LF flow and no epidural flow. (B) LF mid-portion anteroposterior fluoroscopic view.

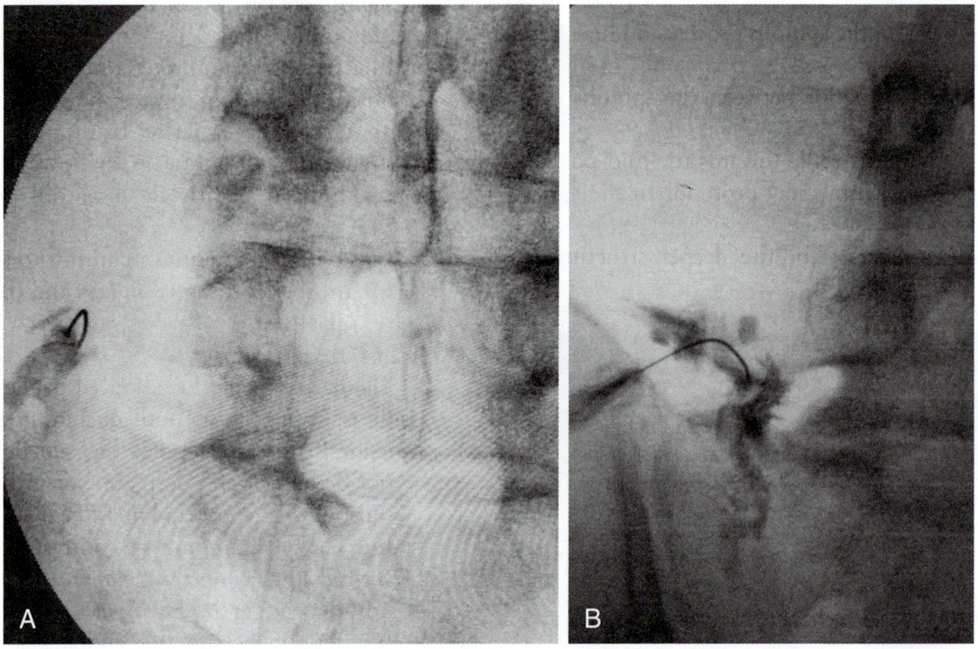

• **Fig. 14.65** (A) Iliolumbar ligament anteroposterior fluoroscopy with contrast inferior band showing connection to superior supraspinous injection (SI) joint capsule. (B) Iliolumbar ligament inferior and transverse bands with contrast also showing flow along the anterior inferior band connecting to anterior SI capsule.

Technique for Lateral Aspect of the Ligamentum Flavum

Patient Position

- Same as for other lumbar procedures.
- Prone with pillow under the waist to decrease lordosis.

Clinician Position

- Standing opposite of the C-arm.

C-Arm Position Fluoroscopy

- True AP view, so the spinous process of the desired level is centered between the vertebral bodies.

- "Square off" endplate of the desired level.
- Make sure the lamina are clearly visualized.
- Use CLO view around 40 degrees or what rotation visualizes the lamina best in order to gauge needle depth.
- Can also use true lateral to gauge needle depth.

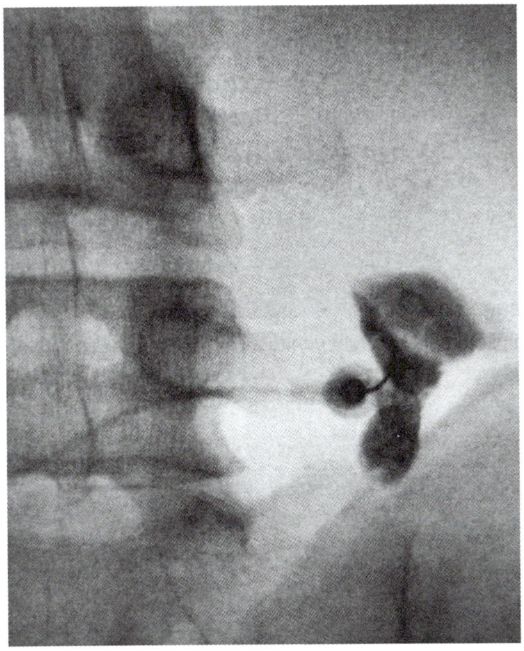

• **Fig. 14.66** Iliolumbar Ligament Anteroposterior Fluoroscopy with Contrast Needle at Superior Band Also Showing Inferior Band Flow.

Needle Position

- Identify the lamina just below the targeted area.

For example, for the L3-4 ligamentum flavum, identify the L4 lamina.

- Start the needle just lateral to the spinous process and mid-portion of the lamina superior to inferior.
- Guide the needle anterior and slightly superior to touch the superior aspect of the lamina.

Target

- Target the ligament flavum by redirecting the needle just superior to the lamina.
- Stop and check the needle depth in the contralateral oblique view or utilize a true lateral view.
- Advance the needle to the spinal laminar line.
- Inject a small amount of contrast to show flow along the ligament in the CLO view or lateral and to make sure no epidural flow. Can confirm in the AP as well.

PEARLS AND PITFALLS

- The starting needle position should always be over the periosteal surface of the lamina and always touch down on the lamina to ascertain depth and for safety prior to advancing the needle into the interlaminar space.
- Theoretically, tightening the ligamentum flavum with prolotherapy or orthobiologics may decrease buckling and hypertrophy, thus widening the epidural space and potentially providing symptomatic relief in patients with central canal stenosis and ligamentum flavum hypertrophy (Figs 14.68 and 14.69).

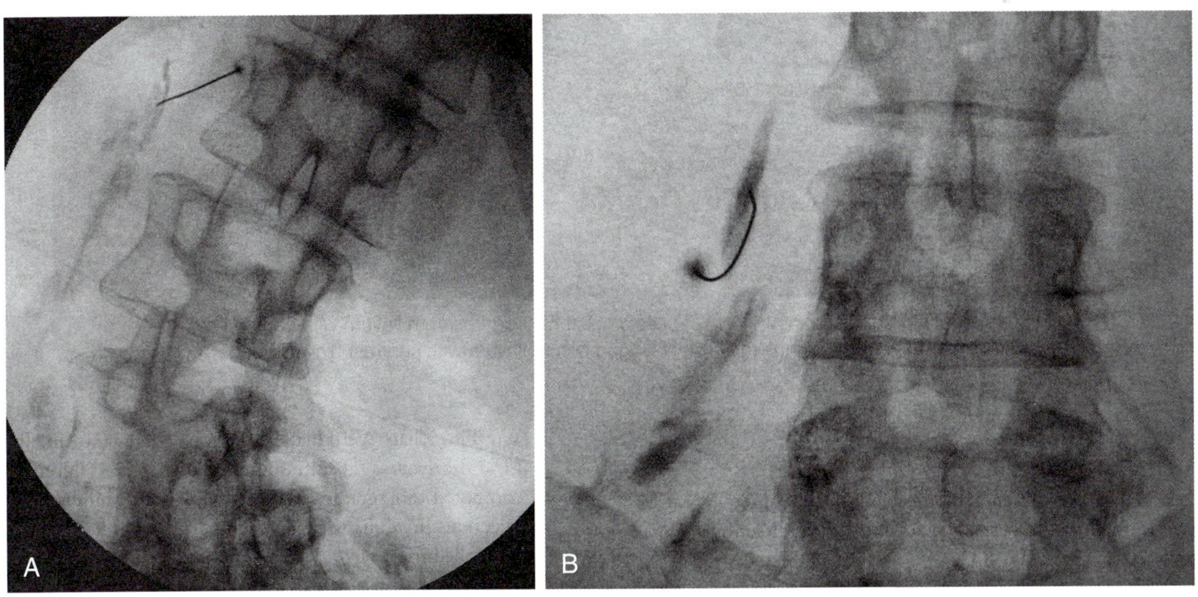

• **Fig. 14.67** (A) Anteroposterior (AP) view of scoliotic patient with needle at the left L1-2 intertransverse ligament (IT) with contrast highlighting the injected IT ligaments. (B) AP view of needle at the L3-4 IT ligament with contrast highlighting the injected IT ligaments.

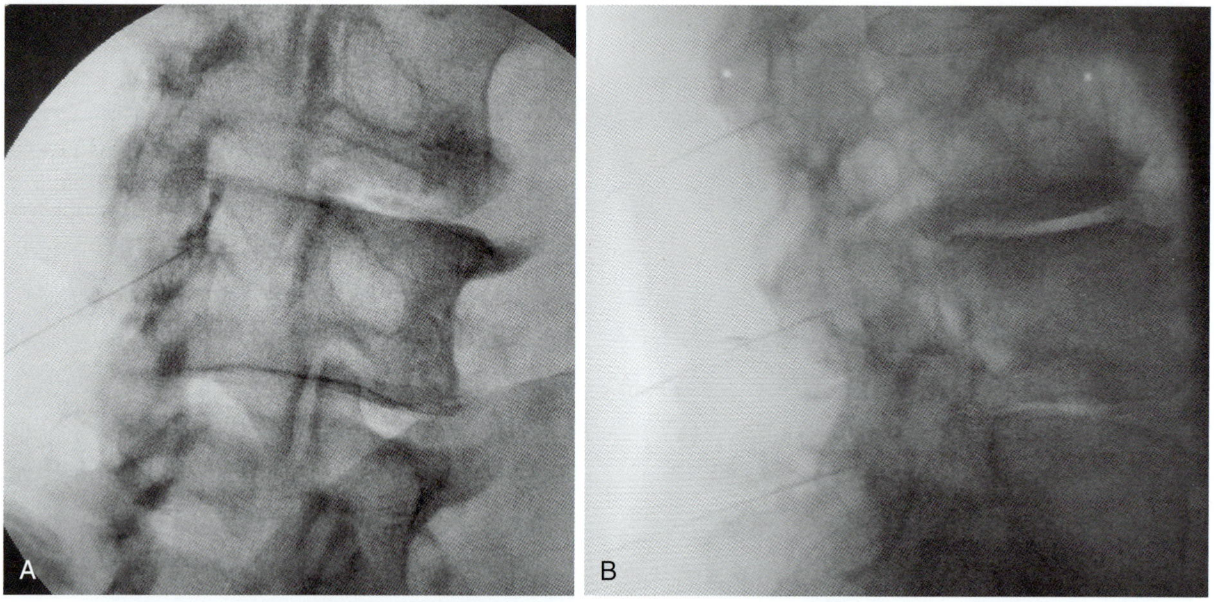

• **Fig. 14.68** (A) Contralateral oblique view of needle at the ligamentum flavum with contrast highlighting. (B) Lateral view of needles at the ligamentum flavum.

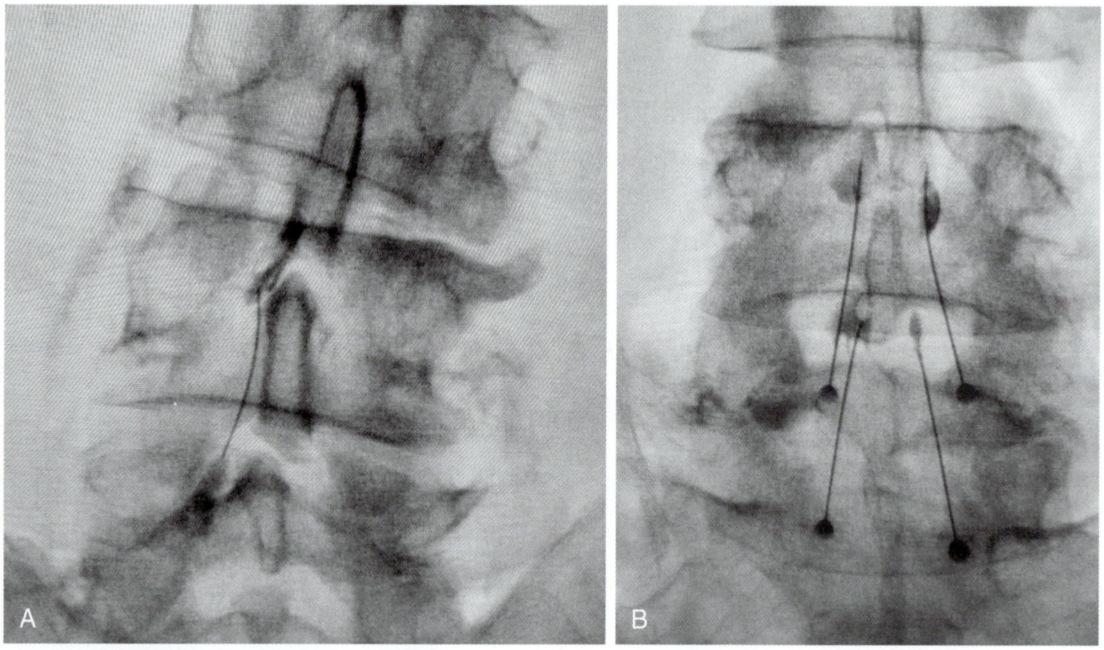

• **Fig. 14.69** (A) Anteroposterior (AP) view of needle at left L3-4 ligamentum flavum with contrast highlighting. (B) AP view of needles at bilateral L3-4, l4-5 ligamentum flavum with contrast highlighting.

References

1. Oxland TR. Fundamental biomechanics of the spine--What we have learned in the past 25 years and future directions. *J Biomech*. 2016;49(6):817–832.
2. Panjabi MM, White 3rd AA. Basic biomechanics of the spine. *Neurosurgery*. 1980;7(1):76–93. https://doi.org/10.1227/00006123-198007000-00014.
3. Wu Tao, Zhao Wei-Hua, Dong Yan, Song Hai-Xin, Jian-Hua Li, Effectiveness of ultrasound-guided versus fluoroscopy or computed tomography scanning guidance in lumbar facet joint injections in adults with facet joint syndrome: a meta-analysis of controlled trials. *Arch Phys Med Rehabil*. 2016;97(9):1558–1563.
4. Galiano K, Obwegeser AA, Walch C, Schatzer R, Ploner F, Gruber H. Ultrasound-guided versus computed tomography-controlled facet joint injections in the lumbar spine: a

prospective randomized clinical trial. *Reg Anesth Pain Med.* 2007;32(4):317–322.

5. Alonso F, Kirkpatrick CM, Jeong W, et al. Lumbar facet tropism: a comprehensive review. *World Neurosurg.* 2017;102:91–96.
6. Kalichman L, Pradeep S, Ali G, Li L, Hunter DJ. Facet orientation and tropism: associations with facet joint osteoarthritis and degeneratives. *Spine (Phila Pa 1976).* 2009;34(16):E579–E585.
7. Liu Ziyang, Duan Yuchen, Rong Xin, Wang Beiyu, Chen Hua, Hao Liu. Variation of facet joint orientation and tropism in lumbar degenerative spondylolisthesis and disc herniation at L4-L5: a systematic review and meta-analysis. *Clin Neurol Neurosurg.* 2017;161:41–47.
8. Cohen SP, Raja SN. Pathogenesis, diagnosis, and treatment of lumbar zygapophysial (facet) joint pain. *Anesthesiology.* 2007;106(3):591–614.
9. Wu Jiuping, Du Zhenwu, Yang Lv, et al. A new technique for the treatment of lumbar facet joint syndrome using intra-articular injection with autologous platelet rich plasma. *Pain Phy.* 2016;19(8):617–625.
10. Karkucak M, Kurt M, Özçakar L. Ultrasound video demonstration for lumbar facet joint injection. *Am J Phy Med Rehabil.* 2016;95(10):e165–e166.
11. Oxland TR. Fundamental biomechanics of the spine--What we have learned in the past 25 years and future directions. *J Biomech.* 2016;49(6):817–832.
12. https://www.imaios.com/en/e-Anatomy/Anatomical-Parts/Supraspinous-ligament.
13. (*Spine: November* 1, 2004 - Volume 29 - Issue 21 - p 2395-2403)
14. https://www.ajronline.org/doi/pdf/10.2214/ajr.175.3.1750661. https://hospitalhealthcare.com/latest-issue-2015/joint-hypermobility-and-lumbar-disc-herniation/.
15. Creze M. Conceptualization, Data curation, Methodology, Resources. The paraspinal muscle-tendon system: its paradoxical anatomy. *PLoS One.* 2019;14(4):e0214812.
16. Gorman N. Multifidus muscle. *Jana Vasković.* 2020.
17. Zhang Shanshan, Xu Yi, Han Xiulan, Wu Wen, Tang Yan, Wang Chuhuai. Functional and morphological changes in the deep lumbar multifidus using electromyography and ultrasound. *Sci Rep.* 2018;8:6539.
18. Hildebrandt M, Fankhauser G, Meichtry A. Hannu L. Correlation between lumbar dysfunction and fat infiltration in lumbar multifidus muscles in patients with low back pain. *BMC Musculoskelet Disord.* 2017;18(1):12.
19. Smuck M, Crisostomo RA, Ryan D, Fitch DS, Kennedy DJ, Geisser ME. Lumbar spine after lumbar medial branch radiofrequency neurotomy: a quantitative radiological study. *Spine J.* 2015;15(6):1415–1421.
20. Bahar S, Hubbard JC, Gibbons MC, et al. Lumbar multifidus muscle degenerates in individuals with chronic degenerative lumbar spine pathology. *J Orthop Res.* 2017;35(12):2700–2706.
21. Park Moon Soo, Moon Seong-Hwan, Kim Tae-Hwan, et al. Paraspinal muscles of patients with lumbar diseases. *J Neurol Surg A Cent Eur Neurosurg.* 2018;79(4):323–329.
22. Goubert D, Van Oosterwijck J, Meeus M, Danneels L. Structural changes of lumbar muscles in non-specific low back pain: a systematic review. *Pain Phys.* 2016;19(7):E985–E1000.
23. Goubert D, De Pauw R, Meeus M, et al. Lumbar muscle structure and function in chronic versus recurrent low back pain: a cross-sectional study. *Spine J.* 2017;17(9):1285–1296.
24. Chon Jinmann, Kim Hee-Sang, Jong Ha Lee, et al. Asymmetric atrophy of paraspinal muscles in patients with chronic unilateral lumbar radiculopathy. *Ann Rehabil Med.* 2017;41(5): 801–807.
25. Dreyfuss P, Stout A, Aprill C, Pollei S, Johnson B, Bogduk N. The significance of multifidus atrophy after successful radiofrequency neurotomy for low back pain. *PM R.* 2009;1(8):719–722.
26. Hu Zhi-Jun, Zhang Jian-Feng, Xu Wen-Bin, et al. Effect of pure muscle retraction on multifidus injury and atrophy after posterior lumbar spine surgery with 24 weeks observation in a rabbit model. *Eur Spine J.* 2017;26(1):210–220.
27. Hu Zhi-Jun, Xu Wen-Bin, Chen Shuai, et al. Accuracy of magnetic resonance imaging signal intensity ratio measurements in the evaluation of multifidus muscle injury and atrophy relative to that of histological examinations. *Spine (Phila Pa 1976).* 2014;39(10):E623–E629.
28. Oxland TR. Fundamental biomechanics of the spine--What we have learned in the past 25 years and future directions. *J Biomech.* 2016;49(6):817–832.
29. Panjabi MM, White 3rd AA. Basic biomechanics of the spine. *Neurosurgery.* 1980;7(1):76–93.
30. Willard FH, Vleeming A, Schuenke MD, Danneels L, Schleip R. The thoracolumbar fascia: anatomy, function and clinical considerations. *J Anat.* 2012;221(6):507–536.
31. Fan Chenglei, Fede Caterina, Nathaly Gaudreault. Anatomical and functional relationships between external abdominal oblique muscle and posterior layer of thoracolumbar fascia. *Clin Anat.* 2018;31(7):1092–1098.
32. Faraj AA, Mehdian H, Thoracolumbar hernia. A rare cause of back pain. *Eur Spine J.* 1997;6(3):203–204.
33. Yan Y, Xu R, Zou T. Is thoracolumbar fascia injury the cause of residual back pain after percutaneous vertebroplasty? A prospective cohort study. *Osteoporos Int.* 2015;26(3):1119–1124.
34. Centeno Chris. *Pain After Back Surgery? Did the Surgeon Leave a Big Hole in Your Fascia?*; 2017.
35. Fullerton Bradley D. Prolotherapy for the thoracolumbar myofascial system. *Phys Med Rehabil Clin N Am.* 2018;29(1):125–138.
36. Kushchayev SV, Glushko T, Jarraya M, et al. ABCs of the degenerative spine. *Insights Imaging.* 2018;9(2):253–274. https://doi.org/10.1007/s13244-017-0584-z.
37. Naeim F, Froetscher L, Hirschberg GG. Treatment of the chronic iliolumbar syndrome by infiltration of the iliolumbar ligament. *West J Med.* 1982;136(4):372–374.
38. Hong JO, Park JS, Jeon DG, Yoon WH, Park JH. Extracorporeal shock wave therapy versus trigger point injection in the treatment of myofascial pain syndrome in the quadratus lumborum. *Ann Rehabil Med.* 2017;41(4):582–588. https://doi.org/10.5535/arm.2017.41.4.582.
39. Phillips S, Mercer S, Bogduk N. Anatomy and biomechanics of quadratus lumborum. *Proc Inst Mech Eng H.* 2008;222(2):151–159. https://doi.org/10.1243/09544119JEIM266.

40. Kennedy DJ, et al. Comparative effectiveness of lumbar transforaminal epidural steroid injections with particulate versus nonparticulate corticosteroids for lumbar radicular pain due to intervertebral disc herniation: a prospective, randomized, double-blind trial. *Pain Med.* 2014;15(4):548.
41. Okubadejo, Gbolahan O, et al. Perils of intravascular methylprednisolone injection into the vertebral artery: an animal study. *JBJS.* 2008;90(9):1932–1938.
42. Kim D, Brown J. Efficacy and safety of lumbar epidural dexamethasone versus methylprednisolone in the treatment of lumbar radiculopathy: a comparison of soluble versus particulate steroids. *Clin J Pain.* 2011;27(6):518–522.
43. El-Yahchouchi C, et al. The noninferiority of the nonparticulate steroid dexamethasone vs the particulate steroids betamethasone and triamcinolone in lumbar transforaminal epidural steroid injections. *Pain Med. 14.* 2013;11:1650–1657.
44. Centeno C, Markle J, Dodson E, et al. The use of lumbar epidural injection of platelet lysate for treatment of radicular pain. *J Exp Orthop.* 2017;4(1):38. https://doi.org/10.1186/s40634-017-0113-5.
45. Furman MB, et al. Injectate volumes needed to reach specific landmarks in lumbar transforaminal epidural injections. *Reeves RS PM R.* 2010;2(7):625–635.
46. Bogduk N, ed. *Practice Guidelines for Spinal Diagnostic and Treatment Procedures.* International Spine Intervention Society; 2013. Artery of Adam.
47. Bogduk N, Aprill CN, Derby R. Epidural steroid injections. In: White AH, Schofferman JA, eds. *Spine Care: Diagnosis and Treatment.* St. Louis: Mosby Year Book. 1995: 322–342.
48. Simon Jeremy I, et al. Intravascular penetration following lumbar transforaminal epidural injections using the infraneural technique. *Pain Med.* 2015;16(8):1647–1649.
49. Sayre PA, Burr Ridge IL, Glaser Scott E. Root cause analysis of paraplegia following transforaminal epidural steroid injections: the "unsafe" triangle. *Pain Phy.* 2010;13:237–244.
50. Kroszczynski AC, et al. Intraforaminal location of thoracolumbar anterior medullary arteries. *Pain Med.* 2013;14(6):808–812.
51. Yoshioka K, et al. MR angiography and CT angiography of the artery of Adamkiewicz: noninvasive preoperative assessment of thoracoabdominal aortic aneurysm. *Radiographics.* 2003;23(5):1215–1225.
52. Bogduk N, et al. Complications of spinal diagnostic and treatment procedures. *Pain Med.* 2008;9(suppl 1):S11–S34.
53. Levi D, Horn S, Corcoran S. The incidence of intradiscal, intrathecal, and intravascular flow during the performance of retrodiscal (infraneural) approach for lumbar transforaminal epidural steroid injections. *Pain Med.* 2016;17(8):1416–1422. https://doi.org/10.1093/pm/pnv067.
54. Ridley LJ, Han J, Ridley WE, Xiang H. Scotty dog: normal anatomy—pars interarticularis. *J Med Imaging Radiat Oncol.* 2018;62(suppl 1):152. https://doi.org/10.1111/1754-9485.26_12786.
54a. Pereira DM, Camino Willhuber GO., Pars interarticularis injury. StatPearls;2021. https://www.ncbi.nlm.nih.gov/books/NBK545191/.
55. Mansfield JT, Wroten M. *Pars Interarticularis Defect. [Updated 2019 Nov 27]. In: StatPearls [Internet].* Treasure Island (FL): StatPearls Publishing; 2020. Available from: https://www.ncbi.nlm.nih.gov/books/NBK538292/.
56. Panteliadis P, Nagra NS, Edwards KL, Behrbalk E, Boszczyk B. Athletic population with spondylolysis: review of outcomes following surgical repair or conservative management. *Global Spine J.* 2016;6(6):615–625. https://doi.org/10.1055/s-0036-1586743.
57. Imam MA, Mahmoud SSS, Holton J, Abouelmaati D, Elsherbini Y, Snow M. A systematic review of the concept and clinical applications of bone marrow aspirate concentrate in orthopaedics. *SICOT J.* 2017;3:17. https://doi.org/10.1051/sicotj/2017007.
58. Marongiu G, Dolci A, Verona M, Capone A. The biology and treatment of acute long-bones diaphyseal fractures: overview of the current options for bone healing enhancement. *Bone Rep.* 2020;12:100249. https://doi.org/10.1016/j.bonr.2020.100249.
59. Lundon K, Bolton K. Structure and function of the lumbar intervertebral disk in health, aging, and pathologic conditions. *J Orthop Sports Phys Ther.* 2001;31(6):291–306. https://doi.org/10.2519/jospt.2001.31.6.291.
60. Aoki Y, Nakajima A, Ohtori S, et al. Increase of nerve growth factor levels in the human herniated intervertebral disc: can annular rupture trigger discogenic back pain? *Arthritis Res Ther.* 2014;16(4):R159. https://doi.org/10.1186/ar4674.
61. Ohtori S, Miyagi M, Inoue G. Sensory nerve ingrowth, cytokines, and instability of discogenic low back pain: a review. *Spine Surg Relat Res.* 2018;2(1):11–17. https://doi.org/10.22603/ssrr.2016-0018.
62. Waxenbaum JA, Reddy V, Futterman B. Anatomy, back, intervertebral discs. In: *StatPearls [Internet].* Treasure Island (FL): StatPearls Publishing; 2020. Available from: https://www.ncbi.nlm.nih.gov/books/NBK470583/.
63. Mirza SK, White 3rd AA. Anatomy of intervertebral disc and pathophysiology of herniated disc disease. *J Clin Laser Med Surg.* 1995;13(3):131–142. https://doi.org/10.1089/clm.1995.13.131.
64. Panjabi MM. A hypothesis of chronic back pain: ligament subfailure injuries lead to muscle control dysfunction. *Eur Spine J.* 2006;15(5):668–676. https://doi.org/10.1007/s00586-005-0925-3.
65. Kushchayev SV, Glushko T, Jarraya M, et al. ABCs of the degenerative spine. *Insights Imaging.* 2018;9(2):253–274. https://doi.org/10.1007/s13244-017-0584-z.
66. Behrsin JF, Briggs CA. Ligaments of the lumbar spine: a review. *Surg Radiol Anat.* 1988;10(3):211–219. https://doi.org/10.1007/BF02115239.
67. Fujiwara A, Tamai K, Yoshida H, et al. Anatomy of the iliolumbar ligament. *Clin Orthop Relat Res.* 2000;380:167–172. https://doi.org/10.1097/00003086-200011000-00022.

68. Rucco V, Basadonna PT, Gasparini D. Anatomy of the iliolumbar ligament: a review of its anatomy and a magnetic resonance study. *Am J Phys Med Rehabil.* 1996;75(6):451–455. https://doi.org/10.1097/00002060-199611000-00010.
69. Naeim F, Froetscher L, Hirschberg GG. Treatment of the chronic iliolumbar syndrome by infiltration of the iliolumbar ligament. *West J Med.* 1982;136(4):372–374.
70. Pool-Goudzwaard AL, Kleinrensink GJ, Snijders CJ, Entius C, Stoeckart R. The sacroiliac part of the iliolumbar ligament. *J Anat.* 2001;199(Pt 4):457–463. https://doi.org/10.1046/j.1469-7580.2001.19940457.x.

15

Sacrococcygeal Injection Techniques

JOANNE BORG-STEIN, CATHERINE MILLS, CAROLYN BLACK, OLUSEUN OLUFADE, AND GIORGIO A. NEGRON

Ultrasound Guided Procedures

Sacroiliac Joint

KEY POINTS

- Ultrasound-guided intra-articular injections can provide both pain relief and diagnostic information in sacroiliac (SI) joint pain

Pertinent Anatomy

- The SI joint is stabilized by the anterior SI ligament, the interosseous ligament, and the short and long posterior SI ligaments. Secondary stabilizers are the sacrospinous and sacrotuberous ligaments (Fig. 15.1).
- The cranial third of the joint is a fibrous joint, the middle third of the joint is fibrocartilaginous and resembles a symphysis, while the caudal third is synovia.[1,2]
- The anterior joint capsule is contiguous resulting in a "true synovial joint", while the posterior joint capsule is thin and non-contiguous, made up of a series of ligaments, allowing for diffusion of larger volumes of injectate around the posterior ligaments and soft tissue structures.[1,2]

Common Pathology

- The SI joint (SIJ) is a common source of axial low back pain, with a prevalence of 25%.[3]
- The pathophysiology of SI joint pain is highly debated. Pain generation may be the result of abnormal movement of the SI joint (either laxity or immobility), malalignment of the SI joint, and osteoarthritis of the SI joint.
- Sacroiliitis may be an early symptom of seronegative spondyloarthropathies. Seronegative spondyloarthropathy should be suspected in younger (<45 years) male patients presenting with SI joint or low back pain of insidious onset that improves with activity.[4,5]
- Increased Doppler signal surrounding the SI joint is seen in sacroiliitis.[6]
- In addition to axial pain, pathology of the SIJ can produce variable referred pain patterns, including pain referred into the buttock, the lower lumbar area, and the thigh.[7]

Equipment

- Needle size: 25–22 gauge and 2 to 3.5-inch needle
- Low frequency curvilinear ultrasound transducer

Common Injectates

- Local anesthetics for diagnostics, corticosteroids
- Prolotherapy, Orthobiologics (PRP, bone marrow concentrate, etc.)

Injectate Volume

- 0.8–2.5 mL[8]

Technique

Patient Position

- Prone with a pillow under the abdomen to flatten the lumbar curvature.
- Lower extremities should be internally rotated while feet are inverted to help flatten the gluteal region.

Clinician Position

- Sitting or standing by the patient's side

Transducer Position

- Transverse orientation to identify the sacral hiatus
- Move the transducer laterally to identify the lateral edge of the sacrum
- Keeping the transducer in the transverse orientation, move cephalad until the contour of the ilium is identified (Fig. 15.2A)
- Transducer should end over the caudal third of the SI joint.[9,10]

Needle Position

- In-plane with the transducer, medial to lateral approach with approximately 45–65 degrees of angulation (see Fig. 15.2B)

Target

- The caudal third of the SI joint is targeted advancing the needle past the posterior SI ligament (see Fig. 15.2).[9,10]
- Alternatively, the middle third or the cranial third of the SI joint can be targeted with comparable pain reduction.[11–13]

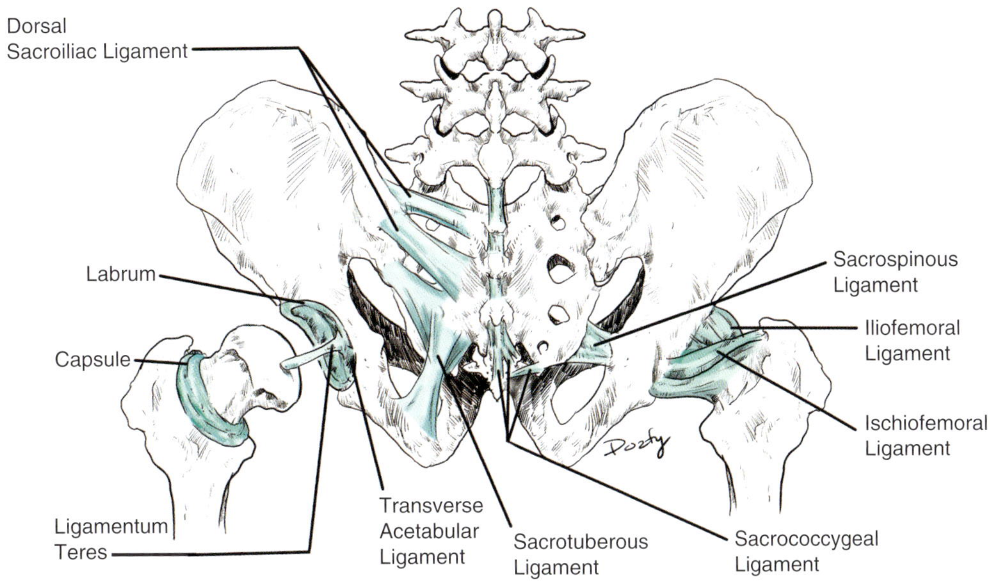

• **Fig. 15.1** Posterior pelvic and sacral ligaments.

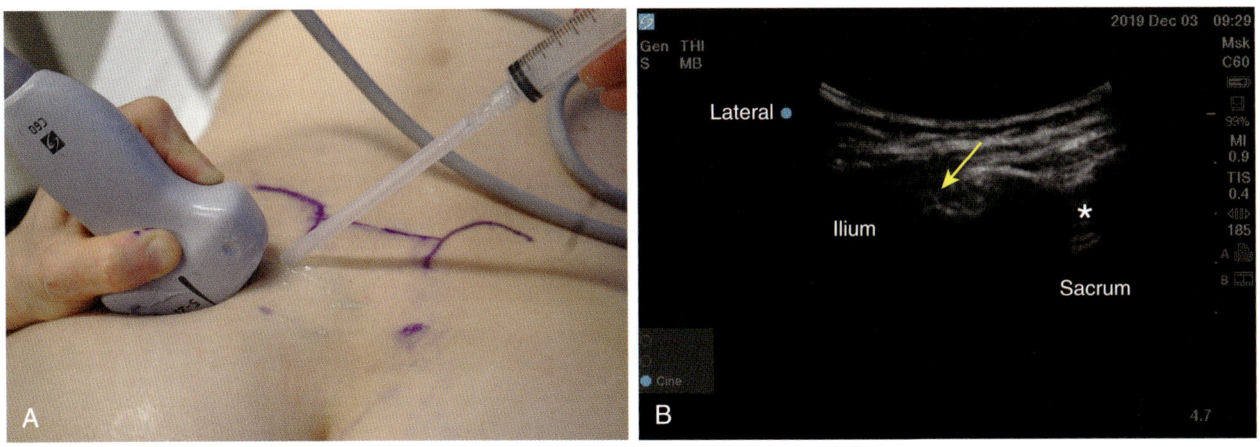

• **Fig. 15.2** Ultrasound guided sacroiliac joint injection (A) Set-up. The posterior superior iliac spine, superior border of the sacrum, and lateral borders of the sacrum are marked on the model for reference during the procedure. (B) A transverse ultrasonic view of the SI joint with the ilium to the left of the screen and sacrum to the right. The needle approach shown from medial to lateral into the boat-shaped SI joint *(arrow)*. Dorsal sacral foramina *(*)*.

PEARLS AND PITFALLS

- A 2%–2.5% rate of vascular uptake in US guided SI joint injection has been reported.[14,15]
- The posterior sacral foramen should be visualized on ultrasound along with the SI joint to confirm injection location lateral to the S2 foramen, and avoid foraminal injection.
- In cadaveric studies, >50% of injections at the caudal third of the SI joint had extra-articular spread.[16] For this reason, it may be worthwhile to consider targeting the cranial third or middle third of the SI joint, as the approach may be technically less challenging with the wider joint space in this area.[13]

The Sacrococcygeal Joint

KEY POINTS

- Ultrasound can be a useful adjunct to fluoroscopy to locate the sacrococcygeal joint (SCJ) for joint injection or set-up for ganglion impar block. Fluoroscopy is required to confirm needle depth and position.

Pertinent Anatomy

- The SCJ contains the sacrococcygeal disc, which may ossify with age and obscure the SCJ on fluoroscopy.
- The ganglion impar is located ventral to the deep sacrococcygeal ligament and can be accessed through the SCJ.

Common Pathology

- Pain can be traumatic or non-traumatic
- Coccydynia more frequently affects women. Compared to males, the female coccyx tends to be shorter, straighter, and more prone to retroversion.[17]

Equipment

- Needle size: 25–22 gauge and 2 to 3-inch needle.
- High-frequency linear ultrasound transducer

Common Injectates

- Local anesthetics for diagnostics, corticosteroids
- Prolotherapy, Orthobiologics (PRP, bone marrow concentrate, etc.)

Injectate volume

- 1–3 mL

Technique

Patient Position

- Prone, with a pillow under the abdomen to flatten the lumbar curve.
- Lower extremities should be internally rotated while feet are inverted to help flatten the gluteal region.

Clinician Position

- Seated or standing next to the patient

Transducer Position

- Start with the transducer transverse across the midline and locate the sacral hiatus.
- Identify the sacral cornua.
- The sacrococcygeal ligament can be identified overlying the sacral hiatus, which is superficial to the base of the sacrum.
- Rotate longitudinally over the SCJ and sacral hiatus, so the proximal part of the transducer rests between the two cornua, and the first cleft caudal to the sacral hiatus is the SCJ (Fig. 15.3A).

Needle position

- In plane with the transducer Fig. 15.3B

Target

- The cleft of the SCJ (the first cleft caudal to the sacral hiatus is the SCJ) (see Fig. 15.3B)

PEARLS AND PITFALLS

- The tip of the needle can be difficult to visualize in the joint space using ultrasound.
- Fluoroscopy is preferred to confirm needle depth and position.
- The same approach is used for ganglion impar block, passing through the joint to reach the ganglion anterior to the ventral sacrococcygeal ligament with fluoroscopy to confirm needle placement.

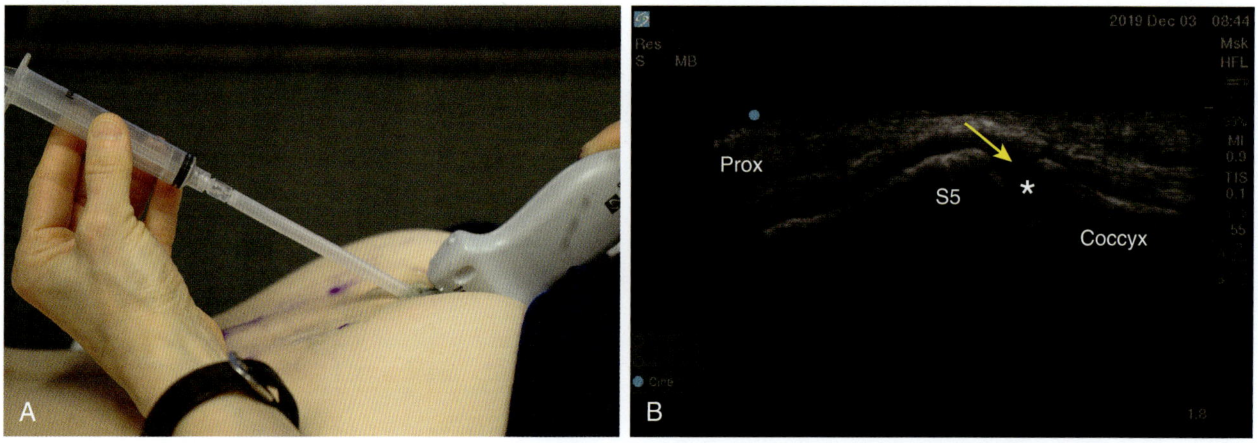

• **Fig. 15.3** Ultrasound guided injection of the sacrococcygeal joint. (A) Set up. (B) Ultrasound view of the sacrum (proximal, *left*), coccyx (distal, *right*), and sacrococcygeal joint (*), with needle path *(arrow)*.

Short and Long Dorsal Sacroiliac Ligaments

KEY POINTS

- The short and long dorsal SI ligaments are able to be visualized superficial to the SI joint using ultrasound guidance and targeted for injection.[18,19]

Pertinent Anatomy

- The SI joint is located in the bony cleft between the sacrum and the contour of the ilium.
- The dorsal ligaments lie within this bony cleft lateral to the sacrum at the S1–S2 level.
- The short dorsal ligament is oriented perpendicular to the joint, while the long ligament runs oblique to it.

Common Pathology

- Disruption or laxity of the ligamentous structures leading to altered joint mechanics is a potential cause of SIJ pain.[20]

Equipment

- Needle size: 25–22 gauge and 2 to 3.5-inch needle.
- High-frequency linear ultrasound transducer

Common Injectates
- Local anesthetics for diagnostics
- Prolotherapy, Orthobiologics (PRP, bone marrow concentrate, etc.)
- Avoid intra-ligamentous corticosteroid injections.

Injectate Volume
- 1–3 mL

Technique

Patient Position
- Prone, with a pillow under the abdomen to flatten the lumbar curvature.
- Lower extremities should be internally rotated while feet are inverted to help flatten the gluteal region.

Clinician Position
- Sitting or standing next to the patient opposite the side to be injected (for a medial to lateral approach).

Transducer Position
- Transverse to the SI joint, long-axis to the short ligament
- Obliquely paralleling the lateral border of the sacrum and long-axis to the long ligament

Needle Position
- In-plane to the transducer, medial to lateral approach with needle oriented 45 to 65 degrees.

Target
- Anechoic or hypoechoic signal within the ligaments.

PEARLS AND PITFALLS

- Marking the posterior superior iliac spine on the skin for reference allows for better transducer positioning during the procedure.

Superficial Posterior Sacrococcygeal Ligament

KEY POINTS

- In 90% of cases, coccydynia responds to conservative treatment.[21]
- In refractory cases, interventional procedures such as injections have been shown to be effective.

Pertinent Anatomy

- The superficial posterior sacrococcygeal ligament runs posteriorly, spanning from the sacral hiatus and inserting distally to the first inter-coccygeal joint.

Common Pathology

- Pain can be traumatic or non-traumatic
- In non-traumatic cases, ligamentous laxity with excessive motion of the 1st intercoccygeal joint is one proposed mechanism of coccydynia (the second intercoccygeal joint is typically fused).[22]

Equipment

- Needle size: 27–25 gauge and 1.5 to 3-inch needle.
- High-frequency linear ultrasound transducer

Common Injectates
- Local anesthetics for diagnostics
- Prolotherapy, orthobiologics (PRP, bone marrow concentrate, etc)
- Avoid intraligamentous corticosteroid injections.

Injectate Volume
- 1–3 mL

Continued

KEY POINTS—cont'd

Technique

Patient Position

- Prone with a pillow under the abdomen to flatten the lumbar curvature.
- Lower extremities should be internally rotated while feet are inverted to help flatten the gluteal region.

Clinician Position

- Seated or standing directly next to the patient

Transducer Position

- Long-axis to the sacrococcygeal ligament (Fig. 15.4A).

Needle Position

- Long-axis to the ligament and in plane to the transducer. A proximal to distal or distal to proximal approach can be used (see Fig. 15.4B).

Target

- Anechoic or hypoechoic signal within the ligament (see Fig. 15.4B).

PEARLS AND PITFALLS

- Interstitial tearing of the ligament can be challenging to identify with imaging. A diagnostic lidocaine injection into the ligament can be used to confirm the ligament as a source of pain, which can guide further workup and treatment decisions.
- Occult interstitial tearing can sometimes be identified during the injection when small aliquots of the injectate are placed in the ligament as the needle is advanced.
- Gauze should be placed in the inter-gluteal or natal cleft just proximal to the rectum to protect the mucosa during skin preparation from the antiseptic cleansing agents.
- Ultrasound allows for direct visualization of the superficial fibers of the sacrococcygeal ligament, but acoustic shadowing from the bone prevents visualization of the deep sacrococcygeal ligament. If there is suspected involvement of the deep sacrococcygeal ligaments (SCL), fluoroscopy guidance should be used to access the superficial and deep fibers[23].

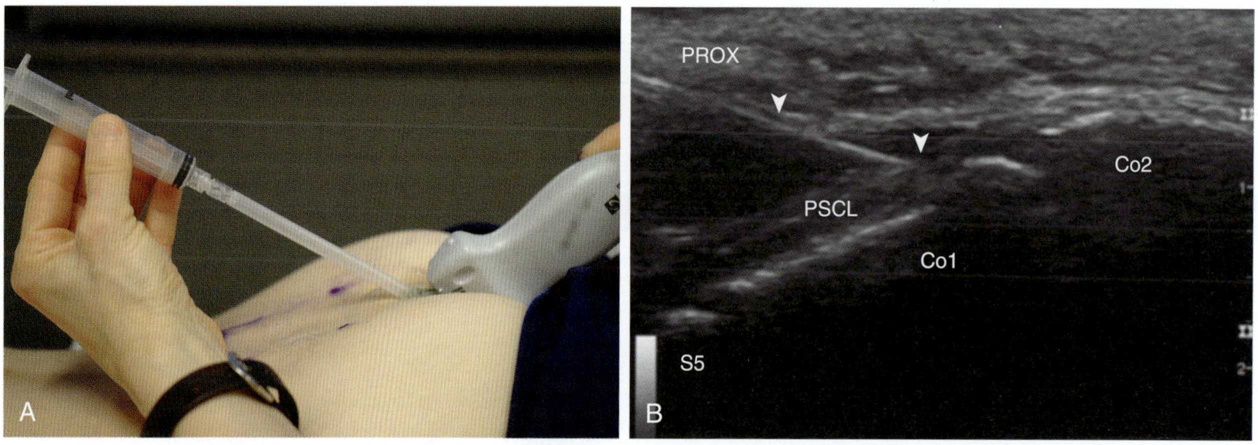

• **Fig. 15.4** Ultrasound guided injection of the sacrococcygeal ligament. (A) Setup. (B) Ultrasound view with proximal to the left. The sacrum *(S5)*, first and second bones of the coccyx *(cox1, cox2)*, posterior sacrococcygeal ligament *(PSCL)*, and needle approach *(arrowheads)* are shown.

Sacrotuberous and Sacrospinous Ligaments

KEY POINTS

- The sacrotuberous ligament is a key point of attachment for the hamstrings and gluteal musculature.

Pertinent Anatomy

- The sacrotuberous and sacrospinous ligaments have a conjoint origin, with interwoven fibers that attach proximally to the posterior superior iliac spine, the long posterior SI ligament, the lateral sacrum, and the coccyx proximally. Fibers of the proximal sacrotuberous ligament serve as attachment sites for the gluteus maximus and piriformis.[24]
- The sacrotuberous ligament narrows and spirals along its length, then broadens toward its distal attachment on the ischial tuberosity. Fibers of the distal sacrotuberous ligament are contiguous with the conjoined tendon of the biceps femoris and semitendinosus.[24,25]
- The sacrospinous ligament attaches distally on the ischial spine.

Common Pathology

- Entrapment between the sacrotuberous and sacrospinous ligaments is a common cause of pudendal neuralgia.[26]
- The sacrotuberous and sacrospinous ligaments are important pelvic stabilizers, and may be injured due to high-energy trau-ma (i.e., motor vehicle collisions, falls, pedestrians struck by a vehicle) with anterior-posterior compression forces across the pelvis.
- Irritation of the sacrotuberous ligament with localized pain, swelling, and reduced echogenicity may be seen at its junction with the conjoined tendon. Fibers of the distal ligament are contiguous with the conjoined tendon of the long head of the biceps femoris and semitendinosus, and they are disrupted in full hamstring tear.[25]

Equipment

- Needle size: 25–22 gauge and 2 to 3.5-inch needle.
- Low frequency curvilinear ultrasound transducer

Common Injectates

- Local anesthetics for diagnostics
- Prolotherapy, Orthobiologics (PRP, bone marrow concentrate, etc.)
- Avoid intraligamentous corticosteroid injections.

Injectate Volume

- 1–3 mL

Technique

Patient Position

- Prone with a pillow under the abdomen to flatten the lumbar curvature.
- Lower extremities should be internally rotated while feet are inverted to help flatten the gluteal region.

Clinician Position

- Seated or standing directly next to the patient

Transducer Position

- Start with one end of the transducer positioned along the lateral border of the sacrum and the other pointed toward the greater trochanter over the piriformis, the probe is then rotated toward the ischial spine (lateral edge greater sciatic notch).
- The sacrospinous ligament is visualized as a hyperechoic line extending medially from the ischial spine.
- The sacrotuberous ligament can be seen as a light hyperechoic line parallel and superficial to the sacrospinous ligament.[26,27]
- The transducer may need to be rotated clockwise/counterclockwise to improve visualization of the ligament.

Needle Position

- In-plane with the transducer

Target

- Anechoic or hypoechoic signal within the ligament.

PEARLS AND PITFALLS

- Patient body habitus is a key factor influencing success visualizing the sacrotuberous and sacrospinous ligaments under ultrasound.
- Resistance can be felt as the needle advances through the sacrotuberous ligament, typically with a loss of resistance as the needle "punches through" the ligament to the soft tissues underneath.
- The sacrotuberous ligament may be confused with the sciatic nerve at the level the sciatic notch. The sciatic nerve can be traced down into the posterior thigh, passing lateral to the ischial spine, while the sacrotuberous ligament can be followed to its attachment on the ischial tuberosity.
- The pudendal nerve is difficult to reliably visualize due to its small size and anatomic variability. One, two, or three nerve trunks may be identified at this level. Doppler ultrasound visualizing the pudendal artery can be a useful guide, although it should be noted that the artery course is highly variable. The pudendal artery may be located medial to the nerve, lateral to the nerve, or with two branches on either side of the nerve.[27]

Caudal Epidural

KEY POINTS

- Ultrasound greatly enhances the accuracy of caudal epidural injection compared to palpation alone, and treatment outcome in ultrasound-guided injection is comparable to fluoroscopy.[28,29]

Pertinent Anatomy

- The sacral hiatus is the open caudal termination of the sacral canal. It is most commonly located at the S4 level[30].
- The sacral cornua border the sacral hiatus laterally and are frequently palpable.
- The dural sac typically terminates between S1 and S2.

Common Pathology

- Caudal approach is frequently preferred in the setting of lumbar stenosis or history of lumbar surgery with altered anatomy.
- Also can be used for:
  - Lumbosacral radiculitis
  - post-laminectomy or post-fusion syndromes
  - epidural fibrosis
  - Nerve block required for posterior hip and lower extremity procedures

Equipment

- Needle size: 25–22 gauge and 2 to 3.5-inch needle
- High-frequency linear ultrasound transducer

Common Injectates

- Anesthetics for lower extremity/sacral nerve block
- Corticosteroids
- Orthobiologics (platelet lysate, PRP).[31]

Injectate Volume

- 10–20 mL

Technique

Patient Position

- Prone, with a pillow under the abdomen to flatten the lumbar curve.
- Lower extremities should be internally rotated while feet are inverted to help flatten the gluteal region.

Clinician Position

- Seated or standing next to the patient

Transducer Position

- Start with the transducer transverse across the midline and locate the sacral hiatus, sacral cornua, and sacrococcygeal ligament superficial to the base of the sacrum (Fig. 15.5A and B)
- Rotate longitudinally over the sacral hiatus so the transducer rests between the two cornua.

Needle Position

- In plane to the transducer distal to proximal approach (Fig. 15.6).

Target

- The needle pierces the SCL into sacral hiatus and advance 0.5 cm deep (Fig. 15.7A)
- Inject under color flow to show epidural flow (see Fig. 15.7B)

PEARLS AND PITFALLS

- Gauze should be placed in the inter-gluteal or natal cleft just proximal to the rectum to protect the mucosa during skin preparation from the antiseptic cleansing agents.
- There should not be much resistance during injection.
- The needle is no longer visualized once it enters the sacral hiatus. In the majority of patients, the hiatus is located at the S4 level (65%–68% of patients). However, in a minority of patients it may be located further cranially (S3 level: 15% of patients, S1 to S2: 3%–5% of patients). A cranial hiatus is located closer to the dural sac, and care must be taken to avoid accidental dural puncture. Don't advance more than 0.5 mm into the hiatus to avoid dural penetration as shortest distance to the dural can be 6 mm.[30,32]
- Avoid injecting air, as there have been reports of portal vein air embolism.[33]
- Ultrasound guided caudal injection technique has been shown to have 96.9%–100% accuracy, however patients with a closed or small sacral hiatus are poor candidates and may have a higher failure rate.[34,35] Unidirectional flow within the sacral hiatus may be visualized on Doppler to confirm successful injection.[28,29]

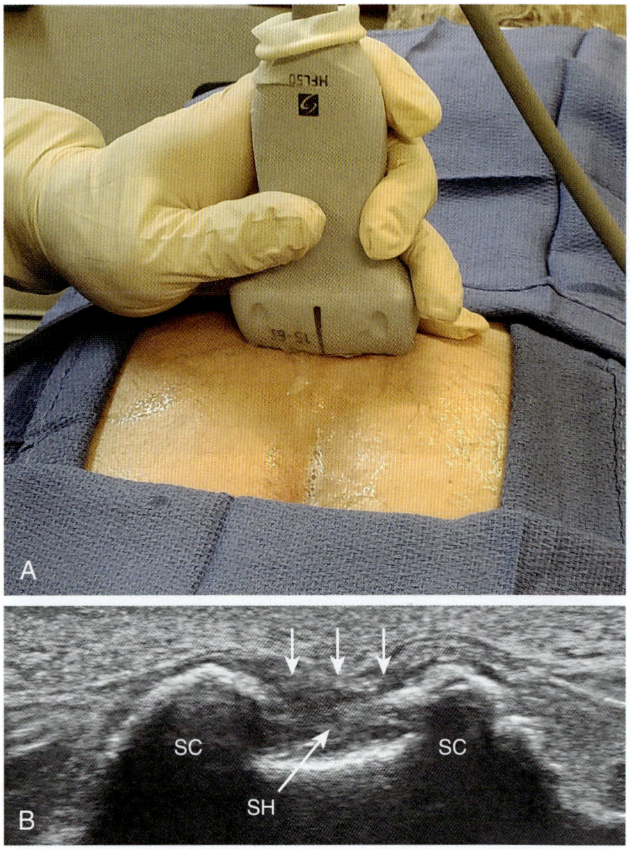

• **Fig. 15.5** (A) Sacral cornua view transducer set up. (B) Sacral cornua ultrasound view. *SC*, sacral cornua; *SH*, Sacral hiatus; *Downward white arrows*, sacrococcygeal ligament.

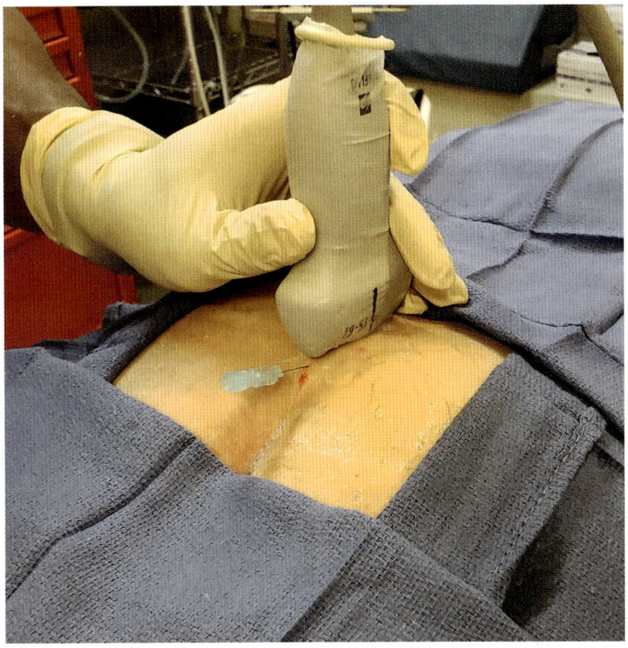

• **Fig. 15.6** Caudal epidural injection under ultrasound needle trajectory.

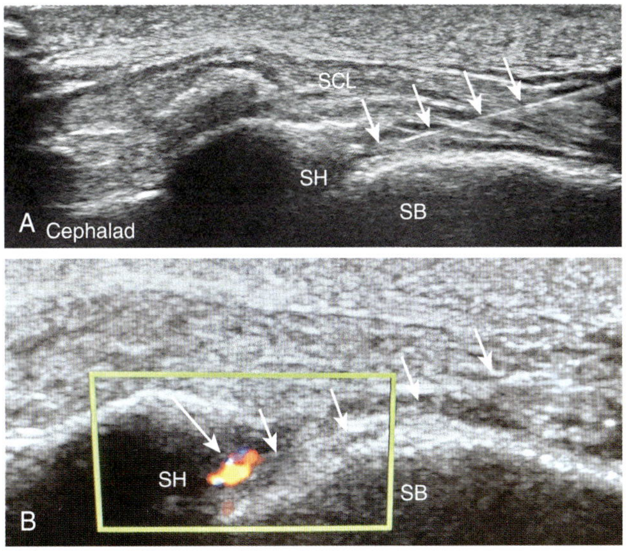

• **Fig. 15.7** (A) Caudal epidural injection under ultrasound needle into sacral hiatus. (B) Injecting under color flow Doppler to ensure epidural flow. *SH*, sacral hiatus; *SB*, sacral base; *SCL*, sacrococcygeal ligament; *White arrows*, needle path.

Fluoroscopic Procedures

S1 transforaminal epidural using the subpedicular approach.

KEY POINTS

- The objective of transforaminal injection is to deliver injectate around the spinal nerve and its nerve root sleeve. It must not be delivered into the thecal sac.

Pertinent Anatomy

- Each lumbar intervertebral foramen is formed between two consecutive vertebrae with the most inferior lumbar articular facet joining with S1 superior articular process.
- The sacrum is made up of five fused vertebrae (S1–S5) with four pairs of ventral and dorsal sacral foramina (left and right).
- S1 foramen is bounded superiorly by L5 pedicles, inferiorly by sacral base, anteriorly by the sacral intervertebral disc (L5–S1) and posterior longitudinal ligament, and posteriorly by the ligamentum flavum.

Common Pathology

- L5–S1 Degenerative disk disease
- Lumbosacral radiculopathy
- Failed back surgery syndrome
- Epidural fibrosis

Equipment

- 25–22 gauge and 3 to 3.5-inch spinal needle
- Connecting tube
- Water soluble, non-ionic radiographic contrast medium (Isovue 300/370 or omnipaque)

Common Injectates

- Local anesthetics for diagnostics, corticosteroids
- Neuroprolotherapy, Orthobiologics (platelet lysate)

Injectate Volume

- 2–5 mL

Technique

Patient Position

- Prone position on a fluoroscopy table

Clinician Position

- Lateral to the patient

Fluoroscopic

- "Square off" the superior endplate of the sacrum using a cephalad tilt in the AP view
- The target dorsal S1 foramen can be difficult to visualize and can be mistaken for the larger, more obvious ventral S1 foramen.
- The dorsal S1 foramen is a more ovoid shape, smaller and located superiomedial to the ventral S1 foramen and inferior to the S1 pedicle at 6 o'clock.
- First, visualize the S1 pedicle and look just inferior to the 6 o'clock position.
- Visualize "Charlie's line," named after Charlie Aprill, which runs along the medial aspect of the S1 pedicle (Fig. 15.8). This can also help localize the dorsal S1 foramen.
- If the dorsal S1 foramen cannot be visualized in the AP view, then oblique the C arm slightly ipsilateral, 5 to 10 degrees.

Needle Position

- Place the needle coaxial to the fluoroscopic beam aiming to be in the **superolateral aspect of the foramen.** This avoids the nerve, which runs inferolaterally.

Continued

KEY POINTS—cont'd

- Depth can be gauged by touching down on the lateral wall of the foramen and then "walking" off the periosteum

Target

- Superior lateral aspect of the foramen in the AP view
- In the lateral view (Fig. 15.9), the tip of the needle should lie about 5 mm short of the floor of the sacral canal (SIS) and should lie just short of the floor of the sacral canal.
- Once the target site is achieved, inject a small amount of contrast already primed and attached to the extension tubing (Fig. 15.10).
- The injection should be done under live fluoroscopy to better identify a vascular filling pattern (Fig. 15.11).
- Ideal flow should outline the S1 nerve and flow medially into the epidural space to the S1 pedicle.

PEARLS AND PITFALLS

- First contact the posterior sacral bone prior to "walking" off the periosteum and entering the S1 foramen
- Do not advance past the iliopectineal line to avoid visceral injuries

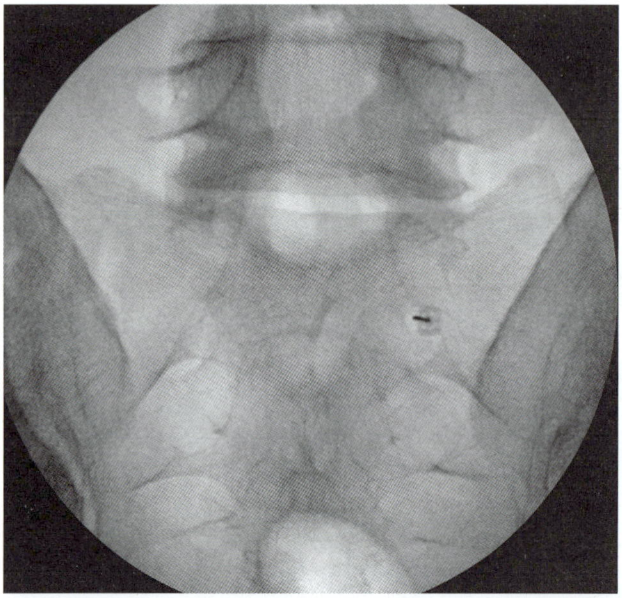

• **Fig. 15.8** Precontrast L S1 transforaminal epidural. Note: Charlie's line.

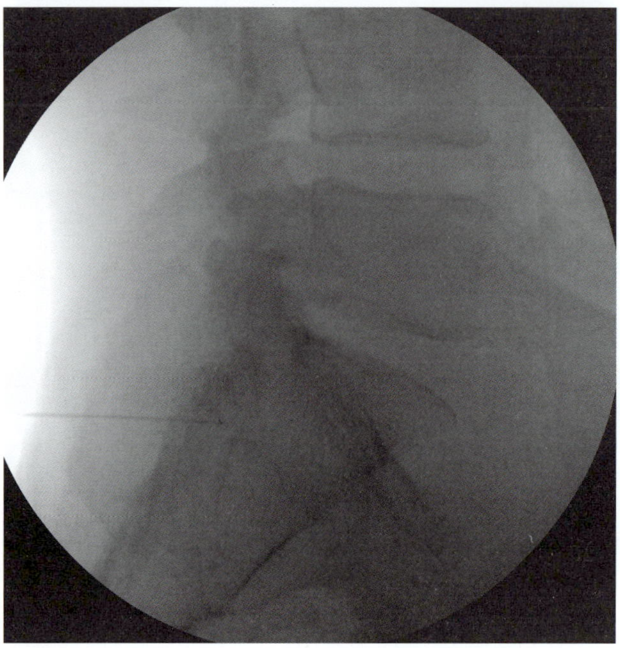

• **Fig. 15.9** Lateral view of S1 TFESI. Note iliopectineal line.

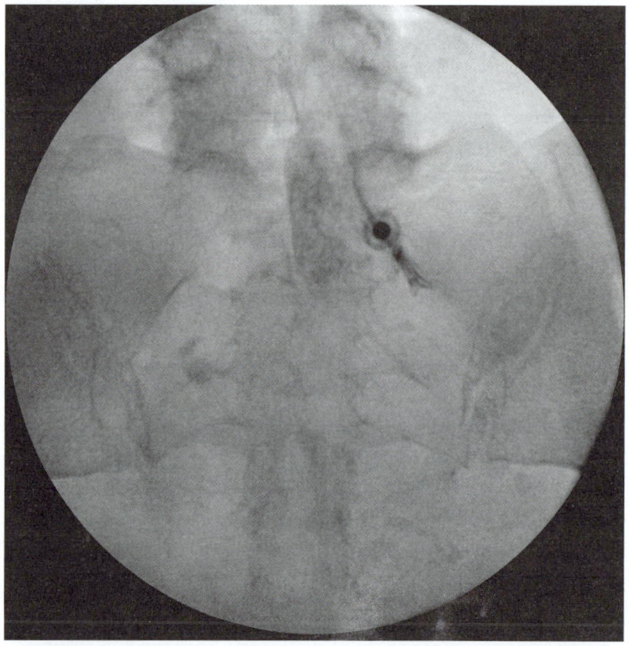

• **Fig. 15.10** Post contrast with S1 nerve root flow and epidural flow.

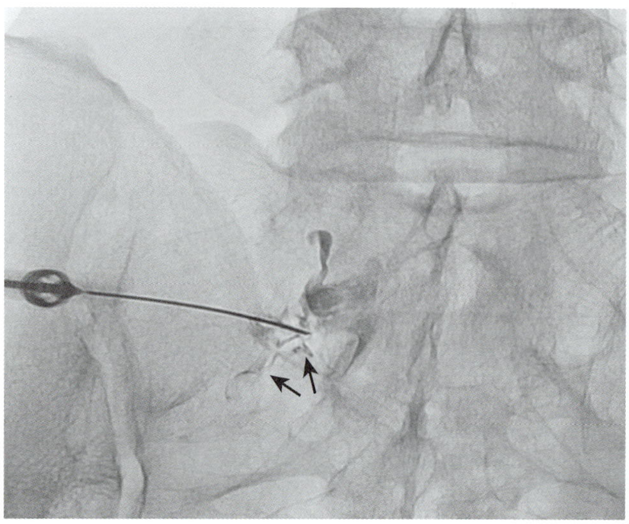

• **Fig. 15.11** Intra-arterial contrast flow during an S1 transforaminal epidural injection showing tortuous filling of the vasculature.

Caudal Epidural Injection

KEY POINTS

- Landmark guided caudal epidural results in incorrect needle placement as high as 38% of procedures.[36]

Pertinent Anatomy

- The sacrum is a triangular bone dorsally convex, that consists of fused 5 sacral vertebra
- Sacral hiatus is an opening in the spinal canal in the lower part of the sacrum formed by the incomplete midline fusion of the lamina at S4 or S5.
- The sacral hiatus is a U-shaped space with the lateral margins formed by the sacral cornu and covered by the sacrococcyeal ligament.
- The sacral canal contains terminal part of the dural sac which generally ends at the S2 but may terminate at the S1 or S3 level

Common Pathology

- Lumbar radiculopathy
- Lumbar stenosis with and without axial low back pain
- Post-laminectomy syndrome
- Epidural fibrosis

Equipment:

- 25–22 gauge and 2 to 3.5-inch spinal needle
- Extension tubing
- Contrast

Common Injectates

- Local anesthetic and non particulate corticosteroids
- Orthobiologics (platelet lysate)
- Avoid particulate steroids

Injectate Volume

- 5–15 mL pending patient tolerance

Technique

Patient Position

- Prone with abdomen on a pillow to reduce lumbar lordosis

Clinician Position

- Lateral to the patient

Fluoroscope Position

- Start in the lateral view to identify the sacral hiatus
- AP view is used to keep the needle midline and avoid advancing too cephalad (Fig. 15.12).

Needle Position

- Palpate the sacral cornuae and start 0.5–1 inch below
- Use the lateral fluoroscopic view to identify needle trajectory. Insert the needle into the skin caudal to cephalad heading towards the sacral hiatus (Fig. 15.13)
- Ensure the needle is in the midline

Target

- Sacral epidural space via the sacral hiatus
- Advance the needle past opening and not higher than the S3 level to avoid dura sac puncture
- Contrast is injected to confirm epidural flow (Figs. 15.14 to 15.16).
- One can visualize how far cephalad the contrast flows after adding an injectate (see Fig. 15.14)

PEARLS AND PITFALLS

- Major complications related to procedure may include infection, hematoma/abscess formation, subarachnoid and subdural injection
- Avoid advancing too ventral and puncturing the bowel.

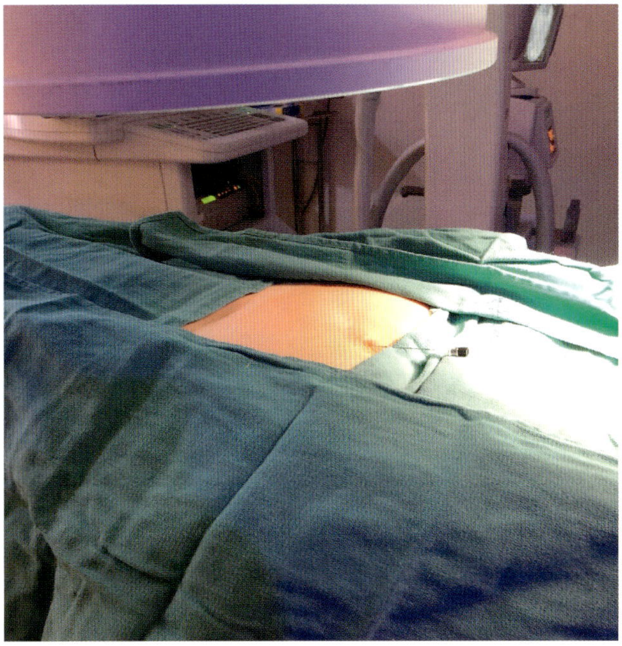

• **Fig. 15.12** AP view of the C-arm at the needle's point of entry into the skin.

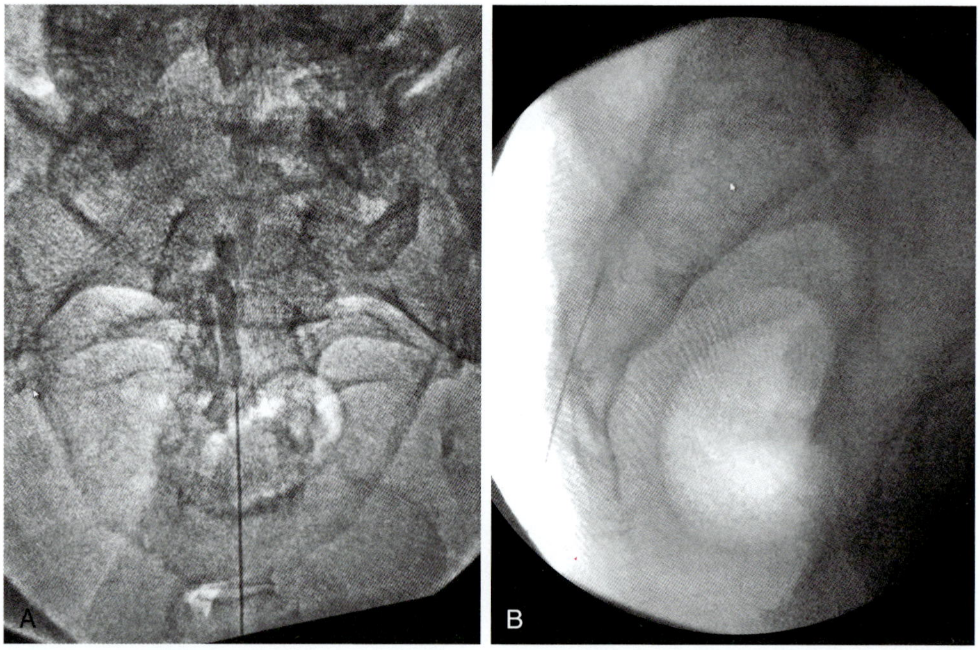

• **Fig. 15.13** Lateral view of the C-arm as the needle approaches the S3 foramen.

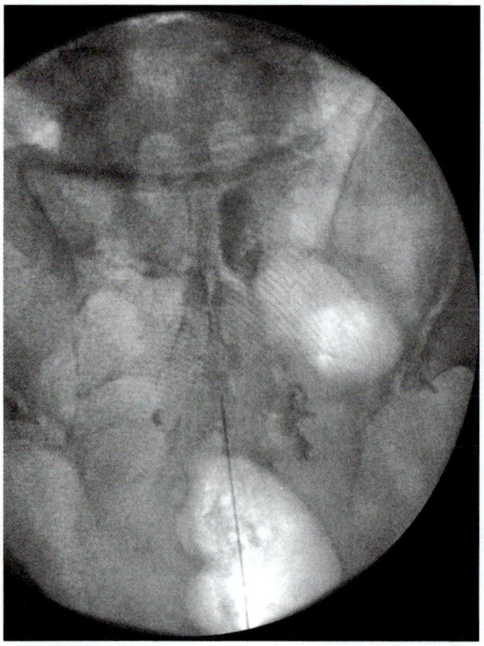

• **Fig. 15.14** AP and lateral view of a caudal epidural injection with and without contrast injection

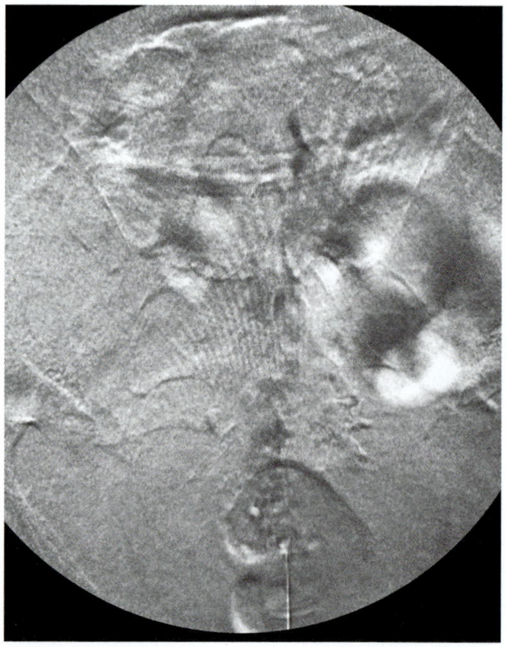

• **Fig. 15.15** AP and lateral view of a caudal epidural injection with and without contrast injection

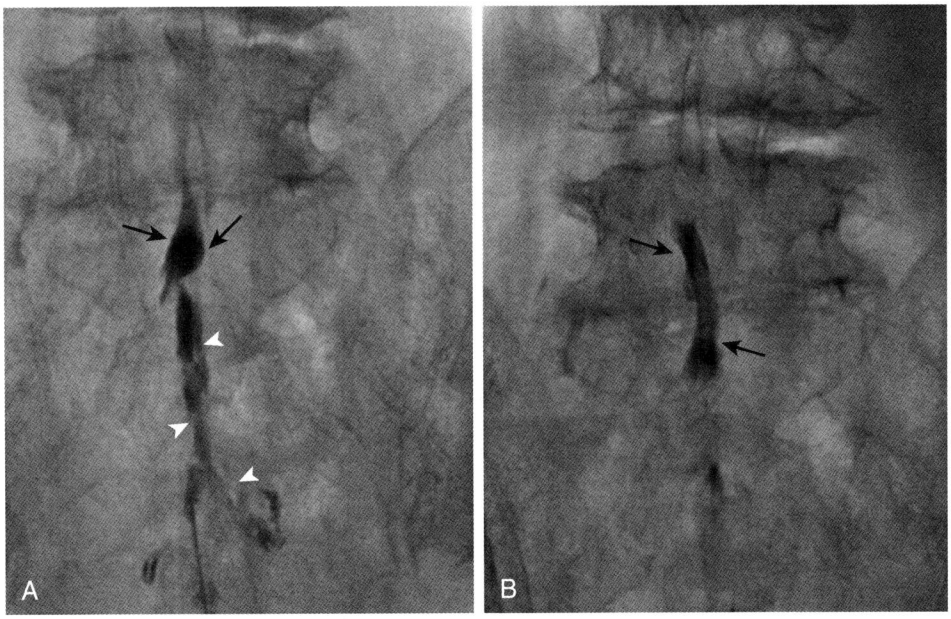

• **Fig. 15.16** Fluoroscopic view during caudal epidural injection with and without contrast.

Sacroiliac Joint

KEY POINTS

- The inferior approach is the author's preferred approach.
- The superior approach is an alternative if the inferior approach is unsuccessful.
- One can use the superior approach to inject the superior SI joint dorsal ligaments.

Pertinent Anatomy

- SI joint is an auricular-shaped di-arthrodial joint with joint capsule and synovial fluid. It has hyaline cartilage on the sacral side and fibrocartilage on the iliac side.
- Multiple ligaments support the SIJ joint; namely the anterior, short, lateral and interosseous ligament.
- The sacrotuberous and sacrospinous ligament stabilize the pelvis.
- The posterior aspect of the joint is innervated by the posterior rami of L4–S3.

Common Pathology

- SIJ dysfunction
- SIJ arthropathy

Equipment

- C arm fluoroscopy
- 25–22 gauge and 3 to 3.5-inch spinal needle
- Contrast

Common Injectates

- Local anesthetic for diagnostics: Corticosteroids
- Prolotherapy and orthobiologics (PRP, bone marrow concentrate, etc.)

Injectate Volume

- 1–2 mL

Technique (Inferior Approach)

Patient Position

- Prone position

Clinician Position

- Lateral to the patient

Fluoroscope Position

- Tilt the fluoroscope cephalad, approximately 10–15 degrees to visualize the lower SI joint effectively
- Under live fluoroscopy, oblique the C-arm to obtain the best view of the dorsal caudal joint opening. Author found that ipsilateral oblique is more common, but the best view may be contralateral oblique as well.
- Watch for the hyperlucency region at the caudal portion of the SIJ.

Needle position

- Start just caudal and medial to the Joint
- Guide the needle to the caudal and medial wall of the joint, and then "walk off" cephalad and laterally to enter the joint.
- As the needle contacts firm tissues on the posterior aspect of the joint, it should be redirected if needed and advanced through the ligaments and capsule into the joint.

Target

- The target is the medial aspect of the SIJ 1–2 cm cephalad to the caudal aspect of the joint (Fig. 15.17).
- Contrast in injected with ideal flow visualized outlining the medial and lateral aspect of the joint (Fig. 15.18).
- If resistance is felt, withdraw or advance the needle and injection contrast again. A tactile sensation of a "giving away" or loss of resistance can often be felt.
- If desired, one can inject just overlying the joint to target the inferior dorsal SI ligaments (Fig. 15.19).

PEARLS AND PITFALLS

- Care should be taken not to advance the needle beyond the ventral joint capsule

Technique (Superior Approach)

Patient Position
- Prone position

Clinician Position
- Lateral to the patient

Fluoroscope Position
- Tilt the fluoroscope cephalad approximately 10–20 degrees to improve the target
- Move the C-arm to 40–50 degrees contralateral oblique to visualize the joint opening (Fig. 15.20A).
- The AP view is used to show the needle advancing lateral and caudal to the joint.

Needle Position
- Start the needle medial and cephalad to the joint.
- The tip of the needle should be advanced laterally and caudally
- Touch on the medial wall of the joint (i.e., sacrum), and then walk off laterally into the joint (see Fig. 15.20B and C).

Target
- Cephalad aspect of the SIJ
- Inject a small amount of contrast to confirm intra-articular flow (see Fig. 15.20 D and E).
- If desired, one can inject just overlying the joint to target the superior dorsal SI ligaments (see Fig. 15.20F).

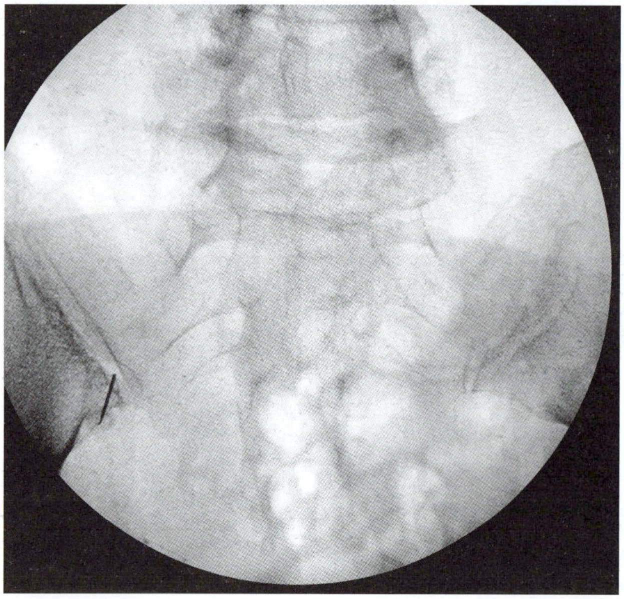

• **Fig. 15.17** Posterior and lateral fluoroscopy view during a left sacroiliac joint injection.

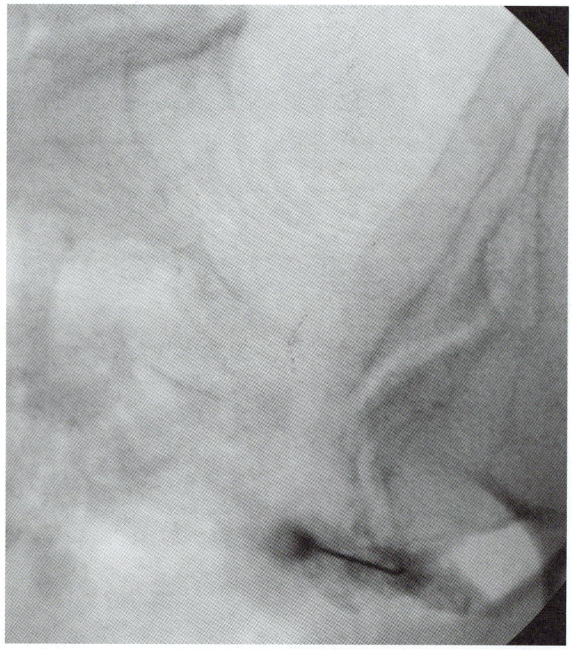

• **Fig. 15.19** Optional figure showing sacrospinous and part of sacrotuberous ligament off inferior SI joint approach.

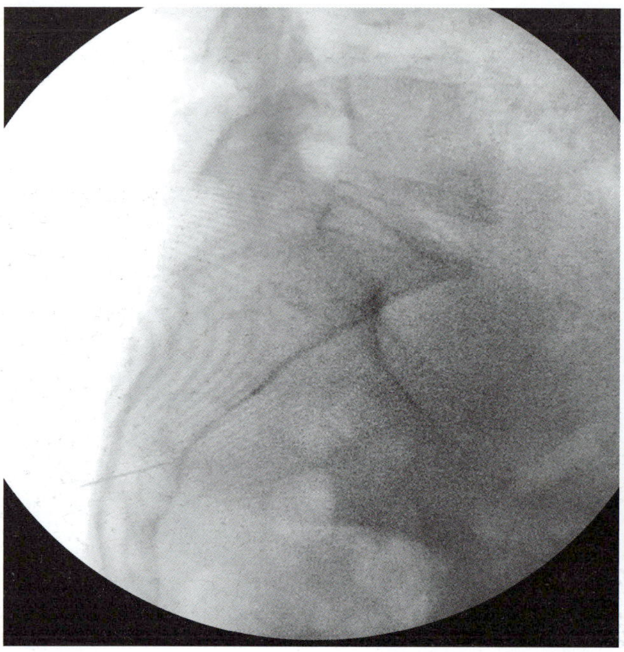

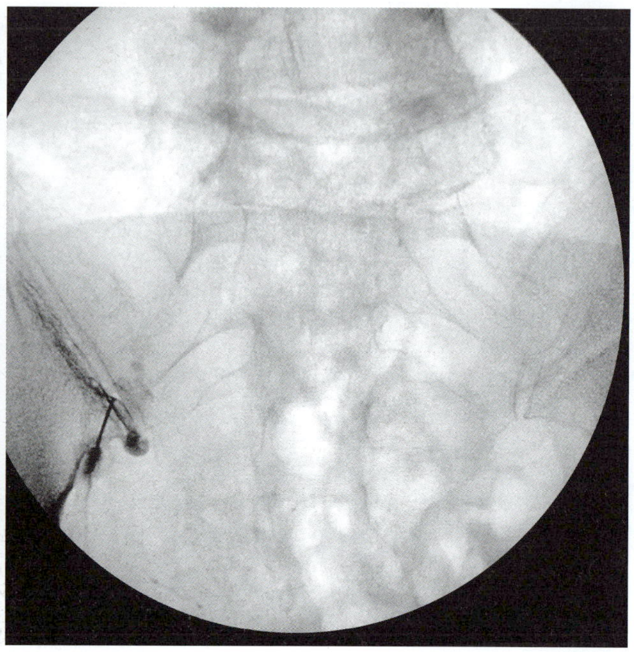

• **Fig. 15.18** Contrast was injected to ensure the joint has been accessed.

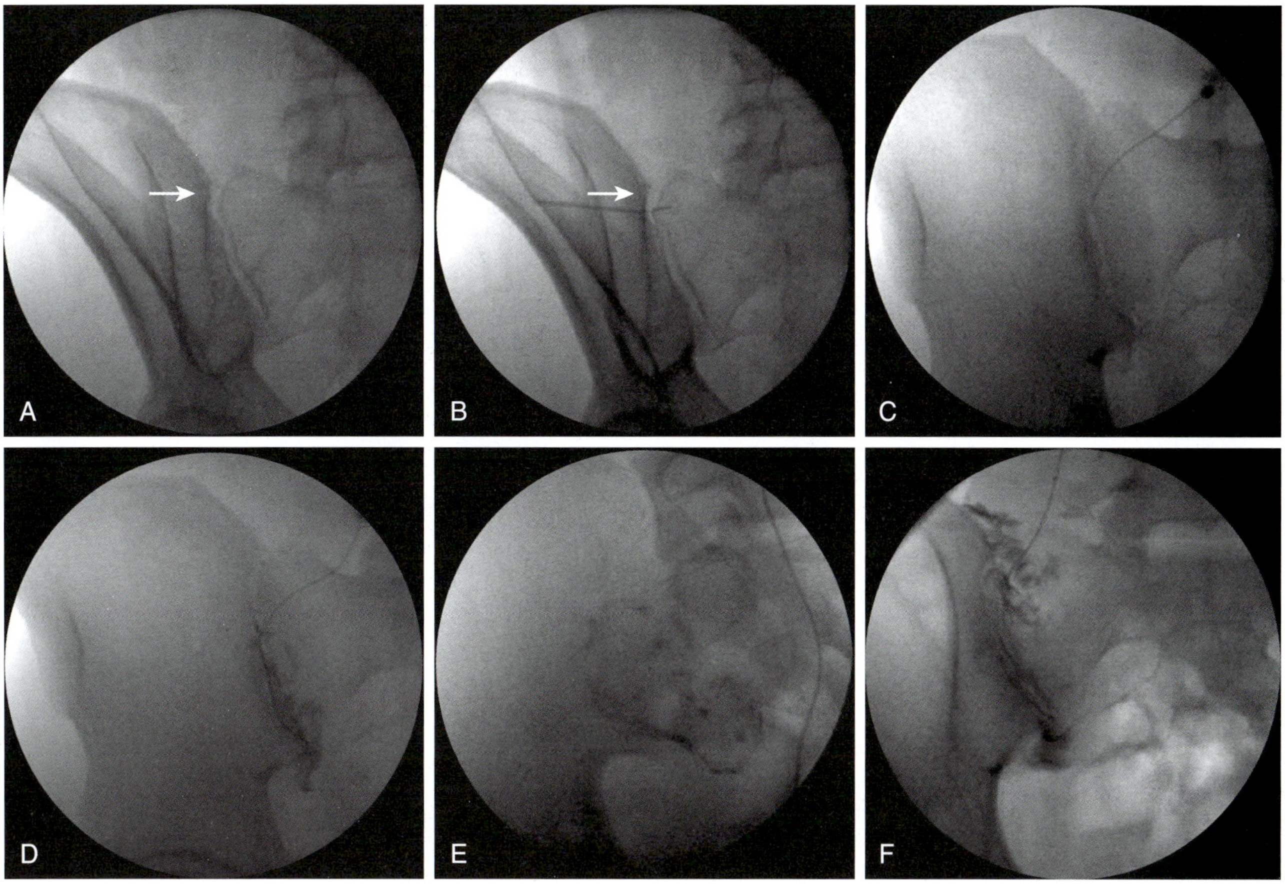

• **Fig. 15.20** Superior approach of SIJ injection showing access to the joint by using (A) contralateral oblique view. The C-arm was positioned at 40–50 degrees (42 degrees in this view) in contralateral oblique view to demonstrate the wedge shape formed by the medial iliac ala and the lateral border of the sacrum *(white arrow)*. (B) Contralateral oblique view. After positioning a guide needle, a 26-gauge curved needle was inserted into the wedge shape and then advanced laterally and inferiorly into the sacroiliac joint. (C) Antero-posterior view showing the needle advanced further laterally and inferiorly into the joint. (D) Antero-posterior view showing an arthrogram of the sacroiliac joint after injecting contrast material. (E) SI joint arthrogram in ipsilateral oblique view. (F) The periarticular injection was performed using the same needle. After withdrawing the needle cranially, needle position was confirmed by contrast injection.

PEARLS AND PITFALLS

- Care should be taken not to advance the needle beyond the ventral joint capsule.[13]
- Though less common, the success rate of the superior approach has been found to be 90%.[37]

Sacroiliac Joint Radiofrequency Ablation

KEY POINTS

- Thermal or conventional radiofrequency (RF) neurotomy produces a RF current through an electrode creating thermal energy and lesions or destroys the targeted nerve by denaturing its constituent proteins. It develops between 60 and 80 °C at interval of 60–90 seconds per lesion.
- Pulsed RF is similar to thermal ablation; however, it uses a higher voltage dissipating heat easily and generating less heat. This can be achieved with a single probe electrode and grounding pad (monopolar) or two parallel probe electrodes (bipolar).
- Cooled RF sends RF current through cooled electrodes, and has a larger lesion size than traditional RF. It relies on keeping the impedance low and allowing alternate current to heat tissues longer. Cooled RF can be delivered for two and a half minutes to achieve target electrode temperature of 60°C[38,39].

Pertinent Anatomy

- The SIJ is innervated by the dorsal rami of L5–S3, dorsal rami and ventral rami of L4–5.

Continued

KEY POINTS—cont'd

Common Pathology

- SIJ dysfunction
- SIJ arthropathy

Equipment

- C-arm fluoroscopy
- Generator that produces a high-frequency, alternating, electric current
- A ground plate that delivers the current
- A needle like electrode whose shaft is insulated but whose tip is exposed, which receives current

Common Injectates

- Local anesthetic

Injectate Volume

- 1–2 mL

Technique

Patient Position

- Prone position

Clinician Position

- Lateral to the patient

Fluoroscope Position

- L5 dorsal rami is identified by obtaining an AP view to visualize the notch between the ala and the superior articular process of the sacrum.
- Using a lateral view, the needle is confirmed to be no deeper than the AP midline of the superior articular process.
- Using the AP view, the S1, S2 and S3 foramen are identified.
- A lateral view is taken to ensure that the probe is not in the sacral canal.

Needle Position

- The introducer is inserted lateral and inferior to the target until bony contact is made.

Target

- For the L5 dorsal rami, aim for the notch between the sacral ala and the superior articular process
- Aim just lateral to the sacral foramen (Figs. 15.21 and 15.22).
- Before RFA, sensory and motor stimulation confirms correct needle position. Muscle contraction in the distal lower extremities indicates the needle is in close proximity to the spinal nerve and needs to be repositioned.
- Stylet of the introducer is removed and a small amount of local anesthetic is administered to the target site.
- RFA is delivered

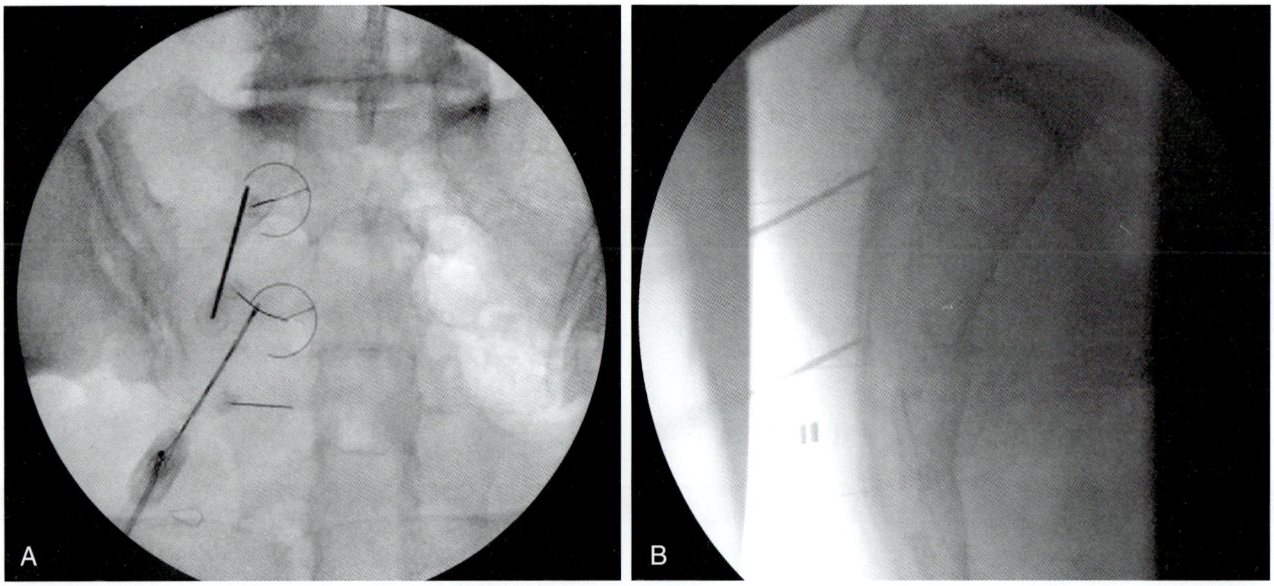

• **Fig. 15.21** Needle placement of the S1 and S2 lateral nerve.

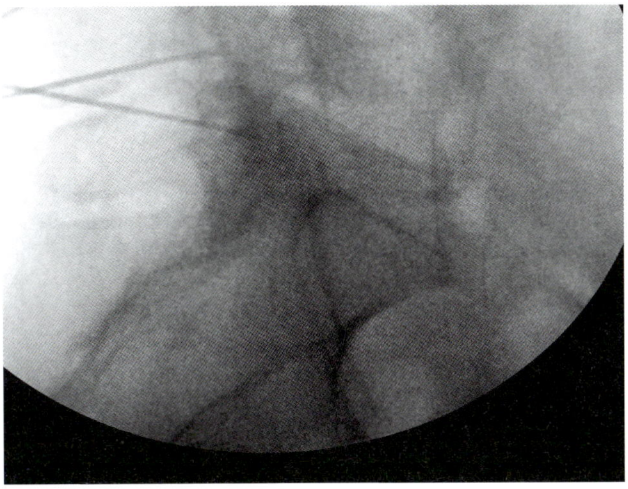

• **Fig. 15.22** Lateral view with the inferior needle at the target position during an L5 dorsal rami RF ablation.

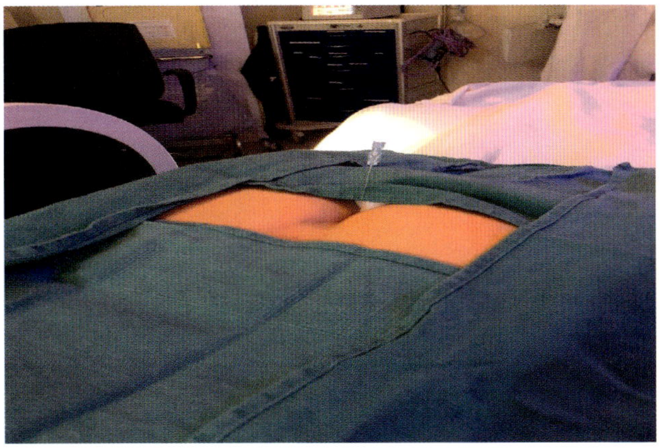

• **Fig. 15.23** Lateral view of C-arm at the point of entry.

PEARLS AND PITFALLS

- Patients should be monitored for groin, anterior thigh, lower leg and foot pain.
- Observational studies noted that success rates for bipolar RFA was 38% compared to 82% for cooled RFA.[40]
- When compared to monopolar RFA technique, bipolar lesions more reliably captured lateral branches with potential of a 100% capture rate on cadaveric studies.[40]

Ganglion Impar Injection

KEY POINTS

Pertinent Anatomy

- Ganglion impar is the most inferior ganglia of the sympathetic nervous system and is the terminal fusion of the 2 sacral sympathetic chains.
- It is located retroperitoneal at the level of the sacrococcygeal junction (SCJ) but can be located between the SCJ and lower segment of the first coccyx.
- The ganglion impar provides nociceptive and sympathetic innervation to pelvic and perineal structures.

Common Pathology

- Coccydynia
- Pelvic pain
- Rectal/perineal pain
- Sympathetically mediated pain (i.e., complex regional pain syndrome)

Equipment

- C-arm fluoroscopy
- 25–22 gauge and 3 to 5-inch spinal needle
- Contrast

Common Injectates

- Local anesthetic plus or minus corticosteroids
- Neuroprolotherapy, Orthobiologics (platelet lysate)

Injectate Volume

- 3–5 mL

Technique

Patient Position

- Prone position

Clinician Position

- Lateral to the patient

Fluoroscope Position

- Use a lateral view and place metallic mark to identify the coccygeal cornu and SCJ
- The C-arm is then brought to AP position to confirm midline
- Use the lateral view to identify needle tip proximity to the anterior coccygeal line

Needle Position

- The needle is inserted midline over the SCJ in the AP view and then advance in the lateral view (Fig. 15.23).

Target

- Needle advanced through the SCJ and disc
- The clinician may feel a subtle loss of resistance when the needle passes through anterior longitudinal ligament
- Inject a small amount of contrast, which should form the "comma sign" in the retroperitoneal space on the lateral view (Figs. 15.24 and 15.25).

PEARLS AND PITFALLS

- Avoid bowel perforation by going too ventral
- If the needle deviates too far from midline, it can block other pelvic nerves
- RF ablation of the ganglion impar can also be performed which has been shown to improve chronic intractable coccydynia through the transacrococcygeal approach[41]

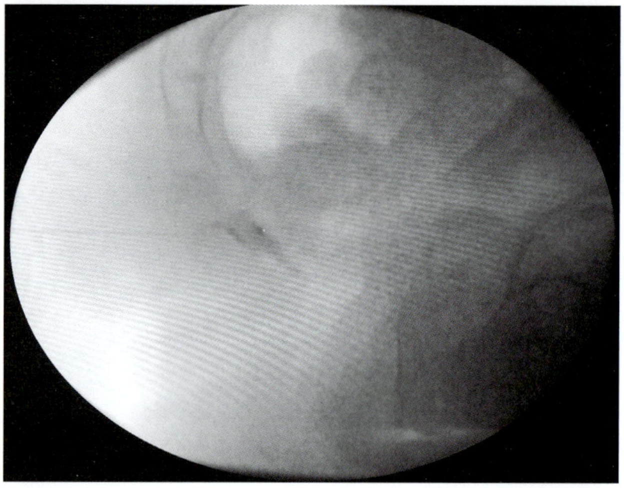

• **Fig. 15.24** Lateral view of the C-arm around contrast is injected.

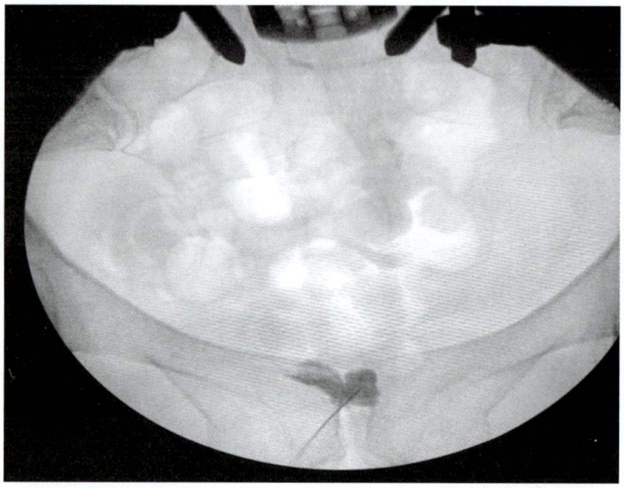

• **Fig. 15.25** AP view of the C-arm around contrast is injected.

References

1. Vleeming A, Schuenke MD, Masi AT, Carreiro JE, Danneels L, Willard FH. The sacroiliac joint: an overview of its anatomy, function and potential clinical implications. *J Anat.* 2012;221(6):537–567. https://doi.org/10.1111/j.1469-7580.2012.01564.x.
2. Cohen SP. Sacroiliac joint pain: a comprehensive review of anatomy, diagnosis and treatment. *Anesth Analg.* 2005;101(5):1440–1453. https://doi.org/10.1213/01.ANE.0000180831.60169.EA.
3. Simopoulos TT, Manchikanti L, Singh V, et al. A systematic evaluation of prevalence and diagnostic accuracy of sacroiliac joint interventions. *Pain Physician.* 2012;15(3):E305–E344.
4. Taurog JD, Chhabra A, Colbert RA. Ankylosing spondylitis and axial spondyloarthritis. *N Engl J Med.* 2016;374(26):2563–2574. https://doi.org/10.1056/NEJMra1406182.
5. Duba AS, Mathew SD. The seronegative spondyloarthropathies. *Prim Care Clin Off Pract.* 2018;45(2):271–287. https://doi.org/10.1016/j.pop.2018.02.005.
6. Gutierrez M, Rodriguez S, Soto-Fajardo C, et al. Ultrasound of sacroiliac joints in spondyloarthritis: a systematic review. *Rheumatol Int.* 2018;38(10):1791–1805. https://doi.org/10.1007/s00296-018-4126-x.
7. Fortin J, Dwyer A, West S, Pier J. Sacroiliac joint: pain referral maps upon applying a new injection/arthrography technique. Part I: asymptomatic volunteers. *Spine (Phila Pa 1976).* 1994;19(13):1475–1482.
8. Zheng P, Schneider BJ, Yang A, McCormick ZL. Image-guided sacroiliac joint injections: an evidence-based review of best practices and clinical outcomes. *Pharm Manag PM R.* 2019;11(S1):S98–S104. https://doi.org/10.1002/pmrj.12191.
9. Chang WH, Lew HL, Chen CPC. Ultrasound-guided sacroiliac joint injection technique. *Am J Phys Med Rehabil.* 2013;92(3):278–279. https://doi.org/10.1097/PHM.0b013e318278d108.
10. Harmon D, O'Sullivan M. Ultrasound-guided sacroiliac joint injection technique. *Pain Physician.* 2008;11(4):543–547.
11. Murakami E, Tanaka Y, Aizawa T, Ishizuka M, Kokubun S. Effect of periarticular and intraarticular lidocaine injections for sacroiliac joint pain: prospective comparative study. *J Orthop Sci.* 2007;12(3):274–280. https://doi.org/10.1007/s00776-007-1126-1.
12. Nacey NC, Patrie JT, Fox MG. Fluoroscopically guided sacroiliac joint injections: comparison of the effects of intraarticular and periarticular injections on immediate and short-term pain relief. *Am J Roentgenol.* 2016;207(5):1055–1061. https://doi.org/10.2214/AJR.15.15779.
13. Park J, Park HJ, Moon DE, Sa GJ, Kim YH. Radiologic analysis and clinical study of the upper one-third joint technique for fluoroscopically guided sacroiliac joint injection. *Pain Physician.* 2015;18(5):495–503.
14. De Luigi AJ. Ultrasound guided sacroiliac joint injections. *Acad Med.* 2019 September. https://doi.org/10.1097/PHM.0000000000001289.
15. De Luigi AJ, Saini V, Mathur R, Saini A, Yokel N. Assessing the accuracy of ultrasound-guided needle placement in sacroiliac joint injections. *Am J Phys Med Rehabil.* 2019;98(8):666–670. https://doi.org/10.1097/PHM.0000000000001167.
16. Perry JM, Colberg RE, Dault SL, Beason DP, Tresgallo RA. A cadaveric study assessing the accuracy of ultrasound-guided sacroiliac joint injections. *Pharm Manag PM R.* 2016;8(12):1168–1172. https://doi.org/10.1016/j.pmrj.2016.05.002.
17. Woon JTK, Perumal V, Maigne JY, Stringer MD. CT morphology and morphometry of the normal adult coccyx. *Eur Spine J.* 2013;22(4):863–870. https://doi.org/10.1007/s00586-012-2595-2.
18. Saunders J, Cusi M, Hackett L, Van Der Wall H. An exploration of ultrasound-guided therapeutic injection of the dorsal interosseous ligaments of the sacroiliac joint for mechanical dysfunction of the joint. 1:1–4.
19. Saunders J, Cusi M, Hackett L, Van Der Wall H. A comparison of ultrasound guided PRP injection and prolotherapy for mechanical dysfunction of the sacroiliac joint. *J Prolotherapy.* 2018;10:e992–e999.
20. Saunders J, Cusi M, Wall HVD. What's old is new again: the sacroiliac joint as a cause of lateralizing low back pain. *Tomography.* 2018;4(2):72–77. https://doi.org/10.18383/j.tom.2018.00011.
21. Thiele GH. Coccygodynia: cause and treatment. *Dis Colon Rectum.* 1963;6:422–436.
22. Postacchini F, Massobrio M. Idiopathic coccygodynia. *J Bone Jt Surg.* 1983;65(8):1116–1124.
23. Montero-Cruz F-R, Aydin S. Platelet-rich plasma injection therapy for refractory coccydynia: a case series. *Interv Pain Manag Reports.* 2018;2(5):183–188.
24. Aldabe D, Hammer N, Flack NAMS, Woodley SJ. A systematic review of the morphology and function of the sacrotuberous ligament. *Clin Anat.* 2019;32(3):396–407. https://doi.org/10.1002/ca.23328.

25. Bierry G, Simeone FJ, Borg-Stein JP, Clavert P, Palmer WE. Sacrotuberous ligament: relationship to normal, torn, and retracted hamstring tendons on MR images. *Radiology*. 2014;271(1):162–171. https://doi.org/10.1148/radiol.13130702.
26. Peng PWH, Tumber PS. Ultrasound-guided interventional procedures for patients with chronic pelvic pain - a description of techniques and review of literature. *Pain Physician*. 2008;11(2):215–224.
27. Rojas-Gómez MF, Blanco-Dávila R, Tobar Roa V, Gómez González AM, Ortiz Zableh AM, Ortiz Azuero A. Regional anesthesia guided by ultrasound in the pudendal nerve territory. *Colomb J Anesthesiol*. 2017;45(3):200–209. https://doi.org/10.1016/j.rcae.2017.06.007.
28. Park Y, Lee JH, Park KD, Ahn JK, Park J, Jee H. Ultrasound-guided vs. fluoroscopy-guided caudal epidural steroid injection for the treatment of unilateral lower lumbar radicular pain: a prospective, randomized, single-blind clinical study. *Am J Phys Med Rehabil*. 2013;92(7):575–586. https://doi.org/10.1097/PHM.0b013e318292356b.
29. Park KD, Kim TK, Lee WY, Ahn J, Koh SH, Park Y. Ultrasound-guided versus fluoroscopy-guided caudal epidural steroid injection for the treatment of unilateral lower lumbar radicular pain: case-controlled, retrospective, comparative study. *Medicine (Baltim)*. 2015;94(50):e2261. https://doi.org/10.1097/MD.0000000000002261.
30. Sekiguchi M, Yabuki S, Satoh K, Kikuchi S. An anatomic study of the sacral hiatus: a basis for successful caudal epidural block. *Clin J Pain*. 2004;20(1):51–54. https://doi.org/10.1097/00002508-200401000-00010.
31. PRP Ruiz-Lopez R, Tsai Y-C. A randomized double-blind controlled pilot study comparing leucocyte-rich platelet-rich plasma and corticosteroid in caudal epidural injection for complex chronic degenerative spinal pain. *Pain Pract*. 2020. https://doi.org/10.1111/papr.12893.
32. Aggarwal A, Kaur H, Batra YK, Aggarwal AK, Rajeev S, Sahni D. Anatomic consideration of caudal epidural space: a cadaver study. *Clin Anat*. 2009;22(6):730–737. https://doi.org/10.1002/ca.20832.
33. Fujikawa T, Murai S. Portal venous gas after a caudal block. *BMJ Case Reports*. 2014;2014. https://doi.org/10.1136/bcr-2014-205381.
34. Chen CPC, Tang SFT, Hsu TC, et al. Ultrasound guidance in caudal epidural needle placement. *Anesthesiology*. 2004;101(1):181–184. https://doi.org/10.1097/00000542-200407000-00028.
35. Chen CPC, Lew HL, Tang SFT. Ultrasound-guided caudal epidural injection technique. *Am J Phys Med Rehabil*. 2015;94(1):82–83. https://doi.org/10.1097/PHM.0000000000000047.
36. Naidoo K, Alazzawi S, Montgomery A. The use of contrast in caudal epidural injections under image intensifier guidance: is it necessary? *Clin Orthop Surg*. 2017;9(2):190–192. https://doi.org/10.4055/cios.2017.9.2.190.
37. Do KH, Ahn SH, Jones R, et al. New sacroiliac joint injection technique and its short-term effect on chronic sacroiliac region pain. *Pain Med*. 2016;17(10):1809–1813.
38. Wolfgang S, Michael A, Dominik S, Valentin S. Use of cooled radiofrequency lateral branch neurotomy for the treatment of sacroiliac joint-mediated low back pain: a large case series. *Pain Med*. 2013;14(1):29–35.
39. Vafi Salmasi, MDa, Gassan Chaiban, MDb, Hazem Eissa, MDb, Application of Cooled Radiofrequency Ablation in Management of Chronic Joint Pain Anesthesiology Institute, Cleveland Clinic, Cleveland, Ohio Department of Pain Management, *Ochsner Health Syst*.
40. Yang AJ, et al. Radiofrequency ablation for posterior sacroiliac joint complex pain: a narrative review. *Pharm Manag PM R*. 2019;11(suppl 1):S105–S113.
41. Adas C, Ozdemir U, Toman H, Luleci N, Luleci E, Adas H. Transsacrococcygeal approach to ganglion impar: radiofrequency application for the treatment of chronic intractable coccydynia. *J Pain Res*. 2016;9:1173–1177. https://doi.org/10.2147/JPR.S105506. Published 2016 Dec 7.

16 Shoulder Injection Techniques

JASON MARKLE AND CLEO D STAFFORD II

Ultrasound Guidance

Glenohumeral Joint: Intra-Articular

KEY POINTS

- Intra-articular ultrasound-guided injections can be done using the anterior rotator interval approach or posterior approach. The posterior technique avoids accidental neurovasculature injury and has lower extra-articular extravasation rates of the injectate compared to the anterior approach.[1]

Pertinent Anatomy

See Fig. 16.1.

- The shoulder joint (glenohumeral joint) is a ball and socket synovial joint between the scapula and the humerus.
- The joint is the major joint connecting the upper limb to the trunk.
- The joint is one of the most mobile joints in the human body, at the cost of joint stability.[2]

Common Pathology

- Intra-articular pathology can present with a joint effusion, and distention of the joint can be seen posterior joint line or inferior axillary recess on magnetic resonance imaging (MRI).[3]
- Patient presents with stiffness, loss of range of motion, and pain described as deep-seated anterior or posterior. Osteoarthritis can result in chronic instability from chronic ligament or tendon pathology.[4]

Equipment

- Linear array ultrasound transducer
- 25 to 22 gauge 2 to 3.5 inch needle

Common Injectates

- Local anesthetics for diagnostics
- Corticosteroids, hyaluronic acid, prolotherapy, orthobiologics (platelet-rich plasma [PRP], bone marrow concentrate, micronized adipose tissue, etc.)
- For capsular distention: High-volume mix of anesthetics, saline (corticosteroids, or orthobiologics: PRP, platelet lysate, platelet-poor plasma)

Injectate Volume

- 2 to 8 mL
- 20 to 60 mL for capsular distention (40 to 50 mL most common per authors' experience). Inject maximum volume as tolerated by pain or stop when getting back flow into the syringe to avoid capsular rupture.[5]

Technique: Glenohumeral Intra-Articular Posterior Approach

Patient Position

See Fig.16.2.

- Lateral recumbent with elbow flexed 90 degrees and shoulder internally rotated (authors' preferred).
- Can also have patient in the seated position with the shoulder internally rotated and hand resting in the patient's lap or contralateral shoulder to open to posterior joint space.

Clinician Position

- Posterior to the patient

Transducer Position

- Long axis to infraspinatus tendon, starting with probe parallel and just inferior to the spine of the scapula
- Visualize the posterior glenohumeral joint line deep to the muscle belly (infraspinatus)

Needle Position

- In-plane: needle visualization from lateral to medial with target between the posterior glenoid labrum and humeral head.
- Out-of-plane: visualize the needle tip as it contacts the humeral head lateral to the posterior labrum

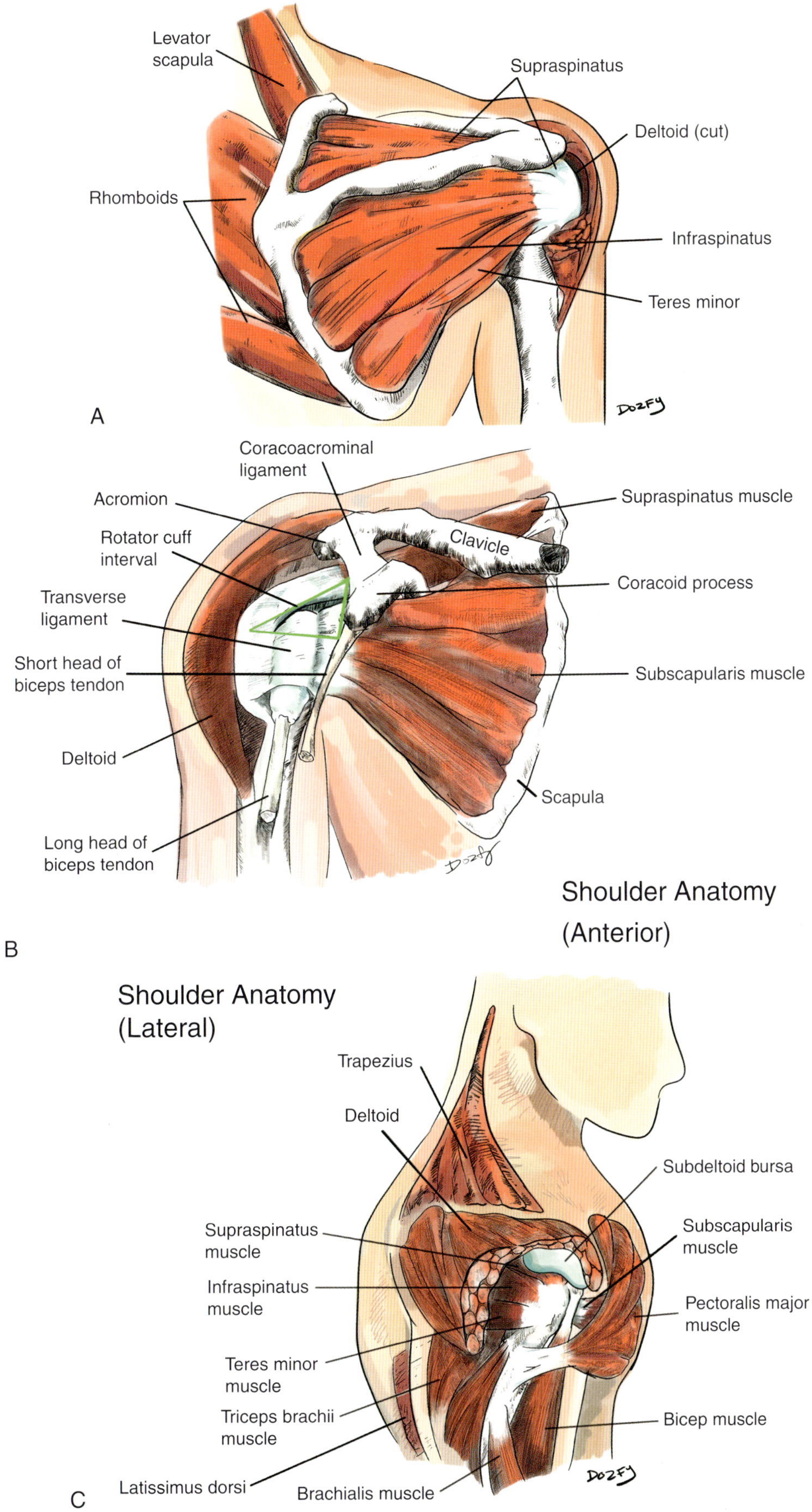

• **Fig. 16.1** Shoulder Anatomy. (A) Rotator cuff musculature, posterior view. (B) Rotator cuff musculature, anterior view. (C) Shoulder girdle musculature, lateral view.

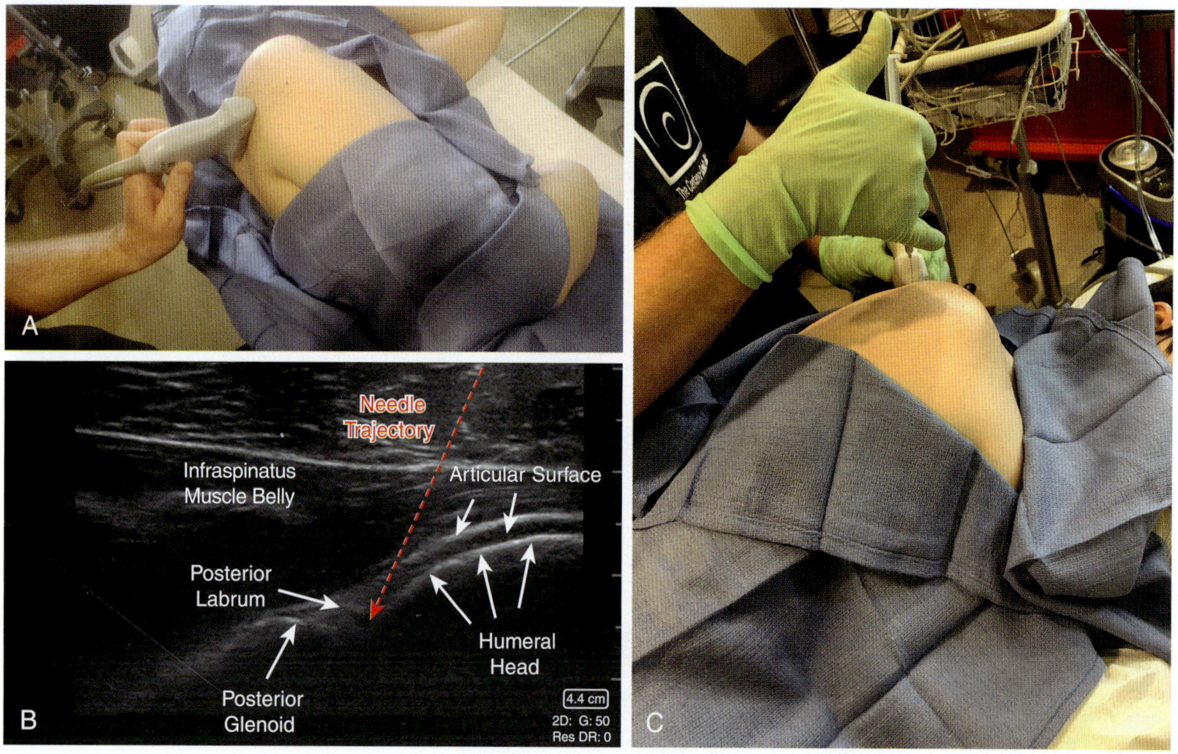

• **Fig. 16.2** (A) Patient positioning and probe position. (B) Ultrasound image and target. (C) Injection.

Target

- Glenohumeral joint space, avoiding the posterior labrum.
- Should visualize injectate flowing over the humeral head without extravagating superficial to the joint line.
- Can use power Doppler imaging to ensure intra-articular flow and no pooling outside of the joint.

PEARLS AND PITFALLS

- For posterior approach the needle angle can be steep, so sometimes gel stand-off can help.
- Keep needle closer to humeral head to avoid labral injury.
- With larger body habitus patient, curved linear probe may be needed.
- With capsular dilations, common to have resistance initially given the thickened capsule but with continued pressure and injectate volume into joint, flow becomes less restrictive.

Technique: Glenohumeral Intra-Articular Anterior Approach Via Rotator Interval

Patient Position

See Fig. 16.3.

- The patient lies supine or semi-supine with the affected shoulder slightly extended, externally rotated with elbow flexed or extended for patient comfort.

Clinician Position

- Side of the affected shoulder

Transducer Position

- The transducer is placed over the anterior shoulder with a transverse view of the rotator interval. The long head of biceps tendon at the center of image and supraspinatus (SS) and subscapularis to either side is obtained.
- The coracohumeral ligament (CHL) is seen draped superiorly over the biceps tendon.

Needle Position

- In-plane: The needle is introduced into the rotator interval using a lateral to medial approach.

Target

- The needle tip is imaged in real time, and the target is the biceps tendon sheath between the CHL above and biceps tendon below.
- Can use power Doppler imaging to ensure intra-articular flow and no pooling outside of the joint.

PEARLS AND PITFALLS

- For frozen shoulders, anterior capsular distention via rotator interval has been shown to be superior to other techniques.[6,7]

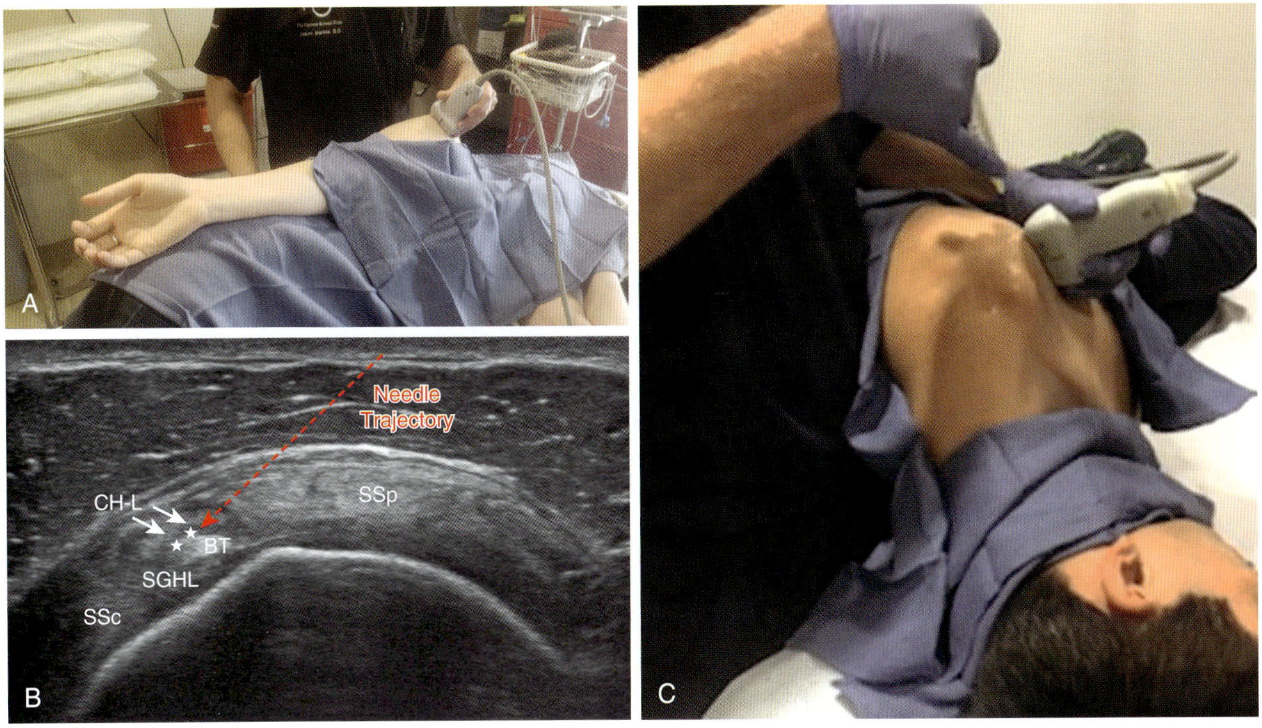

• **Fig. 16.3** (A) Patient positioning and probe position. (B) Ultrasound image and target (*asterisks*). (C) Injection. *BT,* biceps tendon; *CH-L*, Coracohumeral ligament; *SGHL*, superior glenohumeral ligament; *SSc*, subscapularis; *SSp*, supraspinatus.

Subacromial Injection

KEY POINTS

- Impingement syndrome and rotator cuff pathology are a common diagnosis in patients with shoulder pain.[8]
- Ultrasound-guided subacromial bursa injections allow for higher degree of accuracy when compared to landmark-guided injections.[9]
- For adhesive capsulitis, both subacromial and intra-articular glenohumeral corticosteroids have been both shown to be effective.[10]

Pertinent Anatomy

- The subacromial bursa is the largest bursa in the body[11] and lies between the acromion (superiorly) and SS tendon (inferiorly).
- Can extend laterally towards the greater tuberosity and medially towards the acromion-clavicular joint.[11]
- Bursa are synovial line potential space that reduces friction at the tendon-tendon and tendon-bone interface, and there are five potential bursa in the shoulder (subacromial/subdeltoid bursa, subscapularis recess/bursa, subcoracoid bursa, coracoclavicular (CC) bursa, and supra-acromial bursa).[11]

Common Pathology

- Subacromial impingement and rotator cuff tendinosis
- Subacromial and subdeltoid bursitis
- Adhesive capsulitis

Equipment

- Linear array ultrasound transducer
- 25 to 22 gauge 1.5 to 2 inch needle.

Common Injectates

- Local anesthetics for diagnostics
- Corticosteroids, hyaluronic acid, prolotherapy, orthobiologics (PRP, platelet-poor plasma).

Injectate Volume

- 1 to 5 mL

Technique for Subacromial Bursa: Lateral Approach

Patient Position

See Fig. 16.4.

- Seated upright with the shoulder fully adducted and the hand in neutral position with the elbow full extended (author preferred), or the shoulder in a Crass or modified Crass position for better visualization of the SS tendon.
- Can also have patient in the lateral decubitus position with the shoulder fully adducted and the hand in neutral position with the elbow full extended or flexed to 90 degrees.
- Additionally, can place the patient in supine position with the shoulder fully adducted and the hand in neutral or prone position with the elbow full extended.

Clinician Position

- Standing or seated adjacent to the affected shoulder

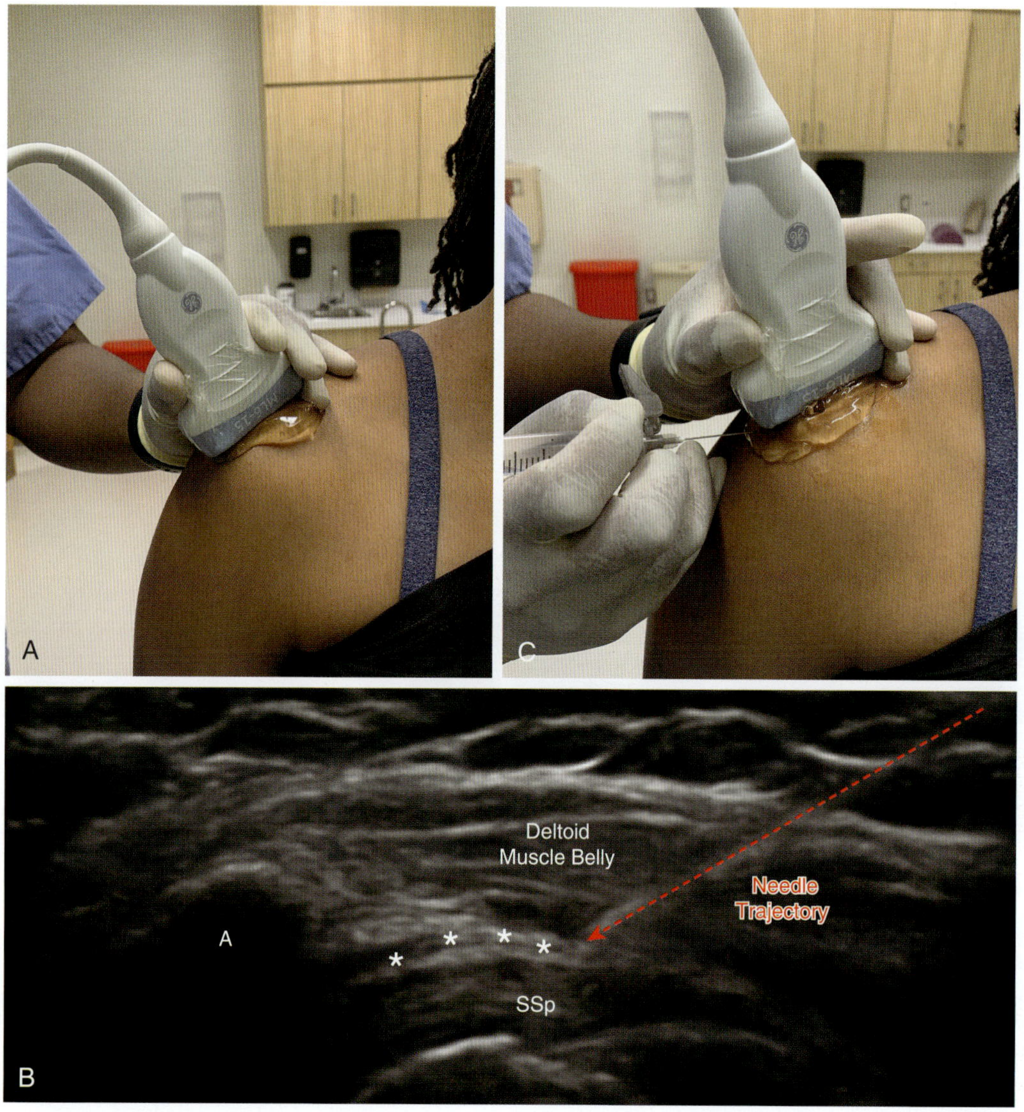

• **Fig. 16.4** Subacrominal Bursa Injection (A) Ultrasound probe and patient positioning (B) Injection (C) Ultrasound image of injection. *A,* acromium; *SSp* supraspinatus tendon; *asterisks*, subacromial bursa target.

Transducer Position

- Long axis to the SS tendon.

Needle Position

- In-plane: needle visualization from lateral to medial

Target

- Subacromial bursa space with target between the undersurface of the deltoid muscle and superior to the SS tendon.

PEARLS AND PITFALLS

- Ensure you visualize a separation between the SS tendon and undersurface of the deltoid muscle when injecting, and your needle tip is not the SS tendon (particularly with corticosteroid injections). [6]
- Consider using a longer needle (2 inches to 2.5 inches) with patients with a larger body habitus to ensure you are not injecting into the deltoid muscle.
- Consider the supine or lateral decubitus position to avoid injury from a potential vasovagal episode.

Rotator Cuff Tendons

KEY POINTS

- Rotator cuff tears are common, and the most commonly affected tendon is the supraspinatus (SS).[12]
- Full-thickness rotator cuff tears are present in 25% individuals over 60% and 50% of individuals over 80.[13]
- Asymptomatic full-thickness tears are common, but 50% will become symptomatic over a 2- to 3-year period.[13]
- The size of the tear increases in 12% to 25% of patients at 18 months,[14] but in 50% of patients who become symptomatic, there is evidence of tear progression.[13]
- Symptomatic full-thickness tears progress in 50% of cases over a 2-year period.[13]
- Long-head biceps tendinopathy can have similar presentation to SS pathology.[15]

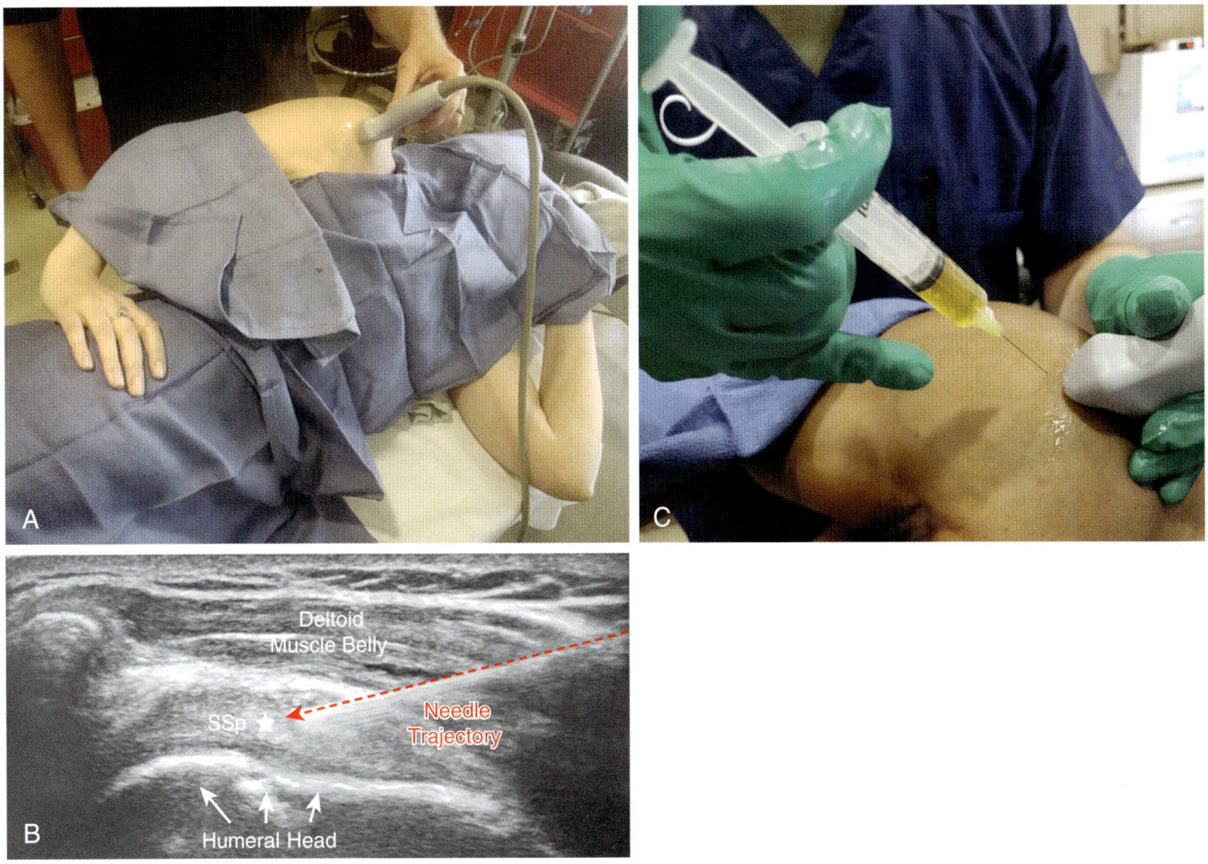

• **Fig. 16.5** (A) Patient positioning and probe position. (B) Ultrasound image and target (*asterisk*): supraspinatus *(SSp)* tendon. (C) Injection.

Pertinent Anatomy

- The footprint of the SS on the greater tuberosity is much smaller compared to the footprint of the infraspinatus.[16]
- Footprint of the SS is triangular in shape, with an average maximum medial-to-lateral length of 6.9 mm and an average maximum anteroposterior width of 12.6 mm.[16]
- The infraspinatus had a long tendinous portion in the superior half of the muscle, which curved anteriorly and extended to the middle facet of the greater tubercle of the humerus.[16]

Common Pathology

- Tendinosis
- Partial-thickness tears
  - Can be interstitial, articular or bursal-sided
- Full-thickness tears
  - Can be incomplete or complete
    - Complete retracted or complete non-retracted
- Calcific tendinopathy

Equipment

- Linear array ultrasound transducer
- 27 to 22 gauge 1.5 to 2 inch needle

Common injectates:

- Local anesthetics for diagnostics
- Prolotherapy, orthobiologics (PRP, bone marrow concentrate, micronized adipose tissue, etc.)
- Avoid intratendinous corticosteroid injections.

Injectate Volume

- 1 to 5 mL

Technique: Supraspinatus Tendon

Patient Position

See Fig. 16.5.

- Seated, supine or lateral recumbent with arm in Crass or modified Crass position (shoulder extended and internally rotated, with the hand on the posterior lateral hip)

Clinician Position

- On the side of the affected shoulder, behind or in front of patient (depending on dexterity and comfort)

Transducer Position

- Long axis to the SS.
- Keeping this orientation, scan the tendon from anterior to posterior to identify locations of pathology. The

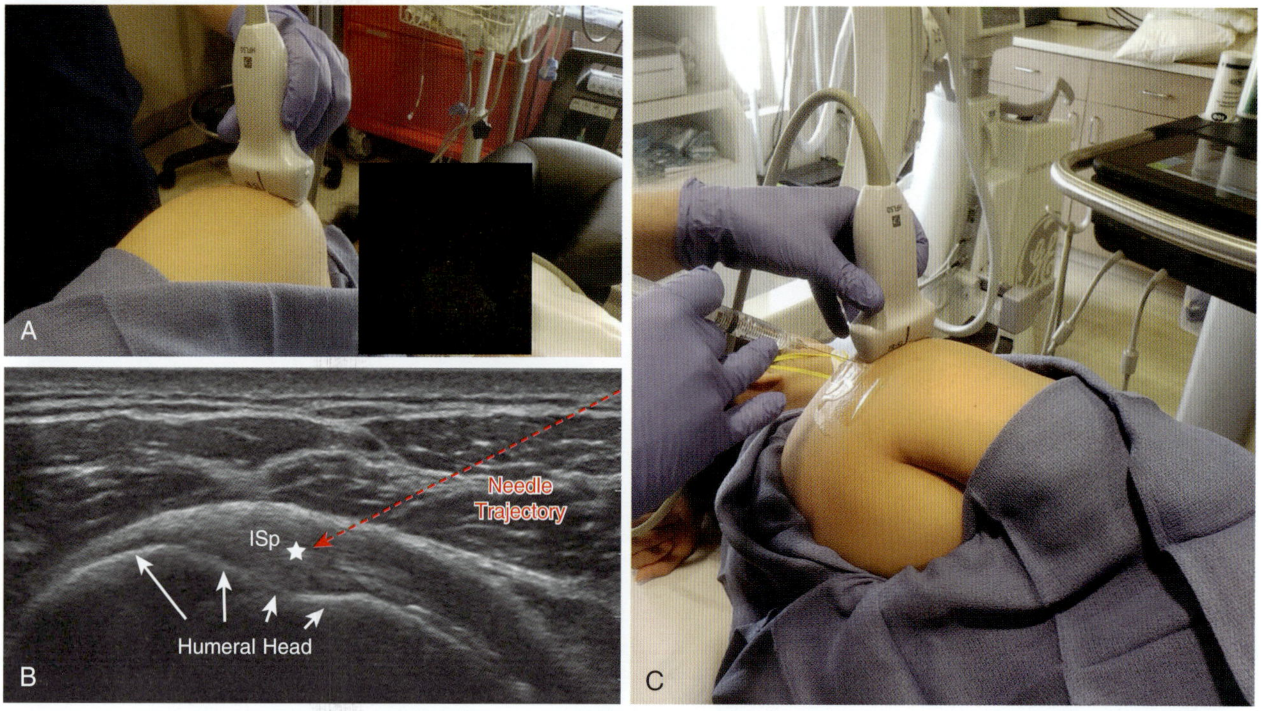

• **Fig. 16.6** (A) Patient positioning and probe position. (B) Ultrasound image and target (*asterisk*). (C) Injection. *ISp,* Infraspinatus tendon.

tendon should also be scanned in transverse to obtain orthogonal views for an accurate assessment.

Needle Position

- In-plane, distal to proximal fibers (lateral to medial) or, alternatively, can inject proximal to distal fibers.
  - Can redirect the needle to get more anterior to posterior fibers.
- Can also inject in the transverse view; can inject in-plane posterior to anterior across the SS fibers.

Target

- Pathologic aspect of SS tendon

Technique: Infraspinatus/Teres Minor Tendons via Ultrasound Guidance

Patient Position

See Fig. 16.6.

- Seated or lateral recumbent with elbow flexed 90 degrees and shoulder internally rotated

Clinician Position

- On the side of the affected shoulder, behind patient

Transducer Position

- Long axis to the tendon, scan anterior-posterior/superior-inferior to identify pathology.
- Continue scanning inferiorly, and you will come to the small footprint of teres minor. The tendon should also be scanned in transverse to obtain orthogonal views for an accurate assessment.

Needle Position

- In-plane, distal to proximal (lateral to medial) approach or proximal to distal approach

Target

- Pathologic aspect of infraspinatus or teres minor

Technique: Subscapularis Tendon via Ultrasound Guidance

Patient Position

See Fig.16.7.

- Lateral decubitus or supine with shoulder externally rotated (instruct patient to turn palm to ceiling)
  - Sometimes easier to have patient flex elbow to 90 degrees and have assistant bedside passively externally rotate shoulder.

Clinician Position

- On the side of the affected shoulder

Transducer Position

- Long axis to the tendon, scan superior-inferior to identify pathology
- The tendon should also be scanned in transverse to obtain orthogonal views for an accurate assessment.

Needle Position

- In-plane, distal to proximal (lateral to medial) approach

Target

- Pathologic aspect of subscapularis

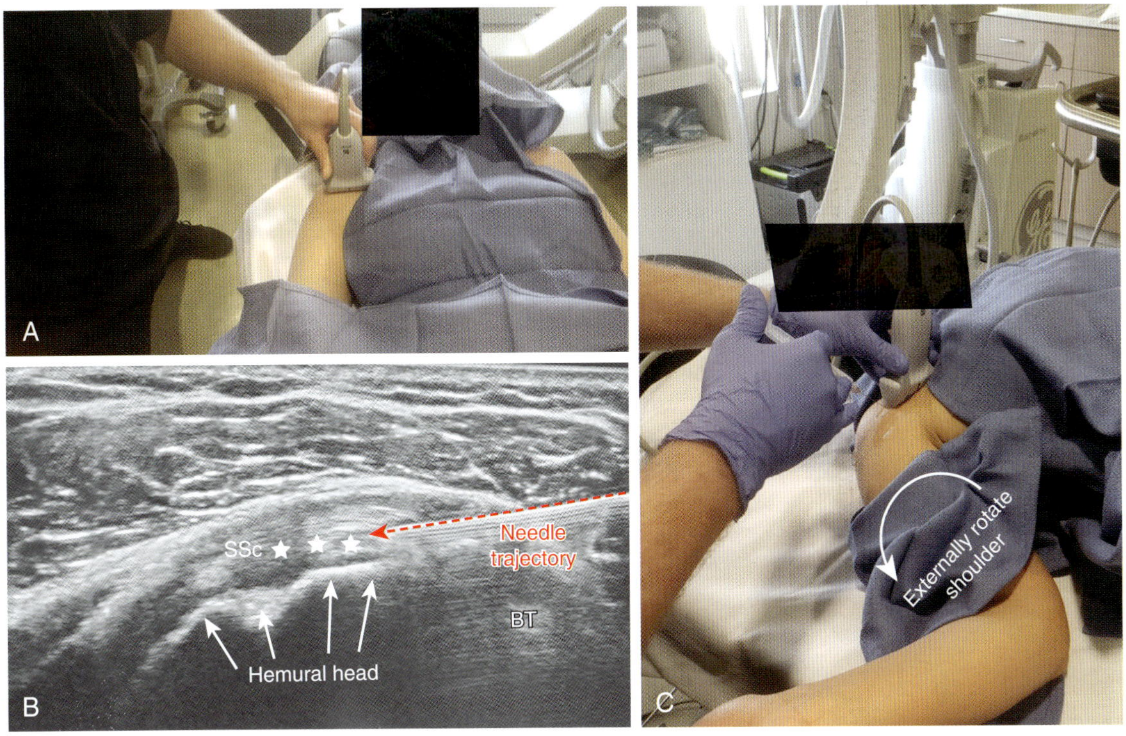

• **Fig. 16.7** (A) Patient positioning and probe position. (B) Ultrasound image and target (*asterisks*). (C) Injection. *BT,* biceps tendon (long head); *SSc,* Subscapularis tendon.

PEARLS AND PITFALLS

- Ultrasound evolution of the rotator cuff is susceptible to anisotropic artifact due to the curved course of the tendons, especially at the insertions, and should not be mistaken for tendinosis or partial-thickness rotator cuff tear.
- The posterior aspect of the SS overlaps with the infraspinatus. The infraspinatus tendon is centrally positioned and surrounded by hypoechoic muscle that can be mistaken for a tendon tear if scanned obliquely.
- The subscapular tendon can have a varied appearance, with hyperechoic tendon fibers interposed with hypoechoic muscle fibers, and can be confused with tendinosis or partial tear.
- Orthogonal views should be used to verify pathology.
- Full Crass position can be difficult for some patients due to pain; modifying with slight shoulder extension and less internal rotation can still bring SS from under the acromion without placing excessive stress on shoulder. If modifying for diagnostic purposes, modified Crass position can result in overestimation of the size of rotator cuff tear.[17]
- Injured areas of tendon may distend with injection and small aliquots of anesthetic before a regenerative procedure can help localize occult or small tears.
- Ultrasound-guided bone marrow concentrate combined with platelet products are a safe and useful alternative to conservative exercise therapy of full thickness, less than 1 cm retracted SS tendons.[18]
- Utilizing a brachial plexus nerve block or suprascapular nerve block can help reduce the discomfort on part of the patient when using bone marrow concentrate or other orthobiologics.
- Patient positioning is best either supine or lateral recumbent. Sitting position risks patient falling if experiencing a vasovagal episode.

Glenohumeral Joint Capsule Ligaments

KEY POINTS

- Anterior capsule can be difficult to visualize under ultrasound in patients with larger body habitus.
- The capsular ligaments provide static stability across the glenohumeral joint.

Pertinent Anatomy

- Anterior capsule is composed of superior glenohumeral ligament (SGHL), middle glenohumeral ligament (MGHL), and anterior band of the inferior glenohumeral ligament (IGHL).
- The SGHL functions to resist inferior translation and external rotation of the humeral head in the adducted arm.[19]
- The MGHL functions primarily to resist external rotation from 0 to 90 degrees and provides anterior stability to the moderately abducted shoulder.[19]
- The anterior band of IGHL functions to resist anteroinferior translation.[19]
- The superior glenohumeral and CHL were shown to be important stabilizers against inferior shoulder motion, even though the CHL is much more robust.[20]
- The MGHL functions to resist external rotation from 0 to 90 degrees and provides anterior stability at 45 to 60 degrees abduction.[21]
- The IGHL complex is the most important stabilizer of the joint, resisting anterior and inferior shoulder

translation. The anterior band prevents anterior dislocation with the shoulder in abduction and external rotation, and is injured in anterior shoulder dislocations.[22]

Common Pathology

- The majority (95%) of traumatic dislocation are anterior.[23]
  - Leads to chronic anterior capsular instability and, if left untreated, eventually leads to need for athroplasty.[24]
- Internal impingement of glenohumeral joint can be a result of deficiencies of glenohumeral capsular ligaments.[25]
  - Excessive repetitive external rotation in throwing athletes (example: baseball pitchers) increases anterior capsule strain, leading to internal impingement syndrome.[26–30]
  - Tightness of the posterior capsule will result in glenohumeral internal rotation deficiencies (GIRDs), leading to internal impingement syndrome.[31]

Equipment

- Linear ultrasound transducer
- Needle size: 25 to 22-gauge 2 to 3.5-inch needle
- 27 to 25 gauge 1.5 to 3 inch needle

Common injectates

- Prolotherapy, orthobiologics (PRP, bone marrow concentrate, etc.)
- Avoid intraligamentous corticosteroids.

Injectate Volume

- 1 to 3 mL per ligament

Technique: Superior Glenohumeral Ligament and Coracohumeral Ligament via Ultrasound Guidance

Patient Position

- The patient lies supine or lateral recumbent with the affected shoulder closest to the physician.
- The shoulder is slightly extended.

Clinician Position

- Side of affected shoulder

Transducer Position

- The transducer is placed over the anterosuperior shoulder transverse view of the rotator interval, with the long head biceps tendon (LHBT) at the center of image in short axis with SS and subscapularis to either side.
- The CHL is draped over the LHBT and SGHL deep to the LHBT, forming a sling around the tendon as it enters the glenohumeral joint.

Needle Position

- Out-of-plane, identify needle tip and redirecting into each structure.
- Alternatively, can inject in long axis lateral to medial approach

Target

- Inject the CHL and SGHL around the LHBT
- See Fig. 16.8

Technique: Middle Glenohumeral Ligament via Ultrasound Guidance

Patient position

See Fig 16.9.

- Supine or lateral recumbent with shoulder externally rotated (instruct patient to turn palm to ceiling)
  - Sometimes easier to have patient flex elbow to 90 degrees and have assistant bedside passively externally rotate shoulder.

Clinician Position

- Side of patient

Transducer Position

- Short axis to LHBT in the bicipital groove
- As patient or assistant externally rotates the shoulder, slide transducer medial to the bicipital groove.

Needle Position

- In-plane needle visualization lateral to medial
  - Out-of-plane optional, visualize needle tip just above humeral head.

Target

- If possible, identify the anterior glenoid and corresponding labrum.
- The MGHL will be just superficial to the labrum traveling from glenoid to humeral head and deep to the subscapularis muscle.
- Inject diffusely along the MGHL

Technique: Inferior Glenohumeral Ligament via Ultrasound Guidance

Patient position

See Figs. 16.10 and 16.11.

- The patient lies supine or lateral decubitus with the affected shoulder closest to the physician.
- The shoulder is flexed and internally rotated.
  - Dorsum of the affected side is just above the patient's head.
  - Goal is to flex and internally rotate the shoulder as much as possible to move neovascular structures out of the needle trajectory.

Clinician Position

- Side of affected shoulder

Transducer Position

- Start distal on humeral shaft in short axis and then slide proximally until the humeral shaft changes into the humeral head (circular structure).

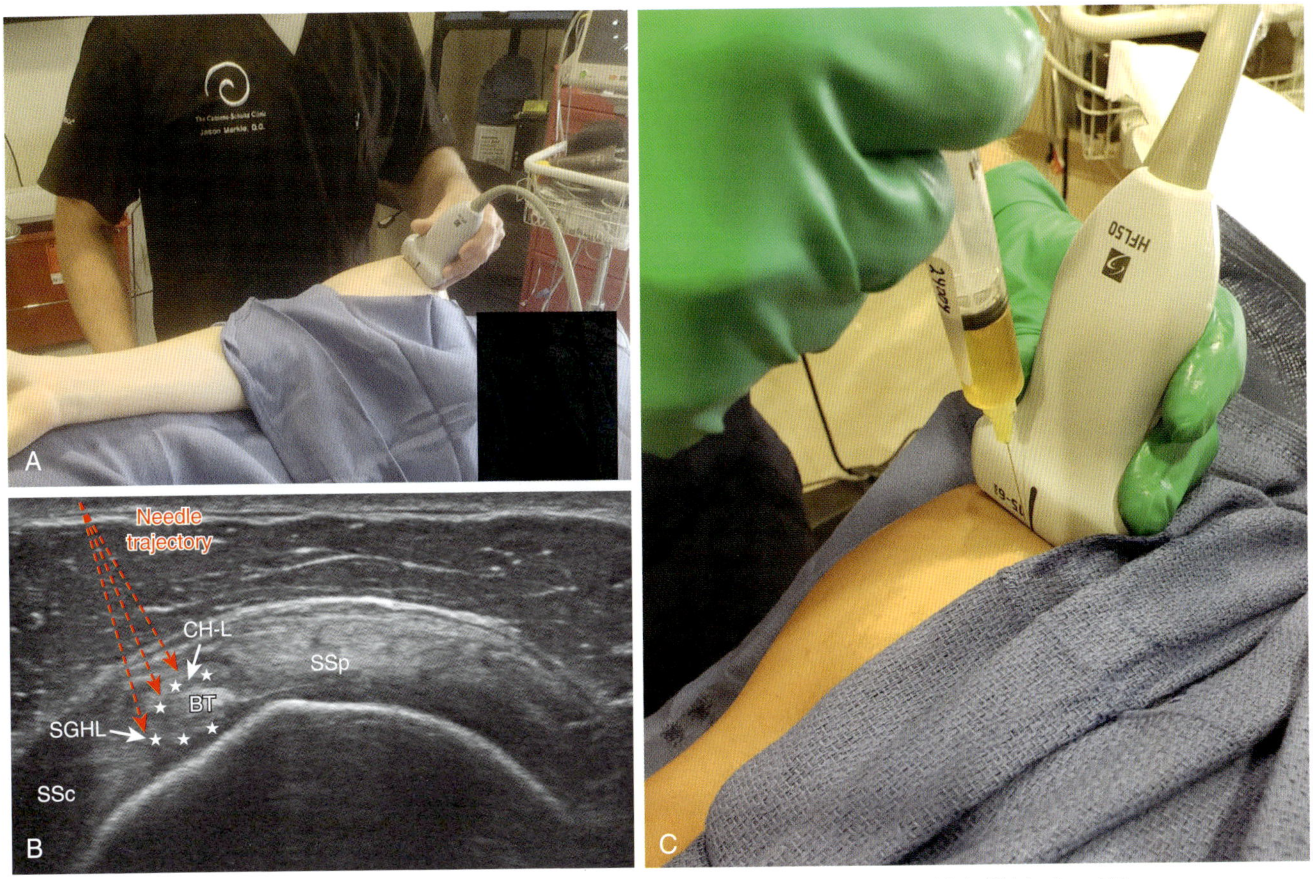

• **Fig. 16.8** (A) Patient and probe position. (B) Ultrasound image with targets (*asterisks*). (C) Injection. *BT,* Biceps tendon; *CH-L,* corahumeral ligament, *SGHL,* superior glenohumeral ligament; *SSc,* subscapularis tendon; *SSp,* supraspinatus tendon.

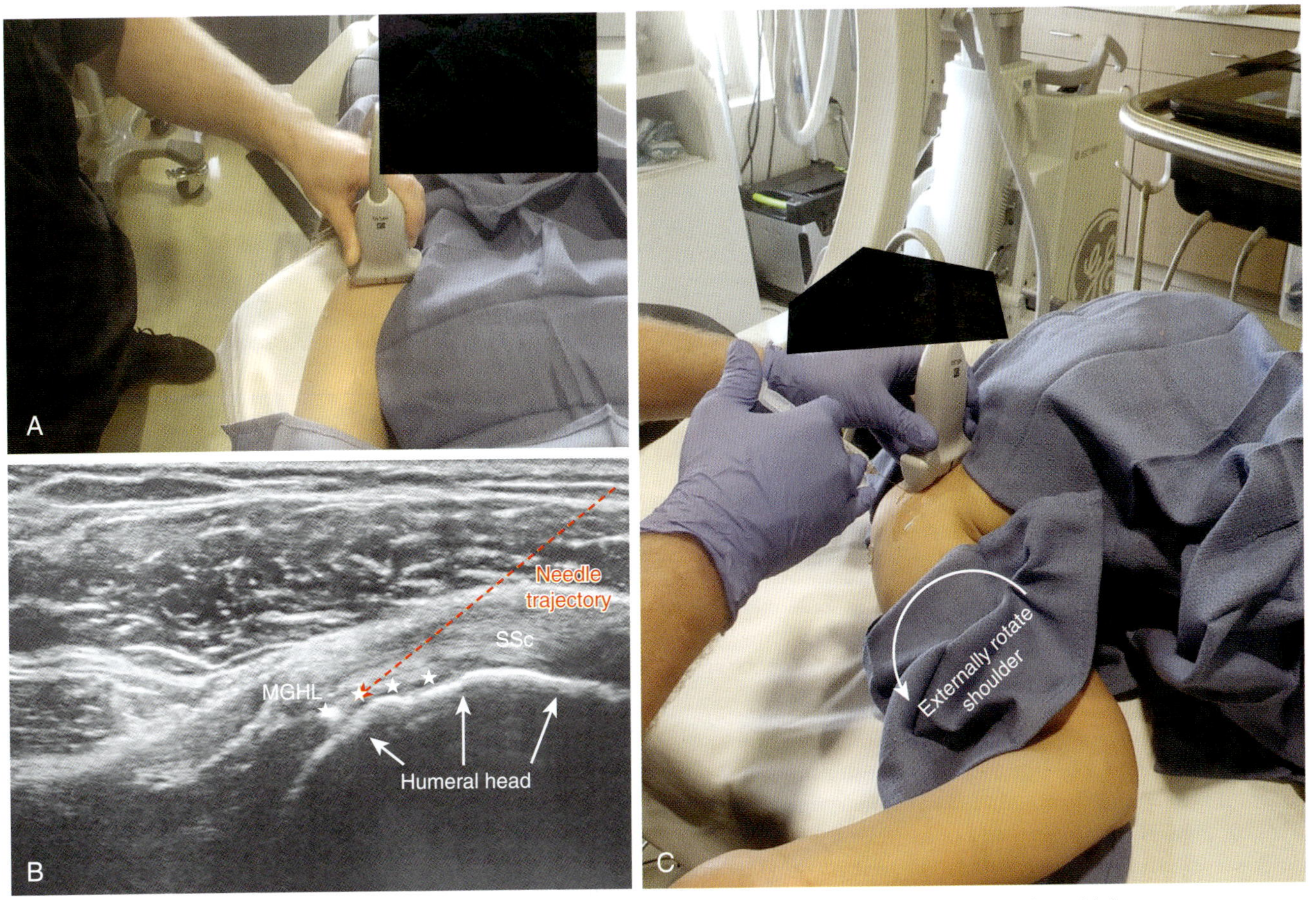

• **Fig. 16.9** In-plane AC joint. (A) Patient and probe position. (B) Ultrasound image with target (*asterisks*). (C) Injection. *SSc,* Subscapularis tendon; *MGHL,* middle glenohumeral ligament.

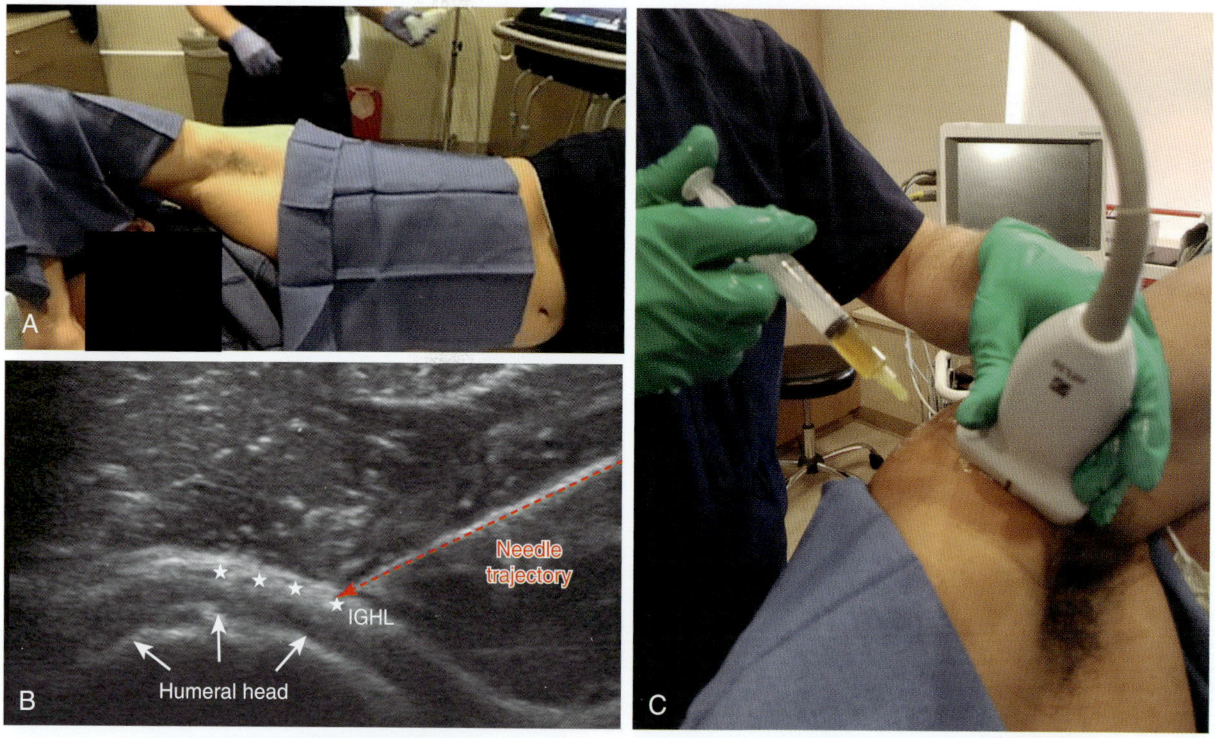

• **Fig. 16.10** IGHL Transverse Approach. (A) Patient and probe position. (B) Ultrasound image with targets (*asterisks*). (C) Injection. *IGHL*, inferior glenohumeral ligament.

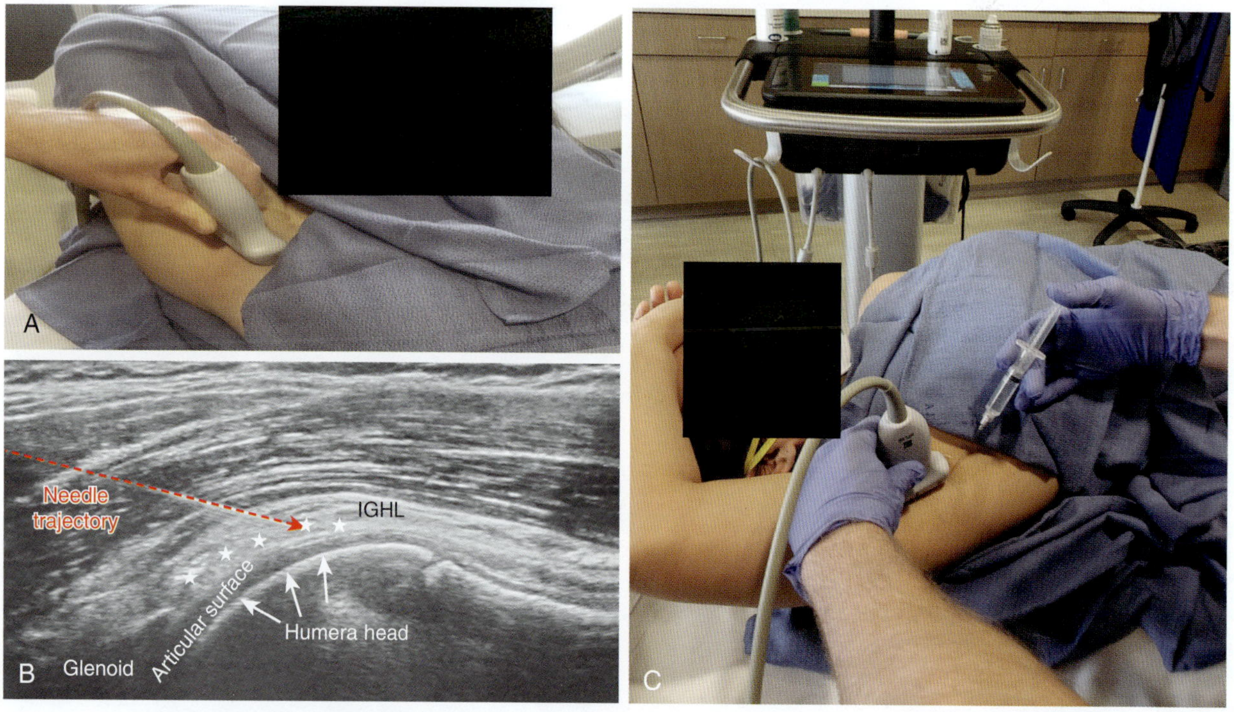

• **Fig. 16.11** IGHL Parallel Approach. (A) Patient and probe position. (B) Ultrasound image with target (*asterisks*). (C) Injection. *IGHL*, inferior glenohumeral ligament.

- The IGHL appears as a hyperechoic thickening over the humeral head as you slide anterior to posterior.
- Should view the ligament in orthogonal views: transducer parallel to humerus and transverse.
- Observe adjacent neovascular structures and avoid them.

Needle Position

- Parallel to humerus view, inject in-plane: from either distal to proximal or proximal to distal.
- Choose the safest approach with regard to neovasculature.
- In the transverse view, in-plane needle approach from posterior/lateral to anterior/medial.

Target

- Inject diffusely along the IGHL fibers surrounding the humeral head.
- Injured areas will easily distend.

PEARLS AND PITFALLS

- When treating the IGHL, utilize Doppler flow to identify and avoid the axillary vessels that run with the axillary nerve.
- After treating the IGHL in the axilla, ensure to discard the needle before targeting other structures in the shoulder and possibly sterilize the probe.
  - *Propionibacterium acnes* mostly colonizes the pilosebaceous follicles in the skin of the upper body, including the head, neck, shoulders, and especially the axilla.[32]

Glenohumeral Joint Labrum

KEY POINTS

- Combination utilizing ultrasound guidance with fluoroscopic guidance is the preferred method for isolating and treating a superior labral tear near or at the biceps anchor.
- Anteroinferior labral injuries, or Bankart lesions, are commonly associated with shoulder dislocations and/or chronic shoulder instability. When treating anterior inferior labrum, co-treating the anterior joint capsule is needed.[33]
- Labral tears that appear to be retracted (types III–IV SLAP tears) off glenoid or in conjunction with fractures (bony Bankart lesion) are considered unstable and unlikely to improve with percutaneous injections, and, if symptomatic, should be managed surgically.[34]

Pertinent Anatomy

- The labrum is a fibrocartilaginous structure rim attached around the margin of the glenoid cavity in the scapula.
- Labrum exists to give additional surface area to the glenoid articulating surface to help maintain stability.[35]
- The long head of biceps brachii tendon (BT) attaches to the glenoid and labrum at the superior anterior aspect (variable in each person) of the glenoid.
- The glenoid labrum runs in a circumferential orientation around the glenoid rim and contributes passive stability to the glenohumeral joint.
- Anteroinferior labrum is in connection with the IGHL.
- Posterior inferior glenohumeral ligament (PIGHL) attaches to the labrum.
- Circumferentially, the labrum deepens the glenohumeral socket by 50%.[36]

Common Pathology

- SLAP tears (superior labral anterior-posterior tear) are common in throwing sport and/or overhead athletes. The deceleration phase of throwing places increased stress on the labrum and biceps tendon compared to other phases of throwing, resulting in repetitive trauma over time with eventual tissue failure.[37]
- Classification of SLAP lesions as types I–IV:
  - Types I and II are classified more degenerative with tearing
  - Types III and IV are characterized by detachment off the glenoid consistent with a bucket handle tear
- Types I and II are candidates for percutaneous treatment with orthobiologics.
- Bankart injuries are common in traumatic dislocations and chronic shoulder instability patients; lesions are typically located in the 3 to 6 o'clock position, where the humeral head dislocates.
- Identification of bony versus fibrous lesion is critical because bony Bankart lesions are treated with surgical management for best outcome.[38] Common injury with repetitive posterior resistive force such as weightlifters (bench press), football players involved with blocking, gymnasts, or swimmers.[39]
- Posterior labral tears are often referred to as "reverse Bankart" lesion, and can have concurrent concealed avulsion fracture of the posteroinferior labrum.

Equipment

- Linear ultrasound transducer
- 25 gauge 3 to 3.5 inch needle (single or multi-needle technique)
- C-arm fluoroscopy (optional)
- Contrast agent (optional)

Common injectates

- Prolotherapy, orthobiologics (PRP, bone marrow concentrate, etc.)
- Avoid intralabral corticosteroids.

Injectate Volume

- 1 to 2 mL

Technique: Superior Glenohumeral Labrum (Biceps Anchor)

Patient Position

See Figs. 16.12 and 16.13.

- Supine
- Shoulder by patient side, externally rotated with palm facing up (brings the BT anterior to allow easier visualization)

Clinician Position

- Standing directly next to the shoulder being injected

MSK Ultrasound Transducer Position

- Short axis to longhead of the biceps
  - Can be long axis to LHBT
    - But ensure you have trajectory that allows to clear the humeral tuberosity with direct path to the glenoid.
- Follow the biceps in short-axis view proximally until lose BT completely; then track distal until visualize again.

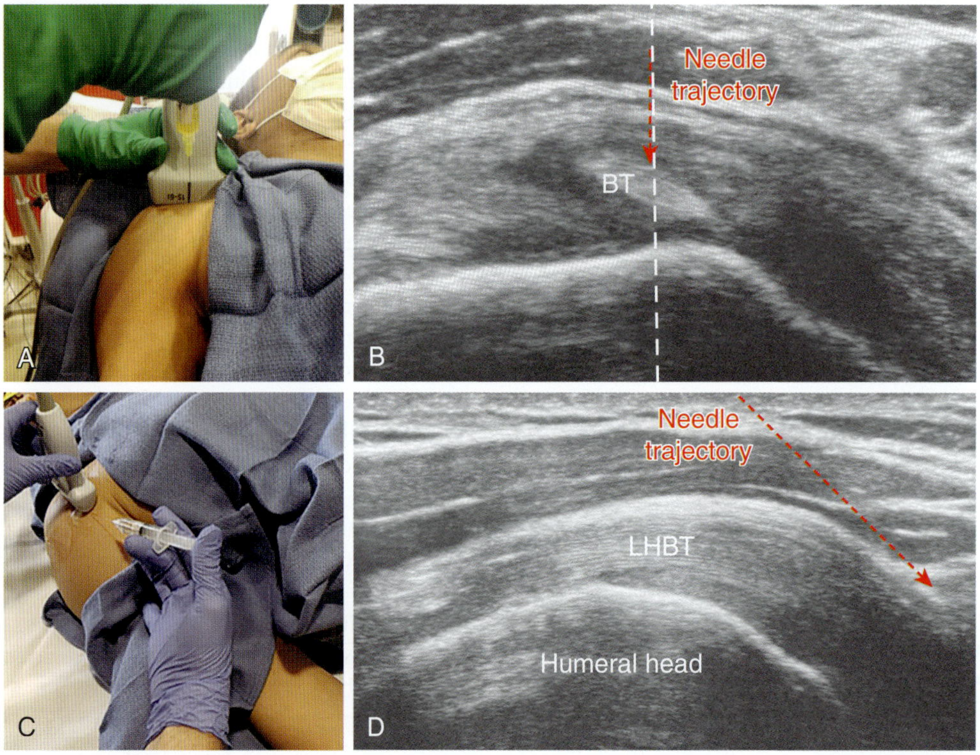

• **Fig. 16.12** (A and B) Short axis to LHBT starting approach. (C and D) Long axis to LHBT starting approach. *BT*, Biceps tendon; *LHBT*, long head biceps tendon.

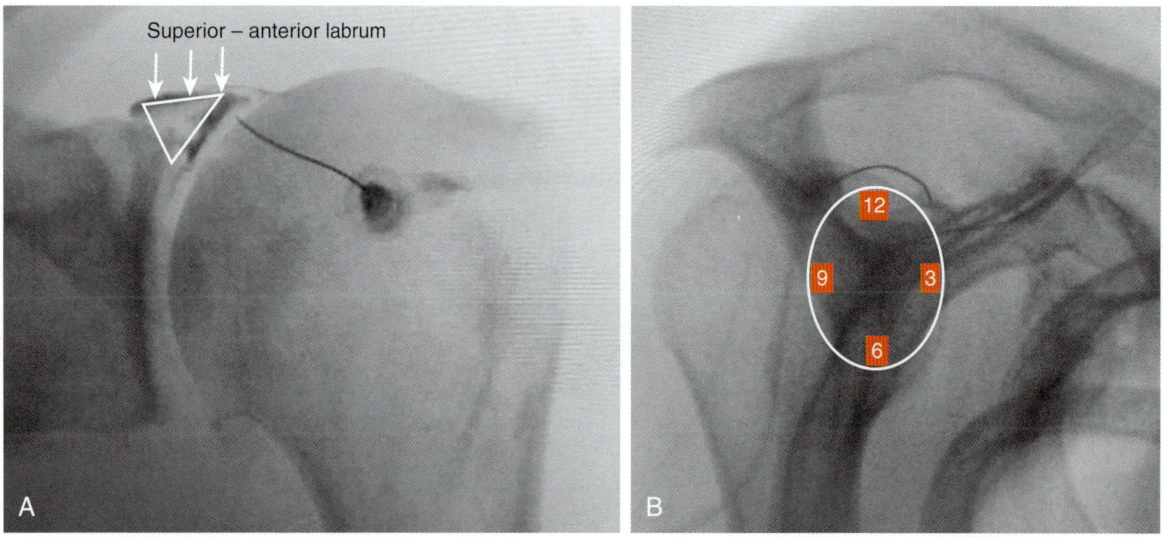

• **Fig. 16.13** Superior-Anterior Labral Injection. (A) AP fluoroscopic image. *Triangle,* labrum. (B) Scapular-Y view. Circle and numbers represent the clock face analogy for the labrum.

C-Arm Position (Biplanar Views)

- AP with contralateral rotation of C-arm to align the anterior and posterior glenoid rim or "true AP", understanding that the shoulder joint is naturally rotated 10 to 30 degrees on the transverse plane (horizontal plane)
  - Evaluates superior/inferior position on glenoid.
- Scapular Y view
  - Evaluates circumferential orientation on the glenoid (where you are in relation to the "clock face").

Needle Position

- Can use MSK ultrasound to identify the BT and guide the needle into the proximal LHBT and direct needle towards the glenoid attachment.
- If available switch to fluoroscopic guidance and advance the needle to the glenoid.
- Once contacting the periosteum, add contrast and check biplanar views to evaluate location on glenoid and contrast flow.

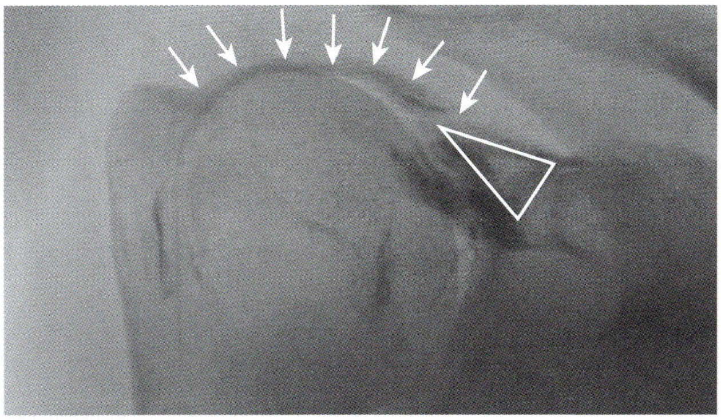

• **Fig. 16.14** Contrast into bicep tendon *(white arrows)*, highlighting attachment to glenoid anchor *(white triangle)*.

- If achieved correct position and contrast flow, then inject and redirect to achieve full coverage of the labral tear.

Target

- Will be based on diagnostic imaging, preferably MRI-arthrogram of shoulder to visualize the tear and extension.
- Utilizing biplanar views (true AP and scapular Y), you can triangulate location on glenoid to ensure covering necessary region of labrum and proximal LHBT.
  - Example: 8 mm intrasubstance labral tear, extending from 11 o'clock to 3 o'clock on the glenoid. Can be confirmed with scapular Y views.

See Fig. 16.14.

PEARLS AND PITFALLS

- Prior to injections, brachial plexus nerve blocks at interscalene or supraclavicular region are advisable for patient comfort.
- Utilizing biplanar views based on MRI
- Placing contrast into the long head of biceps tendon proximally under ultrasound guidance will allow visualization of the root attachment on the biceps to the glenoid and effectively gives you a "target" for the labral anchor.
- If only ultrasound available, utilize the long axis of LHBT approach and attempt to maintain trajectory within the LHBT tendon fibers until contact periosteum.

Technique: Posterior Labrum and Posterior Capsule

Patient Position

See Fig. 16.15.

- Lateral recumbent
- Shoulder by patient side, elbow flexed to 90 degrees and shoulder internally rotated

Clinician position

- Standing posterior side of shoulder

Transducer Position

- Short axis to posterior glenohumeral joint, visualizing the posterior labrum

C-Arm Position

- AP with contralateral rotation of C-arm to align the anterior and posterior glenoid rim or "true AP," understanding that the shoulder joint is naturally rotated 10 to 30 degrees on the transverse plane (horizontal plane)

Needle Position

- Identify the posterior labrum attached to posterior glenoid; guide needle lateral to medial, similar to posterior intra-articular approach.
- Option to confirm with fluoroscopic guidance, true AP view

Target

- Contrast flow should be triangular outlining the labrum.
- Inject pathologic areas of the labrum based on MRI findings.
- Redirect needle based on target location until covered.
  - Under ultrasound guidance, direct needle tip to the superficial layer of labrum (posterior capsule).
- Redirect to achieve full coverage of the labral tear based on MRI findings.
- Will be based on diagnostic imaging, preferably MRI-arthrogram of shoulder to visualize the tear.
- Option to confirm with injection of a small amount of contrast under AP fluoroscopy

PEARLS AND PITFALLS

- When treating inferior posterior labrum, first identify and locate the axillary nerve and posterior circumflex artery.
- Also identify suprascapular nerve and artery descending from the spinoglenoid notch to avoid.

Biceps Tendon

KEY POINTS

- The biceps is a strong supinator of the forearm and serves as a weak elbow flexor.
- The proximal biceps brachii muscle has two heads, a short and long head (LHBT). The LHBT is a well-recognized source of anterior shoulder pain.[44]
- The biceps tendon pathology can be divided into three categories: inflammatory/degenerative (i.e., tendinopathy/tenosynovitis, degenerative tear); instability (subluxation or dislocation); and LHBT anchor abnormalities (SLAP lesions, rupture).
- Shoulder impingement can affect the long head of the biceps tendon, resulting in a spectrum of pathology from tendinosis, degenerative tears, and rupture.
- Due to the impingement mechanism, there is a causal relationship between biceps tendon injures and rotator cuff pathology,[40] but biceps tendon pathology is often overlooked. and partial tears are often missed on MRI (73%).[41]

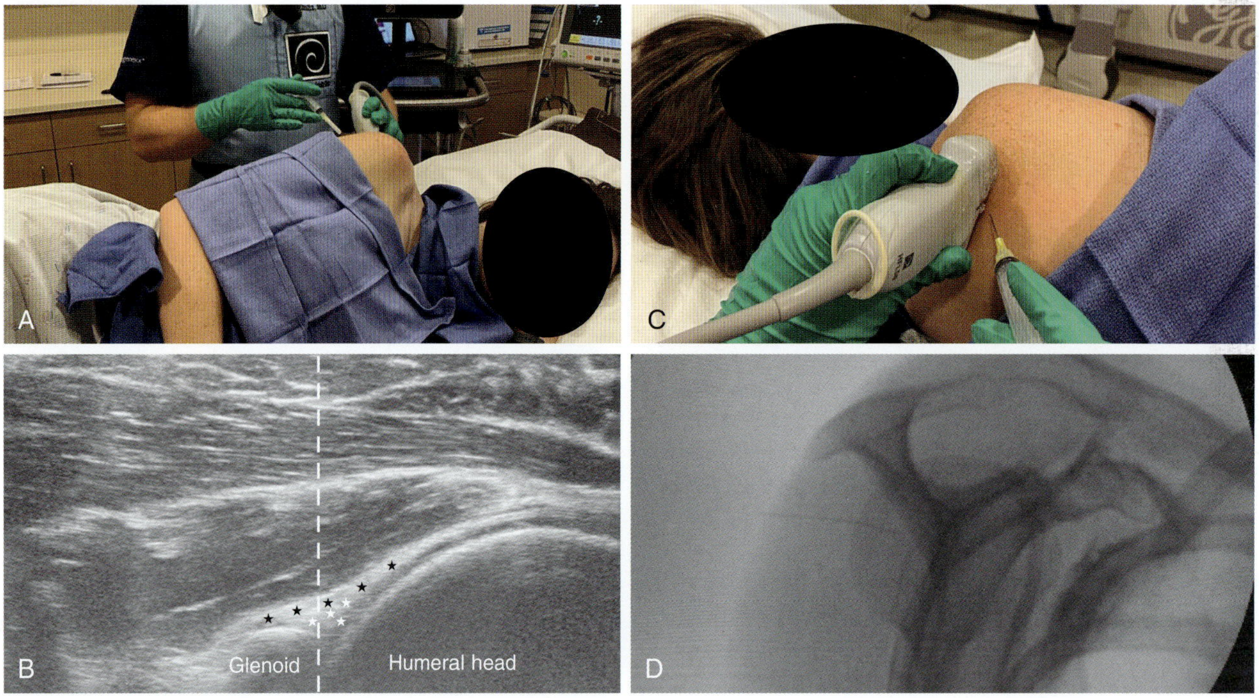

• **Fig. 16.15** (A) Patient positioning. (B) Ultrasound Image: *black asterisk,* posterior capsule; *white asterisk,* posterior labrum. (C) Needle approach. (D) Fluoroscopic image.

Pertinent Anatomy

- Approximately 50% of the long head biceps brachii (LHBT) originates from the supraglenoid tubercle and 50% continuous with the superior portion of the glenoid labrum. The short head originates from the tip of the coracoid process.[42]
- The LHBT exits the joint and passes through the rotator interval and over the anterior shoulder in the bicipital groove. The biceps tendon has a synovial sheath, which is an extension of the synovial lining of the glenohumeral joint.
- The biceps serves to depress the humeral head and diminishes stress on the IGHL. Rupture or surgical detachment decreases the shoulder's resistance to torsion and places a greater strain on the IGHL, impacting anterior shoulder stability,[43] although some evidence refutes any major role of the biceps at the shoulder.[44]

Common Pathology

- Tenosynovitis
- Partial- and full-thickness tears
  - In many cases the MRI will miss a partial biceps tendon. Razmjou et al. showed that 73% of partial biceps tendon tears were missed on an MRI.[41]
- Tendinosis
- Biceps subluxation (transverse humeral ligament injury)

Equipment

- Linear array ultrasound transducer
- 30 to 25 gauge 1 to 2 inch needle

Common Injectates

- Local anesthetics for diagnostics
- Prolotherapy, orthobiologics (PRP, bone marrow concentrate, etc.)
- Avoid intratendinous corticosteroids.

Injectate Volume

- 0.5 to 3 mL

Technique: Long Head of Biceps Tendon

Patient Position

See Figs. 16.16 and 16.17.

- Supine or lateral decubitus with shoulder externally rotated (instruct patient to supinate the forearm)
  - Sometimes easier to have patient flex elbow to 90 degrees and have assistant bedside passively externally rotate shoulder

Clinician Position

- Side of patient

Transducer Position

- Short axis to LHBT in the bicipital groove
- Can also visualize the biceps in long axis.
  - Find pathology in short axis then rotate about the tendon 90 degrees.

Needle Position

- If biceps visualized in short axis, in-plane lateral to medial
- If biceps visualized in long axis, in-plane distal to proximal.

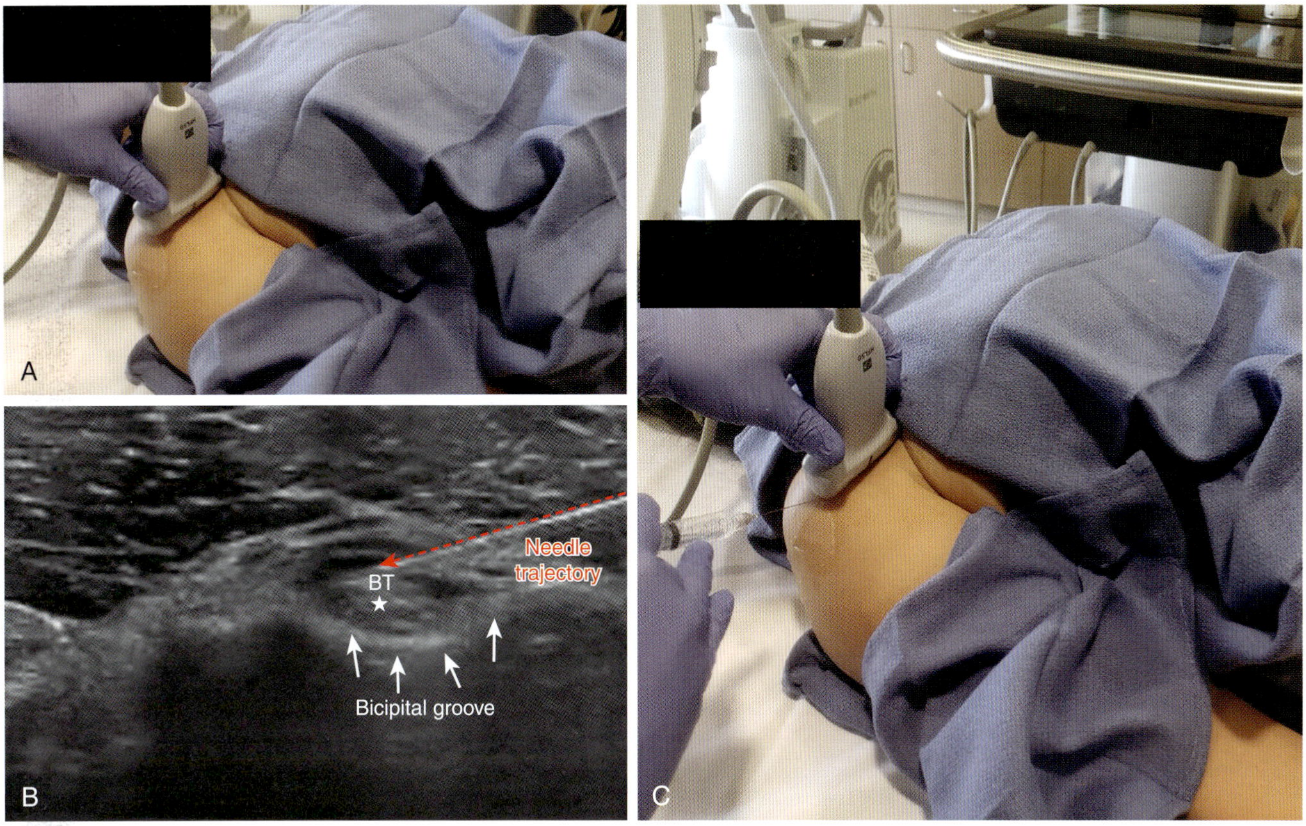

• **Fig. 16.16** Short-Axis Approach. (A) Patient position, (B) ultrasound image, and (C) injection. *Asterisk,* target; *BT*, Biceps tendon.

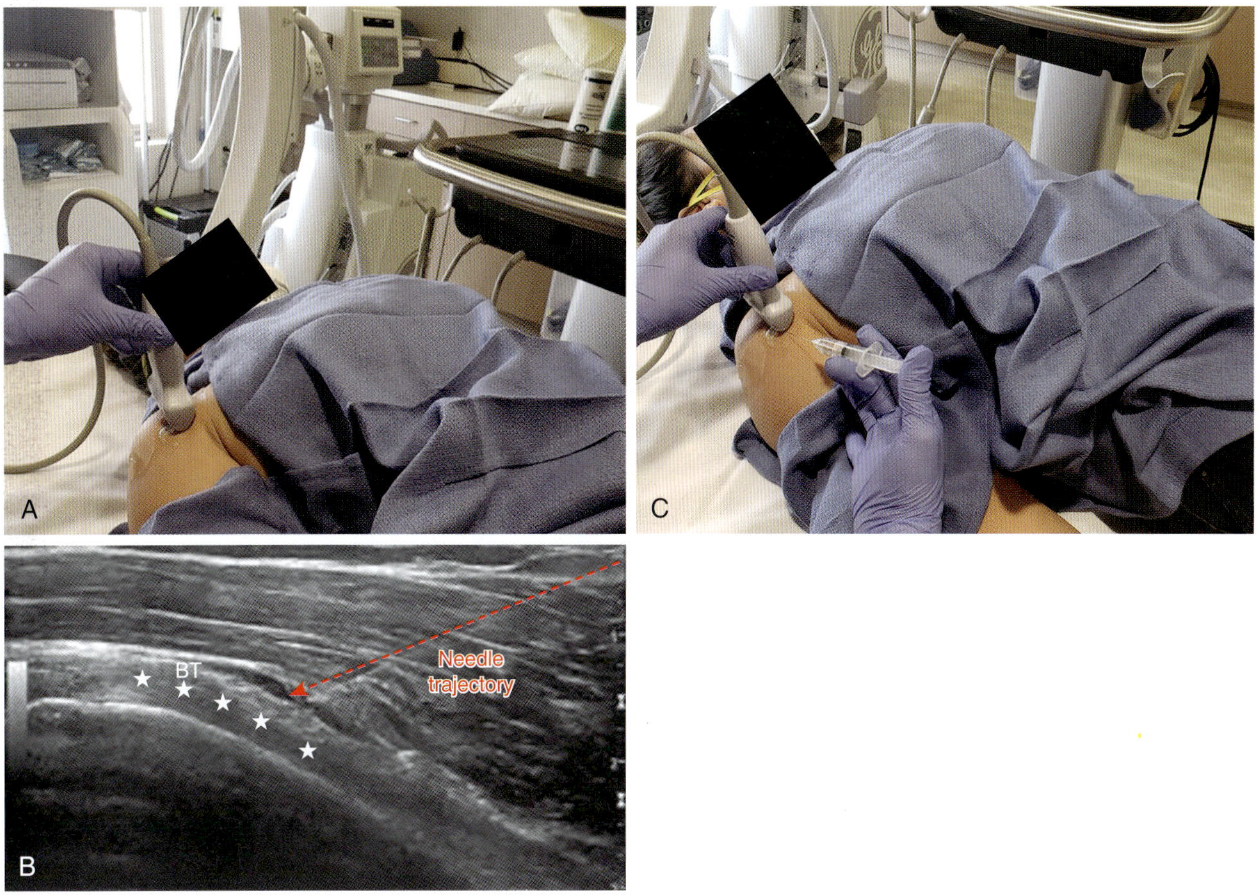

• **Fig. 16.17** Long head of biceps tendon, long-axis approach. (A) Patient position. (B) ultrasound image with target sites along biceps tendon (asterisks). (C) Injection. *BT*, Biceps Tendon.

Target

- Pathologic aspect of LHBT
    - Scan distally to identify the myotendinous junction and then scan proximally until pathology has been identified.
    - The LHBT is approximately 10 cm in length, and pathology can occur proximal to the trochanteric groove, but visualization of the LBBT will be lost as it dives deep into the joint.[45]
- If using corticosteroids, target sheath only.

Technique: Short Head of Biceps Tendon (SHBT), Coracobrachialis and Pectoralis Minor via Ultrasound Guidance

Patient Position

See Fig. 16.18.

- Supine or lateral decubitus with shoulder externally rotated (instruct patient to turn palm to ceiling)
    - Sometimes easier to have patient flex elbow to 90 degrees and have assistant bedside passively externally rotate shoulder

Clinician Position

- Side of patient

Transducer Position

- Short or long axis to the tendon at the insertion on the coracoid process
- Scan distally to identify the myotendinous junction and then scan proximally until pathology has been identified.

Needle Position

- Tendon in short axis, in-plane, lateral to medial
- Tendon in long axis, in-plane, distal to proximal
- Tendon in long axis, out-of-plane, with needle (shortest distance skin to target)

Target

- Pathologic aspects of the tendon or myotendinous junction of SHBT, pec minor, coracobrachialis.

PEARLS AND PITFALLS

- If treating a large partial-thickness tear of LHBT, use the smallest-gauge needle to ensure no additional damage to tendon.
- If the tear located close to proximal origin at labral anchor, utilizing a combination ultrasound and fluoroscopic approach is preferred.
- Pec minor: utilize Doppler flow to identify vasculature as well as the medial and lateral pectoral nerve that supply the muscle and the overlying pec major
- Pec minor: the best approach is out-of-plane because in-plane (medial-lateral) becomes difficult to avoid neuro-vascular structures.

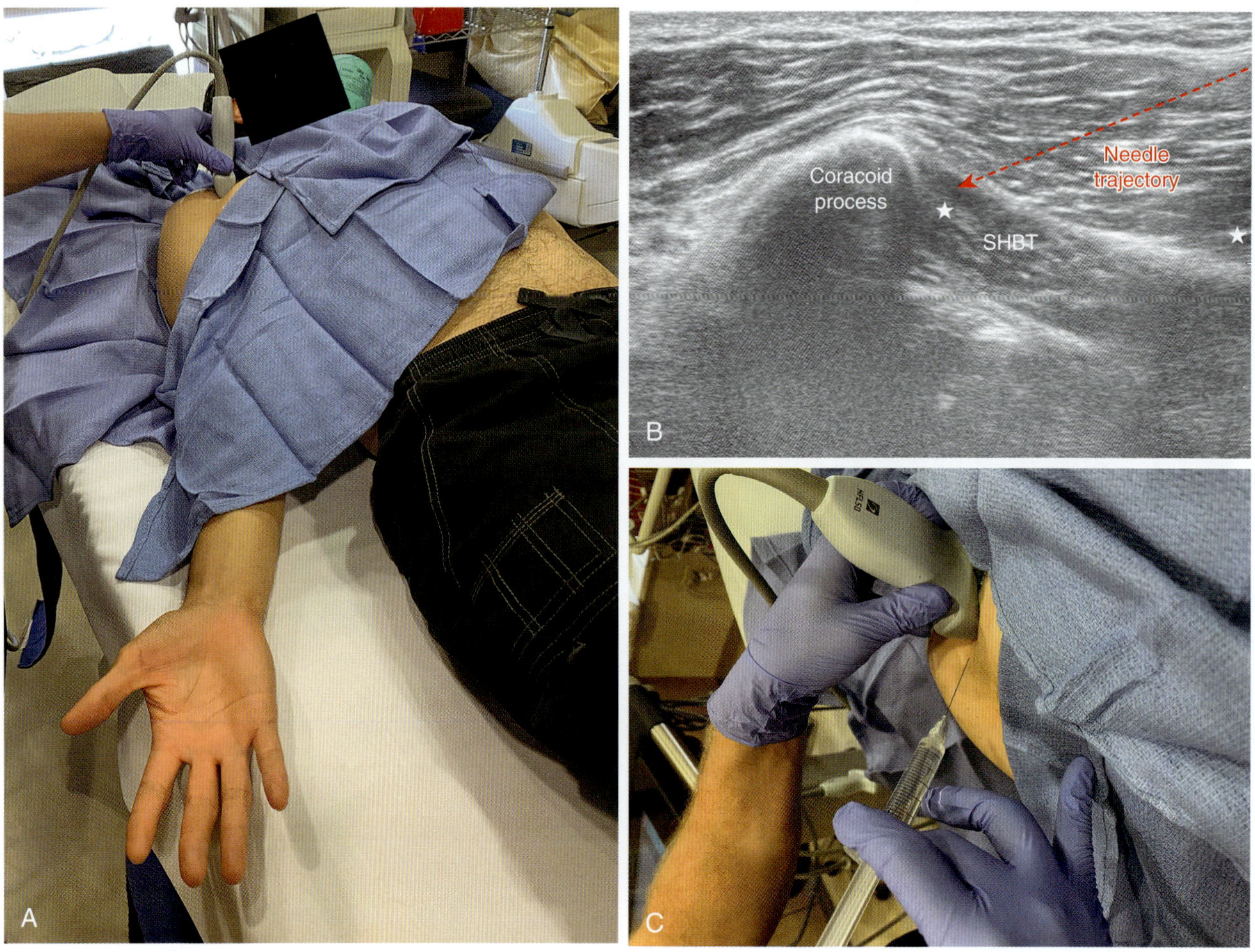

• **Fig. 16.18** Short head of biceps tendon *(SHBT)* approach. (A) patient and probe position. (B) Ultrasound image with target (asterisks) at the SHBT origin. (C) injection.

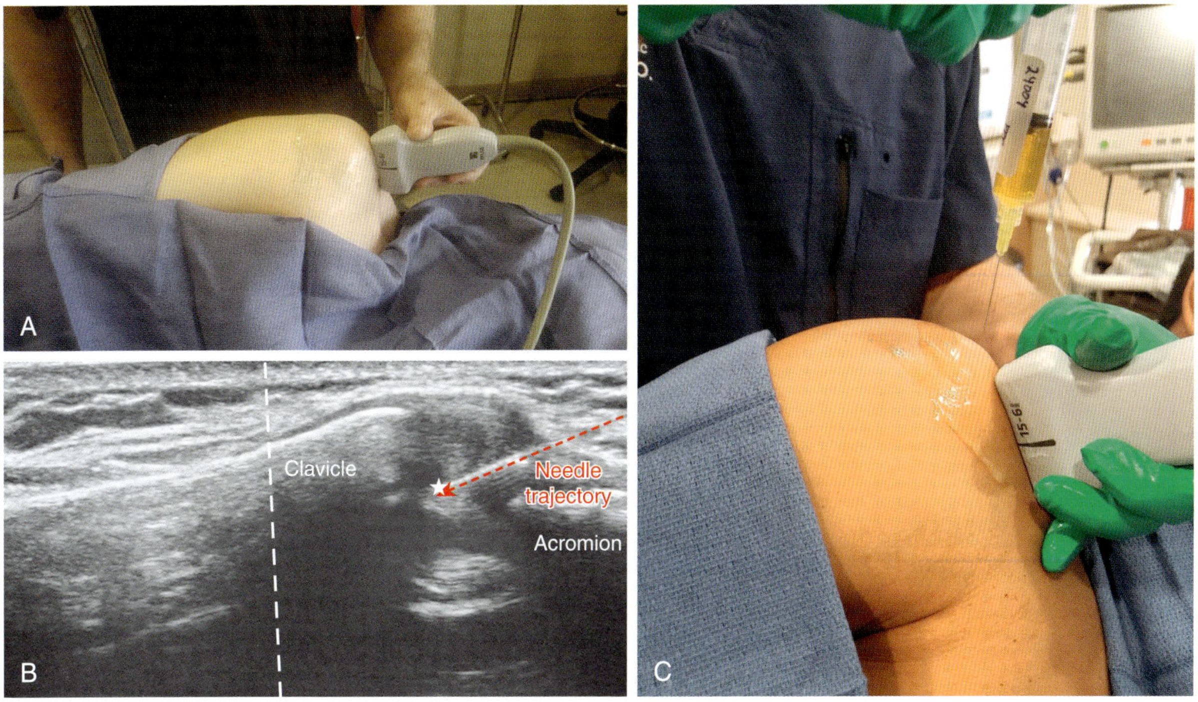

• **Fig. 16.19** In-Plane. (A) Patient and probe positioning, (B) ultrasound image, (C) injection and. *Asterisk*, target.

Acromioclavicular Joint

KEY POINTS

- Acromioclavicular (AC) joint pathology can be classified into acute injuries or degenerative arthropathy.
- The AC joint accounts for over 40% of all shoulder injuries.[46]
- Osteoarthritis of the AC joint with inferior osteophyte lesions may narrow the subacromial space and result in impingement and compression of nearby structures.[46,47]

Pertinent Anatomy

- The articular surface of the AC joint is lined with fibrocartilage and not hyaline cartilage.
- The AC joint is supported by the joint capsule that extends circumferentially around the joint providing. The superior and posterior AC ligaments are the strongest, and mainly provide horizontal stability.[48]
- The CC ligament complex consists of the conoid and trapezoid ligaments providing vertical stability.[49] The conoid and trapezoid ligament insert on the posteromedial and anterolateral region of the undersurface of the distal clavicle, respectively.

Common Pathology

- AC joint sprain and dislocations
  - The AC joint is commonly injured in falls directly on shoulder or falls on an outstretched arm (FOOSH injuries)[50] with disruption of the acromioclavicular and/or CC ligaments.
  - Several classifications describe AC joint injuries, but there continues to be substantial controversy about their management.[51] More severe injuries may require surgery.

Coracoid and distal clavicle fracture can mimic CC ligament and AC injury, respectively.

- AC osteoarthritis
  - Chronic instability can progress to joint arthritis and pain.[52]

Equipment

- Linear array ultrasound transducer
- 30 to 25 gauge 1 to 1.5 inch needle

Common injectates

- Local anesthetics for diagnostics, corticosteroids
- Prolotherapy, orthobiologics (PRP, bone marrow concentrate, etc.)
- Avoid intraligamentous corticosteroids

Injectate Volume

- 0.5 to 1.5 mL intra-articular
- 0.25 to 0.5 mL per joint capsule area
- 0.5 to 1 mL per ligament

Technique: Acromioclavicular Joint Intra-Articular

Patient Position

See Figs. 16.19 and 16.20.

- Lateral recumbent (affected shoulder up)
- Alternatively, the patient can be supine or seated

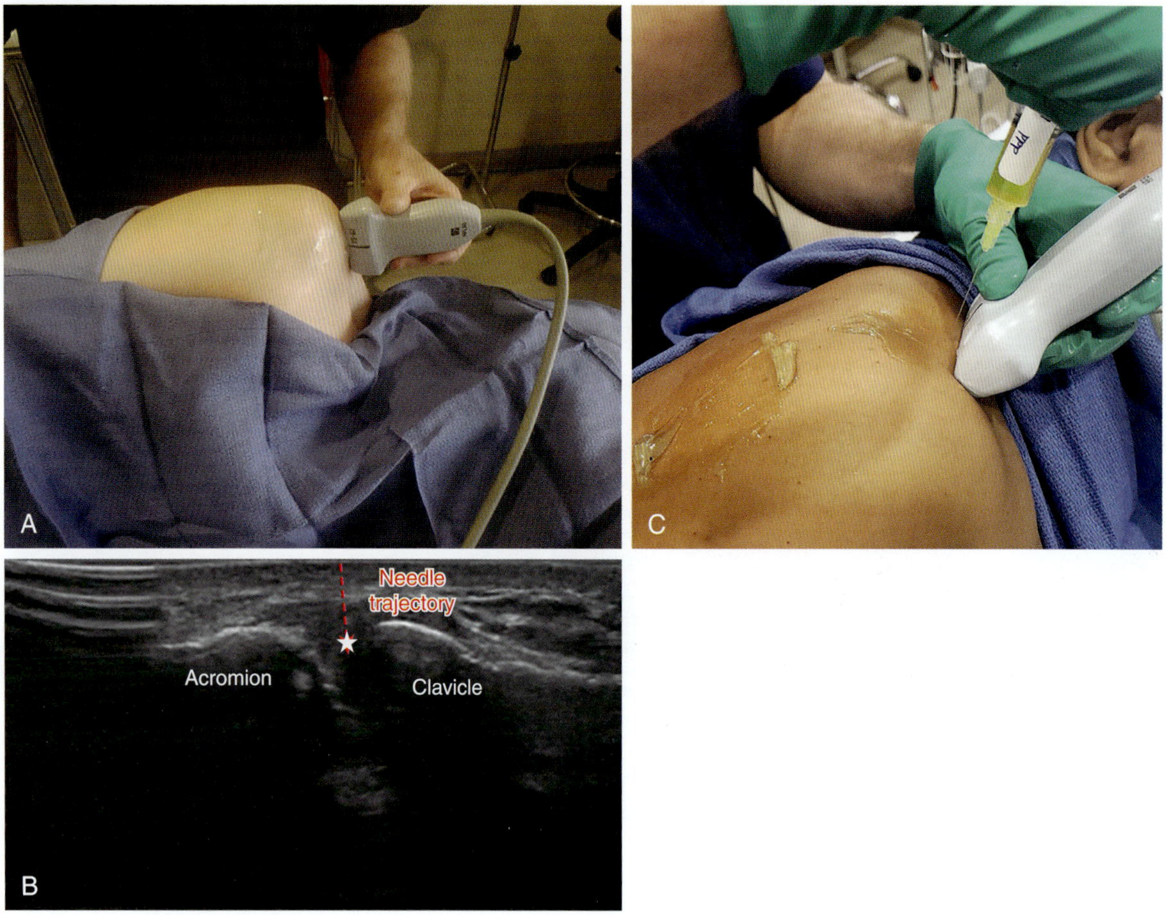

• **Fig. 16.20** AC joint out-of-plane intra articular. (A) patient and probe position. (B) Ultrasound image with target (asterix). (C) injection.

Clinician Position
- Posterior to patient

Transducer Position
- Transverse to the AC joint (visualize acromion and clavicle)

Needle Position
- In plane, from lateral to medial
- Out-of-plane

Target
- AC joint space. As you inject, visualize the injectate flowing into the joint space without extravagating into superficial tissue. Joint should distend slightly with injection.

Technique: Approach for Acromioclavicular Joint Capsule

Patient Position

See Figs. 16.21 and 16.22.
- Lateral recumbent (affected shoulder up) or supine

Clinician Position
- At patient's side

Transducer Position
- Transverse to the AC joint

Needle Position
- In-plane, lateral to medial approach.
- Out-of-plane, joint line in the middle of the probe positioned so that you can visualize the inferior capsule of the joint.

Target
- In-plane can only target superior aspects of the joint capsule.
- Out-of-plane can target all areas: superior, inferior, anterior, and posterior components.
  - Taking a steep angle, visualize needle tip in the deepest aspect of the joint into the inferior joint capsule.

Technique: Conoid and Trapezoid Ligaments via Ultrasound Guidance

Patient Position

See Fig. 16.23.
- Supine or lateral recumbent with affected shoulder up

Clinician Position
- At side of patient

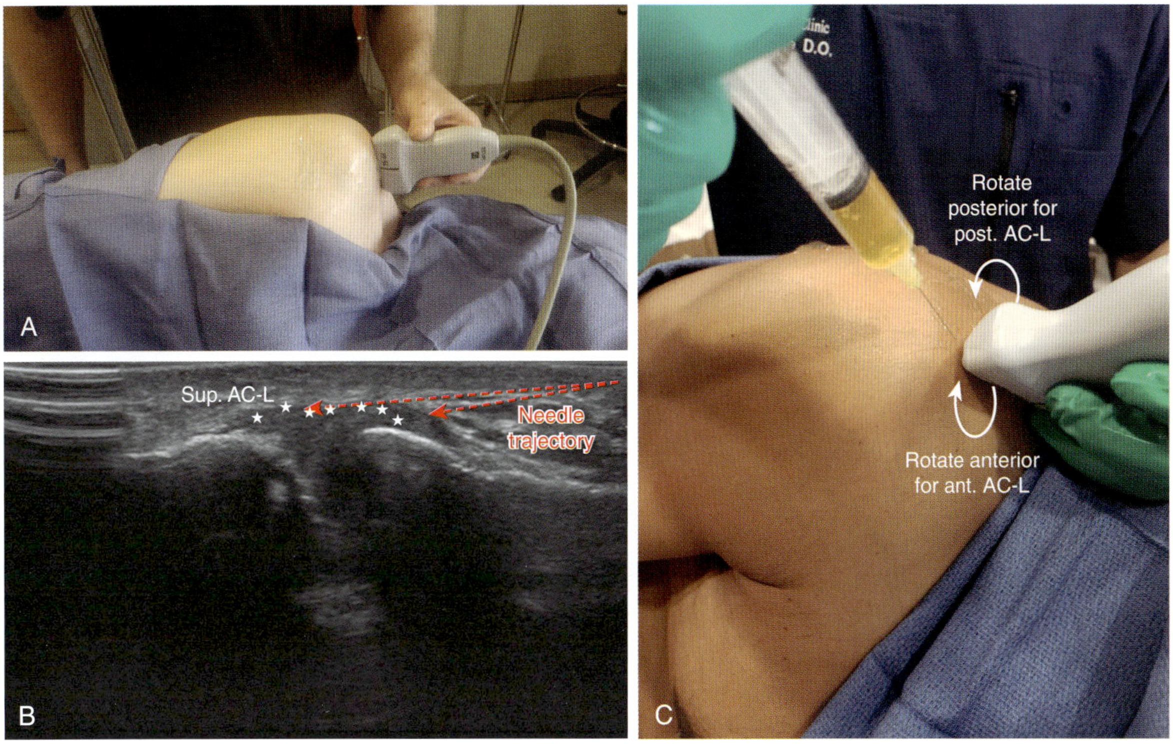

• **Fig. 16.21** Superior, Anterior, and Posterior AC Capsule. (A) Patient and probe positioning, (B) ultrasound image, and (C) injection. *Asterisks*, target; *AC*, Acromioclavicular; *Sup. AC-L,* superior AC joint ligament.

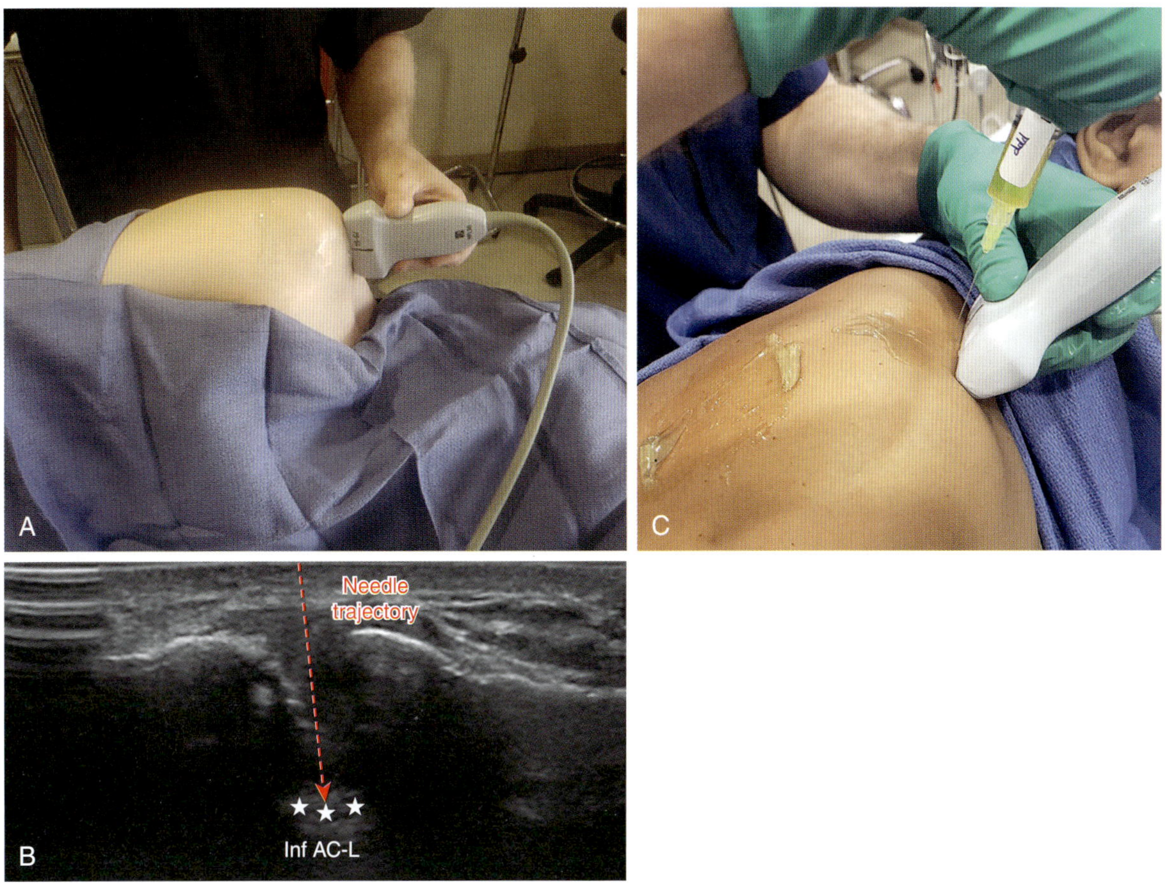

• **Fig. 16.22** Inferior AC Capsule. Inferior AC capsule ligament. (A) patient and probe position. (B) Ultrasound image, and (C) injection. *Asterisks*, target; *inf AC-L*, inferior AC ligament. (C) injection.

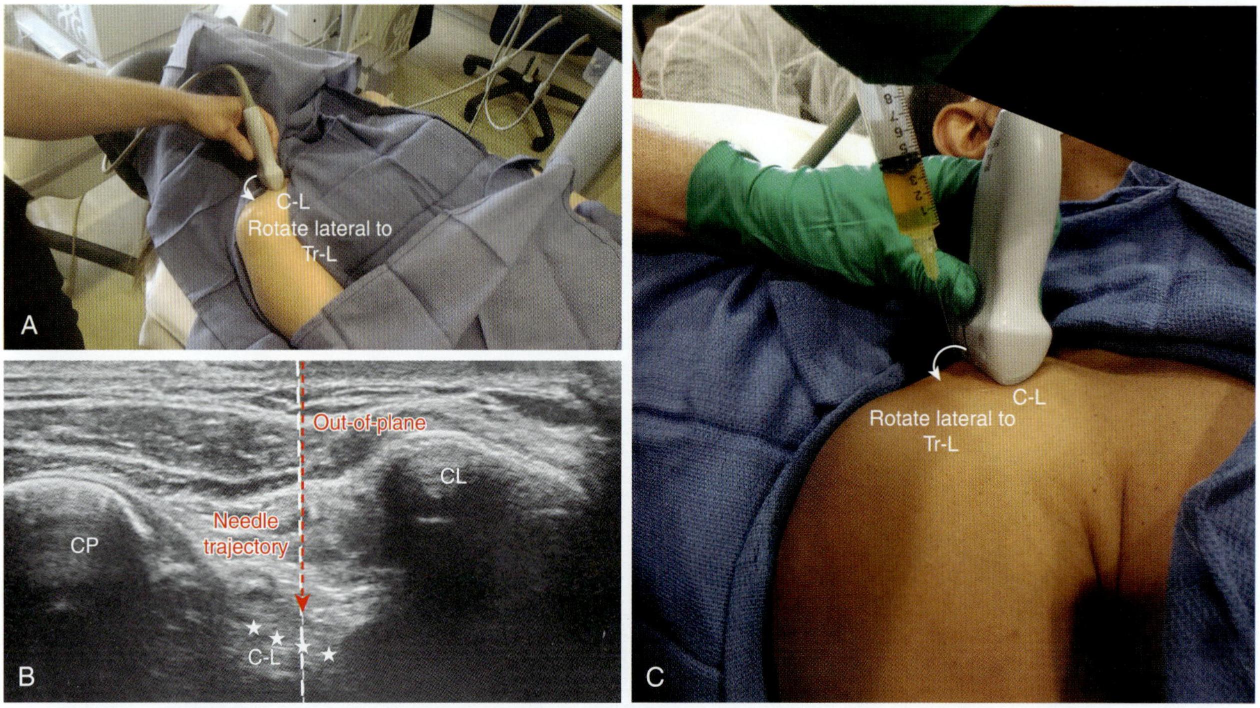

• **Fig. 16.23** (A) Patient and probe positioning, (B) ultrasound image, and (C) injection. *Asterisks*, target; *C-L*, Conoid ligament; *CL*, clavicle; *CP*, coracoid process; *Tr-L*, trapezoid ligament.

Transducer Position

- Identify coracoid process, medial to the biceps tendon.
- Rotate probe so that the clavicle and the coracoid process are visualized in the same field of view.
- For trapezoid, keeping the focal point on the coracoid process, rotate the clavicular end laterally.
- For conoid, keeping the focal point on the coracoid process, rotate medially.

Needle Position

- Out-of-plane, placing the space between clavicle and coracoid process in the middle
  - Can also be done via in-plane

Target

- Advancing needle tip until reaching the anechoic ligaments.
- Target the insertion and origins of the conoid and trapezoid ligaments.
- If no vasculature impeding injection, can also target the mid portion of the ligaments.

PEARLS AND PITFALLS ACROMIOCLAVICULAR JOINT

- Can also target the anterior and inferior AC joint capsule from the same injection point, rotating around the AC joint, allowing visualization of origin, and insertion of capsule on clavicle and acromion, respectfully.
- There can be small vascular bundles overriding the conoid and trapezoid ligaments; using Doppler prior to injecting can help avoid these during injections.

Suprascapular Nerve

KEY POINTS

- Entrapment may present as SS and infraspinatus weakness and pain, and can mimic rotator cuff pain.[53]
- Commonly used nerve for procedural and postprocedural shoulder pain control.[54]
- Ultrasound-guided nerve sheath injections can be a useful diagnostic technique.

Pertinent Anatomy

- Provides motor function to the SS and infraspinatus muscles, and sensory innervation to the posterior capsule and subacromial space.[55]
- Arises from the upper trunk of the brachial plexus (C5, C6) in the majority of patients; however, some have contribution from the C4 nerve root.[56]
- The nerve courses laterally through posterior cervical triangle, then across the superior border of the scapula into the suprascapular notch, where it is accompanied by the suprascapular artery and vein.[57]
- Shortly after passing through the suprascapular notch (underneath the transverse scapular ligament) the nerve innervates the SS muscle. It then courses through the spinoglenoid notch underneath the spinoglenoid ligament, where it innervates the infraspinatus muscle.[56]

Common Pathology

- Suprascapular nerve entrapment and neuropathy

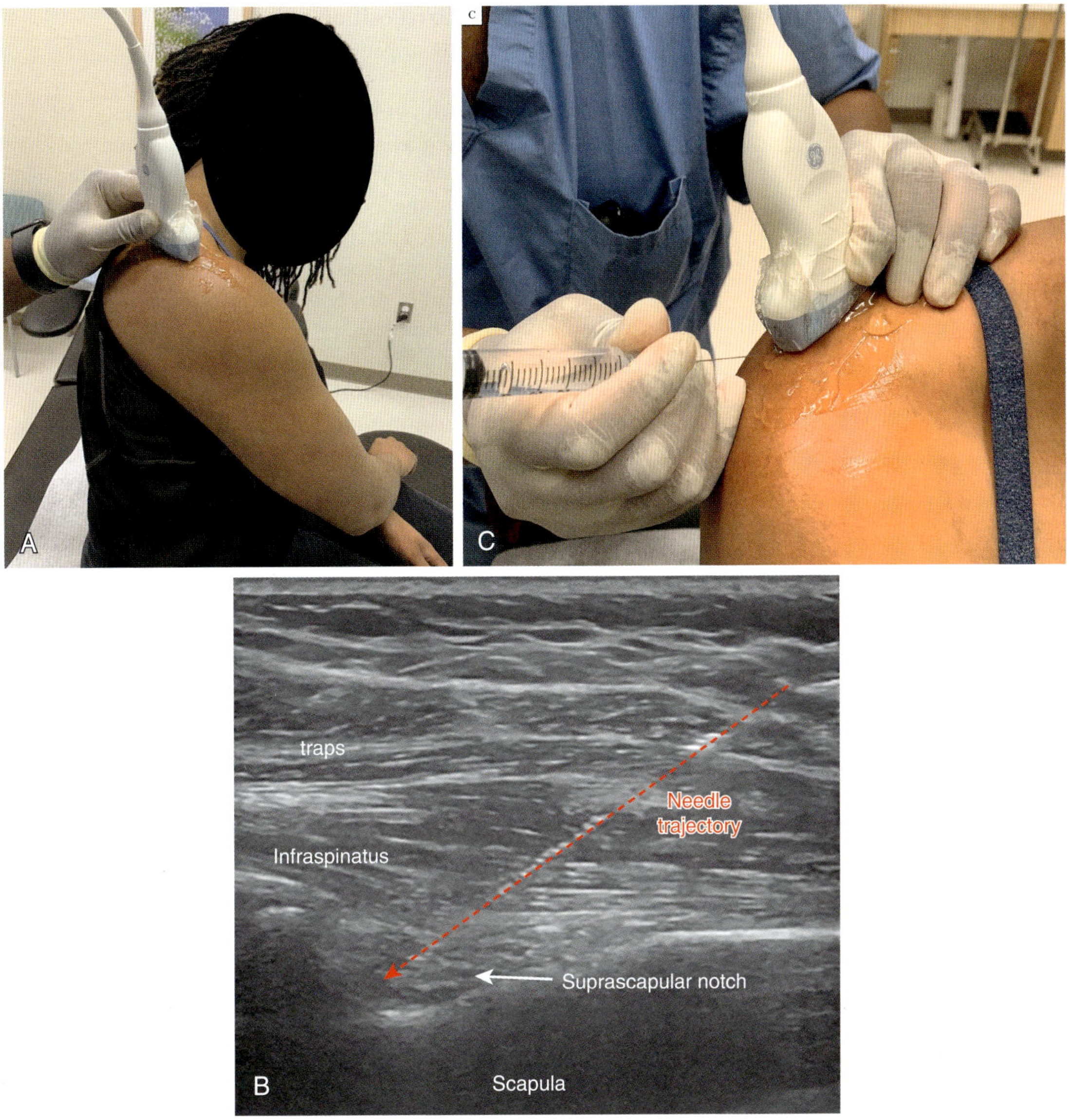

• **Fig. 16.24** In-plane Suprascapular Notch. (A) Patient and probe positioning, (B) ultrasound image, and (C) injection.

Equipment

- Linear array ultrasound transducer
- 25 gauge 1.5 to 2 inch needle.

Common Injectates

- Local anesthetics for diagnostics or preprocedural block
- Corticosteroids, prolotherapy, orthobiologics (PRP).

Injectate Volume

- 1 to 5 mL

Technique: Superior Approach for Suprascapular Nerve Injection

Patient Position

See Fig. 16.24.

- Best if lateral recumbent, seated or prone (can be done seated)

Clinician Position

- Posterior to the patient

Transducer Position

- Start with the probe in long axis over the scapular spine; move in a lateral and cephalad path until the suprascapular notch is identified.
- Identify artery with color flow Doppler prior to injection to avoid.

Needle Position

- In-plane, lateral to medial or medial to lateral
- Alternatively, can inject out-of-plane.

Target

- Just superior to the suprascapular nerve and medial to the suprascapular artery.

PEARLS AND PITFALLS

- Ensure your needle tip is superior to the nerve, and you are able to visualize anechoic halo of fluid around the nerve to ensure the injectate is properly placed.
- Ensure your needle tip is medial to the suprascapular vasculature.[6]
- Consider using a longer needle (2 to 2.5 inches) with patients with a larger body habitus
- Ensure you maintain needle visualization to avoid pleural injury.
- Use color Doppler to identify the suprascapular vascular, and the nerve should lie just medially to it.

Axillary Nerve at Quadrilateral Space

KEY POINTS

- Quadrilateral space is defined by teres minor superiorly, humeral shaft lateral, long head triceps medial, and teres major inferiorly (see Fig. 16.8)

Pertinent Anatomy

- The axillary nerve has fibers from C5 and C6 cervical nerve roots.
- Axillary nerve arises from the upper trunk, posterior division, and posterior cord of the brachial plexus.
- Travels along humeral head with circumflex artery

Common Pathology

- Quadrilateral space (QS) syndrome (QSS) is a relatively rare condition in which the axillary nerve and the posterior humeral circumflex artery are compressed within the QS.[58]
- Due to the low specificity of physical examination maneuvers and lack of a good diagnostic study, local anesthetic blocks often remain as the diagnostic "gold standard."[59]

Equipment

- Linear array ultrasound transducer

Common Injectates

- Local anesthetics for diagnostics
- Corticosteroids, anesthetics, orthobiologics (PRP).

Injectate Volume

- 2 to 4 mL

Technique: Axillary Nerve Entrapment at Quadrilateral Space Hydrodissection

Patient position

See Fig. 16.25.

- Prone
- Shoulder internally rotated with palm facing up

Clinician Position

- Side of patient

Transducer Position

- Long axis to humeral shaft, mid humeral shaft, and slide superiorly until the muscle belly of the teres minor is identified.
- Then slide medially off the humeral head.
- Utilize Doppler flow to identify posterior humeral circumflex artery adjacent to the axillary nerve that will be in short axis.

Needle Position

- Nerve in short axis, in-plane approach, inferior to superior or superior to inferior

Target

- Infiltrating QS

PEARLS AND PITFALLS

- Caution: to avoid vascular injury, utilize Doppler.

Fluoroscopic Guidance

Glenohumeral Joint: Intra-Articular

KEY POINTS

- Intra-articular injections with the use of fluoroscopic guidance can be done using the anterior approach.

Pertinent Anatomy

- See Ultrasound section

Common Pathology

- See Ultrasound section

Equipment

- C-arm fluoroscopy
- Contrast
- 25 to 22 gauge 2 to 3.5 inch needle

Common Injectates

- Local anesthetics for diagnostics
- Corticosteroids, hyaluronic acid, prolotherapy, orthobiologics (PRP, bone marrow concentrate, micronized adipose tissue, etc.)
- For capsular distention: High-volume mix of anesthetics, saline (corticosteroids, or orthobiologics: PRP, platelet lysate, platelet-poor plasma)

Injectate Volume

- 2 to 8 mL

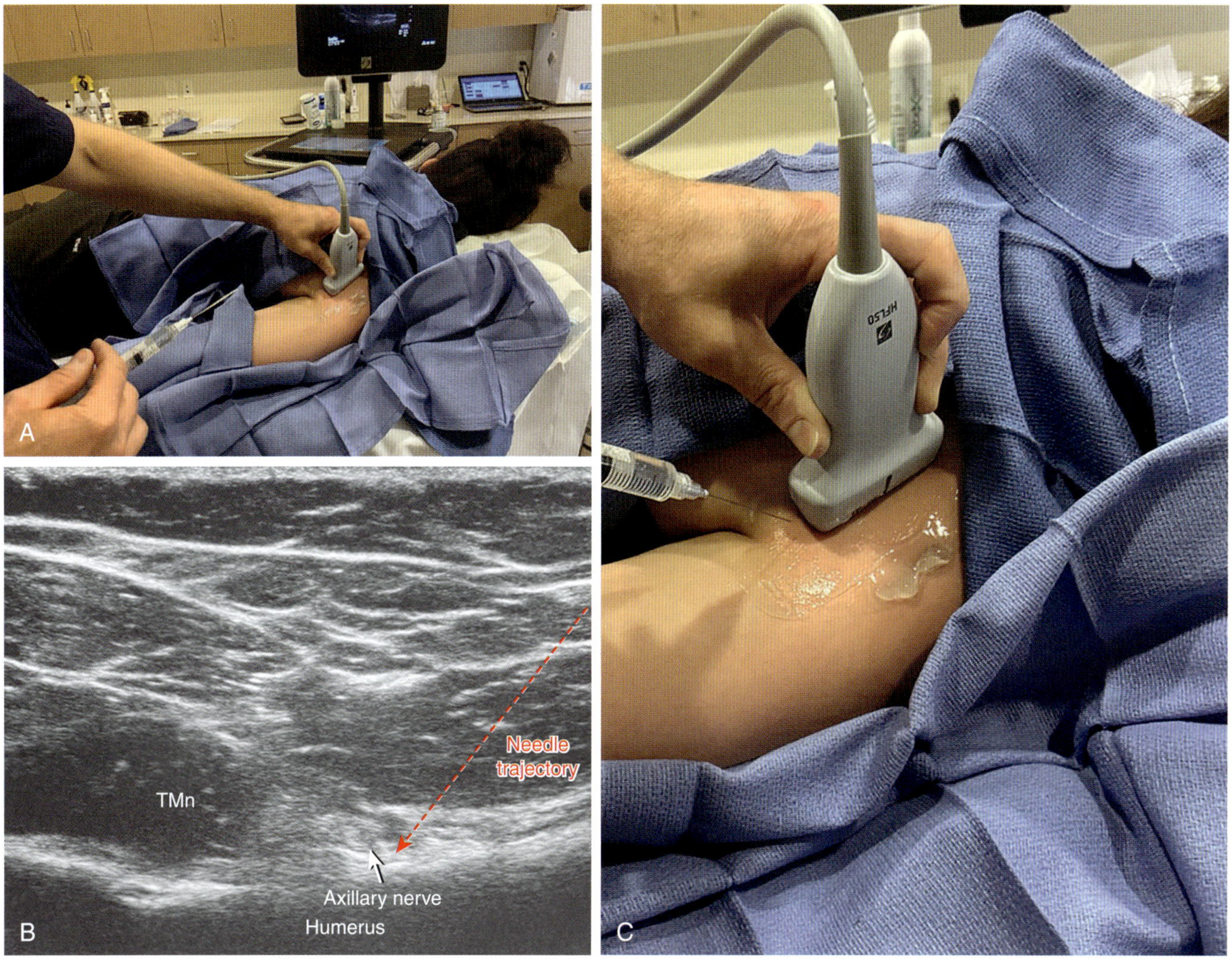

• **Fig. 16.25** Axillary Nerve Hydrodissection. (A) Patient and probe positioning, (B) ultrasound image, and (C) injection.

- 20 to 60 mL for capsular distention (40 to 50 mL most common per authors' experience), Inject maximum volume as tolerated by pain or can stop when getting backflow into the syringe to avoid capsular rupture.[5]

Technique: Glenohumeral Intra-Articular Anterior Approach

Patient Position

See Fig. 16.26.

- Supine
- Shoulder position 10 degrees abduction, externally rotated with forearm supinate, palm facing up

Clinician Position

- Standing directly next to the shoulder being injected

C-Arm Position

- AP with contralateral rotation of C-arm to align the anterior and posterior glenoid rim or "true AP"
- Understanding that the shoulder joint is naturally rotated 10 to 30 degrees contralateral on the transverse plane (horizontal plane)

Needle Position

- Skin entry site over the superior third of humeral head and lateral to the joint line
- With a bent needle tip, off axis with needle tip medial and hub lateral (trajectory lateral to medial)

Target

- Advance needle until contacting the humeral head just lateral to joint line
- Once needle contacts periosteum of humeral head, pull back and advance medially until you feel sensation of needle sliding into the glenohumeral joint
- Inject a small amount of contrast to confirm intra-articular placement with arthrogram of glenohumeral joint (Fig. 16.27)

PEARLS AND PITFALLS

- Caution: starting approach medially and inferior to joint line can risk damaging neurovascular structures.
- Bent needle technique allows for increased maneuverability in tissue.

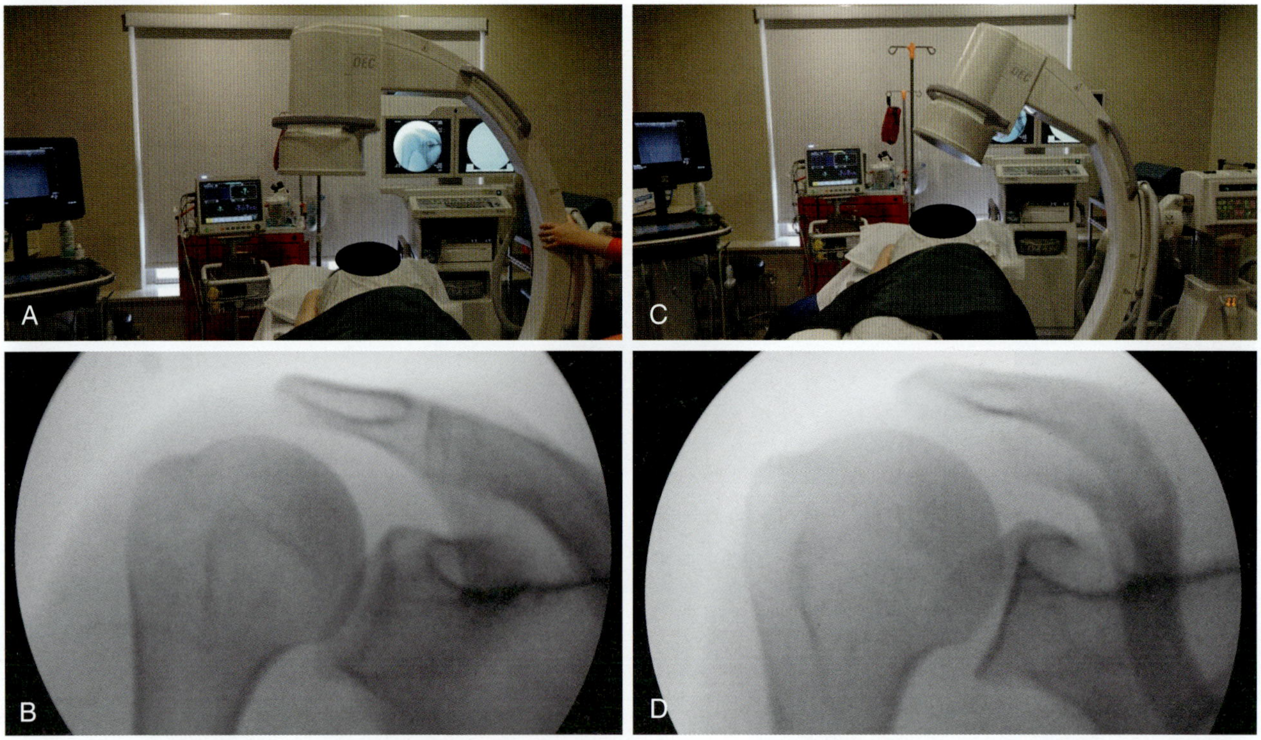

• **Fig. 16.26** Glenohumeral Joint Patient and C-Arm Positioning. (A and B) Fluoroscopic image—not true AP to glenoid; (C and D) true AP to glenoid.

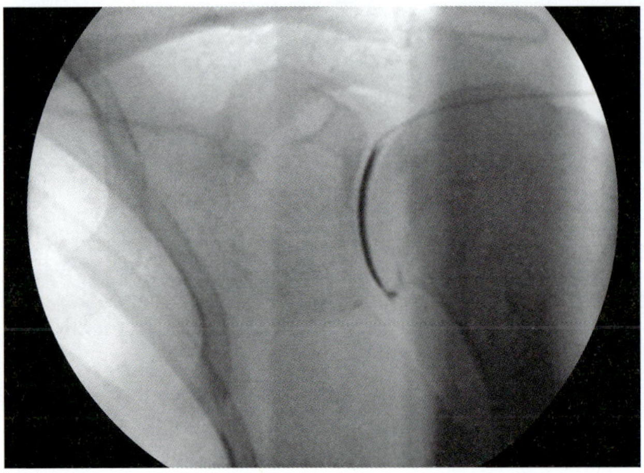

• **Fig. 16.27** Arthrogram of Glenohumeral Joint.

Glenohumeral Joint Capsule Ligaments

KEY POINTS

- You can use bony landmarks to inject the shoulder capsular ligaments with fluoroscopy.

Pertinent Anatomy

- See Ultrasound section

Common Pathology

- See Ultrasound section

Equipment

- C-arm fluoroscopy
- Contrast
- Needle size: 25 to 22-gauge 2 to 3.5-inch needle.
- 27to 25 gauge 1.5 to 3 inch needle

Common injectates

- Prolotherapy, orthobiologics (PRP, bone marrow concentrate, etc.).
- Avoid intraligamentous corticosteroids.

Injectate Volume

- 1–3 mL per ligament

Technique: Anterior Capsule Approach

Patient Position

See Fig. 16.28.

- Supine
- Shoulder position 10 degrees abduction, externally rotated with palm facing up

Clinician Position

- Standing directly next to the shoulder being injected

C-Arm Position

- AP with contralateral rotation of C-arm to align the anterior and posterior glenoid rim or "true AP," understanding that the shoulder joint is naturally rotated 10 to 30 degrees on the transverse plane (horizontal plane)

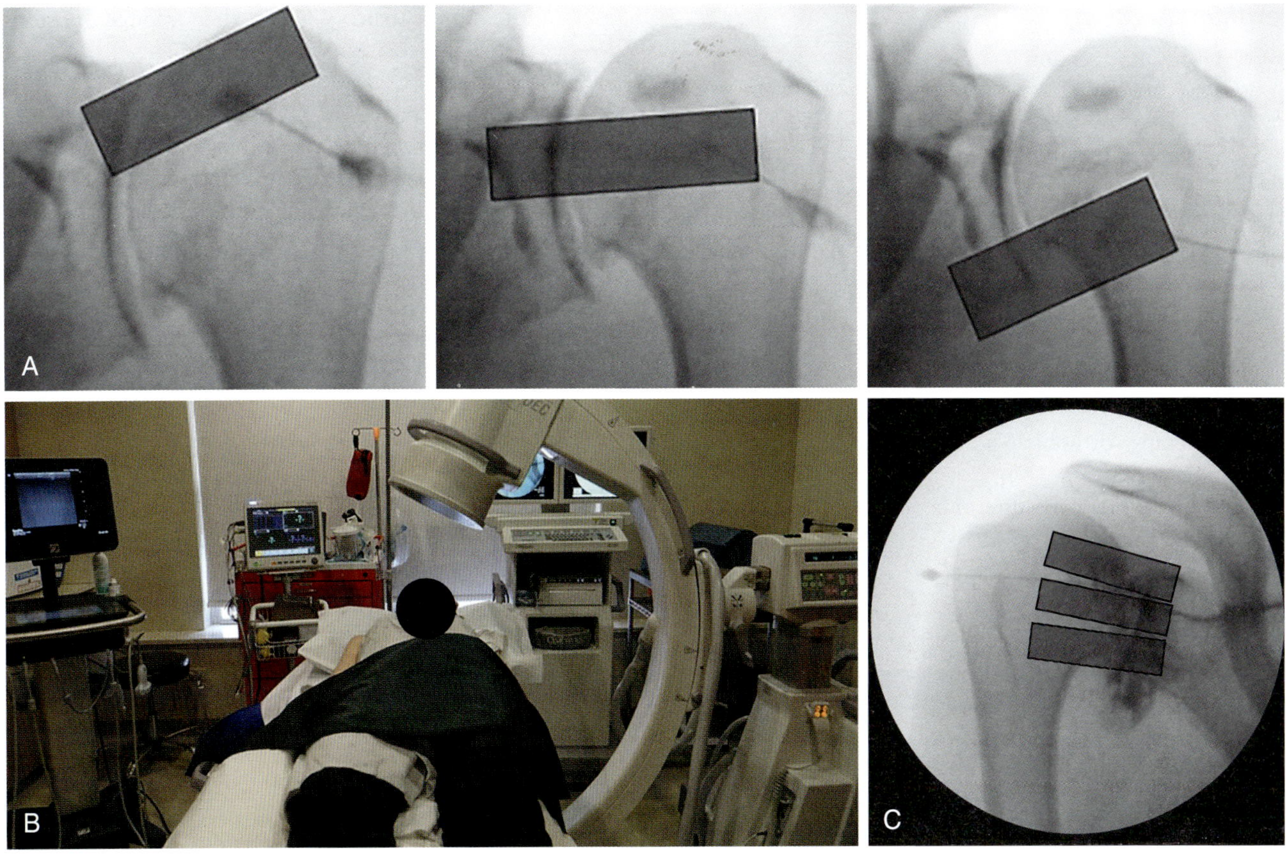

• **Fig. 16.28** (A) Target zone for each band, (B) patient position and C-arm, and (C) contrast spread highlight contour of each ligament.

Needle Position

- Skin entry site is midline on humeral head, lateral to the joint line.
- With bent needle tip, off axis with needle tip medial and hub lateral (trajectory lateral to medial)

Target

- SGHL
  - Starting position at superior aspect of humeral head.
  - Advance needle until contact superior humeral head just lateral to joint line.
  - You can place contrast at humeral head attachment or option to pull back and redirect and advance needle medial until contact glenoid at origin.
  - Contrast flow should be horizontal from humeral head to glenoid.
- MGHL
  - Staring position mid-point on humeral head.
  - Advance needle until contact middle of humeral head just lateral to joint line.
  - You can place contrast at humeral head attachment or option to pull back and redirect and advance needle medial until contact glenoid at origin.
  - Contrast flow should be horizontal from humeral head to glenoid.
- IGHL
  - Starting position mid-point on humeral head (do not start inferior).
  - Advance needle inferior medial until contact just lateral to joint line.
  - Advance needle medial until contact on glenoid.
  - Contrast flow should be horizontal from humeral head to glenoid, highlighting the inferior sling if the IGHL.

PEARLS AND PITFALLS

- Caution: Starting approach medially and inferior to joint line can risk damaging neurovascular structures.

Glenohumeral Joint Labrum

KEY POINTS

- Combination utilizing ultrasound guidance with fluoroscopic guidance is the preferred method for isolating and treating a superior labral tear near or at the biceps anchor, but fluoroscopy alone can be used to inject the labrum directly.

Pertinent Anatomy

- See Ultrasound section

Common Pathology

- See Ultrasound section

Equipment

- 25 gauge 3 to 3.5 inch needle (single or multi-needle technique)
- C-arm fluoroscopy
- Contrast agent

Common Injectates

- Prolotherapy, orthobiologics (PRP, bone marrow concentrate, etc.).
- Avoid intralabral corticosteroids.

Injectate Volume

- 1 to 2 mL

PEARLS AND PITFALLS

- Bent needle tip helps greatly to maneuver needle to the target.
- Avoid the coracoid, which can sometimes affect needle trajectory.
- Though not common or preferred, one can also inject the posterior labrum with the patient in the lateral decubitus position. Use "true" AP C-arm view and target the superior and middle glenoid/labrum in a similar fashion as described above.

Technique: Superior Labrum via Fluoroscopy Only

Patient Position

- Supine
- Shoulder by patient side, externally rotated with palm facing up (brings the BT anterior to allow easier visualization)

Clinician Position

- Standing directly next to the shoulder being injected

C-Arm Position (Biplanar Views)

- AP with contralateral rotation of C-arm to align the anterior and posterior glenoid rim or "true AP," understanding that the shoulder joint is naturally rotated 10 to 30 degrees on the transverse plane (horizontal plane)
  - Evaluates superior/inferior position on glenoid
- Scapular Y view
  - Evaluates circumferential orientation on the glenoid (where you are in relation to the "clock face")

Needle Position

- Start needle over the superior humeral head lateral to the joint line.
- Advance the needle under intermittent fluoroscopy in the AP view and touch down on the humerus.
- Pull the needle back slightly; then redirect posterior medial towards the superior glenoid.

Target

- Needle should touch down on the glenoid.
- Utilizing biplanar views (true AP and scapular Y) can triangulate location on glenoid to ensure covering necessary region of labrum.
- Inject a small amount of contrast in the AP view to ensure triangular labral flow.
- You can sometimes see flow at along the proximal LHBT.
- If only intra-articular flow, redirect the needle just superior to the glenoid.

Technique: Anterior-Inferior Labrum

Patient Position

- Supine
- Shoulder position 10 degrees abduction, externally rotated with palm facing up

Clinician Position

- Standing directly next to the shoulder being injected

C-Arm Position (Biplanar Views)

- AP with contralateral rotation of C-arm to align the anterior and posterior glenoid rim or "true AP," understanding that the shoulder joint is naturally rotated 10 to 30 degrees on the transverse plane (horizontal plane)

Needle Position

- Skin entry site is lower third of the humeral head, lateral to the joint line
- With bent needle tip, off axis with needle tip medial and hub lateral (trajectory lateral to medial)

Target

- Advance needle inferior medial until contact just lateral to joint line
- Advance needle medial until contact on glenoid
- Contrast flow pattern should be triangular shape at the inferior aspect
  - If too superficial, will get the IGHL flow pattern (Fig. 16.29)

PEARLS AND PITFALLS

- Very superficial joint: once you have placed the needle into the skin, check fluoroscopic image to access depth.

Acromioclavicular Joint

Technique: Acromioclavicular Joint Intra-Articular

Patient Position

- Supine
- Shoulder in neutral position

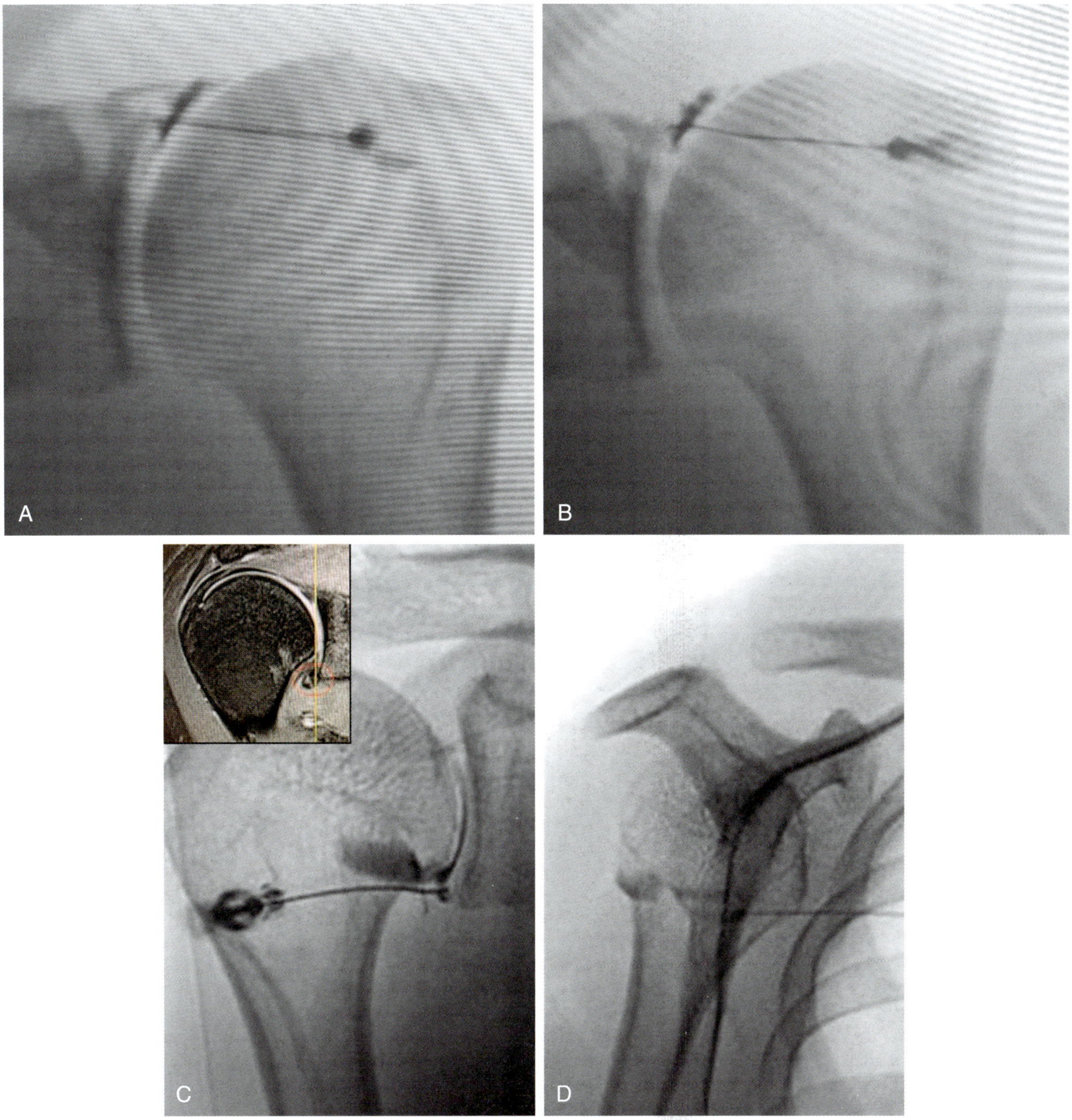

• **Fig. 16.29** Superior-Anterior to Posterior labral approach – SLAP. (A-B) AP fluoroscopic showing contrast spread highlighting labrum. Anterior-Inferior labral approach. (C) AP fluoroscopic image with MRI image of labral tear for reference. (D) Scapular-Y fluoroscopic image showing needle positioning.

Clinician Position

- Standing directly next to the shoulder being injected

C-Arm Position

- True AP view of the AC joint
- May have to rotate ipsilateral or contralateral to visualize AC joint space opening

Needle Position

See Fig. 16.30.

- Palpate the superior aspect of the joint space and place needle into joint

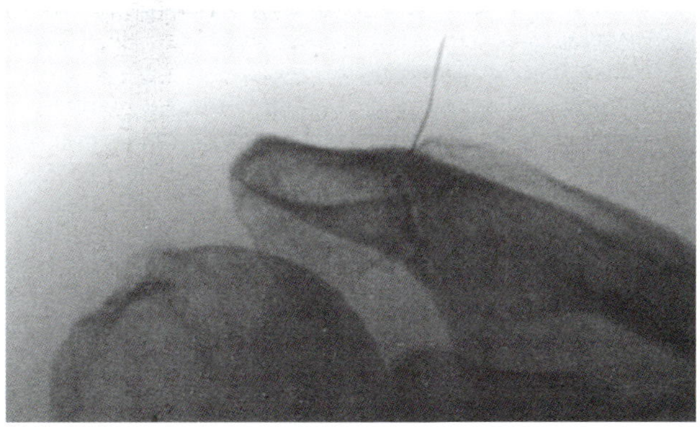

• **Fig. 16.30** Needle Trajectory; Arthrogram of AC Joint.

- Use intermittent fluoroscopy to adjust the needle position until you feel the needle slide into the joint space

Target

- Intra-articular joint space: inject contrast to confirm intra-articular placement

PEARLS AND PITFALLS

- Caution: Avoid starting too inferior on the humerus, approaching medially and inferior to the joint line can risk damaging the neurovascular structures.

References

1. Ogul H, et al. Ultrasound-guided shoulder MR arthrography: comparison of rotator interval and posterior approach. *Clin Imaging.* 2014;38(1):11–17.
2. Cameron KL, Mauntel TC, Owens BD. The epidemiology of glenohumeral joint instability: incidence, burden, and long-term consequences. *Sports Med Arthrosc Rev.* 2017;25(3):144–149.
3. Prendergast N, Rafii M. Magnetic resonance imaging of the shoulder joint. *Curr Opin Radiol.* 1992;4(6):70–76.
4. Warby SA, et al. Multidirectional instability of the glenohumeral joint: etiology, classification, assessment, and management. *J Hand Ther.* 2017;30(2):175–181.
5. Heire RB, Mubashar M, Bhatti W. Ultrasound-guided hydrodilatation for adhesive capsulitis—a step-by-step guide; 2015. https://doi.org/10.1594/ecr2015/C-1817.
6. Yoong P, et al. Targeted ultrasound-guided hydrodilatation via the rotator interval for adhesive capsulitis. *Skeletal Radiol.* 2015;44(5):703–708.
7. Elnady B, et al. In shoulder adhesive capsulitis, ultrasound-guided anterior hydrodilatation in rotator interval is more effective than posterior approach: a randomized controlled study. *Clin Rheumatol.* 2020.
8. van der Windt DA, et al. Shoulder disorders in general practice: incidence, patient characteristics, and management. *Ann Rheum Dis.* 1995;54(12):959–964.
9. Bhayana H, et al. Ultrasound guided versus landmark guided corticosteroid injection in patients with rotator cuff syndrome: randomised controlled trial. *J Clin Orthop Trauma.* 2018;9(suppl 1):S80–s85.
10. Oh JH, et al. Comparison of glenohumeral and subacromial steroid injection in primary frozen shoulder: a prospective, randomized short-term comparison study. *J Shoulder Elbow Surg.* 2011;20(7):1034–1040.
11. Kennedy MS, Nicholson HD, Woodley SJ. Clinical anatomy of the subacromial and related shoulder bursae: a review of the literature. *Clin Anat.* 2017;30(2):213–226.
12. Eljabu W, Klinger HM, von Knoch M. The natural history of rotator cuff tears: a systematic review. *Arch Orthop Trauma Surg.* 2015;135(8):1055–1061.
13. Tashjian RZ. Epidemiology, natural history, and indications for treatment of rotator cuff tears. *Clin Sports Med.* 2012;31(4):589–604.
14. Maman E, et al. Outcome of nonoperative treatment of symptomatic rotator cuff tears monitored by magnetic resonance imaging. *J Bone Joint Surg Am.* 2009;91(8):1898–1906.
15. Brasseur JL, Zeitoun-Eiss D. [Ultrasound of acute disorders of the shoulder]. *JBR-BTR.* 2005;88(4):193–199.
16. Mochizuki T, et al. Humeral insertion of the supraspinatus and infraspinatus. New anatomical findings regarding the footprint of the rotator cuff. *J Bone Joint Surg Am.* 2008;90(5):962–969.
17. Ferri M, et al. Sonography of full-thickness supraspinatus tears: comparison of patient positioning technique with surgical correlation. *AJR Am J Roentgenol.* 2005;184(1):180–184.
18. Centeno C, et al. A randomized controlled trial of the treatment of rotator cuff tears with bone marrow concentrate and platelet products compared to exercise therapy: a midterm analysis. *Stem Cells Int.* 2020;2020:5962354.
19. Yoshida M, et al. Altered shoulder kinematics using a new model for multiple dislocations-induced Bankart lesions. *Clin Biomech.* 2019;70:131–136.
20. Kask K, et al. Anatomy of the superior glenohumeral ligament. *J Shoulder Elbow Surg.* 2010;19(6):908–916.
21. Kuhn JE, et al. External rotation of the glenohumeral joint: ligament restraints and muscle effects in the neutral and abducted positions. *J Shoulder Elbow Surg.* 2005;14(1 suppl S):39s–48s.
22. Burkart AC, Debski RE. Anatomy and function of the glenohumeral ligaments in anterior shoulder instability. *Clin Orthop Relat Res.* 2002;400:32–39.
23. Kane P, et al. Approach to the treatment of primary anterior shoulder dislocation: a review. *Phys Sportsmed.* 2015;43(1):54–64.
24. Pickett A, Svoboda S. Anterior glenohumeral instability. *Sports Med Arthrosc Rev.* 2017;25(3):156–162.
25. Burkhart SS, Morgan CD, Kibler WB. The disabled throwing shoulder: spectrum of pathology Part I: pathoanatomy and biomechanics. *Arthroscopy.* 2003;19(4):404–420.
26. Garving C, et al. Impingement syndrome of the shoulder. *Dtsch Arztebl Int.* 2017;114(45):765–776.
27. Wilk KE, et al. Current concepts in the rehabilitation of the overhead throwing athlete. *Am J Sports Med.* 2002;30:136–151.
28. Burkhart SS, et al. The disabled throwing shoulder: spectrum of pathology: Part I: pathoanatomy and biomechanics. *Arthroscopy.* 2003;19:404–420.
29. Myers J, Laudner K, Pasquale M, Bradley J, Lephart S. Posterior shoulder tightness in throwers with pathologic internal impingement. *Am J Sports Med.* 2006;34:385–391.
30. Mihata T, Gates J, McGarry M, Lee J, Kinoshita M, Lee T. Effect of rotator cuff muscle imbalance on forceful internal impingement and peel-back of the superior labrum: a cadaveric study. *Am J Sports Med.* 2009;37:2222–2227.
31. Myers JB, et al. Glenohumeral range of motion deficits and posterior shoulder tightness in throwers with pathologic internal impingement. *Am J Sports Med.* 2006;34(3):385–391.
32. Kadler BK, Mehta SS, Funk L. *Propionibacterium acnes* infection after shoulder surgery. *Int J Shoulder Surg.* 2015;9(4):139–144.
33. Clavert P. Glenoid labrum pathology. *Orthop Traumatol Surg Res.* 2015;101(1 suppl):S19–S24.
34. Michener LA, et al. National Athletic Trainers' Association position statement: evaluation, management, and outcomes of and return-to-play for overhead athletes with superior labral anterior-posterior injuries. *J Athl Train.* 2018;53(3):209–229.
35. Hester WA, et al. Current concepts in the evaluation and management of type II superior labral lesions of the shoulder. *Open Orthop J.* 2018;12:331–341.
36. Matthew T Provencher AAR. *Shoulder Instability : A Comprehensive Approach*; 2012.

37. Bakshi N, Freehill MT. The overhead athletes shoulder. *Sports Med Arthrosc Rev*. 2018;26(3):88–94.
38. Ruiz Iban MA, et al. Instability severity index score values below 7 do not predict recurrence after arthroscopic Bankart repair. *Knee Surg Sports Traumatol Arthrosc*. 2019.
39. Escobedo EM, et al. Increased risk of posterior glenoid labrum tears in football players. *AJR Am J Roentgenol*. 2007;188(1):193–197.
40. Chen CH, et al. Incidence and severity of biceps long head tendon lesion in patients with complete rotator cuff tears. *J Trauma*. 2005;58(6):1189–1193.
41. Razmjou H, et al. Accuracy of magnetic resonance imaging in detecting biceps pathology in patients with rotator cuff disorders: comparison with arthroscopy. *J Shoulder Elbow Surg*. 2016;25(1):38–44.
42. Vangsness Jr CT, et al. The origin of the long head of the biceps from the scapula and glenoid labrum. An anatomical study of 100 shoulders. *J Bone Joint Surg Br*. 1994;76(6):951–954.
43. Rodosky MW, Harner CD, Fu FH. The role of the long head of the biceps muscle and superior glenoid labrum in anterior stability of the shoulder. *Ame J Sports Med*. 1994;22(1):121–130.
44. Krupp RJ, et al. Long head of the biceps tendon pain: differential diagnosis and treatment. *J Orthop Sports Phys Ther*. 2009;39(2):55–70.
45. Denard PJ, et al. Anatomy of the biceps tendon: implications for restoring physiological length-tension relation during biceps tenodesis with interference screw fixation. *Arthroscopy*. 2012;28(10):1352–1358.
46. Amirtharaj MJ, et al. Trends in the surgical management of acromioclavicular joint arthritis among board-eligible US orthopaedic surgeons. *Arthroscopy*. 2018;34(6):1799–1805.
47. Doyscher R, et al. Acute and overuse injuries of the shoulder in sports. *Der Orthopade*. 2014;43(3):202–208.
48. Chang I-R, Varacallo M. Anatomy, shoulder and upper limb, glenohumeral joint. In *StatPearls*. Treasure Island, FL: StatPearls Publishing, 2020.
49. Hyland S, Varacallo M. Anatomy, shoulder and upper limb, clavicle. In *StatPearls*. Treasure Island, FL: StatPearls Publishing, 2019.
50. Bontempo NA. AD Mazzocca, Biomechanics and treatment of acromioclavicular and sternoclavicular joint injuries. *Br J Sports Med*. 2010;44(5):361–369.
51. Johansen JA, et al. Acromioclavicular joint injuries: indications for treatment and treatment options. *J Shoulder Elbow Surg*. 2011;20(2 suppl):S70–S82.
52. Merrigan B, Varacallo M. Acromioclavicular joint injection. In *StatPearls*. Treasure Island, FL: StatPearls Publishing LLC; 2019.
53. Kostretzis L, et al. Suprascapular nerve pathology: a review of the literature. *Open Orthop J*. 2017;11:140–153.
54. Auyong DB, et al. Comparison of anterior suprascapular, supraclavicular, and interscalene nerve block Approaches for major outpatient arthroscopic shoulder surgery: a randomized, double-blind, noninferiority trial. *Anesthesiology*. 2018;129(1):47–57.
55. Vorster W, et al. The sensory branch distribution of the suprascapular nerve: an anatomic study. *J Shoulder Elbow Surg*. 2008;17(3):500–502.
56. Shin C, et al. Spinal root origins and innervations of the suprascapular nerve. *Surg Radiol Anat*. 2010;32(3):235–238.
57. Bigliani LU, et al. An anatomical study of the suprascapular nerve. *Arthroscopy*. 1990;6(4):301–305.
58. Flynn LS, Wright TW, King JJ. Quadrilateral space syndrome: a review. *J Shoulder Elbow Surg*. 2018;27(5):950–956.
59. Chen H, Narvaez VR. Ultrasound-guided quadrilateral space block for the diagnosis of quadrilateral syndrome. *Case Rep Orthop*. 2015;2015:378627.

17
Elbow Injection Techniques

CHRIS WILLIAMS, WALTER I. SUSSMAN, AND JOHN PITTS

KEY POINTS

- Most injections can be accomplished using a high-frequency linear ultrasound transducer.
- Ultrasound allows evaluation of the three elbow articulations (radiocapitellar, ulnotrochlear, and proximal radioulnar).
- Imaging of the posterior olecranon recess with the elbow in flexion is the most sensitive means to identify pathologic fluid.

Ultrasound Guided

Joint Injections

Pertinent Anatomy

- The elbow joint is a synovial hinged joint consisting of an articulation between the humerus, radius, and ulna.
- The joint allows flexion at the elbow and forearm supination and pronation.
- The joint can be accessed from a medial, lateral, anterior, or posterior approach (Fig. 17.1).

Common Pathology

- Three primary patterns of arthritis can affect the elbow joint: rheumatoid (inflammatory), post-traumatic, and primary osteoarthritis. Intra-articular pathology can present with a joint effusion, synovitis, and associated intra-articular bodies.
- Stiffness, restriction of elbow extension, and painful mechanical symptoms are common symptoms associated with arthritis. Pain is typically deep or diffuse, and may present without any palpable tenderness.

Equipment

- Needle size: 25- or 27-gauge 1- or 1.5-inch needle.
- High-frequency linear ultrasound transducer.

Common Injectates

- Local anesthetics for diagnostics, corticosteroids.
- Prolotherapy, orthobiologics (platelet-rich plasma [PRP] bone marrow concentrate, etc.).

Injectate Volume

- 2 to 3 mL

Technique: Lateral Approach

Patient Position

- Seated or supine.
- Elbow is flexed 40 degrees and the forearm is pronated with palm resting on the table (Fig. 17.2).

Clinician Position

- Seated or standing directly next to the elbow being injected.

Transducer Orientation

- Long-axis to the radius over the radiocapitellar joint.

Needle Orientation

- In-plane to the transducer
- Or out-of-plane and short-axis to the transducer

Target

- In-plane: directed from distal to proximal into the radio-capitellar joint.
- Short axis: start in center of probe and direct into joint directly below transducer.

PEARLS AND PITFALLS

- See the injectate expand the joint without soft tissue distention.

Technique: Posterior Approach

Patient Position

- Prone position.
- Elbow is flexed approximately 90 degrees and the forearm is hanging over the table (Fig. 17.3).

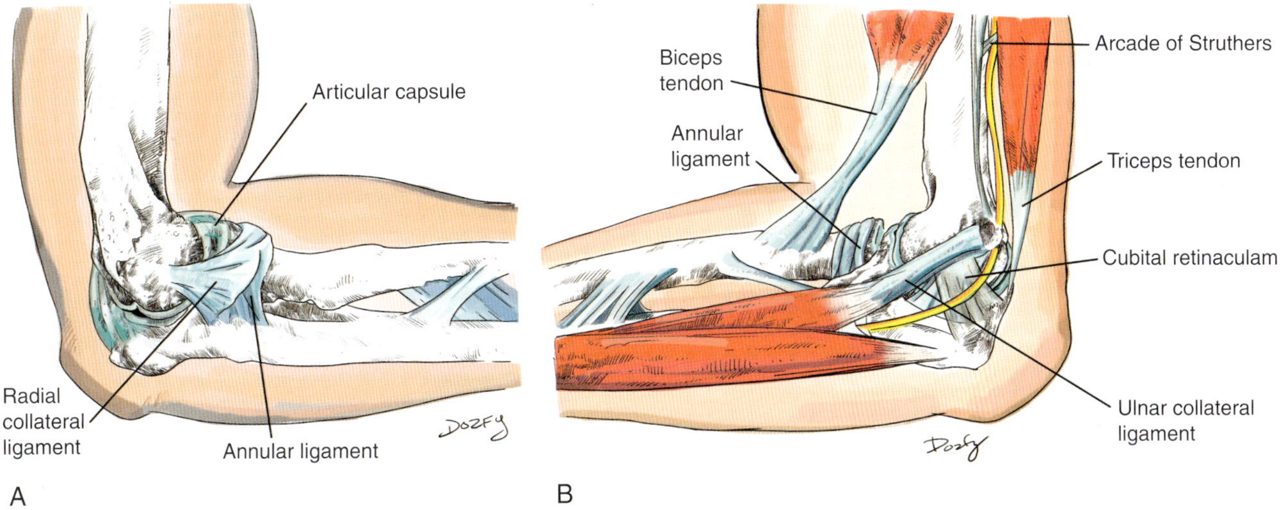

• **Fig. 17.1** (A and B) Illustration of pertinent bony and soft tissue anatomy anatomy of the elbow demonstrating lateral and posterior views.

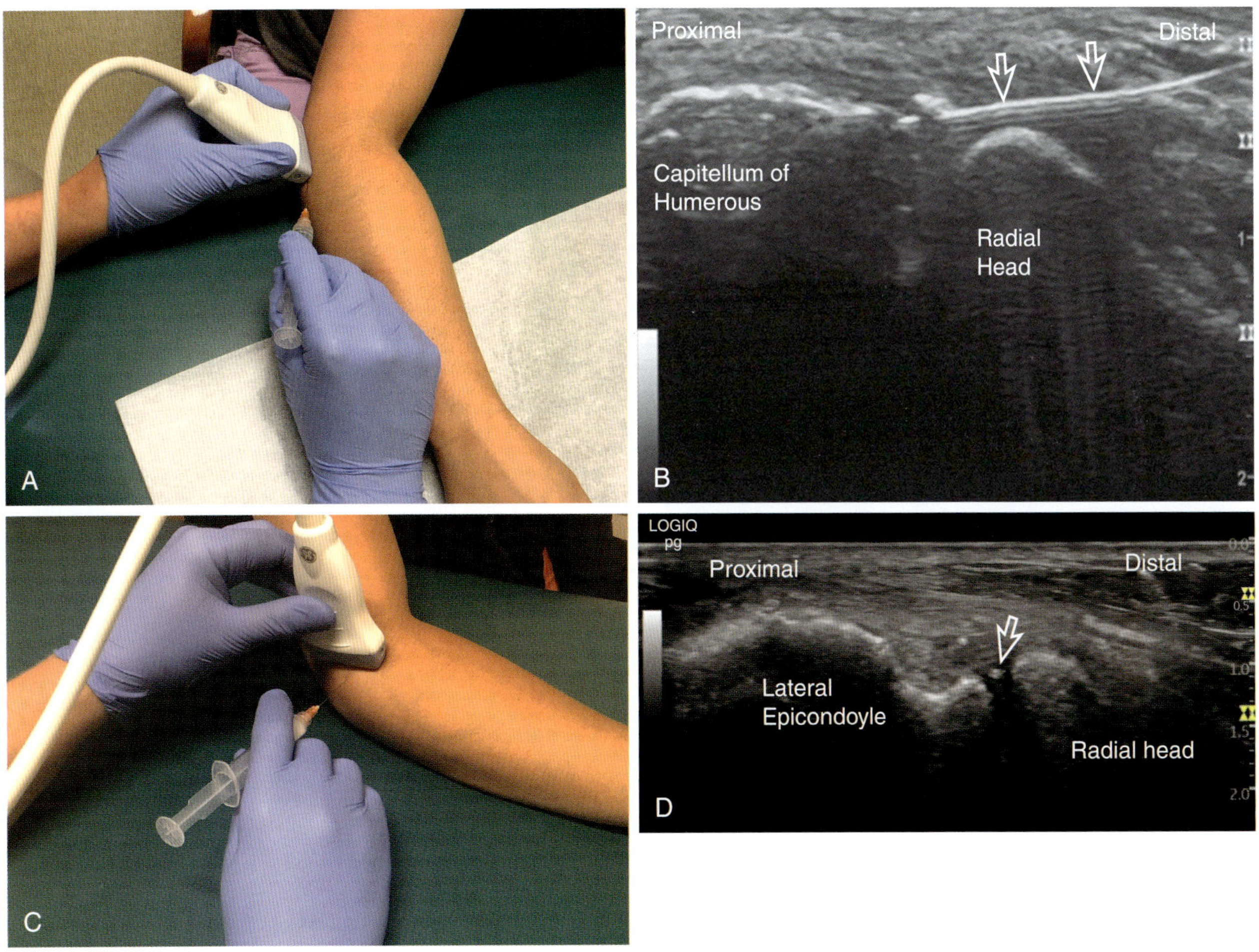

• **Fig. 17.2** Intra-articular injection of the radiocapitellar joint using a 27-gauge needle. (A) Elbow position, transducer position, and needle position for the in-plane approach. (B) Ultrasound shows the needle trajectory *(open arrow)*. (C) Elbow position, transducer position, and needle position for the out-of-plane approach for entry into the lateral elbow joint. (D) Elbow position, transducer position, and needle position for the in-plane approach for entry into the lateral elbow joint. (D) Ultrasound shows the needle out-of-plane in the joint space (*open arrow*). *Dashed circles* indicate needle trajectory. *Solid white arrow* identify the needle trajectory.

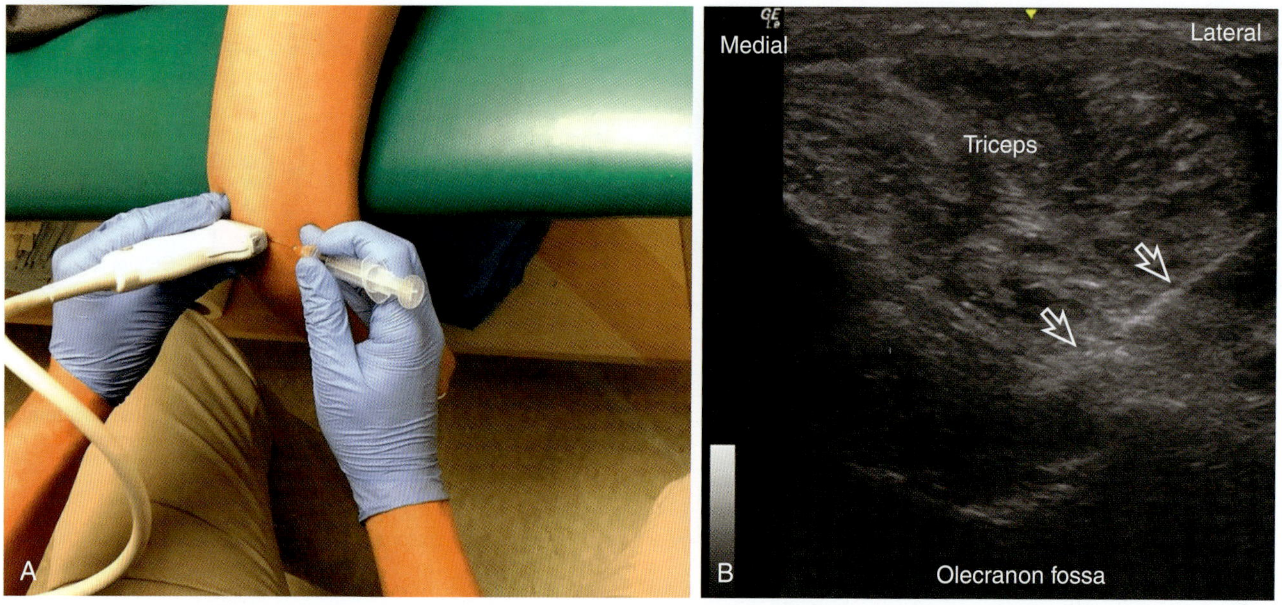

• **Fig. 17.3** Aspiration of the ulnar-olecranon joint using a 22-gauge needle in patient with triceps myositis and septic elbow joint. (A) Elbow position, transducer position, and needle position for the in-plane approach. (B) Ultrasound shows the needle *(open arrow)* trajectory.

Clinician Position

- Seated or standing directly next to the elbow being injected.

Transducer Orientation

- Short-axis to the tendon over the olecranon fossa.

Needle Orientation

- Short-axis to the triceps tendon and in-plane to the transducer from a lateral to medial direction.

Target

- Directed underneath the triceps tendon and into the joint.

PEARLS AND PITFALLS

- The ulnar nerve should be visualized at the medial epicondyle before the injection to avoid nerve injury.

Ligament Injections

Lateral Collateral Ligament Complex

KEY POINTS

- Most injections can be accomplished using a high-frequency linear ultrasound transducer.

Pertinent Anatomy

- Lateral collateral ligament (LCL) complex consists of four ligaments: accessory lateral collateral ligament (ALCL); annular ligament; lateral radial collateral ligament (LRCL); lateral ulnar collateral ligament (LUCL).
- LCUL is the primary stabilizer to varus and external rotation stress to the elbow.

Common Pathology

- Subtle instability of the LCL complex is challenging to identify on examination, but associated ligament injuries have been reported in up to 20% of cases of lateral epicondylitis. There seems to be a correlation with the severity of the injury to the common extension tendon and LUCL injury.[2–3]
- Associated with a traumatic elbow dislocation, significant injury and instability is detected by conventional physical examination and characterized by mechanical symptoms: that is, clicking or catching.

Equipment

- Needle size: 25- or 27-gauge 1- or 1.5-inch needle.
- High-frequency linear ultrasound transducer.

Common Injectates

- Prolotherapy, orthobiologics (PRP, bone marrow concentrate, etc.).
- Avoid intraligamentous corticosteroids.

Injectate Volume

- 2 to 3 cc.

Technique

Patient Position

- Seated or supine position.
- Elbow is flexed approximately 90 degrees and the forearm is pronated.

Clinician Position

- Seated or standing directly next to the elbow being injected.

Transducer Position

- Long-axis or longitudinal to the ligaments.

Needle Position

- Four ligaments comprise the LCL complex and the needle position should be adjusted to be in long-axis to the ligaments and in-plane to the transducer.
- The LRCL and LUCL should be approached from a distal to proximal orientation.
- The ALCL and annular ligament should be approached from a lateral to medial orientation (Fig. 17.4).

Target

- Areas of hypoechogenicity and cortical irregularities.
- Fenestration of tendon and mild excoriation at sites of cortical irregularities until achieve change in the tissue texture.
- Regenerative injection (PRP, adipose-derived stromal cell [ADSC], bone marrow aspirate concentrate [BMAC]) should target areas of hypoechogenicity filling interstitial tears with injectate.

PEARLS AND PITFALLS

- For the ALCL and annular ligament injections, visualize the radial nerve first to avoid injury.
- Post-procedure pain medication should be offered and the patient should be informed that pain in the elbow region would likely be increased.
- Extremes of range of movement (ROM) should be limited in first 10–12 weeks after the procedure, especially repetitive supination.

Medial Ulnar Collateral Ligament

KEY POINTS

- Most injections can be accomplished using a high-frequency linear ultrasound transducer.

Pertinent Anatomy

- Medial ulnar collateral ligament (MUCL) is composed of three bands: anterior band, posterior band, and transverse ligament.
- Anterior band is the primary restraint to valgus stress with the elbow in 30–120 degrees of flexion, coursing from the medial epicondyle to the sublime tubercle.[4]

Common Pathology

- The MUCL is commonly injured in overhead throwing athletes due to valgus stress on the elbow during the late cocking and early acceleration phases.

Equipment

- Needle size: 25- or 27-gauge 1- or 1.5-inch needle.
- High-frequency linear ultrasound transducer

Common Injectates

- Prolotherapy, orthobiologics (PRP, bone marrow concentrate, etc.),
- Avoid intraligamentous corticosteroids

Injectate Volume

- 2 to 3 cc.

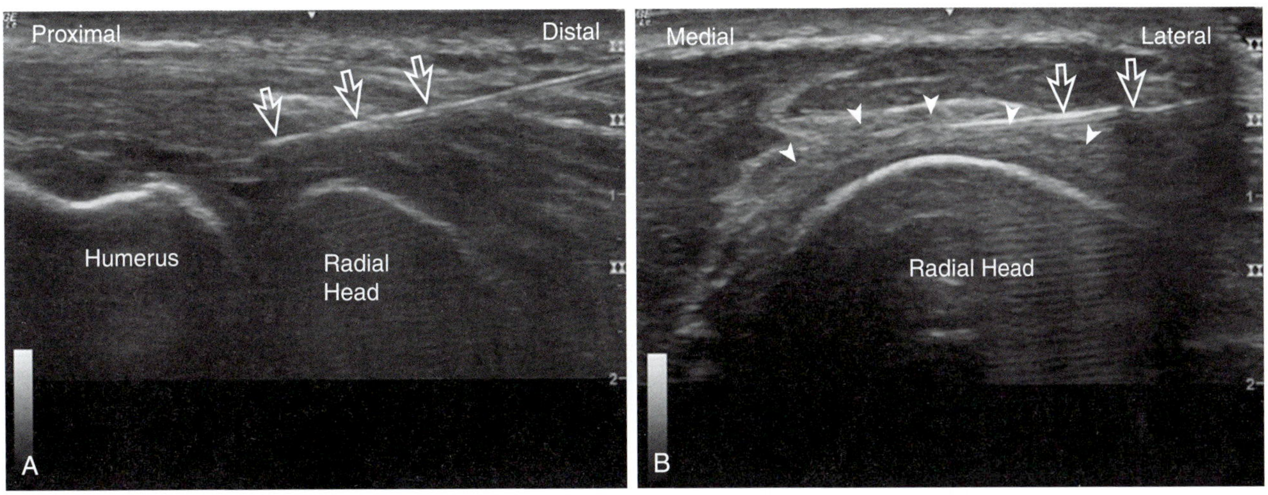

• **Fig. 17.4** Intraligamentous injection of the lateral collateral ligament using a 25-gauge needle. Elbow position, needle position, and transducer placement are similar to the common extensor tendon injection. (A) Needle *(open arrows)* approaching lateral ulnar collateral ligament intraligamentous defect. (B) Needle *(open arrows)* approaching intraligamentous defect in the annular ligament *(arrowheads)*

Technique

Patient Position

- Supine position.
- Elbow and shoulder are flexed to approximately 90 degrees and the forearm is supinated.

Clinician Position

- Seated or standing directly next to the elbow being injected.

Transducer Position

- Long-axis or longitudinal to the ligaments.

Needle Position

- The needle position should be positioned in long-axis to the UCL and in-plane to the transducer.

Target

- Areas of hypoechogenicity within the ligament.
- Regenerative injection (PRP, ADSC, BMAC) should target areas of hypoechogenicity filling interstitial tears with injectate.

PEARLS AND PITFALLS

- Post-procedure pain medication should be offered and the patient should be informed that pain in the elbow region would likely be increased.
- Valgus stress should be limited in first 10–12 weeks after the procedure. Overhead athletes should start a progressive throwing program after the period of rest.
- The ulnar nerve should be visualized before the procedure to avoid accidental nerve injury (Fig. 17.5).

Tendon Injections

Common Extensor Tendon

KEY POINTS

- Most injections can be accomplished using a high-frequency linear ultrasound transducer.

Pertinent Anatomy

- The tendon originates from the lateral epicondyle of the humerus.
- Deep to the common flexor tendon, the radial collateral ligament occupies approximately 50% of the footprint at the lateral epicondyle (Fig. 17.6).[5]

Common Pathology

- Lateral epicondylitis is the most common cause of lateral elbow pain.
- Typically an overuse syndrome.
- Degenerative changes include tendon thickening, intratendinous calcifications, or partial and complete tearing.

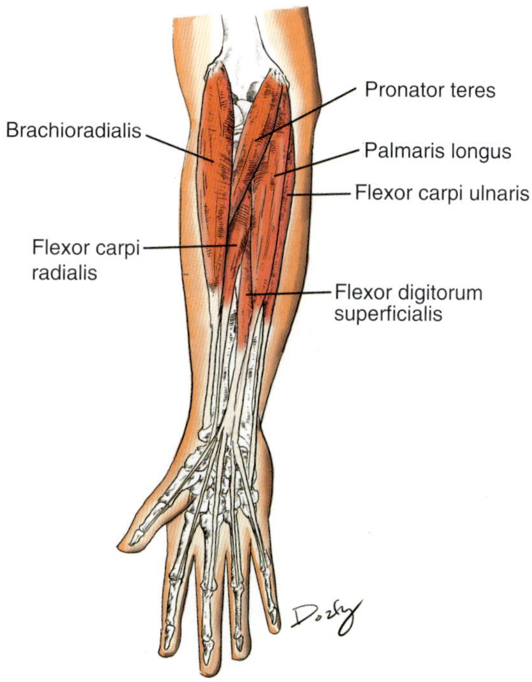

• **Fig. 17.6** Pertinent muscular anatomy of the elbow demonstrating the extensor muscles on the dorsal surface of the forearm and their attachment on the lateral epicondyle of the humerus.

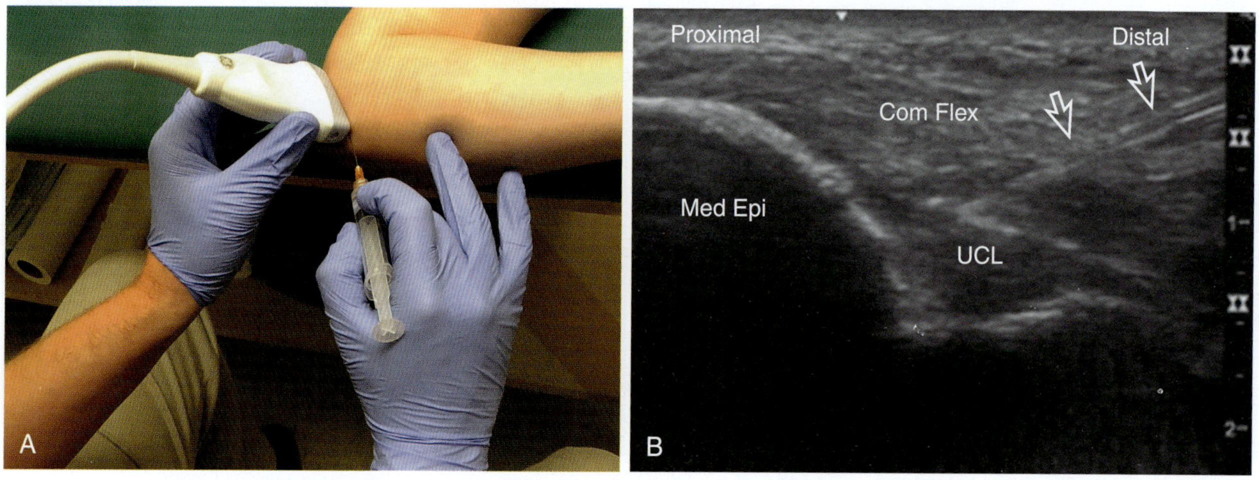

• **Fig. 17.5** Intraligamentous injection of the ulnar collateral ligament (UCL) using a 25-gauge needle. (A) Elbow position, needle position, and transducer placement. (B) Needle *(open arrow)* approaching the UCL.

Equipment

- Needle size: 25- or 27-gauge 1- or 1.5-inch needle.
- High-frequency linear ultrasound transducer.

Common Injectates

- Local anesthetic plus or minus corticosteroids peritendinous.
- Orthobiologics (PRP, bone marrow concentrate, etc.).
- Avoid intratendinous corticosteroids.

Injectate Volume

- 2 to 3 cc.

Technique

Patient Position

- Seated or supine position.
- Elbow is flexed approximately 90 degrees and the forearm is prone (Fig. 17.7).

Clinician Position

- Seated or standing directly next to the elbow being injected.

Transducer Position

- Long-axis or longitudinal to the tendon.

Needle Position

- Long-axis to the tendon and in-plane to the transducer from a distal to proximal orientation.

Target

- Areas of hypoechogenicity and cortical irregularities.
- Fenestration of tendon and mild excoriation at sites of cortical irregularities until achieve change in the tissue texture.
- Regenerative injection (PRP, ADSC, BMAC) should target areas of hypoechogenicity filling interstitial tears with injectate.
- The needle should also be repositioned, moving in a medial to lateral fashion for complete coverage of the enthesis and targeting all areas of hypoechogenicity.

PEARLS AND PITFALLS

- Examine for associated varus instability of lateral collateral complex as associated ligament injuries have been reported in up to 20% of cases of lateral epicondylitis.
- Long-term studies have shown that corticosteroid injections are no more beneficial than observation alone and may even have an inferior outcome with higher recurrence rates at 1 year.[6,7]
- Avoid intratendinous injection of local anesthetics, especially bupivacaine and lidocaine, as these have been shown to have deleterious effects on progenitor cells. If intratendinous anesthesia is required, then a small amount of 0.125% ropivacaine is preferred.

Common Flexor Tendon

KEY POINTS

- Most injections can be accomplished using a high-frequency linear ultrasound transducer.

Pertinent Anatomy

- The tendon originates from the medial epicondyle of the humerus and is shorter and broader than the lateral collateral ligament.

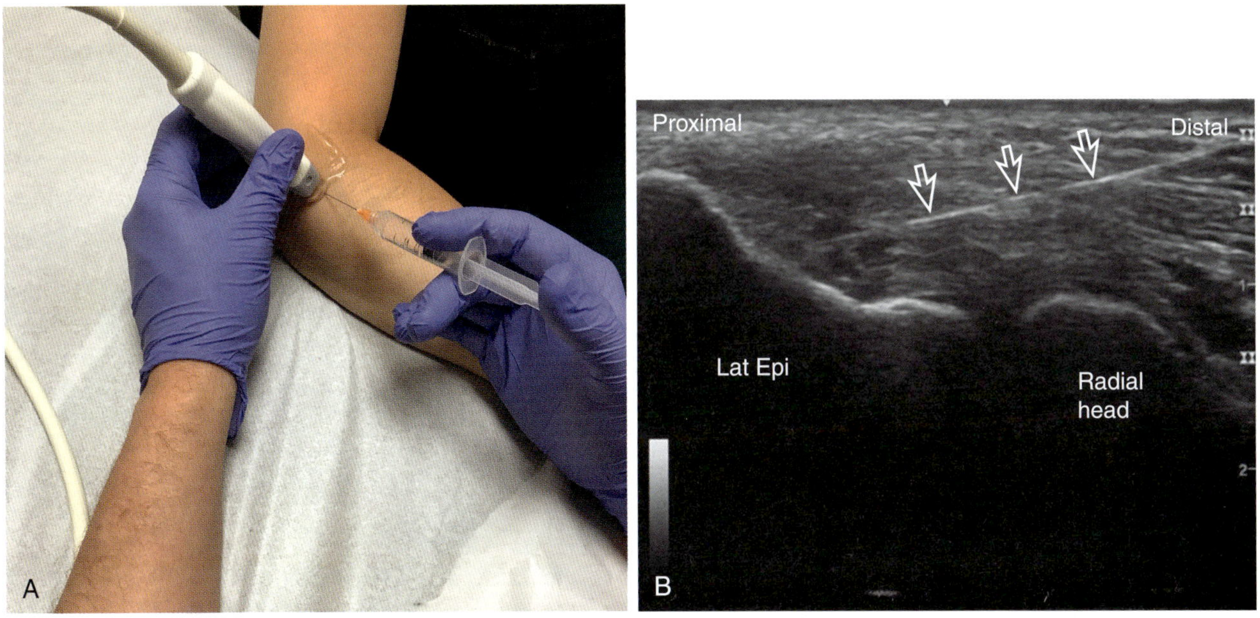

• **Fig. 17.7** Intratendinous injection of the common extensor tendon using a 25-gauge needle. (A) Elbow position, needle position, and transducer placement. (B) Needle *(open arrow)* approaching intratendinous defect.

Common Pathology

- Typically an overuse syndrome.
- 7 to 10 times less common than lateral epicondylitis.[8]
- Degenerative changes include tendon thickening, intratendinous calcifications, or partial and complete tearing.
- Examine for associated valgus instability of UCL and ulnar neuritis.

Equipment

- Needle size: 25- or 27-gauge 1- or 1.5-inch needle.
- High-frequency linear ultrasound transducer.

Common Injectates

- Local anesthetic plus or minus corticosteroids peritendinous.
- Orthobiologics (PRP, bone marrow concentrate, etc.).
- Avoid intratendinous corticosteroids.

Injectate Volume

- 2 to 3 cc.

Technique

Patient Position

- Seated or supine position.
- Elbow is flexed approximately 90 degrees, shoulder abducted to 60 to 90 degrees, and the forearm is supinated (Fig. 17.8).

Clinician Position

- Seated or standing directly next to the elbow being injected.

Transducer Position

- Long-axis or longitudinal to the tendon.

Needle Position

- Long-axis to the tendon and in-plane to the transducer from a distal to proximal orientation.

Target

- Areas of hypoechogenicity and cortical irregularities.
- Fenestration of tendon and mild excoriation at sites of cortical irregularities until achieve change in the tissue texture.
- Regenerative injection (PRP, ADSC, BMAC) should target areas of hypoechogenicity, filling interstitial tears with injectate.
- The needle should also be repositioned, moving in a medial to lateral fashion for complete coverage of the enthesis and targeting all areas of hypoechogenicity.

PEARLS AND PITFALLS

- Post-procedure pain medication should be offered and the patient should be informed that pain in the elbow region would likely be increased.
- The ulnar nerve should be visualized before the procedure to avoid accidental nerve injury.
- Avoid intratendinous injection of local anesthetics, especially bupivacaine and lidocaine as these have been shown to have deleterious effects on progenitor cells. If intratendinous anesthesia is required, then a small amount of 0.125% ropivacaine is preferred.

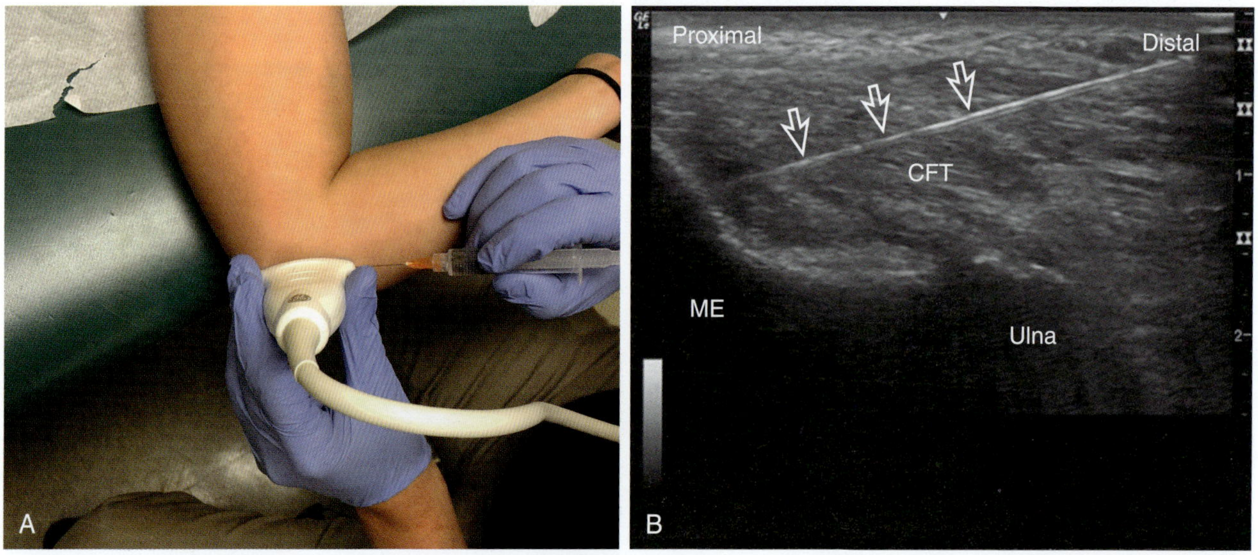

• **Fig. 17.8** Intratendinous injection of the common flexor tendon using a 25-gauge needle. (A) Elbow position, needle position, and transducer placement. (B) Needle *(open arrow)* approaching intratendinous defect.

Distal Biceps Tendon

KEY POINTS

- Most injections can be accomplished using a high-frequency linear ultrasound transducer.

Pertinent Anatomy

- Distal biceps tendon inserts onto the radial tuberosity.
- Brachial artery runs superficial to the distal biceps myotendinous junction. The median, radial, and lateral antebrachial cutaneous nerves travel adjacent to the tendon.

Common Pathology

- Distal biceps tendinopathy often results from repetitive injuries with the elbow flexed and supinated.
- Bicipitoradial bursa and interosseous bursa can occur due to friction irritation and may be more amenable to aspiration and injection by alternative approaches.

Equipment

- Needle size: 25- or 27-gauge 1.5-inch needle.
- High-frequency linear ultrasound transducer.

Common Injectates

- Local anesthetic plus or minus corticosteroids peritendinous.
- Orthobiologics (PRP, bone marrow concentrate, etc.).
- Avoid intratendinous corticosteroids.

Injectate Volume

- 2 to 3 cc.

Technique: Anterior Approach

Patient Position

- Seated or supine position.
- Elbow is fully extended and the forearm is supinated (Fig. 17.9).

Clinician Position

- Seated or standing directly next to the elbow being injected.

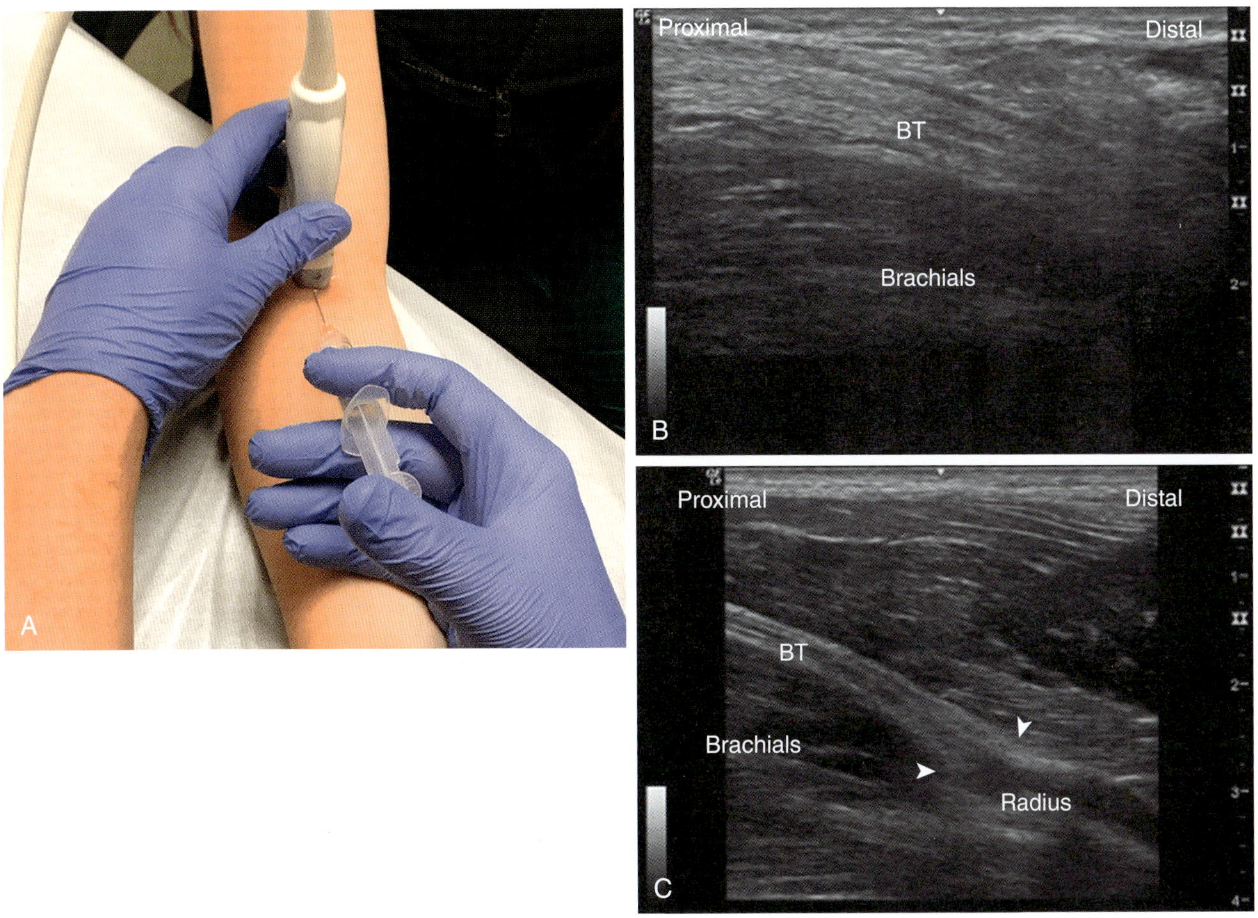

• **Fig. 17.9** Intratendinous injection of the biceps tendon. (A) Elbow position, needle position, and transducer placement. (B) Anterior ultrasound of the biceps tendon demonstrating anisotropy of the tendon limiting visualization of the insertion. (C) Oblique view showing biceps tendon to the insertion site on the radial tuberosity *(arrowhead)*.

Transducer Position

- Long-axis to the tendon.

Needle Position

- Long-axis to the tendon and in-plane to the transducer. A distal to proximal or proximal to distal approach can be used.

Target

- The tendon insertion is difficult to visualize with this approach, and an anterior approach is better suited to target the myotendinous junction.
- Target areas of hypoechogenicity with regenerative injections (PRP, ADSC, BMAC) filling interstitial tears with injectate.

PEARLS AND PITFALLS

- Doppler flow should be used to help identify the anterior elbow vasculature. An anterior approach may be precluded by the brachial artery in some patients.
- There is a theoretical risk of tendon rupture after corticosteroid injections.

Technique: Posterior Approach (Preferred Technique)

Patient Position

- Seated or supine position.
- Elbow is flexed to approximately 120 degrees and the forearm is pronated (Fig. 17.10).

Clinician Position

- Seated or standing directly next to the elbow being injected.

Transducer Position

- Long-axis to the tendon on the dorsal (posterior) forearm.

Needle Position

- The needle is advanced in-plane from a radial to ulnar direction deep to the supinator.

Target

- Intratendinous regenerative injection (PRP, ADSC, BMAC) should target areas of abnormalities (hypoechoic clefts) within the tendon with the injectate.
- Peritendinous injection/bicipitoradial bursa injection of corticosteroids should target the peritendinous space around the biceps tendon.

PEARLS AND PITFALLS

- In one cadaveric intratendinous injectate had a proximal flow of 3.4 cm (range, 3.0 to 4.0 cm). Proximal spread may be enhanced by not maximally pronating the forearm which narrows the interosseous space.[9]
- Theoretical risk of tendon rupture after corticosteroid injection. Avoid intratendinous corticosteroids and local anesthetics besides a small amount of 0.125% ropivacaine, if required.
- Position of the posterior interosseous nerve between the superficial and deep head of the supinator should be identified before injection.

Triceps Tendon

KEY POINTS

- Most injections can be accomplished using a high-frequency linear ultrasound transducer.

Pertinent Anatomy

- Triceps brachii tendon is composed of a superficial layer (lateral and long heads) and a deep layer (medial head)

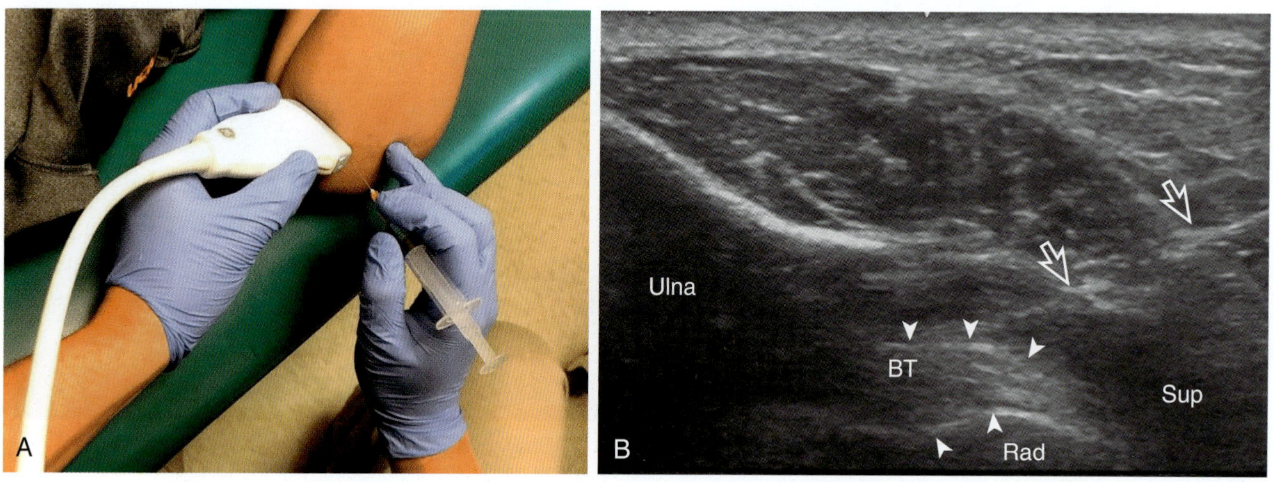

• **Fig. 17.10** Intralegamentous injection of the distal biceps tendon using a 25-gauge needle. (A) Elbow position, needle position, and transducer placement. (B) Needle *(open arrow)* approaching biceps tendon *(arrowheads)*.

that blends with the posterior capsule as it inserts on the olecranon process.

Common Pathology

- Pathologic changes may include disruption of the tendon fibers (as seen with a partial-thickness or full-thickness tear), or hypoechoic thickening of intact fibers (as seen with tendinosis).

Equipment

- Needle size: 25- or 27-gauge 1.5-inch needle.
- High-frequency linear ultrasound transducer

Common Injectates

- Local anesthetic plus or minus corticosteroids peritendinous.
- Orthobiologics (PRP bone marrow concentrate, etc.).
- Avoid intratendinous corticosteroids.

Injectate Volume

- 2 to 3 cc.

Technique: Anterior Approach

Patient Position

- Supine or prone position.
- Elbow is flexed to 90 degrees and forearm resting on the abdomen if patient is supine or hanging off the table if patient is prone (Fig. 17.11).

Clinician Position

- Seated or standing directly next to the elbow being injected.

Transducer Position

- Long-axis to the tendon.

Needle Position

- Long-axis to the tendon and in-plane to the transducer. A distal to proximal or proximal to distal approach can be used.

Target

- Areas of hypoechogenicity and cortical irregularities.
- Fenestration of tendon and mild excoriation at sites of cortical irregularities until achieve change in the tissue texture.
- Regenerative injection (PRP, ADSC, BMAC) should target areas of hypoechogenicity, filling interstitial tears with injectate.
- The needle should also be repositioned, moving in a medial to lateral fashion for complete coverage of the enthesis and targeting all areas of hypoechogenicity.

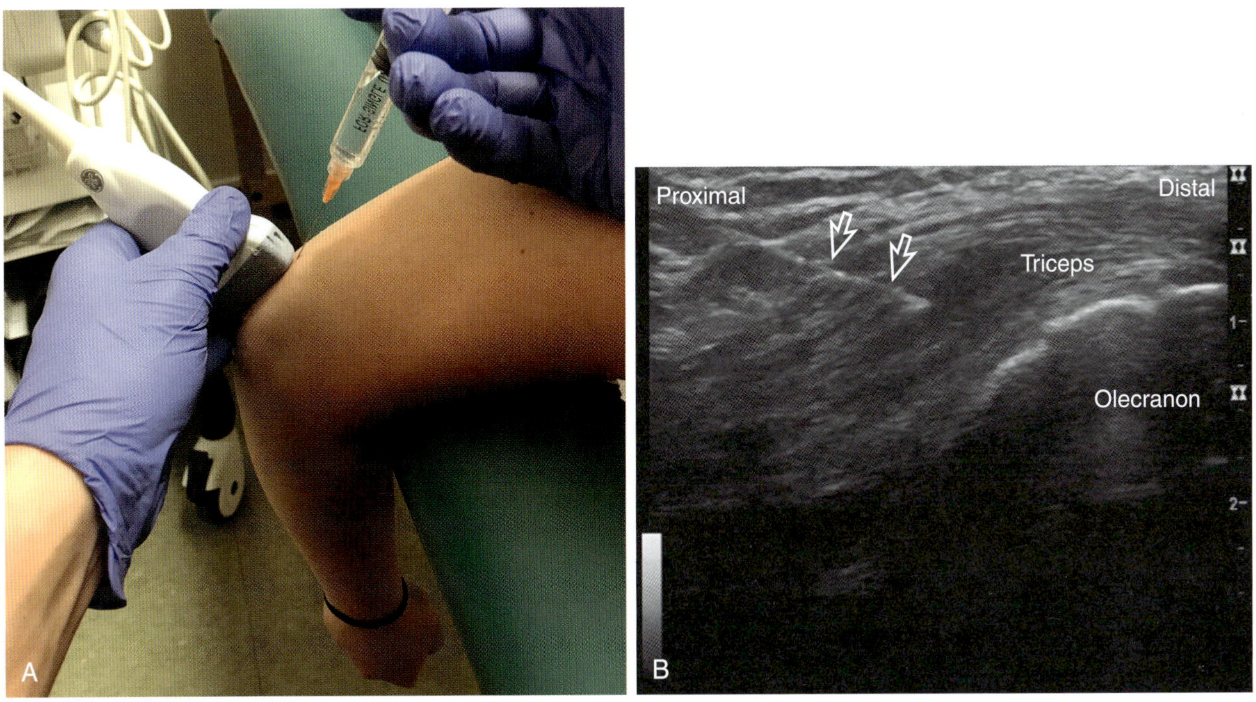

• **Fig. 17.11** Intratendinous injection of the distal triceps tendon. (A) Elbow position, needle position, and transducer placement. (B) Needle *(open arrow)* approaching intratendinous defect.

PEARLS AND PITFALLS

- If clinical suspicion exists, the posterior ultrasound evaluation should include assessment of the olecranon bursa superficial to the olecranon process.
- Local corticosteroid injections have been associated with subsequent rupture of the triceps tendon. Avoid intratendinous corticosteroids and local anesthetics besides a small amount of 0.125% ropivacaine, if required.

Olecranon Bursa

KEY POINTS

- Most injections can be accomplished using a high-frequency linear ultrasound transducer.

Pertinent Anatomy

- The olecranon bursa is an adventitious bursa that is located over the olecranon process. The superficial location of the bursae makes it vulnerable to injury and inflammation.

Common Pathology

- The most common etiology is post-traumatic bursitis. Minor or repetitive trauma can provoke bursitis.
- Olecranon bursitis is associated with diabetes, gout, rheumatoid arthritis, and human immunodeficiency virus (HIV).
- Septic bursitis can also occur and *Staphylococcus aureus* is the most common causative bacteria.

Equipment

- Needle size: 25- to 27-gauge 1.5- to 22-inch needle for anesthetic.
- 18- or 22-gauge for aspiration of the bursa.
- High-frequency linear ultrasound transducer.

Common Injectates

- Aspiration.
- Anesthetic and corticosteroid.
- Sclerosing agents can be used for recurrent bursitis.

Injectate Volume

- 1 to 2 cc.

Technique: Anterior Approach

Patient Position

- Supine or prone position.
- Elbow is flexed to 90 degrees and forearm resting on the abdomen if patient is supine, or hanging off the table if patient is prone (Fig. 17.12).

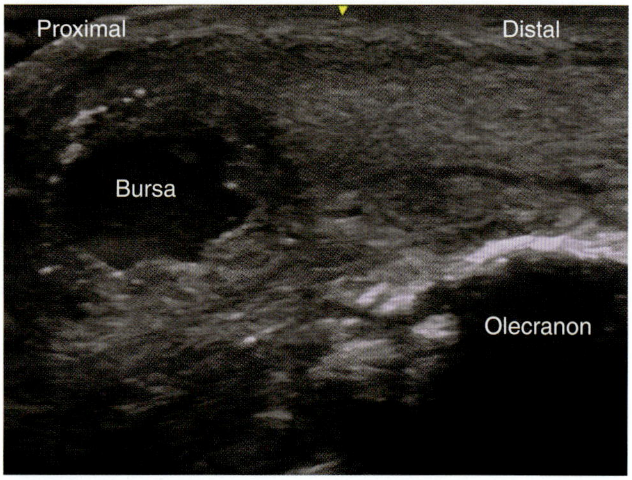

• **Fig. 17.12** Aspiration of traumatic olecranon bursitis. Elbow position, needle position, and transducer placement similar to triceps tendon injection (see *Triceps Tendon* Fig. 17.11 for positioning). Needle *(open arrow)* in the bursa.

Clinician Position

- Seated or standing directly next to the elbow being injected.

Transducer Position

- Long-axis to the tendon.

Needle Position

- Long-axis to the tendon and in-plane to the transducer. A distal to proximal or a proximal to distal approach can be used.

Target

- Anechoic or hypoechoic collection superficial to the olecranon process.

PEARLS AND PITFALLS

- Slight compression can displace the bursa and the ultrasound probe may need to be "floated" on gel and a gel standoff used during the procedure.
- If clinical suspicion exists, aspirate should be sent for culture and sensitivity.
- Neoplastic pathology can mimic simple olecranon bursitis, and rapidly expanding growth, failure of treatment, weight loss, and prior history of neoplasia should prompt further work-up. Aspirate can be sent for cytology.

Perineural Injections

Deep Branch Radial Nerve

KEY POINTS

- Most injections can be accomplished using a high-frequency linear ultrasound transducer.

Pertinent Anatomy

- The radial nerve bifurcates into the deep branch of the radial nerve and superficial radial sensory nerve at the level of the radiocapitellar joint.
- The deep branch of the radial nerve passes through the arcade of Frohse (supinator arch), the tendinous edge of the supinator, and fibrous entrance to the radial tunnel.
- The nerve then passes between the superficial and deep layers of the supinator and becomes the posterior interosseus nerve once it exits the supinator.

Common Pathology

- The arcade of Frohse is thought to be the most frequent site of entrapment, although this is controversial. Entrapment may occur in or at the exit from the radial tunnel (radial head to the inferior border of the supinator muscle).
- Focal or diffuse enlargement of the nerve can help localize site of entrapment.
- Compression of the deep radial branch results in a deep aching pain only, without motor manifestations (although may have weakness due to pain). Symptoms increase with forearm rotation and lifting activities.

Equipment

- Needle size: 25- or 27-gauge 1.5-inch needle.
- High-frequency linear ultrasound transducer.

Common Injectates

- For nerve block: local anesthetic.
- For hydrodissection: mixture of normal saline and local anesthetic solution or 5% dextrose solution, or platelet lysate solution.

Injectate Volume

- For nerve block: 2 to 5 cc.
- For hydrodissection: 5 to 10 cc.

Technique

Patient Position

- Supine or seated position.
- Elbow is flexed approximately 90 degrees and the forearm resting on the table, with the thumb pointed upward (Fig. 17.13).

Clinician Position

- Seated or standing directly next to the elbow being injected.

Transducer Position

- Short-axis to the nerve.

Needle Position

- The needle position should be positioned in-plane to the transducer.
- Medial-to-lateral or distal-to-proximal approach.

Target

- Areas of focal flattening or proximal swelling.

PEARLS AND PITFALLS

- Pre-procedural scanning should be performed to identify surrounding vasculature (recurrent radial artery) and potential anatomic variants.
- The focal zone should be placed at the level of the nerve and gray-scale adjusted to provide the greatest contrast between the nerve and surrounding tissue.
- The needle should not be advanced if the tip is not visible.
- Inject just before approaching the epineurium and advance while injecting slowly to push the nerve away, thus reducing the risk of intraneural injection.
- Creating a halo around the nerve will increase the definition of the nerve borders.

Median Nerve at Pronator Teres

KEY POINTS

- Most injections can be accomplished using a high-frequency linear ultrasound transducer.

Pertinent Anatomy

- The median nerve crosses the elbow and passes beneath the bicipital aponeurosis (lacertus fibrosus) and then between the radial and ulnar heads of the pronator teres.

Common Pathology

- Pronator tunnel syndrome is a rare compressive neuropathy of the median nerve at the elbow and involves entrapment at the level of the pronator teres.
- Neurologic symptoms in the median innervated forearm muscles (flexor carpi radialis, palmaris longus, and flexor digitorum superficialis) and numbness in median distribution in the hand. Vague forearm pain with repetitive pronation-supination.
- Commonly associated with medial epicondylitis.

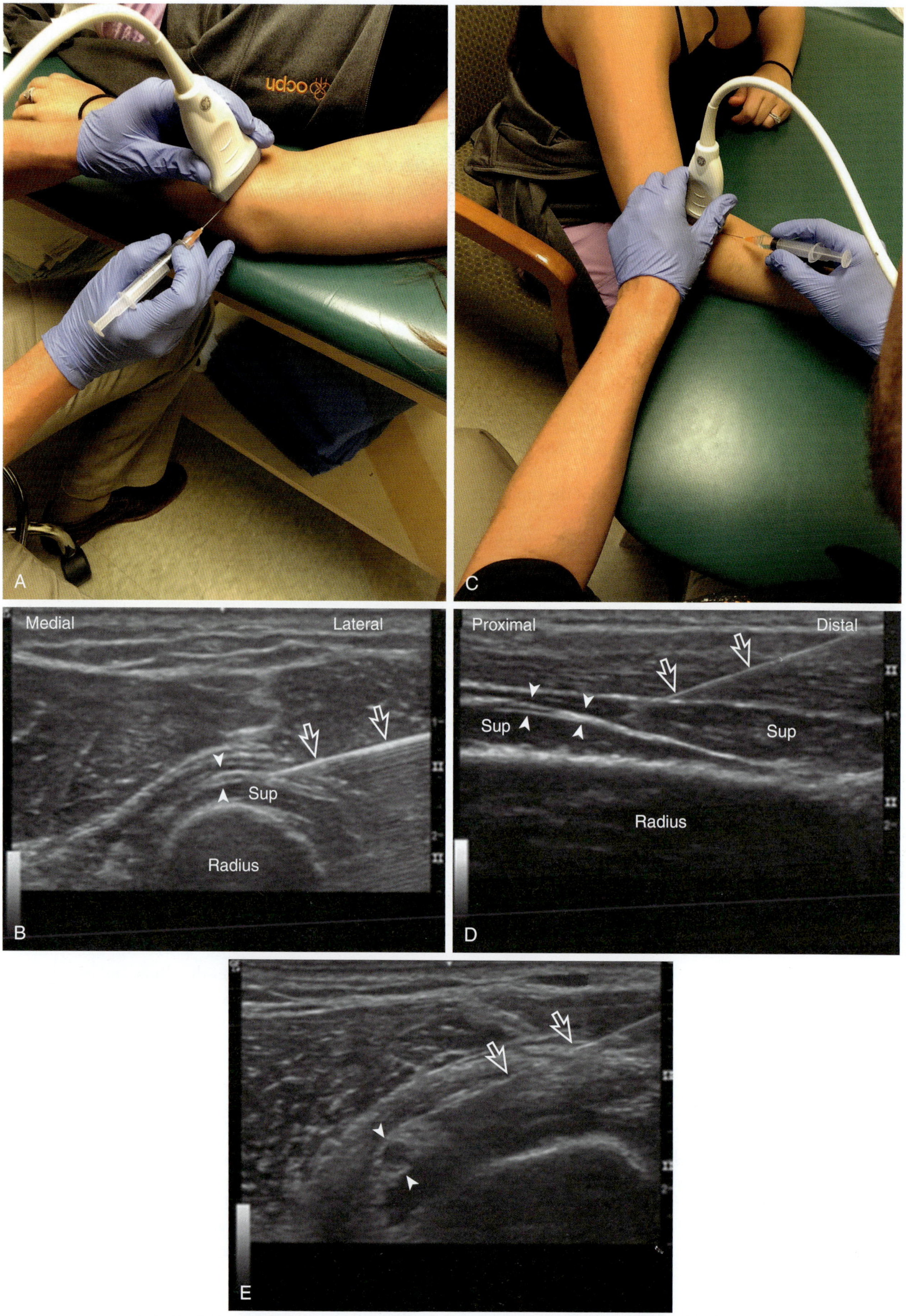

• **Fig. 17.13** Perineural injection of the deep branch of the radial nerve (DBRN) *(arrowheads)*. Elbow position, needle position, and transducer placement for short-axis (A) and long-axis (B) to the nerve. (C) Needle *(open arrow)* in-line to transducer approaching the DBRN in short-axis as it passes through the fascial plane between the superficial and deep heads of the supinator muscle. (D) Long-axis approach to DBRN. (E) Perineural injection of a thickened DBRN at the arcade of Frosch *(arrowheads)*. Needle *(arrow)* is in-line to the transducer and approaching the DBRN in short-axis.

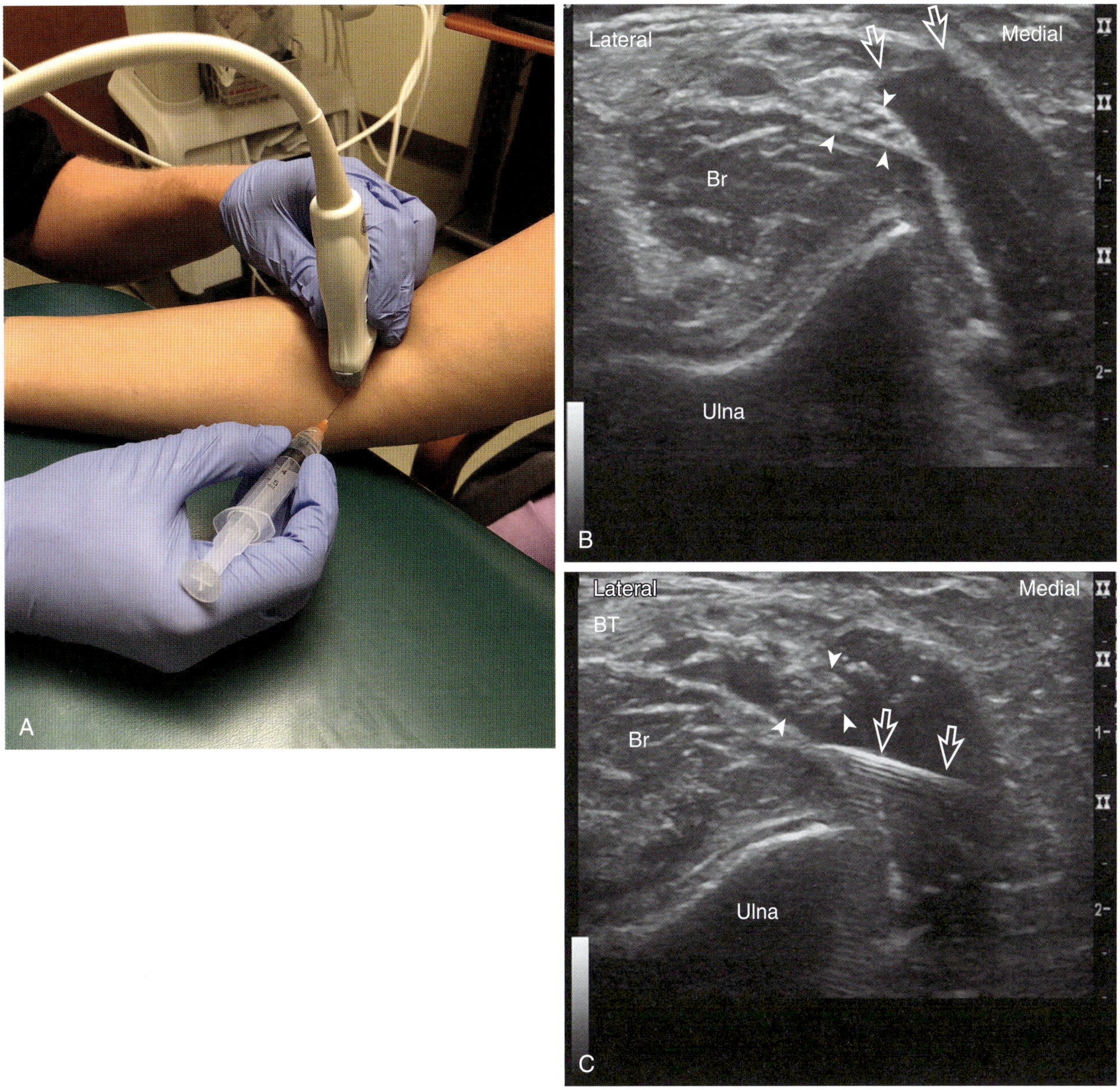

• **Fig. 17.14** Perineural injection of the median nerve *(arrowheads)*. (A) Elbow position, needle position, and transducer placement. (B and C) Needle *(open arrow)* in-line to transducer approaching the median nerve *(arrowheads)*.

Equipment

- Needle size: 25- or 27-gauge 1.5-inch needle.
- High-frequency linear ultrasound transducer.

Common Injectates

- For nerve block: local anesthetic.
- For hydrodissection: mixture of normal saline and local anesthetic solution or 5% dextrose solution, or platelet lysate solution.

Injectate Volume

- For nerve block: 2 to 5 cc.
- For hydrodissection: 5 to 10 cc.

Technique

Patient Position

- Supine or seated position.
- Elbow is extended, with forearm supinated and resting on the table (Fig. 17.14).

Clinician Position

- Seated or standing directly next to the elbow being injected.

Transducer Position

- Short-axis to the nerve.

Needle Position

- The needle position should be positioned in-plane to the transducer.
- Medial-to-lateral or distal-to-proximal approach.

Target

- Areas of focal flattening or proximal swelling.

PEARLS AND PITFALLS

- Pre-procedural scanning should be performed to identify surrounding vasculature and potential anatomic variants. Brachial artery is typically lateral to the nerve proximally, and the ulnar artery adjacent to the distal median nerve.
- The focal zone should be placed at the level of the nerve and the gray scale adjusted to provide the greatest contrast between the nerve and surrounding tissue.
- The needle should not be advanced if the tip is not visible.
- Inject just before approaching the epineurium and advance while injecting slowly to push the nerve away, thus reducing the risk of intraneural injection.
- Creating a halo around the nerve will increase the definition of the nerve borders.

Ulnar Nerve at the Cubital Tunnel

KEY POINTS

- Most injections can be accomplished using a high-frequency linear ultrasound transducer.

Pertinent Anatomy

- The ulnar nerve crosses the elbow in the cubital tunnel posterior to the medial epicondyle.

Common Pathology

- Ulnar neuropathy at the elbow is the second most common entrapment in the upper extremity.
- The most common site of entrapment is between the radial and ulnar heads of the flexor carpi ulnaris (FCU). Less common sites include between Osborne's ligament and the MCL, medial head of the triceps, and anomalous anconeus epitrochlearis.
- Neurologic symptoms include paresthesias of the small finger and ulnar {½} of the ring finger and loss of strength in the ulnar intrinsic muscles.

Equipment

- Needle size: 25- or 27-gauge 1.5-inch needle.
- High-frequency linear ultrasound transducer.

Common Injectates

- For nerve block: local anesthetic.
- For hydrodissection: mixture of normal saline and local anesthetic solution or 5% dextrose solution, or platelet lysate solution.

Injectate Volume

- For nerve block: 2 to 5 cc.
- For hydrodissection: 5 to 10 cc.

Technique

Patient Position

- Supine or seated position.
- Elbow is extended with forearm supinated and resting on the table (Fig. 17.15).

Clinician Position

- Seated or standing directly next to the elbow being injected.

Transducer Position

- Short-axis to the nerve.

Needle Position

- The needle position should be positioned in-plane to the transducer.
- Medial-to-lateral approach.

Target

- Areas of focal flattening or proximal swelling of the ulnar nerve.

PEARLS AND PITFALLS

- Pre-procedural scanning should be performed to identify surrounding vasculature and potential anatomic variants.
- The focal zone should be placed at the level of the nerve and the gray scale adjusted to provide the greatest contrast between the nerve and surrounding tissue.
- The needle should not be advanced if the tip is not visible.
- Inject just before approaching the epineurium and advance while injecting slowly to push the nerve away, thus reducing the risk of intraneural injection.
- Creating a halo around the nerve will increase the definition of the nerve borders.

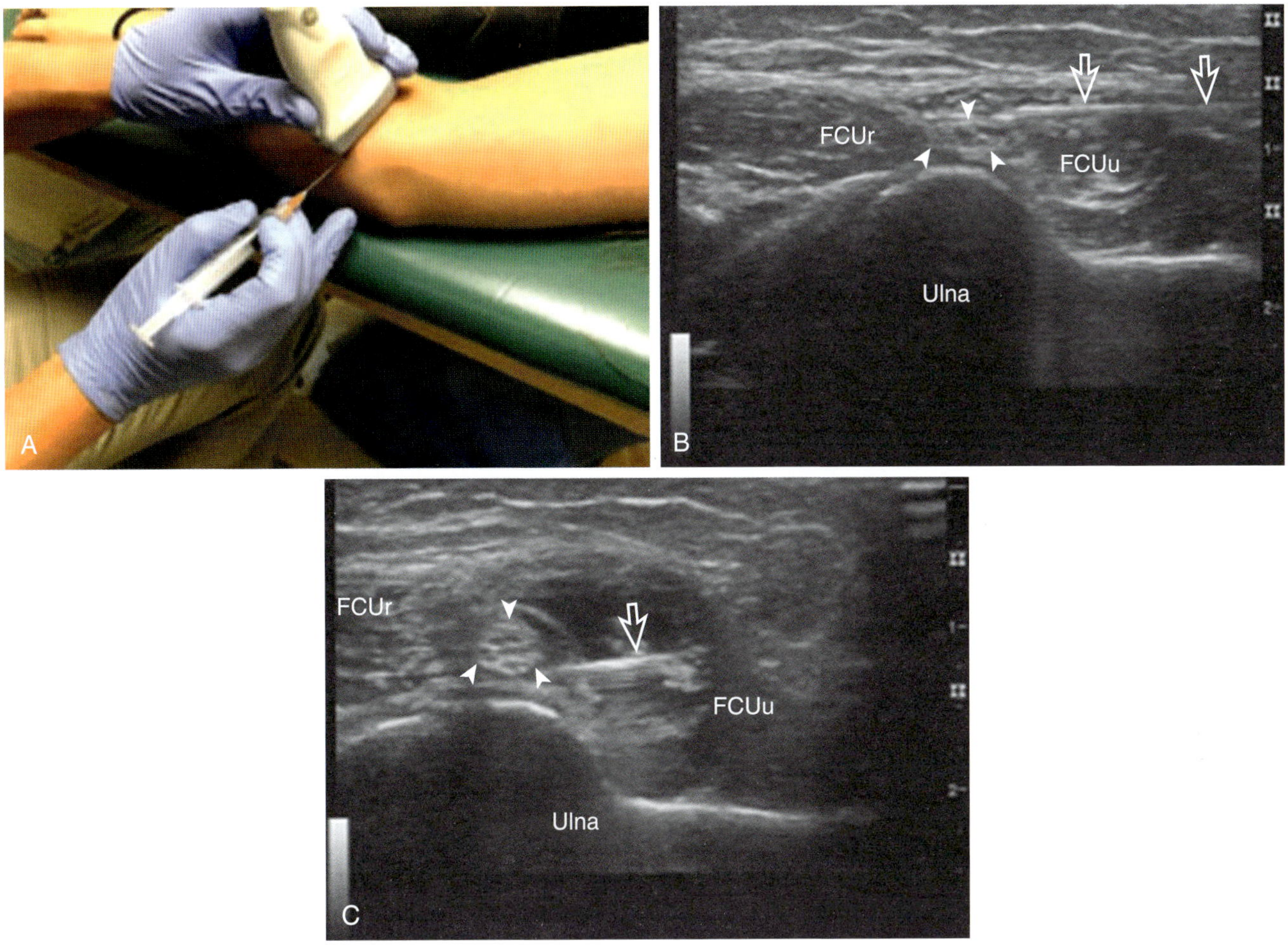

• **Fig. 17.15** Perineural injection of the deep branch of the ulnar nerve. (A) Elbow position, needle position, and transducer placement. (B) Needle *(open arrow)* in-line to transducer approaching the ulnar nerve *(arrowheads)* in short-axis as it passes through the fascial plane between the two heads of the flexor carpi ulnaris . The nerve is hydrodissected (C) above and below the nerve, creating an anechoic halo around the nerve.

Fluoroscopy Injections

Joint Injections

KEY POINTS

- Patient position and C-arm position is key to minimize radiation exposure and increase the likelihood of successful intra-articular needle placement.

Pertinent Anatomy

- The elbow joint is a synovial hinged joint consisting of an articulation between the humerus, radius, and ulna.
- The joint allows flexion at the elbow and forearm supination and pronation.
- The joint can be accessed from a medial, lateral, anterior, or posterior approach.

Equipment

- C-arm fluoroscopy.

Common Injectates

- Local anesthetics for diagnostics, corticosteroids.
- Orthobiologics (PRP, bone marrow concentrate, etc.).

Injectate Volume

- 2 to 3 cc.

Technique: Lateral Approach

Patient Position

- Supine.

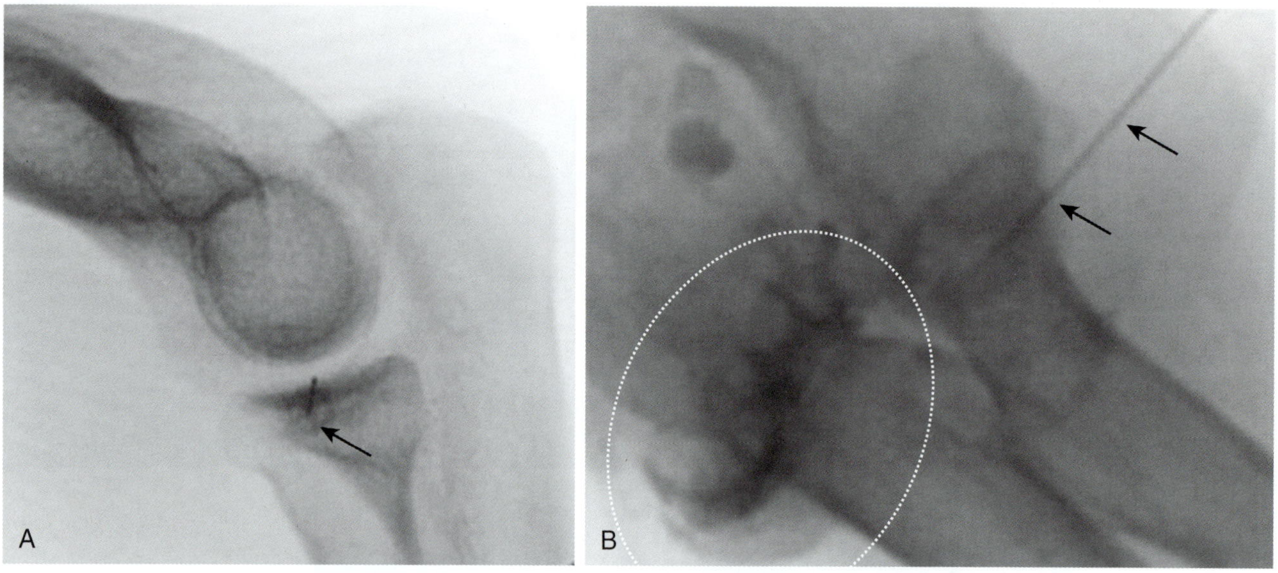

• **Fig. 17.16** Radiocapitellar joint lateral approach under fluoroscopy. (A) Needle directly in the joint space. (B) Intra-articular injection from a lateral approach through the radiocapitellar joint using a 27-gauge needle. *Solid white arrow* identifies the needle. *Dashed line with circle* indicates is showing the intra-articular contrast flow pattern.

- Arm is extended away from the body to allow C-arm positioning. Elbow is extended and forearm supinated.
- Elbow is flexed 40 degrees and the forearm is pronated, with palm resting on the table.

Clinician Position

- Seated or standing directly next to the elbow being injected.

C-Arm Position

- Lateral view of the elbow with visualization of the joint.

Needle Position

- Enter the skin laterally, directly over the joint line.
- Advance the needle until the joint capsule is penetrated (Fig. 17.16).

Target

- Radiocapitellar joint.

PEARLS AND PITFALLS

- Mark sure the C-arm is aligned with the joint.
- Ensure contrast is circulating around the epicondyle without any contrast outside the joint.
- If desired, obtain an anteroposterior (AP) view to see contrast flow lateral to medial. Reposition the arm so that the elbow is extended and supinated.
- Use as little contrast as needed to confirm good flow.

Technique: Posterior Approach

Patient Position

- Prone.
- Shoulder is flexed and abducted. Elbow is flexed 90 degrees and the forearm is pronated with palm resting on the table or arm rest (Fig. 17.17).

Clinician Position

- Seated or standing adjacent to the patient behind the elbow.

C-arm Position

- Lateral view of the elbow, with humeral olecranon joint opened, medial, and lateral epicondyles aligned.

Needle Position

- Start at the skin posterior and superior to the joint.
- Angle and advance the needle under intermittent fluoroscopy toward the joint.

Target

- Humeral olecranon joint just into the posterior capsule.
- Inject contrast to demonstrate intra-articular flow.

PEARLS AND PITFALLS

- Mark sure the C-arm is aligned with the joint.
- Ensure contrast is circulating around the epicondyle without any contrast outside the joint.
- Use as little contrast as needed to confirm good flow.

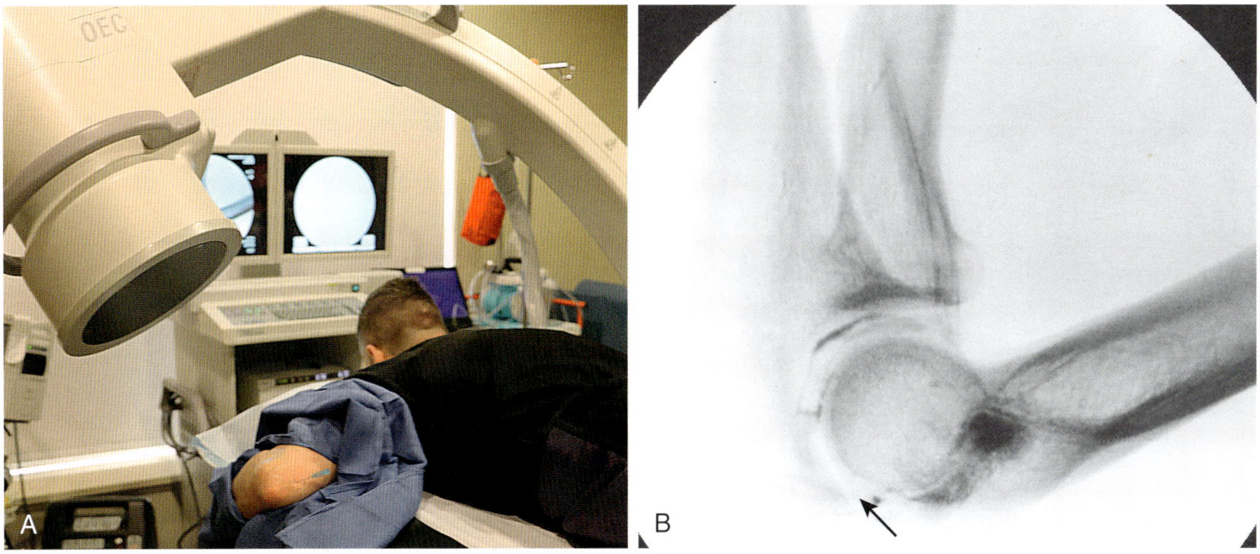

• **Fig. 17.17** (A) Humeral olecranon joint injection fluoroscopy, posterior approach set up. (B) Humeral olecranon joint injection under fluoroscopy, posterior approach using a 25-gauge needle. *Arrow* represents needle trajectory. *Black contrast* fills joint space.

References

1. Potter HG, Hannafin JA, Morwessel RM, DiCarlo EF, O'Brien SJ, et al. Lateral epicondylitis: correlation of MR imaging, surgical, and histopathologic findings. *Radiology*. 1995;196(1):43–46.
2. Bredella M, Tirman P, Fritz R, Feller J, Wischer T, Genant H. MR imaging findings of lateral ulnar collateral ligament abnormalities in patients with lateral epicondylitis. *AJR Am J Roentgenol*. 1999;173(5):1379–1382.
3. Qi L, Zhu Z-F, Li F, Wang R-F. MR imaging of patients with lateral epicondylitis of the elbow: is the common extensor tendon an isolated lesion? *PloS One*. 2013;8(11):e79498.
4. Labott JR, Aibinder WR, Dines JS, Camp CL. Understanding the medial ulnar collateral ligament of the elbow: review of native ligament anatomy and function. *World J Orthop*. 2018;9(6):78–84.
5. Bureau NJ, Destrempes F, Acid S, Lungu E, Moser T, Michaud J, et al. Diagnostic accuracy of echo envelope statistical modeling compared to B-mode and power Doppler ultrasound imaging in patients with clinically diagnosed lateral epicondylosis of the elbow. *J Ultrasound Med*. 2019;38(10):2631–2641.
6. Smidt N, van der Windt DA, Assendelft WJ, et al. Corticosteroid injections, physiotherapy, or a wait-and-see policy for lateral epicondylitis: a randomized controlled trial. *Lancet*. 2002;359(9307):657–662.
7. Bisset L, Beller E, Jull G, et al. Mobilisation with movement and exercise, corticosteroid injection, or wait and see for tennis elbow: randomised trial. *BMJ*. 2006;333(7575):939.
8. Leach RE, Miller JK. Lateral and medial epicondylitis of the elbow. *Clin Sports Med*. 1987;6(2):259–272.
9. Sellon JL, Wempe MK, Smith J. Sonographically guided distal biceps tendon injections: techniques and validation. *J Ultrasound Med*. 2014;33(8):1461–1474.

18

Wrist Injection Techniques

KEVIN CONLEY, YODITI TEFERA, MICHAEL ERICKSON, ADAM M. POURCHO, PHILLIP HENNING, AND OLUSEUN OLUFADE

Ultrasound-Guided Techniques

KEY POINTS

- A hockey stick transducer or small linear/shorter footprint transducer may be beneficial in areas about the hand and wrist due to the nature of the smaller anatomy.
- A gel standoff can be beneficial when doing procedures about the wrist to facilitate better needle visualization.
- As with any procedure, a knowledge of the at-risk structures and common anatomic variants with sonographic identification prior to any procedure is recommended.

Wrist Joint Injections

Pertinent Anatomy

- The wrist region is composed of three noncommunicating synovial joints: the radiocarpal joint, the midcarpal joint, and the distal radioulnar joint (DRUJ) (Fig. 18.1).
- The triangular fibrocartilage complex (TFCC) is a construct between the distal ulna and proximal carpal row. The TFCC is composed of fibrocartilage (meniscal homolog), flexor carpi ulnaris tendon sheath, and radioulnar ligaments, which stabilize the DRUJ.[1,2]

Common Pathology

- Injuries to the wrist include dislocations, chronic instability/ligamentous laxity, inflammatory arthritis, and osteoarthritis.[3–8]
- Prior scaphoid fractures, scapholunate or lunotriquetral ligament (LTL), and TFCC injuries may predispose to post-traumatic arthritis.[4,5,9]
- The anatomic variation of positive ulnar variance may cause abutment of the cartilage and subsequent attritional tearing/degeneration of the TFCC.[10,11]
- Pathologic signs include osteophyte formation, cortical irregularities, articular space narrowing, joint effusions, or thickening of the synovium/synovitis.[6,12]

Equipment

- Injections can be performed using a high-frequency linear array transducer. If available, a hockey stick or shorter footprint transducer may also be helpful.
- 30 to 22 gauge, 1 to 2 inch needle.

Common Injectates

- Local anesthetics for diagnostics, corticosteroids
- Prolotherapy
- Orthobiologics (platelet-rich plasma [PRP], bone marrow concentrate, etc.)

Injectate Volume

- 1 to 3 cc

Technique

Wrist Joint Injections (Radiocarpal, Midcarpal, and Distal Radioulnar Joints)

- Patient position
  - A supine or seated position with the forearm fully pronated and wrist in slight flexion (Fig. 18.2A).
  - Place the wrist on a rolled-up towel; slight wrist flexion opens up the dorsal joint recess.[13,14]
- Clinician position
  - Seated facing the wrist and ultrasound machine monitor.
- Transducer orientation
  - Placing the transducer in the anatomic sagittal plane optimizes visualization of most of the wrist joints, with the exception of the DRUJ, which is best visualized in the anatomic axial plane due to its orientation (see Fig. 18.2).

Radiocarpal Joint (Proximal Carpal Row)

- Transducer orientation: radiocarpal joint
  - The anatomic axial plane over the dorsal radius at the level of Lister's tubercle.
  - Center the transducer over Lister's tubercle; then visualize the radiocarpal joint by rotating the transducer 90 degrees to the anatomic sagittal plane on the longitudinal axis (see Fig. 18.2A).

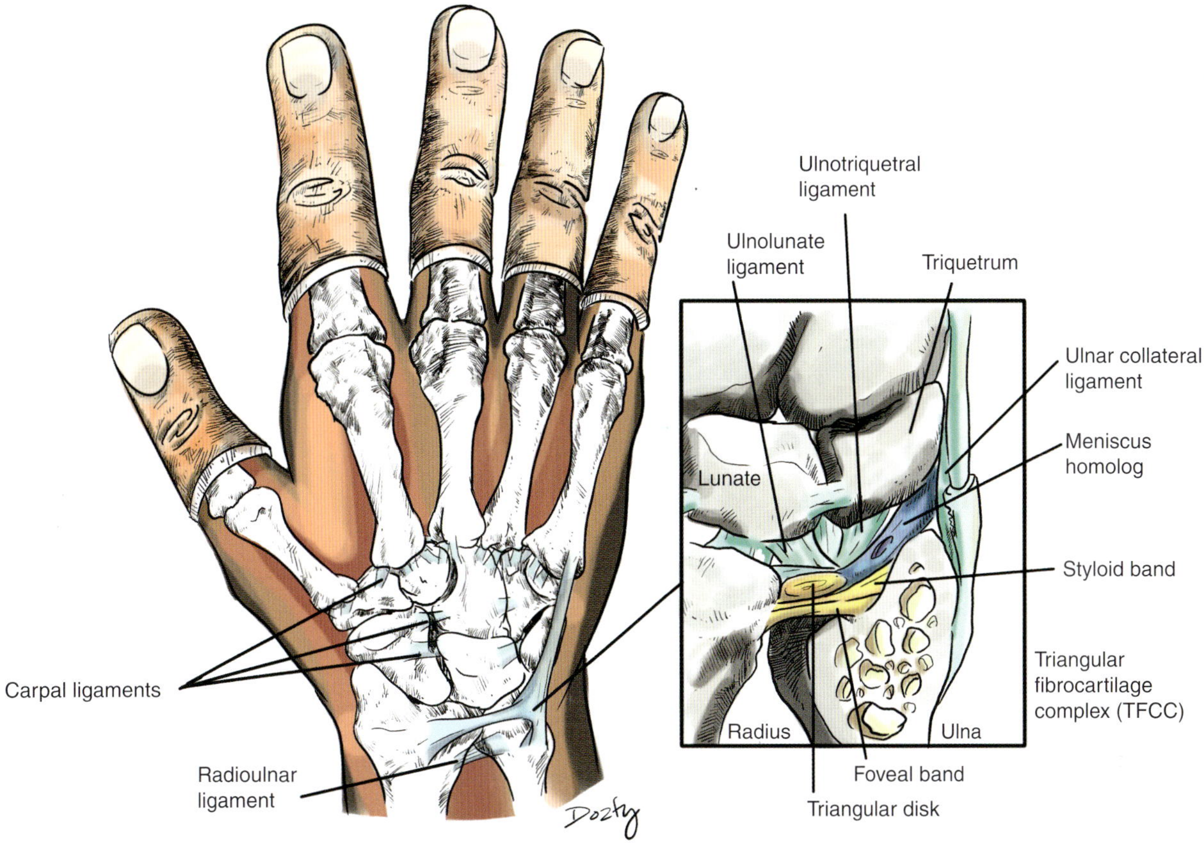

• **Fig. 18.1** Drawing of The Wrist Joint. Note the radiocarpal joint *(green)* between the radius and ulna proximally and proximal carpal row distally. Mid carpal joint *(blue)* lies between the proximal and distal carpal row. The distal radioulnar joint *(yellow)* is the articulation between the distal radius and ulna. The triangular fibrocartilage complex is the fibroligamentous construct between the distal ulna and proximal carpal row.

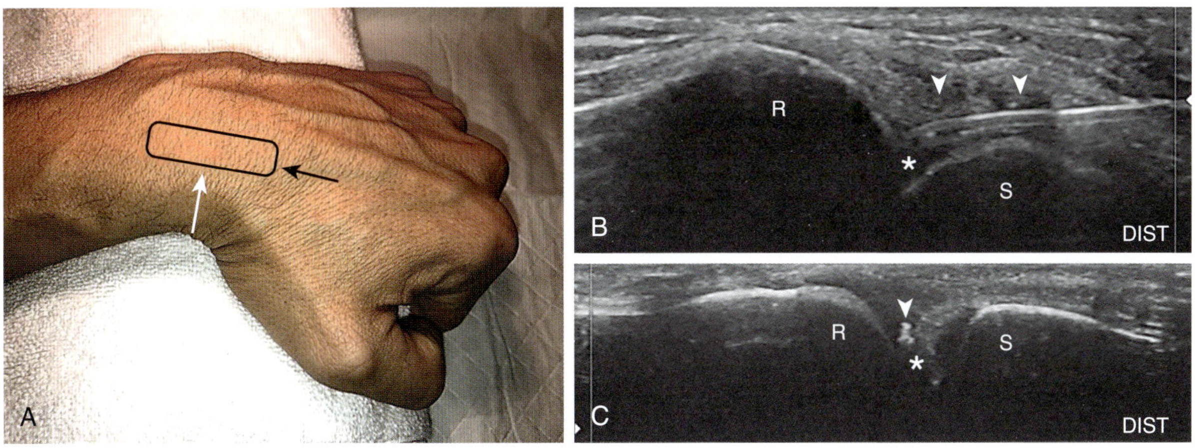

• **Fig. 18.2** Wrist Joint (Radiocarpal Joint [RC]). (A) Transducer placed along the anatomic sagittal plane to optimize visualization of the RC and midcarpal joint. Black arrow represents the direction of needle when using an in plane approach from a distal to proximal direction. White arrow represents path of needle when performing an out of plane injection from ulnar to radial. (B) Needle *(arrowheads)* placed in plane with transducer from distal to proximal direction *(black arrow 2A)*. Asterisk denotes location of joint space. (C) Needle is placed out of plane with transducer from radial to ulnar direction *(white arrow 2A.)*, asterisk denotes location of joint space. *R*, Radius, *S*, scaphoid.

- Needle orientation
  - A needle can then be inserted via an in-plane distal-to-proximal trajectory toward the joint (see Fig. 18.2B).
  - The transducer (Td) can be rotated and translated slightly to create a tendon-free region through which the needle will traverse (see Fig. 18.2B).
  - This can also be performed via an out-of-plane technique with the transducer placed in the anatomic sagittal plane centered over the radioscaphoid joint (see Fig. 18.2A and C).
- Target
  - Due to the paucity of overlying neurovascular structures and ease of access to the joint space, the

radioscaphoid joint is the preferred target in an in-plane approach.[13,14]
- Important to note that the articular hypoechoic scaphoid cartilage may not be easily visualized given the orientation.

Midcarpal Joint Injection

The technique is like the radiocarpal joint, with the exception being the target is the dorsal recess of the midcarpal joint.

Distal Radioulnar Joint Injection

Transducer Orientation
- Centered over the DRUJ and overlying extensor digiti minimi tendon in anatomic axial orientation (Fig. 18.3A).

Needle Orientation

In plane with ulnar-to-radial approach with the tip placed in the dorsal recess of the joint (see Fig. 18.3B).
- Alternatively, an out-of-plane technique can be used when the needle is introduced from a distal-to-proximal direction into the joint (see Fig. 18.3A).

Target
- Joint recess.
- A slight oblique pathway of the needle may be needed to avoid placement of the needle through the overlying extensor digiti minimi tendon or the posterior interosseous nerve (PIN) (see Fig. 18.3C).

PEARLS AND PITFALLS

- The location of the PIN in the fourth dorsal compartment should be identified and monitored during the injection.
- Joint aspiration may help to further delineate pathology and direct treatment for diseases such as inflammatory and crystalline arthropathies.[5,8] If one prefers to initially aspirate the joint, a larger-gauge needle, such as an 18 gauge, would be recommended.
- Reported accuracy rates of palpation-guided and ultrasound-guided injections for these regions range from 25% to 97% and 79% to 94%, respectively.[15-19]

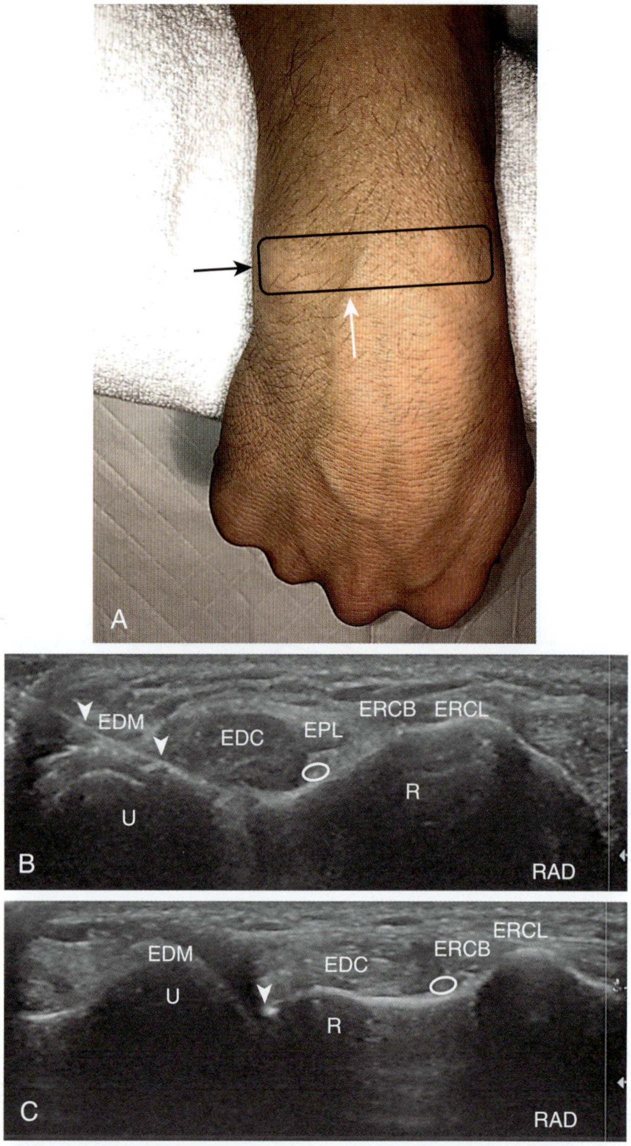

• **Fig. 18.3** Distal Radioulnar Joint (DRUJ) Injection. (A) Transducer is placed along the anatomic axial plane to optimize visualization of the DRUJ. (B) Ultrasound image with needle placed *(arrowheads)* in plane with transducer from ulnar to radial direction *(black arrow* [3A]) into the dorsal recess of the joint. (C) Ultrasound image with needle placed *(arrowhead)* out of plane with transducer from distal to proximal *(white arrow* [3A]). *ECRB*, Extensor carpi radialis brevis; *ECRL*, extensor carpi radialis longus; *EDC*, extensor digitorum communis; *EDM*, extensor digiti minimi; *EPL*, extensor pollicis longus; *white oval* encircles the posterior interosseous nerve; *R*, radius; *U*, ulna.

Scapholunate Ligament, Lunotriquetral Ligament, and TFCC Injections

Pertinent Anatomy

- Scapholunate ligament (SLL) and lunotriquetral ligament LTL are both composed of 3 structurally distinct parts (volar, membranous, and dorsal). The dorsal SLL is the strongest component, while the volar portion is the strongest portion in the LTL.[20]
- The TFCC can be difficult to see in its entirety as the ulnar styloid process blocks the view. Adjacent structures include wrist ulnar collateral ligament (UCL), extensor carpi ulnaris (ECU) tendon, and sheath.
- Easily visualized structures associated with the complex include the UCL and the overlying ECU tendon sheath.[2,6,21]

Common Pathology

- There are Twenty individual ligaments in the wrist, but the SLL and TFCC are more prone to injury.
- SLL and LTL injuries occur with a fall onto an outstretched hand. This can lead to altered arthrokinematics and subsequent development of arthritis.[22] Total disruption of the

SLL and LTL can lead to instability and result in a scapholunate advanced collapse of the wrist. Acute total SLL injuries should be treated surgically.
- TFCC injuries may occur as a result of direct trauma from falls or chronic attrition associated with ulnar abutment syndrome.[1]

Equipment

- Injections can be performed using a high-frequency linear array transducer. If available, a hockey stick or shorter footprint transducer may also be helpful.
- 30 to 22 gauge, 1 to 2 inch needle

Common Injectates

- Local anesthetics for diagnostics
- Prolotherapy
- Orthobiologics (PRP, bone marrow concentrate, etc.)
- Corticosteroids should not be injected directly into a ligament or tendon.

Injectate Volume

- 1 to 3 cc

Technique

Patient Position

- Supine or seated with forearm pronated and resting on table with a towel under the wrist to induce slight wrist flexion (Fig. 18.4A).

Clinician Position

- Standing or seated facing the wrist and ultrasound machine monitor.

TFCC Injection

- Transducer orientation
  - Anatomic axial plane over the distal ulna and radius.
  - Slide the transducer distally to view the ulnar attachment of the TFCC. The transducer may need to be rotated clockwise/counterclockwise to improve visualization of the ligament (see Fig. 18.4A).
- Needle orientation
  - Use an ulnar gel standoff
  - In plane
  - Ulnar-to-radial direction
- Target
  - Dorsal aspect of the TFCC and UCL (see Fig. 18.4B)

Scapholunate and Lunotriquetral Ligament Injection

- Transducer Orientation
  - The SLL is identified by placing the transducer in the anatomic axial plane over the distal radius and sliding the transducer distally (see Fig. 18.4A).
  - The dorsal aspect of the LTL is identified by placing the transducer in the anatomic axial plane over the distal ulna and radius and sliding distally to view the LTL.

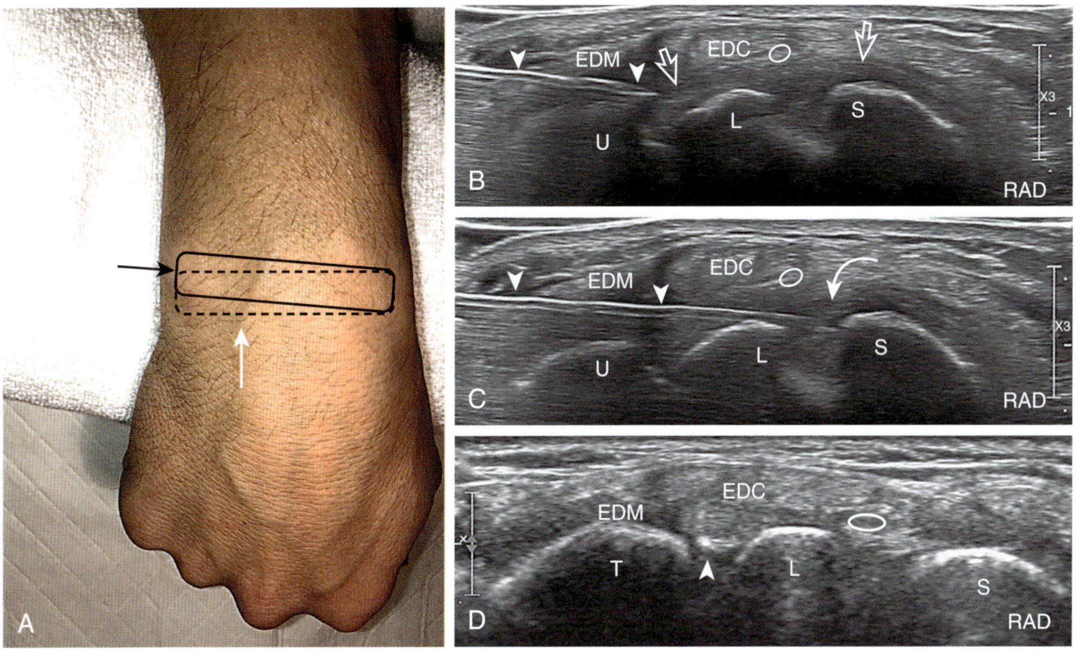

• **Fig. 18.4** Dorsal Wrist Ligament and Triangular Fibrocartilage Complex (TFCC) Injection: (A) Transducer orientation (*black rectangle* for SL and TFCC) (*dashed rectangle* for lunotriquetral ligament [LTL]) axial to dorsal wrist. *Black arrow,* direction of needle placement from ulnar to radial. *White arrow,* out-of-plane needle trajectory for LTL injection. (B) Needle *(arrowheads)* placed into the dorsal TFCC *(open arrow)*. (C) Needle *(arrowheads)* placed into the dorsal scapholunate ligament *(curved arrow)*. Placement of the forearm and wrist in preparation for the dorsal wrist joint injections. Hint: A rolled towel placed under the distal forearm to cause slight wrist flexion aides in visualization of the target and needle. *EDC*, Extensor digitorum communis; *EDM*, extensor digiti minimi; *L*, lunate; *open oval*, posterior interosseous nerve; *S*, scaphoid; *U*, ulna.

- Needle Position
  - Using an ulnar gel standoff, the SLL injection is performed via an in-plane ulnar-to-radial direction with the goal of placing the injectate in the ligament (see Fig. 18.4C).
  - The LTL injection is performed using an out-of-plane distal-to-proximal approach.
  - Caution should be taken to identify and avoid the PIN located on the radial side of the fourth dorsal compartment (see Fig. 18.4C).
- Target
  - Hypoechoic or pathologic areas of the scapholunate or LTL.

PEARLS AND PITFALLS

- Fewer dorsal neurovascular structures are present compared to the volar wrist, but the location of the PIN on the radial side of the fourth dorsal compartment should be noted prior to any procedure using the dorsal approach.

Volar Ligaments: Radioscaphocapitate, Long Radiotriquetral, Short Radiolunate, Radioscapholunate

KEY POINTS

- This is an advanced injection that requires excellent needle visualization skills.
- Must clearly identify and avoid the median nerve, radial, and ulnar arteries.
- One does not have to specifically identify each individual ligament for injection.

Pertinent Anatomy

- The wrist ligaments are generally grouped into the intrinsic (ligaments between the carpal bones) and extrinsic (connecting carpal bone to distal radius or ulna). The volar ligaments can generally be called the palmar extrinsic capsular wrist ligaments, and specific ligaments are named for the bones they originate and insert onto.[20,23]
- Four ligaments originate from the distal radius and attach to the carpal bones.
  - The radioscaphocapitate ligament (RSCL) originates from the volar aspect of the radial styloid to approximately the middle of the scaphoid fossa.
  - The long radiotriquetral ligament (LRLL), which also is known as the palmar radiolunotriquetral or the radiotriquetral ligament, originates from the volar rim of the distal radius, ulnar to the RSCL and spans the remaining part of the scaphoid fossa.
  - The short radiolunate ligament (SRLL) originates from the volar ulnar aspect of the distal radius across the entire width of the lunate fossa and attaches to the radial half of the palmar cortex of the lunate.
  - The radioscapholunate ligament (RSLL) (ligament of Testut and Kuenz) is located just ulnar to the LRLL and radial to the SRLL.

Common Pathology

- Hyperextension of the wrist is a common mechanism.
- While the TFCC and SLL are the most commonly injured structure, any of the 20 wrist ligaments can be injured.

Equipment

- Injections can be performed using a high-frequency linear array transducer. If available, a hockey stick or shorter footprint transducer may also be helpful.
- 30 to 25 gauge, 1 to 2 inch needle.

Common Injectates

- Local anesthetics for diagnostics
- Prolotherapy
- Orthobiologics (PRP, bone marrow concentrate, etc.)
- Corticosteroids should not be injected directly into a ligament or tendon.

Injectate Volume

- 1 to 3 cc

Technique

Patient Position

- Supine, wrist supinated (Fig. 18.5A).
- May have a small towel roll under the wrist for slight extension to "open" the space.

Clinician Position

- Seated or standing on the side of the patient's wrist.

Transducer Orientation

- Short axis to the wrist and carpal tunnel structures.
- Take care to angulate parallel or perpendicular to avoid anisotropy.

Needle Orientation

- The radial and ulnar approaches are necessary to target the desired ligaments.[24]
- Radial approach: the needle will enter medial to the radial artery and radial to the median nerve (see Fig. 18.5B).
- Ulnar approach: the needle will enter radial to ulnar neurovascular structures and medially to the median nerve (see Fig. 18.5C).

Target

- Target the bands overlying (extrinsic ligaments) and between (intrinsic ligaments) the carpal bones.
- Redirect the needle as needed, targeting the ligaments with care to avoid the neurovascular bundle.
- Redirect proximal to target ligaments over the first proximal row and between the first carpal row and the distal radius and ulna as well.

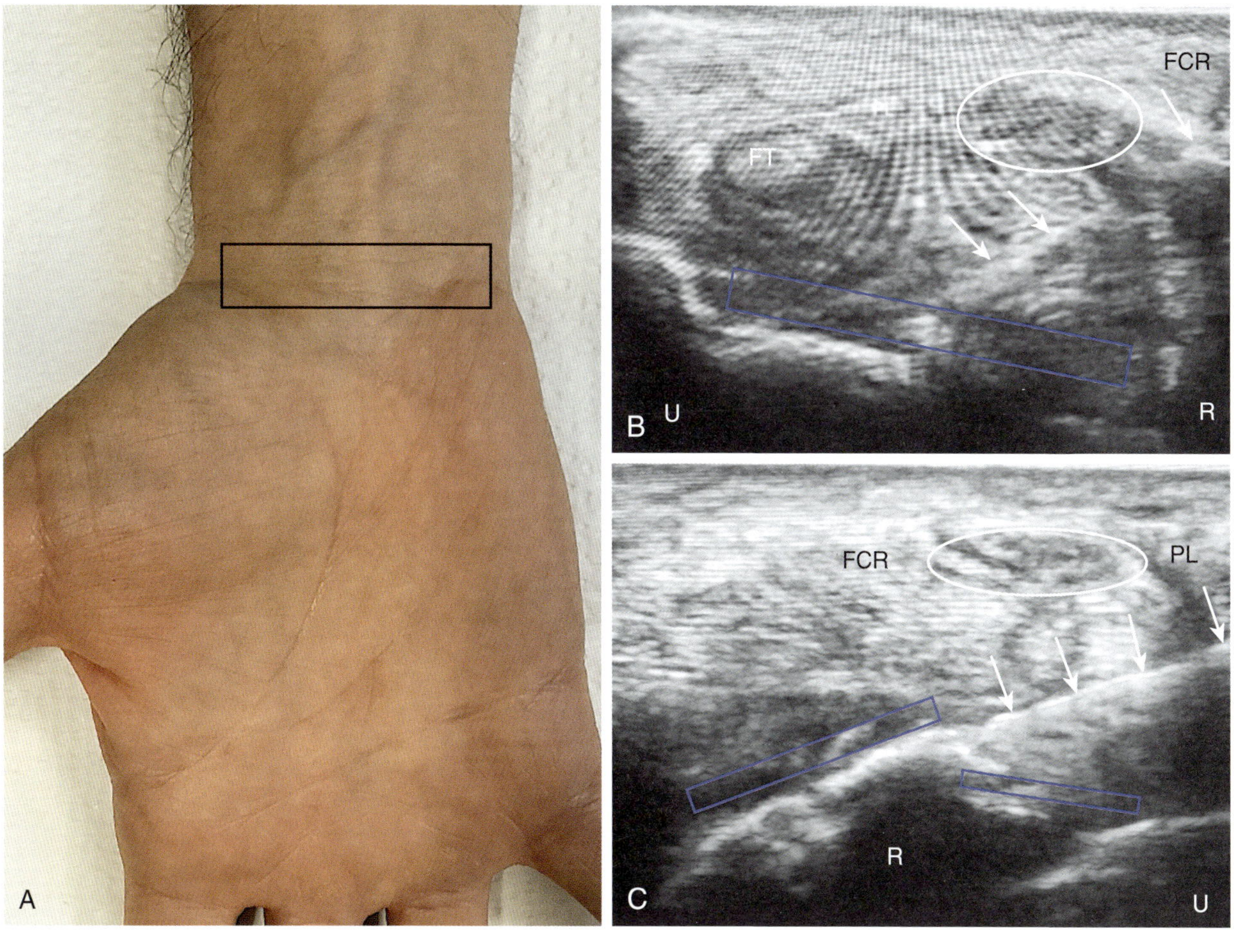

• **Fig. 18.5** Sonographic Images of Volar Wrist Ligament Injections. (A) Transducer placement *(black rectangle)* along the volar wrist. (B) Needle placement along the volar wrist ligaments *(blue rectangles)*, needle *(white arrows)* traversing radial to ulnar. (C) Needle placement *(white arrows)* along the volar wrist ligaments, needle traversing ulnar to radial. *FCR*, Flexor carpi radialis; PL, palmar ligament; *R*, radius; *U*, ulna.

PEARLS AND PITFALLS

- Be sure to always visualize needle tips and avoid the neurovascular structures.
- Variances in anatomy will determine how many of the ligaments will be accessible

Dorsal Compartments of the Wrist (1 to 6) Injection

KEY POINTS

- The first and sixth compartments are most commonly clinically involved.[2]
- The first compartment tendons may have a separate sheath that may require separate injections to adequately resolve pain in this region.[2]

Pertinent Anatomy

- Six compartments on the dorsal side of the wrist house the extensor tendons, and the tendons are held in place by the overlying extensor retinaculum (Fig. 18.6). The compartments are numbered from lateral to medial, and contents include:
  - First–abductor pollicis longus (APL) and extensor pollicis brevis (EPB)
  - Second–extensor carpi radialis longus and brevis (ECRL/ECRB)
  - Third–extensor pollicis longus (EPL)
  - Forth–extensor digitorum and extensor indices (lies deep to digitorum) (EDC, EIP)
  - Fifth–extensor digiti minimi/quinti (EDM/EDQ)
  - Sixth–extensor carpi ulnaris (ECU)
- The superficial radial nerve traverses over the first dorsal compartment and divides into the SR3 and SR2 branches just proximal to the extensor retinaculum (Fig. 18.7A and B).[7] The SR2 branch courses from volar to dorsal over the first compartment, often just proximal to the proximal edge of the retinaculum (see Fig. 18.7A and B).[25]
- The cephalic vein has a branch that is typically located over or slightly dorsal to the first dorsal compartment (see Fig. 18.7D).

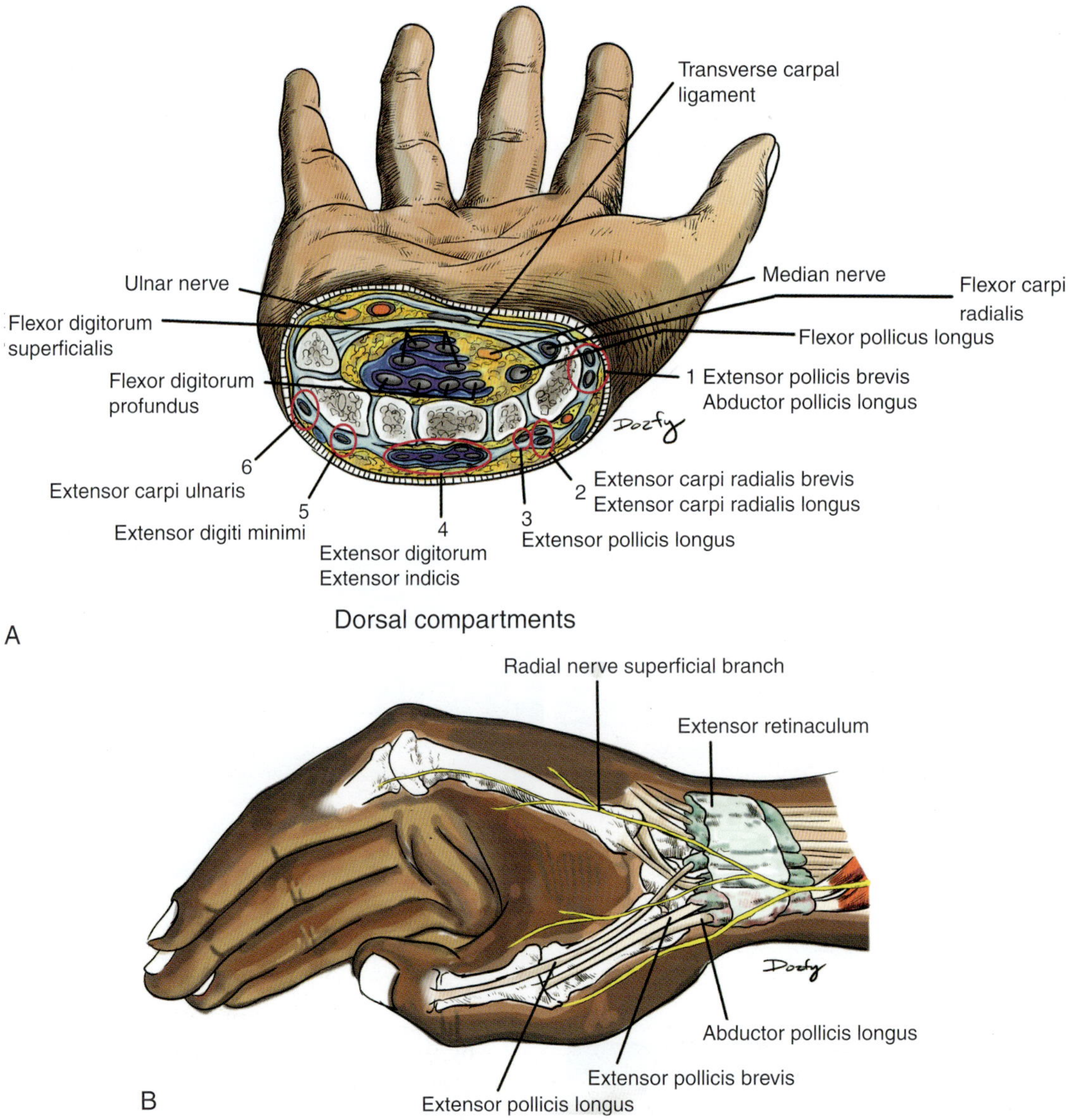

• **Fig. 18.6** The Six Dorsal Compartments of the Wrist. (A) Transverse wrist.

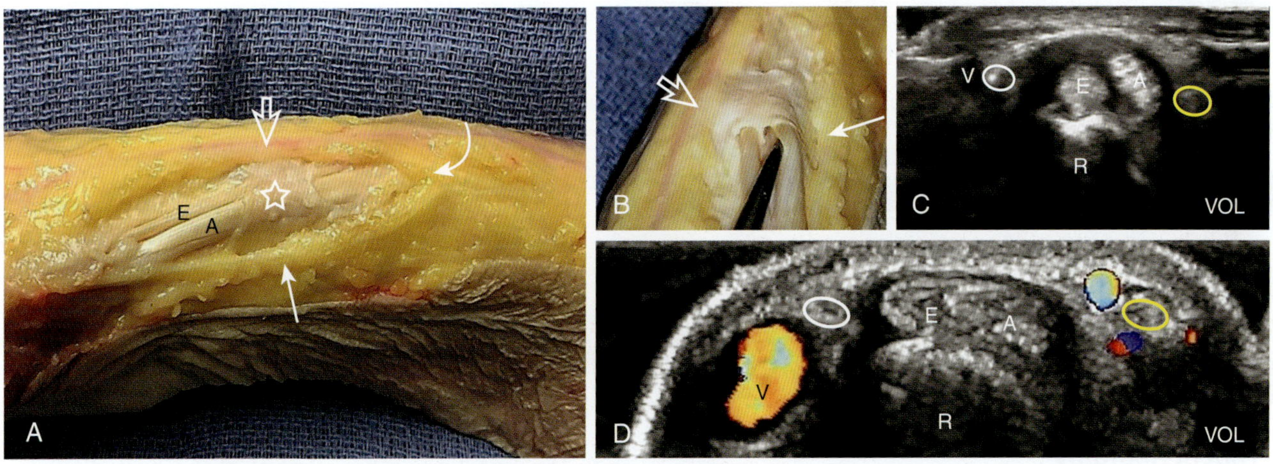

• **Fig. 18.7 Anatomy of the First Dorsal Compartment.** (A and B) Cadaveric dissection of the compartment showing the abductor pollicis longus *(A)*, extensor pollicis brevis *(E)*, retinaculum *(open star)*, the bifurcation of the superficial radial nerve *(curved arrow)* and the SR2 *(open arrow)* and SR3 *(white arrow)* branches. (C and D) Sonographic axial images of the first dorsal compartment. Note the SR2 *(white oval)* and SR3 *(yellow oval)*. *R,* Radius; *V,* adjacent cephalic vein.

- The first compartment can be divided into separate synovial sheaths and compartments for the APL and EPB tendons by an intra-compartment septum in up to 33% of patients. Implications include isolated tenosynovitis of the EPB or APL and may be clinically significant for the treatment of de Quervain's syndrome[7] (see Fig. 18.7B and C).
- The APL tendon often has multiple slips, which can be mistaken as longitudinal split tearing.[12,26]
- Anatomic variations may also be seen in the second dorsal compartment, such as the extensor carpi radialis intermedius, which should not be mistaken for a longitudinal split tear.[8]

Common Pathology

- Stenosing tenosynovitis most commonly involves the first (de Quervain's syndrome) and sixth dorsal compartments.[27,28]
- The mechanism of action is believed to be repetitive microtrauma related to occupation or sporting activities at the distal radial styloid, causing degeneration and inflammation in the APL and EPB tendons.[29,30]
- Tenosynovitis is seen more commonly in those with diabetes mellitus or autoimmune conditions such as rheumatoid arthritis.[4,19,28]
- The first compartment crossing over the second (proximal intersection syndrome) and the third compartment crossing over the second (distal intersection syndrome) can be other areas of pathology.[31]

Equipment

- High-frequency linear array transducer.
- Smaller footprint or hockey stick probes may be easier to use.
- 30 to 25 gauge, 1 to 2 inch needle.

Common Injectates

- Local anesthetics for diagnostics, corticosteroids into tendon sheaths only
- Prolotherapy
- Orthobiologics (PRP, bone marrow concentrate, etc.)

Injectate Volume

- 1 to 2 cc

Technique

Patient Position

- First to second compartments: Seated or supine on the table with the forearm in neutral position (thumb pointed upward) for (Fig. 18.8A and B).
- Third and fifth compartments: Seated or supine on the table with the forearm pronated (see Fig. 18.8C and D).
- Sixth compartment: Supine with the forearm pronated over a pillow on the chest (see Fig. 18.8E and F).

Clinician Position

- Seated or standing on the side of the patient's wrist.

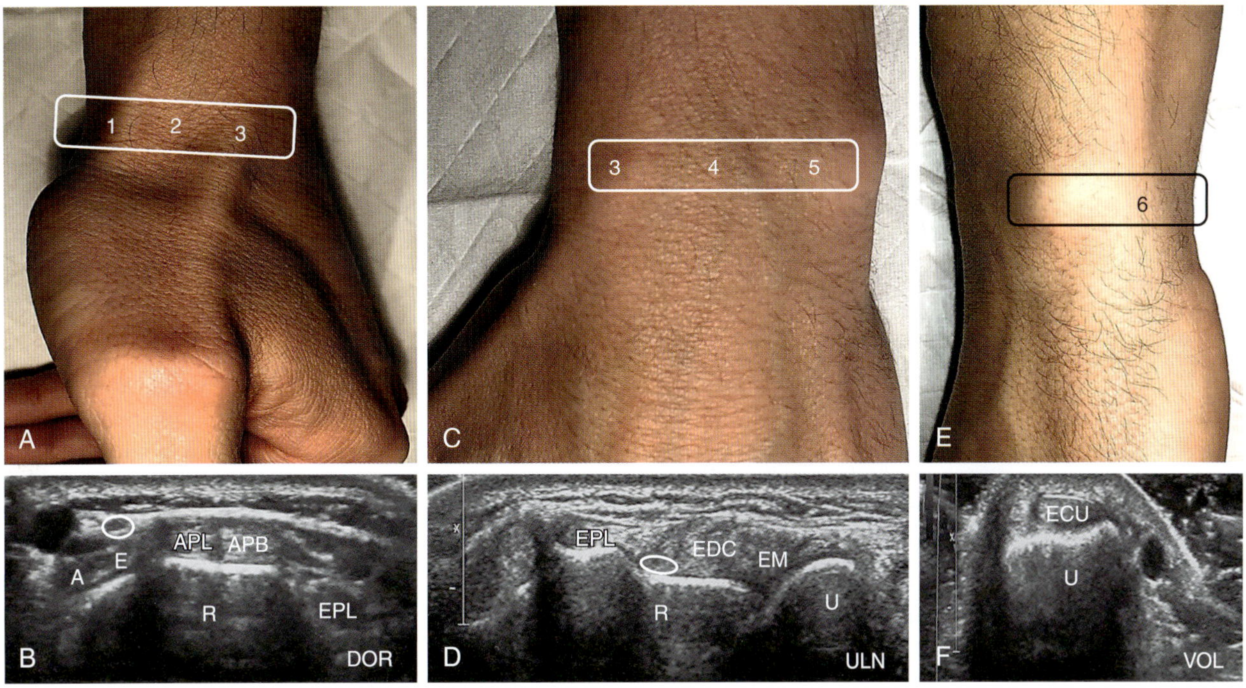

• **Fig. 18.8** Transducer Placement and Sonographic Images of The Six Dorsal Compartments. (A and B) Compartments 1–3, (C and D) Compartments 3–5, (E and F) 6th compartment. A, abductor pollicis longus; E, extensor pollicis brevis; EM, extensor digiti minimi; ECU, extensor carpi ulnaris; *EDC*, Extensor digitorum; *EPL*, extensor pollicis longus; *R*, radius.

Transducer Orientation

- The anatomic axial plane, short axis relative to the desired tendon (in-plane technique) (Fig. 18.9A and B).
- Alternative position: sagittal to the long axis of the distal forearm/tendon (in or out-of-plane technique) (see Fig. 18.9A and C).

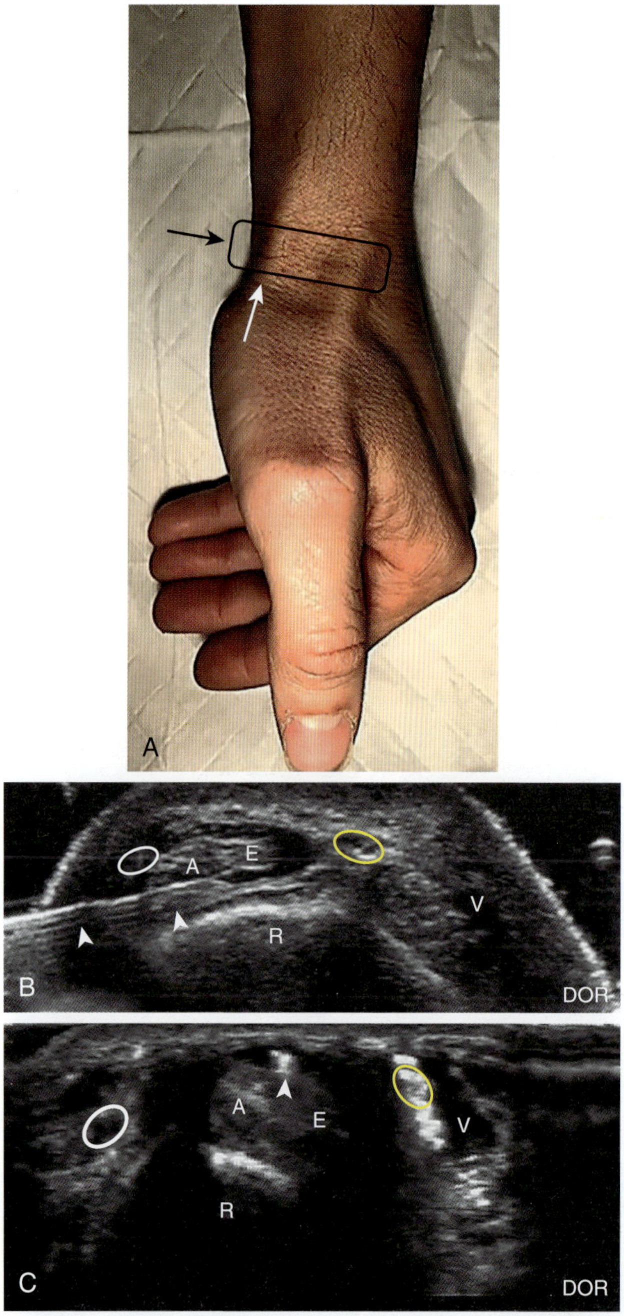

• **Fig. 18.9** Injection Technique for First Dorsal Compartment. (A) Transducer placement *(black rectangle)*; in-plane approach, *black arrow*, out-of-plane approach, *white arrow*. (B) Sonographic image of in-plane injection, needle *(arrowheads)* placed deep to the abductor pollicis longus *(A)* and extensor pollicis brevis *(E)* tendons. (C) Sonographic image of out-of plane approach; note hyperechoic needle tip *(arrowhead)* superficial to the tendons. *Yellow oval,* SR2; *white oval,* SR3; *V,* cephalic vein; *I*, radius.

Needle Orientation

- The needle is introduced via an ulnar-to-radial, radial-to-ulnar, or in the case of the ECU tendon volar-to-dorsal or dorsal-to volar direction.

Target

- Tendon sheath of EPB/APL
- If using prolotherapy or orthobiologics, inject directly into the tendon

PEARLS AND PITFALLS

- It is important to recognize anatomic variants of the first and second dorsal compartment as they may affect treatment outcomes or approaches.
- Note the presence of subcompartmentalization for first dorsal compartment injections, with a septum separating the APL and EPB. In cases with distinct tendon sheaths, injecting only one sheath may be associated with poor treatment outcomes.[27,32-34]
- The use of the gel standoff technique helps with the accurate initial placement of the needle during an in-plane approach.
- Tendon sheath distention during injection ensures accurate placement of the injectate.
- The SR2 and SR3 branches of the superficial radial nerve should be identified and avoided during first compartment procedures.
- The use of particulate corticosteroids can increase the risk of skin depigmentation, especially with superficial injections.[35]

Ultrasound-Guided Ganglia Injection

KEY POINTS

- Ganglion cysts are often associated with joint, joint capsule, or tendon sheath injury. These underlying causes should be evaluated and treats as needed as well.

Pertinent Anatomy

- Location of ganglion cysts can be variable, with a majority (up to 70%) occurring in the dorsal wrist.[36]
- The majority of cysts in the hand originate from the scapholunate joint dorsally, while ventral cysts will originate from the radiocarpal or scaphotrapezial joints (see Fig. 18.11B and C).[24]
- Dorsal cysts arising from the scapholunate joint can impinge on the PIN (see Fig. 18.11B and C).
- On the volar side, the cyst most commonly arises from the radiocarpal joint, the radial artery and superficial radial nerve typically are superficial and radial to the cyst. The median nerve is typically ulnar to the cyst (see Fig. 18.10B and C). A volar cyst can also originate from other areas, such as between the pisiform and triquetrum, with impingement of the ulnar neurovascular structures.

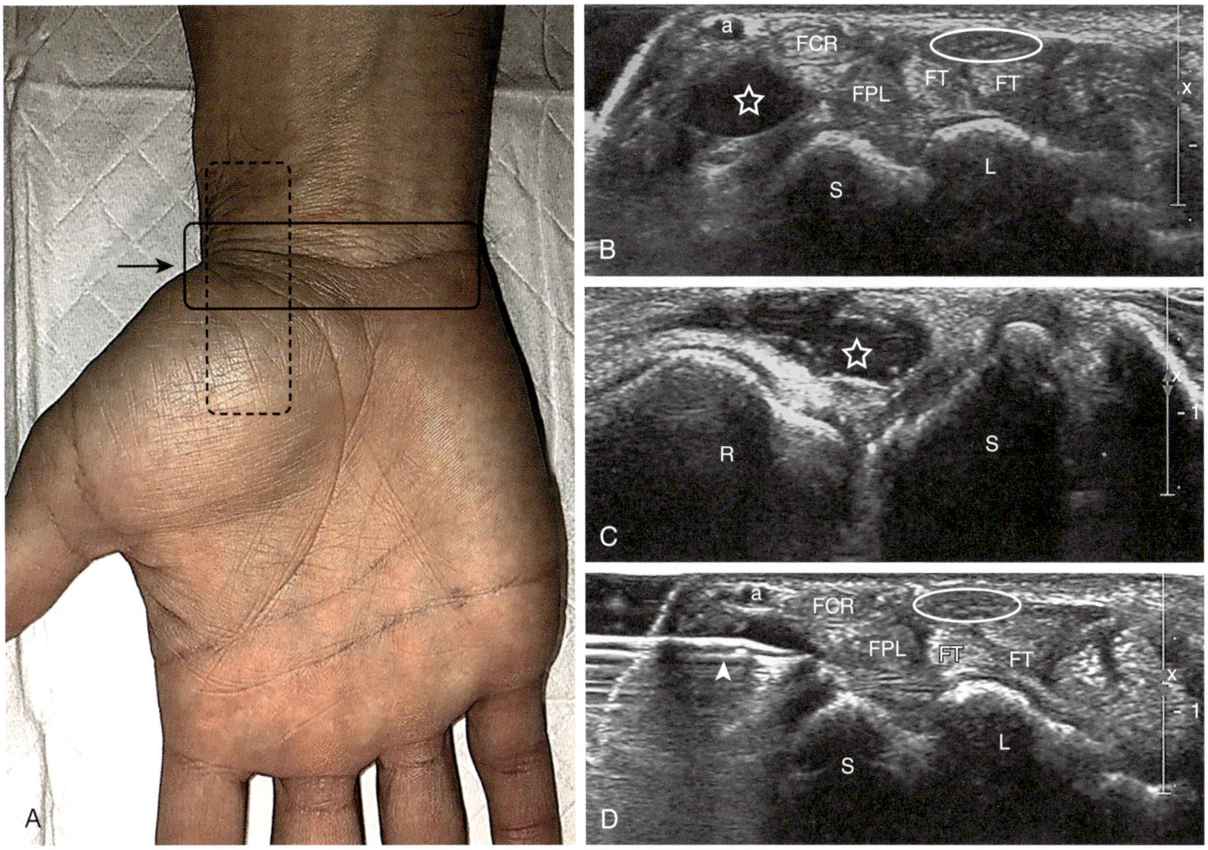

• **Fig. 18.10** Volar Wrist Ganglion Cyst Aspiration/Injection. (A) Transducer placement: axial to wrist, *solid black rectangle*, sagittal to wrist, *dashed rectangle*. (B and C) Sonographic appearance of ganglion cyst *(open star)*. (D) Needle *(arrowhead)* placement into the cyst. *a,* Radial artery; *FCR,* flexor carpi radialis; *FPL,* flexor pollicis longus; *FT,* flexor tendon; *L,* lunate; *R,* radius; *S,* scaphoid; *white oval*, median nerve.

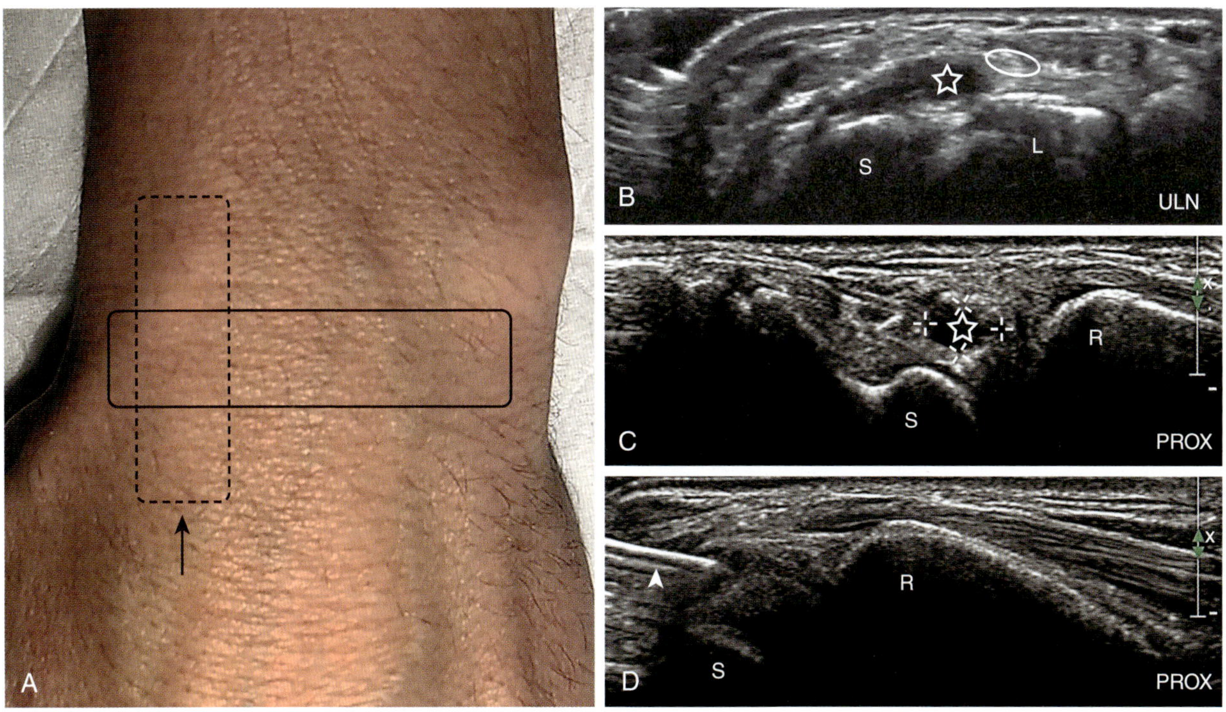

• **Fig. 18.11** Dorsal Wrist Ganglion Cyst Aspiration/Injection. (A) Transducer placement: axial to wrist, *solid black rectangle*, sagittal to wrist, *dashed rectangle*. (B and C) Sonographic appearance of ganglion cyst *(open star)*. (D) Needle *(arrowhead)* placement into the cyst. *L,* Lunate; *R,* radius; *S,* scaphoid; *white oval,* posterior interosseous nerve.

Common Pathology

- Ganglion cysts can average 1 to 2 cm in diameter and can be described as firm, nodular structures connected to a nearby joint capsule or tendon sheath.[37] These synovial cysts are typically lined with a thin connective tissue layer and filled with gelatinous mucoid material.[9]
- Common complaints from the patient include wrist pain aggravated by moving the wrist. Depending on the location, cysts can impinge on the neurovascular structures, causing either pain or paresthesia's.[38]

Equipment

- Anesthetic needle size: 25 or 27 gauge needle, 31.75 and 38 mm
- Cyst penetration and aspiration: 18 gauge, 38 mm needle
- High-frequency linear array ultrasound transducer
- Depending on the location of the cyst, a gel standoff may be used to help needle visualization and access to the cyst

Common Injectates

- Aspirate
- After aspiration:
  - Local anesthetics and corticosteroids
  - Prolotherapy
  - Sclerosing agents
  - Orthobiologics (PRP, bone marrow concentrate, etc.)

Technique

Patient Position

- The wrist may be pronated or supinated based on the location of the ganglion cyst (dorsal or volar, respectively) (Fig. 18.11A; see also Fig. 18.10A).

Clinician Position

- Seated or standing facing the patient's wrist and monitor.

Transducer Orientation

- For a volar ganglion cyst, the transducer is placed axial or sagittal to the ganglion cyst, depending on the safest anatomic window for approach (see Fig. 18.10A and C).
- For a dorsal ganglion cyst, the transducer is placed axial or sagittal to the ganglion cyst, depending on the safest anatomic window for approach (see Fig. 18.11A and C).

Needle Orientation

- Depending on the safest approach, an in-plane radial-to-ulnar or proximal-to-distal trajectory may be used (see Fig. 18.10D).

Target

- The needle tip should be placed in the center of the cyst (see Fig. 18.11A and D).

PEARLS AND PITFALLS

- Gel standoff may be helpful in maintaining contact over the area of interest.
- High-viscosity ganglion fluid can make aspiration difficult unless using a larger-gauge needle. (see Fig. 18.11D).
- Cyst lavage may be necessary with local anesthetic or sterile saline.[39]

Flexor Carpi Radialis Tendon and Sheath Injection

Pertinent Anatomy

- The flexor carpi radialis (FCR) is the most radial and superficial of all the flexor tendons and does not pass through the carpal tunnel. The transverse carpal ligament (TCL) splits around the FCR, dividing into deep and superficial components that create a separate fibro-osseous tunnel for the FCR tendon.[40]
- The radial artery is located just radial to the FCR tendon.
- The palmar cutaneous branch of the median nerve (PCN) is located between the FCR and, if present, the palmaris tendon.[40]
- The FCR inserts into the base of the second and third metacarpal and can be followed longitudinally to its insertion to confirm location.[10]

Common Pathology

- As the FCR passes over the scaphoid, it can develop attritional injuries in patients with radiocarpal, scaphotrapezial trapezoidal, and first carpometacarpal osteoarthritis.[12]
- Pathology is commonly seen in tennis players and golfers.[12]

Equipment

- 27 to 25 gauge, 31.75 and 38 mm needle
- High-frequency linear array ultrasound transducer

Common Injectates

- Local anesthetics for diagnostics, corticosteroids in the sheath only
- Prolotherapy
- Orthobiologics (PRP, etc.)

Injectate Volume

- 1 and 2 cc

Technique

Patient Position

- Elbow flexed, wrist supination with the patient sitting, or lateral recumbent with arm forearm supinated.

Clinician Position

- Seated or standing facing the wrist and monitor.

Transducer Orientation

- With the transducer placed in the anatomic axial plane short axis to the tendon.

Needle Orientation

- In-plane, radial-to-ulnar direction, deep to the FCR tendon at the level of the scaphoid (Fig. 18.12A–C).

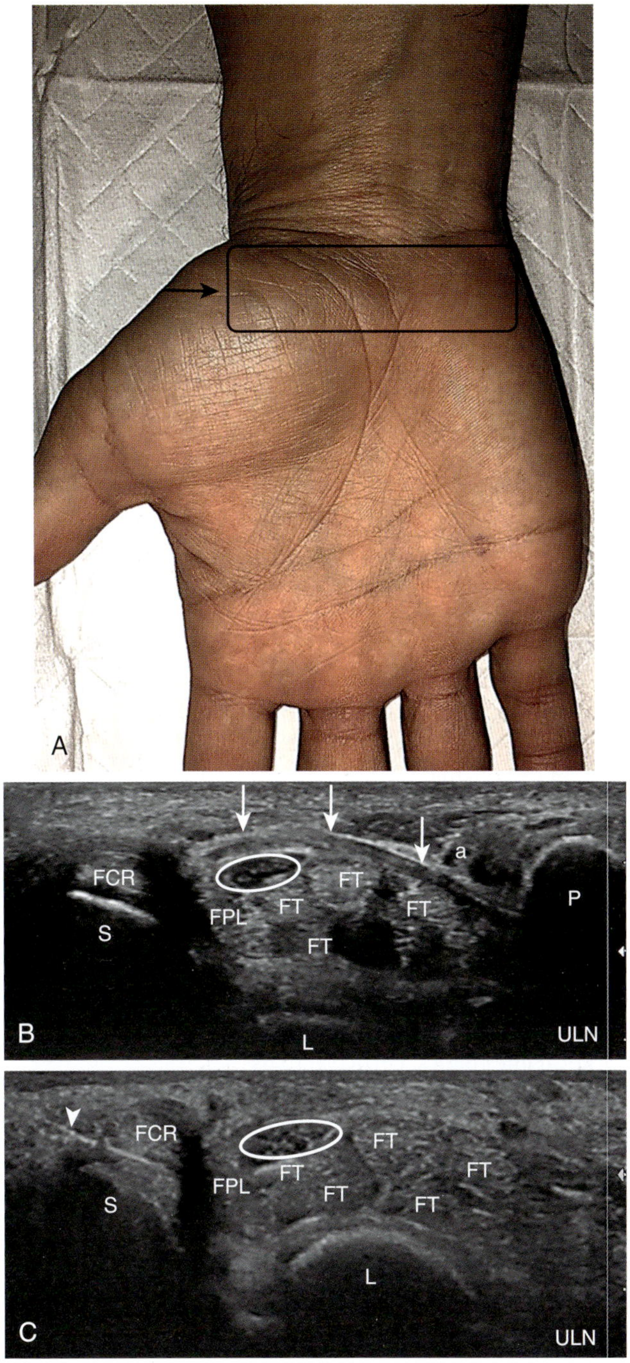

• **Fig. 18.12** Flexor Carpi Radialis *(FCR)* Tendon Sheath Injection. (A) Transducer placement *(black rectangle)*; needle trajectory, *black arrow*. (B) Axial sonographic image of the volar wrist; note FCR tendon superficial to the scaphoid (S). (C) Sonographic image of FCR tendon sheath injection with needle in place (*arrowhead*). *a*, Ulnar artery; *FPL*, flexor pollicis longus; *FT*, flexor tendons; *L*, lunate; *P*, pisiform; *white arrows*, transverse carpal ligament overlying carpal tunnel entrance.

Target

- Tendon sheath if diagnostics or steroids
- Pathologic areas of the tendon if prolotherapy or orthobiologics are utilized

PEARLS AND PITFALLS

- Have the patient flex the wrist against resistance, and the tendon of the FCR will be visualized most proximal to the thumb.[41]
- The palmar cutaneous nerve (PCN), radial artery, and median nerve locations should be identified for avoidance during procedures involving the FCR tendon.

Flexor Carpi Ulnaris Tendon Lavage for Calcific Tendonitis

Pertinent Anatomy

- The ulnar nerve and artery are adjacent and radial to the flexor carpi ulnaris (FCU) tendon when followed from the forearm distally.[2]
- The FCU is innervated by the ulnar nerve and functions to flex, and ulnarly deviate the wrist.[2]
- The FCU does not have a tendon sheath and inserts distally into the pisiform, hamate, and fifth metacarpal.[2]

Common Pathology

- Pathology in the region is relatively rare; however, there are case reports of tendinopathy as well as calcium hydroxyapatite disease involving the FCU.[42]

Equipment

- 30 and 25 gauge needle, 38 mm
- High-frequency linear array ultrasound transducer
- Several syringes of sterile, normal saline may be needed to lavage the calcium deposit if present

Common Injectates

- Anesthetize the skin and tendon with the anesthetic of choice.
- Corticosteroids can be deposited parallel/outside the tendon versus orthobiologics in the sheath or tendon, based on provider preference.

Injectate Volume

- 0.5 and 1 cc

Author's Preferred Technique

Patient Position

- A supine or lateral recumbent with the arm at the side and forearm supinated.

Clinician Position

- Seated or standing facing the wrist and monitor.

Transducer Orientation

- The transducer is placed in the anatomic axial plane, short axis to the FCU tendon proximal to the pisiform (Fig. 18.13A).

Needle Orientation

- The needle is introduced via an in-plane ulnar-to-radial direction.
- A gel standoff is used ulnarly to better visualize the needle.

Target

- The pathologic areas of the tendon for the calcific lavage or injection of the tendon itself (see Fig. 18.13A and B).

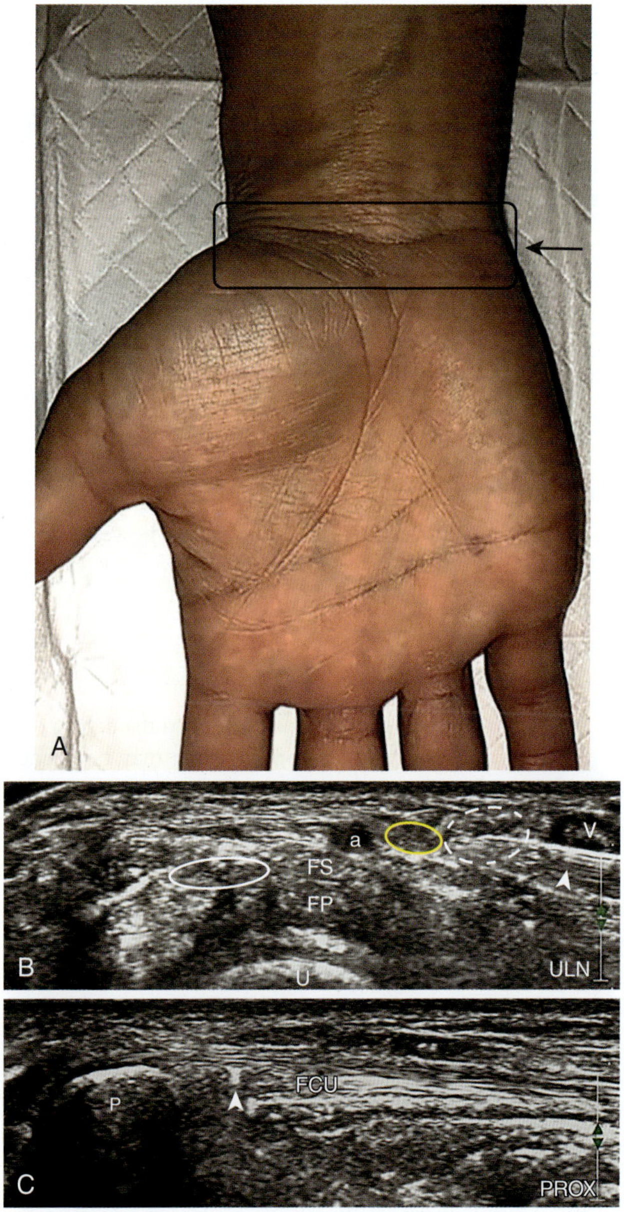

• **Fig. 18.13** Flexor Carpi Ulnaris Injection/Aspiration. (A) Transducer placement *(black rectangle)* and needle trajectory *(black arrow)*. Sonographic images of the needle *(arrowhead)* placed in plane (B) and out of plane (C) within the flexor carpi ulnaris *(FCU)* tendon. *a,* Ulnar artery; *FP,* flexor digitorum profundus; *FS,* flexor digitorum superficialis; *P,* pisiform; *U,* ulna; *yellow oval,* ulnar nerve.

PEARLS AND PITFALLS

- Color Doppler can be used to identify the at-risk ulnar neurovascular structures prior to the procedure.

Carpal Tunnel Injection (i.e., Median Nerve Hydrodissection)

Pertinent Anatomy

- The carpal tunnel is bounded by the scaphoid and pisiform proximally and tubercle of the trapezium and hook of the hamate distally. The TCL overlies the tunnel.[40]
- Contents of the tunnel include the median nerve, flexor pollicis longus, and the tendons of the flexor digitorum superficialis and profundus (Fig. 18.14).[40]

Common Pathology

- Compression of the median nerve can be related to thickening of the TCL, ganglion cysts, tenosynovitis, amyloidosis, joint effusions/synovitis, aneurysms, lipomatous hamartomas, and accessory muscles.[43,44]
- It is the most common site of nerve compression in the upper extremity, with an incidence of 3.5% and 6.2%.[43,45]
- There are many anatomic variants of the median nerve that need to be taken into consideration when doing injections about the carpal tunnel. The most common anatomic variant is that of a persistent median artery with a bifid median nerve.[13,46]
- There are also anatomic variants of the thenar motor branch, which should be identified prior to procedures about the median nerve.[47]
- For further information on anatomic variants, please see Chapter 32.

Equipment

- 30 to 25-gauge needle, 1 and 2 inch
- High-frequency linear array ultrasound transducer

Common Injectates

- Local anesthetics, corticosteroids
- Neuroprolotherapy (5% dextrose)
- Orthobiologics (PRP, platelet lysate)

Injectate Volume

- 1 to 5 cc

Technique

Patient Position

- Seated with the elbow flexed and the wrist supinated, with fingers relaxed.
- An alternate position is lateral recumbent or supine with the arm at the side, on the arm board.

Clinician Position

- Seated or standing facing the patient's wrist and monitor.

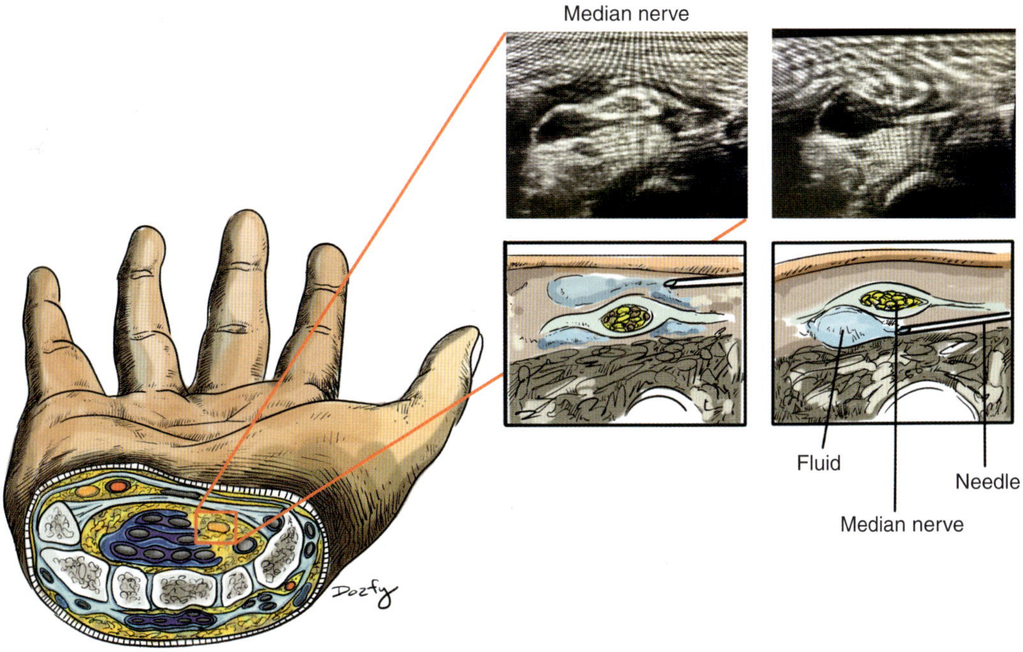

• **Fig. 18.14** Median Nerve Hydrodissection at The Wrist Under Ultrasound Guidance.

Transducer Orientation

- The transducer is placed in the anatomic axial plane, short axis to the median nerve, identifying the proximal and distal carpal tunnel and any anatomic variants that would prohibit a safe injection (Fig. 18.15A–C).

Needle Orientation

- The needle is introduced via an in-plane, ulnar-to-radial approach.
- Alternatively, an out-of-plane, distal-proximal or proximal-to-distal approach can be used with the transducer in the same position (see Fig. 18.15A and E).

Target

- Place the needle both superficial and deep to the median nerve at the level of the proximal carpal tunnel (see Fig. 18.15B and D). Anesthetic and sterile saline is used to create a halo around the nerve for the hydrodissection.
- With the alternative out-of-plane approach, the goal is to stay ulnar to the nerve.

PEARLS AND PITFALLS

- Color Doppler will help visualize the ulnar artery and ensure safe needle placement away from the vasculature.
- An ultrasound can be used for real-time visualization of injectate flow along the nerve by moving the transducer along the length of the nerve.
- A gel standoff is recommended during an in-plane approach to avoid the ulnar artery and nerve.
- Identification of at-risk structures and understanding of possible variant anatomy prior to injection is recommended.

Ulnar Nerve Hydrodissection

Pertinent Anatomy

- Distal to Guyon's canal, the ulnar nerve splits into deep and superficial branches[40] (Fig. 18.16B and see also Fig. 18.15C).
- The ulnar artery travels with the ulnar nerve over the ulnar aspect of the wrist. Color Doppler can be used to help identify neurovascular structures.
- Anatomic variation of the ulnar nerve is present in 1% to 3% of the population, where the nerve travels in an osseo-fibrous canal distinct from Guyon's canal).[40]
  - This is usually situated on the anteromedial portion of the TCL spanning 4 cm from the pisiform to the hook of the hamate bifurcation, which may affect the approach/technique.[40]

Common Pathology

- The ulnar nerve at the wrist is subject to injuries related to hamate fractures, ganglion cysts, arterial aneurysms, nerve sheath tumors, repetitive compression, and ganglion (see Fig. 18.15B and D).[48,49]
- Typically, entrapment of the ulnar nerve at the wrist within or near Guyon's canal may have a positive Tinel sign over the ulnar nerve and decreased sensation over ulnar nerve distribution in the palm. If motor fibers are affected, there may be a positive Wartenberg's sign.[49]

Equipment

- 30 to 25 gauge needle, 1 and 2 inch
- High-frequency linear array ultrasound transducer

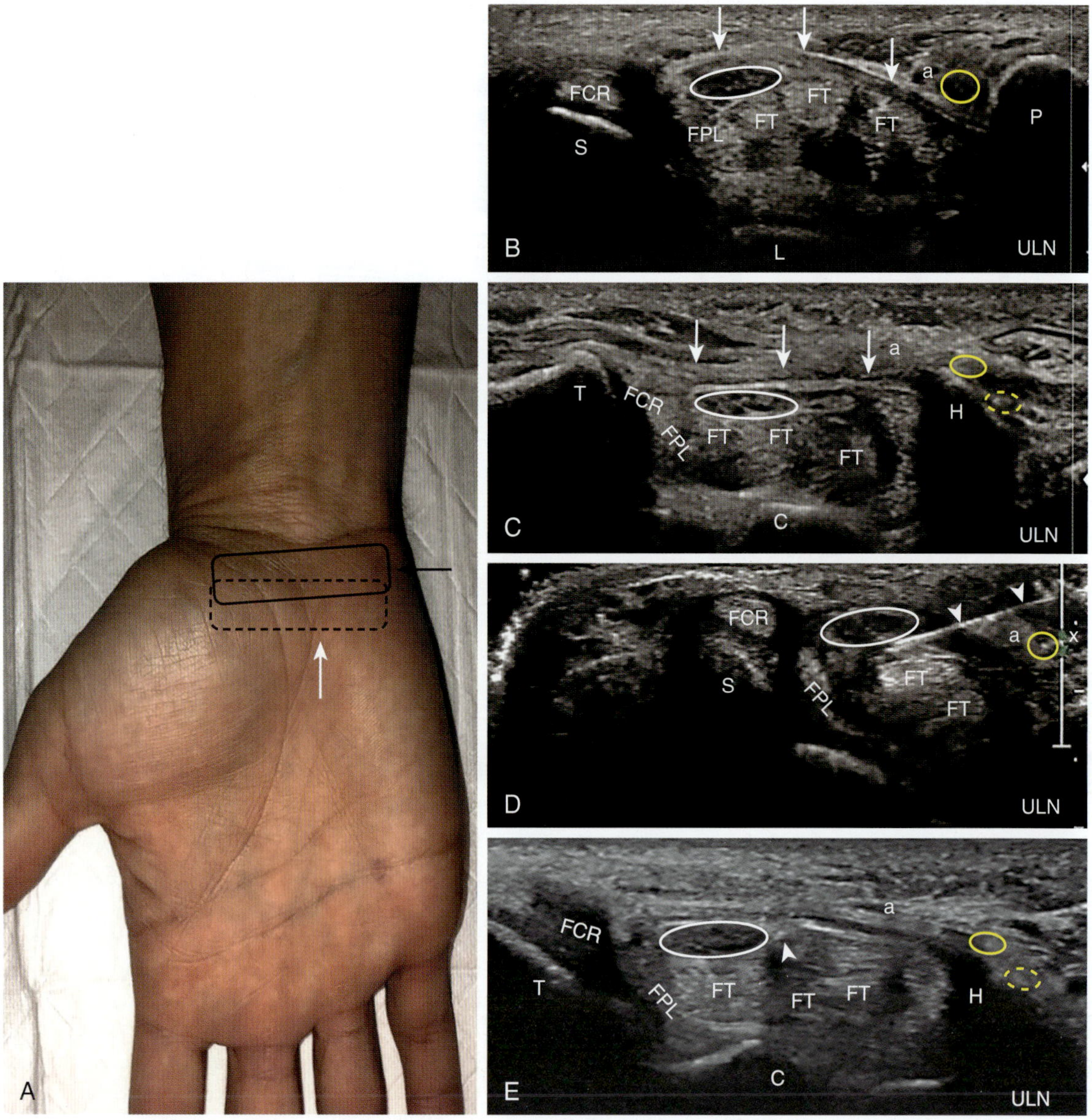

• **Fig. 18.15** Ultrasound-Guided Carpal Tunnel Injection. (A) Transducer placement axial to wrist *(dashed rectangle)*, axial oblique placement of transducer *(solid rectangle)*. Axial sonographic appearance of the proximal (B) and distal (C) portions of the tunnel. (D) In-plane approach. (E) Out-of-plane approach. *a,* Ulnar artery; *arrowhead*, needle; *FCR,* flexor carpi radialis; *FPL,* flexor pollicis longus; *FT,* flexor tendon; *L,* lunate; *H*, hook of hamate; *C*, capitate; *S*, scaphoid; *T,* trapezium; *white arrows,* transverse carpal ligament; *white oval,* median nerve; *yellow ovals,* ulnar nerve (*dashed,* deep motor branch of ulnar nerve).

Common Injectates

- Local anesthetics, corticosteroids
- Neuroprolotherapy (5% dextrose)
- Orthobiologics (PRP, platelet lysate)

Injectate Volume

- 3 to 5 mL of total solution

Technique

Patient Position

- Seated with the elbow flexed, wrist supinated with fingers relaxed (Fig. 18.17A).
- An alternate position is lateral recumbent or supine with the arm at the side, on the arm board.

Clinician Position

- Seated or standing facing the patient's wrist and monitor.

Transducer Orientation

- The transducer is placed in the anatomic axial plane, over the ulnar nerve, under the flexor carpi ulnaris (FCU) tendon (see Fig. 18.17A).
- Color Doppler can be used to identify the ulnar artery.

Needle Orientation

- The needle is introduced via an in-plane ulnar-to-radial direction.

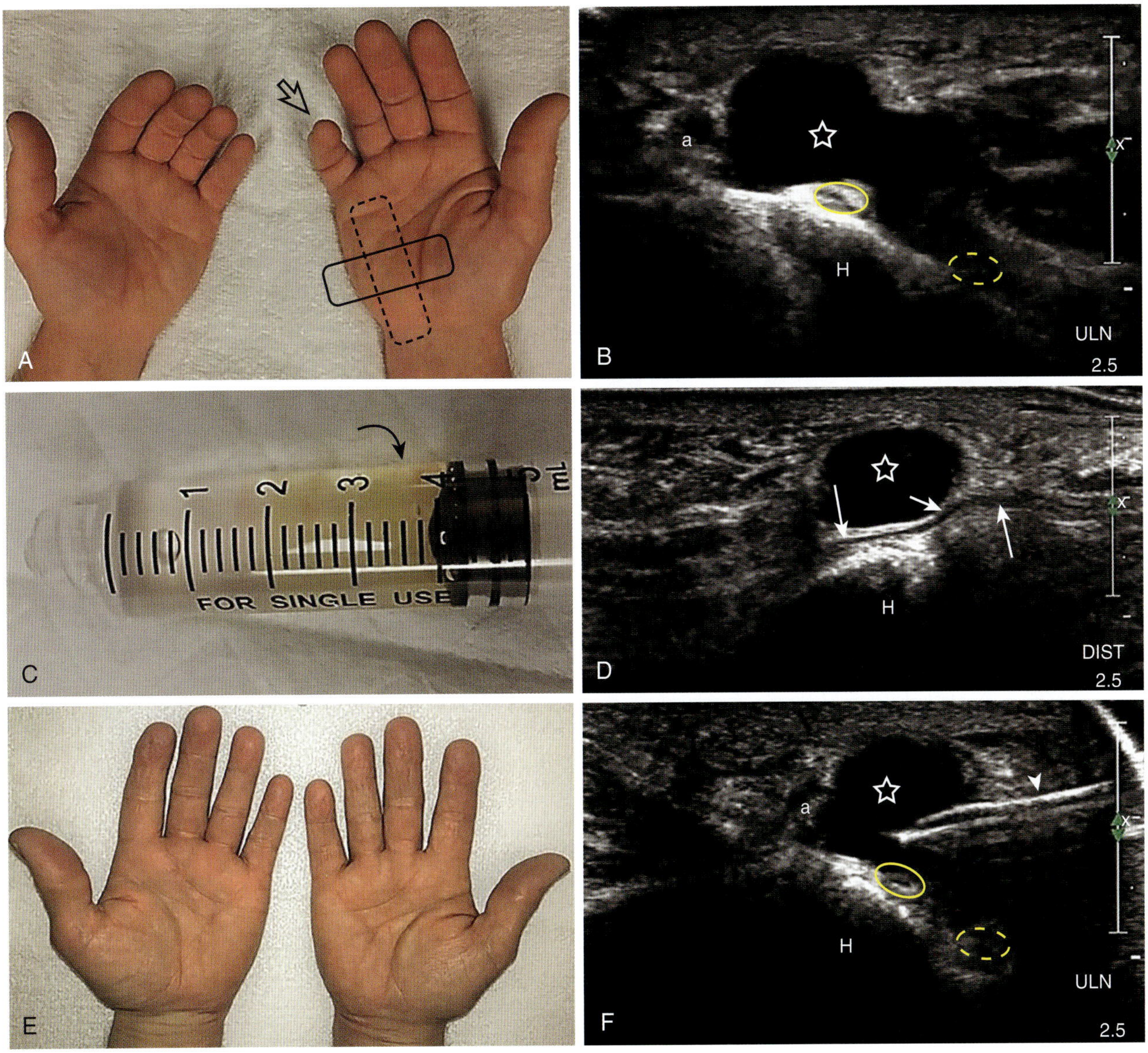

• **Fig. 18.16** Ganglion Cyst Guyon's Canal. (A) Transducer placement, axial *(solid rectangle)* and sagittal *(dashed rectangle)*. (B) Ganglion cyst overlying distal canal *(open star)*; note superficial *(solid yellow oval)* and deep *(dashed yellow oval)* branches of the ulnar nerve overlying the hook of hamate *(H)*. (C) Syringe with aspirated synovial fluid (black curved arrow). (D) Sagittal sonographic image of the ganglion cyst overlying the superficial branch of ulnar nerve *(white arrows)*, (E) Note slight atrophy of the hypothenar eminence. (F) Sonographic image of cyst aspiration\; needle, *white arrowhead; a*, ulnar artery.

Target

- Advance to the perineural space where injectate is used to create a halo surrounding the nerve (see Fig. 18.17A–C).

PEARLS AND PITFALLS

- Color Doppler will help visualize the ulnar artery and ensure safe needle placement away from the vasculature.
- As you are injecting, monitor the flow of solution along the nerve by moving the transducer along the length of the nerve.

Superficial Radial Nerve Hydrodissection/ Block

Pertinent Anatomy

- The superficial radial nerve divides into the SR3 and SR2 branches just proximal to the retinaculum of the first dorsal compartment (Fig. 18.18A and B).[7]
- The SR2 branch courses from volar to dorsal over the first compartment, often just proximal to the proximal edge of the retinaculum (see Fig. 18.18A).[25]
- At the wrist, the superficial radial nerve moves to a subcutaneous location and traverses between the brachioradialis and ECRL tendons.

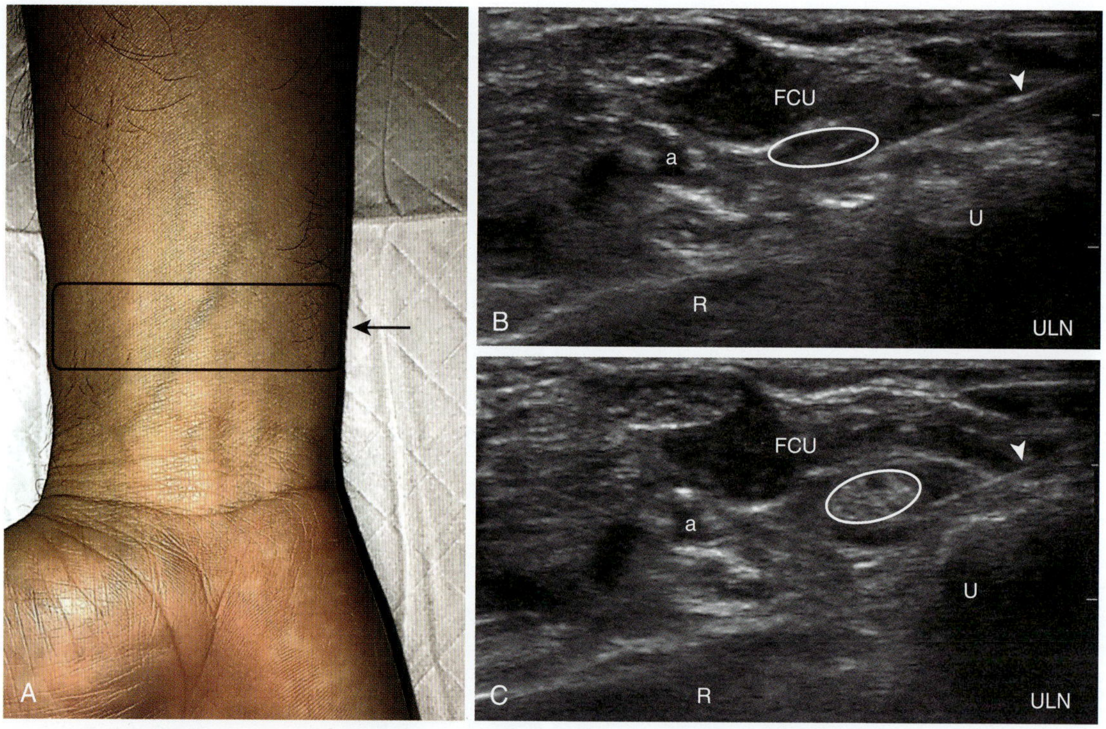

• **Fig. 18.17** Ulnar Nerve Hydrodissection. (A) Axial placement of the transducer *(black rectangle)* along volar distal forearm. (B) Needle *(arrowhead)* placement deep to the ulnar nerve *(white oval)* sitting just deep to the flexor carpi ulnaris *(FCU)* tendon. (C) Note hypoechoic fluid margin/halo around the ulnar nerve post-injection. *a,* Ulnar artery; *R,* radius; *U,* ulna,.

Common Pathology

- The nerve is subject to compression as it moves between the brachioradialis and ECRL tendons or from external compression, such as handcuffs or ligatures.[50]

Equipment

- 27 to 25 gauge needle, 31.75 to 38 mm
- High-frequency linear array ultrasound transducer

Common Injectates

- Local anesthetics, corticosteroids
- Neuroprolotherapy (5% dextrose)
- Orthobiologics (PRP, platelet lysate)

Injectate Volume

- 3 to 5 mL of total solution

Author's Preferred Technique

Patient Position

- Supine with the forearm in a neutral position (see Fig. 18.18A).

Clinician Position

- Seated or standing on the side of the patient's wrist.

Transducer Orientation

- The transducer is placed in the anatomic axial plane, short axis to the nerve proximal to the bifurcation into the SR2 and SR3 branches (see Fig. 18.18A and B).

Needle Orientation

- The needle is introduced via a dorsal-to-volar or volar-to-dorsal direction.

Target

- The needle is advanced to the perineural space with the goal of creating a halo of injectate around the nerve (see Fig. 18.18A and B).

PEARLS AND PITFALLS

- Superficial injection of corticosteroids increases the risk of skin depigmentation.
- As you are injecting, monitor the flow of solution along the nerve by moving the transducer along the length of the nerve.
- Care should be taken to make sure that the injection is performed proximal to bifurcation, thus getting both terminal branches of the nerve.

Dorsal Radioulnar Joint Fluoroscopic-Guided Injection

KEY POINTS

- Ionizing radiation necessitates shielded protection of the patient and staff.

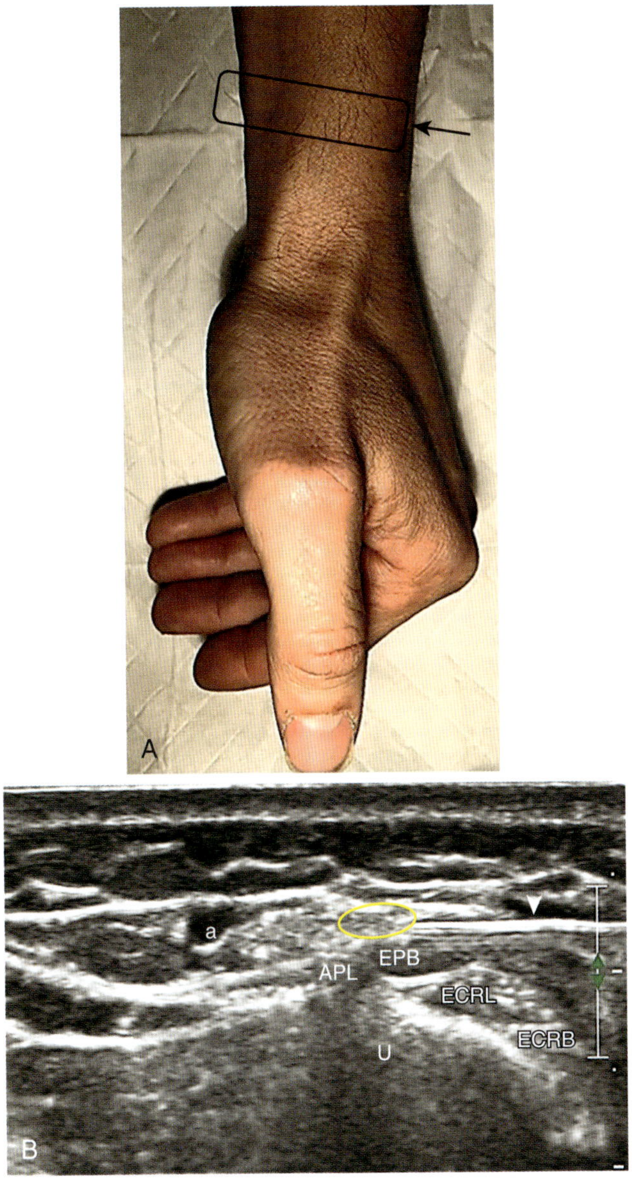

• **Fig. 18.18** Superficial Radial Nerve Hydrodissection. (A) Transducer placement axial to the distal forearm overlying the first dorsal compartment and branches of the superficial radial nerve, *black arrow* shows trajectory of needle. (B) Needle *(arrowhead)* placement deep to the superficial radial nerve *(yellow oval)*. *a,* Radial artery; *APL,* abductor pollicis longus; *ECRB,* extensor carpi radialis brevis; *EPB,* extensor pollicis brevis; *ECRL,* extensor carpi radialis longus.

Pertinent Anatomy

- The complex joint between the distal radius and the ulna.
- The TFC, volar and dorsal radioulnar ligaments, and ulnotriquetral and lunate ligaments, along with the tendon subsheath of the ECU, stabilize the distal radioulnar joint and provide shock absorption between the ulna and the carpus.[51-53]
- Injury typically occurs after a fall on an outstretched hand.[51]

Common Pathology

- TFCC tears are divided into traumatic or degenerative.[53]
- Traumatic tears usually involve a fall onto a pronated hand.
- Degenerative tears are related to repetitive shearing of the structure, and may be seen in conjunction when the ulna is longer than the radius, referred to as positive ulnar variance[53]

Equipment

- C-arm fluoroscopy
- 27 to 22 gauge, 1 and 2 inch needle

Common Injectates

- Local anesthetics for diagnostics, intra-articular corticosteroids only
- Prolotherapy
- Orthobiologics (PRP, bone marrow concentrate, etc.)

Injectate Volume

- 0.5 to 1.5 cc

Technique

Patient Position

- The patient will sit next to the table, with the arm abducted, the elbow flexed, and the placement of the prone wrist flat over a rolled towel.[54]

Clinician Position

- The clinician should be next to the affected hand.

Fluoroscope Position

- PA position centered on the DRUJ.

Needle Position

- Palpate medial to the border of the ulna head on the dorsal aspect.
- Mark the area with a needle tip.
- Slowly insert the needle into the joint (Fig. 18.19C).
- Use a dorsal-to-volar approach.

Target

- Medial border of the ulna head.
- If there is resistance, reposition the needle by advancing or removing it slightly. Confirm intra-articular placement with a small amount of contrast.

PEARLS AND PITFALLS

- To aid in stabilizing the joint, prolotherapy or orthobiologics can be used to target the volar and dorsal radioulnar ligaments, lunotriquetral and ulnolunate ligaments, and the TFC.
- Distal placement of the needle may cause an inadvertent injection in the radiocarpal joint.

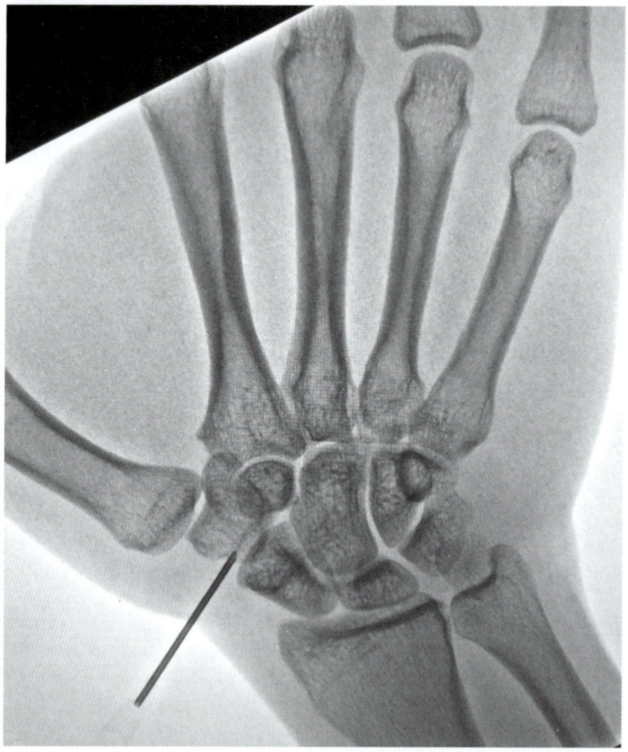

• **Fig. 18.19** Dorsal Fluoroscopic-Guided Injections of the Midcarpal and Distal Radioulnar Joints. (A) Needle position for injection of the midcarpal joint via the scaphotrapezial joint. (B) Needle position along with contrast distribution of the midcarpal joint when injected from the medial side of the joint. (C) Needle position and contrast flow of the distal radioulnar joint. Note contrast flow proximal to the triangular fibrocartilage complex (*white arrow*).

Distal Carpal Rows Fluoroscopic-Guided Injection

KEY POINT

- Ionizing radiation necessitates shielded protection of the patient and staff.

Pertinent Anatomy

- The midcarpal joint is found between the proximal and distal carpal bones.
- It is responsible for 60% of wrist flexion and about two-thirds of wrist extension.[55]
- The radioscaphoid column bridges the proximal and distal carpal rows on the radial side and articulates with the scaphoid fossa of the distal radius, the lunate, the capitate, the trapezium, and the trapezoid.
- The scaphoid distal pole transfers load from the thumb and radial side of the hand to the radioscaphoid and scaphocapitate joints
- The midcarpal joint is stabilized by the scaphocapitate, triquetrocapitatoscaphoid ligaments volarly, and the dorsal intercarpal ligament dorsally.[56]

Common Pathology

- The wrist is a relatively stable complex. Fracture or dislocation can lead to midcarpal joint instability.

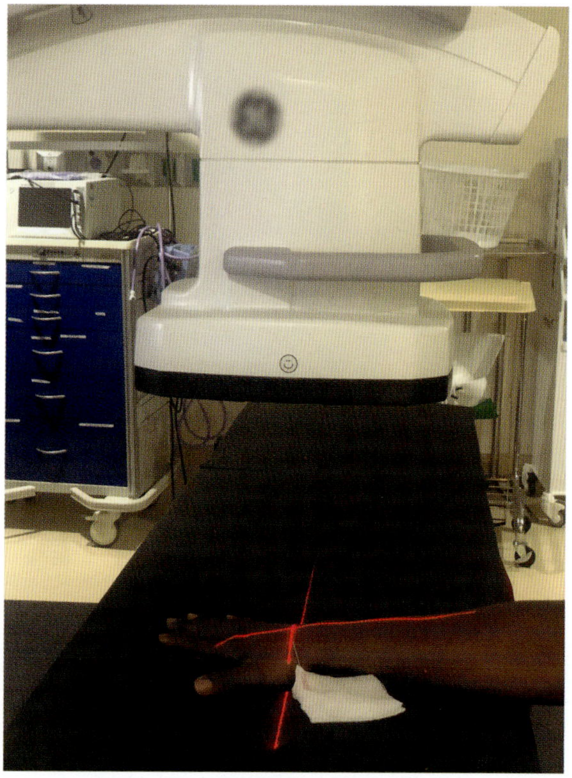

• **Fig. 18.20** Distal carpal setup, PA view.

- Dorsal midcarpal instability is often due to a high-energy injury and can present as subluxation or "clunk." In cases of true subluxation, surgery may be necessary to maintain anatomic position.
- Scaphoid-trapezium-trapezoid arthritis.

Equipment

- C arm fluoroscopy
- 27 to 25 gauge, 1 and 2 inch needle

Common Injectates

- Local anesthetics for diagnostics, intra-articular corticosteroids only
- Prolotherapy
- Orthobiologics (PRP, bone marrow concentrate, etc.)

Injectate Volume

- 0.5 to 1.5 cc

Technique

Patient Position

- A supine position with the elbow flexed, in a neutral positioning, and the wrist in pronation.
- The elbow is supported with the placement of towels.

Clinician position

- The clinician stands next to the affected wrist.

Fluoroscope position

- PA position centered on the scaphoid trapezium joint (Figs. 18.20 and 18.21).

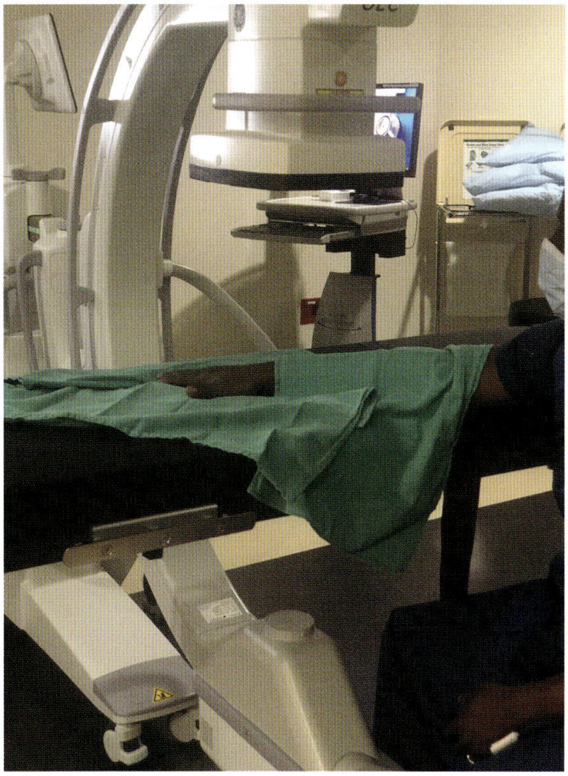

• **Fig. 18.21** Distal carpal setup, PA view.

Needle position

- Palpate for the distal border of the scaphoid bone dorsal aspect, and mark the area with a needle tip.
- Slowly insert the needle into the joint.

Target

- Dorsal to the scaphoid trapezium joint space (see Fig. 18.19A).
- Alternatively, the dorsal joint recess between the triquetrum and hamate allows for flow across the midcarpal joint space (see Fig. 18.19B).
- If there is resistance, reposition the needle by advancing or removing it slightly. Confirm intra-articular placement with the injection of a small amount of contrast.

PEARLS AND PITFALLS

- Monitoring contrast flow while injecting is important to assess for aberrant flow. Normally, contrast will flow into the carpometacarpal recesses of the index through the little fingers.[54,57,58] Contrast will also normally flow to the level of the proximal scapholunate and lunotriquetral joints.[59]

Proximal Carpal Rows Fluoroscopic-Guided Injection

KEY POINTS

- Ionizing radiation necessitates shielded protection of the patient and staff.
- The radiocarpal joint is the articulation between the proximal carpal row and the distal forearm construct: radius, ulnar, and the intervening triangular fibrocartilage complex.
- This joint normally does not communicate with the distal radioulnar or midcarpal joints.[58]

Pertinent Anatomy

- The radiocarpal joint can be palpated just distal to the distal radius in a depression near the scapholunate articulation.
- The SLLT complex is composed of volar, interosseous, and dorsal segments. Injury to the dorsal ligament can lead to instability of the joint.[60]
- Complete disruption of these ligaments will cause the scaphoid to flex relative to the lunate, known as a DISI (dorsal intercalated segment instability) deformity.[56]
- The lunotriquetral joint is stabilized by volar, proximal, and dorsal ligaments.[60]
- Complete injury to the lunotriquetral, ulnotriquetral, and anterior midpalmar ligaments allows the lunate to flex relative to the capitate, known as VISI (volar intercalated segment instability) deformity.[56]
- Radiographic clenched fist views demonstrating more than 2 mm of separation between the scaphoid and lunate signify the potential of a severe ligamentous injury.[61]
- Prolonged instability of the joint(s) can lead to the development of arthritis or scapholunate advanced collapse (SLAC) wrist deformity.[62]

Common Pathology

- Intercarpal ligament injury
- Wrist arthritis

Equipment

- C-arm fluoroscopy
- 27 to 22 gauge, 1 and 2 inch needle

Common Injectates

- Local anesthetics for diagnostics, intra-articular corticosteroids only
- Prolotherapy
- Orthobiologics (PRP, bone marrow concentrate, etc.)

Injectate Volume

- 0.5 to 1.5 cc

Technique

Patient Position

- The patient should be in supine position with the elbow flexed, in a neutral positioning, and the wrist in pronation.
- The elbow is supported with the placement of towels.

Clinician Position

- The clinician stands next to the affected wrist.

Fluoroscope Position

- PA position centered on the scapholunate or triquetrohamate or radiocarpal joint depending on the ligament or joint target, respectively (Figs. 18.22 and 18.23).

Needle Position

- Palpate for the dorsal aspect of the scapholunate or triquetrohamate space, and mark the area with a needle tip.

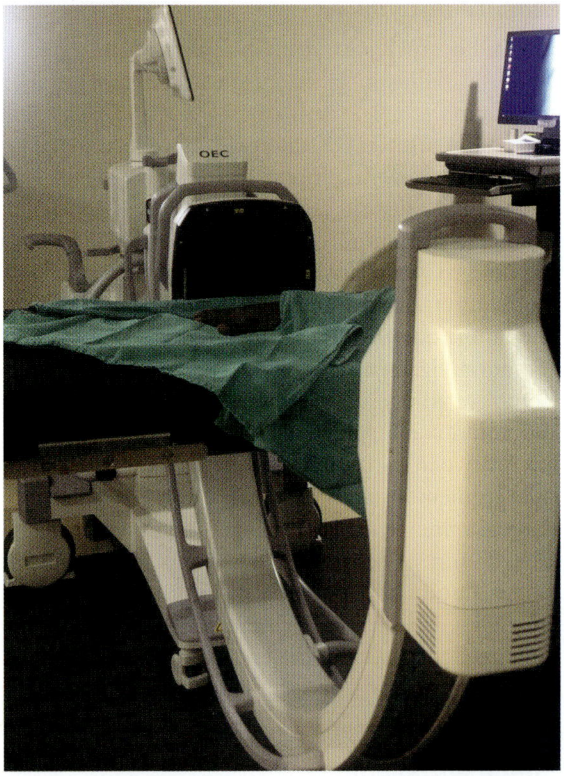

• **Fig. 18.22** Proximal carpal setup, lateral view.

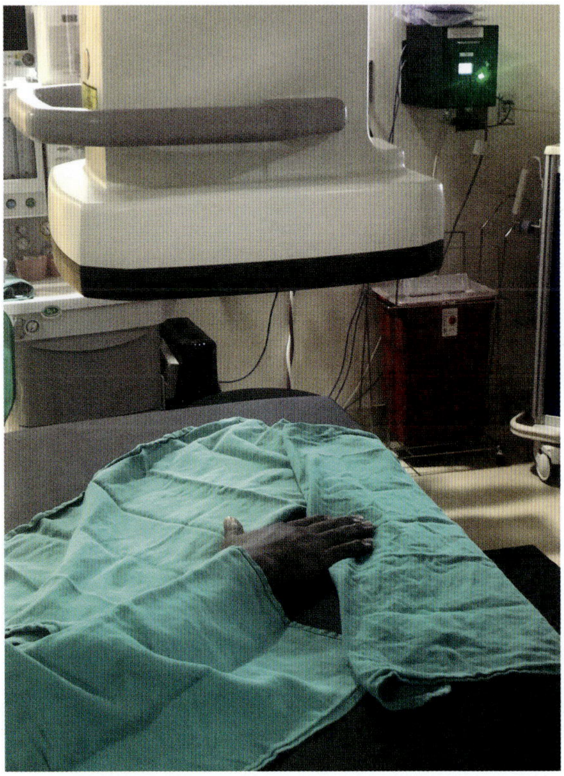

• **Fig. 18.23** Distal carpal injection setup, AP view.

- Slowly insert the needle into the joint space between the proximal carpal row and radius for the radiocarpal joint.
- Dorsal scapholunate and LTLs can be injected by the placement of the needle just superficial to the joint spaces (Fig. 18.24A and B).

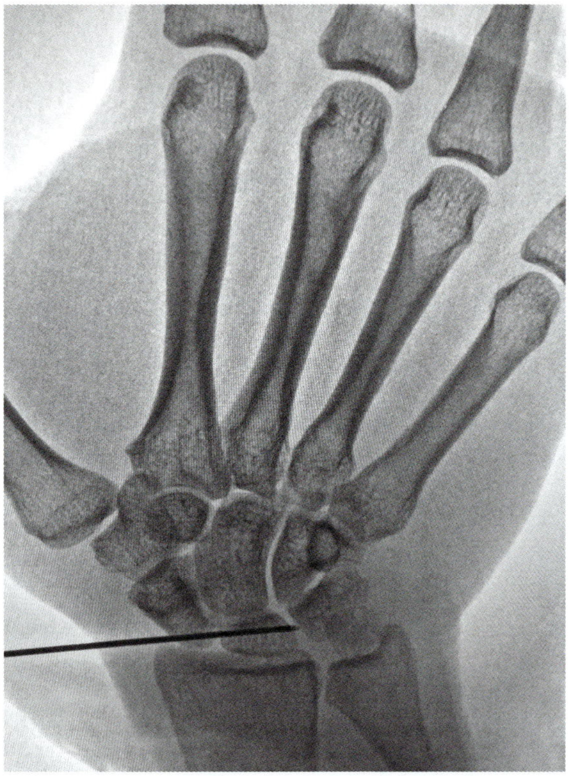

• **Fig. 18.24** Fluoroscopic guided injections of the dorsal scapholunate (A) and lunotriquetral ligaments (B).

Target

- Dorsal scapholunate or triquetrohamate joint space.
- If there is resistance, reposition the needle by advancing or removing it slightly. Confirm with an injection of a small amount of contrast.

PEARLS AND PITFALLS

- There is a good flow of contrast or medication to the proximal carpal bones despite the site of entry.

References

1. Haugstvedt JR, Langer MF, Berger RA. Distal radioulnar joint: functional anatomy, including pathomechanics. *J Hand Surg Eur Vol.* 2017;42(4):338–345.
2. Bianchi S, Martinoli C. *Ultrasound of the Musculoskeletal System.* Springer; 2007.
3. Gaston RG, Loeffler BJ. Sports-specific injuries of the hand and wrist. *Clin Sports Med.* 2015;34(1):1–10.
4. Geissler WB, Burkett JL. Ligamentous sports injuries of the hand and wrist. *Sports Med Arthrosc Rev.* 2014;22(1):39–44.
5. Rosen A, Weiland AJ. Rheumatoid arthritis of the wrist and hand. *Rheum Dis Clin North Am.* 1998;24(1):101–128.
6. Jacobson JAJA. *Fundamentals of Musculoskeletal Ultrasound*; 2013:382.
7. Lee Z-H, Stranix J, Anzai L, Sharma S. Surgical anatomy of the first extensor compartment: a systematic review and comparison of normal cadavers vs. de Quervain syndrome patients. *J Plastic Reconstruct Aesthet Surg.* 2017;70(1):127–131.

8. Smith J, Pourcho AM, Kakar S. Sonographic appearance of the extensor carpi radialis intermedius tendon. *Pharm Manag PM R.* 2015;7(7):789–791.
9. Tagliafico A, Rubino M, Autuori A, Bianchi S, Martinoli C. Wrist and hand ultrasound. *Semin Musculoskelet Radiol.* 2007;11(2):95–104.
10. Luong DH, Smith J, Bianchi S. Flexor carpi radialis tendon ultrasound pictorial essay. *Skeletal Radiol.* 2014;43(6):745–760.
11. Yoshioka H, Tanaka T, Ueno T, et al. Study of ulnar variance with high-resolution MRI: correlation with triangular fibrocartilage complex and cartilage of ulnar side of wrist. *J Magn Reson Imaging.* 2007;26(3):714–719.
12. Chiavaras MM, Jacobson JA, Yablon CM, Brigido MK, Girish G. Pitfalls in wrist and hand ultrasound. *Am J Roentgenol.* 2014;203(3):531–540.
13. Presazzi A, Bortolotto C, Zacchino M, Madonia L, Draghi F. Carpal tunnel: normal anatomy, anatomical variants and ultrasound technique. *J Ultrasound.* 2011;14(1):40–46.
14. Lohman M, Vasenius J, Nieminen O. Ultrasound guidance for puncture and injection in the radiocarpal joint. *Acta Radiol (Stockholm, Sweden:1987).* 2007;48(7):744–747.
15. Balint PV, Kane D, Hunter J, et al. Ultrasound guided versus conventional joint and soft tissue fluid aspiration in rheumatology practice: a pilot study. *J Rheumatol.* 2002;29(10):2209–2213.
16. Bland JDP. Treatment of carpal tunnel syndrome. *Muscle Nerve.* 2007;36(2):167–171.
17. Cunnington J, Marshall N, Hide G, et al. A randomized, double-blind, controlled study of ultrasound-guided corticosteroid injection into the joint of patients with inflammatory arthritis. *Arthritis Rheum.* 2010;62(7):1862–1869.
18. Lohman M, Vasenius J, Nieminen O. Ultrasound guidance for puncture and injection in the radiocarpal joint. *Acta Radiol.* 2007;48(7):744–747.
19. Lopes RV, Furtado RN, Parmigiani L, et al. Accuracy of intra-articular injections in peripheral joints performed blindly in patients with rheumatoid arthritis. *Rheumatology (Oxford).* 2008;47(12): 1792–1794.
20. Stanley J, Trail I. Carpal instability. *J Bone Joint Surgy Brit Vol.* 1994;76(5):691–700.
21. Jacobson JA. In: *Fundamentals of Musculoskeletal Ultrasound.* 2nd ed. Philadelphia: Saunders; 2013.
22. Pin PG, Nowak M, Logan SE, et al. Coincident rupture of the scapholunate and lunotriquetral ligaments without perilunate dislocation: pathomechanics and management. *J Hand Surg Am.* 1990;15(1):110–119.
23. Taljanovic MS, Goldberg MR, Sheppard JE, Rogers LF. US of the intrinsic and extrinsic wrist ligaments and triangular fibrocartilage complex—normal anatomy and imaging technique. *Radiographics.* 2011;31(1):79–80.
24. Chopra A, Rowbotham EL, Grainger AJ. Radiological intervention of the hand and wrist. *Br J Radiol.* 2016;89(1057):20150373.
25. Herma T, Baca V, Yershov D, Kachlik D. A case of a duplicated superficial branch of radial nerve and a two-bellied brachioradialis muscle presenting a potential entrapment syndrome. *Surg Radiol Anat.* 2017;39(4):451–454.
26. Motoura H, Shiozaki K, Kawasaki K. Anatomical variations in the tendon sheath of the first compartment. *Anat Sci Int.* 2010;85(3):145–151.
27. Choi SJ, Ahn JH, Lee YJ, Ryu DS, Lee JH, Jung SM. de Quervain disease: US identification of anatomic variations in the first extensor compartment with an emphasis on subcompartmentalization. *Radiology.* 2011;260(2):480.
28. Rettig AC. Athletic injuries of the wrist and hand: part II: overuse injuries of the wrist and traumatic injuries to the hand. *Am J Sports Med.* 2004;32(1):262–273.
29. Sawaizumi T, Nanno M, Ito H. De Quervain's disease: efficacy of intra-sheath triamcinolone injection. *Int Orthop.* 2007;31(2):265–268.
30. Vuillemin V, Guerini H, Bard H, Morvan G. Stenosing tenosynovitis. *J Ultrasound.* 2012;15(1):20–28.
31. Draghi F, Bortolotto C. Intersection syndrome: ultrasound imaging. *Skeletal Radiol.* 2013;43(3):283–287.
32. Hajder E, de Jonge MC, van der Horst CM, Obdeijn MC. The role of ultrasound-guided triamcinolone injection in the treatment of de Quervain's disease: treatment and a diagnostic tool? *Chir Main.* 2013;32(6):403–407.
33. Jeyapalan K, Choudhary S. Ultrasound-guided injection of triamcinolone and bupivacaine in the management of de Quervain's disease. *Skeletal Radiol.* 2009;38(11):1099–1103.
34. McDermott JD, Ilyas AM, Nazarian LN, Leinberry CF. Ultrasound-guided injections for de Quervain's tenosynovitis. *Clin Orthop Relat Res.* 2012;470(7):1925–1931.
35. Brinks A, Koes BW, Volkers AC, Verhaar JA, Bierma-Zeinstra SM. Adverse effects of extra-articular corticosteroid injections: a systematic review. *BMC Musculoskelet Disord.* 2010;11:206.
36. Gude W, Morelli V. Ganglion cysts of the wrist: pathophysiology, clinical picture, and management. *Curr Rev Musculoskelet Med.* 2008;1(3–4):205–211.
37. Malanga GA, Mautner KR. *Atlas of Ultrasound-Guided Musculoskeletal Injections.* McGraw-Hill; 2014.
38. Paramhans D, Nayak D, Mathur RK, Kushwah K. Double dart technique of instillation of triamcinolone in ganglion over the wrist. *J Cutan Aesthet Surg.* 2010;3(1):29–31.
39. Colio SW, Smith J, Pourcho AM. Ultrasound-guided interventional procedures of the wrist and hand: anatomy, indications, and techniques. *Phys Med Rehabil Clin.* 2016;27(3):589–605.
40. Jayaraman S, Naidich TP. The carpal tunnel: ultrasound display of normal imaging anatomy and pathology. *Neuroimaging Clin N Am.* 2004;14(1):103–113.
41. Iskra T, Mizia E, Musial A, Matuszyk A, Tomaszewski KA. Carpal tunnel syndrome—anatomical and clinical correlations. *Folia Med Cracov.* 2013;53(2):5–13.
42. Torbati SS, Bral D, Geiderman JM. Acute calcific tendinitis of the wrist. *J Emerg Med.* 2013;44(2):352–354.
43. Aboonq MS. Pathophysiology of carpal tunnel syndrome. *Neurosciences.* 2015;20(1):4–9.
44. Siegel DB, Kuzma G, Eakins D. Anatomic investigation of the role of the lumbrical muscles in carpal tunnel syndrome. *J Hand Surg Am.* 1995;20(5):860–863.
45. De Krom MCTFM, Knipschild PG, Kester ADM, Thijs CT, Boekkooi PF, Spaans F. Carpal tunnel syndrome: prevalence in the general population. *J Clin Epidemiol.* 1992;45(4):373–376.
46. Mitchell R, Chesney A, Seal S, McKnight L, Thoma A. Anatomical variations of the carpal tunnel structures. *Can J Plast Surg.* 2009;17(3):e3–e7.
47. Beris AE, Lykissas MG, Kontogeorgakos VA, Vekris MD, Korompilias AV. Anatomic variations of the median nerve in carpal tunnel release. *Clin Anat.* 2008;21(6):514–518.
48. Bianchi S, Santa DD, Glauser T, Beaulieu J-Y, Van Aaken J. Sonography of masses of the wrist and hand. *Am J Roentgenol.* 2008;191(6):1767–1775.
49. Duggal A, Anastakis D, Salonen D, Becker E. Compression of the deep palmar branch of the ulnar nerve by a ganglion: a case report. *Hand.* 2006;1(2):98–101.

50. Ehrlich W, Lee Dellon A, Mackinnon SE. Cheiralgia paresthetica (entrapment of the radial sensory nerve). *J Hand Surg*. 1986;11(2):196–199.
51. Thomas BP, Sreekanth R. Distal radioulnar joint injuries. *Indian J Orthop*. 2012;46(5):494.
52. Haugstvedt J, Langer M, Berger R. Distal radioulnar joint: functional anatomy, including pathomechanics. *J Hand Surg Eur Vol*. 2017;42(4):338–345.
53. Wu W-T, Chang K-V, Mezian K, et al. Ulnar wrist pain revisited: ultrasound diagnosis and guided injection for triangular fibrocartilage complex injuries. *J Clin Med*. 2019;8(10):1540.
54. Gilula LA, Hardy DC, Totty WG. Distal radioulnar joint arthrography. *Am J Roentgenol*. 1988;150(4):864–866.
55. Sarrafian SK, Melamed JL, Goshgarian GM. Study of wrist motion in flexion and extension. *Clin Orthop Relat Res*. 1977;(126):153–159.
56. Schmitt R, Froehner S, Coblenz G, Christopoulos G. Carpal instability. *Eur Radiol*. 2006;16(10):2161–2178.
57. Manaster BJ. Digital wrist arthrography: precision in determining the site of radiocarpal-midcarpal communication. *Am J Roentgenol*. 1986;147(3):563–566.
58. Resnick D, Andre M, Kerr R, Pineda C, Guerra Jr J, Atkinson D. Digital arthrography of the wrist: a radiographic-pathologic investigation. *Am J Roentgenol*. 1984;142(6):1187–1190.
59. Linkous MD, Gilula LA. Wrist arthrography today. *Radiol Clin North Am*. 1998;36(4):651–672.
60. Bateni CP, Bartolotta RJ, Richardson ML, Mulcahy H, Allan CH. Imaging key wrist ligaments: what the surgeon needs the radiologist to know. *Am J Roentgenol*. 2013;200(5):1089–1095.
61. Jones W. Beware the sprained wrist. The incidence and diagnosis of scapholunate instability. *J Bone Joint Surg Br Vol*. 1988;70(2):293–297.
62. Watson HK, Ballet FL. The SLAC wrist: scapholunate advanced collapse pattern of degenerative arthritis. *J Hand Surg*. 1984;9(3):358–365.

19

Hand Injection Techniques

YODIT TEFERA, KEVIN CONLEY, MICHAEL ERICKSON, ADAM M. POURCHO, PHILLIP HENNING, AND OLUSEUN OLUFADE

Ultrasound Guided Injection Techniques

Metacarpophalangeal, Interphalangeal, Proximal Interphalangeal, Distal Interphalangeal Joint Injections

KEY POINTS

- Out-of-plane relative to transducer or short axis to the joint approaches maybe easier for these superficial joints
- A gel stand-off may improve joint and needle visualization
- Understanding and identification of at-risk anatomy is required prior to injection
- A hockey stick transducer may improve ability to do injections.
- Joints often hold relatively small volumes of injectate; therefore, practitioner will often have to limit anesthetic in favor of therapeutic injectate when performing the procedure.
- Use of particulate corticosteroids increases the risk of skin depigmentation, especially in the case of superficial injections[1]

Pertinent Anatomy

- The metacarpophalangeal (MCP), interphalangeal (IP), proximal interphalangeal (PIP), and distal interphalangeal (DIP) joints are small synovial joints that allow for flexion and extension of the fingers and thumb.
- Neurovascular structures run along the relative volar side of each digit (Figs. 19.1 and 19.2B).
- Dorsal recess of the joints extends proximal to each joint allowing for relatively easier access than volar to joint (see Fig. 19.2C and D).

Common Pathology

- Osteoarthritis commonly effects the joints of the hand.[1]
- The MCP and IP joints are commonly affected by disorders of the hand, including dislocations, sprains, fractures, and both osteoarthritis and inflammatory arthropathies.[1]
- The PIP joint is a commonly injured finger joint, often resulting in fractures, collateral ligament injuries, palmar plate injuries, and subsequent post-traumatic osteoarthritis.[1]
- Inflammatory arthritis, such as rheumatoid arthritis, can have a predilection for the joints of the hand[1]
- Common findings of joint space narrowing, osteophyte formation, effusion, joint subluxation or deformity, and erosive changes, in the case of inflammatory arthritis can occur.[1]

Equipment

- High frequency linear array transducer
- Smaller footprint or hockey stick probes maybe easier to use over regions with noncompliant tissue.

Common Injectates

- Local anesthetics for diagnostics, corticosteroids intra-articular (IA) only
- Prolotherapy
- Orthobiologics (PRP, bone marrow concentrate, etc.)
- Corticosteroid should not be injected directly into capsular ligaments

Injectate Volume

- 0.5 to 1.5 mL

Authors Preferred Injection Technique

Patient Position

- Seated or supine on table with forearm pronated (Fig. 19.3A)

Clinical Position

- Standing or seated ipsilateral side of the patient

Transducer Position

- The transducer is placed in the anatomic sagittal plane with the desired target joint centered on the transducer, for out-of-plane approach (see Fig. 19.3A).
- Alternatively, this can be done in the anatomic axial plane for the in-plane approach.

Needle Position

- Needle is introduced in short axis from an ulnar to radial or radial to ulnar direction into the joint (see Fig. 19.3A and B).

Targets

- The desired joint
- Watch distention of the capsule or slight separation of the bones with ultrasound during the injection.
- Can also inject the overlying capsular ligaments (with prolotherapy or orthobiologics) for each joint in the same position with the needle in short axis or in long axis (Fig. 19.4A and B)

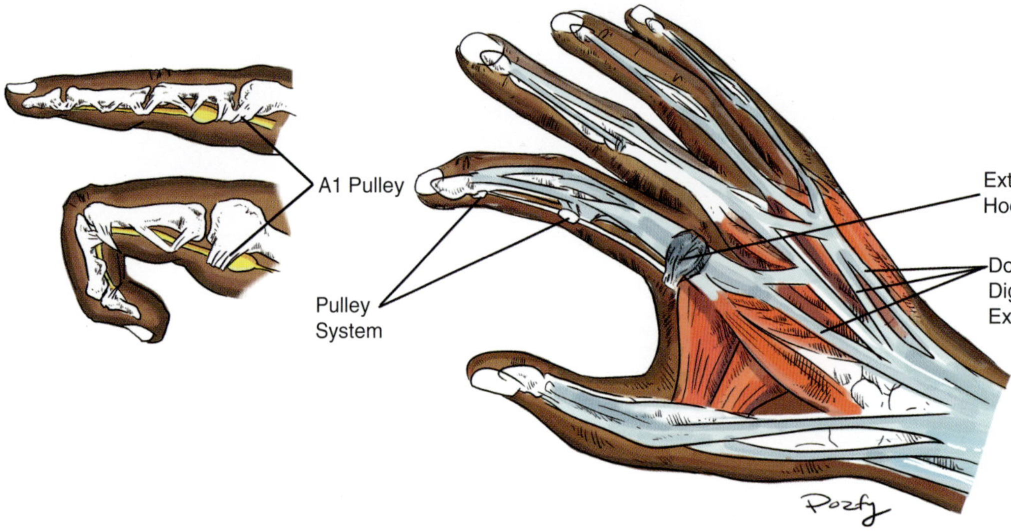

• **Fig. 19.1** Hand Pulley System Anatomy. Note enlarged view of the A1 pully.

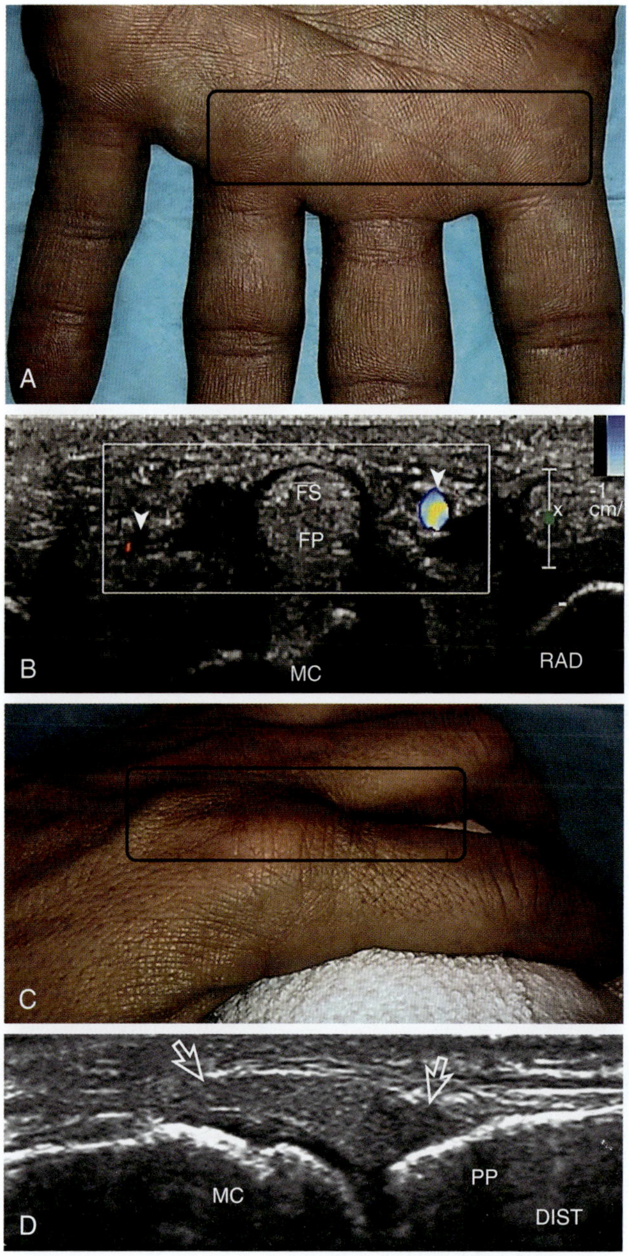

• **Fig. 19.2** Transducer placement and sonographic appearance of volar and dorsal targets for hand injections. (A) Axial position of the transducer (black rectangle) overlying the volar proximal hand with corresponding sonographic (B) sonographic appearance of the anatomy at this level. Note the neurovascular structures (arrowheads) adjacent to the flexor digitorum superficialis (FS) and profundus (FP). (C and D) Sagittal position of the transducer (black rectangle) overlying the dorsal metacarpal phalangeal joint with correlative sonographic image at this level. Note proximal extension of the dorsal recess (open arrows). MC, Metacarpal; PP, proximal phalanx.

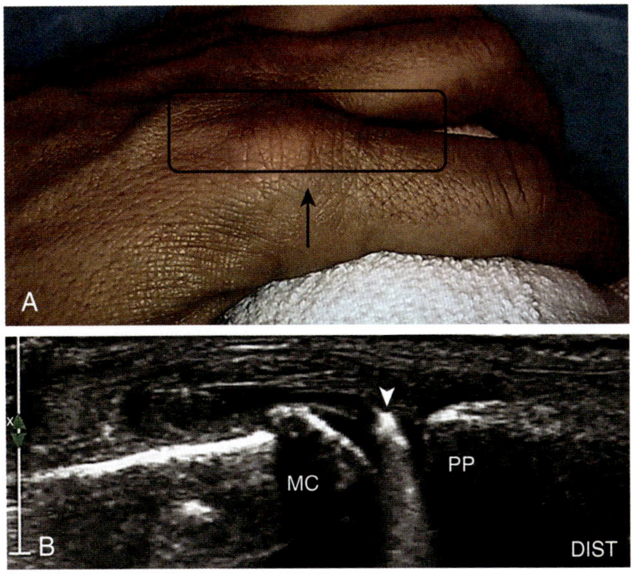

• **Fig. 19.3** Metacarpal or Interphalangeal Joint Injections. (A) Transducer (black rectangle) placement along the dorsal recess of the target joint. *Black arrow*, trajectory of the needle. (B) Sonographic image of the needle tip *(arrowhead)* within the dorsal joint recess. Note reverberation artifact deep to the needle. *MC,* Metacarpal, *PP,* proximal phalanx.

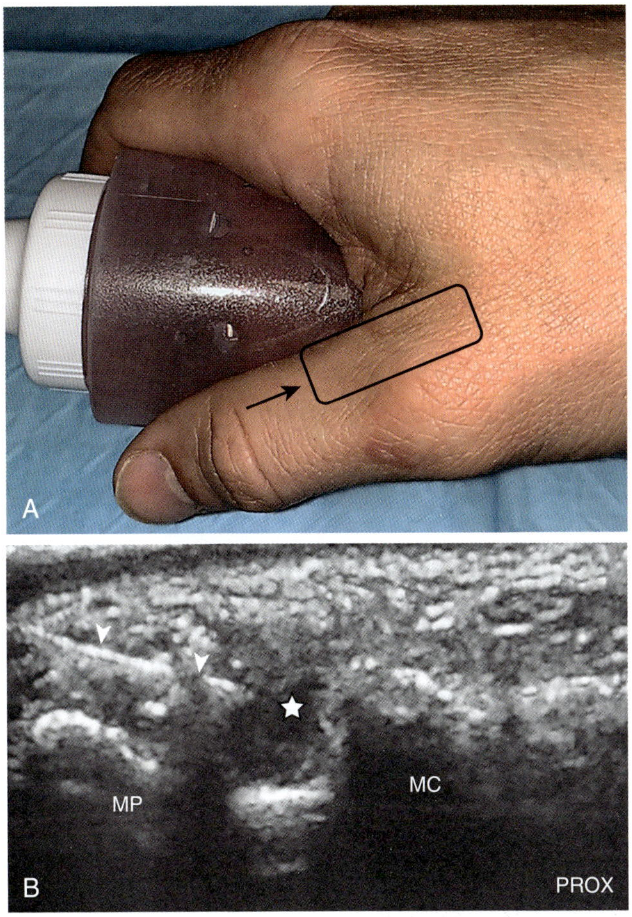

• **Fig. 19.4** Metacarpal Phalangeal Joint and Ulnar Capsular Ligament Injection. (A) Transducer placement *(black rectangle)* for in plane technique with needle traversing from distal to proximal direction *(black arrow)*. (B) Sonographic image of needle *(arrowheads)* injecting along the ulnar capsular ligament, note joint distension *(asterisk)*.

PEARLS AND PITFALLS

- A dorsal approach to the joint effectively avoids the neurovascular bundles, which are volar.
- Needle depth can also be confirmed by turning the transducer 90 degrees to show an in-plane view of the needle.
- When injecting the ulnar collateral ligament of the first MCP joint, it may be helpful to have the patient hold onto a rolled- up towel or other cylindrical object to help position and stabilize the joint during the injection (see Fig. 19.4A).

Carpometacarpal and Scaphotrapeziotrapezoid Joints and Carpometacarpal Capsular Ligaments

KEY POINTS

- When using orthobiologics it is recommended to address the joint instability/mechanical symptoms in addition to the condition being treated.

Pertinent Anatomy

- The carpometacarpal (CMC) joint is a saddle shaped synovial joint between the trapezium and first metacarpal.
- The scaphotrapeziotrapezoid (STT) joint is a dome-shaped articulation composed of scaphotrapezial and/or scaphotrapezoidal articulation[2]
- The terminal SR2 and SR3 branches of the superficial radial nerve border the volar and dorsal sides of the STT and CMC joints.[2]
- Also just proximal to the STT and CMC joints the radial artery branches into superficial and deep palmar arteries (Fig. 19.5A and B).[3]
- The flexor carpi radialis (FCR) tendon is just palmar and ulnar to the CMC and STT joints.
- The palmar cutaneous nerve usual resides between the FCR tendon and the palmaris on the palmar side of the wrist.[4]

Common Pathology

- Observed in up to 15% of radiographic studies and 83.3% of cadaveric specimens, degenerative arthritis of the CMC and STT joint are the first and second most common cause of degenerative changes in the wrist.[5]
- Injuries to the scaphotrapezial ligament, the major anatomic stabilizer of the STT joint, can lead to post-traumatic arthritic changes.[3]
- Other theories for injury to the STT joint include disruption of the scapholunate interosseous ligament and cartilage erosion in the STT joint.[5]
- Common pathologic US findings include joint effusions, synovitis, loss of articular space, cortical irregularities, and osteophyte formation.[6]
- STT and CMC arthropathy have been associated with tendinopathy of the FCR tendon which lies anatomically just palmar and ulnar to the STT joint.[7-9]

Equipment

- Injections can be performed using a high-frequency linear array transducer. If available, a hockey stick or shorter foot-print transducer may also be helpful.
- 30 to 25-gauge 1 to 1.5 inch needle

Continued

KEY POINTS—cont'd

Common Injectates
- Local anesthetics for diagnostics, corticosteroids IA only
- Prolotherapy
- Orthobiologics (PRP, bone marrow concentrate, etc.)
- Corticosteroid should not be injected directly into capsular ligaments

Injectate Volume
- 1 to 2 mL

Technique: CMC and STT Joints Intra-Articular

Patient Position
- Supine (Fig. 19.5A)
- For both joints, wrist supinated supported by towels
- For dorsal approach to the CMC joint, the wrist can be in neutral position.

Clinician Position
- Standing or seated ipsilateral side of the patient

Transducer Position
- Identify CMC joint in the transverse plane palmer aspect
- Transducer angled near parallel with the metacarpal bone
- Scaphotrapeziotrapezoid joint set up similar except the transducer is positioned more proximal

Needle Position
- Short-axis injection

Targets
- The desired joint (see Fig. 19.5A, C and D)
- Watch distention of the capsule or slight separation of the bones with ultrasound during the injection.
- Can also inject the overlying palmer capsular ligaments for both joints in the same position

PEARLS AND PITFALLS

- Volar and dorsal approaches can be used, these authors suggest a dorsal approach with needle as it tends to be less painful.
- In patients with severe osteoarthritis it may help to extend the wrist and ulnar or radially deviate the wrist to open the joint. Also, it can help to pull the thumb to extend the joint opening.
- Toggling the transducer palmar or dorsal can be used of osteophytic formation blocks the desired path to the joint.
- The terminal branches of the superficial radial nerve as well as the deep and superficial branches of the radial artery, should be identified and avoided during procedures involving the STT and CMC joints.
- Color Doppler can be used to help identify the vascular structures.

Technique: CMC Capsule Ligaments: Palmer, Deep Palmer, and Dorsal

Patient Position
- Supine
- Wrist supinated or neutral position supported by towels for palmer ligaments (Fig. 19.6A)

Clinician position
- Standing or seated ipsilateral side of the patient

Transducer position
- Palmer ligaments: place transducer over palmer CMC joint in the transverse plane. Identify more radial (superficial) and deep more medial aspect (see Fig. 19.6A).
- Transducer angled close to parallel with the metacarpal bone
- Dorsal ligaments: identify radial artery to avoid then visualize the joint in the transverse plane over the dorsal aspect (see Fig. 19.6B)

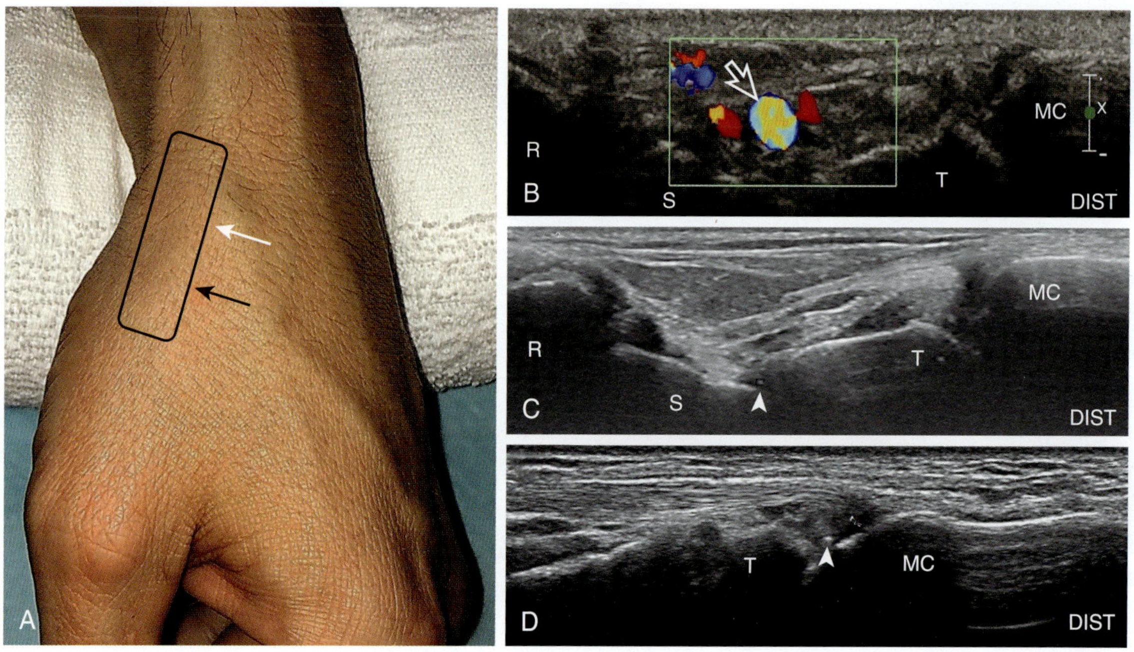

• **Fig. 19.5** Carpometacarpal (CMC) and/or Scaphotrapziotrapezoidal (STT) Joint Injection. (A) Visualization of the CMC or STT joint can be optimized by placement of the transducer *(black rectangle)* sagittal to the hand along the dorsal surface. (B) Sonographic image showing the location of the radial artery *(open arrow)* relative to the STT and CMC joints. (C and D) Sonographic images of the needle *(arrowhead)* within the STT and CMC joints respectively. *MC,* metacarpal; *R,* radius; *S,* scaphoid; *T,* trapezium.

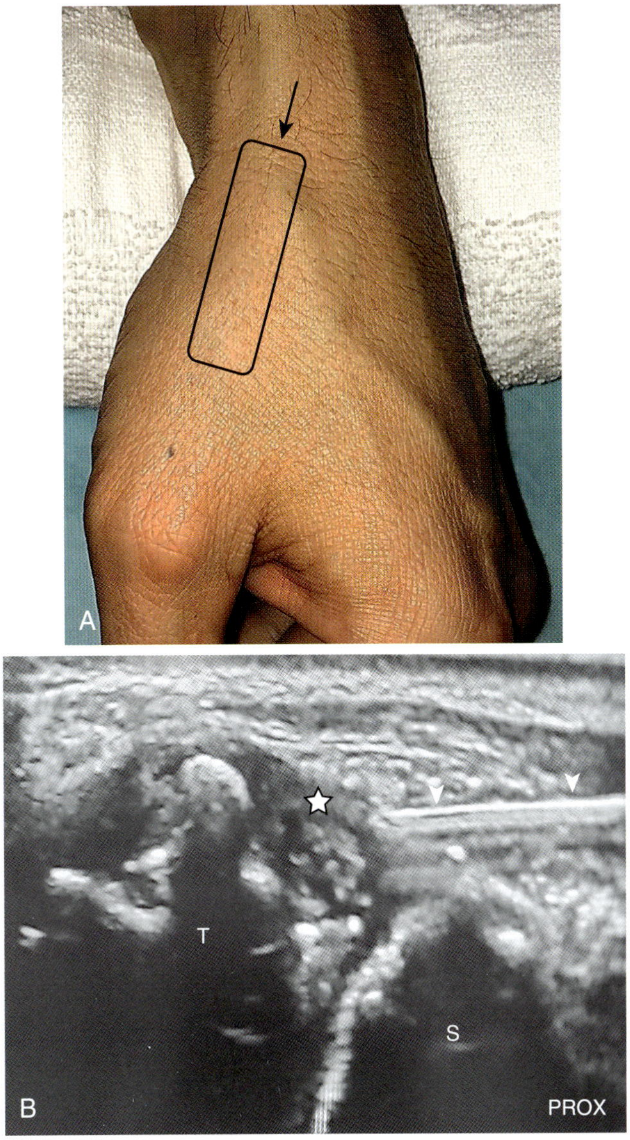

• **Fig. 19.6** Carpometacarpal Capsular Ligament Injections. (A) Transducer *(black rectangle)* and needle placement *(black arrow)* targeting the palmer ligaments. (B) Needle placement targeting the dorsal ligaments. *Arrowhead,* Needle location; *asterisk*, region of the ligaments.

PEARLS AND PITFALLS—cont'd

Needle Position
- Short-axis injection for the superficial and deeper ligaments
- Long axis distal to proximal for the superficial ligaments.

Targets
- Capsular ligament just overlying the joint distal and proximal.
- With short-axis injections redirect to inject the ligaments direct over the joint and distal and proximal.

PEARLS AND PITFALLS

- Deeper capsule is more difficult to inject in long axis due to the anatomy
- Only inject 0.5 to 1 mL per ligament.

A1 Pulley Injection

KEY POINTS

- When injecting steroids it has been found to be more clinically effective if you remain superficial to the pulley.[10]

Pertinent Anatomy
- Flexor tendon sheath contains the tendons of both the flexor digitorum superficialis (FDS) and flexor digitorum profundus (FDP).
- There are five fibro-osseous bands called annular pulleys (A1-A5), that keep the FDS and FDP tendons from bowstringing with finger flexion (Fig, 19.7).[11]
- The A-1 pulley is located just proximal to the MCP joint, superficial to the palmar plate, and can located by surface anatomy using the distal palmar crease.[11]
- The neurovascular bundles, containing the digital nerves, are located just radial and ulnar to the pulley on the palmar side (see Fig. 19.2B).[11]

Common Pathology
- Stenosing tenosynovitis involves thickening/ stenosis of the A1 pulley, with or without a Nodus nodule (Fig. 19.8A and B).[12,13]
- In some cases, there is tenosynovitis involving the tendon and tendon sheath, with low flow color Doppler on ultrasound.[12,13]
- Common risk factors for development of stenosing tenosynovitis include post-partum, diabetes, prior transverse carpal ligament release, rheumatoid arthritis and gout.[12-14]
- Patients will often complain of "triggering" and catching of their fingers.[12,13]

Equipment
- 25 to 30-gauge 1 to 2 inch needle
- Linear array transducer, hockey stick or short footprint transducer maybe preferable if available

Common Injectates
- Corticosteroids with local anesthetics
- Orthobiologics (platelet lysate, etc.)

Injectate Volume
- 1 to 2 mL

Technique

Patient Position
- Supine with forearm supinated and wrist placed in mild extension over towel (Fig. 19.9A)

Clinician position
- Clinician should be lateral to the affected hand

Transducer position
- The pulley is first identified in its short axis by sliding the transducer down the flexor tendons until the relative anechoic shadow of the pulley is visualized.
- Once the pulley is identified, the transducer can be turned 90 degrees relative to the transducer to create a short-axis view of the A1 pulley and long-axis view of the flexor tendons beneath (see Fig. 19.9B).

Continued

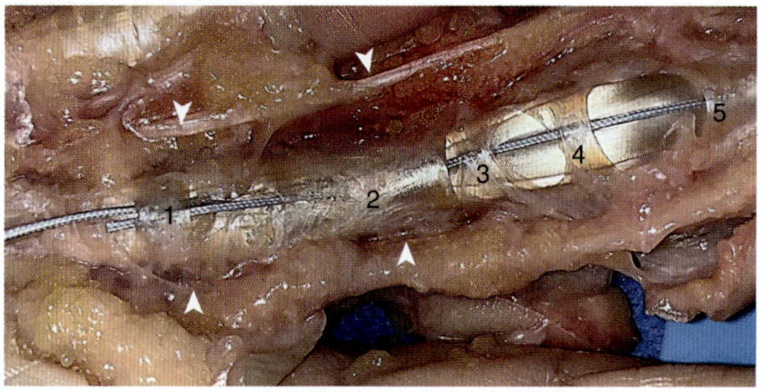

• **Fig. 19.7** Cadaveric Dissection of the Pulley System of the Finger. *1*, A1, *2*, A2, *3*, A3, *4*, A4, *5*, A5. *Arrowheads* note the location of the neurovascular structures relative to the pulley system.

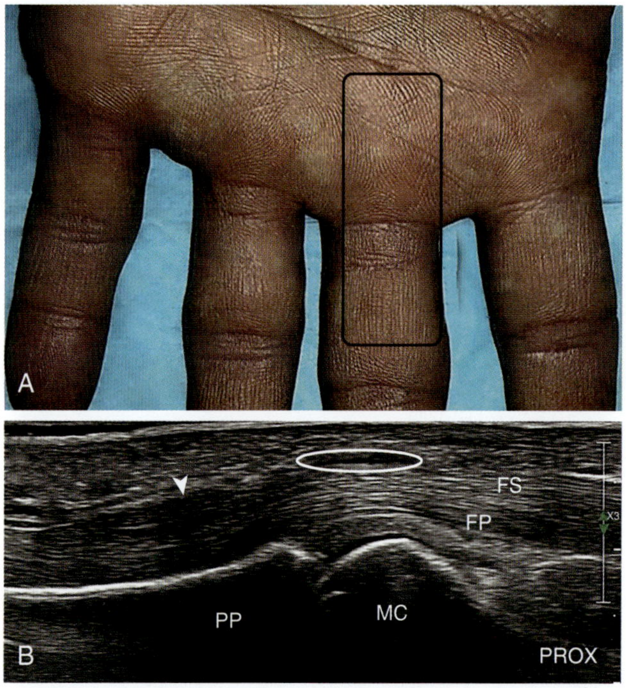

• **Fig. 19.8** Sonographic Evaluation of the A1 Pulley. (A) Transducer (black rectangle) placement sagittal to the involved digit. (B) Sonographic image of the A1 pulley (white oval). Note the thickening in the tendon (arrowhead) distal to the pulley. *FP,* Flexor digitorum profundus; *FS,* flexor digitorum superficialis; *MC*, metacarpal; *PP,* proximal phalanx.

KEY POINTS—cont'd

- Dynamic flexion and extension of the finger can be used prior to injection to identify the pulley superficial to the flexor tendons.

Needle Position

- Needle with slight bend in direction of the bevel, is introduced from either distal-to-proximal or proximal-to-distal direction toward the A1 pulley.

Target

- Target the needle between the pulley and the FDS tendon (see Fig. 19.9A and B).
- The transducer can be turned 90 degrees before injection to confirm centralized placement of the needle relative to the pulley (se Fig. 19.9B and C).

PEARLS AND PITFALLS

- The digital nerves can be visualized both ulnar and radial to the pulley in the anatomic axial view and should be avoided during the injection.
- Dynamic motion, with flexion and extension of the finger, prior to injection can help with the identification of the pulley.

Digital Nerve Block

KEY POINTS

- Goal to anesthetize the digit prior to procedures such as fracture/joint reduction or laceration repair.

Pertinent Anatomy

- At the distal palm, the proper digital nerves are found on the ulnar and radial volar aspect of each digit (Fig. 19.10A and B).

Common Pathology

- The nerve is subject to laceration from penetrating injury or compression from digital swelling of a finger with a ligature or ring in place.[15]

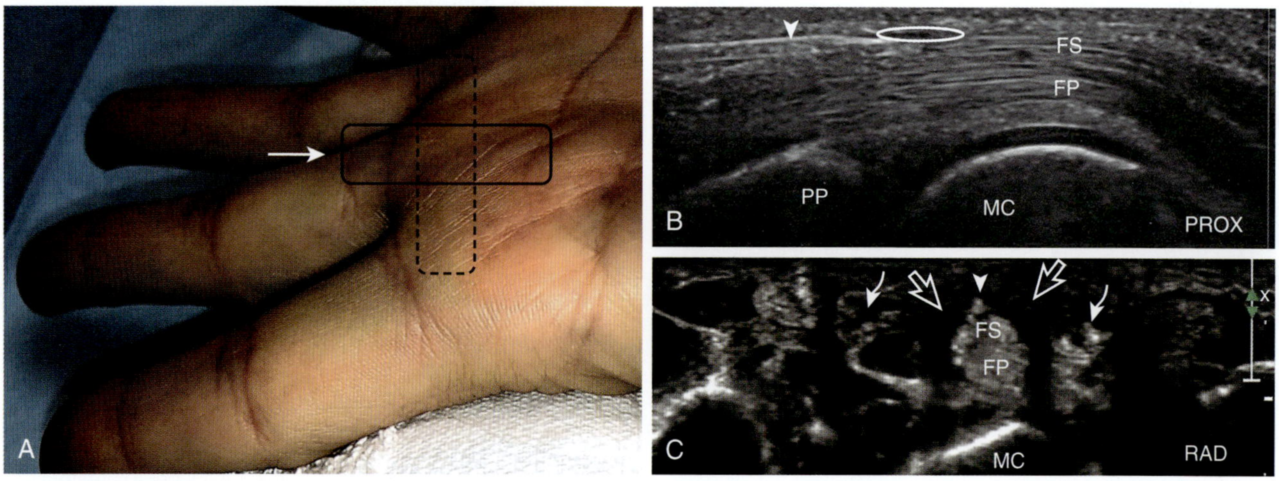

• **Fig. 19.9** Trigger Finger Injection. (A) Transducer placement for in plane *(solid black rectangle)* and out of plane *(dashed black rectangle)* techniques, trajectory of needle (white arrow). (B) Needle *(arrowhead)* placement in plane with transducer adjacent to the A1 pulley. (C) Needle *(arrowhead)* placed out of plane to transducer superficial to the tendons adjacent to the pulley. *Open arrows,* anisotropy of the sides of the A1 pulley, *curved arrows,* neurovascular bundles, *FP,* flexor digitorum profundus; *FS,* flexor digitorum superficialis; *MC,* metacarpal; *PP,* proximal phalanx,.

KEY POINTS—cont'd

Equipment

- 30 to 27-gauge needle, 1 to 1.5 inch
- High frequency linear array ultrasound transducer

Common Injectates

- Local anesthetics

Injectate Volume

- 0.5 to 1.5 mL

Technique: Palmar Proper Digital Nerve Block

Patient position

- Supine with forearm supinated

Clinician position

- Standing or seated ipsilateral side of the patient

Transducer position

- The transducer is placed in the anatomic axial plane, creating a short-axis view of the digital nerve (see Fig. 19.10A).
- Color Doppler can be used to identify the neurovascular bundle

Needle Position

- The needle is introduced via an in-plane approach from both an ulnar-to-radial and radial-to-ulnar direction (see Fig. 19.10A and B).

Targets

- Target the nerves and create a halo of anesthetic is created around each digital nerve to ensure complete block.

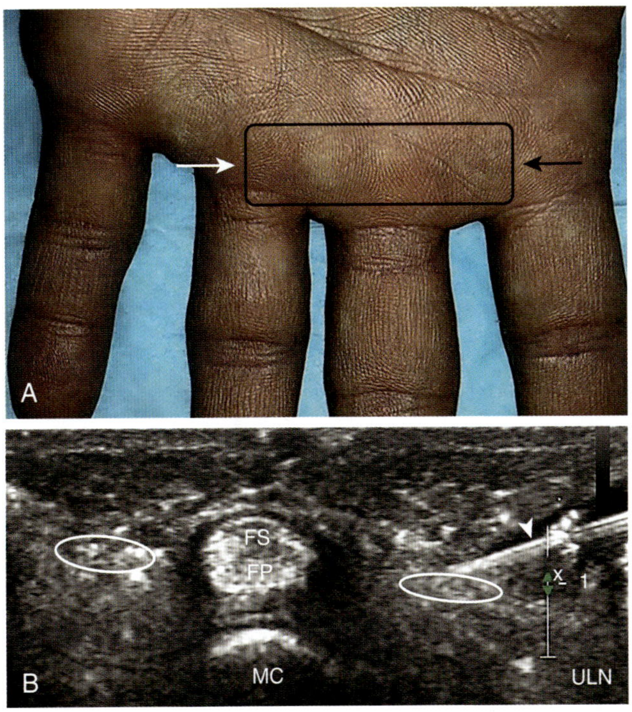

• **Fig. 19.10** Digital Nerve Block. (A) Transducer *(black rectangle)* placement axial to proximal hand overlying the neurovascular structures, ulnar to radial needle course (white arrow), radial to ulnar needle course (black arrow). (B) Needle *(arrowhead)* placement adjacent to the common digital nerve *(white oval)*. *FP,* Flexor digitorum profundus; *FS,* flexor digitorum superficialis; *MC,* metacarpal.

PEARLS AND PITFALLS

- It is recommended that epinephrine is avoided during these blocks to avoid end artery vasoconstriction to the finger.

Fluoroscopy-Guided Injection Techniques

Thumb Carpometacarpal Joint Fluoroscopic Guided Injection

KEY POINTS

- Ionizing radiation necessitates shielded protection of the patient and staff

Pertinent Anatomy

- This joint articulates the trapezium and the 1st metacarpal bone

Common Pathology

- CMC synovitis/osteoarthritis

Equipment

- C-arm fluoroscopy
- 27 to 25-gauge 1 to 2 inch needle

Common Injectates

- Local anesthetics for diagnostics, corticosteroids
- Prolotherapy
- Orthobiologics (PRP, bone marrow concentrate, etc.)

Injectate Volume

- 0.5 to 1.5 mL

Technique

Patient position

- Patient should be in supine position with the wrist held in neural position between supination and pronation
- The wrist is supported with towels

Clinician position

- Clinician should be seated next to the affected hand

Fluoroscope position

- PA position centered on the CMC joint (Fig. 19.11A and B)

Needle position

- Place needle or marker over the joint and confirm with fluoroscopy
- Position the needle perpendicular to the skin with the needle tip directed ulnarly toward the CMC joint

Target

- Intra-articular joint space. If there is resistance, reposition the needle by advancing or removing slightly
- Confirm intra-articular placement with a small amount of contrast. The joint is small and want to make sure contrast does not limit the ability to place the injectate, especially if using orthobiologics.

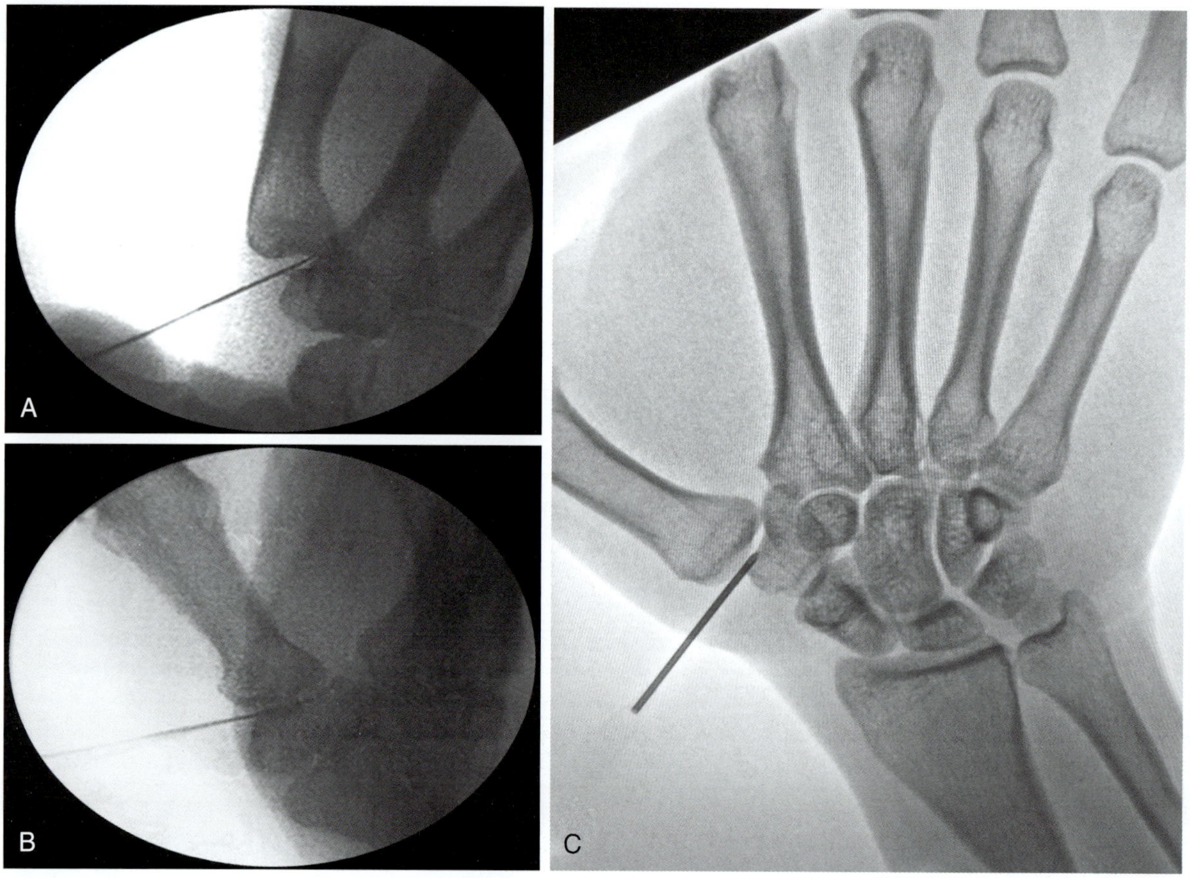

• **Fig. 19.11** Fluoroscopic Guided Carpometacarpal Joint Injections. (A) Fluoroscopic image with needle in the CMC joint. (B) Fluoroscopic image showing distension of the joint. (C) Needle.

PEARLS AND PITFALLS

- Traction to the thumb can help make the joint space more conspicuous to accommodate the injectate.
- The thumb CMC joint can be approached on the extensor side taking care to avoid the radial artery and extensor pollicis tendons.

Metacarpal, Proximal and Distal Interphalangeal Fluoroscopic Guided Joint Injections

KEY POINTS

- Ionizing radiation necessitates shielded protection of the patient and staff

Pertinent Anatomy

- The metacarpophalangeal joints are between the metacarpal bones and the proximal phalanges of the fingers.
- IP joint lines are best palpated with the digit in slight flexion, just lateral to the midline extensor tendon.
- Passive flexion and extension of the joint during palpation may facilitate identification.

Common Pathology

- MCP synovitis/osteoarthritis
- PIP joint osteoarthritis, gout, rheumatoid arthritis
- DIP joint osteoarthritis and gout

Equipment

- C arm fluoroscopic device
- 30 to 25-gauge 1 to 2-inch needle

Common Injectates

- Local anesthetics for diagnostics, corticosteroids
- Prolotherapy
- Orthobiologics (PRP, bone marrow concentrate, etc.)

Injectate Volume

- 0.5 to 1.5 mL

Technique

Patient position

- Patient should be in supine position with the wrist held in pronation and patient making a loose fist
- The hand is supported with placement of towels

Clinician position

- Clinician should be seated next to the affected hand

KEY POINTS—cont'd

Fluoroscope position

- PA position centered on the target joint

Needle position

- Position the needle perpendicular to the skin with the needle tip directed towards the desired joint (Fig. 19.12)
- Identify point of entry on the joint line on either side of the dorsal extensor tendon midline and the neurovascular bundles
- Direct the needle towards the middle of the IP joint (see Fig. 19.12C)
- DIP joints may require a more vertical needle approach (Fig. 19.13)
- Slowly insert needle into the joint

Target

- Point of entry is over the MCP joint, just radial, or ulnar to the extensor tendon
- If there is resistance, reposition the needle by advancing or removing slightly.
- Confirm intra-articular placement with a small amount of contrast. The joint is small and want to make sure contrast does not limit the ability to place the injectate, especially if using orthobiologics

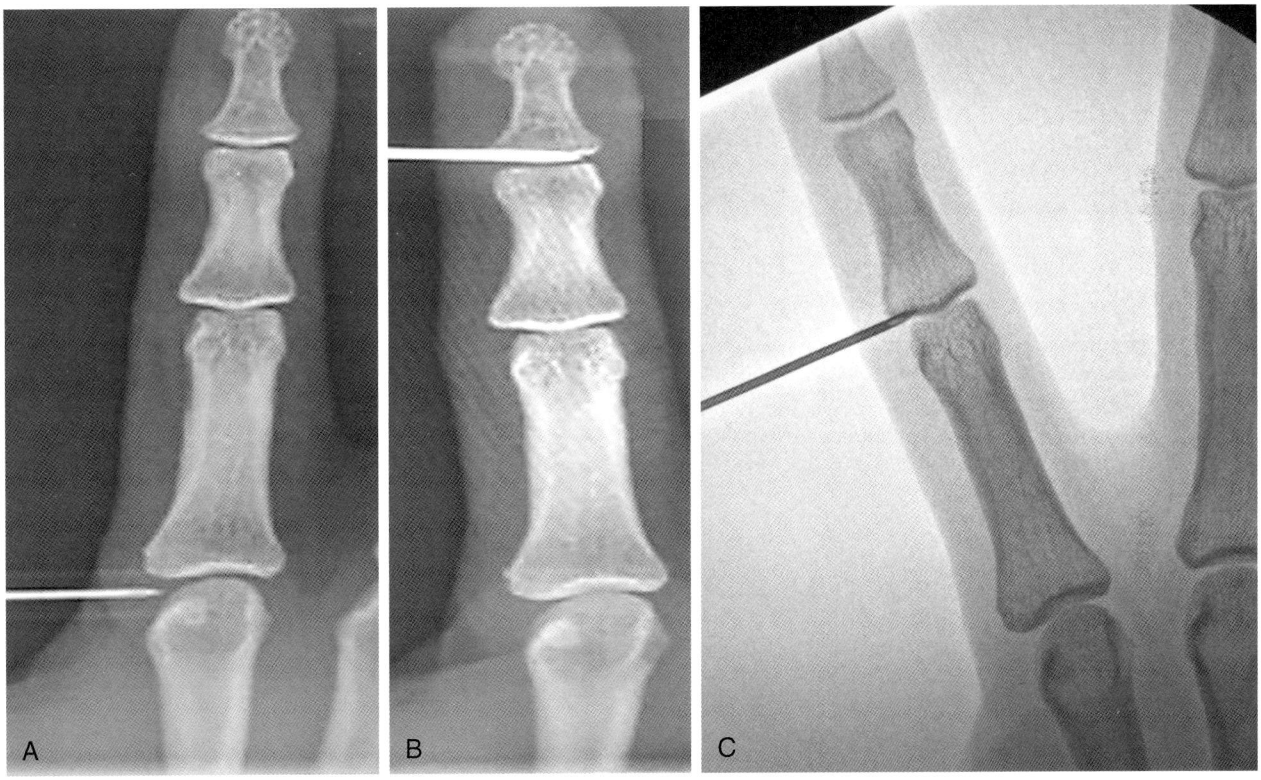

• **Fig. 19.12** Fluoroscopic Guided Metacarpophalangeal (MCP) and Interphalangeal Joint Injections. (A) Note needle traversing from radial to ulnar direction along the dorsal region of the joint space of the MCP joint. (B) Distal interphalangeal joint injection shown here, the proximal interphalangeal joint (C) would be approached in a similar fashion.

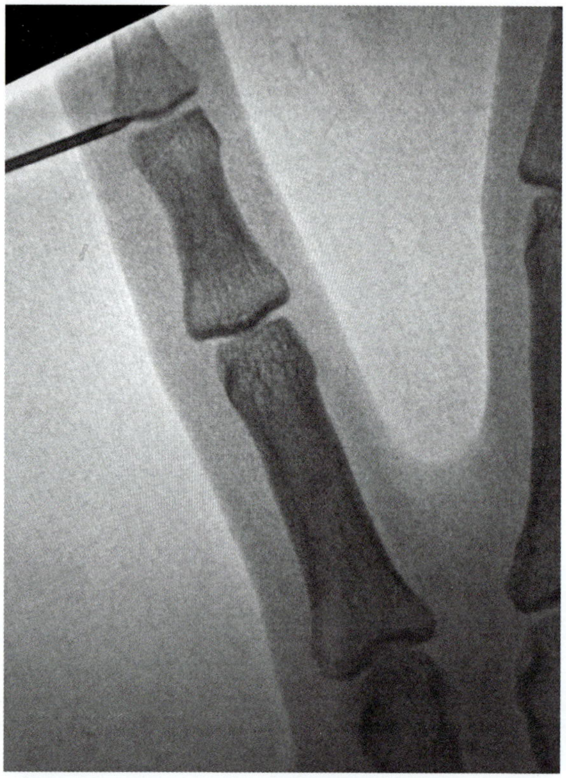

• **Fig. 19.13** Fluoroscopic image of distal interphalangeal joint injection. Note the needle traversing from radial to ulnar direction into the dorsal recess of the joint.

PEARLS AND PITFALLS

- Approach the MCP joint dorsally but avoid placing the needle through the extensor tendon or extensor hood.
- The clinician's non-injecting hand can be used to apply traction to distract the joint
- Slight joint flexion can also facilitate opening of the joint space

References

1. Leung GJ, Rainsford KD, Kean WF. Osteoarthritis of the hand I: aetiology and pathogenesis, risk factors, investigation and diagnosis. *J Pharmacy Pharmacol.* 2014;66(3):339–346.
2. Swigart CR. Arthritis of the base of the thumb. *Cur Rev Musculoskeletal Med.* 2008;1(2):142–146.
3. Coari AIG. Usefulness of high resolution US in the evaluation of effusion in osteoarthritic first carpometacarpal joint. *Scandinavian J Rheumatol.* 2000;29(3):170–173.
4. DaSilva MF, Moore DC, Weiss AP, Akelman E, Sikirica M. Anatomy of the palmar cutaneous branch of the median nerve: clinical significance. *J Hand Surg Am.* 1996;21(4):639–643.
5. Hazani R, Engineer NJ, Cooney D, Wilhelmi BJ. Anatomic landmarks for the first dorsal compartment. *Eplasty.* 2008;8: e53–e53.
6. Bianchi S, Martinoli C. *Ultrasound Musculoskeletal System.* Springer; 2007.
7. Chiavaras MM, Jacobson JA, Yablon CM, Brigido MK, Girish G. Pitfalls in wrist and hand ultrasound. *Am J Roentgenol.* 2014;203(3):531–540.
8. Luong DH, Smith J, Bianchi S. Flexor carpi radialis tendon ultrasound pictorial essay. *Skeletal Radiol.* 2014;43(6):745–760.
9. Smith J, Kakar S. Combined flexor carpi radialis tear and flexor carpi radialis brevis tendinopathy identified by ultrasound: a case report. *PM&R.* 2014;6(10):956–959.
10. Taras JS, Raphael JS, Pan WT, Movagharnia F, Sotereanos DG. Corticosteroid injections for trigger digits: is intrasheath injection necessary? *J Hand Surg Am.* 1998;23(4):717–722.
11. Fiorini HJ, Santos JBG, Hirakawa CK, Sato ES, Faloppa F, Albertoni WM. Anatomical study of the A1 pulley: length and location by means of cutaneous landmarks on the palmar surface. *J Hand Surg.* 2011;36(3):464–468.
12. Fiorini HJ, Santos JB, Hirakawa CK, Sato ES, Faloppa F, Albertoni WM. Anatomical study of the A1 pulley: length and location by means of cutaneous landmarks on the palmar surface. *J Hand Surg Am.* 2011;36(3):464–468.
13. Vuillemin V, Guerini H, Bard H, Morvan G. Stenosing tenosynovitis. *J Ultrasound.* 2012;15(1):20–28.
14. Park I-J, Lee Y-M, Kim H-M, et al. Multiple etiologies of trigger wrist. *J Plastic Reconstruct Aesthetic Surg.* 2016;69(3):335–340.
15. Kay S, Werntz J, Wolff TW. Ring avulsion injuries: classification and prognosis. *J Hand Sur.* 1989;14(2):204–213.

20

Hip Injection Techniques

KEN MAUTNER, JOHN PITTS, OLUSEUN OLUFADE, HEATHER LYNN SAFFEL, AND ADAM STREET

Ultrasound Guided

Joint

Femoroacetabular

KEY POINTS

- The accuracy of ultrasound-guided intra-articular (IA) hip injections is 97%–100%[1–3] in the literature.

Pertinent Anatomy

- The hip joint is a ball and socket synovial joint formed by the femoral head and acetabulum.
- It is surrounded by a thick articulate capsule that is made up of the iliofemoral, ischiofemoral (Y ligament of Bigelow), and pubofemoral ligaments that extend over the femoral head and neck.
- The capsule extends from the acetabulum to the intertrochanteric line. It folds back from this point on itself and inserts on the femoral head-neck junction. Thus, from the acetabulum to the femoral head-neck junction, the capsule has one layer, and from the head-neck junction to the intertrochanteric line, the capsule is composed of two layers.
- The synovial folds are referred to as the retinaculum of Weitbrecht (Fig. 20.1).[4]
- The acetabulum is surrounded circumferentially by the labrum, which is composed of fibrocartilage. The hyaline cartilage on the femoral head articulates with the labrum. The labrum will appear hyperechoic and triangular on ultrasound.
- The femoral neurovascular bundle descends medially from the pelvis into the leg. It exits the pelvis through the femoral triangle, which is lined laterally by the sartorius, medially by the adductor longus, and superiorly by the inguinal ligament. The iliopsoas separates the bundle from the hip joint.
- The lateral and medial circumflex arteries surround and supply the femoral head. They arise from the deep femoral artery, a branch of the femoral artery. Hip joint innervation comes from branches of the femoral, obturator, and sciatic nerves (Figs. 20.2 and 20.3).

Common Pathology

- Hip osteoarthritis, labral degeneration, labral tears, adhesive capsulitis, and can be a source for inflammatory arthropathies.

Equipment

- Needle size: 22- to 25-gauge, 2.5- to 5.0-inch spinal needle
- Low-frequency curvilinear ultrasound transducer

Common Injectates

- Local anesthetics for diagnostics, corticosteroids
- Prolotherapy, hyaluronic acid, orthobiologics (platelet-rich plasma [PRP], bone marrow concentrate, micronized adipose tissue, etc.)
- For capsular distention. local anesthetic and normal saline +/− corticosteroid, and/or orthobiologics, such as platelet-poor plasma, platelet lysate, etc.

Injectate Volume

- For weight-bearing intra-articular (IA) injection: 2 to 5 mL.
- For capsular distention 10 to 20 mL. Stop when getting back flow into the syringe to avoid capsular rupture. Most hip capsules max out close to 16 mL, but some may tolerate close to 20 mL.

Technique: Anterior Approach

Patient Position

- Supine with a pillow under the knees for comfort and to relax the superficial structures around the joint

Clinician Position

- Standing or sitting on affected side of patient

Transducer Position

- Anteriorly in the oblique sagittal plane, parallel with the femoral neck (Fig. 20.4)

Centeno/Schultz Hip Cadaver Dissection

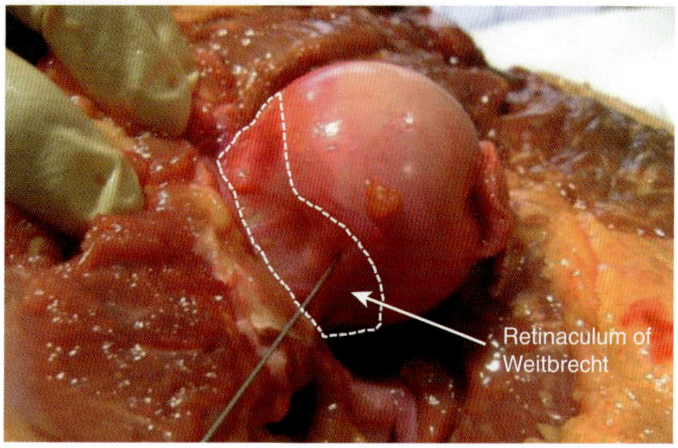

• **Fig. 20.1** Retinaculum of Weitbrecht Dissection. (Courtesy Christopher Centeno and John Schultz.)

- Alternatively, anteriorly, slightly oblique with transducer in plane to the femoral neck (Fig 20.5)

Needle Position

- In plane
- Caudolateral to cephalomedial

Target

- Anterior synovial recess, located at or just proximal to the junction of the femoral head and neck (Fig 20.6).
- For IA biologics, optimal needle placement may be closer to the weight-bearing portion of the joint at the junction of the femoral head and the acetabulum (Fig. 20.7B).
- It is helpful to tilt the transducer so that the needle is parallel to the probe. Placing a gel standoff can eliminate ultrasound dead space (see Fig. 20.7A). A slight bend to the needle tip can help for redirecting, with the goal

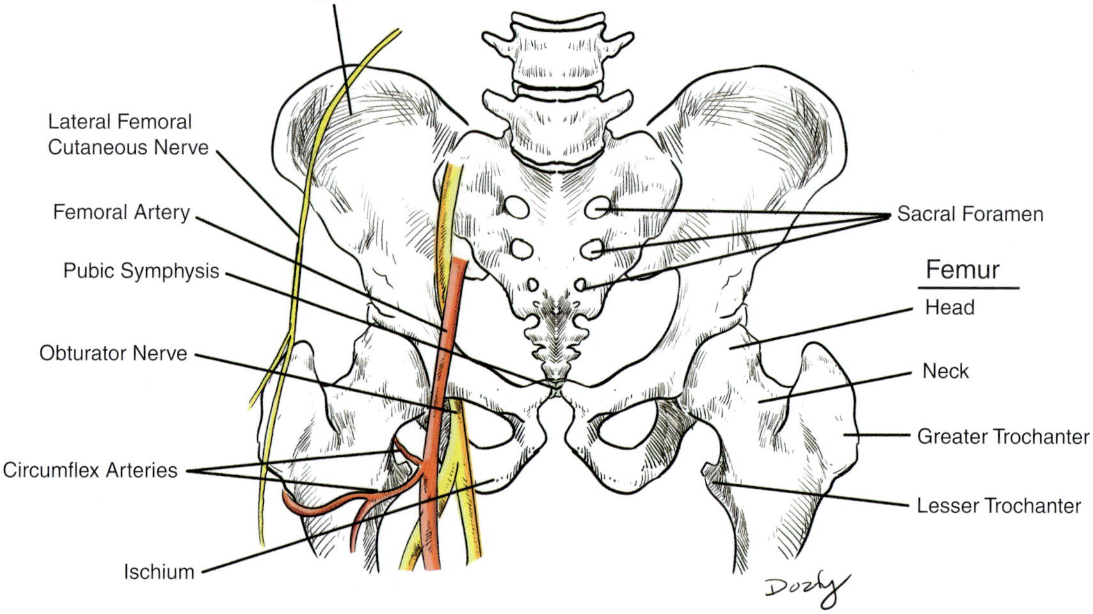

• **Fig. 20.2** Posterior Pelvic Large Neurovascular and Bony Anatomy.

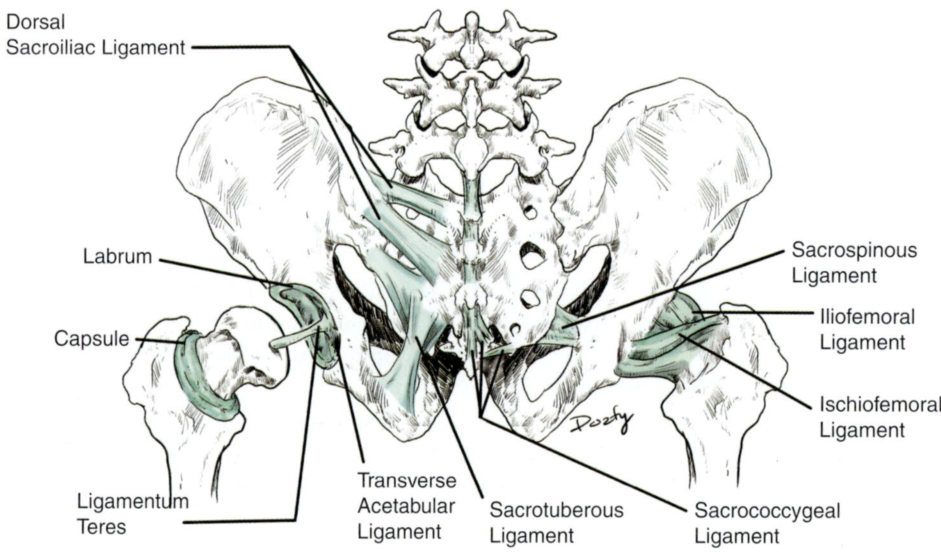

• **Fig. 20.3** Posterior View of Sacropelvic Ligaments.

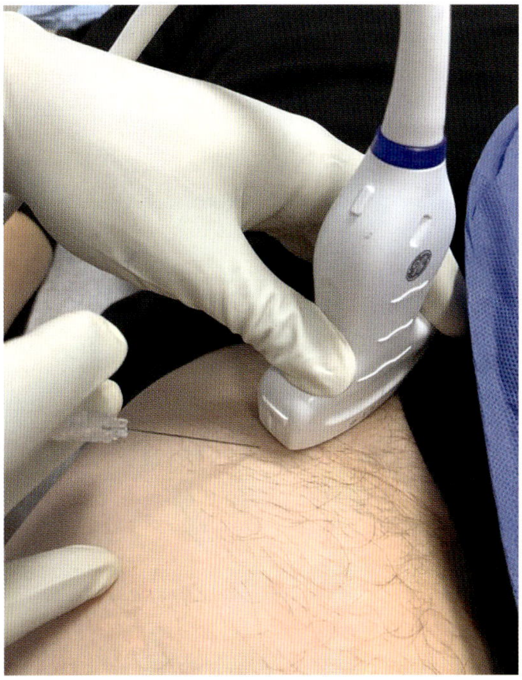

• **Fig. 20.4** Anterior Sagittal Oblique Approach. Transducer in position for in-plane approach to hip joint.

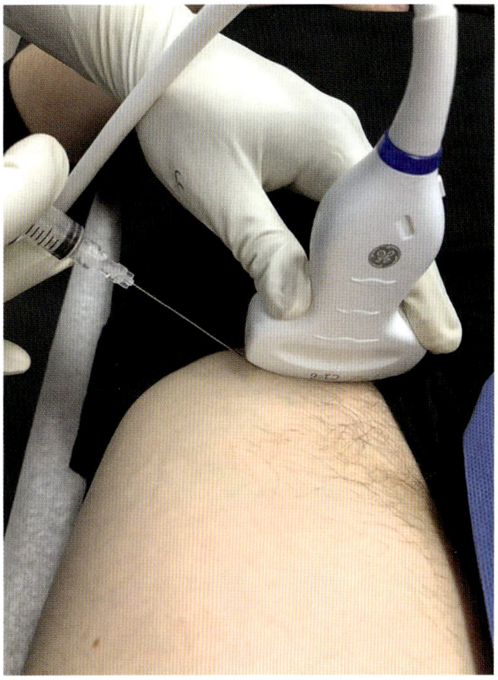

• **Fig. 20.5** Anterior Transverse Approach. Transducer position for alternate approach to hip joint.

being to keep the needle closer to the femoral neck and avoid potential harm to the acetabular labrum.

- Having an assistant apply distal traction on the leg can help open the joint more to allow for easier flow of injectate and open more space to avoid labral injection.

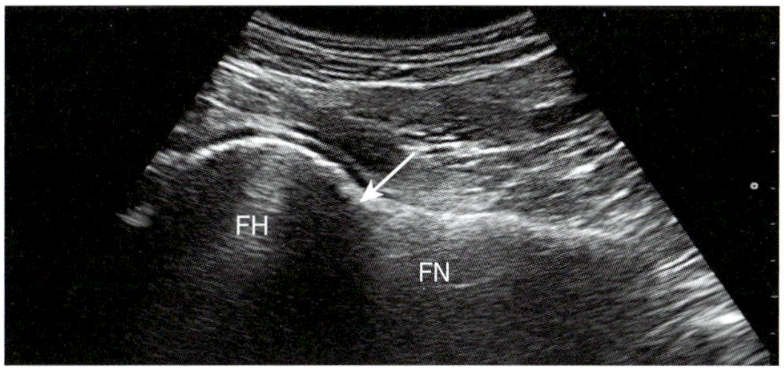

• **Fig. 20.6** Anterior Sagittal Oblique Approach. Ultrasound image with target being the anterior recess of the joint capsule at or just proximal to the femoral head-neck junction. *Arrow* indicates desired path of needle into hip joint and head-neck junction. *FH*, Femoral head; *FN*, femoral neck.

PEARLS AND PITFALLS

- Use lower-frequency probe for better visualization.
- Identify the location of the lateral circumflex femoral artery, as it will often be in the projected trajectory of the needle and the femoral neurovascular bundle medially.
- Needle visualization may be difficult in deeper structures, especially if significant subcutaneous tissue is present, reducing the conspicuity of the target.
- For injecting a collapsed joint recess, it is often helpful to first inject local anesthetic to ensure accurate IA needle placement before final injection.

Adhesive Capsulitis of the Hip

Adhesive capsulitis can occur in the hip similar to the shoulder and can be associated with arthritis. It can be treated first conservatively with physical therapy. Other interventions include steroid injection, capsular dilation, manipulation under anesthesia, and open or arthroscopic synovectomy, lysis of adhesions, and capsular release.[5–7]

Capsular distention can help for adhesive capsulitis. There are small reports in the literature.[8]

- Pitts-Williams A through D criteria for capsular distention:
  A. Utilize color flow to ensure that flow is confined to the capsule and not flowing into the surrounding soft tissue structures.
  B. Inject 5 mL of 0.25% ropivacaine initially, followed by an additional 5–15 mL of injectate connected to the syringe with a T-connector.
  C. Maximal distention volume is reached when there is significant anterior thigh pressure reported by the patient or observed backflow from the T-connector once the syringe is removed. We recommend checking for backflow while injecting in 2–3 mL increments.
  D. Hip range-of-motion (ROM) techniques (i.e., proprioceptive neuromuscular facilitation, muscle energy, muscle activation technique [MAT], etc.) should be performed within 15 min of the distention while the joint is anesthetized. For optimal results, record a side-to-side comparison prior to the distention. Patients should be given a home stretching program to implement three times daily until they can start physical therapy.

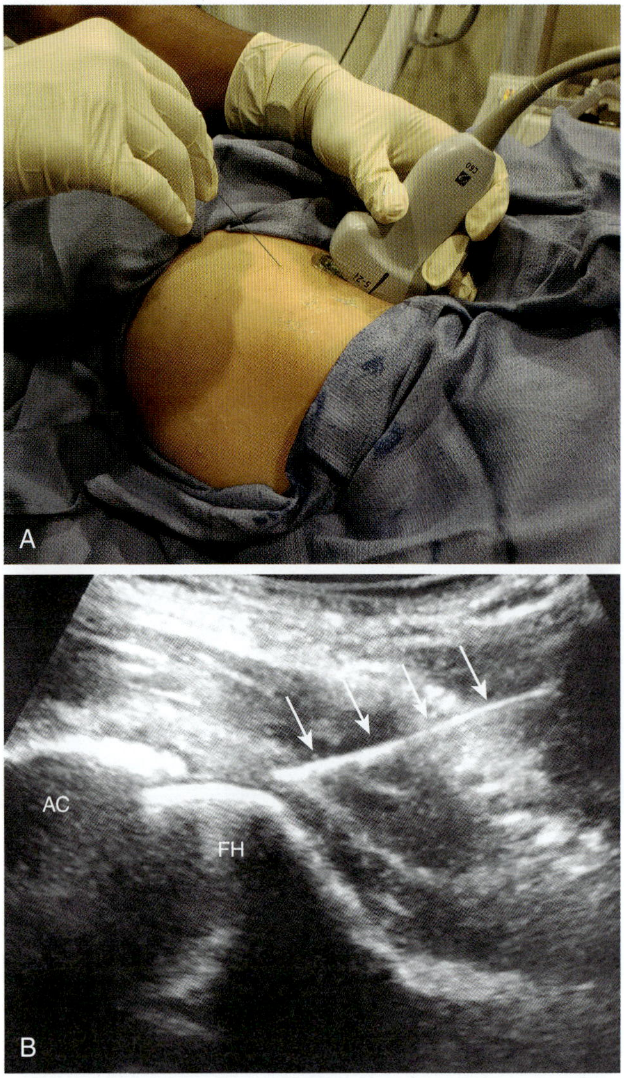

• **Fig. 20.7** (A) Hip intra-articular injection setup with heel toe maneuver and gel standoff. (B) Hip intra-articular injection femoral acetabular junction for weight-bearing flow. *AC*, Acetabulum; *arrows*, needle; *FH*, femoral head.

Technique: Lateral Approach

Alternative approach for patients that have difficulty lying supine

Patient Position

- Lateral decubitus with pillow between the knees

Clinician Position

- Positioned behind the patient

Transducer Position

- Parallel with the femoral neck; often will need to angle and rock the probe to keep the bony cortex parallel or near parallel to the probe

Needle Position

- In-plane, lateral-to-medial approach

Target

- Synovial recess at or just proximal to the junction of the femoral head and neck

PEARLS AND PITFALLS

- Probe positioning and needle must be positioned to clear the greater trochanter on the initial approach. Often, the angle trajectory can be steep, making needle visualization challenging.

Technique: Posterior Approach

Patient Position

- Prone
- Will likely need the hip internal rotated to move the greater trochanter out of the needle trajectory. To achieve this, bend the patient's leg at the knee and rotate from the lower leg outward (Fig. 20.8A)
- Alternatively, patient can be in the lateral decubitus position (see Fig. 20.8B)

Clinician Position

- Standing ipsilateral to the symptomatic hip

Transducer Position

- Posteriorly in the oblique sagittal plane, parallel with the femoral neck

Needle Position

- In plane inferiolateral to superiomedial approach

Target

- Posterior synovial recess, located at or just proximal to the junction of the femoral head and neck (see Fig. 20.8C)

PEARLS AND PITFALLS

- There is more acetabular coverage posterior, so this approach is more difficult to obtain good weight-bearing flow. As such, this is not the preferred approach for IA biologics.
- This is the preferred approach when there is a desire to distend posterior hip capsule due to tightness and adhesions that limit hip internal rotation and hip flexion.

Pubic Symphysis

KEY POINTS

- Commonly underdiagnosed area of pain or instability, and often associated with sacroiliac joint dysfunction and instability.[11,12]
- The pubic symphysis is widest anteriorly.
- There will be some resistance while injecting the fibrocartilage disc in the joint.

Pertinent Anatomy

- The pubic symphysis is a non-synovial amphiarthrodial joint connecting each pubis bone of the pelvis.
- It consists of a fibrocartilaginous disc between the articular surfaces of the pubic bones. It resists tensile,

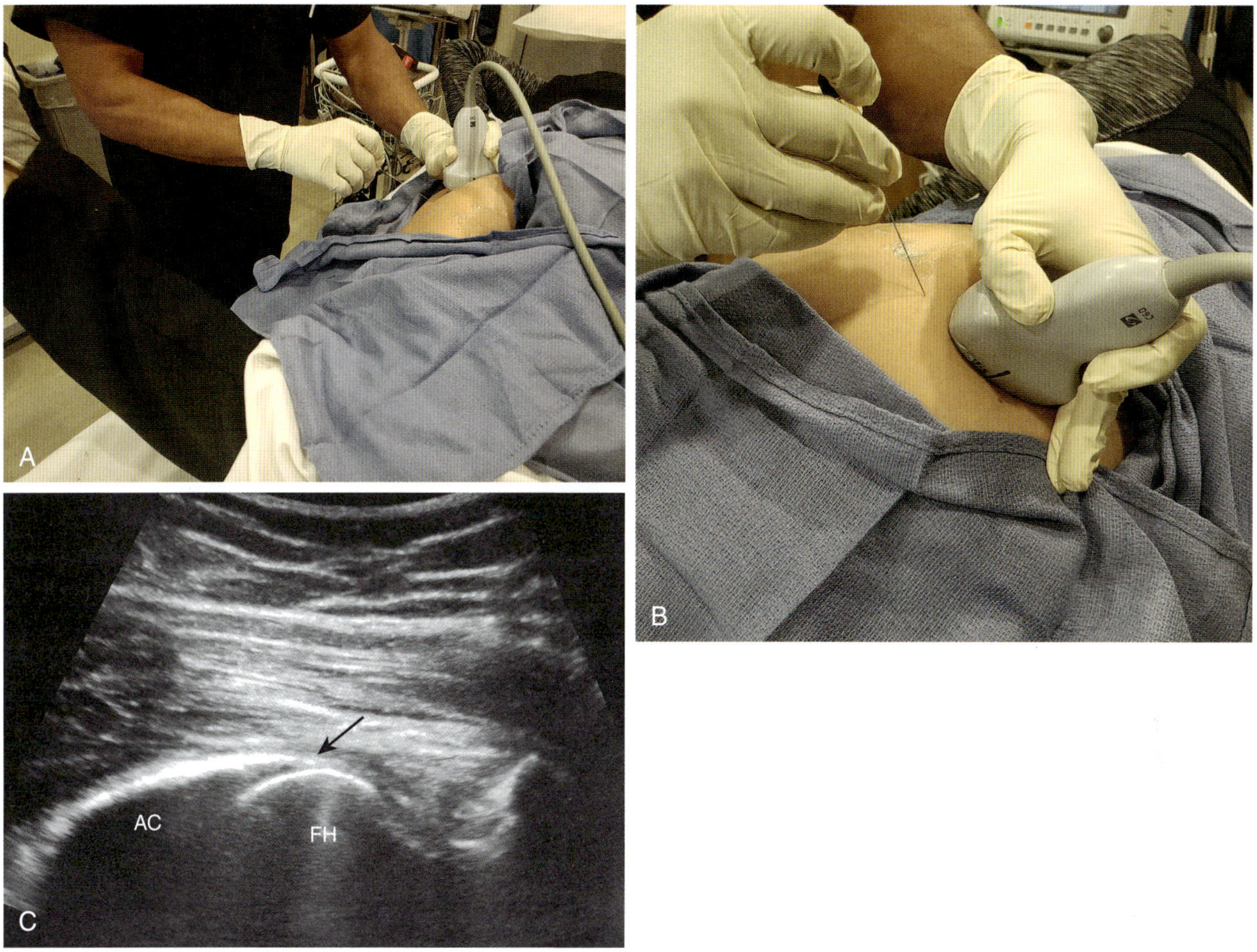

• **Fig. 20.8** (A) Posterior hip joint and capsule injection prone setup. (B) Posterior hip joint and capsule lateral decubitus setup. (C) Posterior hip joint injection ultrasound view. *AC,* Acetabulum; *arrow*, needle tip trajectory; *FH*, femoral head.

shearing, and compressive forces, and is capable of a small amount of movement under physiologic conditions in most adults (up to 2 mm shift and 1 degree rotation).[13]

- Four ligaments reinforce the joint: superior and inferior pubic ligaments, along with the anterior and posterior pubic ligaments.[14]
- The anterior portion of the joint is 3 to 5 mm wider than the posterior portion (see Fig. 20.3).

Common Pathology

- Degenerative of the pubic symphysis syndesmosis,
- Chronic anterior pelvic instability
  - Rare but underdiagnosed. Most common causes of instability include pregnancy and parturition, which often resolves but can persist. External causes of instability include direct trauma, insufficiency fractures, athletics, prior surgery, and osteitis pubis.[15]
- Osteitis pubis
  - Stress injury most commonly seen in athletes that participate in sports involving quick changes of direction, such as football, soccer, ice hockey, etc.[16]
- Secondary pubic symphysis disorder due to sacroiliac joint dysfunction.[17]

Equipment

- Needle size: 22- to 25-gauge, 1.5- to 2.5 inch needle
- High-frequency linear ultrasound transducer

Common Injectates

- Anesthetics for diagnostics.
- Orthobiologics: (PRP, bone marrow concentrate, etc.) and prolotherapy

Injectate Volume

- For IA injection: 0.5 to 1 mL
- For ligamentous injection: 1 to 3 mL

Technique

Patient Position

- Supine with a pillow under knees for comfort (if needed) and to relax the superficial structures around the joint

Clinician Position

- Standing to side of patient

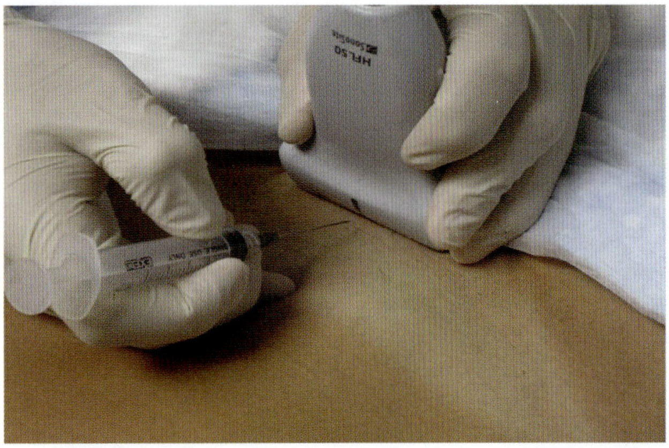

• **Fig. 20.9** Patient supine, with transducer in the transverse plane over the anterior aspect of the pubic symphysis for an out-of-plane approach.

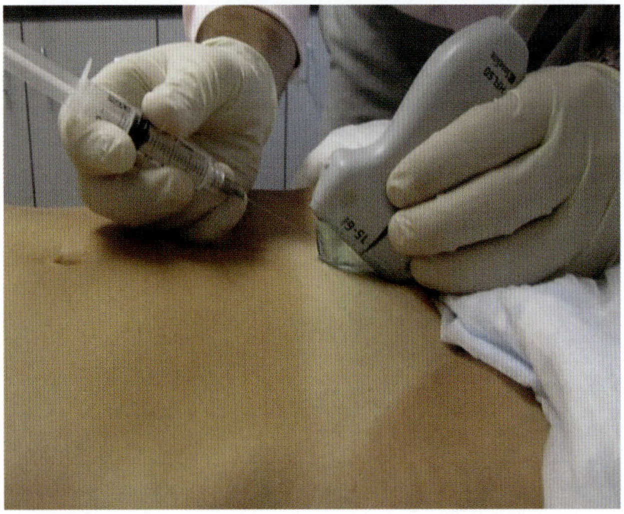

• **Fig. 20.10** Patient supine, with transducer in the sagittal plane over the anterior aspect of the pubic symphysis for an in-plane approach.

Transducer Position

- Out-of-plane approach (Fig. 20.9), anatomic transverse plane over the anterior aspect of the pubic symphysis, with the joint space midline on the monitor
- In-plane approach (Fig. 20.10), anatomic sagittal or transverse plane over the anterior aspect of the pubic symphysis

Needle Position

- Out of plane, needle starting midline over the joint space
- In-plane, from lateral to medial (preferred approach to target the anterior ligaments) (Fig. 20.11)

Target (Fig. 20.12)

- Pubic symphysis fibrocartilaginous disc (Fig. 20.13)
- Anterior ligaments
  - Can inject along the ligament lateral to medial and fan out superiorly and inferiorly (Fig. 20.14)

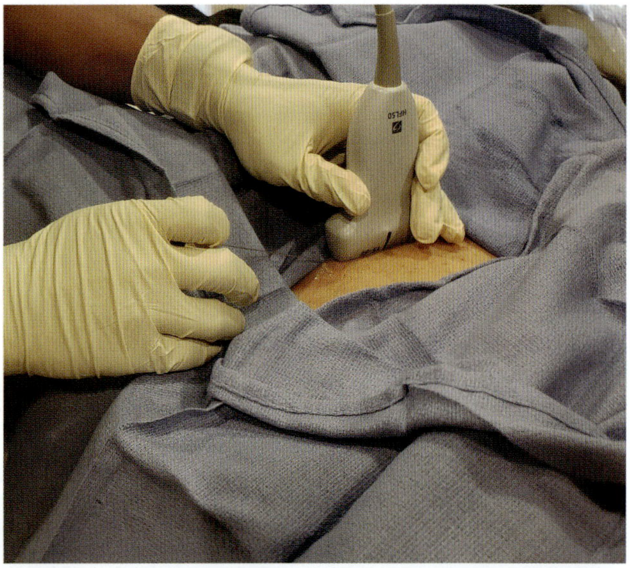

• **Fig. 20.11** Pubic Symphysis Anterior Ligament Injection In-Plane Setup.

PEARLS AND PITFALLS

- Because this joint is a non-synovial joint, it is important to inject the fibrocartilage disc within the joint. There will be some resistance while injecting the fibrocartilage disc. A 25-gauge needle may be used to anesthetize the soft tissue down to the joint; however, a 22-guage needle is often needed to enter the joint.
  - An anterosuperior to posteroinferior approach or lateral in-plane approach is recommended to avoid vascular structures of the genitalia that are inferior to the joint.
  - Be sure not to puncture posterior to the joint as this may cause injury to the bladder. A distended bladder can be positioned above the superior margin of the joint and is susceptible to puncture there, as well.

Hip Capsular Ligaments

Hip Capsular Ligaments

KEY POINTS

- Injection technique is very similar to IA injections except just superficial to the joint, and the goal is to inject multiple sites along the ligaments/capsule.
- Prolotherapy and biologics can be used to stabilize a loose hip, especially in the presence of labral tears, traumatic injuries, connective tissue disorders, and joint arthritis.

Pertinent Anatomy

- Anterior ligaments include:
  - Pubofemoral: originates on iliopectineal eminence of the pubic rami and attaches triangularly to the femoral head, capsule, and ischiofemoral ligament, and

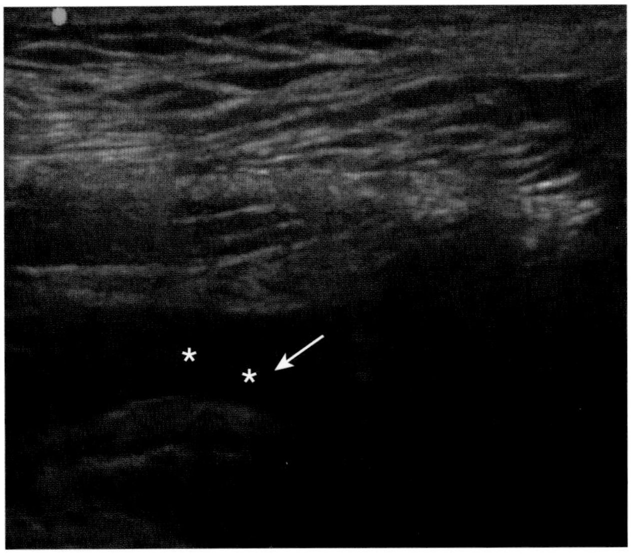

• **Fig. 20.12** Short-Axis View of Pubic Symphysis Joint. *Arrow* indicates needle entry into the joint space. Note the absence of cortical bone in the picture, as this indicates the best view of the pubic symphysis joint for this technique. *Stars* indicate joint space.

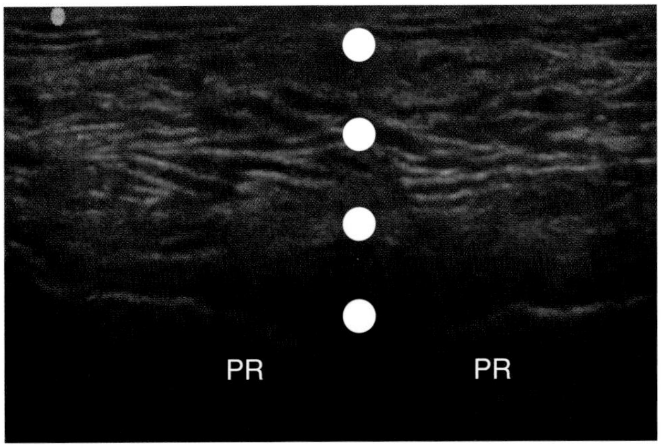

• **Fig. 20.13** Long Axis View of Pubic Symphysis Joint. *Dots* represent walk-down technique into the joint space for out-of-plane injection. *PR*, Pubic ramus.

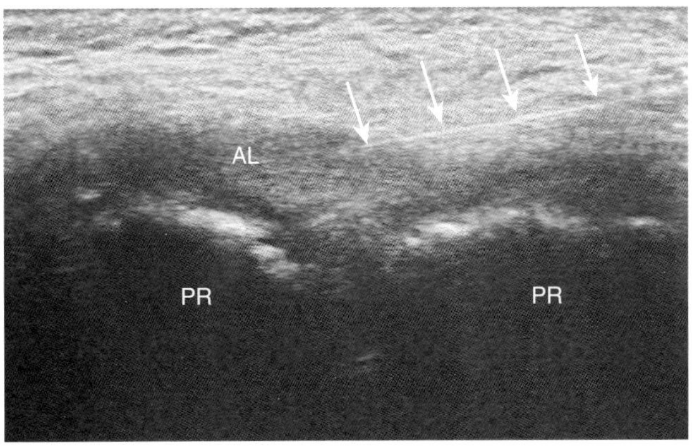

• **Fig. 20.14** Pubic Symphysis Anterior Ligaments In-Plane Injection. *AL*, Anterior ligament; *arrows*, needle; *PR*, pubic rami.

orients more transverse. Limits excess external rotation. Weakest hip ligament.
  - Iliofemoral ligament (Y ligament of Bigelow): the strongest ligament in the body. Inverted Y shape originates vastly along the anterior femur and inserts around the base of the anterior inferior iliac spine (AIIS). Supports standing posture, which limits excessive hip extension
- Lateral ligaments include:
  - Iliofemoral ligament and ischiofemoral ligament
- Posterior ligaments include:
  - Ischiofemoral runs mostly transverse from the ischial acetabular margin to broadly at the base of the greater trochanter. It prevents excessive extension and internal rotation (see Fig. 20.3)

Common Pathology

- Hip instability.[18]
  - Causes include traumatic (post subluxation); iatrogenic, i.e., anterior dislocation after arthroscopy from traction or capsulotomy; developmental dysplasia of the hip; connective tissue/hypermobility disorders; and repetitive microtrauma

Equipment

- Low-frequency curvilinear ultrasound transducer
- Typically, 25- or 22-gauge, 3.5-inch spinal needle is sufficient.
- In larger or taller patient, a 25-gauge, 4.69-inch needle or 22-gauge, 5-inch needle is required

Common Injectates

- Prolotherapy, orthobiologics (PRP, bone marrow concentrate, etc.).
- Steroids should not be used as they can potentially injure ligaments when injected directly.

Injectate Volume

- 2 to 4 mL

Technique: Anterior Approach

Patient Position

- Supine, leg extended, same as IA approach

Clinician Position

- Standing on side of the affected hip

Transducer Position

- Anteriorly in the oblique sagittal plane, parallel with the femoral neck

Needle Position

- In plane, caudolateral to cephalomedial

Target

- Multiple areas along the capsule/iliofemoral and pubofemoral ligaments (Fig. 20.15)
- Adjust transducer to inject multiple points along the joint capsule

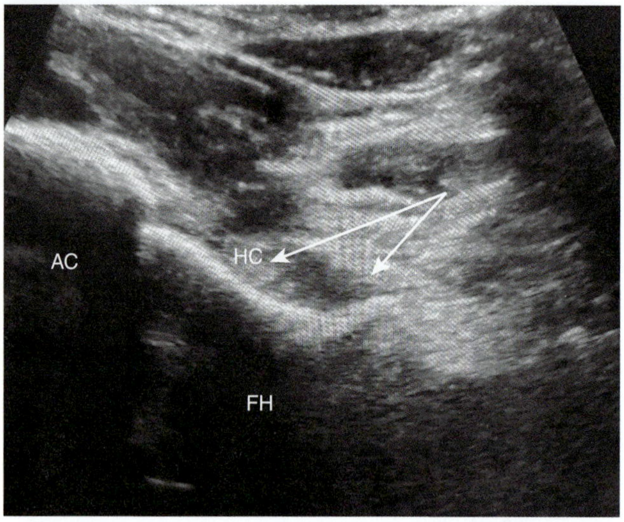

• **Fig. 20.15** Hip Anterior Capsule Injection. *AC,* Acetabulum; *FH,* femoral head; *HC,* hip capsule. *Arrows*, needle trajectory.

PEARLS AND PITFALLS

- Observe injectate flow to ensure injectate is within the ligaments and not IA.
- Should have slightly more resistance than with IA injection, with resistance similar to tendons and other ligaments.

Technique: Posterior Approach

Patient Position

- Prone
- Internally rotate the hip to move the greater trochanter out of the needle trajectory. To achieve this, bend the patient's leg at the knee and rotate from the lower leg outwards (see Fig. 20.8A)

Clinician Position

- Standing ipsilateral to the affected hip

Transducer Position

- Posteriorly in the oblique sagittal plane, parallel with the femoral neck

Needle Position

- In plane, inferolateral to superomedial approach

Target

- Multiple areas along the capsule/ischial femoral ligaments (Fig. 20.16).
- Adjust transducer to inject multiple points along the joint capsule.

PEARLS AND PITFALLS

- Similar approach to intra-articular posterior approach, but injection is into the ligaments. Should have slightly more resistance than intra-articular injection.

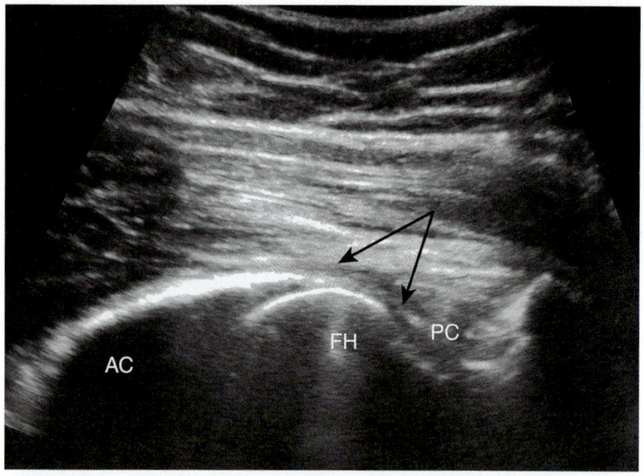

• **Fig. 20.16** Posterior Hip Joint Capsular Ligament Injection. *AC,* Acetabulum; *arrows*, needle trajectories; *FH,* femoral head; *PC*, posterior capsule.

Tendons and Bursae

Rectus Femoris/Sartorius Tendons

KEY POINTS

- Potential site of anterior hip pain.

Pertinent Anatomy

- The quadriceps muscle group is made up of the rectus femoris, and three vastus muscles (medialis, lateralis, and intermedius).
- The rectus crosses two joints and, thus, allows for hip flexion and knee extension.
- The rectus femoris has two origins: a direct head, which originates from the AIIS; and an indirect, which originates inferior and posterior to the AIIS from the superior acetabular ridge.
- The sartorius originates from the anterior superior iliac spine (ASIS) of the pelvis.

Common Pathology

- The quadriceps can be injured by a muscle strain pattern during knee flexion and hip extension. The rectus femoris is the most commonly injured,[19,20] as it is the most superficial and crosses two joints.

Equipment

- Needle size: 22- to 25-gauge, 1.5- to 3.5-inch (depends on body habitus)
- High-frequency linear ultrasound transducer or low-frequency curvilinear transducer

Common Injectates

- Anesthetics for diagnostics
- Prolotherapy, orthobiologics (PRP, bone marrow concentrate, etc.)

Injectate Volume

- 2 to 4 mL in total

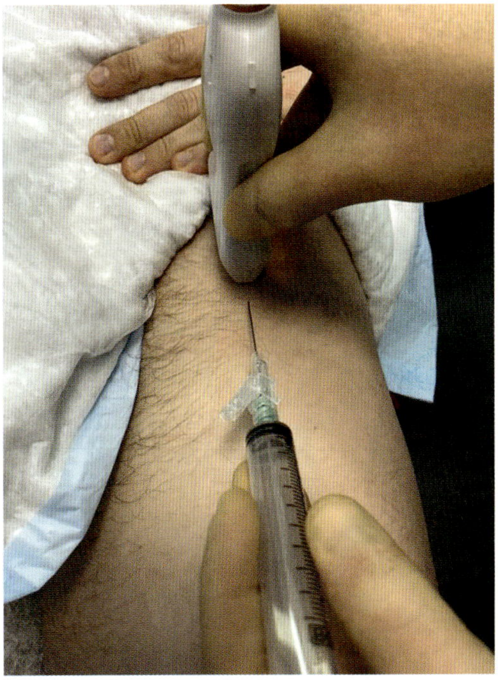

• **Fig. 20.17** Patient and Needle Position. Anterior sagittal approach. Transducer position for in-plane approach to rectus femoris or sartorius tendons.

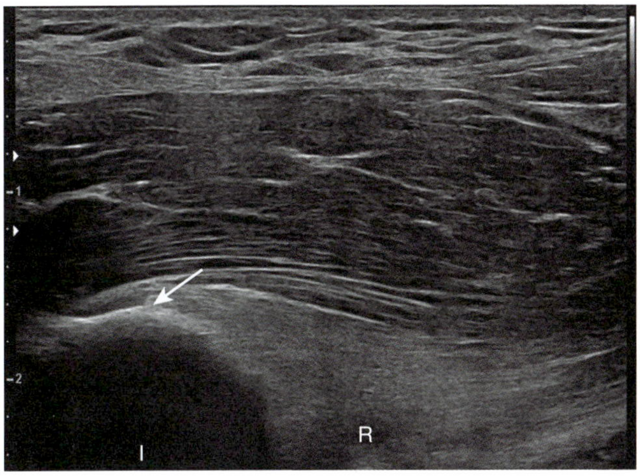

• **Fig. 20.18** Ultrasound image in sagittal plane shows the direct head of the rectus femoris in long axis for an in-plane injection with path of needle directly to tendon pathology. *I*, Anterior inferior iliac spine; *R*, rectus femoris; *arrow*, path of needle.

Technique

See Fig. 20.17.

Patient Position

- Supine with a pillow under knees for comfort (if needed) and to relax the superficial structures

Clinician Position

- Standing or sitting on affected side of patient

Transducer Position

- Long axis to the tendon

Needle Position

- In plane, distal to proximal approach

Target

- Pathologic tendon, usually at or just distal to attachment (Figs. 20.18 and 20.19)

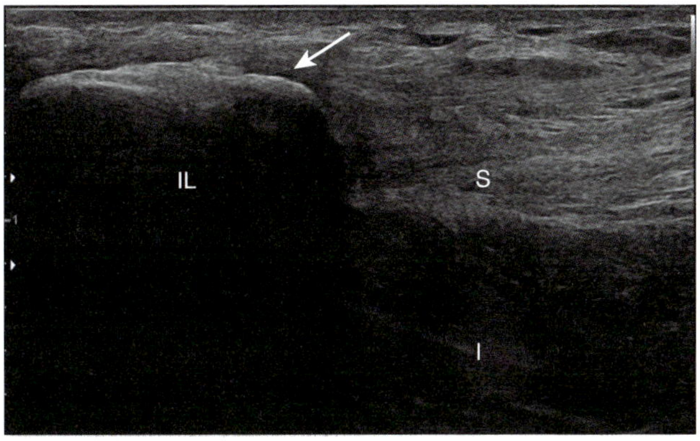

• **Fig. 20.19** Ultrasound image shows long axis of the sartorius for an in-plane injection with path of needle directly to tendon pathology. *I*, Iliopsoas complex; *IL*, anterior superior iliac spine of ilium; *S*, sartorius; *arrow*, path of needle.

PEARLS AND PITFALLS

- Since there is no tendon sheath in this area, avoid corticosteroids, as they could have harmful effects on the tendon.
- If performing fenestration, with or without biologic, be sure to visualize and treat all damaged areas of the tendon.

Adductor Tendons

KEY POINTS

- The adductor longus is the most commonly injured[21] adductor tendon.

Pertinent Anatomy

- The hip adductors are a powerful group of muscles that consist of the adductor magnus/minimus, adductor longus, adductor brevis, and the gracilis and pectineus muscle groups.
- The adductor longus, brevis, and magnus originate from the ischium and pubis of the pelvis.
  - The adductor longus shares a common aponeurosis with the rectus abdominus muscle on the pubis.
- Superficial and medial to the adductors, the gracilis originates from the inferior pubic ramus (Fig. 20.20).

Common Pathology

- Rectus abdominus-adductor longus aponeurotic plate injury
- Adductor tendon injury (acute or chronic)
  - Acute injuries—change of direction, push-off, or stop-and-go movements (i.e., as in soccer, football, hockey, lacrosse, basketball, tennis, etc.), and report a "pop" or "pull" at the time of injury
  - Chronic overuse or repetitive movements, and athletes often complain of a dull ache with these injuries but are often able to continue to play
- Athletic pubalgia—spectrum of related pathology conditions causing groin pain

Equipment

- Needle size: 22-to 25-gauge, 1.5 to 3-inch needle
- High-frequency linear ultrasound transducer

Common Injectates

- Anesthetics for diagnostics
- Prolotherapy, orthobiologics (PRP, bone marrow concentrate, etc.)

Injectate Volume

- 2 to 4 mL

Technique

Patient Position

See Fig. 20.21.

- Supine, with the hip externally rotated and abducted with the knee flexed.
- Patient's arms folded across the abdomen.

Clinician Position

- Standing on affected side.

Transducer Position

See Fig 20.22**.**

- Long axis to the adductor longus tendon.

Needle Position

- In plane.
- Distal-to-proximal approach.

Target

- Adductor tendon where pathology is noted, most often at insertion to pubic symphysis at the insertion of the common aponeurosis of the rectus abdominus-adductor longus (Fig. 20.23)

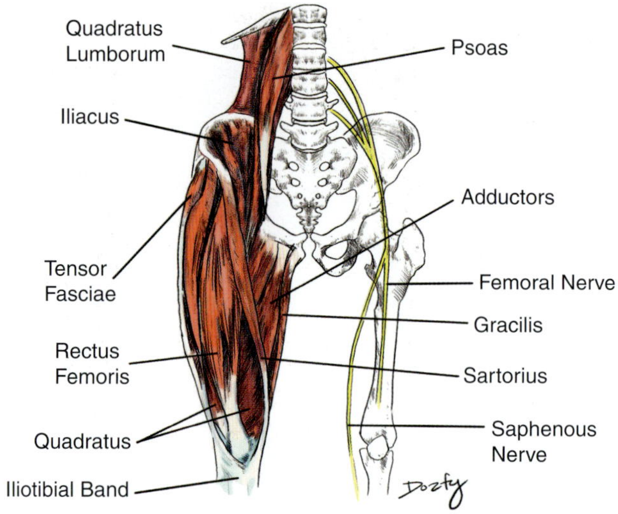

• **Fig. 20.20** Hip Anterior Musculature Anatomy and Large Neuroanatomy.

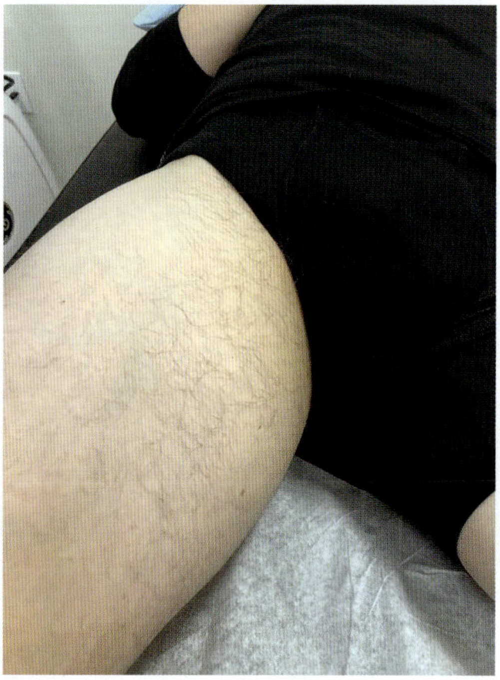

• **Fig. 20.21** Patient Position. The patient is supine with the hip abducted, externally rotated and knee slightly flexed.

PEARLS AND PITFALLS

- Must rotate the transducer to short axis during the procedure to ensure that the entire width of diseased tendon is treated.
- Identify the adductor longus tendon by palpation and place the transducer over it in order to properly identify the entire group of tendons.
- A distal-to-proximal approach for this injection decreases the risk of intravascular injection, as the needle is moving away from the major neurovascular bundle.

Iliopsoas Tendon and Bursa

KEY POINTS

- Dynamic ultrasound evaluation for iliopsoas snapping should be considered.
- Injury to the iliopsoas in this location can occur with total hip arthroplasty or hip arthroscopy.
- Iliopsoas impingement has been associated with anterior labral tears and should be targeted with the same procedure.

Pertinent Anatomy

- The iliopsoas musculotendinous unit is composed of the psoas major, iliacus, and psoas minor, and inserts on the lesser trochanter, with some fibers inserting on the proximal femur.
- The psoas major originates from T12 to L5 transverse processes, vertebral bodies, and intervertebral discs.
- The iliacus originates from the iliac crest and the thoracolumbar spine, and joins the psoas muscles, forming the iliopsoas tendon.
- The psoas minor (which is absent in approximately 40% of the population) attaches at T12 and L1 for its origin, courses anterior to psoas major, and merges to form the iliopsoas tendon.
- The myotendinous junction occurs at the level of the superior pubic ramus.

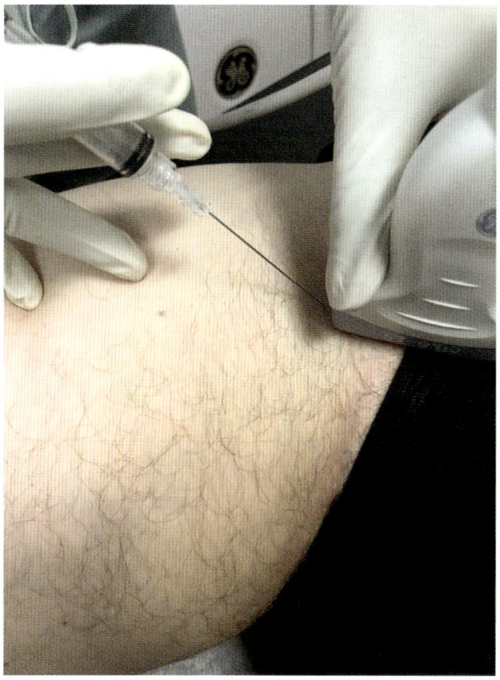

• **Fig. 20.22** Patient and Needle Position. Long-axis, in-plane from distal-to-proximal approach for adductor longus tendon and sheath.

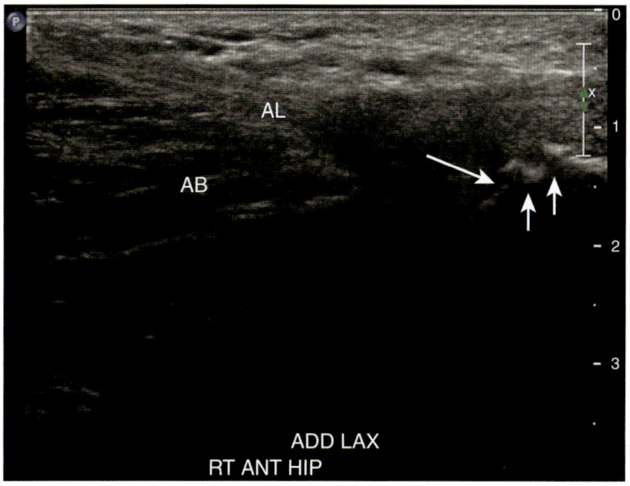

• **Fig. 20.23** Ultrasound image of adductor longus *(AL)* tendinosis with cortical irregularities *(small arrows)* seen at insertion to the pubic ramus. *Long arrow* indicates needle angle and position for tenotomy procedure with long-axis, in-plane approach. *AB*, Adductor brevis muscle; *P*, pubic ramus.

- The iliopsoas bursa is located between the anterior capsule of the hip joint and the iliopsoas tendon.

Common Pathology

- Iliopsoas tendinosis or, less commonly, tendon tear
- Iliopsoas tendon impingement in the setting of a hip replacement and the anterior aspect of the acetabular cup or femoral collar, causing impingement
- Lesser trochanter avulsion fracture
    - Lesser trochanter avulsion in the adult should raise concern for pathologic fracture
- Snapping iliopsoas tendon
    - Seen with dynamic ultrasound when moving the hip from flexion-external rotation or frog leg position to a straightened position
- Iliopsoas bursitis
    - Distention may coincide with iliopsoas tendinosis but is more likely related to an IA hip pathologic process due to continuous synovium between the joint and iliopsoas bursa

Equipment

- Needle size: 22-gauge, 2.5- to 3.5-inch needle
- Medium- to low-frequency linear ultrasound transducer, depending on patient body habitus

Common Injectates

- Anesthetics for diagnostics
- Corticosteroids for bursa only; should not be injected intratendinous
- Prolotherapy, orthobiologics (PRP, bone marrow concentrate, etc.)

Injectate Volume

- 2 to 4 mL
    - Technique iliopsoas bursa or tendon at the femoral head

Patient Position

- Supine
- Hip in neutral position

Clinician Position

- Standing on affected side

Transducer Position

See Fig. 20.24.

- Oblique axial plane parallel to inguinal ligament and iliopectineal eminence (just superior to femoral head)
- Alternatively, sagittal plane in line with the iliopsoas tendon as it crosses the femoral head (Fig. 20.25A)

Needle Position

- In-plane, lateral-to-medial approach

Target

- Intratendinous pathology of the iliopsoas tendon, targeting areas of hypoechogenicity or occult tears
- Target: Iliopsoas bursa if it is distended (Fig 20.26). Otherwise, injection should be deep to the iliopsoas tendon and superficial to the ilium at the iliopectineal eminence

Technique

- Alternative approach distally and insertional iliopsoas tendon

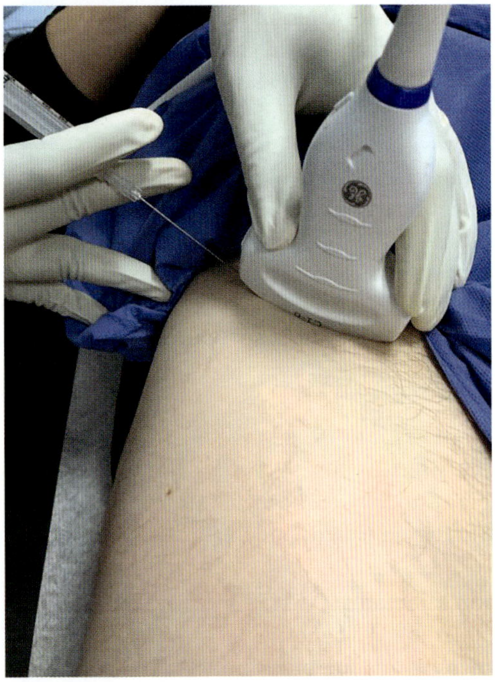

• **Fig. 20.24** Patient and Needle Position. Patient lies supine with the hip in neutral position. Transducer in short axis to the iliopsoas tendon, which is approximately parallel to the inguinal ligament. Needle is in plane to the transducer.

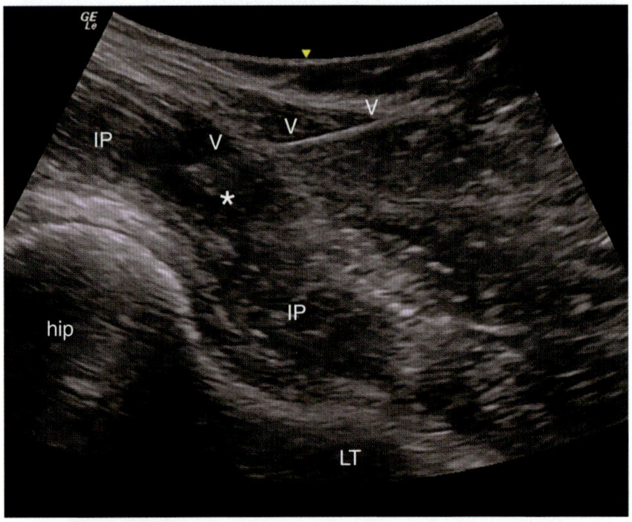

• **Fig. 20.25** (A). Iliopsoas tendon at the femoral head in-plane injection setup. (B) Iliopsoas at femoral head long-axis, in-plane injection. *IP,* Iliopsos at the femoral head long-axis, in-plane ultrasound injection. Hypoechoic interstitial tendon tear (*asterisk*); *LT,* lesser trochanter. Needle *(arrowheads).*

PEARLS AND PITFALLS

- Due to the curvilinear course of the iliopsoas tendon, it is susceptible to anisotropy. Adjust the ultrasound probe to eliminate anisotropy and improve visualization of the tendon.
- Limited ultrasound evaluation of the hip prior to the procedure is essential to screen for snapping hip syndrome and other causes for anterior hip pain, such as paralabral cyst.
- Visualize the femoral neurovascular bundle in relation to the iliopsoas tendon before proceeding with the injection to avoid injury.
- The tendon can require several repositionings of the needle to target all pathologic areas.
- Anesthetic can be used to anesthetize the tendon sheath and small aliquots can be used within the tendon to assess for occult tears and plan where to place the orthobiologic.

Patient Position
- Supine
- Knee flexed and hip externally rotated

Clinician Position
- Standing on affected side

Transducer Position
- Long axis to the tendon
- Scan distal along the tendon to visualize the insertion on the lesser trochanter

Needle Position
- Out-of-plane, lateral-to-medial approach (Fig 20.28A)
  - Alternative: in-plane, proximal-to-distal approach (see Fig. 20.28B)

Target
- Distal iliopsoas tendon, at or just proximal to the lesser trochanter (see Fig. 20.28C and D)

PEARLS AND PITFALLS

- Have to do pre-procedural scan to identify the femoral artery and avoid neurovascular injury.
- Proceduralist has to have good experience with out-of-plane approach as the target can be deep at close to the femoral artery that needs to be avoided.
- The iliopsoas tendon is a long tendon. Anesthetic injections into the tendon can help localize symptomatic pathology tendon at the iliopectineal eminence, superficial to the femoral or at the insertion, and guide future biologic injections.

Iliopsoas Bursa-Technique: Lateral Approach

Patient Position
- Supine, hip in neutral position

Clinician Position
- Seated or standing adjacent to the affected hip.

Transducer Position

See Fig. 20.29.
- Short axis to the iliopsoas tendon, oblique axial plane, parallel to inguinal ligament and cephalad to femoral head

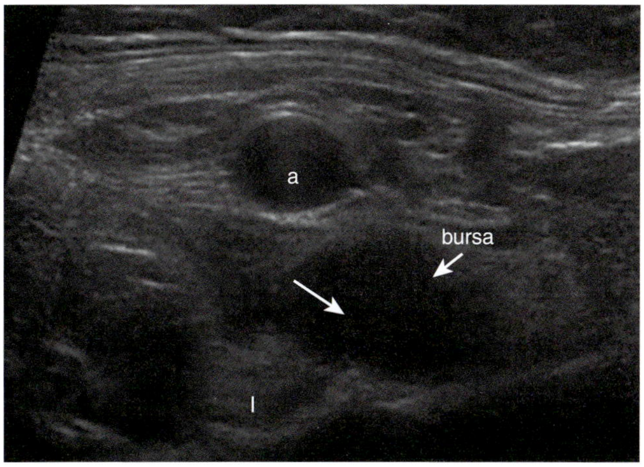

• **Fig. 20.26** Short-axis ultrasound image to iliopsoas tendon *(I)* shows hypoechoic iliopsoas bursal distention *(short arrow)*. *Long arrow* indicates path of needle to iliopsoas bursa injection. The left side of image is lateral. *a*, Femoral artery.

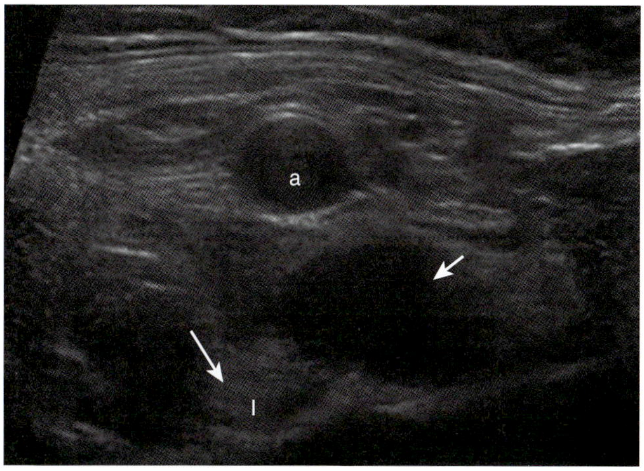

• **Fig. 20.27** Short-axis ultrasound image to iliopsoas tendon *(I)* shows hypoechoic iliopsoas bursal distension (*short arrow*). Long arrow indicates path of needle to iliopsoas tendon injection. The right side of image is medial. *a*, Femoral artery.

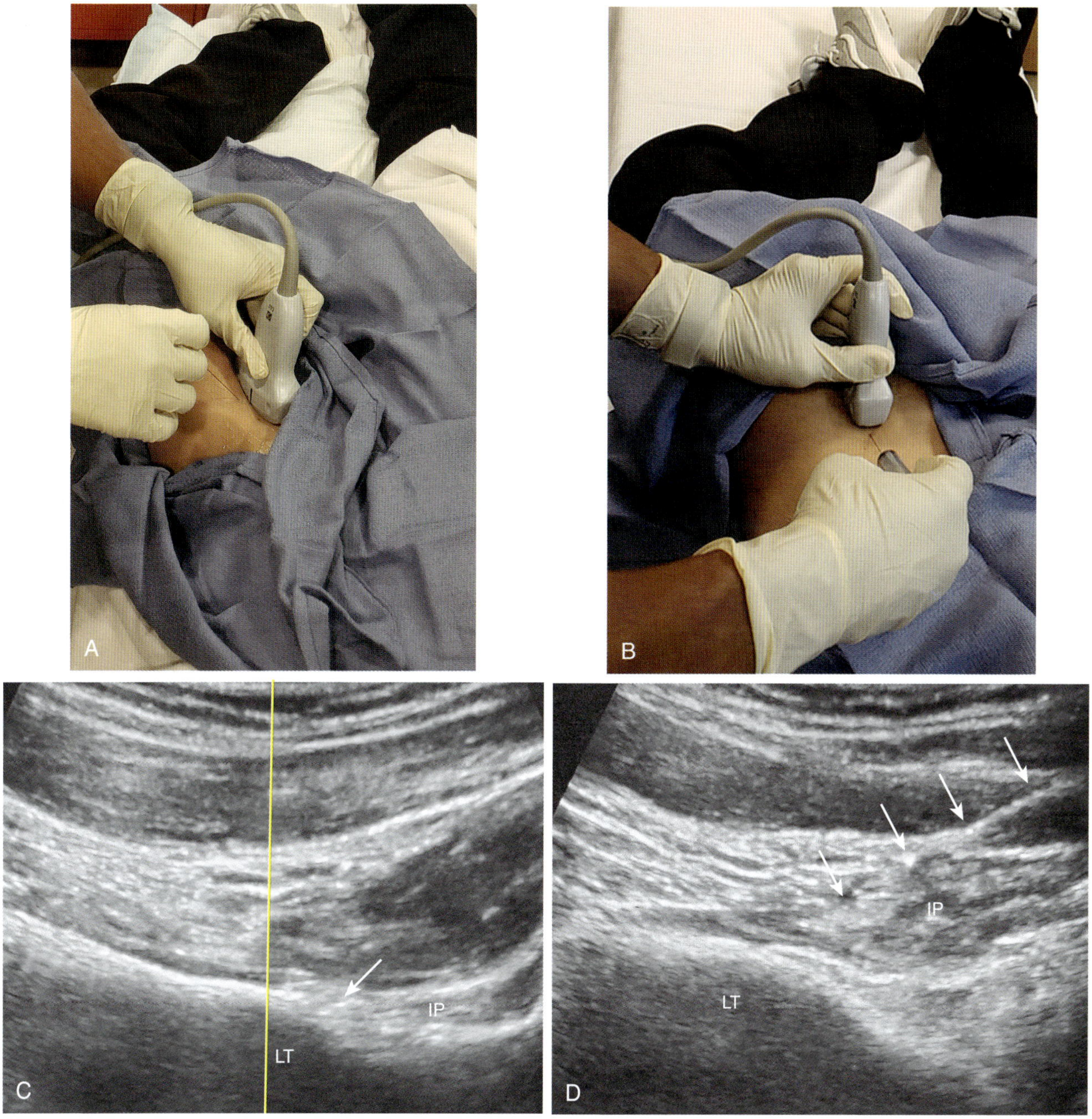

• **Fig. 20.28** (A) Distal iliopsoas tendon out-of-plane injection setup. (B) Distal iliopsoas injection in-plane setup. (C) Distal iliopsoas long-axis, out-of-plane injection. (D) Distal iliopsoas injection long-axis, in-plane injection. *Arrows*, needle; *IP*, Iliopsoas; *LT*, lesser trochanter.

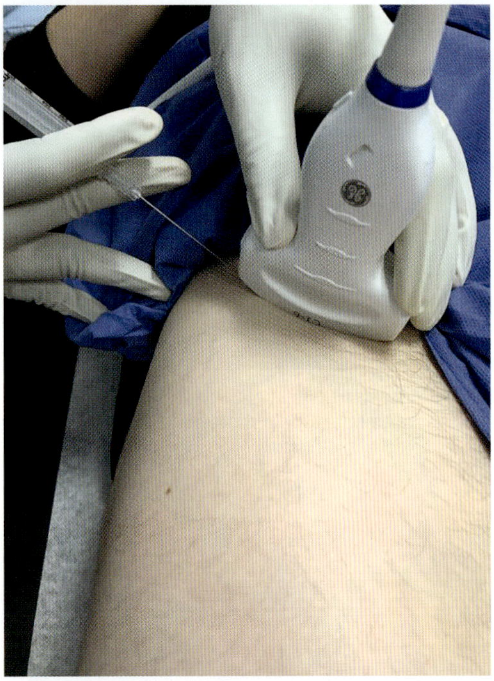

• **Fig. 20.29** Patient and Needle Position. Patient lies supine with the hip in neutral position. Transducer in short axis to the iliopsoas tendon, which is approximately parallel to the inguinal ligament. Needle is in plane to the transducer.

Needle Position
- In-plane, lateral-to-medial approach

Target
- Iliopsoas bursa (see Fig. 20.26)
  - If the bursa is not clearly distended, the injection should be deep to the iliopsoas tendon and superficial to the ilium at the iliopectineal eminence.
- In post-arthroplasty patients, if the bursa is not clearly distended, the target should be directly over the hip joint.

PEARLS AND PITFALLS

- When injecting deep to the iliopsoas tendon, the femoral head should not be in view. This will ensure that the injectate is located within the iliopsoas bursa and not accidently injected into the hip joint

Tensor Fascia Lata Tendon and Proximal Iliotibial Band Injections

KEY POINTS

- The proximal tensor fascia lata (TFL) tendon and iliotibial band are common sites of overuse injuries in runners with pain at the ASIS attachment.

Pertinent Anatomy
- The Tensor fascia lata (TFL) originates from the ASIS and anterior aspect of the iliac crest, and assists with hip flexion, internal rotation, abduction, and stabilization of both the hip and knee.
  - The iliotibial band (ITB) is a dense fibrous band of connective tissue that runs laterally from the iliac crest to the lateral knee.
  - The ITB is a three-layer structure that originates, as the fascia lata, from the iliac tubercle and superficial to the TFL. As it traverses distally, at the site of the greater trochanter, the fascia lata gains thickness (~1.9 mm total) from a fibrous expansion of the gluteus maximus (gluteal aponeurosis) and the TFL to form the ITB.
- The ITB continues to run distally in the lateral portion of the thigh, superficial to the vastus lateralis. The distal insertion point is Gerdy's tubercle, where it merges with biceps femoris and vastus lateralis (see Fig. 20.20).

Common Pathology
- The TFL can become clinically significant in cases of tightening and overuse at its origin, or through its attachment to the ITB
- The TFL is a secondary hip abductor, and pathology may be secondary to underlying gluteal medius weakness.
  - Strain injuries of the ITB (or, more specifically, the fascia lata) at the iliac tubercle have been documented and referred to as proximal iliotibial band syndrome. It is described as a strain injury to the ITB enthesis, where it attaches to the iliac tubercle.
  - Abnormalities of the ITB at the level of the greater trochanter are typically not considered part of proximal iliotibial band syndrome.

Equipment
- High-frequency linear transducer
- Needle size: 22-gauge, 1.5- to 2.5-inch needle

Common Injectates
- Anesthetics for diagnostics and needle fenestration/tenotomy
- Prolotherapy, orthobiologics (PRP, bone marrow concentrate, etc.)

Injectate Volume
- 2 to 4 mL in total

Technique
Patient Position
- Side-lying with affected side upwards, and hip/knee flexed

Clinician Position
- Seated or standing behind the patient

Transducer Position (Fig. 20.30)
- Long axis to the origin of the TFL at the ASIS

Needle Position
- In plane, distal to proximal

Target
- Site of pathology, often at origin of TFL on the anterior iliac crest to the ASIS (Fig. 20.31)

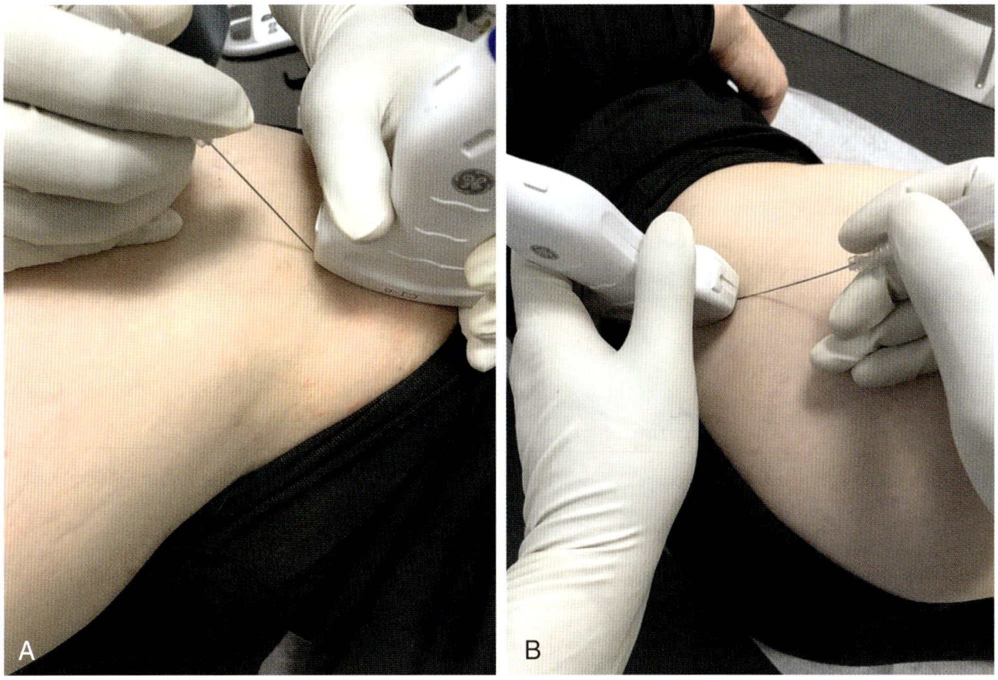

• **Fig. 20.30** (A) Anterolateral sagittal approach. Patient is side-lying and the transducer is in the in-plane sagittal approach, long axis to the tensor fascia lata, on the posterior aspect of the anterior superior iliac spine. (B) Lateral coronal approach. Patient is side-lying and the transducer is long axis to the iliotibial band in the lateral plane at the superior portion of the iliac crest with in-plane needle approach.

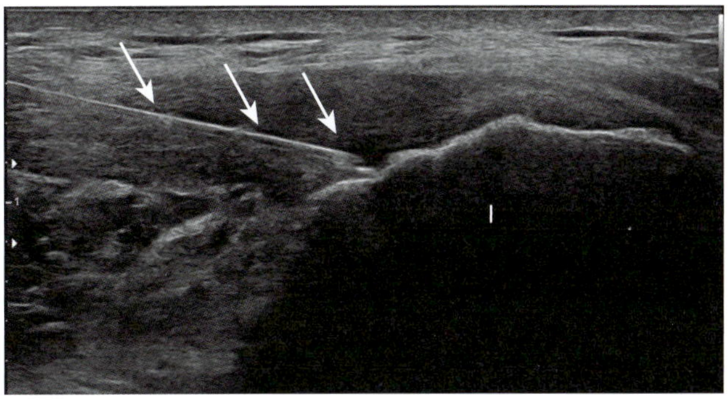

• **Fig. 20.31** Ultrasound image in long axis to the proximal tensor fascia lata shows 20-gauge needle and needle tip *(arrows)* within tendon segment. *I*, Ilium.

PEARLS AND PITFALLS

- Pathology of the TFL is probably underdiagnosed, especially in running athletes.[22–24]
- Would consider needle fenestration with or without PRP injection into the tendon with ultrasound guidance. The number of passes through the tendon during fenestration should be enough until there is a change in tissue resistance.[25]

- Superior portion of the anterolateral iliac crest at the attachment of the proximal ITB (fascia lata), or at the site of defect or fascial injury

Proximal Hamstring Tendon and Ischiogluteal Bursa Injections

KEY POINTS

- The hamstring tendons are deep and curved, making them susceptible to anisotropy. Adjust the ultrasound probe to eliminate anisotropy and improve visualization of the tendon.
- The sciatic nerve should be localized during prescanning, and injection approach should be medial to the nerve.
- For ischial bursa injection, the ischial bursa is not always visible on ultrasound, and the approach for the injection can be difficult, making patient positioning important.

Pertinent Anatomy

- There are four hamstring muscles. Three of the muscles (semimembranosus, semitendinosus, and the long head of the biceps femoris) originate from the ischial tuberosity and cross both the hip and knee joint to flex the knee and extend the hip. The fourth muscle is the short head of the biceps femoris, and it originates from the linea aspera and inserts with the long head on the proximal fibula.
- The long head of the biceps femoris and semitendinosus originate from a conjoint tendon.
- The origin of the semimembranosus is deeper and more lateral on the ischial tuberosity, and then runs deep and

medial to the conjoint tendon. The proximal semimembranosus is mostly aponeurosis, and the muscle mass has a more distal origin. The muscle belly runs medially to the semitendinosus. The insertion is made of five tendinous attachments to the medial tibial condyle, posterior oblique ligament, and the posterior joint capsule.
- The majority of the semitendinosus muscle belly is proximal, with a long, thin tendon located superficial to the semimembranosus that inserts with the sartorius and gracilis tendons forming the pes anserine.
- The long head of the biceps femoris runs laterally and attaches distally to the fibular head.
- The sciatic nerve is located slightly lateral to the conjoint tendon and is critical to locate when performing proximal hamstring injections.
- The ischiogluteal bursa is located superficial to the hamstring tendons and ischial tuberosity, and deep to the gluteus maximus.

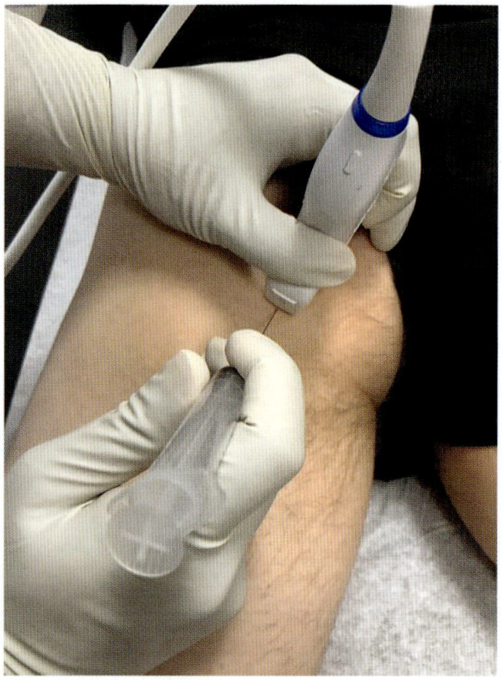

• **Fig. 20.32** Patient is prone, for a long-axis, in-plane approach.

Common Pathology
- The proximal hamstring is a common location for tendinopathy. This is most common in distance runners and starts gradually. Acute injury can occur, particularly with a violent motion of kicking.
- Sonography findings will typically demonstrate thickened tendons, the loss of fibrillation architecture, and hypoechoic areas within the tendon. Cortical irregularities, hyperechoic areas, and tendon calcifications may also be present.
- Ischiogluteal bursitis is often associated with an underlying hamstring tendinopathy.

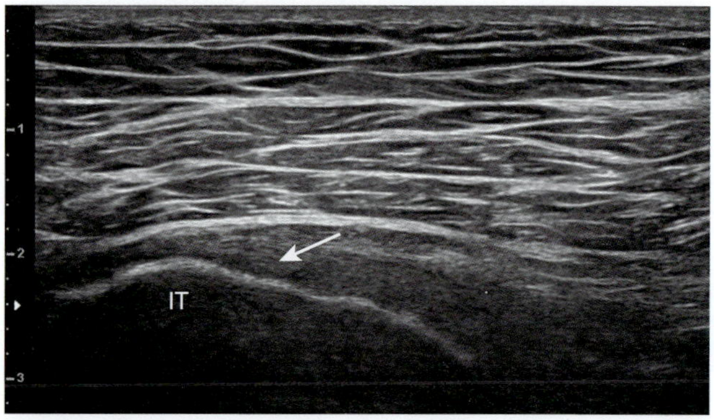

• **Fig. 20.33** Ultrasound image, with patient prone, long axis to the proximal hamstring tendon origin on the ischial tuberosity. *IT*, Ischial tuberosity. *Arrow*, path of needle.

Equipment
- Needle size: 22-gauge, 2.5- to 3.5-inch needle.
- High-frequency linear transducer or low-frequency curvilinear transducer

Common Injectates
- Anesthetics for diagnostics
- Corticosteroids for bursa only, should not be injected intratendinous
- Prolotherapy, orthobiologics (PRP, bone marrow concentrate, etc.)
- Alternate technique to injectates: percutaneous needle fenestration with an 18- to 20-gauge, 1.5- to 2-inch needle. The number of passes would depend on the size of the defect and tactile feedback

Injectate Volume
- 2 to 5 mL

Technique
Patient Position
- Prone (Fig. 20.32): patient's hips propped up with pillows to reduce angle between buttock and upper leg (Fig. 20.33)
- Alternate (Fig. 20.34): side-lying with affected side up and hip and knee flexed (Fig. 20.35)

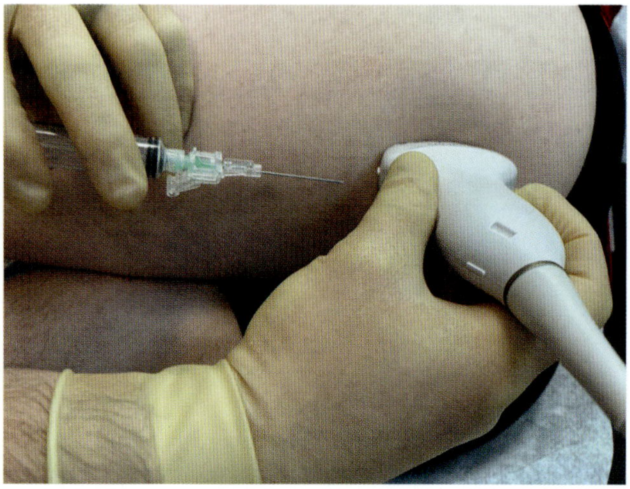

• **Fig. 20.34** Patient is side-lying, for a long-axis, in-plane approach.

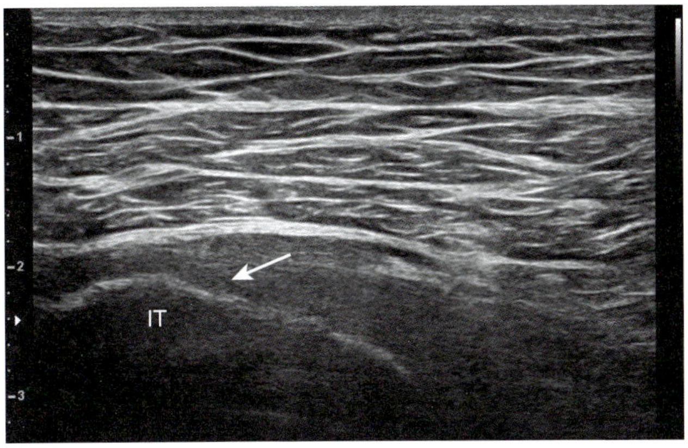

• **Fig. 20.35** Ultrasound image, with patient side-lying, long axis to the proximal hamstring tendon origin on the ischial tuberosity. *Arrow*, needle; *IT*, Ischial tuberosity.

Clinician Position

- Seated or standing on the side of the leg targeted for injection if prone. If side-lying position, in front of the patient.

Transducer Position

- Long axis to the hamstring tendon/conjoint tendon
- Also, can visualize in transverse to inject across the width of the tendon (Fig. 20.36A)

Needle Position

- If long axis to the hamstring, in plane to the transducer, distal to-proximal approach
- If short axis (transverse) to the hamstring, in plane to the transducer, lateral-to-medial approach (see Fig. 20.36B)

Target

- Hamstring tendon origin at site of defect or tendinopathy
- If injecting the bursa: peritendinous hamstring injection at origin or ischial bursa if visible. (Long axis would be the alternate technique; see below for the preferred approach.)

PEARLS AND PITFALLS

- Care should be taken to avoid the sciatic nerve, which is just lateral to the hamstring tendon insertion on the ischial tuberosity.
- While performing the injection, the probe can be changed to short axis (out of plane to the needle) to visualize the medial-to-lateral location of the needle.
- Peritendinous corticosteroid injections can provide short-term pain relief, but symptoms tend to recur and can be more severe.[29,30] Corticosteroids should not be injected into the tendon, but can be used to inject the adjacent and superficial ischiogluteal bursa.

Gluteal Attachments

Gluteal Tendon Origin (Iliac Crest) Injections

KEY POINTS

- This is an underdiagnosed area for tendinopathy, especially in patients with low back pain and radiculitis.

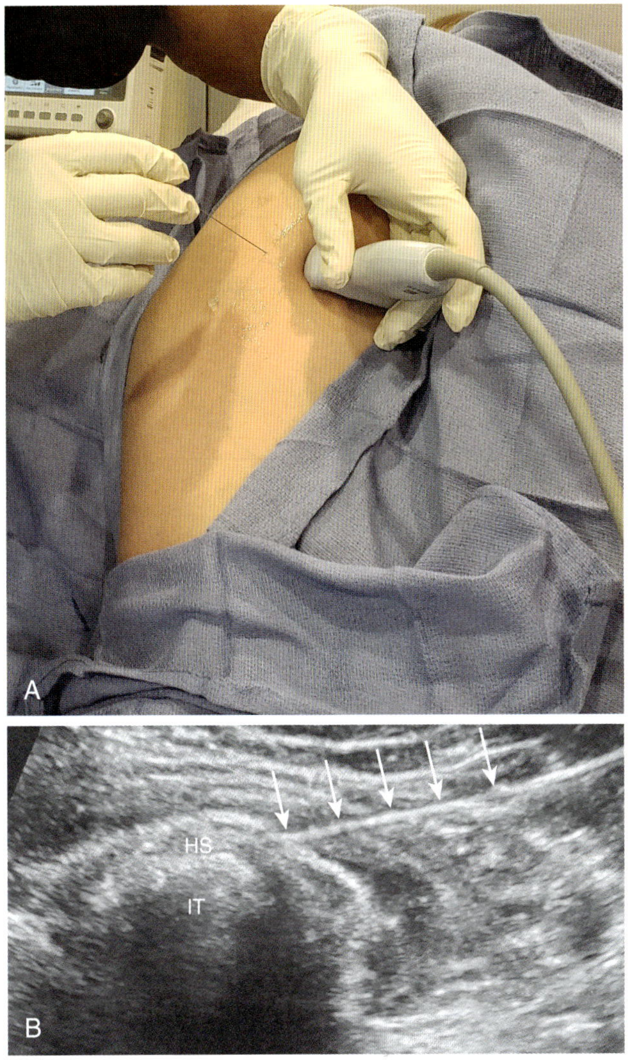

• **Fig. 20.36** (A) proximal hamstring transverse view setup. (B) Proximal hamstring injection transverse view in-plane needle approach lateral to medial. *HS,* Hamstring in transverse; *IT,* ischial tuberosity. *Arrows,* Needle.

Pertinent Anatomy

- The gluteus maximus originates from the sacrum, posterior sacroiliac ligaments, and a small portion of the ilium near the posterior superior iliac spine (PSIS). Some of its fibers insert on the fascia lata and iliotibial tract, and others insert on the proximal posterior femur on the gluteal tuberosity, which is located just distal to the trochanters and the femoral head.
- The gluteus medius originates from the superolateral surface of the posterior iliac wing. The posterior portion of the muscular origin is covered by the gluteus maximus. The anterior portion of the muscle inserts on the lateral facet of the greater trochanter, while the posterior portion inserts on the superoposterior facet.
- The gluteus minimus also originates on the lateral iliac wing, inferior to the gluteus medius, and runs deep to the gluteus medius, inserting on the anterior facet of the greater trochanter.

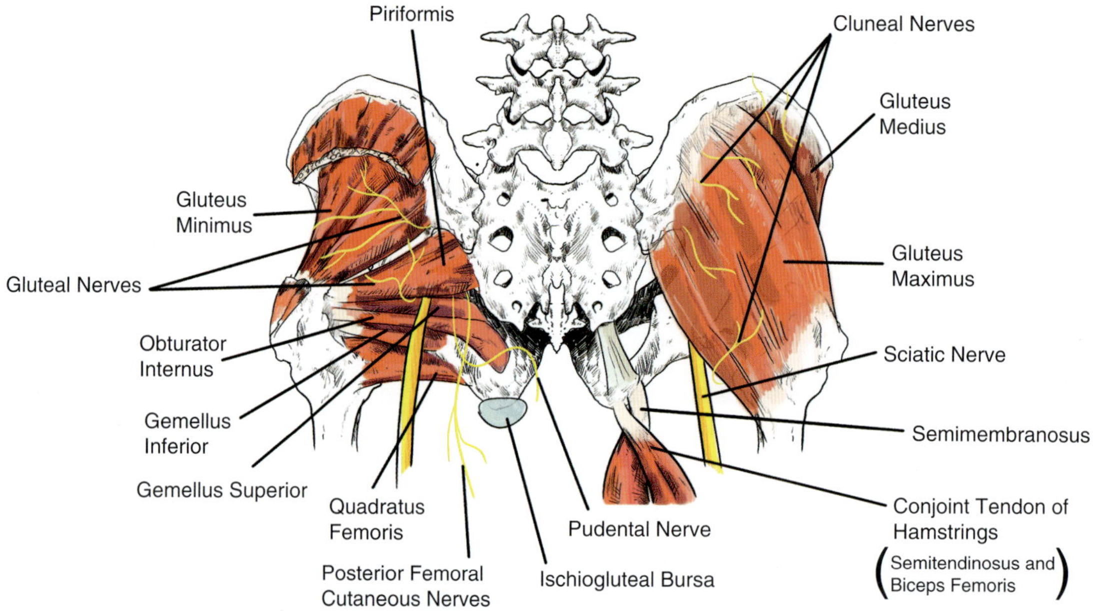

• **Fig. 20.37** Posterior Pelvic/Hip Neuromuscular Anatomy.

- The gluteal aponeurotic fascia covers the gluteal medius and a portion of the gluteus maximus, and serves at the tendon of origin of the gluteus medius (Fig. 20.37).[31]

Common Pathology

- Pathology at the origin of the gluteus maximus, gluteus medius, gluteus minimus, or TFL muscle appears as hypoechoic abnormalities (interstitial tears, tendinopathic changes) or hyperechoic (enthesophytes, calcifications) abnormalities on sonographic evaluation.[32]
- Tearing and discontinuity of the gluteal aponeurotic fascia has also been reported as a source of pain.[31]

Equipment

- Needle size: 22- to 25-gauge, 2.5- to 3.5-inch needle
- Medium- to high-frequency linear transducer; if needed, low-frequency curvilinear transducer

Common Injectates

- Anesthetics for diagnostics and needle fenestration/tenotomy
- Prolotherapy, orthobiologics (PRP, bone marrow concentrate, etc.)

Injectate Volume

- 2 to 4 mL in total

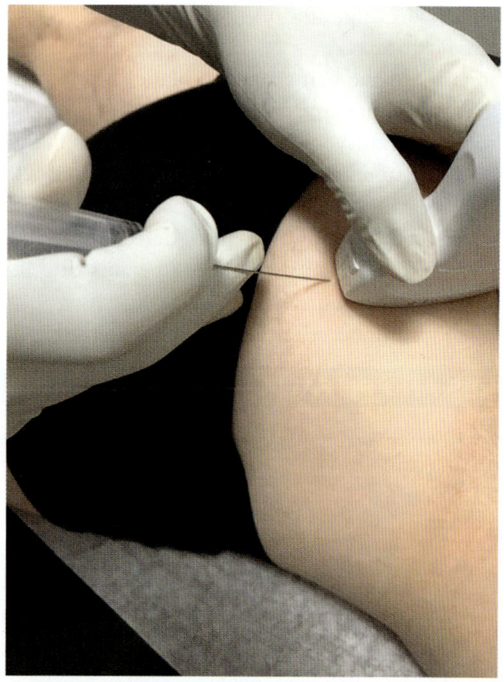

• **Fig. 20.38** Oblique Sagittal Approach. Short axis to the iliac crest, starting at the posterior superior iliac spine with in-plane needle approach.

Technique

Patient Position

- Prone

Clinician Position

- Seated or standing directly next to the hip being treated

Transducer Position

See Fig. 20.38.

- Short axis to the iliac crest, starting at the PSIS. To change target on crest or orientation, operator will fan transducer in superior or inferior direction, maintaining the crest in picture and in short axis

Needle Position

- In plane to the transducer, and lateral-to-medial or distal-to-proximal approaches, depending on the muscle being treated

Target

- Gluteal muscle origin site pathology

PEARLS AND PITFALLS

- Care should be taken to avoid the needle slipping superior or medial off the iliac crest.

From Atlas; Jacobson MSK US, Hollinshead's[9,33]

Gluteus Tendon Insertion (Greater Trochanter) and Trochanteric Bursal Injections

KEY POINTS

- Rotation of hip during scanning identifies the plane between the gluteus medius and gluteus maximus.
- Subgluteus maximus bursitis (trochanteric bursitis) is much less common than gluteal tendon tears and tendinosis.

Pertinent Anatomy

- The greater trochanter has four facets: anterior, lateral, superoposterior, and posterior.
- The gluteus medius originates from the iliac crest. The anterior portion inserts on the lateral facet, and the posterior portion inserts on the superoposterior facet. The gluteus minimus originates on the ilium, runs deep to the gluteus medius, and inserts on the anterior facet.
- The trochanteric (or subgluteus maximus) bursa is located between the gluteus maximus/medius and iliotibial band, overlying much of the posterior facet.
- The hip abductor muscles—the gluteus medius and gluteus minimus—support and level the pelvis during the single leg stance of ambulation or running.
- Sonographic evaluation may demonstrate intratendinous calcification, hypoechoic or anechoic areas within the tendon, cortical irregularities, tendon enlargement, or absence of visible tendon, indicating partial or full-thickness tears (see Fig. 20.37).

Common Pathology

- Excessive friction between the tendon layers can cause inflammation, thickening, and fluid accumulation in the subgluteus maximus bursa. This is commonly referred to as trochanteric bursitis, and has fallen out of favor as a source of greater trochanteric pain as it is exceedingly rare.[34]
- The more common findings at the greater trochanter are interstitial, partial-thickness, or full-thickness tears of the gluteus medius and minimus tendons.
- The most common location of these tears or tendinopathies is the anterior gluteus medius tendon.

Equipment

- Needle size: 22- to 25-gauge, 2- to 3.5-inch needle
- Medium- to high-frequency linear transducer. If needed, a low-frequency curvilinear transducer may be used due to body habitus

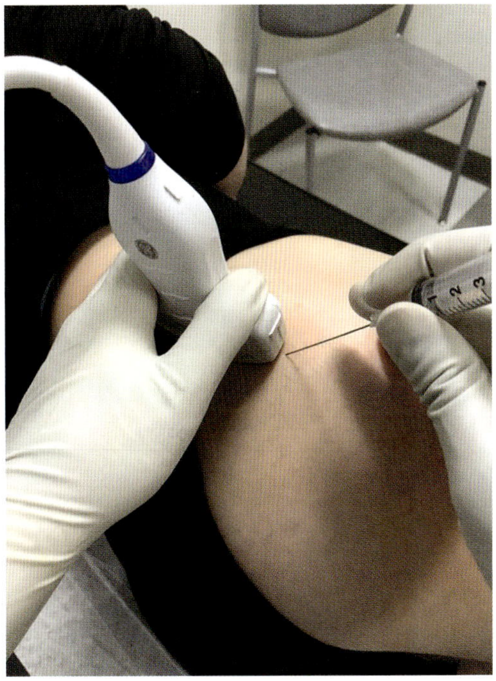

• **Fig. 20.39** Patient Side-Lying With the Hip in Neutral Position. Transducer is long axis to the targeted tendon for an in-plane, distal-to-proximal approach.

Common Injectates

- Anesthetics for diagnostics
- Corticosteroids for bursa only, should not be injected intratendinous
- Prolotherapy, orthobiologics (PRP, bone marrow concentrate, etc.)

Injectate Volume

- 2 to 5 mL in total

Technique: Lateral Approach

Patient Position

- Side-lying with affected hip up, pillows under head and between legs

Clinician Position

- Seated or standing directly next to and posterior to hip being injected

Transducer Position

- Long axis to the gluteal tendon, distal or proximal approach (Fig. 20.39)
- Short axis to the gluteus tendon, posterior-to-anterior approach
- For trochanteric bursa, superficial and slightly posterior to the lateral facet, approximately 37 degrees posterior rotation relative to the long axis of femur (Fig. 20.40)

Needle Position

- In plane to the transducer
- Needle approach: distal to proximal, proximal to distal, or posterior to anterior

Target

- Abnormal gluteus medius, gluteus minimus tendon, or adjacent bursa (Figs. 20.41 and 20.42)

PEARLS AND PITFALLS

- If the subgluteus maximus bursa is not visible, its location in the potential space between the gluteus aponeurosis and gluteus medius tendon layer can be better identified by external hip rotation.
- Corticosteroids for gluteal pain are controversial and may have limited long-term benefits.[35] Corticosteroids may help with bursitis, but intratendinous injection of corticosteroids into the gluteal tendons should be avoided.
- The trochanteric bursa is uncommonly distended and rarely inflamed as an isolated cause of symptoms. If bursitis is present, be extra careful scanning for presence of gluteal tendon pathology, which is more common.[34]
- Alternate technique to injectates: percutaneous needle fenestration with 18- to 20-gauge needle. The number of passes would depend on the size of the defect and tactile feedback

From: Atlas, Jacobson MSK US.[9,10]

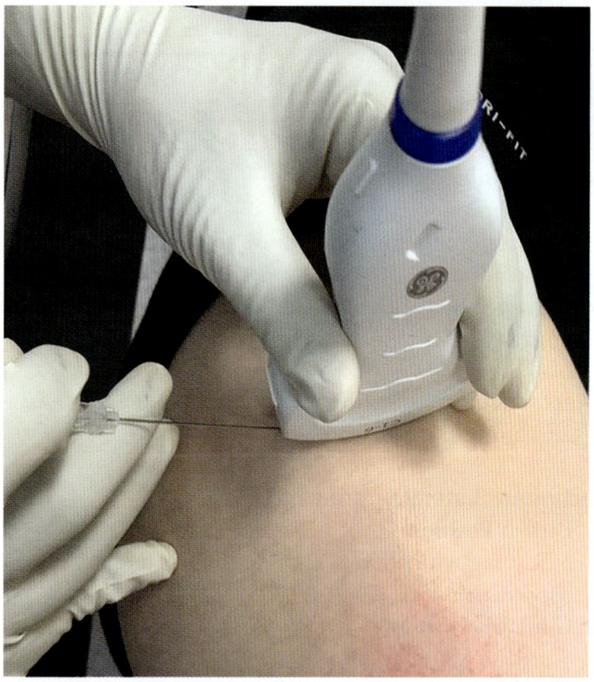

• **Fig. 20.40** In-plane approach, short axis and slightly oblique to the tendon and slightly posterior to the lateral facet.

External Rotators

Piriformis Muscle/Tendon

KEY POINTS

- The sciatic nerve must be identified during pre-procedure scanning and is most commonly deep to the piriformis muscle.
- The ascending branches of the inferior gluteal artery should be identified prior to the procedure and are located underneath the gluteus maximus muscle.

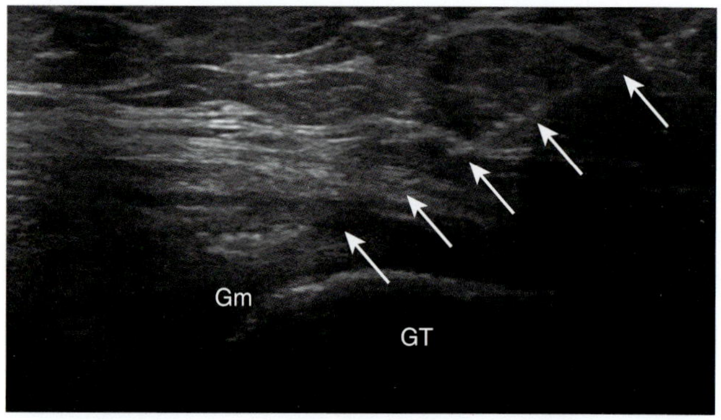

• **Fig. 20.41** Gluteus Medius Fenestration. Ultrasound image long axis to the gluteus medius over the superoposterior facet of the greater trochanter shows needle within hypoechoic and thickened tendon segment (left side of image is superior). *arrows*, needle; *Gm*, Gluteus medius; *GT*, greater trochanter.

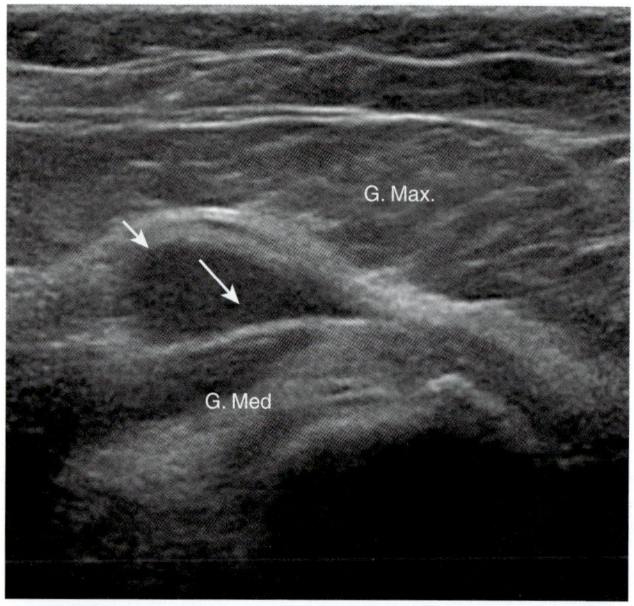

• **Fig. 20.42** Long-axis view of subgluteus maximus bursal fluid collection with needle directed at bursa *(arrow)*.

Pertinent Anatomy

- The piriformis muscle is a relatively small muscle that lies deep to the gluteus maximus muscle.
- Its main function is to externally rotate the hip, although it also abducts the hip when the hip is flexed.
- The sciatic nerve is normally found deep to the piriformis muscle, but anatomic variability exists and, occasionally, the sciatic nerve may pierce or run superficial to the piriformis muscle.

Common Pathology

- The piriformis muscle is a potential cause of myofascial pain in patients presenting with gluteal pain.
- The diagnosis of piriformis syndrome is often a diagnosis of exclusion.

Equipment

- Needle size: 22-gauge, 3.5-inch needle

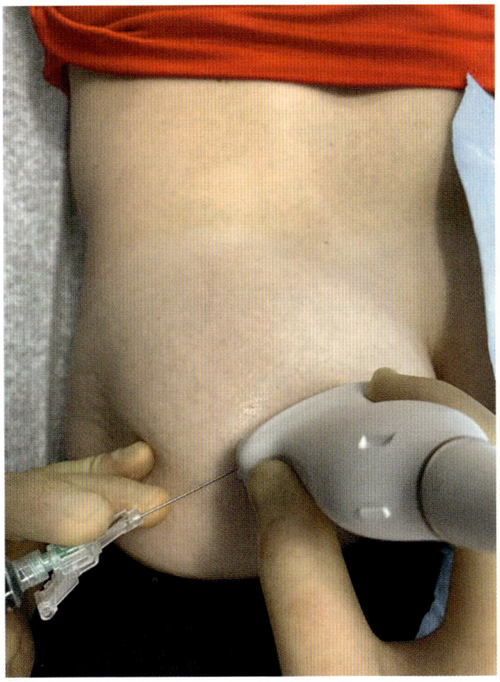

• **Fig. 20.43** Patient prone, with transducer positioned from cephalomedial to caudolateral for a lateral-to-medial, in-plane approach. *ADD*, transducer "long axis to piriformis" positioned.

- Medium-frequency linear transducer or low-frequency curvilinear transducer, depending on body habitus and desired field of view

Common Injectates

- Anesthetics for diagnostics or trigger points
- Corticosteroids for sheath only
- Prolotherapy, orthobiologics (PRP, bone marrow concentrate, etc.)
- Botulinum toxin

Injectate Volume

- 2 to 4 mL in total

Technique

Patient Position

- Prone

Clinician Position

- Standing or sitting on affected side

Transducer Position

See Fig. 20.43.

- Long axis of piriformis muscle, axial oblique from cephalomedial to caudolateral over the piriformis muscle

Needle Position

- In-plane, lateral-to-medial (or medial-to-lateral) approach

Target

- Piriformis muscle sheath and/or piriformis muscle (trigger point) (Fig. 20.44)
- Precise location of injection has not been proven in the literature, but considerations include intramuscular, deep, and superficial to the piriformis

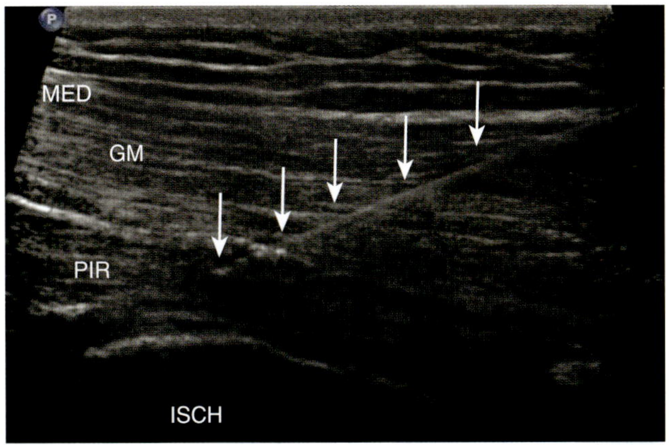

• **Fig. 20.44** Long-Axis Ultrasound Image of Piriformis Muscle Needle Placement. *Arrows* indicates needle. *GM*, Gluteus maximus muscle; *ISCH*, ischium; *MED*, medial; *PIR*, piriformis muscle.

PEARLS AND PITFALLS

- The sciatic nerve position relative to the piriformis muscle should be identified during pre-procedure scanning.
- The sciatic nerve will most often be found deep to the piriformis muscle, but anatomic variations exist in which the nerve or its peroneal division passes through or is superficial to the piriformis.
- Passive hip internal and external rotation may assist in identifying the piriformis muscle because of the relative movement of the muscle compared to the overlying gluteus maximus muscle.

Gemelli-Obturator Internus Complex and Obturator Internus Bursa Injection

KEY POINTS

- Care should be taken to identify the sciatic nerve during pre-procedure scanning, as it should lie just superficial to the obturator internus and gemellar muscles.
- It may be difficult to discern obturator and gemellar muscles apart, as they may look like a single myotendinous unit along with the obturator internus muscle.
- The obturator internus can also be found superficial to the proximal ischium, as it "rotates" around the ischium with internal and external rotation of the hip.

Pertinent Anatomy

- The gemelli muscles are a pair of muscles that bookend the obturator internus, inferiorly and superiorly, in a parallel fashion. The inferior gemellus originates on the superior aspect of the ischial tuberosity, coursing inferior to the obturator internus and superior to the quadratus femoris. The superior gemellus originates from the ischial spine, and courses superior to the obturator internus and inferior to the piriformis muscle. Both of the gemelli insert on the medial aspect of the greater trochanter with the obturator internus tendon.

- The three muscles—inferior gemellus, obturator internus, and superior gemellus—are often viewed as a single functional unit.[9]
- The sciatic nerve normally is found superficial to the lateral part of the tendon.
- The obturator internus bursa is located between the obturator internus tendon and the surface of the ischium.

Common Pathology

- Gemellar and obturator internus myofascial pain, tendinitis, tendinosis, and bursitis have been reported to be associated with gluteal and posterior hip pain. Symptoms are often vague and poorly localized. The deep location of the structures, small size, and close proximity of the other external rotators makes diagnosis difficult. Diagnostic injection of the muscle, tendon sheath, or bursa may be helpful to localize the pain generator.[36,37]

Equipment

- Needle size: 22-gauge, 2.5- to 3.5-inch needle
- Low-frequency curvilinear transducer or a medium-frequency linear transducer, depending on body habitus

Common Injectates

- Anesthetics for diagnostics or trigger points
- Corticosteroids for bursa or sheath only
- Prolotherapy, orthobiologics (PRP, bone marrow concentrate, etc.).

Injectate Volume

- 2 to 4 mL in total

Technique

Patient Position

- Prone

Clinician Position

- Seated or standing on the side of the leg targeted for injection if prone. If side-lying position, in front of the patient.

Transducer Position

See Fig. 20.45.

- Long axis to the gemelli in the transverse plane

Needle Position

- In-plane to the transducer, lateral to medial

Target

- Inferior or superior gemellus muscle, at its insertion on femur or site of pathology (Figs. 20.46 and 20.47)
- Obturator internus bursa deep to the obturator internus muscle on the ischium

PEARLS AND PITFALLS

- The sciatic nerve must be identified and avoided during injection. The nerve will most commonly be found superficial to the gemelli.

From: Atlas of US MSK Inj–Mautner, Fundamentals of MSK US–Jacobson, Grays Anatomy[9,10,38]

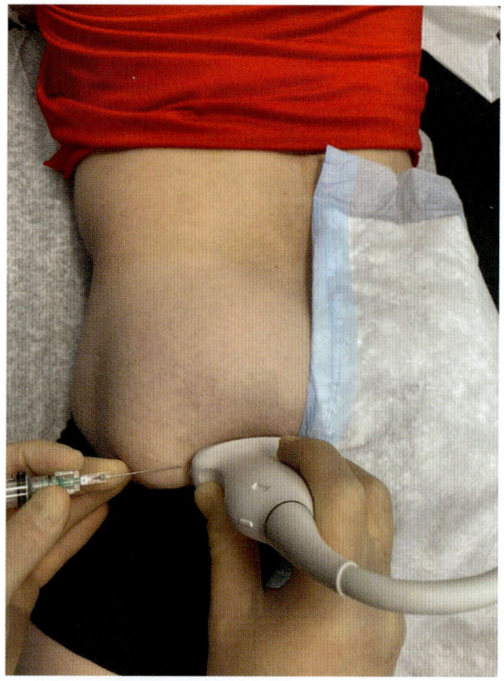

• **Fig. 20.45** Patient is prone, and transducer is placed in the transverse plane, long axis to the obturator internus, quadratus femoris, and gemelli muscles. They should be approached in plane from lateral to medial.

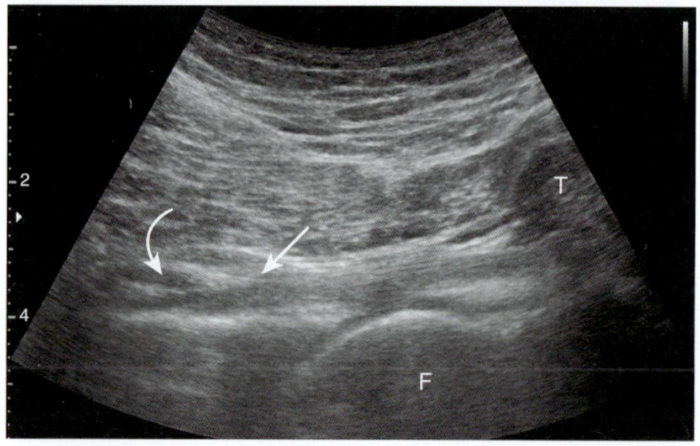

• **Fig. 20.46** Ultrasound image, with patient prone, long axis to the gemelli muscles. *Straight arrow* shows in-plane path of the needle. *Curved arrow,* Sciatic nerve; *F,* proximal femur; *T,* greater trochanter.

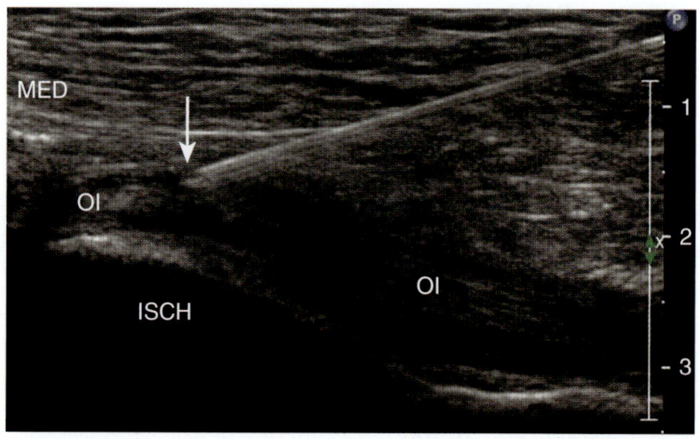

• **Fig. 20.47** Long-axis Ultrasound Image of Obturator Internus Tendon Sheath Injection. *Arrow* indicates needle tip. *ISCH*, Ischium; *MED*, medial; *OI*, obturator internus tendon.

Quadratus Femoris Injection

KEY POINTS

- The sciatic nerve must be identified prior to injection; it will always be just superficial to the quadratus femoris muscle.

Pertinent Anatomy

- The quadratus femoris is a muscle that sits in the posterior pelvis between the lateral ischial tuberosity and the proximal femur at the quadrate tubercle of the posterior intertrochanteric line.
- Once the ischial tuberosity, at the level of the hamstring origin, is visualized under ultrasound, the quadratus is the first muscle lateral to the femur.

Common Pathology

- The quadratus femoris muscle can become impinged between the ischial tuberosity and lesser trochanter of the femur, resulting in ischiofemoral impingement syndrome. Narrowing of the distance between the two bony landmarks of the ischiofemoral space is a risk factor for impingement.

Equipment

- Needle size: 22- to 25-gauge, 2- to 3.5-inch needle
- Low-frequency curvilinear transducer or a medium-frequency linear transducer, depending on body habitus

Common Injectates

- Anesthetics for diagnostics or trigger point
- Corticosteroids in sheath
- Prolotherapy, orthobiologics (PRP, bone marrow concentrate, etc.)
- Botulinum toxin[39]

Injectate Volume

- 2 to 4 mL in total

Technique

Patient Position

- Prone

Clinician Position

- Seated or standing on the side of the leg targeted for injection if prone

Transducer Position

- Long axis to the quadratus femoris muscle (Fig. 20.45)

Needle Position

- In plane to the transducer, lateral-to-medial approach

Target

- Quadratus femoris muscle belly or site of pathology (Fig. 20.48)

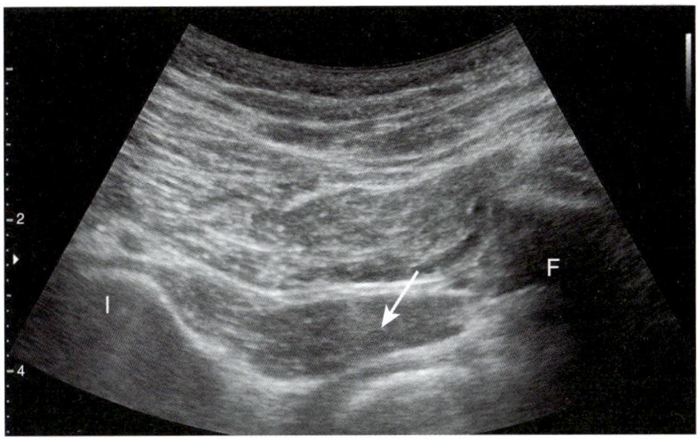

• **Fig. 20.48** Ultrasound image, with patient prone, long axis to the quadratus femoris running between the ischium and proximal femur. Needle in plane from lateral to medial. *Arrow*, Path of needle; *F*, proximal femur; *I*, Ischium.

PEARLS AND PITFALLS

- Quadratus femoris pathology is often due to ischiofemoral impingement.
- A small amount of local anesthetic into the quadratus femoris can help to confirm the ischiofemoral impingement.
- Care must be taken to avoid the sciatic nerve just superficial to the quadratus femoris muscle, but its exact location can vary to some degree.

From: Atlas of US MSK Inj–Mautner; Fundamentals of MSK US–Jacobson; *American Journal of Roentgenology*. 2011;197:1:170–174 (Issue publication date: July 2011) https://doi.org/10.2214/AJR.10.5898 [40]

Labrum

KEY POINTS

- The injection technique is similar to IA, except you want to target the labrum and the specific area of tear based on magnetic resonance imaging (MRI) findings.

Pertinent Anatomy

- The fibrocartilage labrum appears as a hyperechoic triangular structure on ultrasound, extending from the margins of the acetabulum.
- An intact labrum and joint capsule function to seal the joint-enhancing lubrication by maintaining a fluid layer providing lubrication between the articular surfaces, reducing friction and shear on the cartilage, and distributing forces more evenly across the joint (see Fig. 20.3).

Common Pathology

- Labral tears are classified as anterior, posterior, or superior-lateral, with the most common location being in the anterior part of the labrum. Labral tears may be acute/traumatic or degenerative, and may be seen in conjunction with hip dysplasia, femoral-acetabular impingement,

capsular laxity, and osteoarthritis. Labral tears can be asymptomatic or result in symptoms of groin, buttock, or lateral hip pain and clicking.
- Paralabral cysts occur in the presence of labral tears or a weakened joint capsule and are caused by a leakage of joint fluid through the tear. They can be asymptomatic or present with nonspecific or nonfocal symptoms. In some cases, the cysts can impinge on adjacent structures, such as the iliopsoas tendon, causing internal snapping hip, or the femoral or sciatic nerve.

Equipment
- Needle size: 22- to 25-gauge, 2.5- to 3.5-inch spinal needle
- Low-frequency curvilinear ultrasound transducer

Common Injectates
- Anesthetics for diagnostics.
- Prolotherapy, orthobiologics (PRP, bone marrow concentrate, etc.).
- Steroids should not be used as they can potentially injure cartilage/labrum when injected directly.

Injectate Volume
- 1 to 3 mL directly into the labrum. Extra can be placed intra-articularly.

Technique Anterior (Indication: Anterior Tears)
Patient Position
- Supine with pillow under the head and appropriate draping to expose the inguinal region

Clinician Position
- Standing or sitting on affected side of patient

Transducer Position
- Aligned with the long axis of the thigh for an inferior approach (Fig. 20.49), the femoral neck for an inferior-oblique approach, or transverse to the thigh for a lateral approach

Needle Position
- In plane, inferior or inferior-lateral to superior or superior-medial approaches, depending on the target area

Target
- Cleft or defect most commonly visualized at the junction of the acetabulum and the hyperechoic labrum in the anterior portion of the joint (Fig. 20.50)

PEARLS AND PITFALLS
- In the setting of osteoarthritis (OA) of the hip, coexisting "labral tears" are commonly asymptomatic and not the cause of a patient's pain.

Technique Lateral (Indication: Superior Lateral and Posterior Superior Tears)
Patient Position
- Lateral decubitus with pillow between the knees

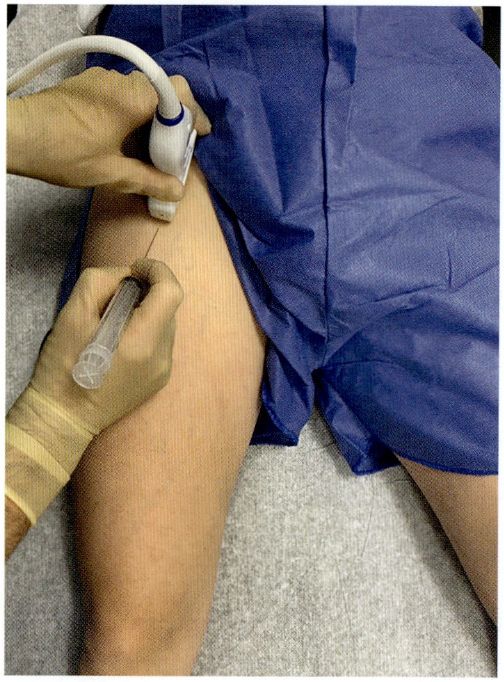

• **Fig. 20.49** Anterior Sagittal Approach. Transducer in position for in-plane approach to hip joint.

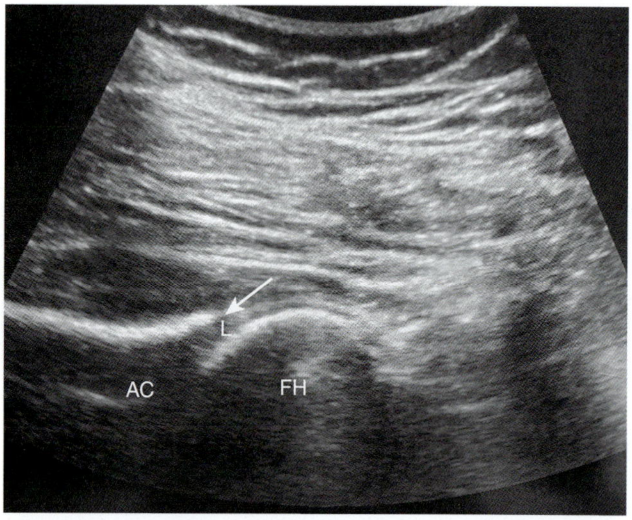

• **Fig 20.50** Ultrasound image with patient supine, transducer aligned with long axis of thigh, and in-plane injection approach with path of needle directed at labrum. Needle *(arrow)*, normal acetabulum *(AC)*, labrum *(L)* and femoral head *(FH)*.

Clinician Position
- If lateral, standing behind the patient

Transducer Position
- Aligned with the long axis of the lateral greater trochanter (Fig. 20.51A)
- For superior-lateral target, position the probe just anterior and superior to the greater trochanter
- For posterior-superior target, position the probe just posterior and superior to the greater trochanter

Needle Position

- In plane, inferior lateral-to-superior medial approach

Target

- Cleft or defect most commonly visualized at the junction of the acetabulum and the hyperechoic labrum in the anterior-lateral or posterior-lateral portion of the joint (see Fig. 20.51B)

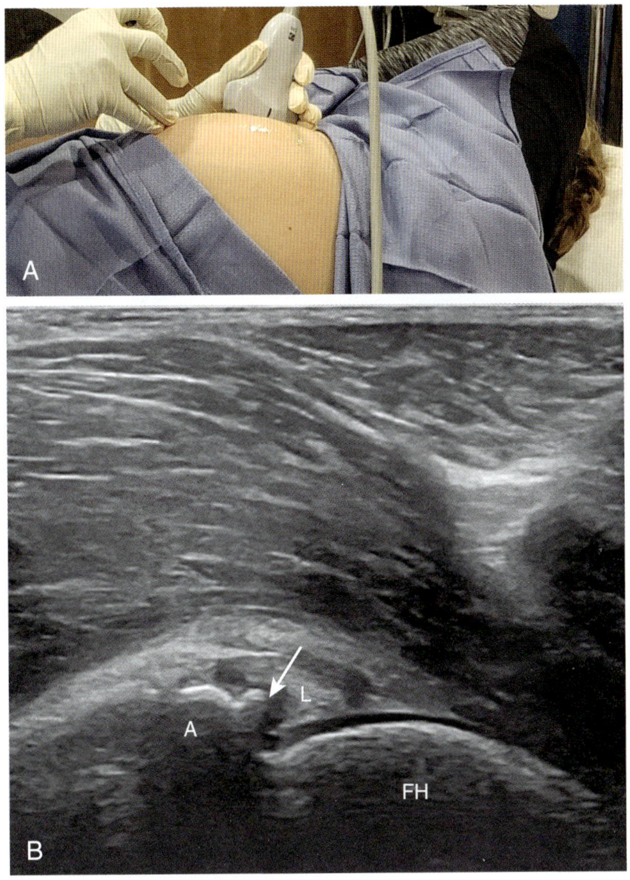

• **Fig. 20.51** (A) Lateral labrum ultrasound setup. (B) Lateral labrum ultrasound injection in plane. Needle *(arrow)*, normal acetabulum *(A)*, labrum *(L)*, and femoral head *(FH)*.

PEARLS AND PITFALLS

- Having the probe slightly anterior or posterior to the greater trochanter will provide better needle clearance to access the labrum.

Perineural

Sciatic Nerve

KEY POINTS

- Sciatic tunnel syndrome refers to entrapment and neuralgia of the sciatic nerve in the gluteal triangle. Sciatic tunnel may result in chronic neuralgic pain in the posterior thigh.
- Care should be taken to avoid intraneural or intravascular injection.
- With expertise, circumferential hydrodissection could be attempted.

Pertinent Anatomy

- The sciatic nerve is formed from the anterior divisions of L4-S3.
- The nerve exits through the greater sciatic foramen, and traverses below (or sometimes through) the piriformis and gluteus maximus muscles. It then courses superficial to the quadratic femoris, lateral to the ischial tuberosity.
- The sciatic nerve runs distally in the posterior thigh, anterior to the biceps femoris, prior to entering the popliteal triangle, where the sciatic nerve divides into the common fibular and tibial nerves branch apart (see Fig. 20.37).

Common Pathology

- Entrapment of the sciatic nerve in the gluteal triangle can occur at the greater sciatic notch, ischial tunnel (between the quadratus femoris and proximal hamstring), and at the level of the piriformis. Associated pathology at these sites of entrapment can diminish the sciatic nerve's mobility, resulting in sciatic neuropathy.
- Piriformis syndrome, ischiofemoral impingement, and hamstring pathology can cause symptoms related to sciatic nerve entrapment.

Equipment

- Needle size: 22- to 25-gauge, 2- to 3.5-inch needle
- Medium-frequency linear transducer or low-frequency curvilinear transducer, as appropriate for the individual's body habitus

Common Injectates

- For nerve block: local anesthetic, plus or minus corticosteroid
- For hydrodissection: mixture of normal saline and local anesthetic solution, 5% dextrose solution, or platelet lysate solution

Injectate Volume

- For nerve block: 5 to 15 mL
- For hydrodissection: 10 to 15 mL

Technique

Patient Position

- Prone (Fig. 20.52)
- Alternate: side-lying with hip flexed, internally rotated and adducted

Clinician Position

- Seated or standing on the side of the intended injection

Transducer Position

- Short axis to the sciatic nerve, at the subgluteal level. Nerve should be identified between the gluteus maximus and the quadratus femoris

Needle Position

- In plane to the transducer, lateral-to-medial approach

Target

- Sciatic nerve perineural sheath. Should see perineural spread surrounding the nerve circumferentially (Fig. 20.53)

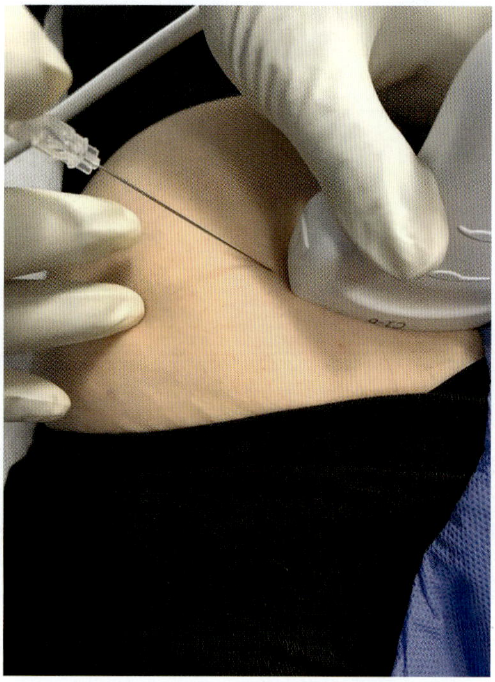

• **Fig. 20.52** Transverse Approach. Prone with transducer in position for in-plane sciatic perineural injection.

PEARLS AND PITFALLS

- The lateral recumbent position may allow improved access to the nerve in individuals with larger body habitus.
- The sciatic nerve is located in the medial subgluteal region with the inferior gluteal artery, and the lateral-to-medial approach is less likely to have unintentional intravascular injection.
- If needed, the sciatic nerve can also be approached long axis to the nerve, in plane.

Lateral Femoral Cutaneous Nerve Block

KEY POINTS

- The lateral femoral cutaneous nerve (LFCN) is a purely sensory nerve, and entrapment or injury to the nerve results in meralgia paresthetica.

Pertinent Anatomy

- The lateral femoral cutaneous nerve (LFCN) is a purely sensory nerve formed by the L2–L3 nerve roots and arises directly from the lumbar plexus.
- The nerve traverses along the lateral border of the iliopsoas muscle into the pelvis. It exits the pelvis under the inguinal ligament, typically 1–4 cm medial to the ASIS. After exiting the pelvis, it enters the thigh, typically piercing the fascia lata.

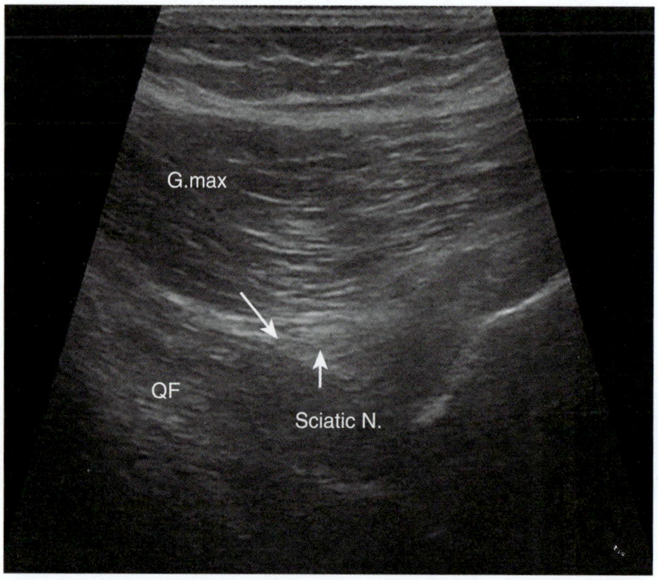

• **Fig. 20.53** Short-axis ultrasound image of the sciatic nerve *(Sciatic N)*, between the gluteus maximus *(G.Max.)* and quadratus femoris *(QF)* muscles. *Arrow* demonstrates the needle path in plane for sciatic nerve block.

- The LFCN can vary in its course, and, in some cases, will cross the iliac crest lateral to the ASIS. The LFCN typically divides into an anterior and posterior branch distal to the inguinal ligament. However, the nerve can be found to form branches proximal to the ligament.
- After the nerve travels under the inguinal ligament, the LFCN or the anterior branch will travel in the superficial triangular space between the sartorius and TFL.
- The most common entrapment site is at the inguinal ligament (see Fig. 20.2).

Common Pathology

- Meralgia paresthetica is a solely sensory mononeuropathy of the LFCN. The nerve is commonly entrapped as it exits the pelvis under the inguinal ligament. Common symptoms include paresthesias, anesthesia, or dysesthesias.
- Scanning from the lateral-to-medial direction in the short axis can help locate the hyperechoic round or elliptical nerve. It is typically best visualized between the sartorius and TFL, just lateral to the ASIS.
- This nerve can often be injured/compressed following anterior approach for a total hip replacement (THR).

Equipment

- Needle size: 22- to 25-gauge, 1.5- to 3.5-inch needle
- Medium- to high-frequency linear transducer

Common Injectates

- For nerve block: local anesthetic, plus or minus corticosteroid
- For hydrodissection: mixture of normal saline and local anesthetic solution, 5% dextrose solution, or platelet lysate solution

Injectate Volume

- For nerve block: 2 to 5 mL
- For hydrodissection: 5 to 10 mL

Technique

Patient Position

- Supine

Clinician Position

- Seated or standing on the side of the intended injection

Transducer Position

- Short axis to the LFCN, transverse to the body (Fig. 20.54). Alternation between short axis and long axis is helpful to confirm needle tip location.

Needle Position

- In plane to the transducer, lateral-to-medial or distal-to-proximal approach

Target

- Nerve sheath, may alternate between long and short axis to confirm perineural spread during hydrodissection of the nerve (Fig. 20.55)

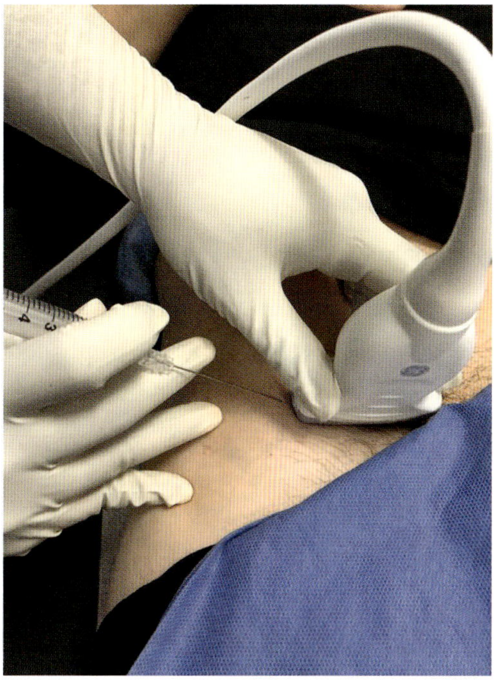

• **Fig. 20.54** Patient is supine, transducer short axis to nerve, a few centimeters distal to the ASIS, for in-plane lateral-to-medial LFCN nerve block. *ASIS*, Anterior superior iliac spine; *LFCN*, lateral femoral cutaneous nerve.

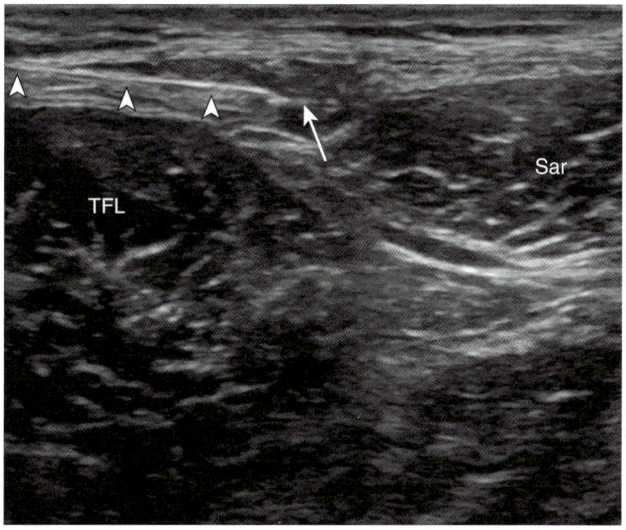

• **Fig. 20.55** Ultrasound image, with patient supine, short axis to the distal anterior superior iliac spine with needle in plane approaching lateral femoral cutaneous nerve (LFCN; *arrow*). *Arrowheads*, needle; *Sar,* sartorius muscle; *TFL,* tensor fascia lata.

PEARLS AND PITFALLS

- The nerve is located just deep to the fascial plane, typically between the sartorius and TFL. Given the very superficial nature or the course of the nerve, do not look too deep when performing sonographic evaluation.
- When performing the injection, care must be made to not approach too steeply.

From: Atlas, Furman[41] Atlas, Jacobson.[9,10]

Obturator Nerve Hydrodissection

KEY POINTS

Entrapment of the obturator nerve is an under-recognized cause of groin, thigh, and knee pain.

Pertinent Anatomy

- The obturator nerve receives contribution from the L2 to L4 nerve roots. It is both a sensory and motor nerve.
- The obturator nerve divides in the pelvis into the anterior and posterior branches.
- The anterior branch traverses between the adductor longus and adductor brevis muscles, and innervates the gracilis, adductor longus, and adductor brevis.
- The posterior branch travels between the adductor longus and adductor magnus, and innervates the adductor magnus.

Common Pathology

- The obturator nerve is susceptible to injury or entrapment in the obturator foramen, particularly in the setting of pelvic fracture. Large adductor strains can also result in nerve injury or compression neuropraxia.
- Adductor spasticity often results from various neurologic diseases, which can interfere with function, mobility, and activities of daily living (ADLs). Neurolysis of the obturator nerve is often an effective treatment.

Equipment

- Needle size: 22-gauge, 2- to 3.5-inch needle
- Medium- to high-frequency linear transducer. Low-frequency curvilinear transducer, as appropriate for the individual's body habitus.

Common Injectates

- For nerve block: local anesthetic, plus or minus corticosteroid
- For hydrodissection: mixture of normal saline and local anesthetic solution, or 5% dextrose solution or platelet lysate solution

Injectate Volume

- For nerve block: 2 to 5 mL
- For hydrodissection: 5 to 10 mL

Technique

Patient Position

Supine with hip externally rotated and flexed, with knee flexed, as well

Clinician Position

- Seated or standing on the side of the intended injection

Transducer Position

- Short axis to the obturator nerve and parallel to the inguinal ligament, making sure to stay medial to the femoral vessels and nerve (Fig. 20.56)

Needle Position

- In plane to the transducer

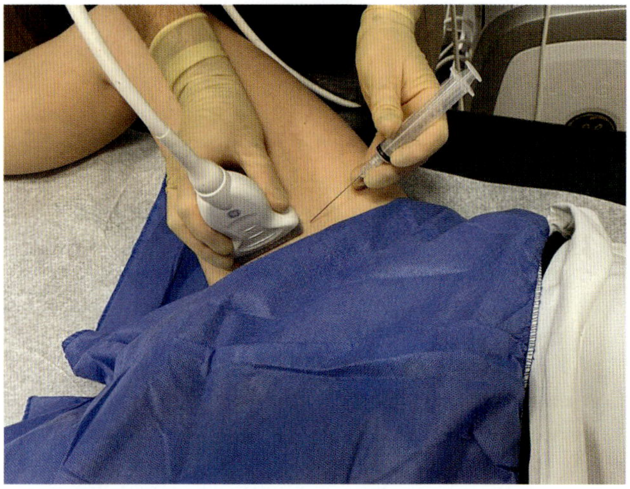

• **Fig. 20.56** Supine Position With Hip Externally Rotated and Flexed. Transducer positioned in transverse plane for lateral-to-medial in-plane approach.

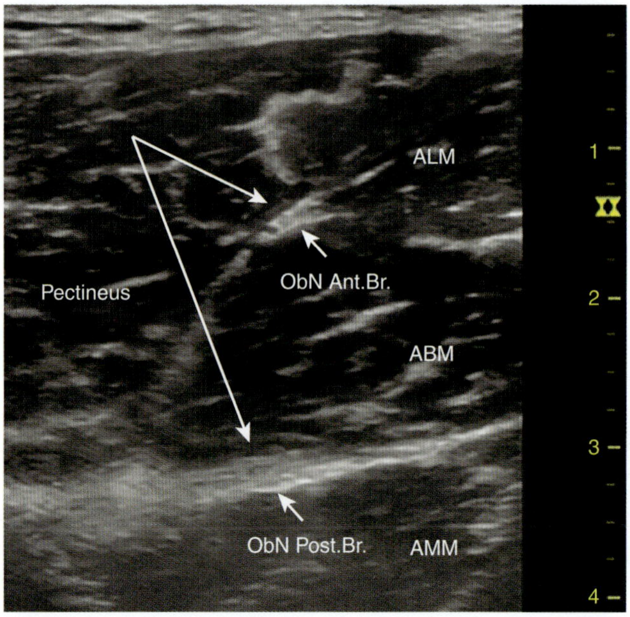

• **Fig. 20.57** Ultrasound image represents a short-axis view of the obturator nerve branches *(ObN Ant.Br.)* in the medial inguinal region: anterior and posterior branches. *Long arrows* demonstrate the in-plane path of needle for a perineural injection of each nerve branch. *ABM,* Adductor brevis muscle; *ALM,* adductor longus muscle; *AMM,* adductor magnus muscle.

- Needle approach: lateral to medial or medial to lateral
- Target: anterior and posterior branches of the obturator nerve. Should note perineural spread surrounding the nerve circumferentially in the planes between the muscles (Fig. 20.57).

PEARLS AND PITFALLS

- The obturator artery must be identified and avoided during the injection.
- Nerve stimulation, in addition to ultrasound, can aid in localization of the nerve, particularly in phenol neurolysis for spasticity.
- Injections can be performed to the anterior branch, posterior branch, or both branches, as indicated.

Posterior Femoral Cutaneous Nerve

KEY POINT

- Could be an overlooked cause of ischial or "sit-bone" pain.

Pertinent Anatomy

- The posterior femoral cutaneous nerve is a small sensory nerve that innervates the posterior thigh.
- The nerve is deep to the gluteus maximus muscle, and superficial to the sciatic nerve and biceps femoris. The nerve travels in close proximity and medial to the sciatic nerve. The nerve is seen departing from the sciatic nerve and gradually surfacing up to the cutaneous layer when the transducer is relocated distally (see Fig. 20.37).

Common Pathology

- The nerve will often have a normal appearance but could be considered painful for those patients who have ischial (sit-bone), pain with or without associated proximal hamstring pathology.

Equipment

- Needle: 22-gauge, 2.5- to 3.5-inch
- Curvilinear or linear transducer, depending on body habitus

Common Injectates

- For nerve block: local anesthetic, plus or minus corticosteroid
- For hydrodissection: mixture of normal saline and local anesthetic solution, or 5% dextrose solution or platelet lysate solution

Injectate Volume

- For nerve block: 2 to 5 mL
- For hydrodissection: 5 to 10 mL

Technique

Patient Position

- Prone with a pillow under the head and under the pelvis (Fig. 20.58)
- Alternatively, side-lying on unaffected side, with hip flexion to bring the structure more superficial and in better view

Clinician Position

- Standing or seated on affected side of patient or behind the patient if side-lying

Transducer Position

- Transverse near the gluteal crease at the level of the ischial tuberosity, similar to proximal hamstring imaging (see Fig. 20.58)

Needle Position

- In plane
- Lateral-to-medial approach

Target

- Perineural to the posterior femoral cutaneous nerve (Fig. 20.59)

PEARLS AND PITFALLS

- Nerve can be injected with very small volume of anesthetics for diagnostic confirmation.
- Nerve can be treated with larger-volume hydrodissection.

Pudendal Nerve Block

KEY POINTS

- Internal pudendal artery should be visualized prior to the procedure; it is located lateral to the pudendal nerve.

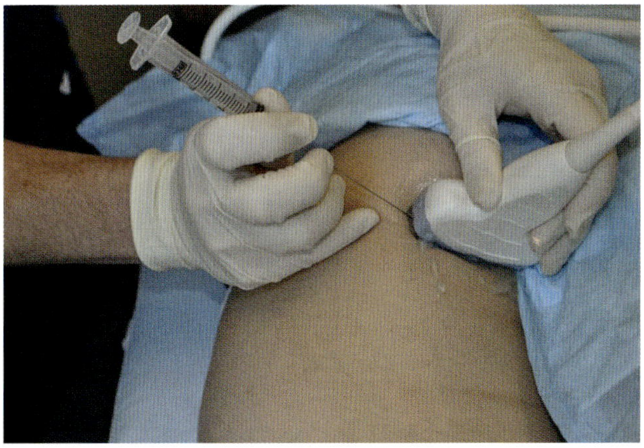

• **Fig. 20.58** Prone or Side Lying Position. Transducer transverse to gluteal crease at the level of the ischial tuberosity for in-plane approach.

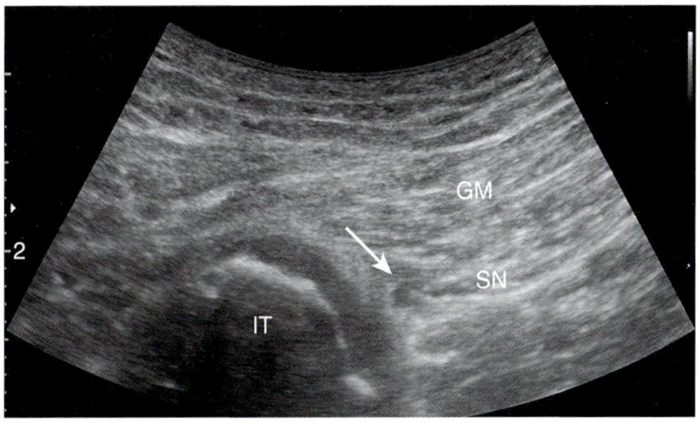

• **Fig. 20.59** Ultrasound in long axis showing *long arrow* as needle path of posterior femoral cutaneous nerve injection. *GM*, Gluteus maximus; *IT*, ischial tuberosity; *SN* sciatic nerve.

Pertinent Anatomy

- The nerve is deep to the gluteus maximus muscle and sacrotuberous ligament, and superficial to the sacrospinous ligament. The ischial spine is found lateral to those structures.

Common Pathology

- Entrapment of the pudendal nerve may cause pain and numbness in the genital area. There are four subtypes of entrapment based on possible sites of entrapment: (1) below the piriformis muscle as the pudendal nerve exits greater sciatic notch; (2) between the sacrospinous and sacrotuberous ligaments (this is the most common cause of nerve entrapment); (3) inside Alcock's canal; and (4) at the terminal branches.[42]

Equipment

- Needle: 22-gauge, 2.3- to 3.5-inch needle
- Linear or curvilinear ultrasound transducer, depending on the patient's body habitus

Common Injectates

- For nerve block: local anesthetic, plus or minus corticosteroid
- For hydrodissection: mixture of normal saline and local anesthetic solution or 5% dextrose solution, or platelet lysate solution

Injectate Volume

- For nerve block: 2 to 5 mL
- For hydrodissection: 5 to 10 mL

Technique

Patient Position

- Side-lying with the area to be blocked facing upwards and knees slightly flexed; pillows under the head and between the legs
- Prone with soft support under the pelvis (Fig. 20.60)

Clinician Position

- Standing or seated

Transducer Position

- Transverse along the ischial spine

Needle Position

- In-plane, medial-to-lateral approach or posterior/transgluteal approach

Target

- Space interposed by the sacrotuberous and sacrospinous ligaments (most common site of entrapment) (Fig. 20.61)
- Alcock's canal, also called pudendal canal (second most common site of entrapment)
- Anywhere along pudendal nerve at possible entrapment sites, beginning with pudendal nerve exiting from greater sciatic notch to the terminal branches

PEARLS AND PITFALLS

- Sciatic nerve should be visualized prior to procedure; it is located lateral to pudendal nerve.
- Internal pudendal artery should be visualized prior to procedure; it is located lateral to the pudendal nerve.

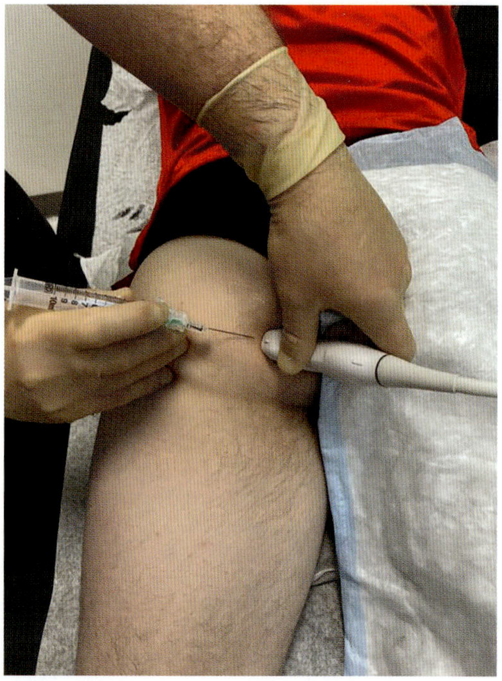

• **Fig. 20.60** Patient is prone, for a short-axis, in-plane approach. Transducer transverse to nerve at the level of the ischial spine.

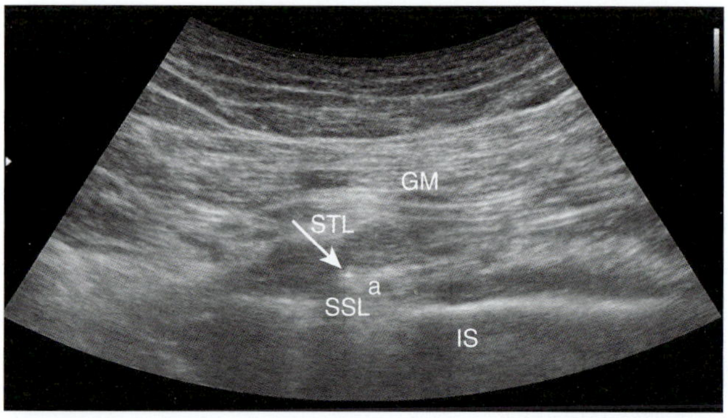

• **Fig. 20.61** Ultrasound in long axis showing *long arrow* as needle path of pudendal nerve injection. The left side of the picture is medial. *a*, Artery; *GM*, gluteus maximus; *IS*, ischial spine; *SSL*, sacrospinous ligament; *STL*, sacrotuberous ligament.

Hip Injection Techniques

Fluoroscopy Guided

Femorocetabular Joint

KEY POINTS

- Authors' preferred approach is placing the needle using ultrasound guidance with the curvilinear transducer and confirming with fluoroscopy.
- For osteoarthritis, ideally, you want to inject to obtain weight-bearing flow into the joint.
- For adhesive capsulitis, intra-articular capsular flow is preferred.
- Weight-bearing IA injection can be used for labral degeneration; however, for symptomatic labral tears, direct labral injection is preferred.
- Avoid placing injectate in the retinaculum of Weitbrecht (see Fig. 20.1). Injecting here may limit weight-bearing articular flow.

Pertinent Anatomy and Common Pathology

- Refer to ultrasound section

Equipment

- C-arm fluoroscopy
- Typically, 25- or 22-gauge, 3.5-inch spinal needle is sufficient
- In larger or taller patients, may require a 25-gauge, 4.69-inch needle or 22-gauge, 5-inch needle
- Contrast

Common Injectates

- Local anesthetics for diagnostics, corticosteroids
- Prolotherapy, hyaluronic acid, orthobiologics (PRP, bone marrow concentrate, micronized adipose tissue, etc.).
- For capsular distention. local anesthetic and normal saline +/– corticosteroid, and/or orthobiologics such as platelet-poor plasma, platelet lysate, etc.

Injectate Volume

- For weight-bearing IA injection: 2 to 5 mL.
- For capsular distention: 10 to 20 mL. Stop when getting backflow into the syringe to avoid capsular rupture. Most hip capsules max out close to 16 mL, but some may tolerate close to 20 mL.

Technique: Anterior Approach

Patient Position

- Supine leg extended (Fig. 20.62).

Clinician Position

- Standing on ipsilateral side of the patient

C-Arm Position Fluoroscopy Technique

- Anteroposterior (AP) projection where the greater trochanter, femoral head, and joint space are visualized

Needle Position

- For diagnostic and therapeutic injections, can start over the lateral-inferior femoral head, needle in a direct anterior-to-posterior approach directed toward the lateral-inferior femoral head or mid-femoral neck
- For weight-bearing flow: start anterior and slightly medial to the greater trochanter (see Fig. 20.62B)
- Advance the needle with a superior, slightly medial trajectory

Target

- For capsular flow (diagnostic and therapeutic intra-articular injections), can aim at lateral-inferior femoral head or, for the superior, mid-femoral neck (see Fig. 20.62D)
- For weight-bearing flow: advance the needle to the bone cortex on the inferior/central-lateral femoral head below the acetabulum. Then, "walk" the needle along the femur superior to enter the joint under the acetabulum (see Fig. 20.62C).

PEARLS AND PITFALLS

- For weight-bearing placement, having a slight bend in the needle can help with redirecting the needle.
- Using 10–15 lb of inferior traction from an assistant during needling guidance and injection can help expand the joint space and improve weight-bearing flow. This can also improve patient comfort.
- Loss of resistance once under the acetabulum can be felt and a small amount of contrast can confirm IA flow. If there is a significant amount of resistance during the injection or a soft tissue contrast dye pattern, then advance the needle further and/or add slightly more traction.
- For capsular distention discussion, see anterior hip capsule distention in ultrasound section.

Technique: Lateral Approach

Patient Position

- Lateral decubitus with pillow between the knees (Fig. 20.63A)
- An alternative approach is to have the patient supine with the legs extended

Clinician Position

- If lateral, standing behind the patient
- If supine, standing on ipsilateral side of the patient

C-Arm Position Fluoroscopy Technique

- AP projection visualizing the femoral acetabular joint, the greater trochanter, and lateral soft tissue
- May use lateral projection to make sure needle is maintained in central plane from anterior to posterior. Option to align both the left and right joints completely or offset them with rotation of the C-arm. If they are offset, then the smaller joint is the joint being injected due to its closer position to the transducer

Needle Position

- Start just anterior and superior to the greater trochanter, but below the lateral acetabular rim
- Needle trajectory should be from inferior to superior toward the lateral joint opening

Target

- Touch the needle onto the bone cortex on the lateral femur just under the acetabulum. The needle should be viewed directly lateral to the femur once the needle touches down onto the periosteum surface
- Advance or "walk" the needle with the bevel pointed upward under the acetabulum, superior to the lateral femoral head for IA flow on the weight-bearing surface of the joint (see Fig. 20.63B)

Technique: Posterior Approach

Patient Position

- Prone
- Will likely need hip internal rotation to move the greater trochanter out of the needle trajectory. To achieve this,

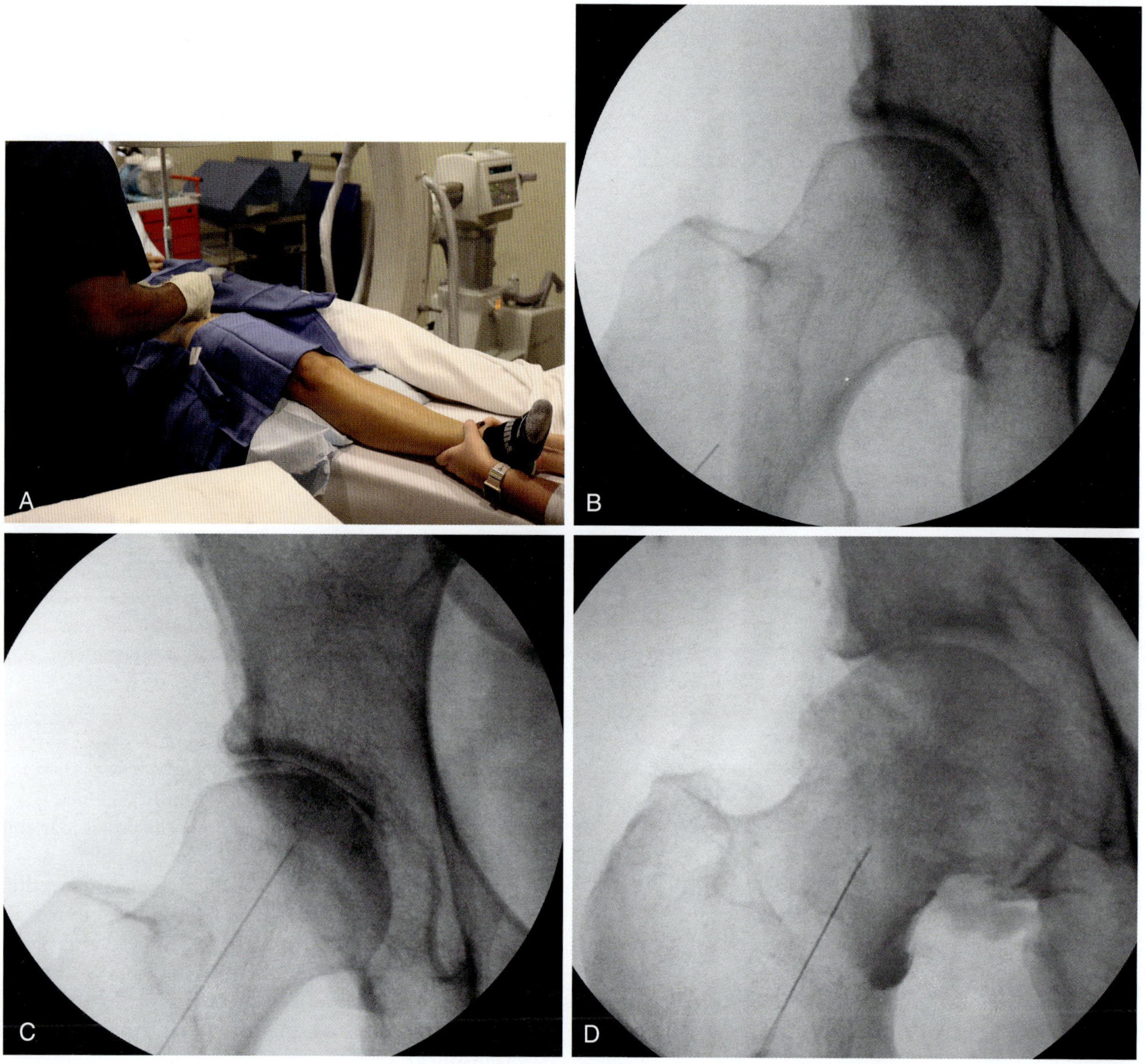

• **Fig. 20.62** (A) Hip anterior fluoroscopy setup. (B) Hip anterior fluoroscopy needle start point. (C) Hip anterior fluoroscopy weight-bearing target with contrast. (D). Hip anterior fluoroscopy target capsular distention.

PEARLS AND PITFALLS

- For weight-bearing placement, having a slight bend in the needle can help with redirecting the needle.
- This is a great approach to get weight-bearing flow. Inferior traction here can help to open the joint, after which a small amount of contrast can be injected to confirm flow.
- Needle placement is key to ensure there is not much anterior or posterior advancement of the needle until it reaches the periosteum. Can use the lateral projection of the joint with the C-arm to confirm the needle trajectory and adjust as needed.
- Consider the use of ultrasound for the needle placement; then make final adjustments with fluoroscopy and confirm an IA flow pattern.
- This is not an ideal approach for hip capsular distention.

bend the patient's leg at the knee and rotate from the lower leg outwards (Fig. 20.64A)

Clinician Position

- Standing ipsilateral side of the patient

Transducer Position or C-Arm Position Fluoroscopy Technique

- AP projection where the greater trochanter, femoral head, and joint space are visualized

Needle Position

- Start posterior and slightly medial to the greater trochanter. Start a little more inferior than the anterior approach (see Fig. 20.64B)
- Needle trajectory should be superior and slightly medial

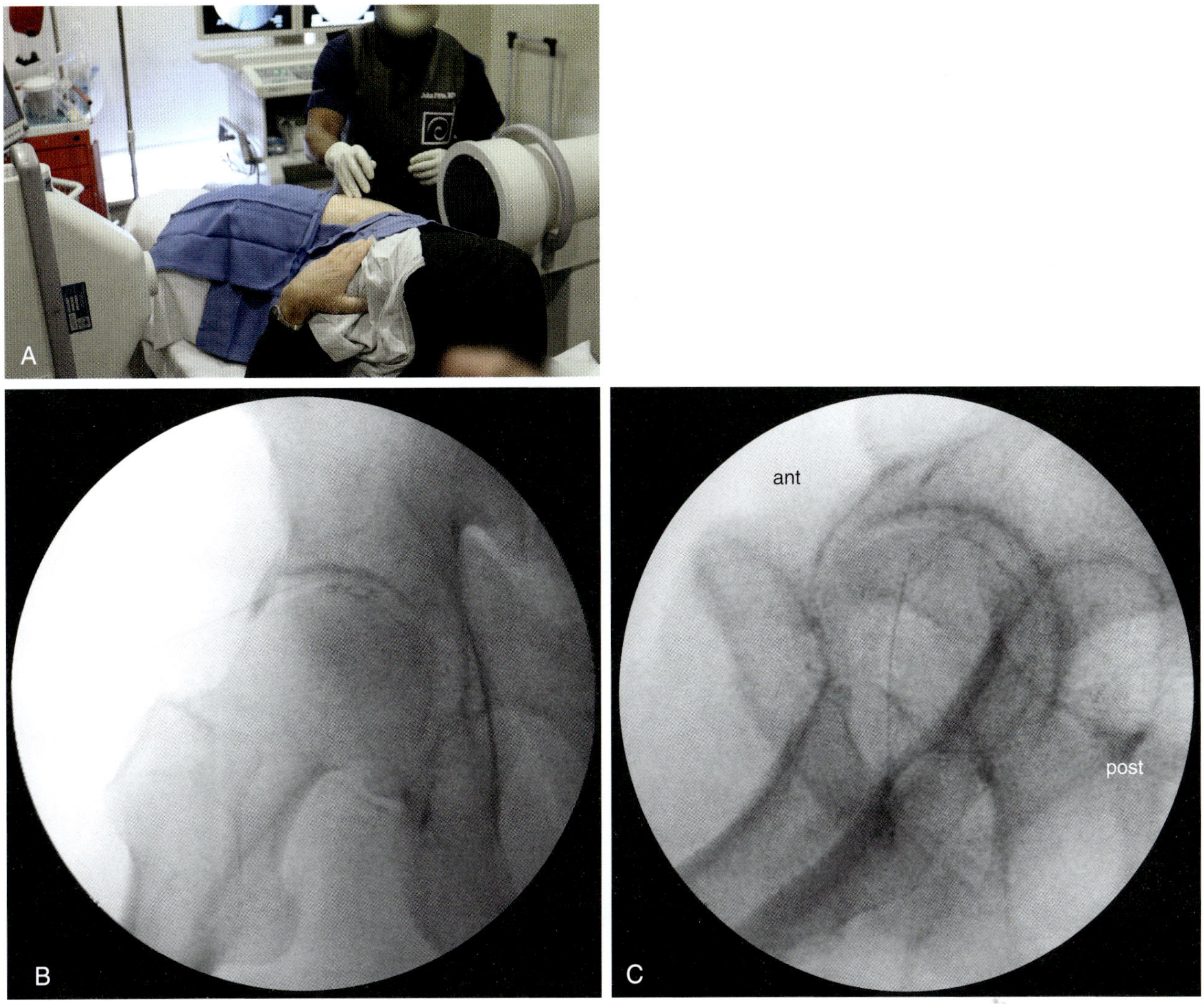

• **Fig. 20.63** (A) Hip fluoroscopy lateral IA setup. (B) Hip fluoroscopy lateral IA target AP. (C) Hip fluoroscopy lateral IA target lateral.

Target

- For IA flow: aim to touch the periosteum on the inferior/central-lateral femoral head below the acetabulum. Then, advance or "walk" the needle along the femur superior to enter the joint under the acetabulum (see Fig. 20.64C).
- For capsular flow, aim for the superior femoral neck mid portion from lateral to medial.

PEARLS AND PITFALLS

- There is more acetabular coverage posterior, so this approach is more difficult to obtain good weight-bearing flow. As such, this is not the preferred approach for IA biologics.
- This is the preferred approach when there is a desire to distend posterior hip capsule due to tightness and adhesions that limit hip internal rotation and hip flexion.
- Having a slight bend in the needle can help with redirecting the needle.

Pubic Symphysis

Key Points and Pertinent Anatomy and Common Pathology

- Refer to ultrasound section

Equipment

- C-arm fluoroscopy
- 25- gauge, 2-inch spinal needle

Common Injectates

- Orthobiologics (PRP, bone marrow concentrate) and prolotherapy

Injectate Volume

- For IA injection: 0.5 to 1 mL
- For ligamentous injection: 1 to 3 mL

Technique

Patient Position

- Supine

Clinician Position

- Standing on either side of the patient

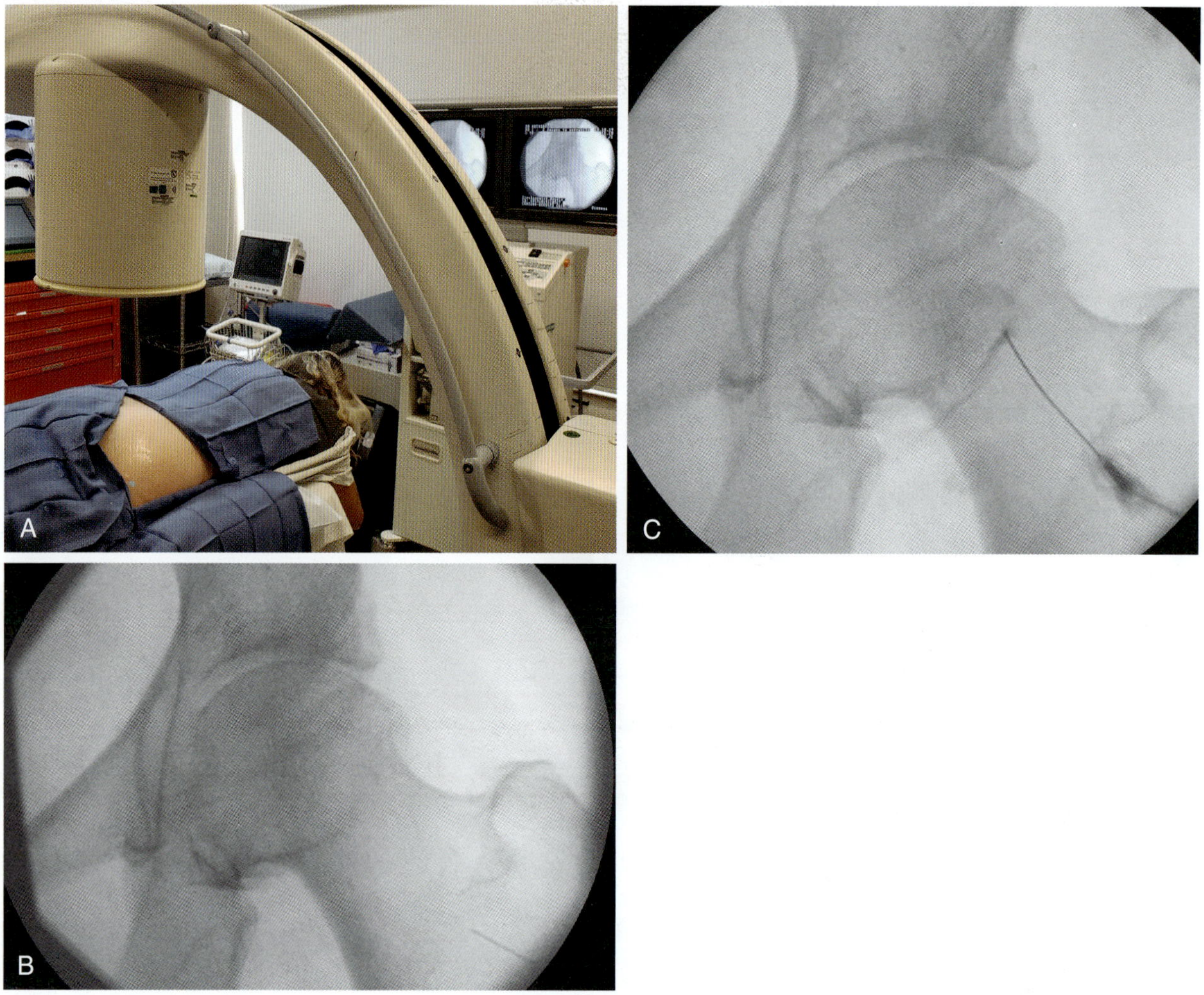

• **Fig. 20.64** (A) Hip posterior fluoroscopy setup. (B) Hip posterior fluoroscopy needle start point. (C) Hip posterior fluoroscopy weight-bearing target with contrast.

Transducer Position or C-Arm Position Fluoroscopy Technique

- AP projection with the pubic symphysis centered

Needle Position

- For IA or intradiscal injection, start directly over the joint space in the middle from superior and anterior positions (Fig. 20.65A).
- For the surrounding ligaments, you can use the same starting position and redirect the needle superior or inferior down to the periosteum and ligamentous attachments.

Target

- For intradiscal needle placement, guide the needle directly into the center of the disc under intermittent fluoroscopy. The depth can vary, but is typically less than 2 cm. To confirm, inject a small amount of contrast to show IA flow. Should notice tissue resistance changes (see Fig. 20.65B).
- For ligament targets, touch down on the joint capsule as described above.
    - Anterior pubic ligament: Inject the anterior surface of the joint and "pepper" the area by moving superior, inferior, and lateral attachments on the pubic rami.
    - Superior and inferior pubic ligaments: Start at the far inferior or superior aspect of the joint. Advance the needle to the superior or inferior edge of the joint. Can be advanced slightly deep to the joint, but not more than a few millimeters (see Fig. 20.65C).
    - Posterior pubic ligament: We do not recommend injecting for safety. A lateral fluoroscopic view would be required to ascertain depth but is difficult to visualize.

PEARLS AND PITFALLS

- Pubic symphysis dysfunction is usually a problem of stability; so targeting the ligaments in addition to IA injection alone is usually recommended.
- Be sure to keep the needle over the joint capsule or bony surfaces. If in the disc, do not advance the needle more than 1–2 cm to avoid infiltrating the pelvis.
- Advancing through or past the joint can result in infiltration of the bladder. Ultrasound can be used for the initial needle placement to prevent injury to the bladder.
- Assess for associated sacroiliac pathology.

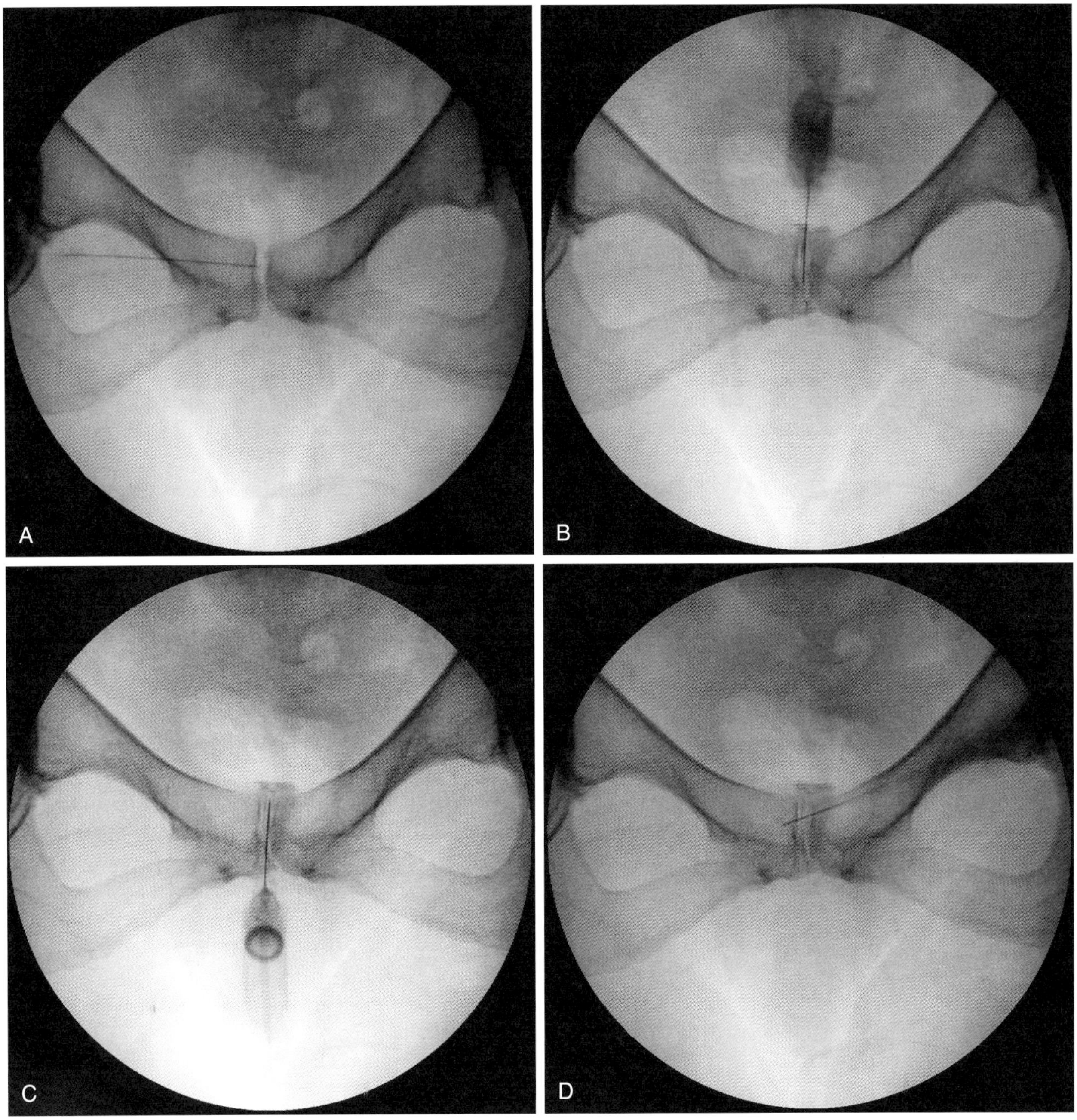

• **Fig. 20.65** (A) Pubic symphysis fluoroscopy needle start. (B) Pubic symphysis IA. (C) Pubic symphysis fluoroscopy superior ligaments. (D) Anterior ligaments.

Ligamentum Teres and Transverse Acetabular Ligament

KEY POINTS

- This is a highly advanced injection that requires both ultrasound and fluoroscopy to inject safely and accurately. Only the injectionist who has significant experience with using both imaging modalities should attempt this injection.
- This ligamentum teres origin is off the transverse acetabular ligament, and both are often treated at the same time, as the injection techniques are similar.

Pertinent Anatomy

- The ligamentum teres is also known as the ligament of the head of the femur or round ligament of the femur. It is a pyramidal ligament that originates on the posteroinferior acetabulum and the transverse ligament. It inserts on the central femoral head at the fovea. It has two bands and is surrounded by a synovial sheath similar to the anterior cruciate ligament (ACL) in the knee.
- The ligament acts as a secondary stabilizer of the hip, and prevents subluxation at extremes of motion, particularly in mid-flexion, abduction/adduction, and rotation.
- Branches of the obturator artery enter inferomedial and penetrate the middle third of the ligament. The ligament

does have proprioceptive and nociceptive free nerve endings throughout.[54]

- The ligamentum teres origin is off the transverse acetabular ligament—a strong band of tissue at the inferior acetabulum that is essentially an extension of the acetabular labrum and provides part of the load-bearing surface for the femoral head (see Fig. 20.3).[55]

Common Pathology

- Injury to the ligamentum teres and transverse acetabular ligament can be traumatic, iatrogenic, or associated with hyperlaxity or acetabular morphology.
  - Trauma can be acute, such as a fall or motor vehicle accident, or repetitive, and injury to the ligamentum teres has been associated with certain sports or activities such as ballet, figure skating, gymnastics, and martial arts.
  - Iatrogenic injury has been reported with hip arthroscopy, which requires a traction force on the hip and can cause ligamentum teres and other capsular ligamentous injury.
  - Hip dysplasia, in which the hip socket is shallower, can cause more stress on the ligamentum teres.
- One study found that, in over 2000 hip arthroscopies for femoral acetabular impingement, the ligamentum teres was found to be frayed or partially torn in 88% and completely torn in 1.5%, suggesting that ligamentum teres injury can be associated with labral tears.[56]

Equipment

- Curvilinear ultrasound probe
- C-arm fluoroscopy
- Typically, a 22-gauge, 5-inch spinal needle is sufficient.
- Contrast media

Common Injectates

- Local anesthetics for diagnostics
- Prolotherapy, orthobiologics (PRP, bone marrow concentrate, etc.)
- Corticosteroids should not be injected directly into a ligament

Injectate Volume

- 1 to 3 mL

Technique

Patient Position

- Supine, leg extended, externally rotate the hip as much as the patient is able (Fig. 20.66A).

Clinician Position

- Standing on ipsilateral side of the patient.

Transducer Position or C-Arm Position Fluoroscopy Technique

- Set up the fluoroscopy image. Obtain a true AP projection with contralateral obliquity of the C-arm, in which the femoral head, acetabulum, and joint space are visualized and the posterior and anterior rims of the acetabulum are aligned (see Fig. 20.66A and B).
- With curvilinear ultrasound transducer, identify the inferior aspect of the femoral acetabular joint. Identify the femoral artery, vein, and nerve.

Needle Position

- Having a curve at the needle tip can help with redirecting the needle.
- Start 2 to 3 cm lateral to the femoral nerve to pass deep to the nerve and vessels when advanced to the trajectory (see Fig. 20.66C).
- Mark the trajectory by placing a needle on the skin or using a surgical marker. Before piercing the skin, take an AP image using the C-arm to ensure that the ultrasound image corresponds with the inferior half of the femur (see Fig. 20.66B).
- Ensure that the needle is staying in the transverse plane in relation to the hip. Check this relationship by taking an AP fluoroscopy picture periodically as you advance the needle under ultrasound guidance.
- Once the needle tip is in the joint as far as you can see with ultrasound, go to the fluoroscopic view.
- Keep the needle close to the femoral head, with the curve going posterior to insure going deep into the joint while also avoiding significant contact with the articular surface to prevent damage to the cartilage.

Target

- Ligamentum teres: Under AP fluoroscopy, advance or "walk" the needle along the femoral head and aim at the inferior aspect of the acetabular wall at the level of the fovea on the femur or just slightly inferior. Once the needle is at the target against the acetabular wall, pull back about 1 to 2 mm.
  - Obtain a lateral view where the needle should be about halfway across the femoral head.
  - A small amount of contrast should be injected showing central flow along the ligament in lateral and AP views without any IA contrast flow (see Fig. 20.66D and E).
- Transverse acetabular ligament: Aim at the inferior aspect of the acetabular wall.
  - Obtain a lateral view in which the needle should be in the central anterior third of the femoral head from anterior to posterior.
- A small amount of contrast should be injected, showing central flow along the ligament in lateral and AP views without any significant joint disbursement (Fig. 20.67B).

PEARLS AND PITFALLS

- This is an advanced injection, so do not attempt unless you have good hip ultrasound and fluoroscopy-guided needle experience.
- It is much safer to use ultrasound to identify the neurovascular structures.
- The patient needs to have good external rotation of the hip, and if unable to, position the hip (i.e., patients with severe hip arthritis, bone spurs, or lack of external rotation); this injection can be difficult or impossible to perform.
- Make sure that the needle stays along the femoral head to ensure that it does not travel into the joint space. The curved needle helps to advance deep into the joint.
- When injecting into the ligament, patients will often have reproduction of some of their typical pain if the ligament is injured.

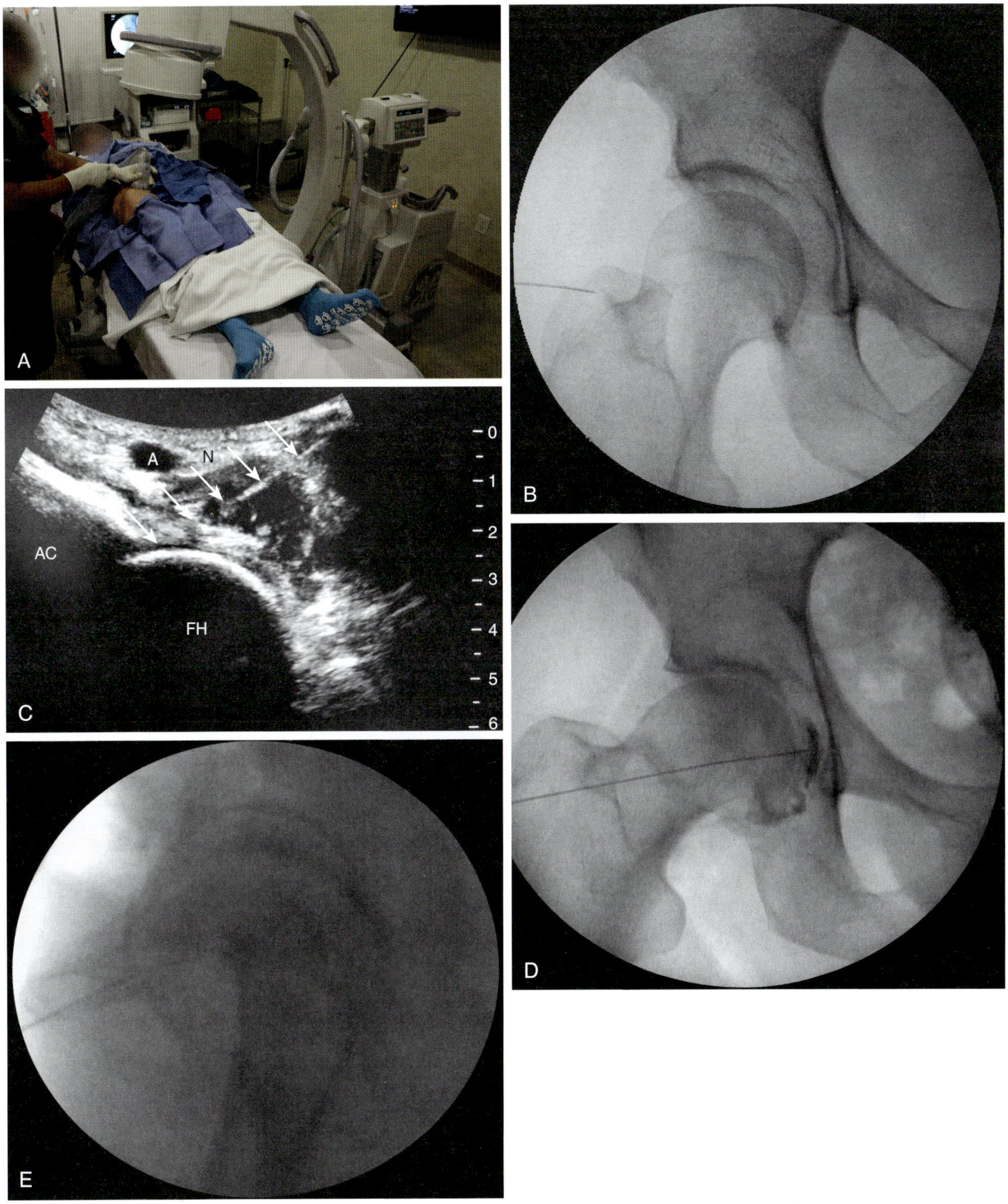

• **Fig. 20.66** (A) Ligamentum teres setup. (B) Ligamentum teres needle trajectory. (C) Ligamentum teres ultrasound. (D) Ligamentum teres fluoroscopy target AP with contrast. (E) Ligamentum teres fluoroscopy target lateral with contrast. *AC*, Acetabulum, *FH*, femoral head.

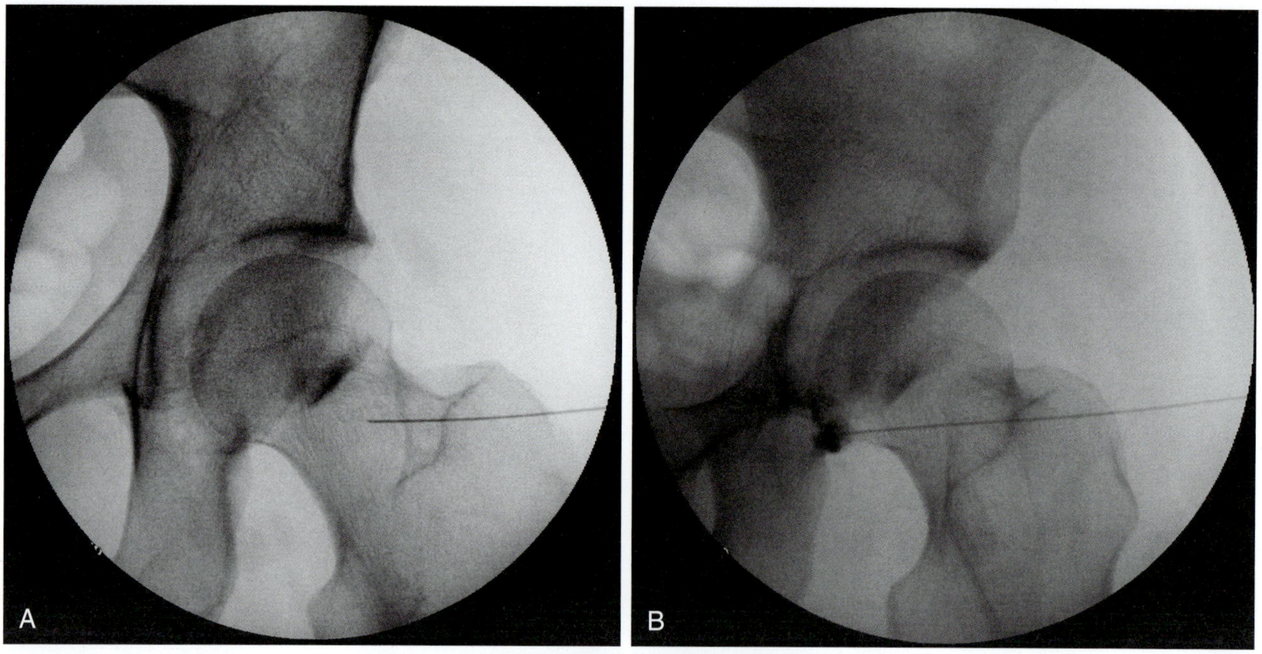

• **Fig. 20.67** (A) Transverse acetabular ligament needle trajectory. (B) Transverse acetabular ligament target.

Hip Capsular Ligaments

KEY POINTS

- Can be used to manage ligament laxity, especially in the presence of labral tears, traumatic injuries, connective tissue disorders, and joint arthritis.
- Injection technique is very similar to IA injections, except just superficial to the joint. The goal is to inject multiple sites along the ligaments/capsule.

Pertinent Anatomy and Common Pathology

- Refer to ultrasound section

Equipment

- C-arm fluoroscopy
- Typically, 25- or 22-gauge, 3.5-inch spinal needle is sufficient. In larger or taller patient, a 25-gauge, 4.69-inch needle or 22-gauge, 5-inch needle is required
- Contrast dye

Common Injectates

- Prolotherapy, orthobiologics (PRP, bone marrow concentrate, etc.).
- Steroids should not be used as they can potentially injure ligaments when injected directly.

Injectate Volume

- 2 to 4 mL

Technique: Anterior Approach

Patient Position

- Supine, leg extended.

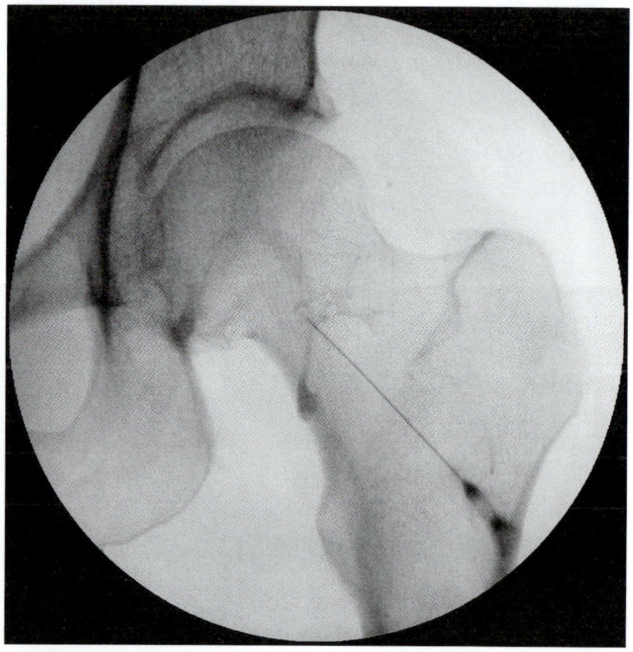

• **Fig. 20.68** Anterior Capsule Target.

Clinician Position

- Standing on ipsilateral side of the patient.

Transducer Position or C-Arm Position Fluoroscopy Technique

- AP projection in which the greater trochanter, femoral head, and joint space are visualized.

Needle Position

- Start anterior and slightly medial to the greater trochanter.

Target

- Femoral neck and inferior portion of femoral head (Fig. 20.68).

- Advance needle to bone; then withdraw 1 mm and inject, "peppering" a broad area of the capsule.

PEARLS AND PITFALLS

- Be sure to always keep the needle over the femoral neck.
- Avoid injecting too far medially in order not to injure the neurovascular structures.
- Can inject a small amount of contrast to make sure that no vascular uptake is observed and to ensure that there is no IA flow.

Technique: Lateral Approach

Patient Position

- Lateral decubitus, with pillow between the knees
- Alternative: supine, legs extended

Clinician Position

- If lateral decubitus, standing behind the patient
- If supine, standing on ipsilateral side of the patient

Transducer Position or C-Arm Position Fluoroscopy Technique

- AP projection visualizing the femoral acetabular joint, the greater trochanter, and the lateral soft tissue.
- May use lateral projection to make sure needle is maintained in central plane from anterior to posterior. Option to align both acetabulum completely or offset them. If they are offset, then smaller joint will be closest to the transducer.

Needle Position

- Start just anterior and superior to the greater trochanter, but below the lateral acetabular rim. Needle trajectory should be from superior to inferior toward the lateral femoral neck.

Target

- Femoral neck and inferior portion of femoral head (Fig. 20.69).
- Advance needle to bone, then withdraw 1 mm and inject, "peppering" a broad area of the capsule.

PEARLS AND PITFALLS

- Be sure to always keep the needle over bone.
- Can inject a small amount of contrast to make sure that no vascular uptake is observed and to ensure that there is no IA flow.

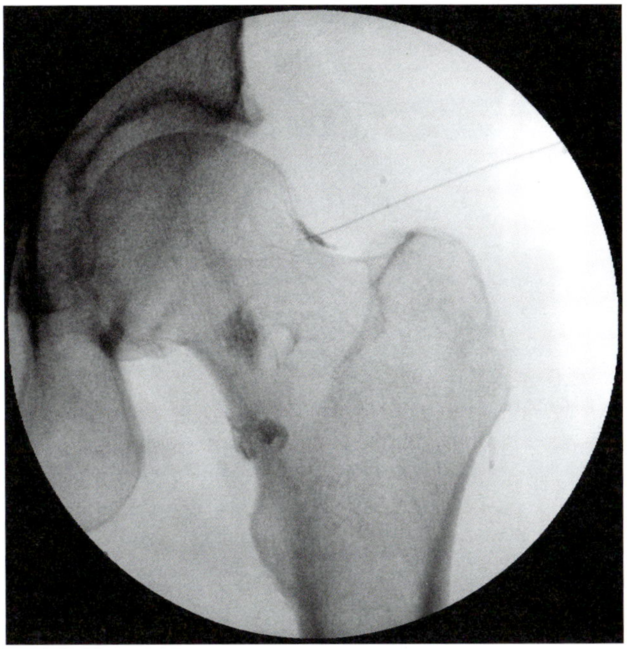

• **Fig. 20.69** Lateral Capsule Target.

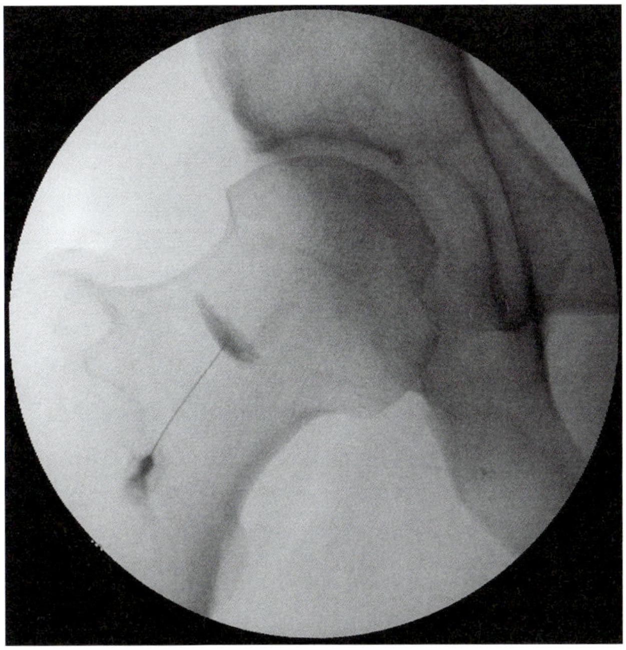

• **Fig. 20.70** Posterior Capsule Target.

Technique: Posterior Approach

Patient Position

- Prone
- Will likely need hip internal rotation to move the greater trochanter out of the needle trajectory. To achieve this, bend the patient's leg at the knee and rotate from the lower leg outwards.

Clinician Position

- Standing ipsilateral side of the patient

Transducer Position or C-Arm Position Fluoroscopy Technique

- AP projection in which the greater trochanter, femoral head, and joint space are visualized

Needle Position

- Start posterior and slightly medial to the greater trochanter

Target

- Femoral neck and inferior portion of femoral head (Fig. 20.70).

- Advance needle to bone, then withdraw 1 mm and inject, "peppering" a broad area of the capsule.

PEARLS AND PITFALLS

- Be sure to always keep the needle over the femoral neck.
- Avoid injecting too far medially in order not to injure the neurovascular structures.
- Can inject a small amount of contrast to make sure that no vascular uptake is observed and to ensure that there is no IA flow.

Femoroacetabular Labrum

KEY POINTS

- Authors' preferred approach is placing the needle under ultrasound guidance and confirming needle placement with fluoroscopy.
- The injection technique is similar to IA, except you want to target the acetabulum and the specific area of tear based on MRI findings.
- Will want to target the location of the labral tear (anterior, superior, or posterior), depending on the location of the labral tear on diagnostic MRI or ultrasound.

Pertinent Anatomy and Common Pathology

- Refer to ultrasound section

Equipment

- C-arm fluoroscopy
- Typically, 25- or 22-gauge, 3.5-inch spinal needle is sufficient. In larger or taller patients, a 25-gauge, 4.69-inch needle or 22-gauge, 5-inch needle is required
- Contrast dye

Common Injectates

- Anesthetics for diagnostics, prolotherapy, orthobiologics (PRP, bone marrow concentrate, etc.).
- Steroids should not be used, as they can potentially injure cartilage/labrum when injected directly.

Injectate Volume

- 1 to 2 mL directly into the labrum

Technique: Anterior Approach

Patient Position

- Supine leg extended.

Clinician Position

- Standing on ipsilateral side of the patient.

Transducer Position or C-Arm Position Fluoroscopy Technique

- AP projection in which the greater trochanter, femoral head, and joint space are visualized.

Needle Position

- Start anterior and slightly medial to the greater trochanter.

Target

- Target the pathology in the superior anterior acetabulum (Fig. 20.71).

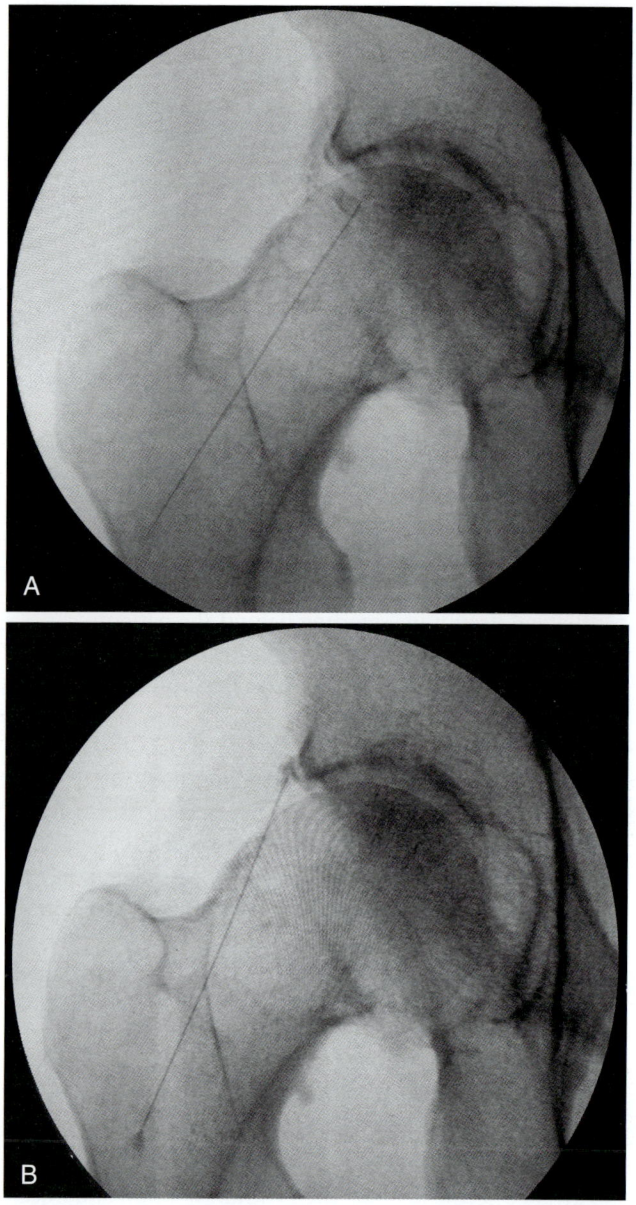

• **Fig. 20.71** (A) Hip fluoroscopy anterior superior labrum. (B) Hip fluoroscopy anterior lateral labrum.

- Aim to touch the needle on the bone cortex on the inferior femoral head and then "walk" the needle along the femur superiorly to end at the acetabulum.
- Once the needle is touching the acetabulum, withdraw the needle 1 mm to inject the labrum.
- Confirm labral flow with a small amount of contrast.

PEARLS AND PITFALLS

- Injectionist can often feel more tissue resistance when injecting the labrum versus IA.
- Inject a small amount of contrast to confirm desired flow.
- There may be significant resistance and patient discomfort when trying to inject more than 1–2 mL into a labrum. Can place any extra injectate into the joint.

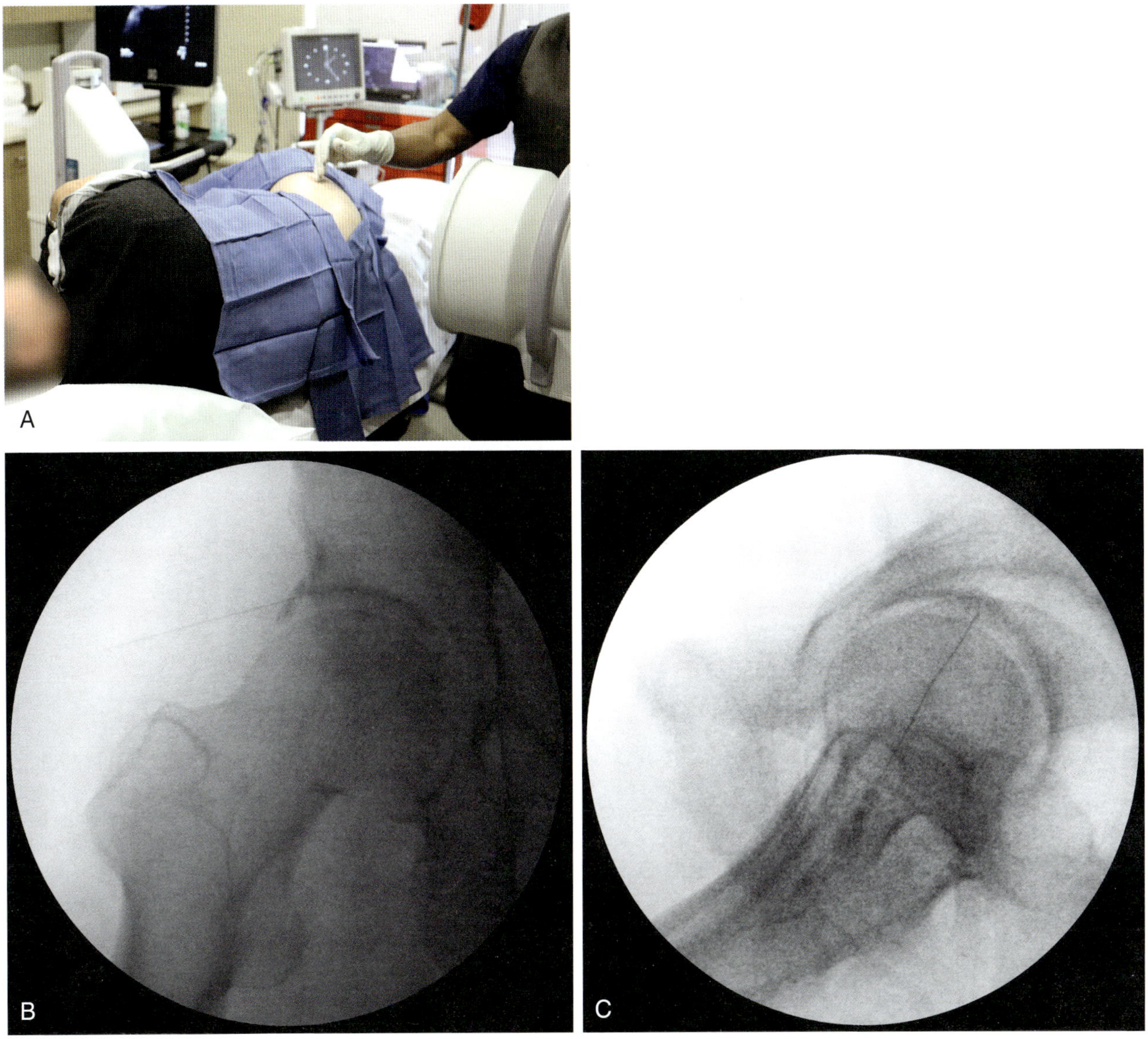

• **Fig. 20.72** (A) Hip fluoroscopy lateral labrum setup. (B) Hip fluoroscopy lateral labrum and superior capsule target in AP. (C) Hip fluoroscopy lateral labrum and superior capsule target in the lateral position.

Technique: Lateral Approach for Superior and Posterior Lateral Labrum

Patient Position

- Lateral decubitus, with pillow between the knees (Fig. 20.72A).
- Alternative is to have the patient supine, legs extended.

Clinician Position

- If lateral, standing behind the patient.
- If supine, standing on ipsilateral side of the patient.

Transducer Position or C-Arm Position Fluoroscopy Technique

- AP projection visualizing the femoral acetabular joint, the greater trochanter, and the lateral soft tissue.
- May use lateral projection to make sure needle is maintained in central plane from anterior to posterior. Option to align both acetabulum completely or offset them. If they are offset, then the smaller joint will be closest to the transducer.

Needle Position

- In the lateral view, ensure that the needle starting position is central, anterior, or posterior, depending on where the labral injury is from diagnostic MRI or ultrasound.
- In the AP view, start just anterior and superior to the greater trochanter, but below the lateral acetabular rim. Needle trajectory should be from inferior to superior toward the lateral joint opening. Having a slight curve in the needle can help guide the needle.

Target

- Superior lateral labrum.
- Advance the needle down to the periosteum on the lateral acetabulum, just above the joint opening.
- Inject a small amount of contrast to ensure accurate flow (see Fig. 20.72B and C).
- Confirm accurate needle placement and contrast flow in AP and lateral projections.

PEARLS AND PITFALLS

- See anterior approach.

References

1. Jay S, Mark FBH, Toby NW. Accuracy of sonographically guided intra-articular injections in the native adult hip. *J Ultrasound Med.* 2009;28(3):329–335. https://doi.org/10.7863/jum.2009.28.3.329.
2. Pourbagher MA, Ozalay M, Pourbagher A. Accuracy and outcome of sonographically guided intra-articular sodium hyaluronate injections in patients with osteoarthritis of the hip. *J Ultrasound Med.* 2005;24:1391–1395.
3. Levi DS. Intra-articular hip injections using ultrasound guidance: accuracy using a linear array transducer. *Pharm Manag PM R.* 2013;5:129–134.
4. Bartoníček J, Naňka O. Josias Weitbrecht, the founder of syndesmology, and the history of the retinacula of Weitbrecht. *Surg Radiol Anat.* 2019;41:1103–1111. https://doi.org/10.1007/s00276-018-2172-4.
5. Looney CG, Raynor B, Lowe R. Adhesive capsulitis of the hip: a review. *J Am Acad Orthop Surg.* 2013;21(12):749–755. https://doi.org/10.5435/JAAOS-21-12-749.
6. de Sa D, Phillips M, Catapano M, et al. Adhesive capsulitis of the hip: a review addressing diagnosis, treatment and outcomes. *J Hip Preserv Surg.* 2015;3(1):43–55. https://doi.org/10.1093/jhps/hnv075.
7. Luukkainen R, Asikainen E. Frozen hip. *Scand J Rheumatol.* 1992;21(2):97.
8. Luukkainen R, Sipola E, Varjo P. Successful treatment of frozen hip with manipulation and pressure dilatation. *Open Rheumatol J.* 2008;2:31–32.
9. Malanga GA, Mautner KR. *Atlas of Ultrasound-Guided Musculoskeletal Injections.* New York: McGraw-Hill; 2014.
10. Jacobson JA. *Fundamentals of Musculoskeletal Ultrasound.* Philadelphia, PA: Elsevier; 2018.
11. Becker S, Capobianco R, Seita M. Is sacroiliac joint pain associated with changes in the pubic symphysis? A radiographic pilot study. *Eur J Orthop Surg Traumatol.* 2015;25(suppl 1):S243–S249.
12. Phieffer LS, Lundberg WP, Templeman DC. Instability of the posterior pelvic ring associated with disruption of the pubic symphysis. *Orthop Clin North Am.* 2004;35(4):445-v.
13. Becker I, Woodley SJ, Stringer MD. The adult human pubic symphysis: a systematic review. *J Anat.* 2010;217(5):475–487. https://doi.org/10.1111/j.1469-7580.2010.01300.x.
14. Becker I, Woodley SJ, Stringer MD. The adult human pubic symphysis: a systematic review. *J Anat.* 2010;217(5):475–487.
15. Stover MD, Edelstein AI, Matta JM. Chronic anterior pelvic instability: diagnosis and management. *J Am Acad Orthop Surg.* 2017;25(7):509–517.
16. Beatty T. Osteitis pubis in athletes. *Curr Sports Med Rep.* 2012;11(2):96–98. https://doi.org/10.1249/JSR.0b013e318249c32b.
17. Becker S, Capobianco R, Seita M. Is sacroiliac joint pain associated with changes in the pubic symphysis? A radiographic pilot study. *Eur J Orthop Surg Traumatol.* 2015;25(suppl 1):S243–S249.
18. Shu B, Safran MR. Hip instability: anatomic and clinical considerations of traumatic and atraumatic instability. *Clin Sports Med.* 2011;30(2):349–367. https://doi.org/10.1016/j.csm.2010.12.008.
19. Hughes 4th C, Hasselman CT, Best TM, Martinez S, Garrett Jr WE. *Am J Sports Med.* 1995;23(4):500–506.
20. Cross TM, Gibbs N, Houang MT, et al. Acute quadriceps muscle strains: magnetic resonance imaging features and prognosis. *Am J Sports Med.* 2004;32:710–719. https://doi.org/10.1177/0363546503261734.
21. McNeilan RJ, Rose M, Mei-Dan O, Genuario J. Open repair of acute proximal adductor magnus avulsion. *Arthrosc Tech.* 2018;8(1):e75–e80. https://doi.org/10.1016/j.eats.2018.09.003.
22. Bass CJ, Connell DA. Sonographic findings of tensor fascia lata tendinopathy: another cause of anterior groin pain. *Skeletal Radiol.* 2002;31:143–148.
23. Bradberry DM, Sussman WI, Mautner KR. Ultrasound-guided percutaneous needle tenotomy for chronic tensor fascia lata tendinopathy: a case series and description of sonographic findings. *PM&R.* 2018;10(9):979–983.
24. Deshmukh S, Abboud SF, Grant T, Omar IM. High-resolution ultrasound of the fascia lata iliac crest attachment: anatomy, pathology, and image-guided treatment. *Skeletal Radiol.* 2019;48(9):1315–1321.
25. Hung CY, Chang KV. Ultrasound-guided percutaneous needle tenotomy with platelet-rich plasma injection for an uncommon case of proximal gluteus medius tendinopathy. *J Med Ultrasound.* 2019;27(2):111–112.
26. Sher I1, Umans H, Downie SA, Tobin K, Arora R, Olson TR. *Skeletal Radiol.* 2011;40(12):1553–1556. https://doi.org/10.1007/s00256-011-1168-5. Proximal iliotibial band syndrome: what is it and where is it?.
27. Brady K. Huang , Juliana CCampos, Philippe Ghobrial Michael Peschka, Michael LPretterklieber, Abdalla YS kaf, Christine BChung, Mini N. Pathria. Injury of the Gluteal Aponeurotic Fascia and Proximal Iliotibial Band: Anatomy, Pathologic Conditions, and MR Imaging
28. Yu D, Bradley MJ. Bristol/UK. Proximal iliotibial band syndrome; An uncommon cause of hip pain found on ultrasound. Educational Poster. https://doi.org/10.1594/essr2014/P-0045. ESSR 2014 / P-0045.
29. Zissen MH, Wallace G, Stevens KJ, Fredericson M, Beaulieu C. High hamstring tendinopathy: MRI and ultrasound imaging and therapeutic efficacy of percutaneous corticosteroid injection. *AJR Am J Roentgenol.* 2010;195(4):993–998.
30. Lempainen L, Sarimo J, Mattila K, Vaittinen S, Orava S. Proximal hamstring tendinopathy: results of surgical management and histopathologic findings. *Am J Sports Med.* 2009;37(4):727–734.
31. Huang BK, Campos JC, Michael Peschka PG, et al. Injury of the gluteal aponeurotic fascia and proximal iliotibial band: anatomy, pathologic conditions, and MR imaging. *Radiographics.* 2013;33(5):1437–1452. https://doi.org/10.1148/rg.335125171.
32. Mehta P, Telhan R, Burge A, Wyss J. Atypical cause of lateral hip pain due to proximal gluteus medius muscle tear: a report of 2 cases. *PMR.* 2015;7(9):1002–1006. https://doi.org/10.1016/j.pmrj.2015.05.017.
33. Jenkins D. *Hollinshead' Functional Anatomy of the Limbs and Back*; 1993.
34. Suzanne SL, David ES, Levon N. Sonography of greater trochanteric pain syndrome and the rarity of primary bursitis. *Nazarian Am J Roentgenol.* 2013;201(5):1083–1086.
35. Nissen MJ, Brulhart L, Faundez A, Finckh A, Courvoisier DS, Genevay S. Glucocorticoid injections for greater trochanteric

pain syndrome: a randomised double-blind placebo-controlled (GLUTEAL) trial. *Clin Rheumatol.* 2019;38(3):647–655. https://doi.org/10.1007/s10067-018-4309-6.

36. Hwang JY, Lee SW, Kim JO. MR imaging features of obturator internus bursa of the hip. *Korean J Radiol.* 2008;9(4):375–378. https://doi.org/10.3348/kjr.2008.9.4.375.
37. Chen B, Rispoli L, Stitik T, Leong M. Successful treatment of gluteal pain from obturator internus tendinitis and bursitis with ultrasound-guided injection. *Am J Phys Med Rehabil.* 2017;96(10):e181–e184.
38. Drake RL, Vogl W, Mitchell AWM, Gray H. *Grays Anatomy for Students.* Philadelphia, PA: Elsevier; 2020.
39. Yin-Ting C, Keyonna MJ. Ultrasound finding of ischiofemoral impingement syndrome and novel treatment with Botulinum toxin chemodenervation: a case report. *PM&R.* 2018;10(6):665–670.
40. Kassarjian, A., Tomas, X., Cerezal, L., et al. MRI of the Quadratus Femoris Muscle: Anatomic Considerations and Pathologic Lesions *American J Roentgenol.* 197(1):170–174. https://doi.org/10.2214/AJR.10.5898
41. Furman MB, Berkwits L. *Atlas of Image-Guided Spinal Procedures.* Philadelphia, PA: Elsevier, Inc; 2018.
42. Kaur J, Singh P. Pudendal nerve entrapment syndrome. In: *StatPearls [Internet].* Treasure Island (FL): StatPearls Publishing; 2020. Available from: https://www.ncbi.nlm.nih.gov/books/NBK544272/
43. Bendtsen TF, Parras T, Moriggl B, et al. Ultrasound-guided pudendal nerve block at the entrance of the pudendal (Alcock) canal. *Regional Anesthesia Pain Med.* 2016;41(2):140–145. https://doi.org/10.1097/aap.0000000000000355.
44. Gray AT. *Atlas of Ultrasound-Guided Regional Anesthesia.* Philadelphia, PA: Elsevier; 2019.
45. Huang BK, Campos JC, Peschka PGM, et al. Injury of the gluteal aponeurotic fascia and proximal iliotibial band: anatomy, pathologic conditions, and MR imaging. *Radiographics.* 2013;33(5):1437–1452. https://doi.org/10.1148/rg.335125171.
46. Johnson CS, Johnson RL, Niesen AD, Stoike DE, Pawlina W. Ultrasound-guided posterior femoral cutaneous nerve block: a cadaveric study. *J Ultrasound Med.* 2017;37(4):897–903. https://doi.org/10.1002/jum.14429.
47. Kassarjian A, Tomas X, Cerezal L, Canga A, Llopis E. MRI of the quadratus femoris muscle: anatomic considerations and pathologic lesions. *Am J Roentgenol.* 2011;197(1):170–174. https://doi.org/10.2214/ajr.10.5898.
48. Luukkainen R, Sipola E, Varjo P. Successful treatment of frozen hip with manipulation and pressure dilatation. *Open Rheumatol J.* 2008;2(1):31–32. https://doi.org/10.2174/1874312900802010031.
49. Rojas-Gomez MA, Blanco-Davila R, Tobar Roa V, Gomez Gonzalez AM, Ortiz Zableh AM, Ortiz Azuero A. Regional anesthesia guided by ultrasound in the pudendal nerve territory. *Colombia J Anesthesiol.* 2017;45(3):200–209. https://doi.org/10.1016/j.rcae.2017.06.007.
50. Sa DD, Phillips M, Catapano M, et al. Adhesive capsulitis of the hip: a review addressing diagnosis, treatment and outcomes. *J Hip Preservation Surg.* 2015;3(1):43–55. https://doi.org/10.1093/jhps/hnv075.
51. Topcu I, Aysel I. Ultrasound guided posterior femoral cutaneous nerve block. *Ağrı—J Turkish Society Algol.* 2014;26(3):145–148. https://doi.org/10.5505/agri.2014.26122.
52. Trammell AP, Pilson H. Anatomy, bony pelvis and lower limb, tensor fasciae latae muscle. In: *StatPearls [Internet].* Treasure Island (FL): StatPearls Publishing; 2020. Available from: https://www.ncbi.nlm.nih.gov/books/NBK499870/
53. Yeap PM, Robinson P. Ultrasound diagnostic and therapeutic injections of the hip and groin. *J Belgian Society Radiol.* 2017;101(S2). https://doi.org/10.5334/jbr-btr.1371.
54. O'Donnell JM, Devitt BM, Arora M. The role of the ligamentum teres in the adult hip: redundant or relevant? A review. *J Hip Preserv Surg.* 2018;5(1):15–22.
55. Beverland D. The transverse acetabular ligament: optimizing version. *Orthopedics.* 2010;33(9):631.
56. Larson CM. Editorial commentary: ligamentum teres tears and femoroacetabular impingement: complex coexistence of impingement and instability. *Arthroscopy.* 2016;32(7):1298–1299.

21

Knee Injection Techniques

JOSH HACKEL, TODD HAYANO, JOHN PITTS, AND
MAIRIN A. JEROME

Ultrasound Guided

Intra-Articular

KEY POINTS

- The superolateral approach is preferred for intra-articular knee injections, especially when an effusion is present[1,2]

Pertinent Anatomy

- The knee joint is an encapsulated hinge-type synovial joint
- The knee joint is composed of four major bones: distal femur, proximal tibia, proximal fibula, and patella (Fig. 21.1)
- The bones form three articulations:
  - Femorotibial (medial and lateral compartments)
  - Patellofemoral
  - Tibiofibular
- Primarily function is to allow for knee flexion and extension

Common Pathology

- The knee is susceptible to several arthritides including osteoarthritis (most common), rheumatoid arthritis, crystal arthropathies, and other inflammatory arthropathies.
- It is also vulnerable to direct trauma, particularly in sports-related injuries or motor vehicle accidents.
- Intra-articular pathology can present with a joint effusion or synovitis.

Equipment

- High-frequency linear array transducer
- 22 to 18 gauge 1.5 to 2 inch needle for aspiration
- 27 to 22 gauge 1.5 to 2 inch needle for injection only
- For aspirations:
  - 10 mL or 20 mL syringe—for small effusions
  - 30 mL or 60 mL syringe—for large effusions

Common Injectates

- Local anesthetics for diagnostics, corticosteroids
- Hyaluronic acid
- Prolotherapy
- Orthobiologics (platelet-rich plasma [PRP], bone marrow concentrate, micronized adipose tissue, etc.)

Injectate Volume

- 2 to 10 mL total

Technique for Suprapatellar Recess (Author Preferred)

Patient Position

- Supine or seated

PEARLS AND PITFALLS

- If aspirating the knee, consider 1–3 mL of local anesthetic with smaller-gauge needle (27 or 30 gauge) for numbing the needle track.
- Directly target the hypoechoic space between the prefemoral and suprapatellar fat pads. Start 1–3 cm below the probe using the ultrasound to estimate depth of the suprapatellar recess and align needle to be as close to parallel to the probe.
- The procedure becomes more difficult without an effusion:
  - Can have the patient contract the quad muscle to bring forth any fluid or more easily see the bursa
  - Can push against medial soft tissue to visualize interval between prefemoral and suprapatellar fat pads
  - Even in a dry knee joint, fluid can often be clearly seen at the lateral midpatella gutter (between the patella and lateral femoral condyle). The joint capsule can be traced proximally as it communicates with the suprapatellar recess
  - Float the transducer on gel, as downward pressure can compress the recess and make it more difficult to visualize.
- Avoid injecting into the quad tendon or fat pads.
- A midpatella lateral approach can also be used targeting the lateral midpatella gutter. This can create a sense of fullness or pressure, and for some will be more uncomfortable than the suprapatella (see Fig. 21.2D). This approach is also less accurate than the superolateral.[3]

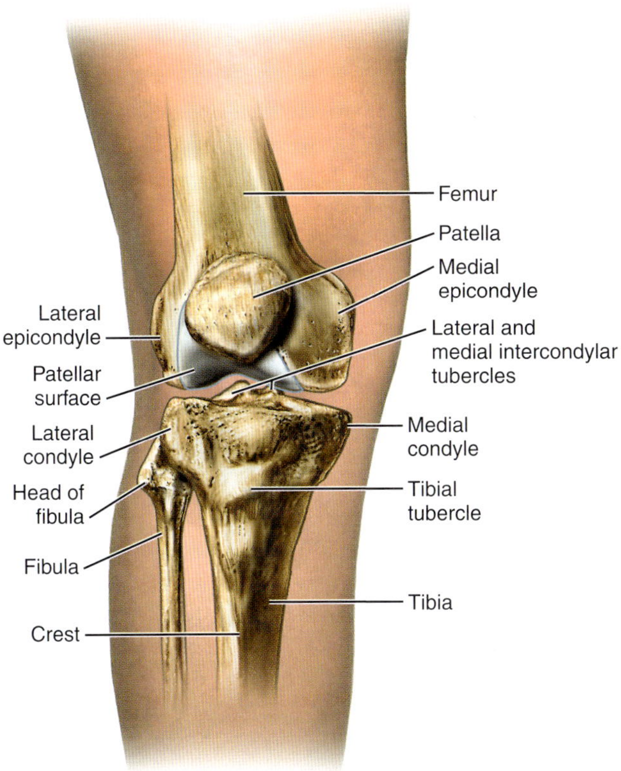

• **Fig. 21.1** Bony Landmarks of the Anterior Knee. (From Detterline A, Babb J, Noyes FR, et al. *Noyes' Knee Disorders: Surgery, Rehabilitation, Clinical Outcomes.* 2017:2–22.)

- Knee flexed to 30 degrees with towel roll or bump under the affected knee

Clinician Position

- Standing or seated on the side of the affected knee

Transducer Position

- Short axis to the quadriceps tendon (Fig. 21.2A)

Needle Position

- In-plane/long axis
- Lateral to medial approach

Target

- Suprapatellar recess (see Fig. 21.2B and C)

Technique for Anterolateral Approach

Patient Position

- Seated or supine with the knee bent 60 to 90 degrees/hook-lying. Can place booster pillow under the knee for support (see Fig. 21.3A)

Clinician Position

- Seated or standing on the side of the affected knee

Transducer Position

- Sagittal plane directly over lateral condyle.
    - Find the patellar tendon in long axis; then maintaining the same probe orientation, move laterally to visualize the trochlear groove deep to the tendon.

Needle Position

- Out of plane (similar to landmark-guided lateral infrapatellar knee injections) (see Fig. 21.3A).

Target

- Deep to the synovial membrane covering the medial or lateral femoral condyle. Care should be taken to visualize the needle tip deep to anterior (Hoffa's) fat pad and confirm intra-articular fluid flow (see Fig. 21.3B)

PEARLS AND PITFALLS

- There should not be any resistance when injecting. If there is resistance the needle may be in the capsule or extra-articular. Pain may indicate the needle is within the anterior fat pad.
- Use color Doppler when injecting to confirm intra-articular flow.
- Medial approach risks incidental injury to the saphenous nerve.[4]
- The anterolateral approach may be less painful than the superolateral approach.[5,6]
- This approach can also be performed with the transducer oriented in short axis to the patellar tendon and the needle in plane. The target can be just superficial to the articular cartilage of the medial or lateral trochlea depending on the anatomy and needle visualization.
- No significant difference in success rates between targeting the lateral or medial femoral condyle using the lateral infrapatellar approach.[7]

Technique for Medial or Lateral Directed Knee Joint Injection

Patient Position

- Supine with the knee bent 60 to 90 degrees/hook-lying. Can place booster pillow under the knee for support (Fig. 21.4A and B)

Clinician Position

- Standing on either side of the patient.

Transducer Position

- Sagittal plane directly over the medial or lateral condyle (depending on target).
- Find the patella; then maintaining the same probe orientation, move medially or laterally to the condyle and tibial plateau.

Needle Position

- Long axis to the transducer proximal to distal (see Fig. 21.4A and B).
- Needle will have a steep angle headed past the femoral chondral surface towards the tibial in the anterior one-third of the joint.

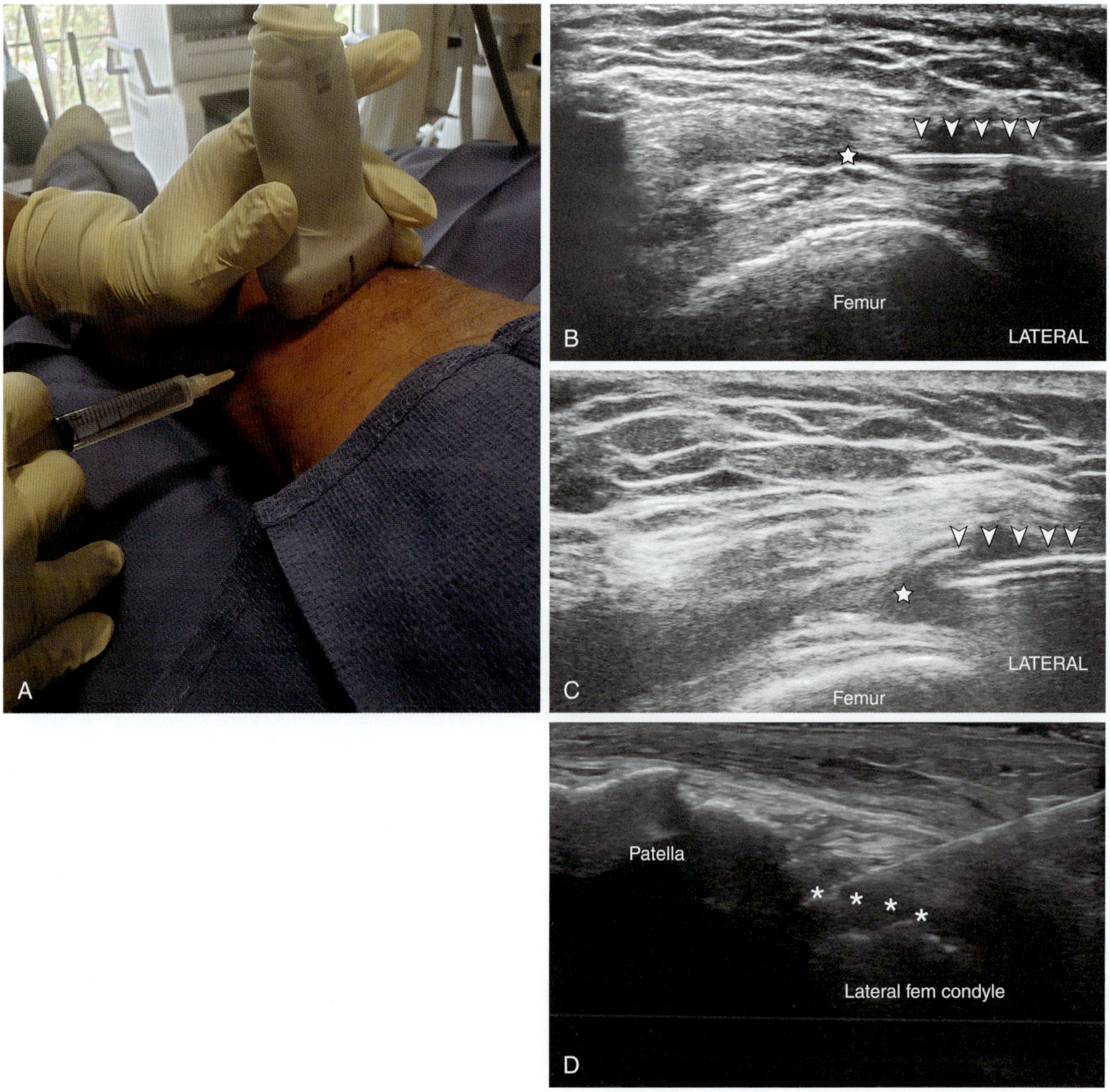

• **Fig. 21.2** (A) Suprapatellar bursa injection setup. (B) Suprapatellar bursa injection. (C) Suprapatellar bursa aspiration. (D) Midpatella gutter.

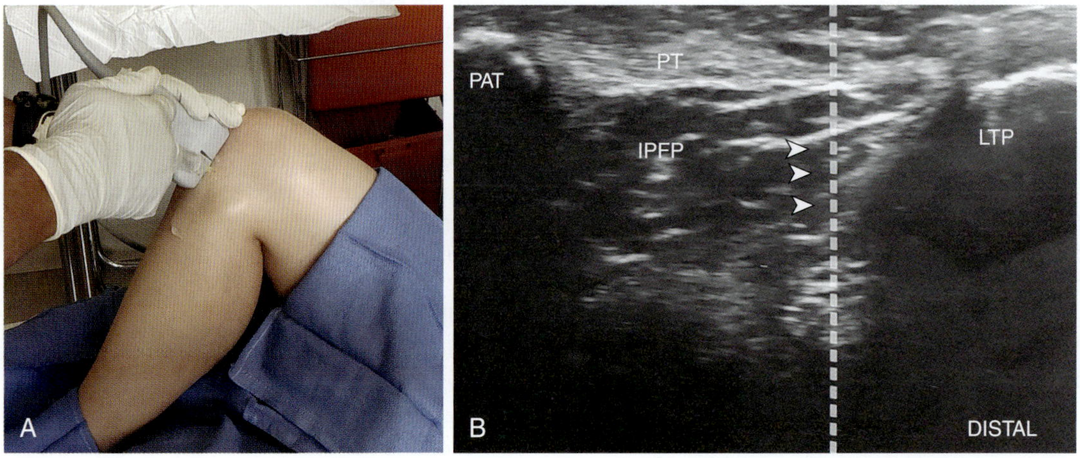

• **Fig. 21.3** (A) Anterolateral knee joint injection hook-lying setup. (B) Anterolateral knee joint injection out of plane.

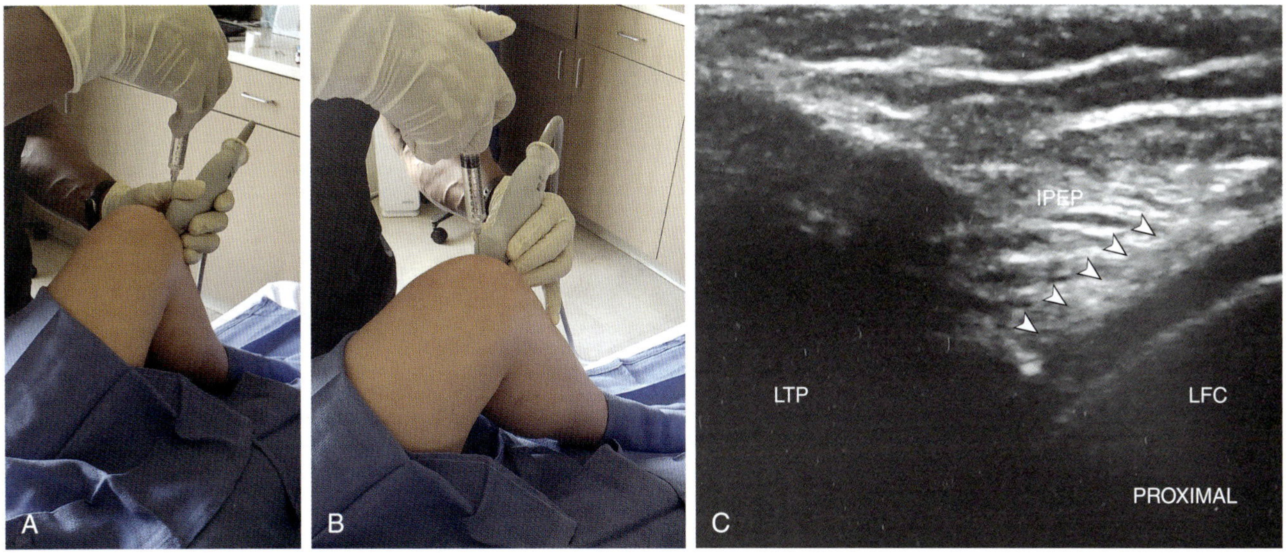

• **Fig. 21.4** (A) Medial knee joint directed injection setup in plane. (B) Lateral knee joint directed setup in plane. (C) Lateral knee joint directed injection in-plane ultrasound injection.

Target

- Between the femoral condyle and the tibial plateau just superficial to the meniscus or the chondral surface (see Fig. 21.4C)

PEARLS AND PITFALLS

- Good approach if want to target specifically medial or lateral compartments but not a commonly used technique, and it is a little more challenging.
- Be careful not to scrape the needle along the chondral surfaces. Visualize needle tip at all times.
- There should not be any resistance when injecting; if so. needle may be in the capsule or meniscus or cartilage. Pain may indicate the needle is within one of those structures.
- Use color Doppler when injecting to ensure intra-articular flow.

Technique for Weightbearing Trochlea Groove Chondral Surfaces

Patient Position

- Supine, hip and knee each flexed 90 degrees. Rest the leg on a block or bolster (Fig. 21.5A and B)

Clinician Position

- Standing on left side of the patient for right-handed injection, right side of patient for left-handed injection.

Transducer Position

- Parallel to the leg/sagittal plane directly over desired condyle medial or lateral.
- Find the patella; then maintaining the same probe orientation, move medially or laterally.
- Scan slightly superior to visualize medial or lateral femoral condyle. The patella can be partially covering the lateral femoral condyle so may have to scroll a little more laterally but stay over weight-bearing surface.

Needle Position

- Long axis, distal to proximal approach (see Fig. 21.5A and B).
- Can inject local anesthetic first from skin to just above the joint capsule.
- If the aiming for lateral condyle and patella is overlapping, angle probe and needle medially to slide needle under the patella but still toward weight-bearing lateral chondral surface.

Target

- Medial or lateral femoral condyle:
    - Aim for the anterior one-third of the chondral surface with the bevel facing the surface (see Fig. 21.5C).
    - Gently touch chondral surface and inject. May have to pull back very slightly to get flow intra-articularly. Should see flow of injectate. Avoid injecting into the capsule.

PEARLS AND PITFALLS

- This is not a common technique, but the authors' preferred approach when using mesenchymal stem cells (MSCs). The 90/90 position can allow for gravity-dependent cell adhesion after 10 min.[8] Inject very slowly over 3–5 min to allow for cell adhesion and to avoid flushing the injectate off of the chondral surface.
- It is unknown if there is any advantage for this position with other biologics besides MSCs.
- Use a smaller-gauge needle where possible to avoid damaging the cartilage. Guide the needle very slowly and barely touch down on the chondral surface. Make sure the bevel is facing the surface to decrease chances of cartilage injury and inject directly on chondral surface.
- Aiming for the more anterior aspect of the condyle helps achieve a more diffuse flow along the cartilage surface.
- Only use 1–3 mL of injectate here. Any extra can be placed intra-articular with above-described techniques.

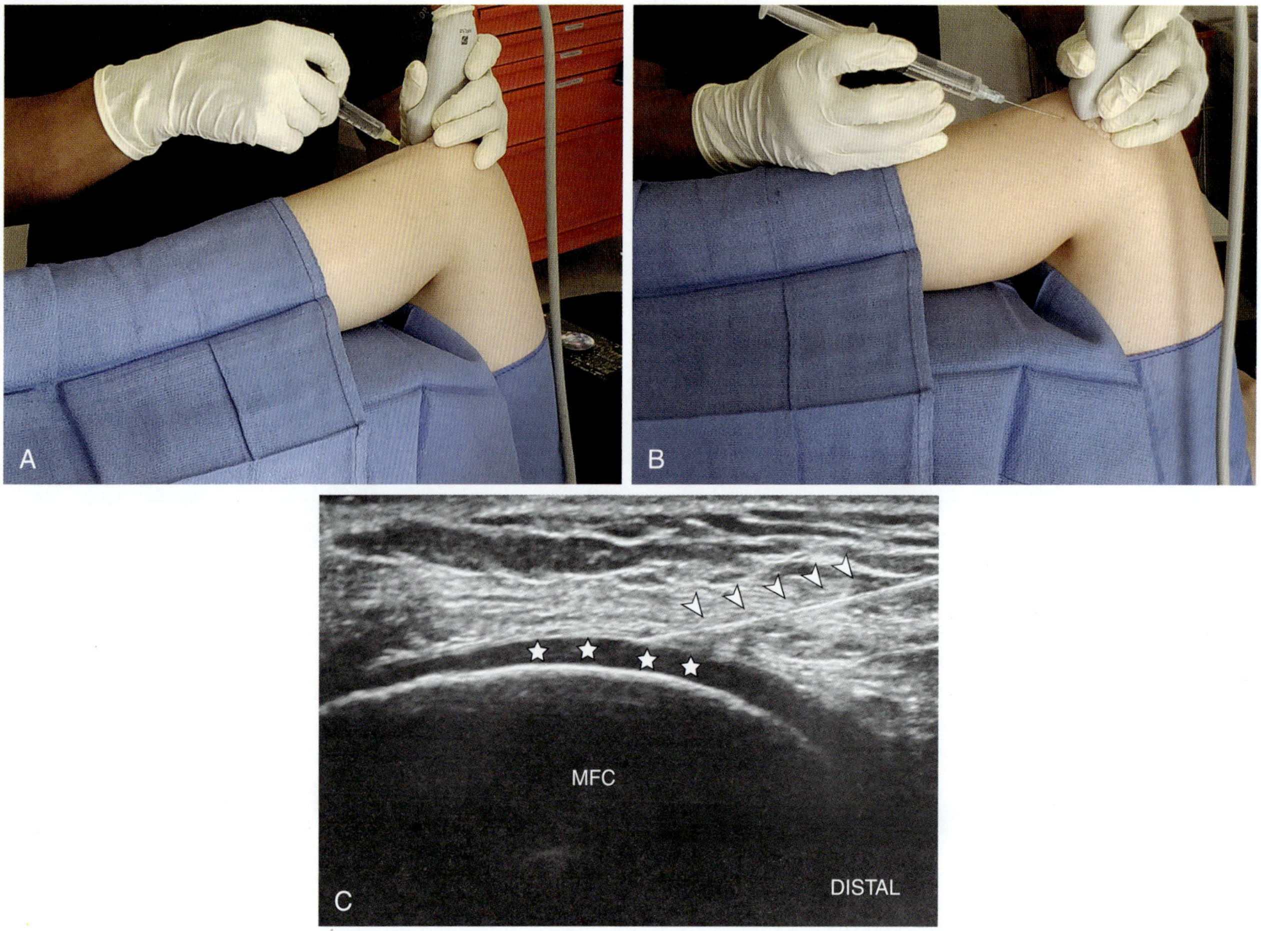

• **Fig. 21.5** (A) Medial femoral condyle intra-articular in-plane setup. (B) Lateral femoral condyle intra-articular in-plane setup. (C) Medial femoral condyle *(MFC)* in-plane injection.

Proximal Tibiofibular Joint Injection

KEY POINTS

- The tibiofibular joint is an often overlooked cause of lateral knee pain.
- The posterolateral corner structures should be evaluated when assessing this region.
- There is significant anatomic variability in the angulation of the proximal tibiofibular joint (PTFJ), which may cause the transducer to be oriented in an anatomic transverse oblique plane for best visualization.
- The PTFJ is a small joint, and injectate volume is typically only 1–2 mL.

Pertinent Anatomy

- The tibiofibular joint is a planar diarthrodial synovial joint consisting of the fibular head facet and the articular facet on the lateral tibial condyle.
  - It is surrounded by a fibrous capsule, which is thicker anteriorly, and stabilized by the tibiofibular ligaments.[9,10]
  - In some patients (10% to 64% of cases)[11] the proximal tibiofibular joint (PTFJ) is contiguous with the femorotibial joint, and can be considered a "4th" compartment of the knee joint.[9,12]
- Vascular supply: circumflex fibular artery wraps laterally the head of the femur and anastomoses with the recurrent branch of the anterior tibial artery (inferomedial to the PTFJ),[10] and the inferior lateral genicular artery (superomedial to the PTFJ).[13]
- Nerves: the common peroneal nerve courses along the lateral aspect of the popliteal fossa and wraps laterally and anterior around the fibular head-neck junction.[14]

Common Pathology

- Degenerative osteoarthritis or direct traumatic injury
- Ganglion cyst, which in some cases can compress the common peroneal nerve
- Posterolateral (PL) corner injury with subsequent instability of the PTFJ (requires co-treatment of surrounding injured/lax structures)

Equipment

- High-frequency linear array transducer
- 25 to 30 gauge 1.5 to 2 inch needle

Common Injectates

- Local anesthetics for diagnostics, corticosteroids
- Prolotherapy
- Orthobiologics (PRP, bone marrow concentrate, etc.).

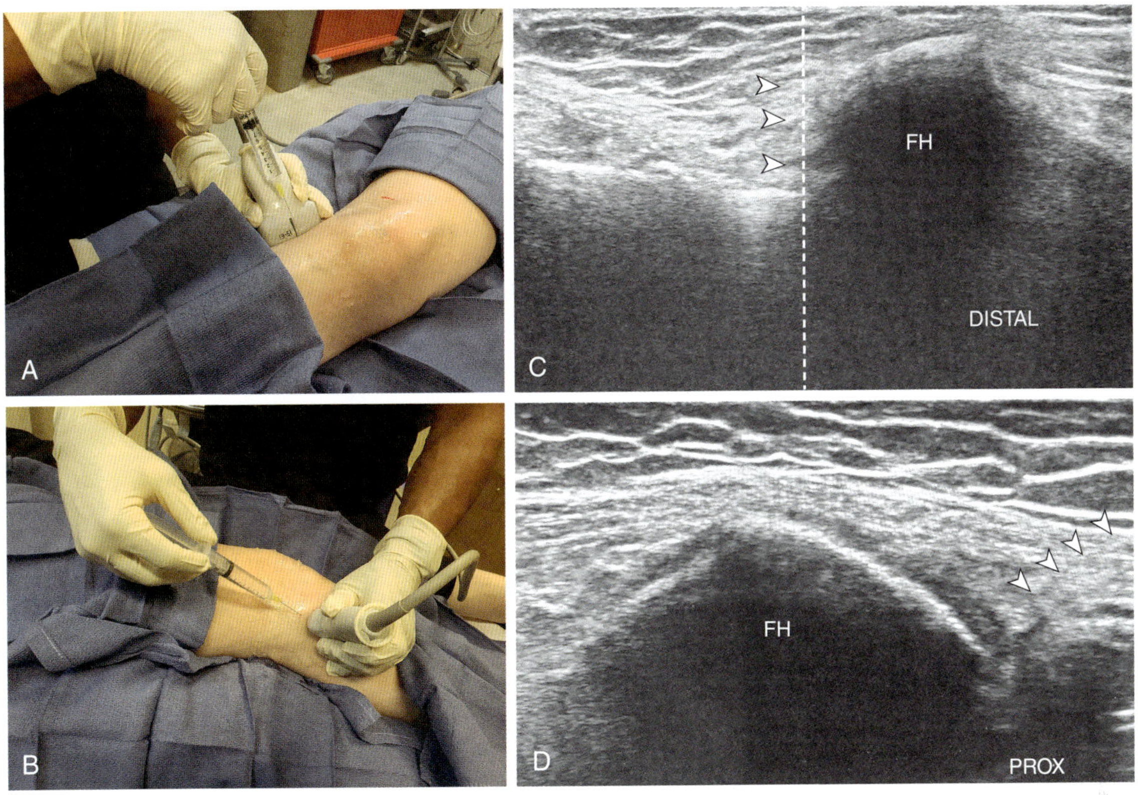

• **Fig. 21.6** (A) Tibiofibular joint out-of-plane setup. (B) Tibiofibular joint in-plane setup. (C) Tibiofibular joint out-of-plane injection. (D) Tibiofibular joint in-plane injection. *FH,* Fibular head.

Injectate Volume

- 1 to 3 mL total

Technique

Patient Position

- Side-lying with affected side facing toward the ceiling
- Knee flexed 20 to 30 degrees with towel roll or bump to place in between legs (Fig. 21.6A and B)

Clinician Position

- Seated facing the anterior PTFJ

Transducer Position

- Transverse oblique plane over the anterior PTFJ

Needle Position

- Out-of-plane anterior to posterior (see Fig. 21.6A)
- Can touch down and the tibia and walk-down posterior
- Alternatively, in-plane proximal to distal approach (see Fig. 21.6B)

Target

- Anterior superior PTFJ (see Fig. 21.6C and D)

PEARLS AND PITFALLS

- Identify the surrounding neurovascular structures such as the common, superficial, and deep peroneal nerves prior to performing injection

Popliteal/Baker's Cyst Injections

KEY POINTS

- Usually result of underlying intra-articular pathology (i.e., osteoarthritis, inflammatory arthritis, meniscus tear, chondral lesions) and increased synovial fluid within the knee joint. Communication between the joint and cyst behaves as a unidirectional or one-way valve, with fluid leaking into and forming the synovial cyst
- Intra-articular pathology should be addressed with the Baker's cyst.

Pertinent Anatomy

- Baker's cyst, also known as popliteal cyst or gastrocnemius-semimembranosus bursa, is located[15] between the medial head of the gastrocnemius and tendon of the semimembranosus
- Typically found posteromedially in the calf at or below the joint line

Common Pathology

- Can occur from blunt/direct trauma, repetitive microtrauma, or inflammation
- Indicative of intra-articular pathology
- Posterior medial meniscus tear can present with similar symptoms as a Baker's cyst without sonographic findings of Baker's cyst

Equipment

- High-frequency linear array transducer
- 30 to 25 gauge 1 to 2 inch needle for local anesthetic
- 18 to 22 gauge 1.5 to 2 inch needle for aspiration
- For aspirations:
  - 10 mL or 20 mL syringe—for small effusions
  - 30 mL or 60 mL syringe—for large effusions

Common Injectates

- Local anesthetic for numbing track with a 25 to 27 gauge 2-inch needle
- Aspiration
- Post-aspiration
- Corticosteroids
- Prolotherapy (typically 25% dextrose solution)
- Sclerosing agents
- Orthobiologics (PRP, bone marrow concentrate, micronized adipose tissue, etc.)

Injectate Volume

- 2 to 3 mL total post-aspiration

Technique

Patient Position

- Prone

Clinician Position

- At foot of patient or along affected side

Transducer Position

- Longitudinal/long axis to the bursa

Needle Position

- In-plane, long axis
- Distal to proximal approach (Fig. 21.7A)

Target

- Middle portion of largest area of the cavity (see Fig. 21.7B)
- Can redirect needle to aspirate into any septations or loculations

PEARLS AND PITFALLS

- Identify all neurovascular structures in the popliteal fossa prior to aspiration/injection.
- If Baker's cyst in an atypical location, must check Doppler to rule out tumor or vascular malformation.

Common mimics:
  - Myxoid liposarcoma
  - Popliteal artery aneurysm
  - Peri-meniscal cysts
- Recurrence is common in adults with underlying intra-articular pathology; consider identifying and addressing primary contributor.
- The semimembranosus tendon may appear hypoechoic from anisotropy; be aware to avoid injecting directly into the tendon.
- Ruptured cysts may mimic symptoms of a deep vein thrombosis.

- After aspiration, can switch out syringe, keeping the needle tip within the collapsed cyst, and inject (see Fig. 21.7C and D)

Medial and Lateral Menisci

KEY POINTS

- Musculoskeletal (MSK) ultrasound by an experienced examiner has similar accuracy identifying medial and lateral meniscus injuries as compared to magnetic resonance imaging (MRI),[16–18] and easy to target and inject peripheral tears of the menisci with ultrasound.

Pertinent Anatomy

- The menisci are crescent-shaped fibrocartilage structures with a peripheral vascular border *(red zone)*, middle inner poorly vascular zone *(red-white zone)*, and avascular zone *(white zone)*.[19,20]
- The thicker convex outer border is attached to the joint capsule, tapering to a thin free-edged innermost border.
- There are a number of meniscal ligaments, which can be variable amongst patients[21]:
  - Coronary ligaments (meniscotibial),[22] which act to anchor the menisci to the tibia both anteriorly and posteriorly.[23,24]
  - Posterior meniscofemoral ligament (ligament of Wrisberg) connects the posterior horn of the lateral meniscus to the medial femoral condyle and the posterior cruciate ligament (PCL).[25]
  - Anterior meniscofemoral ligament (ligament of Humphry) connects posterior horn of lateral meniscus, but lies anterior to the PCL and inserts at the femoral PCL.[25]
  - Anterior intermeniscal ligament, which connects the anterior horns of the medial and lateral menisci (Fig. 21.8).[25]
  - Root attachments:
    - The medial meniscus posterior root attachment is PL to the medial tibial eminence.
    - The lateral meniscus root attachment is posterior and medial to the lateral tibial eminence.
    - The medial meniscus anterior root attachment is anteromedial (AM) to the anterior cruciate ligament (ACL) tibial insertion and inserts into the anterior intercondylar crest of the tibia.
    - The lateral meniscus anterior root is anterolateral to the ACL tibial insertion.[26,27]
  - See Figs. 21.8 and 21.9.

Common Pathology

- Meniscal tears can be traumatic and degenerative, with traumatic injuries usually associated with an injury and sudden onset of pain, and a degenerative lesion without a history of acute injury. Traumatic lesions can occur in isolation but are common in conjunction with ligament injuries.

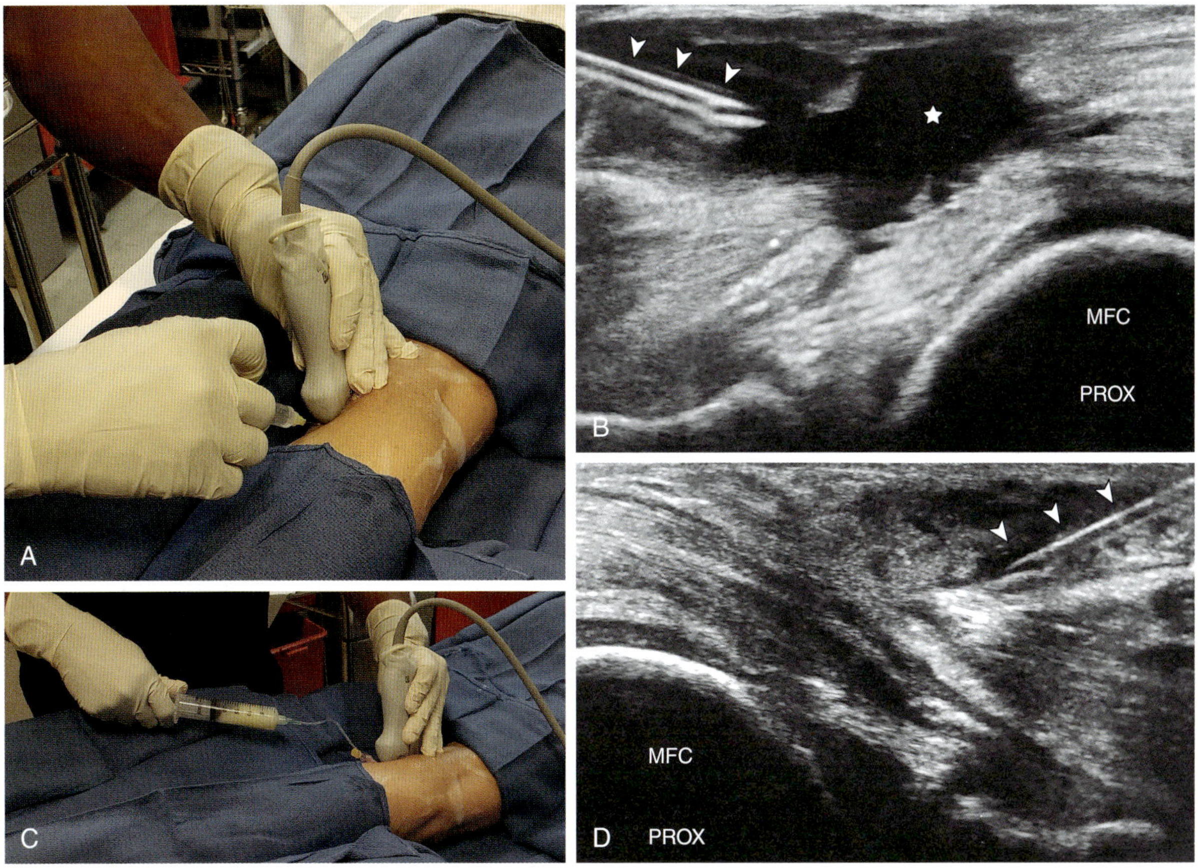

• **Fig. 21.7** (A) Baker's cyst aspiration setup. (B) Bakers cyst in-plane injection. (C) Baker's cyst aspiration. (D) Baker's cyst ultrasound view post-aspiration. *MFC,* Medial femoral condyle.

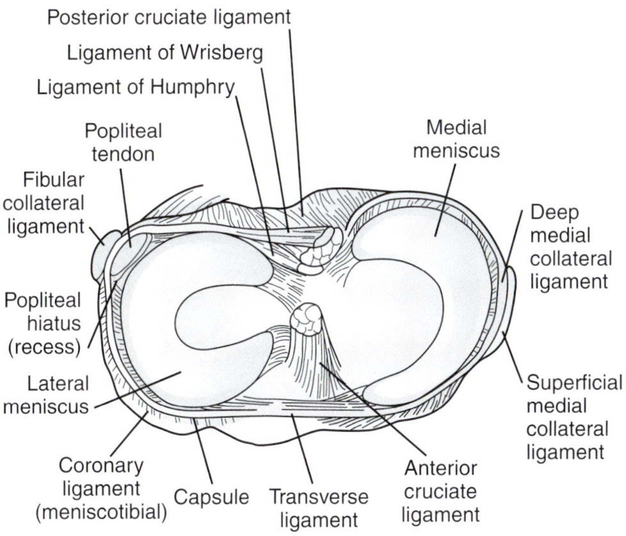

• **Fig 21.8** Meniscal Ligaments. (From Rakel R. *Textbook of Family Medicine*. 7th ed. Philadelphia: Saunders; 2007.)

- Medial meniscus tears should be characterized by the location (e.g., anterior portion, body, posterior portion, or root) and morphologies (e.g. radial, horizontal, vertical, flap, bucket handle, or complex)(Fig. 21.11).[25,28]
- Horizontal and oblique tears are more commonly asymptomatic. Vertical, complex, radial, and displaced tears have a stronger association with pain.[29]
- Medial meniscus posterior horn tears are commonly associated with ACL injury,[23] as are lateral meniscus root tears.[27]

Meniscal ramp tear may not affect the actual meniscus tissue, and generally occur at the ligamentous connection between the posterior horn of the medial meniscus and tibial plateau. Injury to the posterior medial meniscus coronary ligament is associated with increased tibial internal rotation.[23]

Equipment

- High-frequency linear array transducer
- 22 to 27 gauge 1.5 to 2 inch needle

Common Injectates

- Prolotherapy
- Orthobiologics (PRP, bone marrow concentrate, micronized adipose tissue, etc).

Injectate Volume

- 1 to 2 mL total

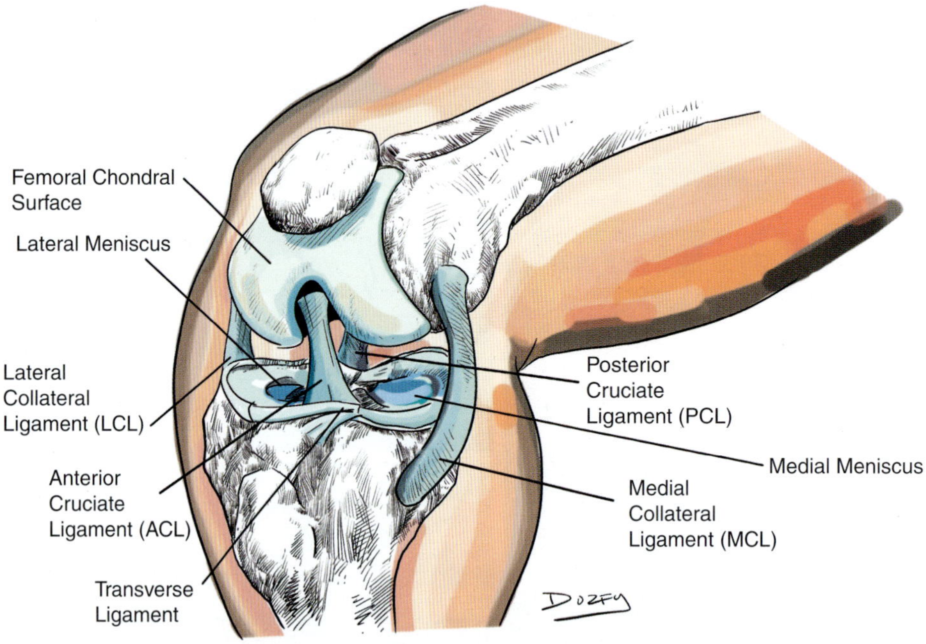

• **Fig. 21.9** Knee Major Ligamentous Anatomy. Note close relation to the menisci.

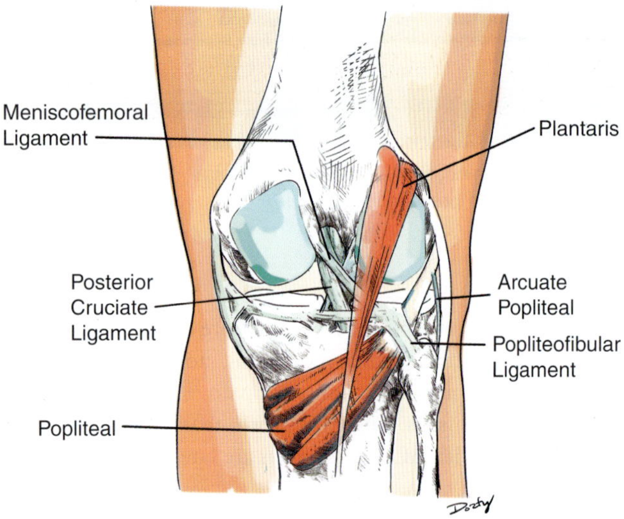

• **Fig. 21.10** Knee Posterior Anatomy: Ligaments and Tendons.

Technique

Patient Position

- Supine with slight knee bend (Fig. 21.12A)

Clinician Position

- Seated or standing on affected side

Transducer Position

- Short axis to the joint line

Needle Position

- In-plane, distal to proximal approach (see Fig. 21.12A)
- Alternatively can inject out of plane with needle centered over the meniscus (see Fig. 21.12B)

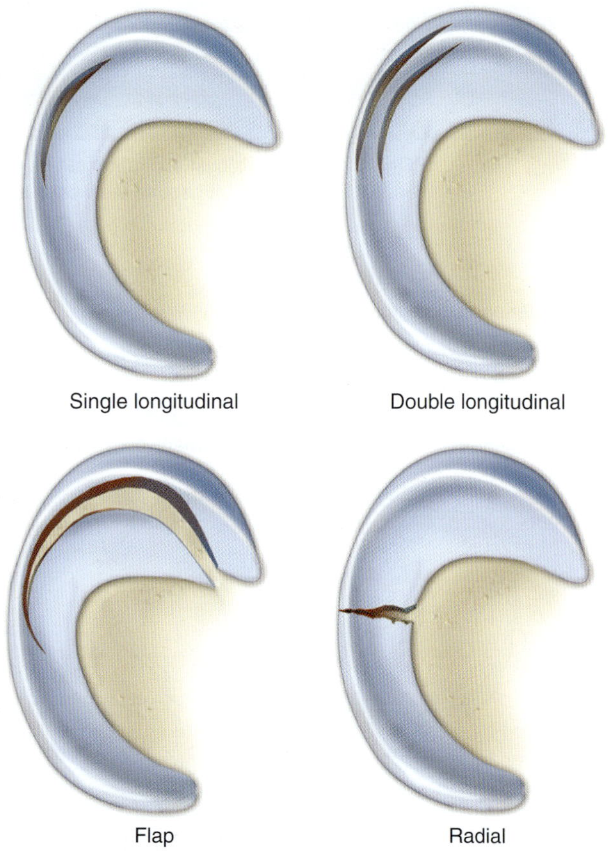

• **Fig. 21.11** Meniscus Tears. (From Detterline A, Babb J, Noyes FR, et al. *Noyes' Knee Disorders*: *Surgery, Rehabilitation, Clinical Outcomes*. 2017:2–22.)

Target

- Areas of hypoechogenicity within the medial or lateral meniscus corresponding to tear of the meniscus (Fig. 21.13C and D; see Fig. 21.12C and D).

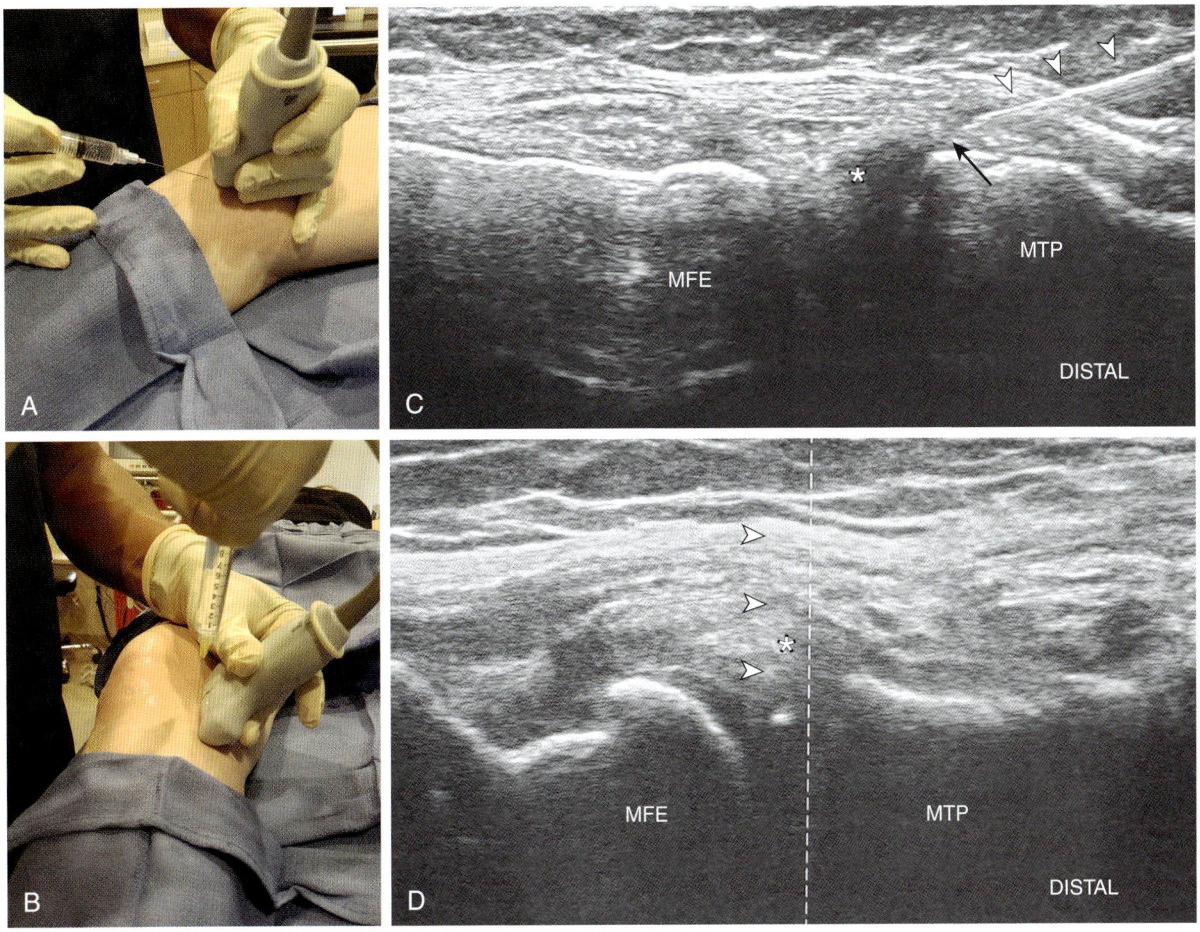

• **Fig. 21.12** (A) Medial meniscus and coronary ligaments in-plane setup. (B) Medial meniscus out-of-plane setup. (C) Medial meniscus coronary ligament in-plane ultrasound injection. (D) Medial meniscus out-of-plane injection.

  - If possible, you can redirect inferior or superior to inject more portions of the capsule.
  - You can adjust to inject along the meniscus to target the length of the tear; this may require coming out, repositioning the probe, and a second injection location.
- Meniscal coronary ligament (see Fig. 21.12C).

PEARLS AND PITFALLS

- Identify the surrounding neurovascular structures prior to injection/aspiration; in particular, the lateral geniculate artery typically runs just superficial to the lateral meniscus.
- The meniscal tissue is dense, and there can be quite a bit of resistance to the injectate. There will be less resistance in areas where the meniscus is. Slightly adjust needle to torn parts if meeting more resistance. A slightly larger-gauge needle can help to inject.
- Perform stress ultrasound of the meniscus to see if the meniscus is extruding with stress. This would suggest possible coronary ligament injury, and the ligament injected as well.
- This approach is best for tears that extend to the periphery where the tear can be visualized with ultrasound guidance.

Technique Alternate for Posterior Horn of the Menisci and Posterior Capsules

Patient Position

- Prone

Clinician Position

- Seated or standing on affected side

Transducer Position

- Short axis to the joint line

Needle Position

- In-plane/long axis, distal to proximal approach (see Fig. 21.13A)
- Can redirect needle to aim for more medial or lateral aspects.
- Alternatively, can inject out of plane, needle centered of the meniscus (see Fig. 21.13B).
- If possible, redirect inferior or superior to inject more portions of the capsule.
- Adjust out-of-plane angle to inject more medial or lateral aspects.

Target

- Areas of hypoechogenicity within the peripheral and central aspects of the posterior horn of the medial or lateral meniscus (see Fig. 21.13C and D).
- Meniscal root.
- Posterior medial or lateral capsules.

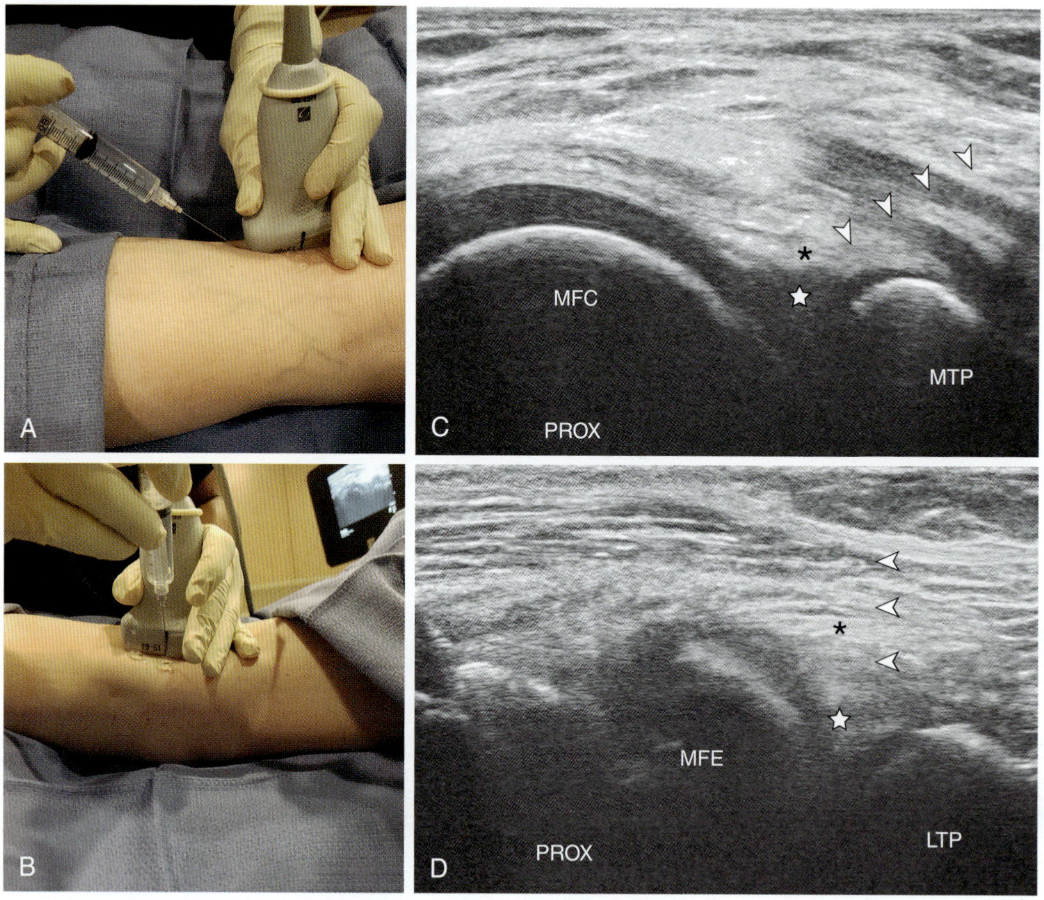

• **Fig. 21.13** (A) Posterior medial meniscus and capsule in-plane setup. (B) Posterior lateral meniscus and capsule out-of-plane setup. (C) Posterior medial capsule injection approaches. (D) Posterior lateral capsule injection approaches. *MFC*, Medial femoral condyle.

PEARLS AND PITFALLS

- Identify the surrounding neurovascular structures prior to injection/aspiration.
- In particular, the lateral geniculate artery typically runs just superficial to the lateral meniscus.
- The meniscus is dense, so there can be quite a bit of resistance. Torn areas may be slightly less dense. Using a slightly large needle gauge can help to inject. Slightly adjust needle to torn parts if meeting more resistance.

Parameniscal Cyst Aspiration/Injection

KEY POINTS

- Parameniscal cysts are typically associated with injuries to the adjacent meniscus.
- Cysts can be multilobulated with viscous, gelatinous material extruded outside the meniscus. (Perimeniscal cysts are due to small lesions and fluid within the cyst.)

Pertinent Anatomy

- Medial and lateral menisci are made of fibrocartilage located along the articular surface between the femoral condyles and tibial plateaus.
- Menisci are typically crescent-shaped structures that are thicker peripherally and thinner centrally.

Common Pathology

- Most commonly, meniscal cysts are associated with horizontal tears of the adjacent meniscus[30] with communication of synovial fluid into the meniscocapsular complex and adjacent soft tissues.
- Three to 10 times [31] more commonly with lateral meniscus tears than medial meniscus tears.

Equipment

- High-frequency linear array transducer
- 30 to 25 gauge 1 to 2 inch needle for local anesthetic
- 18 to 22 gauge 1.5 to 2 inch needle for aspiration
- For aspirations:
  - 10 mL or 20 mL syringe—for small effusions
  - 30 mL or 60 mL syringe—for large effusions

Common Injectates

- Local anesthetic (25 to 27 gauge 1.5 to 2 inch needle) prior to aspiration (18 gauge 1.5 inch needle)
- Post-aspiration
- Corticosteroids
- Prolotherapy, 25% dextrose solution
- Sclerosing agents

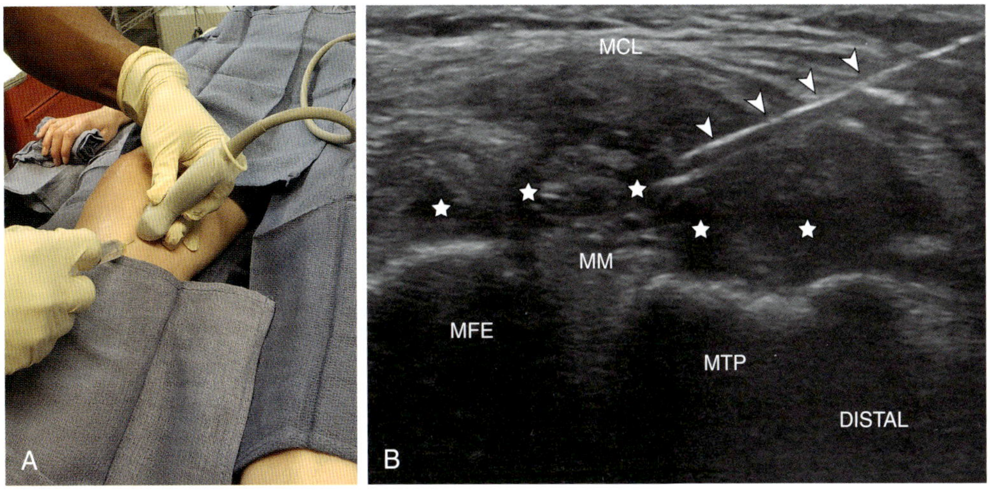

• **Fig. 21.14** (A) Medial meniscal cyst setup. (B) Medial meniscal cyst in-plane injection.

- Orthobiologics (PRP, bone marrow concentrate, micronized adipose tissue, etc.).

Injectate Volume

- 2 to 3 mL total post-aspiration

Technique

Patient Position

- Supine or side-lying

Clinician Position

- Seated or standing on affected side

Transducer Position

- Short axis to the joint line

Needle Position

- In-plane/long axis
- Distal to proximal approach (Fig. 21.14A)

Target

- Middle of largest portion of meniscal cyst (see Fig. 21.14B)

PEARLS AND PITFALLS

- Identify the surrounding neurovascular structures prior to injection/aspiration.
- Take care to avoid compressing the cyst with pressure from the transducer. In some cases compression can decompress the fluid back through the meniscal tear into the joint.[32]
- Cysts may be multilobulated and/or contain thick, viscous, gelatinous material. If material cannot be aspirated, can consider fenestration of cyst.
- Meniscal cysts have been described in the absence of meniscal tears,[33] but in the absence of an associated meniscal tear, alternative diagnoses should be considered, including malignancy.[34]

Tendon Injections

Distal Quadriceps Tendon Injection/ Tenotomy/Barbotage

KEY POINTS

- For percutaneous needle tenotomy, repetitive fenestration should be performed until the needle passes through all of the abnormal tissue with ease.
- We recommend 20- to 22-gauge needles for refractory percutaneous needle tenotomy in quadriceps tendon.
- Since there is no tendon sheath in this area, we would not recommend corticosteroids as they could have harmful effects on the tendon.

Pertinent Anatomy

- The quadriceps tendon (Fig. 21.15) is a conjoined tendon of the rectus femoris, vastus medialis, vastus lateralis, and vastus intermedius muscles, forming a trilaminar tendon that inserts on the superior pole of the proximal of the patella.
- As with most tendons, the quadriceps tendon is typically hypovascularized with a watershed[35] zone just proximal to its insertion.

Common Pathology

- Overuse injuries and the continuum of tendon pathology, include partial tearing
- Calcific tendinopathy of the quadriceps.

Complete tears (direct trauma or hyperflexion of the knee causing rupture of the extensor mechanism). Complete tears require prompt diagnosis and surgical repair.

Equipment

- High-frequency linear array transducer
- 27 to 30 gauge 1.5 to 2 inch needle for anesthesia (stay superficial outside of tendon/lesion)
- 22 to 27 gauge 1.5 to 2 inch needle for injection
- 18 to 22 gauge 1.5 to 2 inch needle and 10 mL syringe flushes for barbotage

Common Injectates

- Local anesthetics for diagnostics
- Prolotherapy
- Orthobiologics (PRP, bone marrow concentrate, etc.) injections
- Saline for barbotage in calcific tendinopathy

Injectate Volume

- 2 to 3 mL of regenerative agent or 10 mL saline (for barbotage)

Technique

Patient Position

- Supine with knee flexed to 30 degrees with towel roll or bump to place under affected knee

Clinician Position

- On side of affected knee

Transducer Position

- Long or short axis to the quadriceps tendon (Fig. 21.16A and B)

Needle Position

- In plane with probe (long axis to tendon), proximal to distal approach (see Fig. 21.16C)
- Alternate position: in plane with probe (short axis to the tendon), lateral to medial approach (see Fig. 21.16D)

Target

- Pathologic tendon (hypoechoic area of tendinopathy or interstitial tear, calcification).
- For percutaneous needle tenotomy, repetitive fenestration should be performed until the needle passes through all of the abnormal tissue with ease and can also target areas of cortical irregularity/enthesophytes at the superior pole of the patella.
- Calcification for barbotage procedure (see Chapter—barbotage Chapter 24)

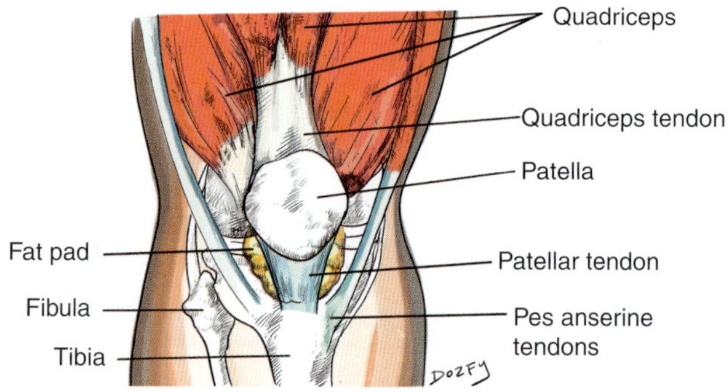

• **Fig. 21.15** Anterior Knee Anatomy. Note knee extensor mechanism

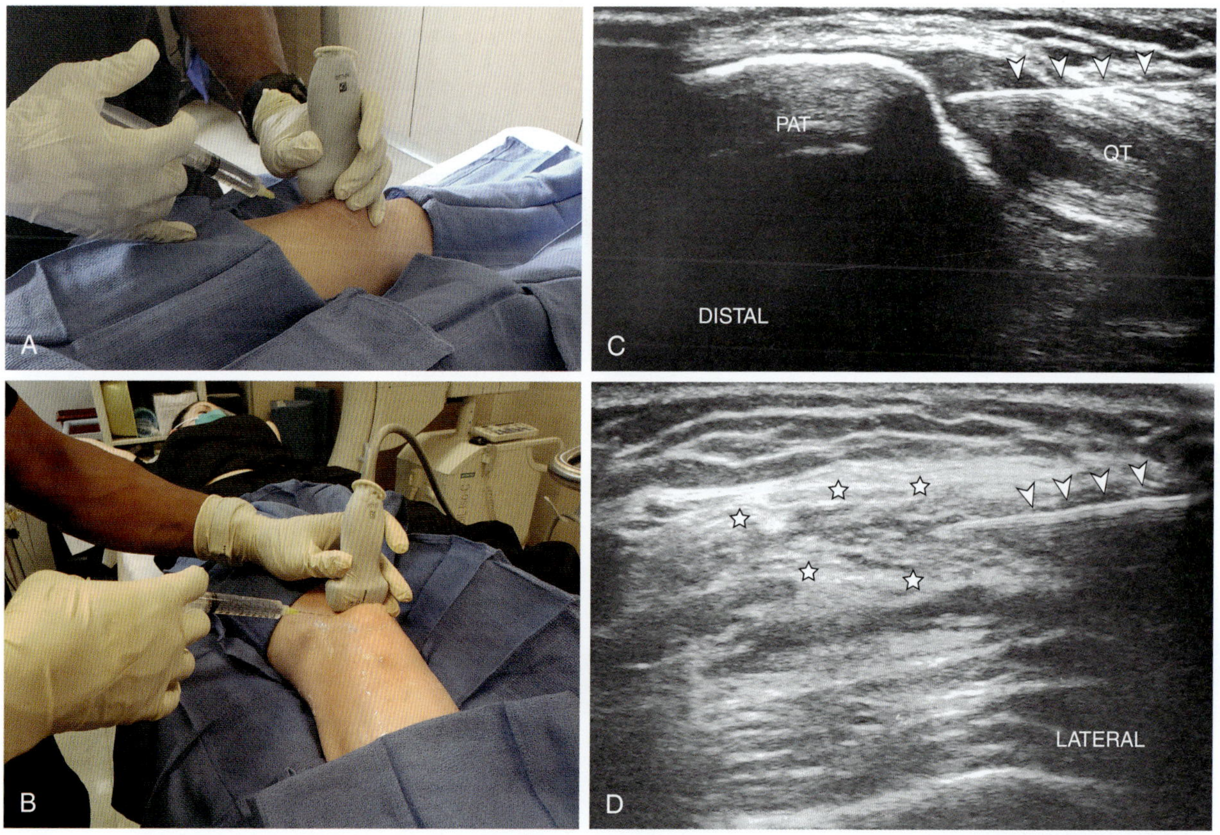

• **Fig. 21.16** (A) Distal quad injection setup. (B) Distal quad long-axis in-plane injection. (C) Distal quad transverse setup. (D) Distal quad transverse in-plan injection.

PEARLS AND PITFALLS

- Proper visualization and planning prior to the procedure will allow for accuracy and efficiency of targeting of the focal lesion and avoid normal tendon.
- Fenestrating or needling the enthesis for insertional tendinosis is recommended to encourage angiogenesis from the periosteum.

Patellar Tendon Injection and Tenotomy/ Barbotage

KEY POINTS

- For percutaneous needle tenotomy, repetitive fenestration should be performed until the needle passes through all of the abnormal tissue with ease.
- We recommend 18–22 gauge needles for percutaneous needle tenotomy in patella tendinosis refractory to conservative treatment options.
- Corticosteroids are not recommended as they could have harmful effects on the tendon.

Pertinent Anatomy

- The patellar tendon is a continuation of the deep fibers of the rectus femoris of the quadriceps tendon, and technically is a ligament attaching the distal pole of the patella to the tibial tuberosity.

Common Pathology

- Overuse injuries and the continuum of tendon pathology include partial tearing. The most common location of pain and pathology is the proximal patellar tendon; however, the distal insertion and mid tendon can also be affected.[36]
- Calcific tendinopathy of the patellar tendon.
- Complete tears (direct trauma or hyperflexion of the knee causing rupture of the extensor mechanism). Complete tears require prompt diagnosis and surgical repair.
- Infrapatellar fat pad impingement can present similar to patellar tendinopathy.

Equipment

- High-frequency linear array transducer
- 27 to 30 gauge 1.5 to 2 inch needle for numbing track (stay superficial outside of tendon/lesion)
- 22 to 27 gauge 1.5 to 2 inch needle for injection
- 18 to 22 gauge 1.5 to 2 inch needle and 10 mL syringes flushes for barbotage

Common Injectates

- Local anesthetics for diagnostics
- Prolotherapy
- Orthobiologics (PRP, bone marrow concentrate, etc.) injections
- Saline for barbotage in calcific tendinopathy

Injectate Volume

- 1 to 3 mL of regenerative agent
- 10 mL saline (for barbotage)

Technique

Patient Position

- Supine
- Knee flexed to 30 degrees with towel roll or bump to place under affected knee

Clinician Position

- On side of affected leg

Transducer Position

- Patellar tendon in long axis (Fig. 21.17A and B)
- Alternative approach with tendon in short axis

Needle Position

- In-plane/long axis
- Proximal to distal for distal lesions and enthesopathy; distal to proximal approach for proximal lesions/myotendinous junction (see Fig. 21.17C and D)
- Alternate approach (probe short axis to the tendon): needle in plane, lateral to medial

Target

- Pathologic tendon (hypoechoic area of tendinopathy or interstitial tear, calcification).
- For percutaneous needle tenotomy, repetitive fenestration should be performed until the needle passes through all of the abnormal tissue with ease and can also target areas of cortical irregularity/enthesophytes at the superior pole of the patella.
- Calcification for barbotage procedure (see Chapter 24)

PEARLS AND PITFALLS

- Proper visualization and planning prior to the procedure will allow for accuracy and efficiency of targeting of the focal lesion and avoid normal tendon.
- Needling the enthesis for insertional tendinosis is recommended to encourage angiogenesis from the periosteum.
- Hoffa's fat pad hydrodissection or high-volume injection between the deep patellar fibers and Hoffa's fat pad may provide some therapeutic benefit. (See chapter 27.)

Prepatellar Bursal Injection

KEY POINTS

- Prepatellar bursitis are common. Up to one-third of cases can be septic and two-thirds non-septic. In cases of suspected septic bursitis, fluid should be sent for analysis.[37]

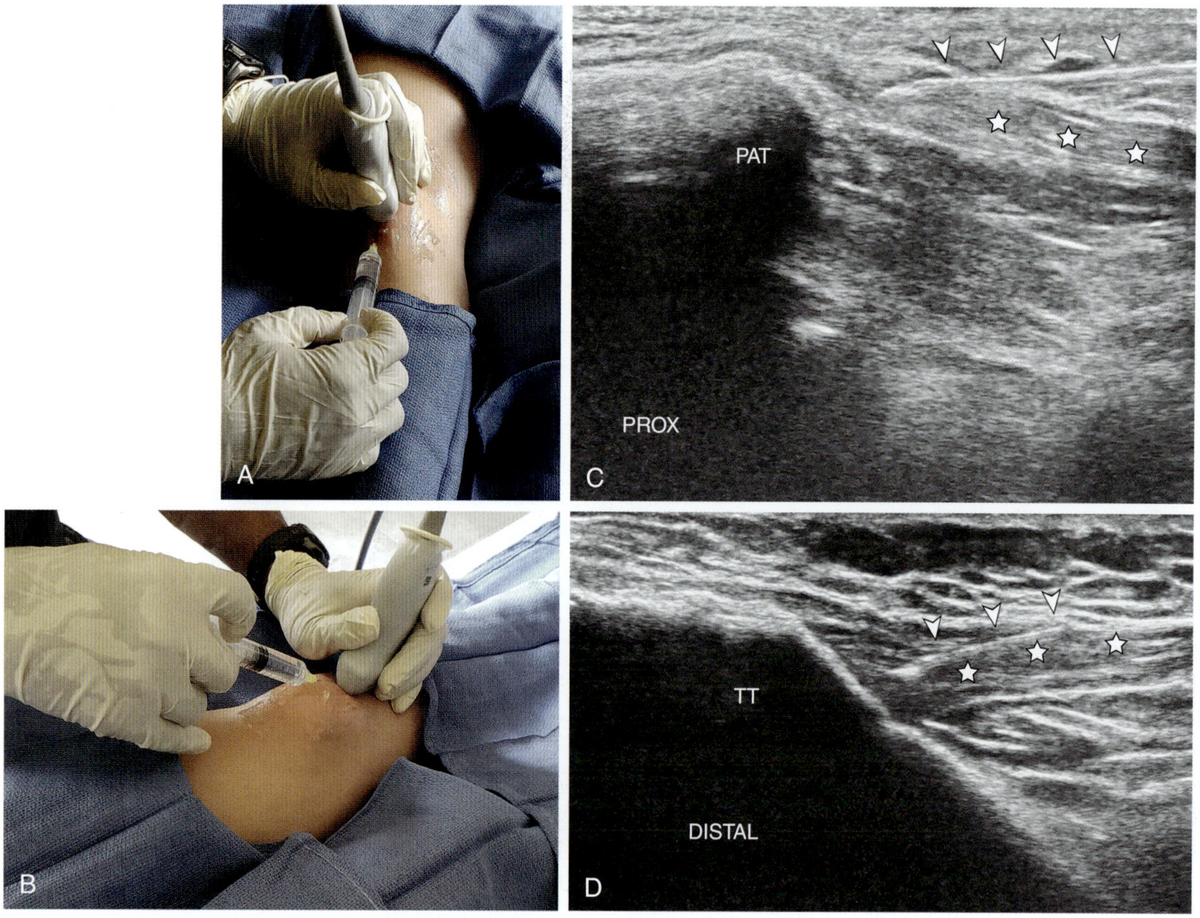

• **Fig. 21.17** (A) Proximal patellar tendon setup. (B) Distal patellar tendon setup. (C) Proximal patellar tendon long-axis in-plane injection. (D) Distal patellar tendon long-axis in-plane injection.

Pertinent Anatomy

The prepatellar bursa is generally superficial and centered over the patella but can have lateral and medial extension.

Common Pathology

- Typically associated with chronic trauma from prolonged or repeated kneeling. Direct trauma or fall on the knee can result in a prepatellar bursa hematoma.
- Septic bursitis.
- Rule out other potential etiologies such as patellar fracture or Morel-Lavallée lesion.

Equipment

- High-frequency linear array transducer
- 22 to 27 gauge 1.5 to 2 inch needle for injection
- 18 to 22 gauge 1.5 to 2 inch needle for aspiration

Common Injectates

- Local anesthetics for diagnostics
- Corticosteroids
- Sclerotherapy or prolotherapy
- Orthobiologics (PRP, bone marrow concentrate, etc.) injections

Injectate Volume

- 1 to 2 mL

Technique

Patient Position

- Supine with knee flexed to 30 degrees with towel roll or bump to place under affected knee

Clinician Position

- On affected side of leg

Transducer Position

- Over the patella bursa and patella in short or long axis (Fig. 21.18A and B)

Needle Position

- In-plane (distal to proximal [Fig. 21.18C]; lateral to medial approach [see Fig. 21.18D])

Target

- Prepatellar bursa

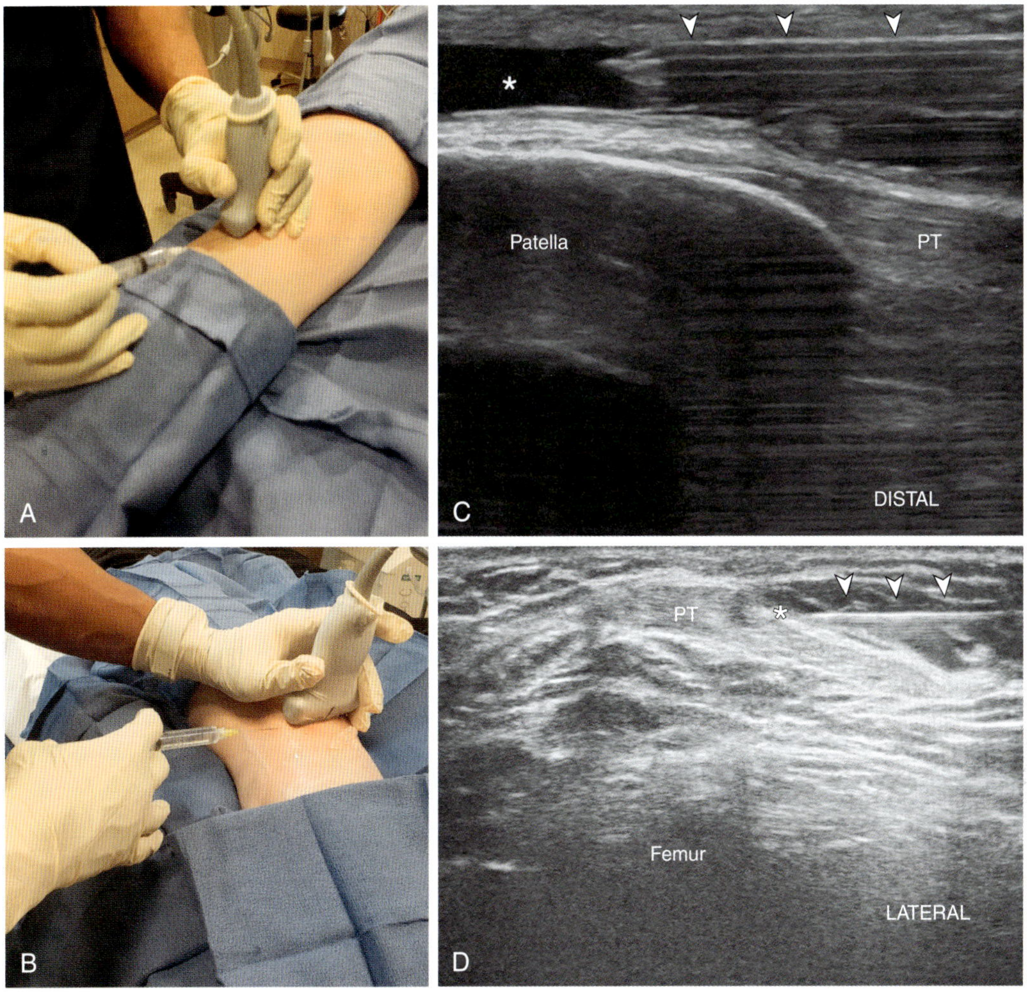

• **Fig. 21.18** (A) Prepatellar bursa long-axis setup. (B and C) Prepatellar bursa in-plane injection distal aspect. (D) Prepatellar bursa in-plane injection proximal aspect.

PEARLS AND PITFALLS

- Septic bursitis is common, and any cases of suspected infectious bursitis should be aspirated and sent for analysis.
- Applying too much pressure with the transducer may decrease bursal fluid and make evaluation and needle placement more difficult.
- Sclerotherapy with polidocanol has been reported, but other sclerosing agents can be considered.[38]

Infrapatellar Superficial/Deep Bursal Injection

KEY POINTS

- Infrapatellar bursa can be superficial or deep.
- Some fluid in the deep infrapatellar bursa is considered physiologic.

Pertinent Anatomy

- The superficial infrapatellar bursa is located between the tibial tubercle and the overlying skin. The deep infrapatellar bursa is located between the posterior aspect of the patellar tendon and the tibia.
- Fluid within the deep infrapatellar bursa can be physiologic (present in up to 68% of knees), and should be distinguished from bursitis.[39]
- No communication exists between the deep infrapatellar bursa and the knee joint.

Common Pathology

- Typically associated with chronic trauma from prolonged or repeated kneeling.
- May also be seen in gout, syphilis or association with rheumatologic conditions.
- Superficial infrapatellar bursitis should be differentiated from subcutaneous edema.

Equipment

- High-frequency linear array transducer
- 27 to 22 gauge 1.5 to 2 inch needle for injection
- 22 to 18 gauge 1.5 to 2 inch needle for aspiration

Common Injectates

- Local anesthetics for diagnostics

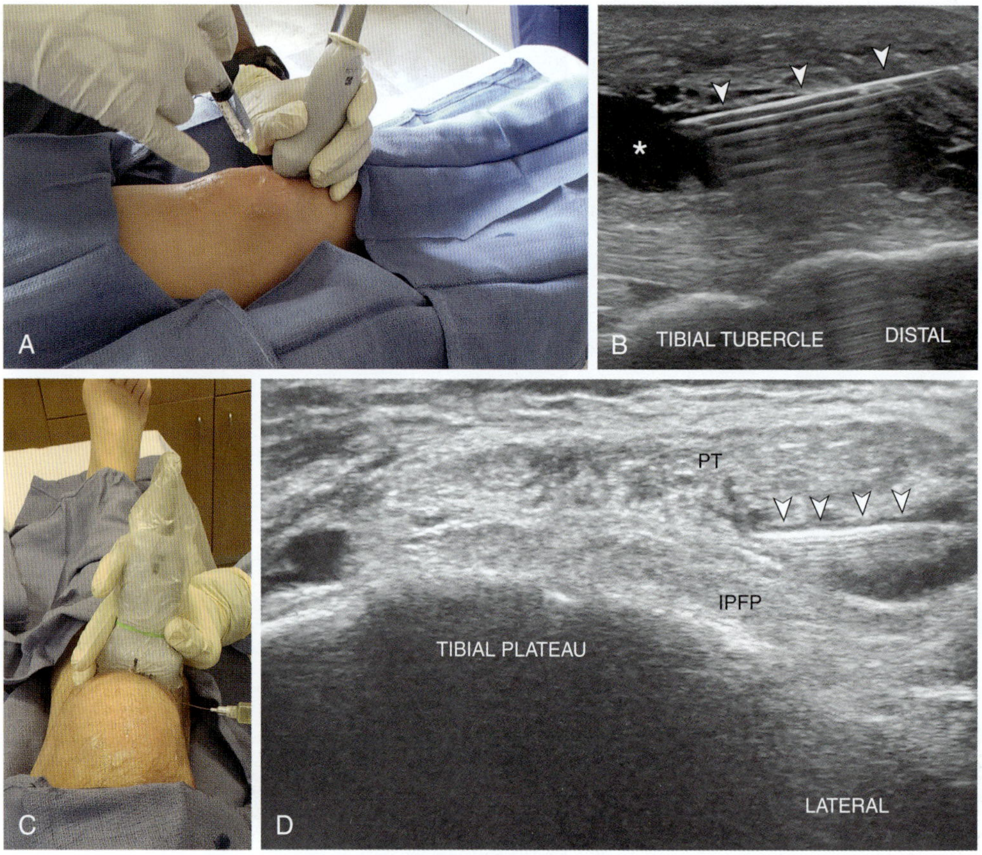

• **Fig. 21.19** (A) Infrapatellar bursa long-axis setup proximal to distal. (B) Prepatellar bursa long-axis distal to proximal approach in-plane injection. (C) Deep Infrapatellar bursa transverse view in-plane injection setup. (D) Deep infrapatellar bursa transverse view in-plane ultrasound injection.

- Corticosteroids
- Sclerotherapy or prolotherapy
- Orthobiologics (PRP, bone marrow concentrate, etc.) injections

Injectate Volume

- 1 to 2 mL

Technique

Patient Position

- Supine with knee flexed to 30 degrees with towel roll or bump to place under affected knee

Clinician Position

- On affected side of leg with a lateral to medial approach

Transducer Position

- Infrapatellar region with the patellar tendon in short or long axis to the bursa

Needle Position

- Superficial infrapatellar: in plane, proximal to distal or distal to proximal approach (Fig. 21.19A)
- Deep infrapatellar bursa: in plane, lateral to medial approach (see Fig. 21.19C)

Target

- Superficial infrapatellar bursa (see Fig. 21.19B)
- Deep infrapatellar bursa (see Fig. 21.19D)

PEARLS AND PITFALLS

- Applying too much pressure on the transducer may disperse bursal fluid and make evaluation and needle placement more difficult.
- If infection is clinically suspected, the fluid should be aspirated and sent for analysis.

Distal Iliotibial Band Bursa and Peritendinous Injection

KEY POINTS

- Use of corticosteroid injectate is only indicated for bursal procedures.
- The iliotibial band comes in closest proximity to the lateral femoral condyle at ≈30 degrees flexion of the knee, which causes friction/impingement.
- Be sure to identify and avoid the common peroneal nerve prior to any procedure due to its proximity to these structures.

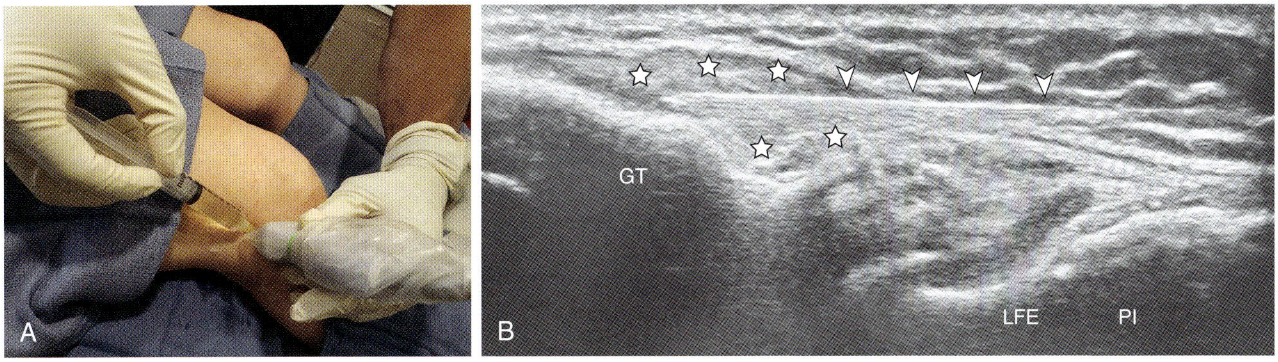

• **Fig. 21.20** (A) Distal iliotibial band (ITB) injection setup. (B) Distal ITB injection.

Pertinent Anatomy

- The iliotibial band (ITB) is a dense, thick band of connective tissue formed by the tensor fascia lata and gluteus maximus proximally and runs distally over the vastus lateralis and lateral femoral condyle to attach to Gerdy's tubercle on the lateral proximal tibia.
- At 30 degrees of knee flexion, the ITB is taut and moves over the lateral femoral condyle, which can often be the cause of friction and symptoms of bursitis/impingement syndrome.

Common Pathology

- Often susceptible to overuse/repetitive-type injuries, which may include partial- or full-thickness tearing, inflammation to the surrounding bursa or irritation to the adipose tissue.

Equipment

- High-frequency linear array transducer
- 27 to 30 gauge 1.5 to 2 inch needle for numbing track
- 22 to 27 gauge 1.5 to 2 inch needle for injection

Common Injectates

- Local anesthetics for diagnostics
- Prolotherapy
- Orthobiologics (PRP, bone marrow concentrate, etc.) injections

Injectate Volume

- 1 to 3 mL of corticosteroid or regenerative agent

Technique

Patient Position

- Side-lying with knee flexed to 20 to 30 degrees with towel roll or bump in between the knees

Clinician Position

- Behind the patient

Transducer Position

- Long axis to the ITB (authors' preferred approach for percutaneous tenotomy [Fig. 21.20A])
- Alternative approach: transverse to the ITB

Needle Position

- Long axis to the ITB: in plane to probe, proximal to the distal (see Fig. 21.20B)
- Alternative approach (probe transverse to the ITB): in-line, posterior to anterior approach

Target

- Thickened fascia at the level of the lateral femoral condyle
- Enthesopathy of the tendon at Gerdy's tubercle
- Inflamed bursa adjacent to the ITB

PEARLS AND PITFALLS

- Identify and avoid the common peroneal nerve and lateral collateral ligament.

Popliteus Tendon/Tendon Sheath Injection/ Tenotomy

KEY POINTS

- Recommend 18–22 gauge needles for percutaneous needle tenotomy in popliteus tendinosis refractory to conservative treatment options.
- Be sure to identify and avoid the common peroneal nerve prior to any procedure due to its proximity to these structures.

Pertinent Anatomy

- The popliteus muscle originates from the posteromedial tibia and courses obliquely and inserts proximally along the PL femoral condyle.
- The action of the popliteus is to "unlock" the knee as it goes from extension into flexion

Common Pathology

- Isolated injuries to the popliteus muscle are rare but can occur with hyperextension or twisting injuries.
- Susceptible to overuse/repetitive-type injuries which may include partial- or full-thickness tearing or calcinosis of the tendon.
- Pathology of the popliteus tendon is often associated with other PL corner injuries.

Equipment

- High-frequency linear array transducer
- 27 to 30 gauge 1.5 to 2 inch needle for numbing track (stay superficial outside of tendon/lesion)
- 22 to 27 gauge 1.5 to 2 inch needle for injection

Common Injectates

- Local anesthetics for diagnostics, corticosteorids for the sheath only
- Prolotherapy
- Orthobiologics (PRP, bone marrow concentrate, etc.) injections

Injectate Volume

- 1 to 3 mL

Technique

Patient Position

- Side-lying with the knee flexed to 20 to 30 degrees with towel roll or bump in between the knees
- Add slight internal rotation

Clinician Position

- Behind or in front of the patient, depending on the approach

Transducer Position

- Oblique to the popliteus tendon
- Alternative position: long axis to the popliteus tendon, visualizing the tendon at the insertion at the popliteus sulcus on the lateral femoral condyle

Needle Position

- In plane (probe in oblique axis to the tendon) distal to proximal (Fig. 21.21A and B)
- Out of plane (probe in oblique axis to the tendon) (see Fig. 21.21C and D)
- In plane (probe in long axis to the tendon) posterior to anterior approach (see Fig. 21.21E and F) (preferred for needle tenotomy or if calcifications).
- Alternatively, can inject anterior to posterior for musculotendinous junction pathology.

Target

- Within the tendon sheath along the popliteal fossa overlying the lateral femoral condyle.
    - Can trace posteriorly and distally in an oblique angle to follow the course of the popliteal tendon to assess defective areas.
- For percutaneous needle tenotomy, can also target calcific or tendinopathic lesions.

PEARLS AND PITFALLS

- Avoid normal tissue if possible.
- Identify and avoid the common peroneal nerve and lateral collateral ligament.
- For tenotomy, repetitive fenestration should be performed until the needle passes through all of the abnormal tissue with ease.

Pes Tendon and Bursa Injection

KEY POINTS

- Avoid the inferior geniculate artery and nerve, which are located in close proximity.

Pertinent Anatomy

- The pes anserine is a confluence of tendons which insert along the proximal AM tibia approximately 4 cm below the tibial plateau.
- The pes anserine consists of the sartorius, gracilis, and semitendinosus tendons, and they run proximal to distal in a linear fashion.[40]
- The tendons form the anserinus plate as the tendons fuse with the fascia of the leg, with the superficial layer formed by the sartorius and the deep layer formed by the gracilis and semitendinosus.[41]
- These tendons can have individual insertion, but there can be significant variations of the tendons, with accessory tendons and fascial bands arising from any of the tendons with separate insertions.
- The pes anserinus bursa is situated between the pes anserinus and the medial collateral ligament (MCL) and does not communicate with the knee joint.[40]

Common Pathology

- Often associated with pain related to knee osteoarthritis, the mean thickness of pes anserine tendons in knees with osteoarthritis have been shown to be significantly greater than controls.[42] This may be due to valgus knee deformity often associated with knee osteoarthritis.[43]
- Medial meniscus protrusion and displacement of the MCL can result in localized inflammation.
- Overuse injuries can result in tendinopathy or pes anserinus bursitis.
- Injury from acute trauma and iatrogenic injury have been reported. Pes anserinus snapping syndrome can occur when the semitendinosus or gracilis tendon snaps over the posteromedial knee during knee flexion/extension.

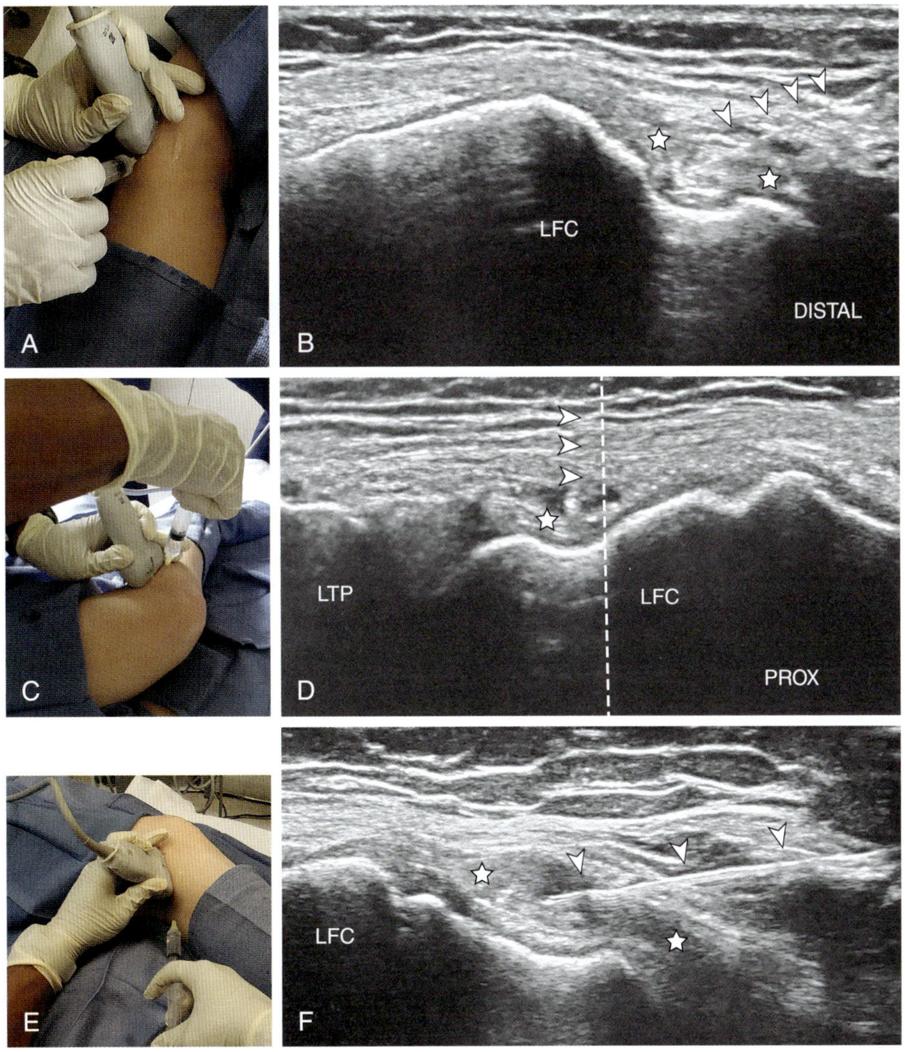

• **Fig. 21.21** (A) Popliteus in-plane setup lateral decubitus. (B) Popliteus out-of-plane setup. (C) Popliteus short-axis in-plane ultrasound (US) injection. (D) Popliteus short-axis in-plane US injection. (E) Popliteus long-axis in-plane injection. (F) Popliteus long-axis in-plane injection.

Equipment

- High-frequency linear array transducer
- 22 to 27 gauge 1.5 to 2 inch needle for injection

Common Injectates

- Local anesthetics for diagnostics
- Prolotherapy
- Orthobiologics (PRP, bone marrow concentrate, etc.) injections

Injectate Volume

- 1 to 2 mL

Technique

Patient Position

- Supine
- Knee flexed to 30 degrees with towel roll or bump to place under affected knee
  - Can obtain better exposure with slight external rotation of the hip

Clinician Position

- At the foot of the patient

Transducer Position

- Short axis to the pes anserine tendons
- Alternative approach: rotate probe to position-affected tendon in long axis to tendon (preferred approach for intratendinous orthobiologic injection).

Needle Position

- In-plane (oblique to pes anserine tendon/bursa), distal to proximal or proximal to distal approaches (Fig. 21.22A and C)
- Alternative approach: in plane (long-axis to tendon)

Target

- Pes anserine tendon sheath or bursa (between pes anserine tendons and MCL) (Fig. 21.23).
- For orthobiologics, target the thickened pes anserine tendon. Interstitial tears will often be occult and open up with the intratendinous injection (see Fig. 21.22B and D).

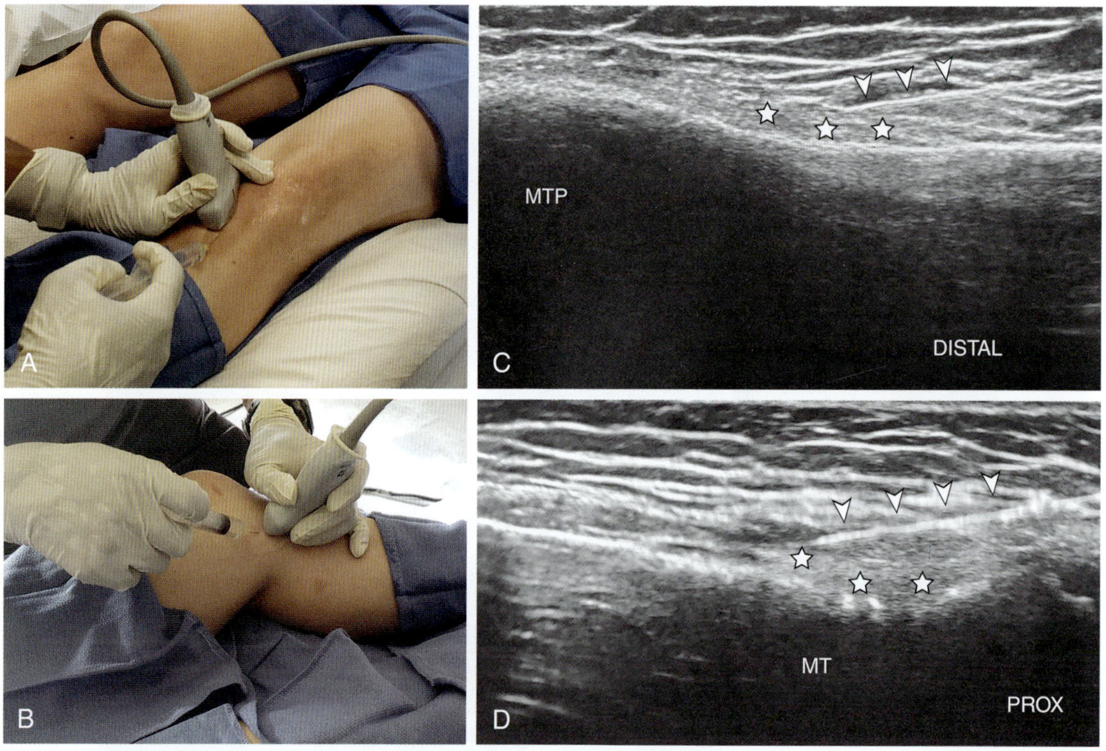

• **Fig. 21.22** (A) Pes tendon/bursa distal to proximal setup. (B) Pes tendon/bursa proximal to distal setup. (C) Pes tendon distal to proximal in-plane injection (D) Pes tendon in plane proximal to distal injection.

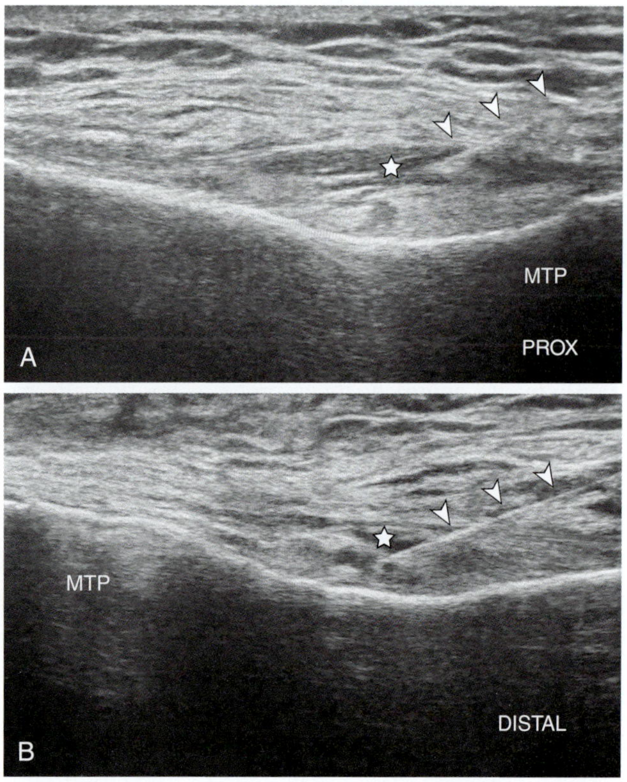

• **Fig. 21.23** (A) Pes anserine bursa in-plane proximal to distal ultrasound injection. (B) Pes anserine bursa in-plane distal to proximal ultrasound injection.

PEARLS AND PITFALLS

- Color flow Doppler should be used to identify and avoid injecting the inferior geniculate artery and nerve.
- Avoid injecting corticosteroids into the pes anserine tendons or medial collateral ligament (MCL).
- Distinguish between the pes anserine tendons and the semimembranosus tendon or MCL to ensure the correct target site. Sonopalpation and differential lidocaine injections can help localize the source of pain.

Distal Biceps Femoris Injection/Tenotomy

KEY POINTS

- We recommend 18–22 gauge needles for percutaneous needle tenotomy in distal biceps femoris tendinosis refractory to conservative treatment options.
- Use of corticosteroid injectate is not indicated for intratendinous procedures.
- Be sure to identify and avoid the common peroneal nerve prior to any procedure due to its proximity to these structures.

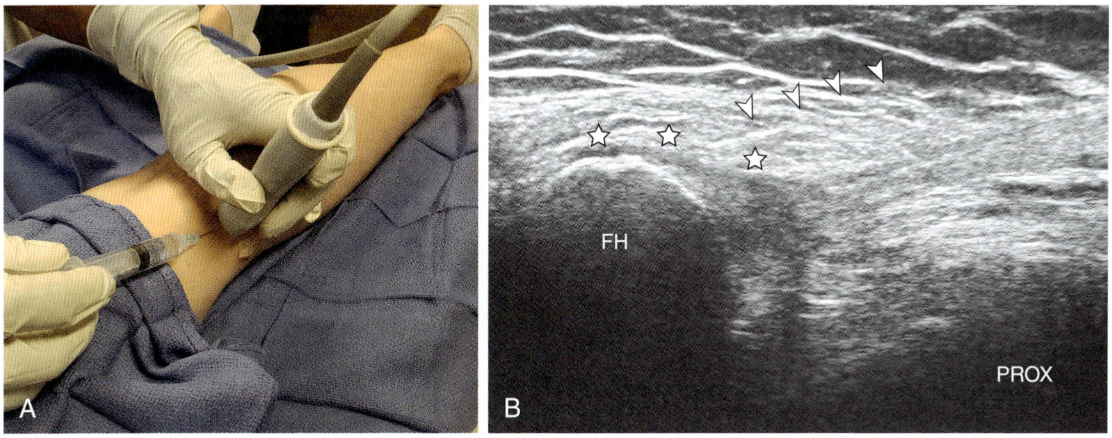

• **Fig. 21.24** (A) Distal biceps in-plane setup. (B) Distal biceps long-axis in-plane injection.

Pertinent Anatomy

- The distal biceps femoris tendon complex is composed of the lateral hamstring muscle (the long and short head of the biceps femoris).
- The tendon inserts in a fan-like fashion with multiple attachments, including attachments on the fibula and tibia.
- The tendon bifurcates into superficial and deep portions that encompass the lateral collateral ligament (LCL), otherwise known as the distal fibular collateral ligament.
- The fibular collateral ligament-biceps femoris bursa is a small bursa that exists between the superficial fibers and the LCL.
- The common peroneal nerve and posterior lateral geniculate artery run along the distal biceps femoris tendon complex.

Common Pathology

- Susceptible to overuse/repetitive-type injuries; pathology includes partial- or full-thickness tearing or calcinosis of the tendon.
- Fibular collateral ligament-biceps femoris bursitis.

Equipment

- High-frequency linear array transducer
- 27 to 30 gauge 1.5 to 2 inch needle for numbing track (stay superficial outside of tendon/lesion)
- 22 to 27 gauge 1.5 to 2 inch needle for injection

Common Injectates

- Local anesthetics for diagnostics
- Prolotherapy
- Orthobiologics (PRP, bone marrow concentrate, etc.) injections

Injectate Volume

- 1 to 3 mL

Technique

Patient Position

- Prone or side-lying
- Knee slightly flexed to 10 degrees with towel roll or bump under the ankle or shins

Clinician Position

- Along the affected side of the patient

Transducer Position

- Long axis to the biceps femoris tendon.
  - Be sure to visualize its insertion onto the proximal fibula to ensure correct structure, and clearly identify the fibular collateral ligament between the superficial and deep fibers of the distal biceps tendon.

Needle Position

- In-plane (long axis to biceps femoris tendon complex), proximal to distal (Fig. 21.24A) or distal to proximal approach

Target

- Distal insertion of the biceps femoris at the proximal fibular head (see Fig. 21.24B)
- For percutaneous needle tenotomy, you can also target calcific or tendinopathic lesions.

PEARLS AND PITFALLS

- Avoid normal tissue if possible. Caution should be used when interpreting the anatomy in long-axis imaging as the divergent superficial and deep heads of the biceps femoris can simulate the appearance of tendinopathy due to thickening and anisotropy. The biceps femoris and fibular collateral ligament should be examined in multiple acoustic windows to help control for anisotrophy.[44]
- Sonopalpation can be useful to help correlate potential pathologic findings with sonographic findings.
- Identify and avoid the common peroneal nerve and fibular collateral ligament.
- For tenotomy, repetitive fenestration should be performed until the needle passes through all of the abnormal tissue with ease.

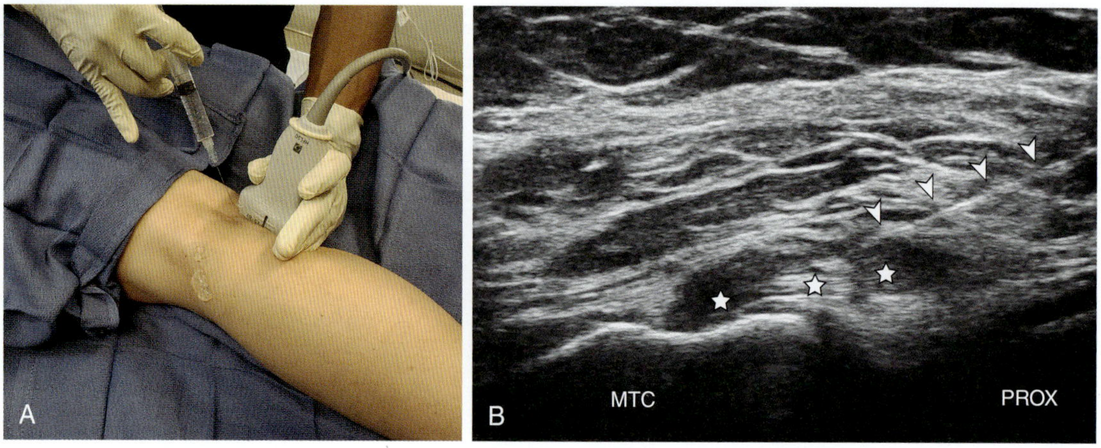

• **Fig. 21.25** (A) Distal semimembranosus in-plane injection setup. (B) Distal semimembranosus long-axis in-plane ultrasound injection.

Distal Semimembranosus Tendon Injection/ Tenotomy

KEY POINTS

- We recommend 18–22 gauge needles for percutaneous needle tenotomy in distal semimembranosus tendinosis refractory to conservative treatment options.
- Use of corticosteroid injectate is not indicated for intra-tendinous procedures.
- Identify the pes anserine tendons, which are located anterior and distal to the semimembranosus tendon insertion.

Pertinent Anatomy

- The distal semimembranosus tendon has five different insertions along the medial knee.[45,46]
- The main tendon inserts into the posterior medial tibial condyle
- The anterior arm (pars reflexa) inserts onto the tibia, runs deep to the MCL inserting distal to the medial joint line.
- There is some evidence of insertion onto the medial meniscus in some patients, which likely functions to pull the meniscus posteriorly with deep knee flexion.[47]

Common Pathology

- Overuse/repetitive-type injuries, which may include partial- or full-thickness tearing or calcinosis of the tendon.
- Association between MCL pathology, knee osteoarthritis, and semimembranosus tendon pathology[46]
- Often injured from valgus stress to the knee causing strains, tears, avulsions, and contusions.

Equipment

- High-frequency linear array transducer
- 27 to 30 gauge 1.5 to 2 inch needle for numbing track (stay superficial outside of tendon/lesion)
- 22 to 27 gauge 1.5 to 2 inch needle for injection

Common Injectates

- Local anesthetics for diagnostics
- Prolotherapy
- Orthobiologics (PRP, bone marrow concentrate, etc.) injections

Injectate Volume

- 1 to 3 mL

Technique

Patient Position

- Prone or side-lying
- Knee fully extended

Clinician Position

- Along the affected side of the patient

Transducer Position

- Long axis to the semimembranosus tendon.
    - Be sure to visualize its insertion onto the posterior medial tibial condyle to ensure correct structure.

Alternate position

- Short axis to the semimembranosus tendon

Needle Position

- In-plane (long axis to semimembranosus tendon), proximal to distal approach (Fig. 21.25A)
- Alternate approach: short-axis approach

Target

- Distal insertion of the semimembranosus tendon at the posterior medial tibial condyle (see Fig. 21.25B)

PEARLS AND PITFALLS

- Avoid normal tissue if possible.
- Distinguish between the semimembranosus tendon and the medial collateral ligament or pes anserine tendons to ensure the correct target.

- For percutaneous needle tenotomy, you can also target calcific or tendinopathic lesions.

Ligaments

Anterior Cruciate Ligament Injection

KEY POINTS

- Can be difficult to visualize. Hyperflexion of the knee can help, but may be limited due to ROM.
- Often used in treatment of distal partial ACL injuries, mostly for orthobiologic use.
- For more severe partial injuries or proximal injuries, fluoroscopy technique is required.

Pertinent Anatomy

- The two bundles (AM and PL) of the ACL course from lateral to medial, attaching the femur to the tibia to prevent excessive anterior translation of the tibia.
- Main stabilizer of anterior tibial translation.
- Main arterial supply is the middle geniculate artery.

Common Pathology

- Susceptible to acute tear/rupture from a non-contact injury or indirect contact resulting in valgus loading of the knee. A direct contact blow to the lateral aspect of the knee can also injure the ACL.
- May be associated with other injuries such as medial or lateral meniscus, PCL, LCL, or posterolateral corner (PLC) injuries.

Equipment

- High-frequency linear array transducer
- 22 to 25 gauge 2 to 3 inch needle for injection

Common Injectates

- Prolotherapy
- Orthobiologics (PRP, bone marrow concentrate)

Injectate Volume

- 1 to 3 mL

Technique

Patient Position

- Supine
- Knee flexed to at least 90 degrees with tibia in slight internal rotation to further increase tension on ACL
  - Can obtain better exposure with more hyperflexion of the knee

Clinician Position

- On affected side of patient knee

Transducer Position

- Long axis to the ACL
  - Start transducer in the sagittal plane over the patella in long axis. Slide the transducer just medial to the patella and orient oblique along the axis of the ACL. This may be about 30 degrees but can vary.
  - The distal ACL seen in long axis ≈1 to 1.5 cm deep to the anterior tibial cortex.
- ACL will often appear hypoechoic due to anisotropy.

Needle Position

- In-plane (long or oblique axis to ACL), distal/anterior to proximal/posterior approach (Fig. 21.26A)
- Alternative position: can inject out of plane from medial to lateral (see Fig. 21.26B)

Target

- The ACL distal and mid substance (see Fig. 21.26C and D)

PEARLS AND PITFALLS

- For in-plane injection, doing a gel stand-off can help clear the needle between the tibia and the transducer.

Posterior Cruciate Ligament Injection

KEY POINTS

- Be aware of proximity to the popliteal artery and tibial nerve, which lie superficial to approach.
- Often used in treatment of partial posterior cruciate ligament (PCL) injuries, mostly for orthobiologic use, or aspiration of PCL cysts.

Pertinent Anatomy

- The two bundles (anterolateral and posteromedial) PCL course from medial to lateral, attaching the femur to the tibia to prevent excessive posterior translation of the tibia.
- Main stabilizer in posterior tibial translation (primarily anterolateral bundle).
- Main arterial supply is the middle geniculate artery.

Common Pathology

- Susceptible to acute tear/rupture from a direct blow to a flexed knee (dashboard injury) or hyperextension injury.
- May be associated with other injuries such as PLC, multiligamentous, or knee dislocation injuries.
- PCL ganglion cysts are uncommon, and often incidental, but can mimic meniscal or chondral lesions.

Equipment

- Curvilinear or high-frequency linear array transducer
- 22 to 25 gauge 2 to 3.5 inch needle for injection

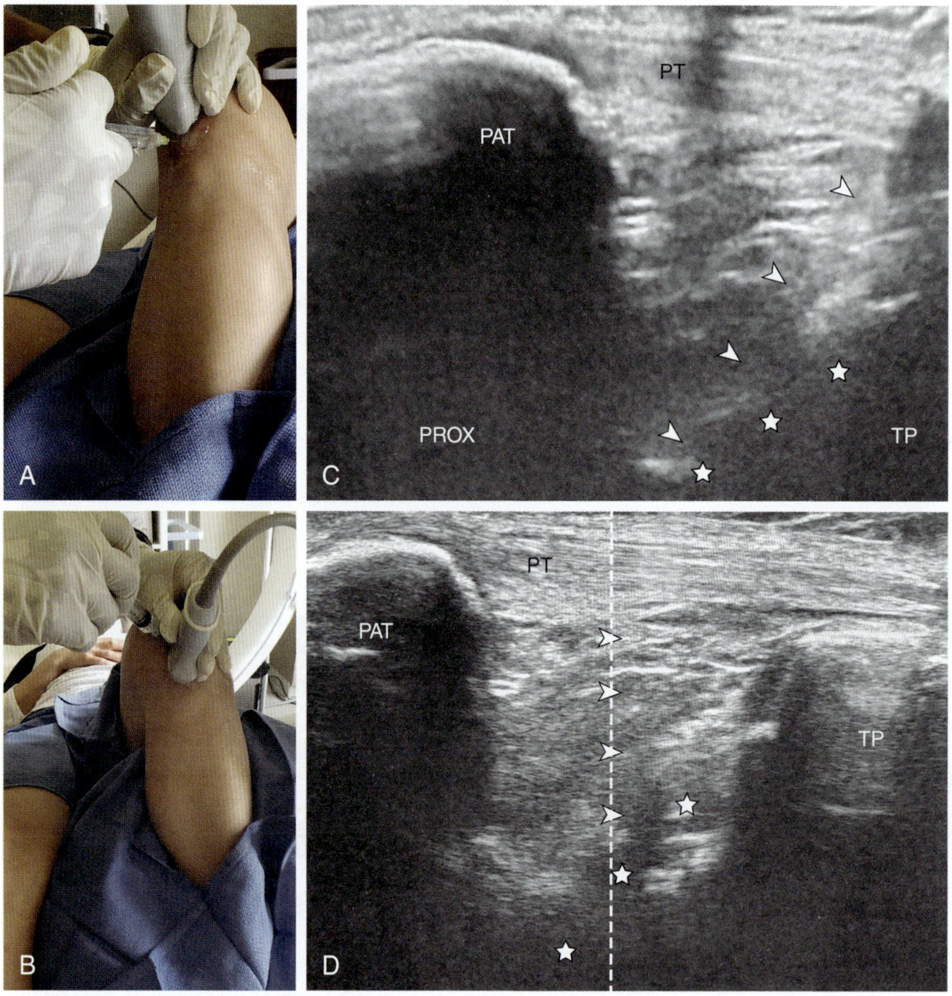

• **Fig. 21.26** (A) Anterior cruciate ligament (ACL) in-plane injection setup. (B) ACL out-of-plane injection setup. (C) ACL in-plane ultrasound injection. (D) ACL out-of-plane ultrasound injection.

Common Injectates

- Prolotherapy
- Orthobiologics (PRP, bone marrow concentrate, etc.)

Injectate Volume

- 1 to 2 mL

Technique

Patient Position

- Prone
- Knee in full extension with tibia in slight external rotation to further increase tension on PCL

Clinician Position

- On affected side of patient knee

Transducer Position

- Long axis to the PCL.
    - Rotate from coronal plane toward sagittal plane from medial to lateral direction until PCL seen in long axis deep to the posterior tibial cortex.

Needle Position

- In-plane (long axis to PCL), distal/anterior to proximal/posterior approach (Fig. 21.27A)
- Alternative approach: out of plane from medial to lateral (see Fig. 21.27B)

Target

- PCL distal or mid substance (see Fig. 21.27C and D)

PEARLS AND PITFALLS

- The posterior cruciate ligament will often appear hypoechoic due to anisotropy.
- Gel stand due to the anatomy of the popliteal fossa can improve visualization of the needle under the transducer.
- Be sure to identify the popliteal vessels and nerves, and make sure the needle stays medial to those structures.

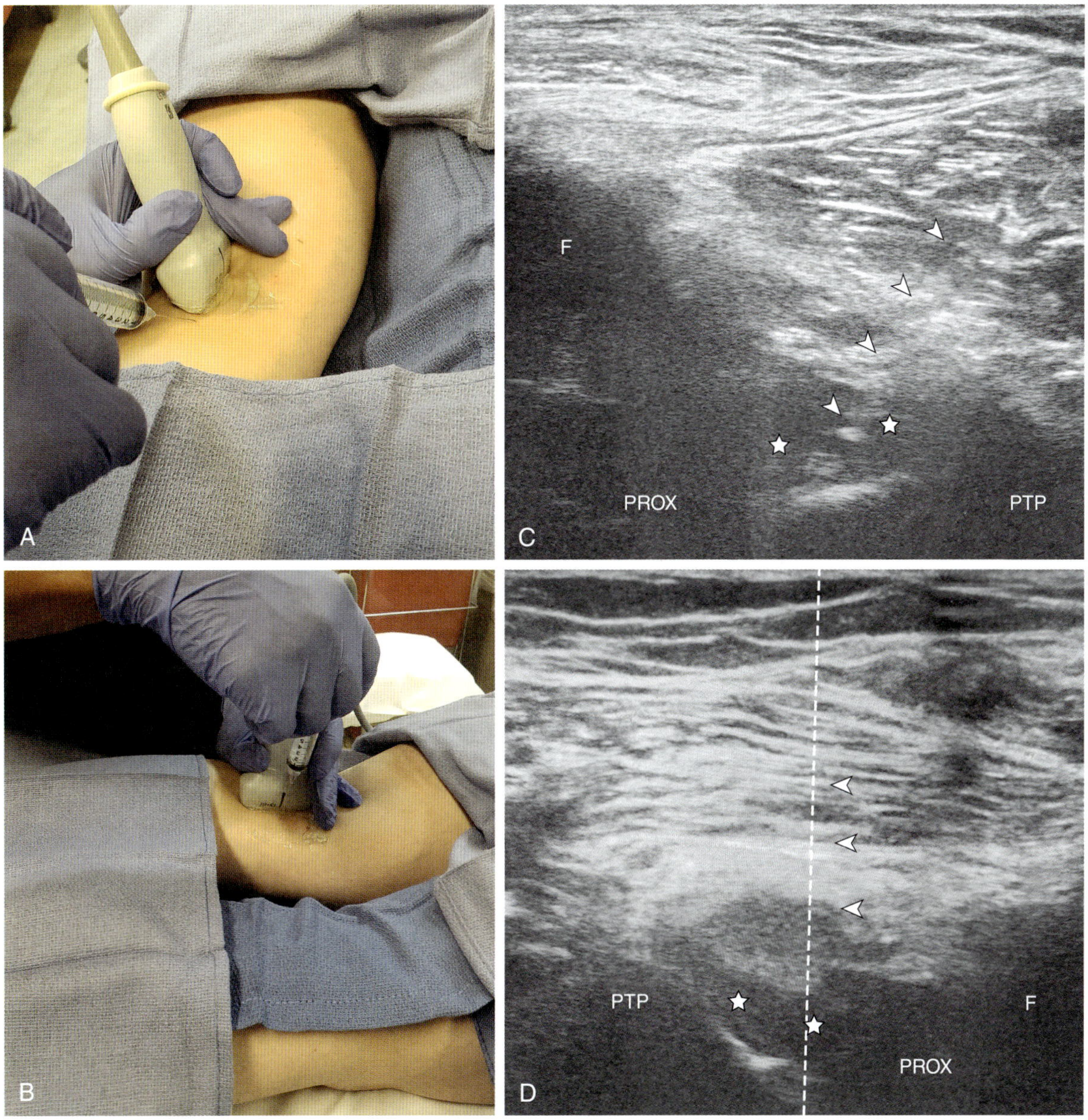

• **Fig. 21.27** (A) Posterior cruciate ligament (PCL) in-plane injection setup. (B) PCL out-of-plane injection setup. (C) PCL long-axis in-plane injection. (D) PCL out-of-plane ultrasound injection.

Medial Collateral Ligament and Bursal Injection

KEY POINTS

- The bursa is located between the superficial and deep layers of the medial collateral ligament.
- Avoid the saphenous nerve or intra-articular joint, which may be inadvertently affected due to its proximity.

Pertinent Anatomy

- The MCL is part of the capsuloligamentous complex of the medial knee and is a primary static stabilizer to valgus stress and external rotation, particularly with the knee in flexion.
- It has three layers:
  - The superficial layer is composed of sartorius and the investing fascia, which forms part of the patellar retinaculum.
  - The middle layer includes semimembranosus, the superficial MCL, the medial patellofemoral ligament (MPFL), and the posterior oblique ligament.
  - The deep layer includes the deep MCL, the posterior medial capsule, and the meniscotibial ligament.
- The MCL originates at the posterior aspect of the medial femoral epicondyle and attaches distally to the medial condyle of the tibia 5 to 7 cm below the joint line and posterior to the pes anserinus insertion.[48]
- The MCL bursa, when present, is located between the superficial and deep layers of the MCL.

Common Pathology

- MCL injuries are common after valgus injury and classified by the degree of injury.
- A subset of patients with incomplete MCL injuries may fail conservative management, with deep MCL often the source

of ongoing symptoms. The meniscofemoral ligament is more commonly affected than the meniscotibial ligament.[49]

- MCL bursitis can be due to overuse/repetitive- or direct trauma-type injuries, which may cause inflammation to the bursa.
- Calcification of the MCL and MCL bursa have both been reported, and are distinct from the Pellegrini-Stieda process.[50,51]

Equipment

- High-frequency linear array transducer
- 22 to 27 gauge 1.5 to 2 inch needle for injection

Common Injectates

- Prolotherapy
- Orthobiologics (PRP, bone marrow concentrate, etc.)

Injectate Volume

- 1 to 3 mL

Technique

Patient Position

- Supine
- Knee flexed to 30 degrees with towel roll or bump to place under affected knee
    - Can obtain better exposure with slight external rotation of the hip

Clinician Position

- At the foot of the patient

Transducer Position

- Long axis to the MCL

Needle Position

- In-plane, distal to proximal approach for proximal portion of the MCL or MCL bursa, proximal to distal for the distal portion of the MCL (Fig. 21.28A and B).

Target

- MCL: the affected areas of the MCL (proximal mid-portion deep fibers [see Fig. 21.28C and D])
- MCL bursa: target between the superficial and deep MCL fibers (Fig. 21.29B)

PEARLS AND PITFALLS

- It is helpful to use color flow Doppler to identify small vessels to which the nerves travel adjacently in order to avoid injecting branches of the saphenous nerve.
- Chronic pathology of the medial collateral ligament (MCL) more often will involve the deep fibers.[49]
- The bursa can be small, and applying direct pressure may disperse the bursal fluid, making evaluation and needle placement difficult,
- Fluid extravasation from the bursa may anesthetize the saphenous nerve due to its proximity.
- Calcification of the MCL and MCL bursa can be treated with a percutaneous barbotage procedure.

Lateral (Fibular) Collateral Ligament and Bursa Injection

KEY POINTS

- The lateral collateral ligament courses longitudinally across the knee joint.
- Avoid the common peroneal nerve, which may be inadvertently affected due to its proximity.

Pertinent Anatomy

- The LCL is the primary restraint to varus stress with the knee in flexion, originating from the lateral femoral condyle adjacent to the popliteus tendon, and inserting on the proximal fibular head.
- The LCL inserts on the fibular head between the superficial and deep heads of the biceps femoris.
- The fibular collateral ligament-biceps femoris bursa is a small bursa that exists between the superficial fibers of the biceps femoris and the LCL.

Common Pathology

- The LCL is susceptible to varus injury to the knee.
- Isolated LCL injury is uncommon, and LCL injury is more commonly associated with PL corner injury.[52]
- Calcification of the LCL and fibular collateral ligament-biceps femoris calcific bursitis have been reported.[53,54]

Equipment

- High-frequency linear array transducer
- 22 to 27 gauge 1.5 to 2 inch needle for injection

Common Injectates

- Prolotherapy
- Orthobiologics (PRP, bone marrow concentrate, etc.)

Injectate Volume

- 1 to 2 mL

Technique

Patient Position

- Lateral decubitus position with knee flexed 30 degrees OR supine with knee flexed to 30 degrees with towel roll or bump to place under affected knee and hip in slight internal rotation of the hip

Clinician Position

- Standing on either side of the patient

Transducer Position

- Long axis to the LCL over area of pathology

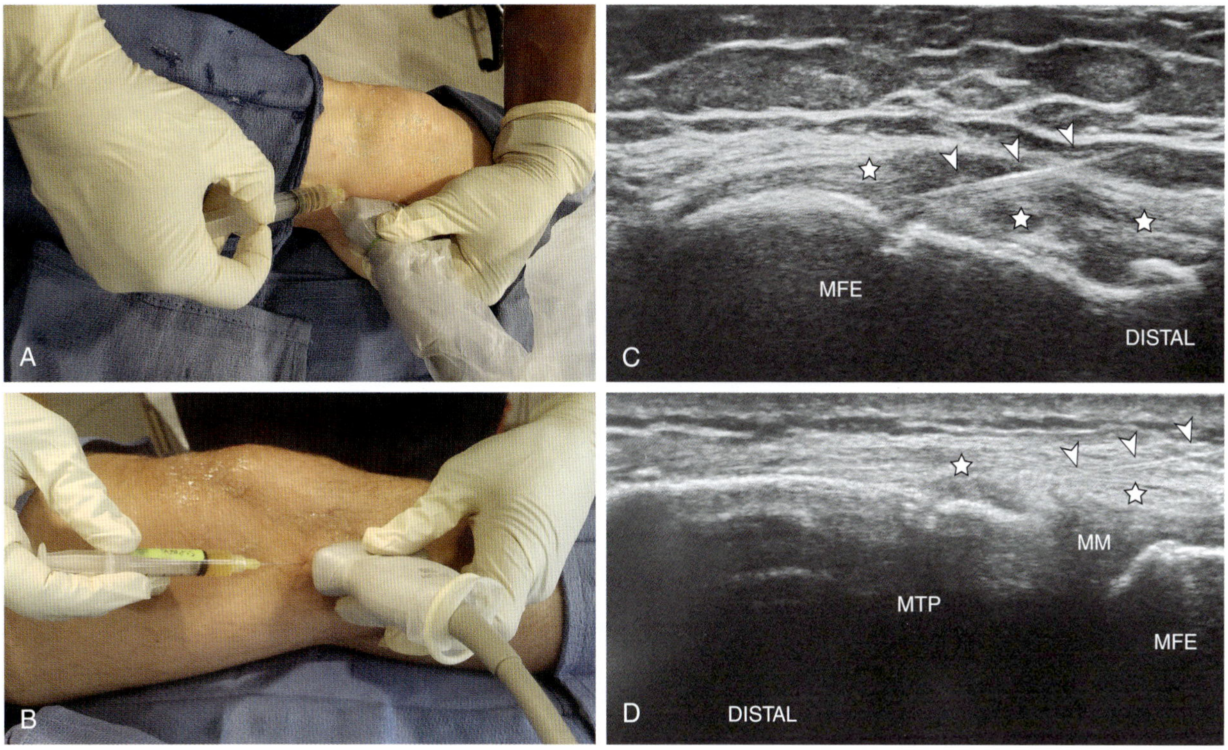

• **Fig. 21.28** (A) Proximal medial collateral ligament (MCL) setup. (B) Distal MCL setup. (C) Proximal MCL long-axis in-plane injection. (D) Distal MCL injection long-axis in-plane injection.

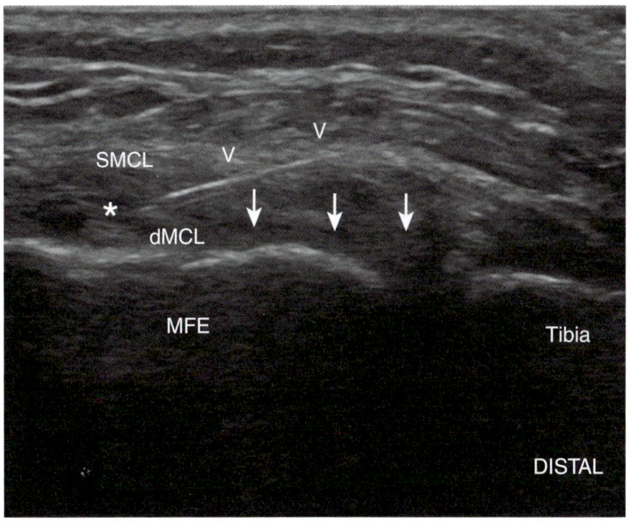

• **Fig. 21.29** Medial Collateral Ligament Bursa In-Plane Ultrasound Injection.

Needle Position

- In-plane (long axis to LCL), distal to proximal for the proximal portion of the LCL or proximal to distal approach for the distal areas of the LCL (Fig. 21.30A and B)

Target

- Pathologic areas of the LCL (see Fig. 21.30C and D)

PEARLS AND PITFALLS

- Avoid normal tissue if possible. Caution should be used when interpreting the anatomy in long-axis imaging as the divergent superficial and deep heads of the biceps femoris can simulate the appearance of tendinopathy due to thickening and anisotropy. The biceps femoris and fibular collateral ligament should be examined in multiple acoustic windows to help control for anisotrophy.[44]
- Sonopalpation can be useful to help correlate potential pathologic findings with sonographic findings.
- Fluid extravasation external to the bursa may anesthetize the common peroneal nerve due to its proximity.

It is helpful to use color flow Doppler to identify small vessels to which the nerves travel adjacently in order to avoid injecting branches of the geniculate nerves.

Anterolateral Ligament Injection

KEY POINTS

- The anterolateral ligament is a thickening of the anterolateral capsule, and has often been disregarded.
- Associated with anterior cruciate ligament (ACL) injuries.

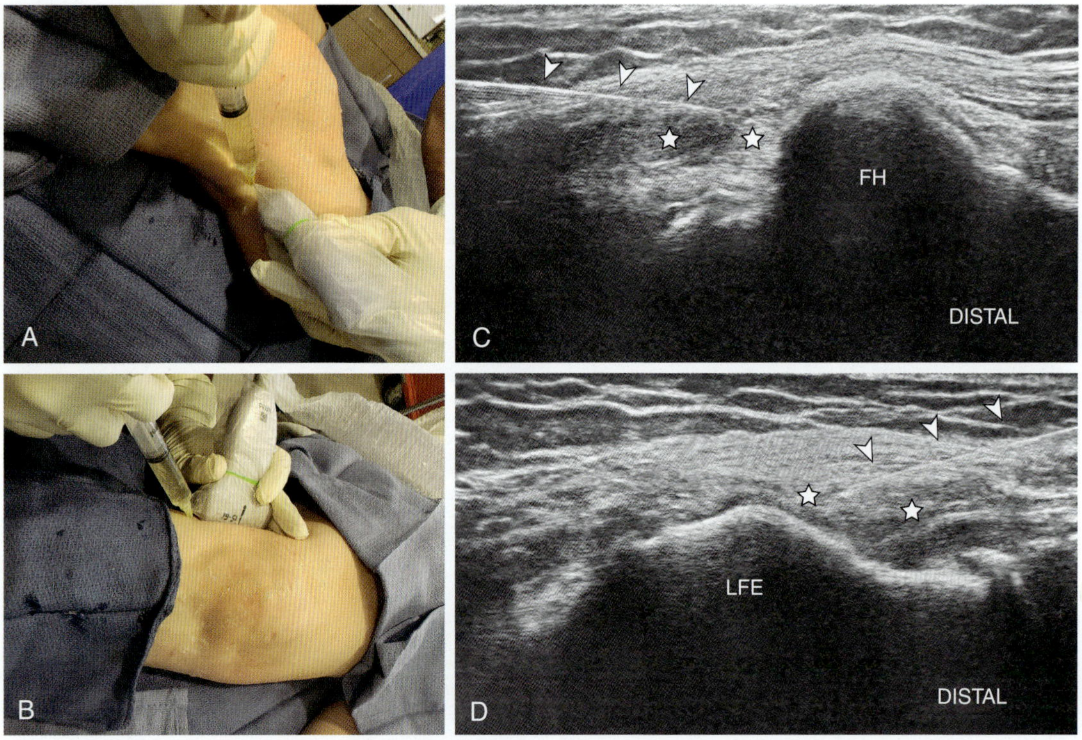

• **Fig. 21.30** (A) Distal lateral collateral ligament (LCL) in long-axis setup. (B) Proximal LCL long-axis setup. (C) Distal LCL long-axis in-plane injection. (D) Proximal LCL long-axis in-plane injection.

Pertinent Anatomy

- The anterolateral ligament (ALL) is an important stabilizer against internal rotation, with the knee in greater than 35 degrees of flexion,[55] and against anterior translation of the tibia on the femur.
- Fanlike origin at the prominence of the lateral femoral epicondyle anterior to the proximal LCL, and insertion on the tibia between Gerdy's tubercle and the tip of the fibular head. The ALL takes an oblique course over the anterolateral knee, with firm attachments to the lateral meniscus.[56]

Common Pathology

- Susceptible to overuse/repetitve- or direct trauma (varus directed blow)-type injuries, which may cause partial tear or rupture.
- Similar mechanism to injury as ACL and ITB injuries.[57]

Equipment

- High-frequency linear array transducer
- 22 to 27 gauge 1.5 to 2 inch needle for injection

Common Injectates

- Prolotherapy
- Orthobiologics (PRP, bone marrow concentrate, etc.)

Injectate Volume

- 1 to 2 mL

Technique

Patient Position

- Supine with knee flexed to 30 degrees with towel roll or bump to place under affected knee
    - Can obtain better exposure with slight internal rotation of the hip

Clinician Position

- At the foot of the patient

Transducer Position

- Long axis in oblique angle to the ALL (Fig. 21.31A).
- Find the ITB, which is easily identifiable; then scan to the LCL. The ALL are the thin bands between the two.

Needle Position

- In-plane, proximal to distal approach (see Fig. 21.31B)

Target

- The affected areas of the ALL fibers

PEARLS AND PITFALLS

- It is important to consider the anterolateral ligament for therapy in ACL injuries, lateral meniscus, and ITB injuries.

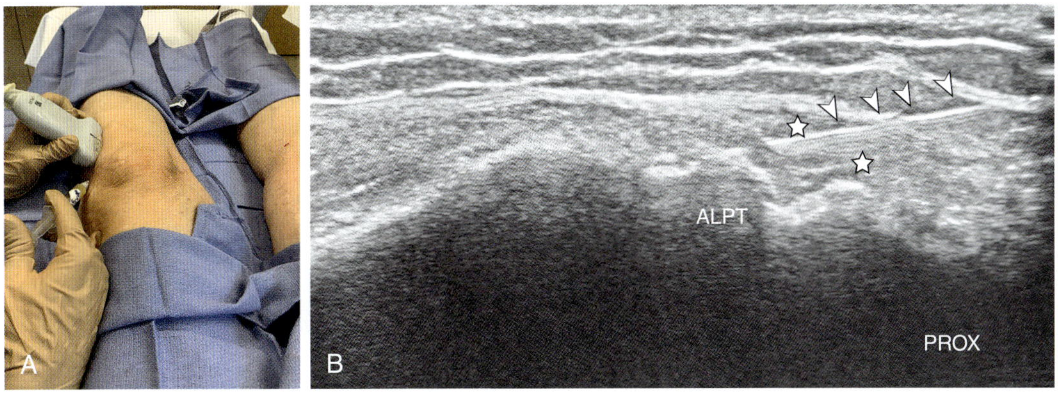

• **Fig. 21.31** (A) Anterolateral ligament (ALL) long-axis setup. (B) Distal ALL long-axis in-plane injection.

Medial and Lateral Patellar Ligament Injection

KEY POINTS

- The medial patellofemoral ligament (MPFL) is the primary medial patellar stabilizing ligament, and the medial patellotibial ligament (MPTL) and medial patellomeniscal ligament (MPML) are secondary restraints.
- It is important to examine patellar stability in 20–30 vs. 5–10 degrees of knee flexion to distinguish between MPFL vs. MPML or MPTL laxity.

Pertinent Anatomy

- The medial patellofemoral ligament (MPFL) and medial patellomeniscal ligament (MPML) are important in maintaining stability of the patellofemoral joint, particularly in the final phases of extension when they oppose lateral traction of the quadriceps associated with recurrent lateral patellar dislocations
- The medial patellar retinaculcum is composed of three layers, the deepest of which contains three medial patellar ligaments.[58]
  1. MPFL[58]
     - Primary medial restraint against lateral subluxation of patella[58]
     - Origin is between adductor tubercle and medial epicondyle[59] and insertion at the superior border of the medial patella.
     - Lateral glide/translation is best assessed for laxity at 20 to 30 degrees of flexion[60]
  2. MPML[58]
     - Secondary stabilizer
     - MPML origin at the medial meniscus anterior to the MCL and tibia through the coronary ligaments, and insertion at the inferomedial border of the patellar[60]
     - Lateral glide/translation is best assessed for laxity at 5 to 10 degrees of flexion[60]
  3. Medial patellotibial ligament (MPTL)[58]
     - Thinnest of the layers[58] and not as clinically relevant
     - Lateral patellar retinaculum
     - Lateral patellofemoral ligament (LPFL)
     - Origin is anterior and distal to the lateral epicondyle, and inserts on the middle third of the lateral patella[61]

Common Pathology

- MPFL and MPML are typically injured in lateral patellar dislocations, and rupture or injury of the ligament can lead to patellofemoral joint instability[58,60,62]
- Rupture of the MPFL has also been associated with ACL injury[58]
- LPFL laxity, tearing or insufficiency:
  - Medial patellofemoral joint instability (rare)[61]
  - Prior aggressive lateral retinaculum surgical release[61]

Equipment

- High-frequency linear array transducer
- 25 to 27 gauge 1.5 to 2 inch needle for injection

Common Injectates

- Prolotherapy
- Orthobiologics (PRP, bone marrow concentrate, etc.)

Injectate Volume

- 0.5 to 1 mL per site

Techniques

Patient Position

- Supine with knee flexed to 15 to 30 degrees with towel roll or bump to place under affected knee

Clinician Position

- MPFL and MPML
  - Standing at the contralateral side of the affected leg
- LPFL
  - Standing at the ipsilateral side of the affected leg

Transducer Position

- MPFL (Fig. 21.32A): long axis to the ligament, position over the insertion at proximal medial patella at an oblique angle with fibers in view in the direction of the medial condyle.

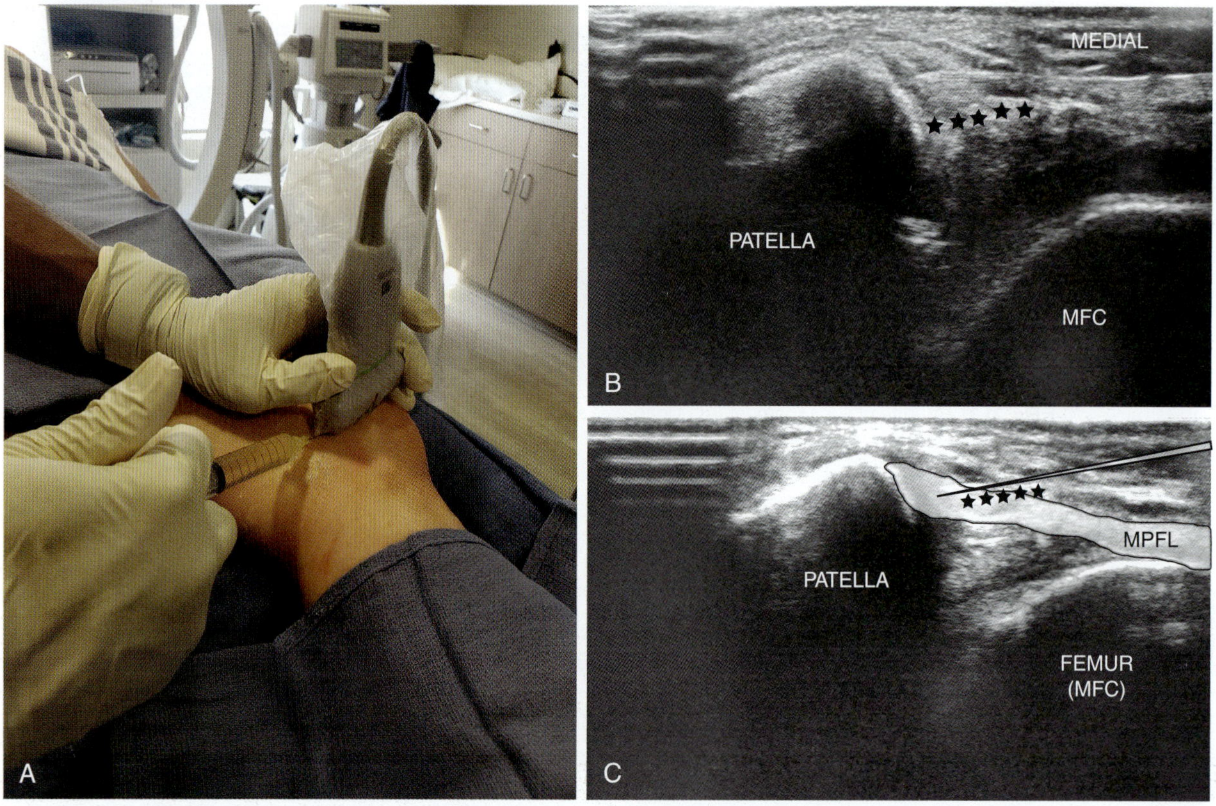

• **Fig. 21.32** (A) Setup for medial patellofemoral ligament (MPFL) injection. (B) Long-axis ultrasound-guided injection of MPFL. (C) Illustration overlying ultrasound to highlight MPFL. *MFC*, Medial femoral condyle; *MPFL*, medial patellofemoral ligament; *stars* indicate needle.

- MPML: reposition probe to the inferomedial patella.
- LPFL (Fig. 21.33A): long axis the ligament, position over insertion at middle third of the lateral patella at an oblique angle with fibers in view in the direction lateral epicondyle.

Needle Position

- MPFL (Fig. 21.32B and C): in-plane, medial posterior to lateral anterior approach
- LPFL (Fig. 21.33B and C): in-plane, lateral posterior to medial anterior approach

Target

- Pathologic ligament (area of hypoechogenicity and disorganization)

PEARLS AND PITFALLS

- Visualize the needle and target the ligaments and not the adjacent fat pad.
- It is important to localize and target the ligaments involved by examining for patellar instability in 20–30 vs. 5–10 degrees of knee flexion to distinguish between medial patellofemoral ligament and medial patellomeniscal ligament involvement

Perineural Injections

Tibial Nerve Injection

KEY POINTS

- An approach too far cephalad before bifurcation targeting the sciatic nerve will affect the peroneal nerve fibers.
- Use a medial to lateral approach to avoid the peroneal nerve.

Pertinent Anatomy

- The popliteal artery is located deep and medial to the tibial nerve near the knee joint line.
- The medial cutaneous sural nerve branches off of the tibial nerve within the popliteal fossa to join with the lateral cutaneous sural nerve from the common peroneal nerve.

Common Pathology

- Occasionally used to perform tibial nerve blocks for lower extremity procedures or for the treatment of complex regional pain syndrome of the lower extremity.

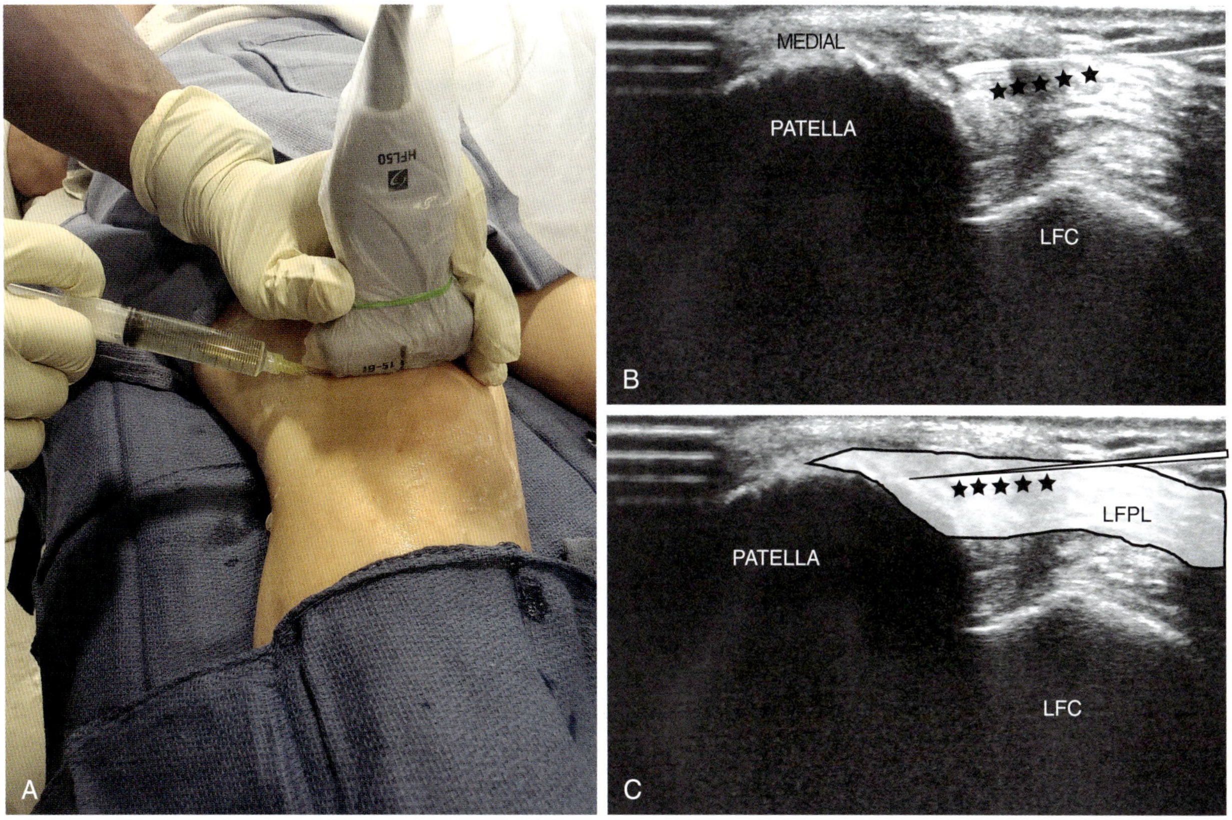

• **Fig. 21.33** (A) Setup for lateral patellofemoral ligament (LPFL) injection. (B) Long-axis ultrasound-guided injection of LPFL. (C) Illustration overlying ultrasound to highlight LPFL. *LFC*, Lateral femoral condyle; *LPFL*, lateral patellofemoral ligament; *stars* indicate needle.

- Typically, the popliteal fossa is not a site of entrapment, but may develop entrapment from post-traumatic or post-procedural scar tissue formation.

Equipment

- High-frequency linear array transducer
- 25 to 22 gauge 2 to 3 inch needle
- Electromyography stimulator, if required for confirmation

Common injectates

- Local anesthetics for diagnostics or nerve block
- For hydrodissection, anesthetics, corticosteroids, 5% dextrose solution, orthobiologics (platelet lysate, platelet-poor plasma, PRP, etc.)

Injectate volume

- 5 to 20 mL

Technique

Patient Position

- Prone

Clinician Position

- Along the opposite lower extremity of the patient or at the foot of the patient

Transducer Position

- Short axis to the tibial nerve at the middle of the popliteal fossa
  - Start transverse to the distal thigh and find the sciatic nerve; then follow the sciatic nerve inferior until it bifurcates into the tibial branch

Needle Position

- In-plane, medial to lateral approach (Fig. 21.34A)

Target

- Perineural sheath, can target above and below the nerve to confirm adequate spread (see Fig. 21.34B).

PEARLS AND PITFALLS

- The needle should not be advanced if the tip is not visible.
- Avoid the neurovascular structures which lie deep to and lateral to the tibial nerve in the popliteal fossa.
- A lateral approach may pose risk to peroneal nerve injury.
- A tibial nerve block at this location may affect the motor function of the tibial nerve and should be anticipated prior to the procedure.
- Inject as the needle is approaching the epineurium and advance while injecting slowly to push the nerve away, thus reducing the risk of intraneural injection.
- For hydrodissection, creating a halo around the nerve will increase the definition of the nerve borders.

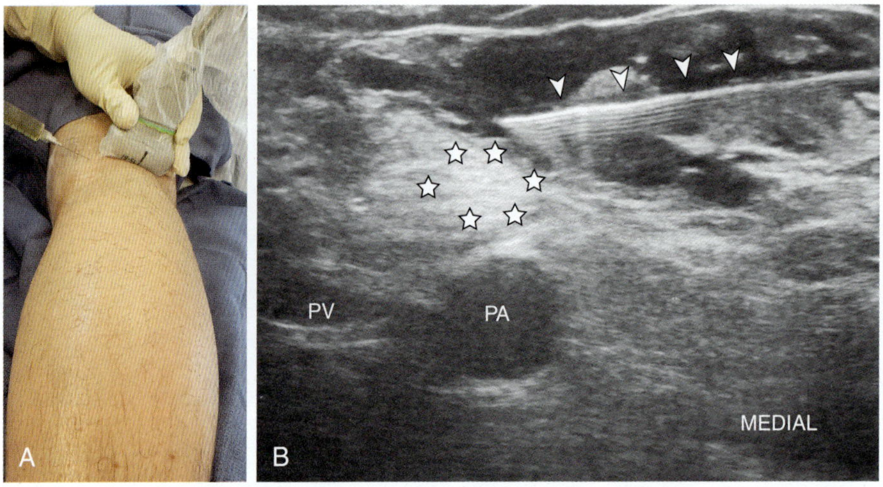

• **Fig. 21.34** (A) Tibial nerve block setup. (B) Tibial nerve block transverse in-plane injection.

Common Peroneal Nerve Injection

KEY POINTS

- Approaches to cephalad (prior to the bifurcation of the tibial nerve) or caudal (too distal after the bifurcation of the lateral sural cutaneous nerve) may have undesired effects on nerve function.

Pertinent Anatomy

- The common peroneal nerve is the lateral branch of the sciatic nerve. While in the popliteal fossa, the common peroneal nerve gives off the lateral genicular branches to the knee joint and the lateral cutaneous sural nerve prior to coursing around the fibular head and dividing into the superficial and deep peroneal nerve.

Common Pathology

- Can be a common site of entrapment between the fibular head and external pressure from the tendinous origin of the peroneus longus.
- Injury associated with fracture of the proximal fibula, post-traumatic or iatrogenic from positioning during a procedure compression.

Equipment

- High-frequency linear array transducer
- 22 to 25 gauge 2 to 3 inch needle
- Electromyography stimulator, if required for confirmation

Common Injectates

- Local anesthetics for diagnostics or nerve block
- For hydrodissection, anesthetics, corticosteroids, neuroprolotherapy, orthobiologics (platelet lysate, platelet-poor plasma, PRP, etc.)

Injectate Volume

- 5 to 20 mL

Technique

Patient Position

- Side-lying with contralateral side closest to the table with knee flexed to 30 degrees with pillow or towel roll or bump placed in between the knees

Clinician Position

- In front of the patient

Transducer Position

- Short axis to the common peroneal nerve posterior to the knee joint line and directed laterally towards the fibular head
  - Start transverse to the distal thigh and find the sciatic nerve; then follow the sciatic nerve inferior until it bifurcates into the tibial and peroneal branches

Needle Position

- In-plane, distal to proximal approach (Fig. 21.35A)

Target

- Perineural sheath, can target above and below the nerve to confirm adequate spread (see Fig. 21.35B and C)

PEARLS AND PITFALLS

- Avoid the neurovascular structures which lie posterior and deep to the common peroneal nerve within the popliteal fossa.
- An approach too far cephalad may affect the tibial nerve prior to the bifurcation.
- A common peroneal nerve block at this location may affect the motor function of the peroneal nerve and should be anticipated prior to procedure.
- The needle should not be advanced if the tip is not visible.
- Inject just before approaching the epineurium and advance while injecting slowly to push the nerve away, thus reducing the risk of intraneural injection.
- For hydrodissections, creating a halo around the nerve will increase the definition of the nerve borders.

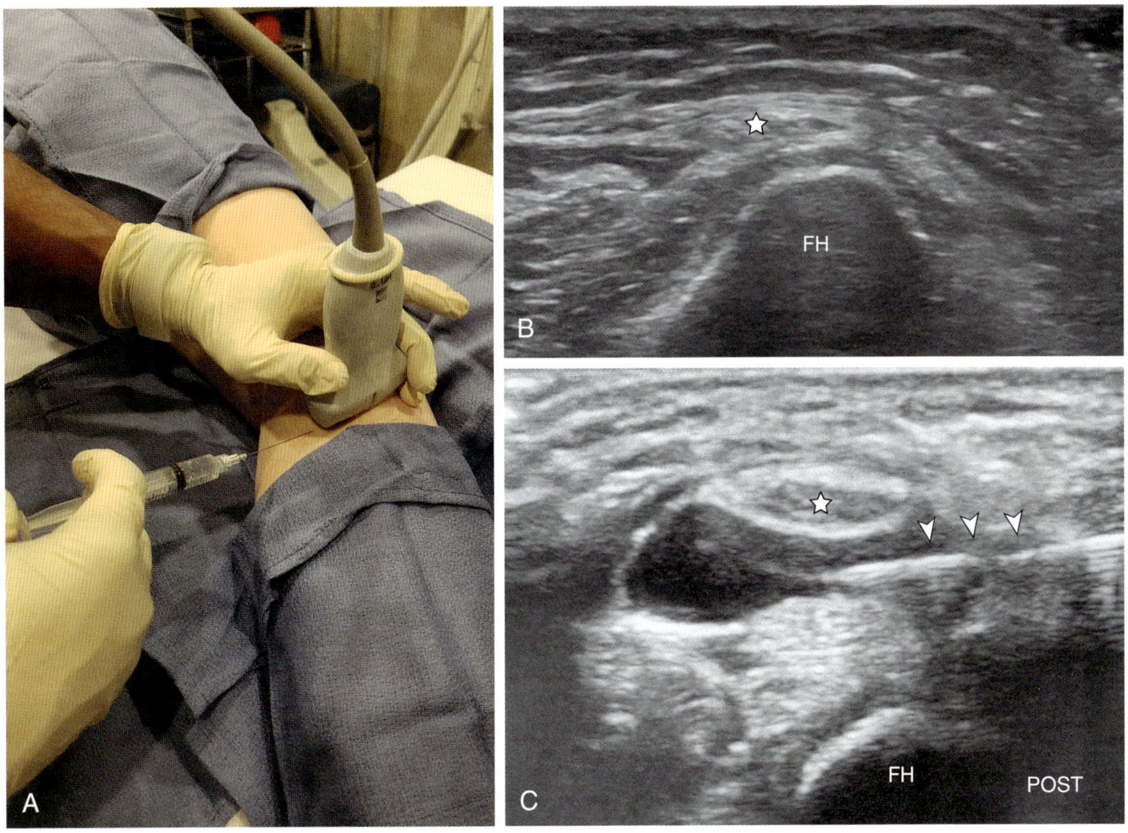

• **Fig 21.35** (A) Common peroneal nerve at fibular head setup. (B) Common peroneal nerve short-axis in-plane injection. (C) Common peroneal nerve at the fibular head hydrodissection.

Saphenous Nerve Injection and Infrapatellar Branch of Saphenous Nerve Injection

KEY POINTS

- Anesthetize above and below the saphenous or infrapatellar branch of the saphenous nerve within the perineural sheath to ensure adequate effect.

Pertinent Anatomy

- The saphenous nerve is a pure sensory branch of the femoral nerve, which innervates the medial knee and foot.
- The infrapatellar division can be a vulnerable to injury due to its proximity to the prominence of the medial femoral condyle, and the nerves superficially course through the sartorius muscle.

Common Pathology

- Associated with direct trauma or associated muscle/tendon injury of the adductor and medial thigh.
- Vulnerable to entrapment, inflammation or injury anywhere along its long course.
  - Saphenous nerve syndrome refers to symptomatic entrapment of the nerve as it courses through the adductor canal.
- Iatrogenic injury may occur post-procedurally during hamstring tendon harvest and total knee arthroplasty.[63,64]

Equipment

- High-frequency linear array transducer
- 25 to 27 gauge 2 to 3 inch needle
- Electromyography stimulator, if required for confirmation

Common Injectates

- Local anesthetics for diagnostics or nerve block
- For hydrodissection, anesthetics, corticosteroids, neuroprolotherapy, orthobiologics (platelet lysate, platelet-poor plasma, PRP, etc.)

Injectate Volume

- 5 to 20 mL

Technique

Patient Position

- Supine with lower extremity externally rotated for better exposure of the nerve

Clinician Position

- Along the affected side of the patient

Transducer Position

- Saphenous nerve: short axis to the saphenous nerve just inferior to the adductor canal

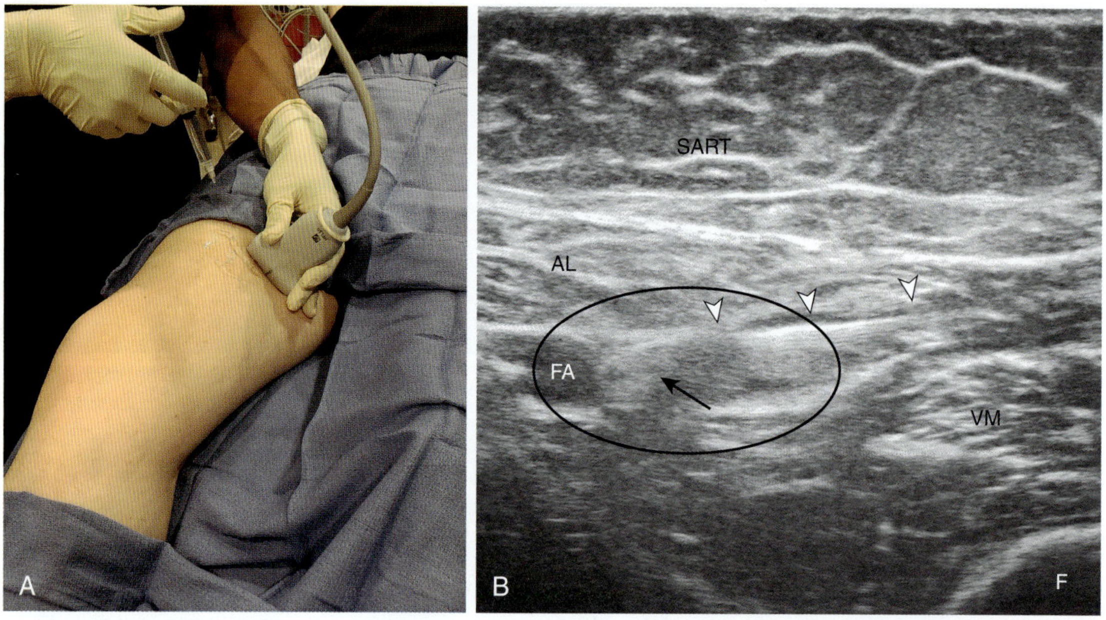

• **Fig. 21.36** (A) Saphenous nerve block just inferior to the adductor canal. (B) Saphenous nerve block in plane.

- Infrapatellar branch: long axis to the infrapatellar branch at the proximal tibia or short axis to the infrapatella adjacent to the metaphysis of the proximal tibia

Needle Position

- Saphenous nerve: in-plane, anterior lateral to posterior medial approach (Fig. 21.36A)
- Infrapatellar branch: in-plane, anterior lateral to posterior medial approach (Fig. 21.37A)
  - Alternative: out-of-plane, anterior to posterior approach (see Fig. 21.37B)

Target

- Perineural sheath, can target above and below the nerve to confirm adequate spread
  - Saphenous (see Fig. 21.36B)
  - Infrapatellar branch (see Fig. 21.37C and D)

PEARLS AND PITFALLS

- High-frequency linear array or curvilinear transducer may be used, depending on the patient's body habitus. If it is difficult to visualize the nerve, so you may consider injecting the fascial plane adjacent to the nerve.
- Femoral vessels and small vessels around the infrapatellar saphenous nerve may serve as a landmark for a poorly visualized nerve. Use color flow Doppler to identify the vessels as the nerve often travels adjacent to those. Avoid intravascular injection.
- The needle should not be advanced if the tip is not visible.
- Inject just before approaching the epineurium and advance while injecting slowly to push the nerve away, thus reducing the risk of intraneural injection.
- For hydrodissections, creating a halo around the nerve will increase the definition of the nerve borders.

Genicular Nerve Block

KEY POINTS

- The nerves run adjacent to the corresponding genicular arteries, which should be identified and used as landmarks for injection. Utilize Doppler to identify vasculature prior to injection.
- These nerves are typically blocked or ablated for knee pain, but also be injured or entrapped with knee surgeries.

Pertinent Anatomy

- The knee is innervated by articular branches of several nerves, including the femoral, obturator, saphenous, common peroneal, and posterior tibial nerves.
- Superolateral genicular nerve (SLGN)
  - Located at the junction of the lateral condyle and femoral shaft[65]
- Superomedial genicular nerve (SMGN)
  - Located at the junction of the medial condyle and femoral shaft.[65] Lies beneath the adductor magnus tendon.[66]
- Inferomedial genicular nerve (IMGN)
  - Located between the medial tibial condyle and the tibial insertion of the MCL.[66]
- Inferolateral genicular nerve (ILGN)
  - Located superficial to the lateral tibial plateau and superior and anterior to the fibular head.[67]

Common Pathology

- Injury to the genicular nerves is uncommon in the literature.
- Interventional procedures for the genicular nerves are primarily to treat intra-articular pathology, including knee

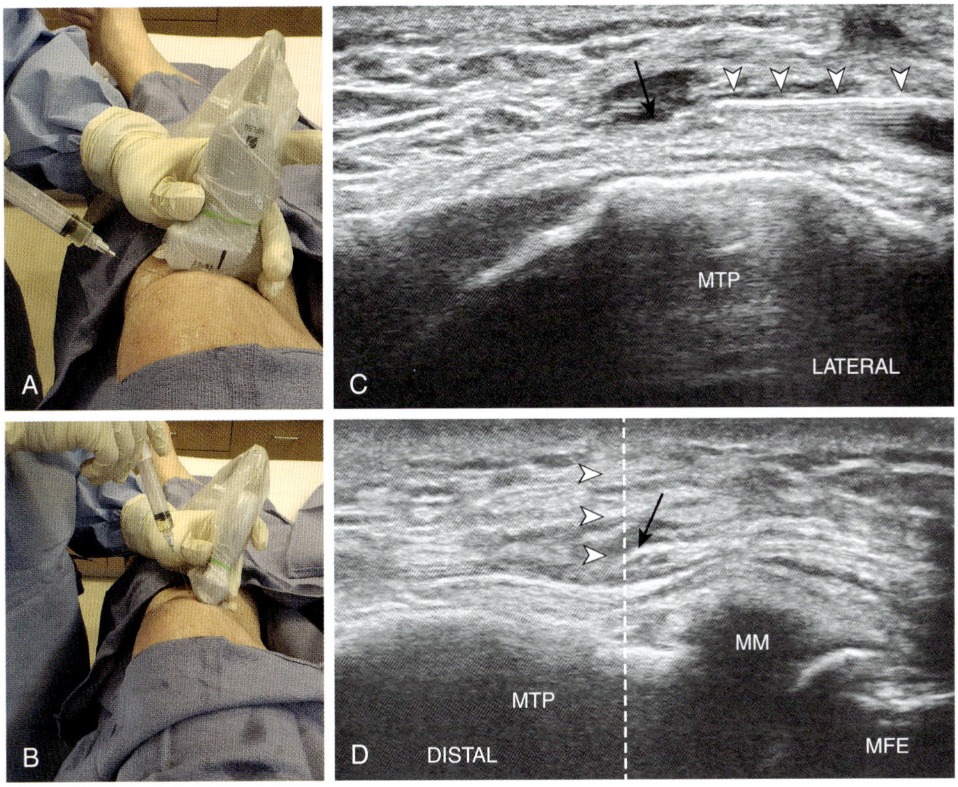

• **Fig. 21.37** (A) Infrapatellar branch of saphenous nerve injection in-plane setup. (B) Infrapatellar branch of saphenous nerve out-of-plane setup. (C) Infrapatellar branch of saphenous nerve injection transverse in plane ultrasound injection. (D) Infrapatellar branch of saphenous nerve transverse out-of-plane ultrasound injection.

osteoarthritis[66-68] postoperative pain following total or partial knee replacement[66,68]

Equipment

- High-frequency linear array transducer
- 25 to 27 gauge 1.5 to 2 inch needle for injection

Common Injectates

- Local anesthetics, plus or minus corticosteroids
- 5% dextrose (neuroprolotherapy)
- Platelet lysate
- Radiofrequency ablation is also used but not discussed here

Injectate Volume

- 1 to 1.5 mL per site

Technique

Patient Position

- Supine and knee flexed to 15 to 30 degrees with towel roll or bump to place under the popliteal fossa of the affected knee

Clinician Position

- SLGN and ILGN
  - Clinician ipsilateral to affected knee
- SMGN and IMGN
  - Clinician contralateral to affected knee

Transducer Position

- Short axis to the nerves. Confirm with color flow Doppler. The nerves are adjacent to the arteries and may be hard to visualize. To help identify each:
- SLGN (Fig. 21.38A)
  - Place the transducer in long axis to identify the quadriceps tendon.
  - Slide the transducer laterally to the intersection of the lateral femoral shaft and the lateral epicondyle.
  - Identify the superolateral genicular artery above the periosteum.
- SMGN (Fig. 21.39A)
  - Place the transducer in long axis to identify the quadriceps tendon.
  - Slide the transducer medially to the intersection of the medial femoral shaft and the medial epicondyle.
  - Identify the superomedial genicular artery adjacent to the periosteum, proximal to the adductor tubercle, and deep to the adductor magnus tendon.
- IMGN (Fig. 21.40A)
  - Place the transducer in long axis to identify the intersection of the medial tibial shaft and the medial epicondyle.
  - Identify the inferomedial genicular artery adjacent to the periosteum between the medial tibial epicondyle and the tibial insertion of the MCL fibers.

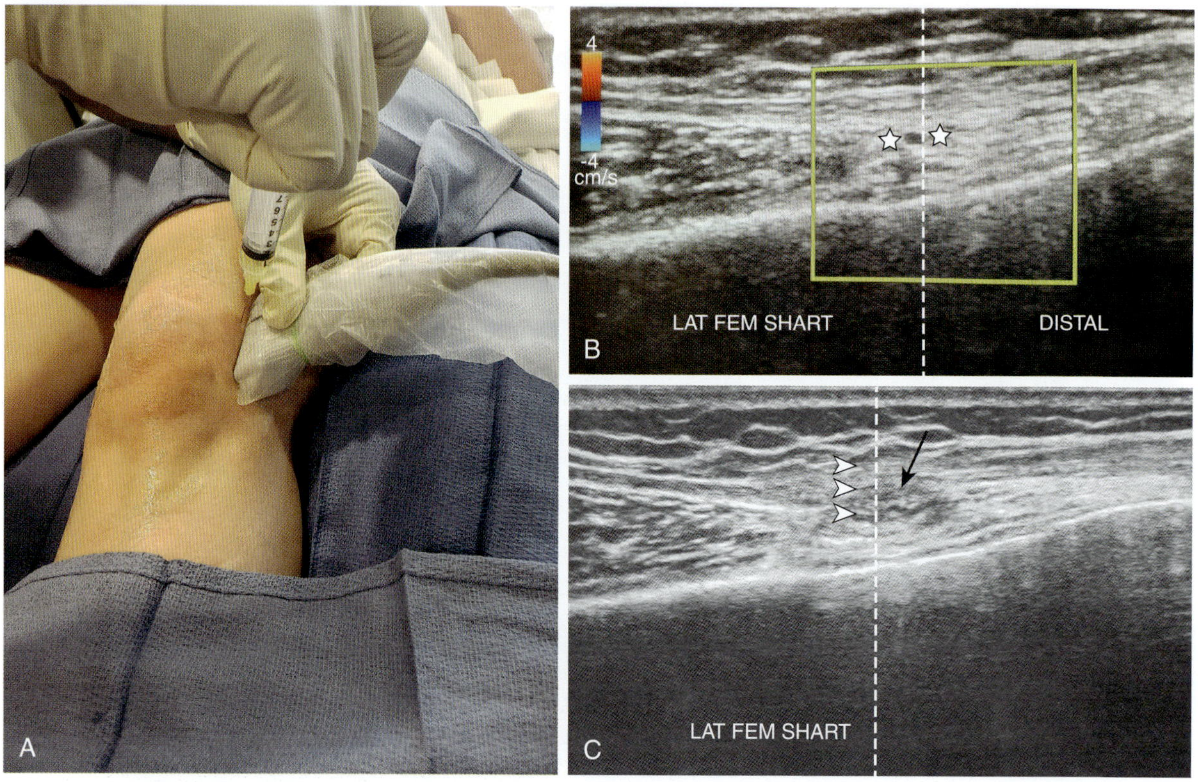

• **Fig. 21.38** (A) Setup for superolateral genicular nerve (SLGN) injection. (B) Identification of superolateral genicular artery. (C) Out-of-plane ultrasound-guided perineural injection of SLGN.

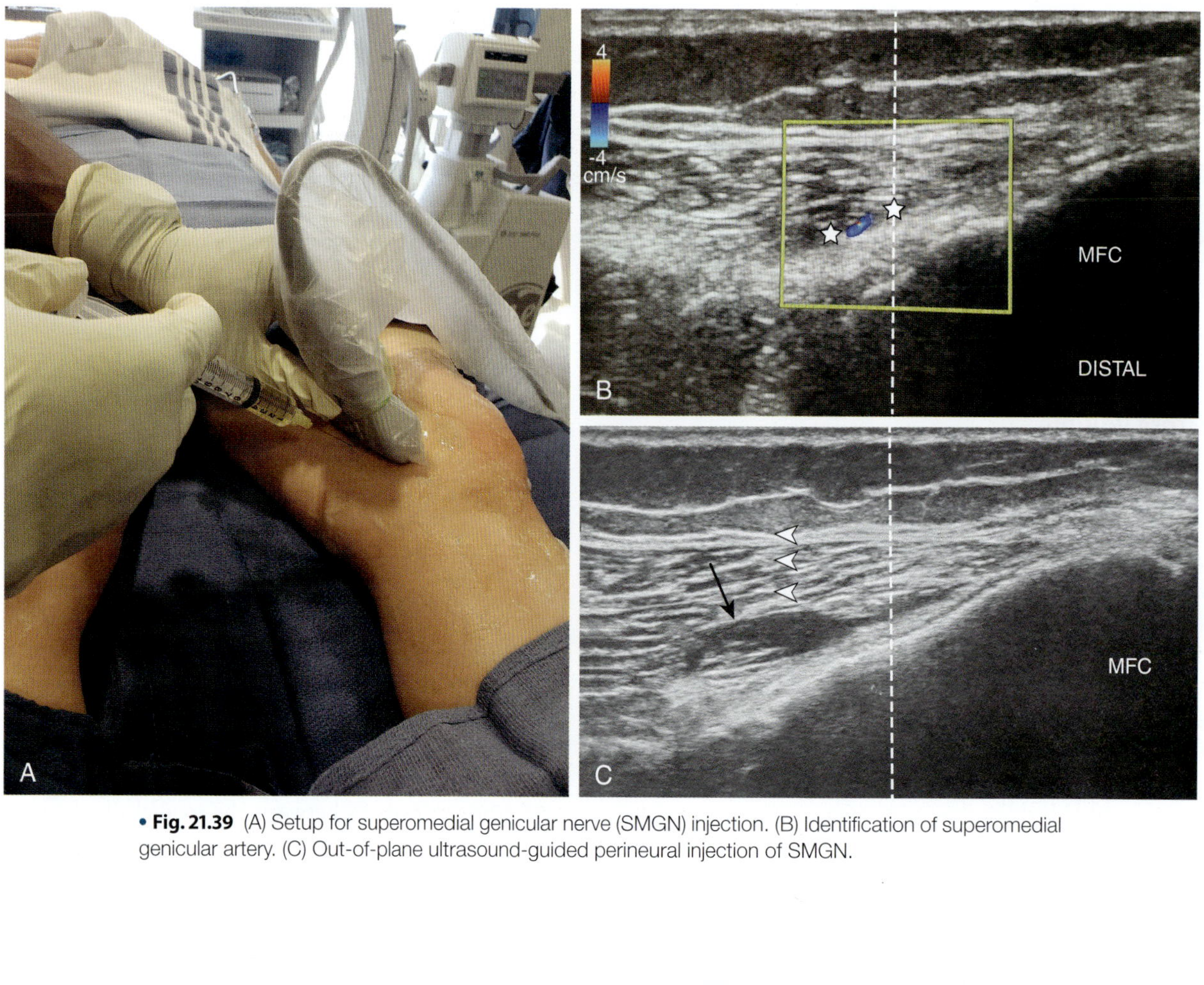

• **Fig. 21.39** (A) Setup for superomedial genicular nerve (SMGN) injection. (B) Identification of superomedial genicular artery. (C) Out-of-plane ultrasound-guided perineural injection of SMGN.

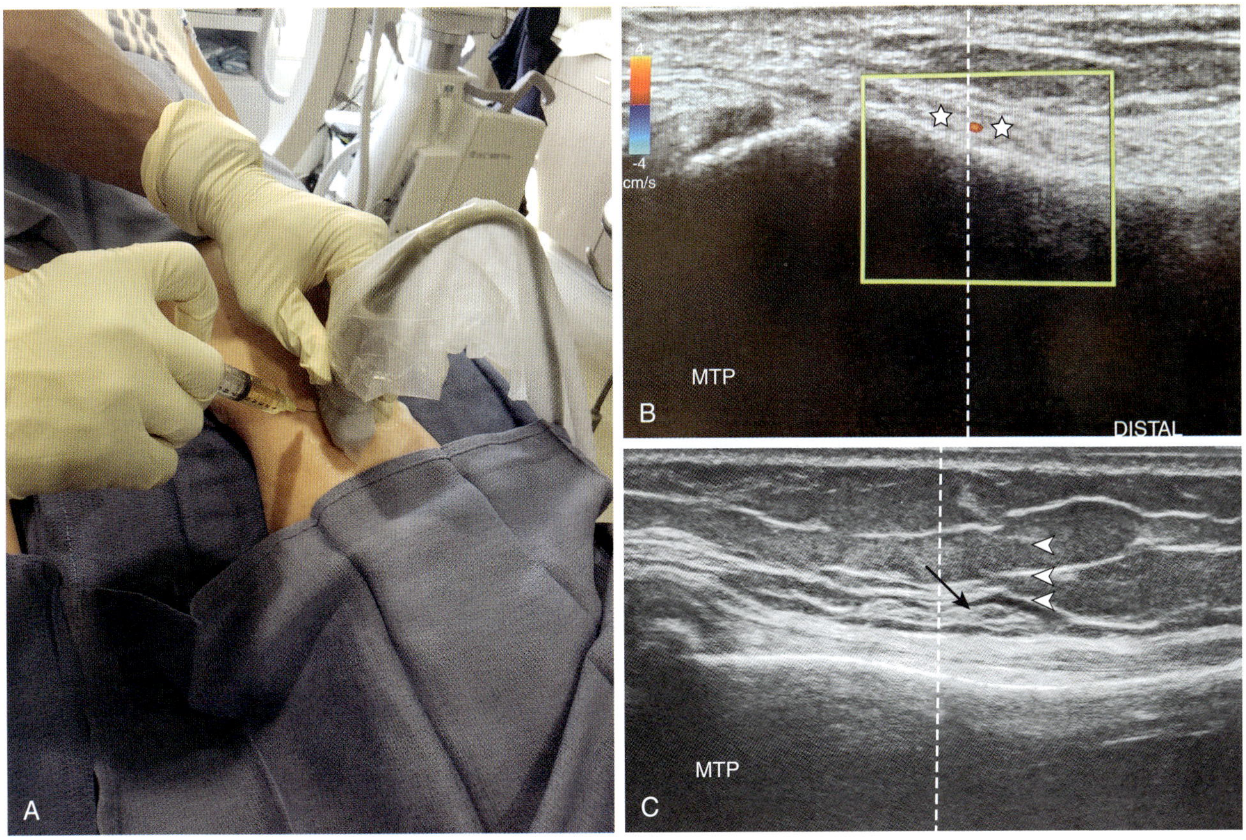

• **Fig. 21.40** (A) Setup for inferomedial genicular nerve (IMGN) injection. (B) Identification of inferomedial genicular artery. (C) Out-of-plane ultrasound-guided perineural injection of IMGN.

- ILGN (Fig. 21.41A)
  - Place the transducer in long axis to the knee, and identify the lateral meniscus and lateral tibial plateau.
  - Slide the transducer distally, proximal to fibular head, and anteriorly until the inferolateral genicular artery is identified, which may be at the lateral border of the tibial plateau or superficial to the lateral meniscus.

Needle Position

- SLGN
  - Out of-plane, lateral to medial approach (Fig. 21.38B and C)
- SMGN
  - Out of-plane, medial to lateral approach (Fig. 21.39B and C)
- IMGN
  - Out of-plane, medial to lateral approach (Fig. 21.40B and C)
- ILGN
  - Out of-plane, lateral to medial approach (Fig. 21.41B and C)
- Alternately, for all, inject inject in-plane, proximal to distal approach

Target

- Adjacent to corresponding genicular artery or perineurally, if nerve is visible.

PEARLS AND PITFALLS

- Be sure to use Doppler to identify the genicular arteries.
- Use the quadriceps tendon as a landmark to identify the superomedial and superolateral nerves.
- For the inferolateral genicular nerve block, be sure to identify and avoid the common peroneal nerve.

Knee Fluoroscopy Injection

Joints

Femorotibial Joint: Medial and Lateral

KEY POINTS

- Fluoroscopy can be used to confirm placement of injectate in specific area of the knee joint.
- You can ensure flow directly along the specific chondral surface.
- For accurate anterior, posterior, and lateral fluoroscopic views, be sure to align femoral condyles and tibial plateaus.

Pertinent Anatomy

See Ultrasound section.

Common Pathology

See Ultrasound section.

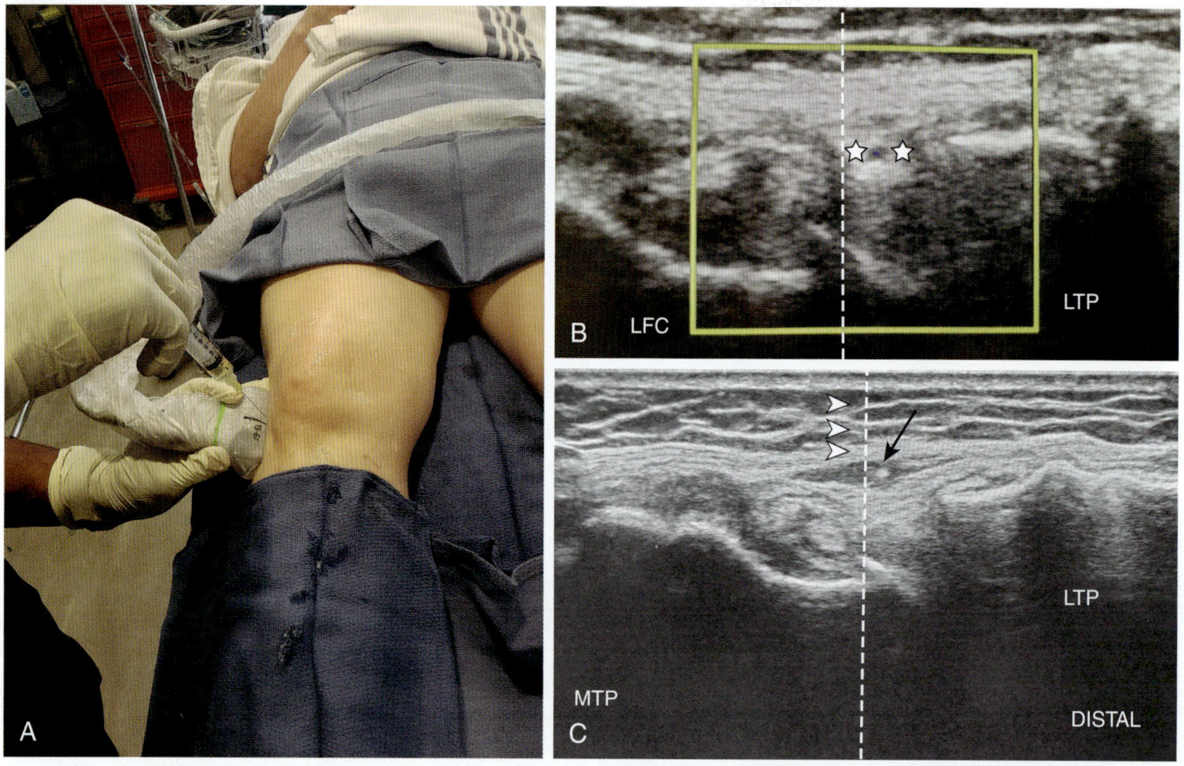

• **Fig. 21.41** (A) Setup for inferolateral genicular nerve (ILGN) injection. (B) Identification of inferolateral genicular artery. (C). Out-of-plane ultrasound-guided perineural injection of ILGN.

Equipment

- C-arm fluoroscopy
- 18 to 27 gauge 1.5 or 3.5 inch needle depending on injectate and body habitus. Micronized adipose tissue will require 18 to 22 gauge needle. Bone marrow concentrate or aspirate will require 22 to 25 gauge needle. Other therapeutic injectates usually performed with 25-gauge needle.
- Contrast dye

Common Injectates

- Local anesthetics for diagnostics, corticosteroids, hyaluronic acid, prolotherapy, orthobiologics (PRP, bone marrow concentrate, micronized adipose tissue, etc.)

Injectate Volume

- 2 to 10 mL total

Technique for Medial and Lateral Joint Compartments

Patient Position

- Supine hook-lying. Can place booster pillow under the knee for support (Fig. 21.42).

Clinician Position

- Standing on ipsilateral side of the patient.

C-Arm Position

- True anteroposterior (AP) projection, where anterior and posterior femur and tibia are aligned.
- Lateral projection, where medial and lateral femoral condyles and medial and lateral tibial plateaus are aligned.

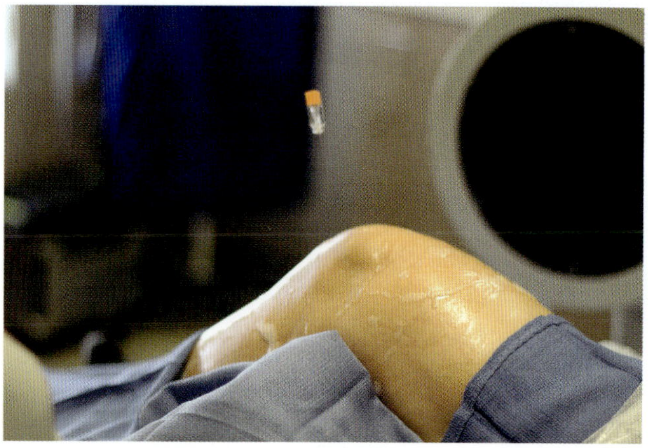

• **Fig. 21.42** Knee Hook-Lying Position.

Needle Position

- Use AP projection to identify mid portion of medial femoral condyle or lateral femoral condyle.
- Then, in lateral position, start needle entry about 1 cm above the tibial plateau.
- Under intermittent fluoroscopy, advance needle from superior to inferior, anterior to posterior towards the middle of the tibial plateau.
- Avoid hitting the femoral condyle articular cartilage.

Target

- Medial or lateral joint compartments
  - Aim to gently touch down on the desired tibial plateau or the meniscus in the middle third of the joint from anterior to posterior (Fig. 21.43).

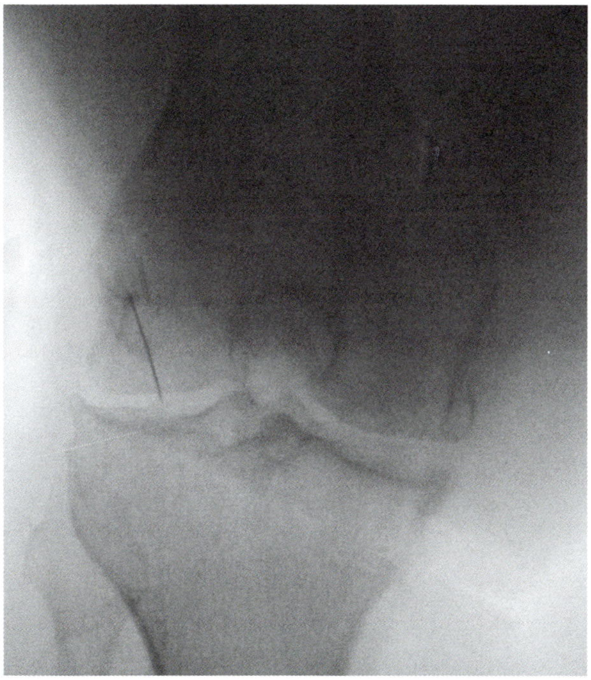

• **Fig. 21.43** Knee lateral compartment intra-articular injection fluoroscopy AP view with contrast.

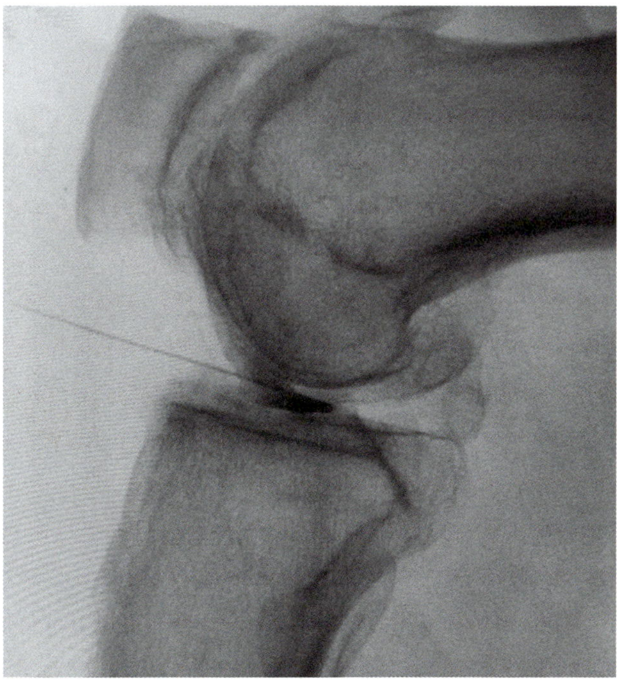

• **Fig. 21.44** Knee medial compartment intra-articular injection fluoroscopy lateral view with contrast.

- Contrast in lateral should spread anterior and posterior above the tibial surface, perhaps making a "U" shape under the medial femoral condyle (Fig. 21.44).
- In the AP view the contrast should be spread medial and lateral through the medial compartment (Fig. 21.45).

PEARLS AND PITFALLS

- Use a smaller-gauge needle where possible and avoid hitting the femoral surface to avoid cartilage injury.
- Needle trajectory should be slightly angled superior to inferior instead of parallel to the tibial plateau. The angled approach helps avoid damage to the meniscus and tibial or femoral cartilage. Also, this can allow for the needle to have adequate depth to get into the joint if there is less joint space or osteophytes.
- Osteophytes can be seen on the x-ray and should be avoided by a more lateral or medial starting point, or angling the needle to avoid them.
- Use minimal contrast (⅛ to ¼ mL) to limit cytotoxic effects.
- If contrast is pooling in the soft tissues rather than easily flowing along the chondral surfaces, then placement is likely extra-capsular within Hoffa's fat pad. In this case, advance the needle.
- If the injection is painful, the needle is likely not intra-articular.

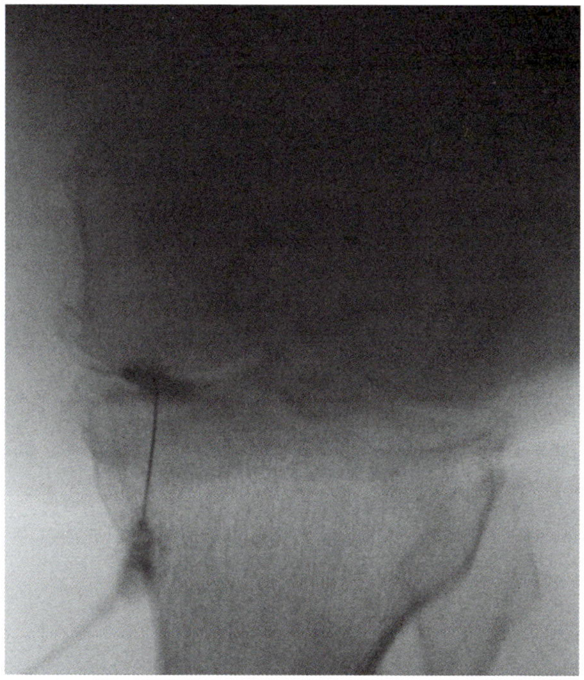

• **Fig. 21.45** Knee medial compartment intra-articular injection fluoroscopy AP view with contrast.

Technique for Weightbearing Medial and Lateral Femoral Chondral Surfaces

Patient Position

- Supine, hip, and knee each flexed 90 degrees. Rest the leg on a block or bolster (Fig. 21.46)

Clinician Position

- Standing on the side of the patient

C-Arm Position

- Lateral projection with the femoral condyles and tibial plateau aligned.

Needle Position

- Palpate the patellar tendon. Move medial or lateral depending on target to palpate the mid portion of the desired femoral condyle.
- Start needle entry about 1 cm distal to the medial or lateral aspect of the patella.
- Aim slightly proximally with bevel facing the chondral surface.

Target

- Medial or lateral femoral condyle
  - Aim for the one-third of the chondral surface with the bevel facing the surface. Gently touch os.
  - Inject a small amount of contrast. There should be no resistance and easy flow if intra-articular. If not, pull the needle back usually about 1 mm or less while injecting until resistance is loss.
  - In the lateral view, contrast should flow directly along the desired chondral surface (Fig. 21.47).

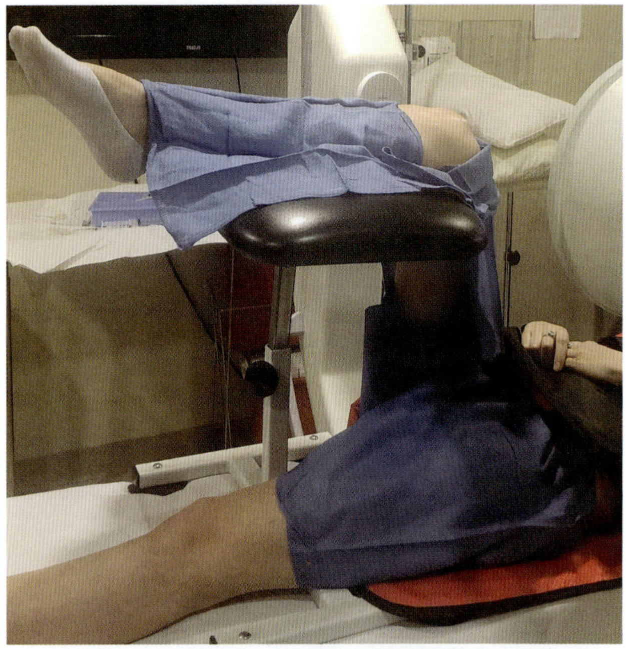

• **Fig. 21.46** Knee setup for weightbearing femoral chondral surface (90/90) position.

PEARLS AND PITFALLS

- This is the preferred approach when using mesenchymal stem cells (MSCs). The 90/90 position (hip and knee flexed 90 degrees each) can allow for gravity-dependent cell adhesion after 10 min.[8] Inject very slowly over 3–5 min to allow for cell adhesion and to avoid flushing the injectate off of the chondral surface.
- It is unknown if there is any advantage for this position (?approach) with other biologics besides MSCs.
- Use a smaller-gauge needle where possible to avoid damaging the cartilage. Guide the needle very slowly and barely touch down on the chondral surface. Make sure bevel is facing the surface to decrease chances of cartilage injury and inject directly on chondral surface.
- Contrast pool indicates extra-articular flow and the needle may need to be redirected.
- Aiming for the more anterior aspect of the condyle helps achieve a more diffuse flow along the cartilage surface.
- If treating a femoral osteochondral defect or cartilage defect using x-ray or previous diagnostic MRI, you can specifically aim for the defect to inject.
- Only use 1–3 mL of injectate here. Any extra can be placed intra-articular with traditional techniques.

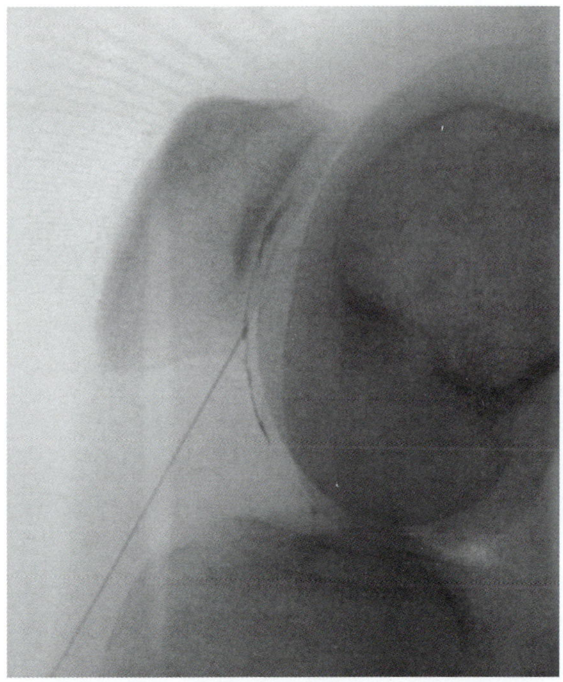

• **Fig. 21.47** Injection of weightbearing femoral chondral surface fluoroscopic lateral view.

Patellar Facets Intra-Articular: Medial and Lateral

KEY POINTS

- Direct targeting of patellar facets is optimal for patients with patellofemoral pain or chondral defects when targeting with cellular therapy.

Pertinent Anatomy

- The patellofemoral joint: the cartilaginous articulation between the undersurface of the patella and the trochlea
- The patella: it is composed of two main facets, medial and lateral, separated by a vertical ridge.[69] It is further subdivided into seven facets: three medial and three lateral that articulate with the femoral groove and an odd facet at the medial border that articulates with the medial femoral condyle in deep knee flexion due to patellar rotation in this position (Fig. 21.48A).[70,71]
- Vascular supply to the patella consists of the geniculate arteries: superolateral, inferolateral, superomedial, and inferomedial (see Fig. 21.48B).

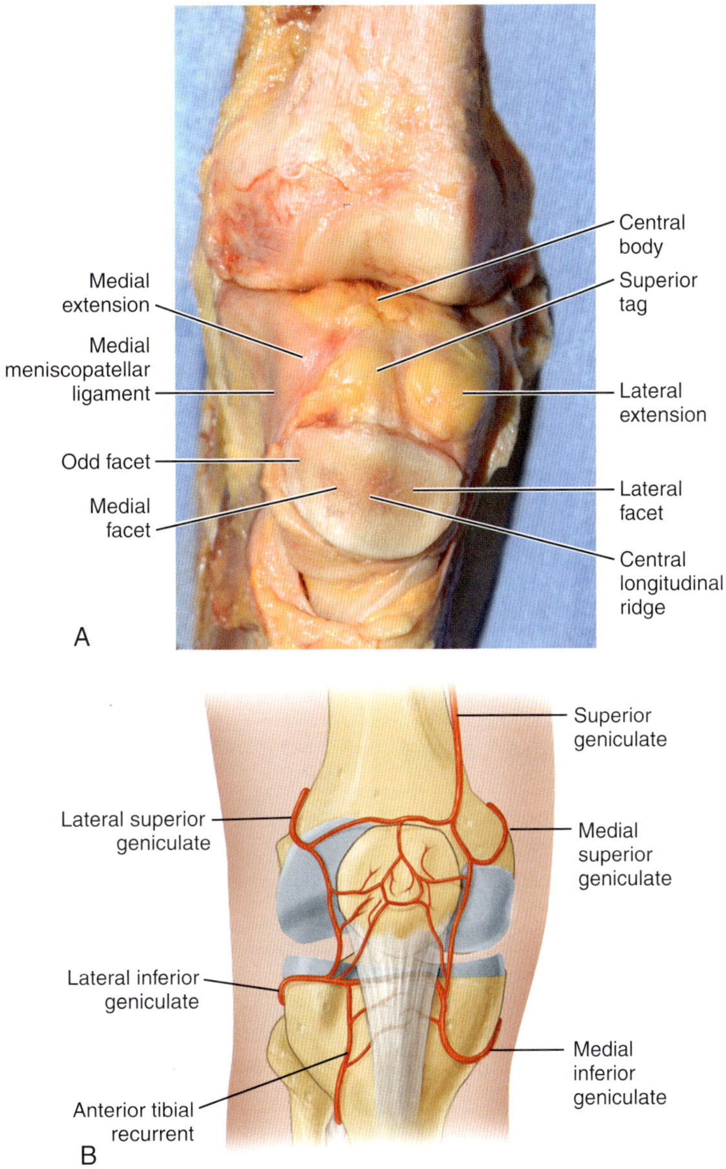

• **Fig. 21.48** (A) Patella. (B) Patella vascular supply. (*A*, Detterline A, Babb J, Noyes FR, et al. *Noyes' Knee Disorders: Surgery, Rehabilitation, Clinical Outcomes.* 2017:2–22. *B*, From Miller. *DeLee & Drez's Orthopaedic Sports Medicine.* 5th ed.)

Common Pathology

- Focal patellofemoral chondral defects
- Osteochondral defects
- Chondromalacia patellae
- Patellofemoral osteoarthritis

Equipment

- C-arm fluoroscopy
- 22 to 27 gauge 2 inch needle
- Contrast

Common Injectates

- Local anesthetics for diagnostics, corticosteroids, hyaluronic acid, prolotherapy, orthobiologics (PRP, bone marrow concentrate, micronized adipose tissue, etc.)

Injectate Volume

- 2 to 10 mL total

Technique

Patient Position

- Patient prone with pillows, block, or sheets placed under the hip flexors and under the chin. The goal is to elevate the knee a few inches above the bed/table (Fig. 21.49).

Clinician Position

- Standing on ipsilateral side of the patient.

C-Arm Position

- True lateral projection with femoral condyles aligned and clear visualization of the patellofemoral space. The C-arm will likely be angled rather than parallel to the floor, as elevating the knee as described will cause some external rotation of the leg.

- Anterior posterior view angling the beam to be parallel to posterior patellar surface.

Needle Position

- Palpate the superior lateral pole of the patella. Use your hand to push from the medial aspect of the patella to slide the patella laterally.
  - Start needle about 1 cm posterior/above the superior pole of the patella.
- Lateral patellar facet:
  - Needle will have steep trajectory aiming distal, medial, and inferior toward the lateral facet.
- Medial patellar facet:
  - Needle will have less steep trajectory. Aim just above the middle ridge of the patella.

Target

- Lateral patellar facet:
  - Target superior middle portion of the facet. In the lateral view, the needle will be just above the cartilage surface in the superior half of the patella.
  - Contract will flow along the patella surface proximal and distal with a linear appearance (Fig. 21.50).
  - In the AP view, the needle will be on the lateral patellar facet superior aspect. Contrast will spread in a slightly circular fashion from the needle tip (Fig. 21.51).
- Medial patellar facet:
  - Same approach as lateral but needle will continue to over superior middle portion of the medial facet. The middle ridge of the patella can block needle entry, and if contact is felt, redirect slightly above the ridge and then reangle back to the target.
  - In the AP view, the needle will be on the superior aspect of the medial patellar facet. Contrast will spread in slightly circular fashion from the needle tip

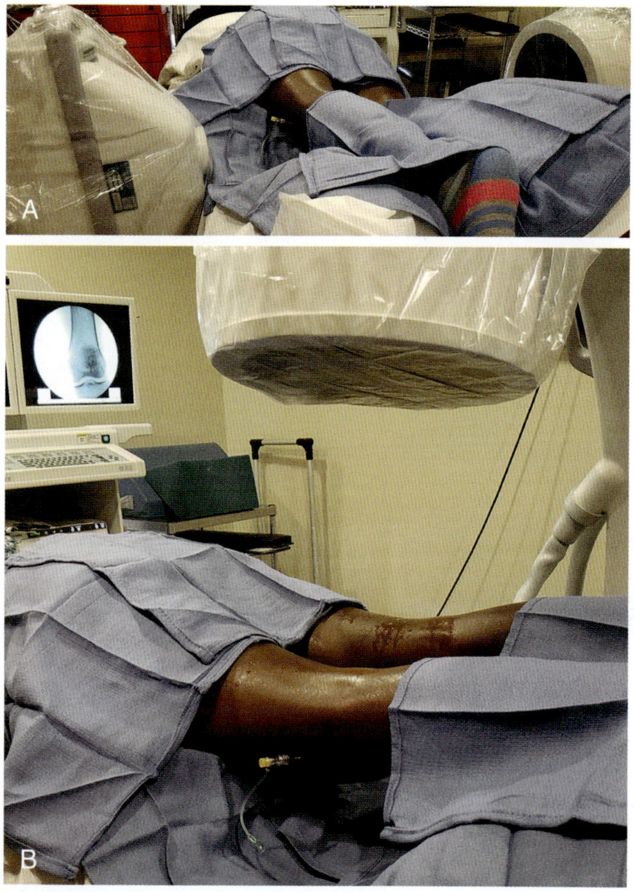

• **Fig. 21.49** (A) Patient positioning and lateral fluoroscopic setup. (B) Patient positioning and AP fluoroscopic setup.

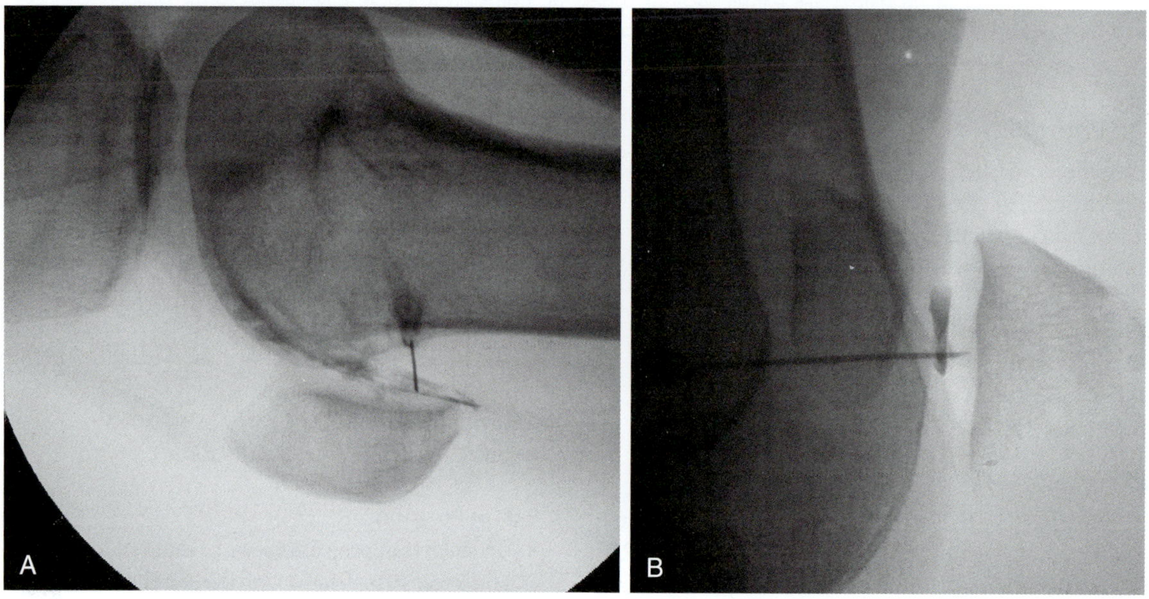

• **Fig. 21.50** Lateral patellar facet injection lateral fluoroscopic view with contrast.

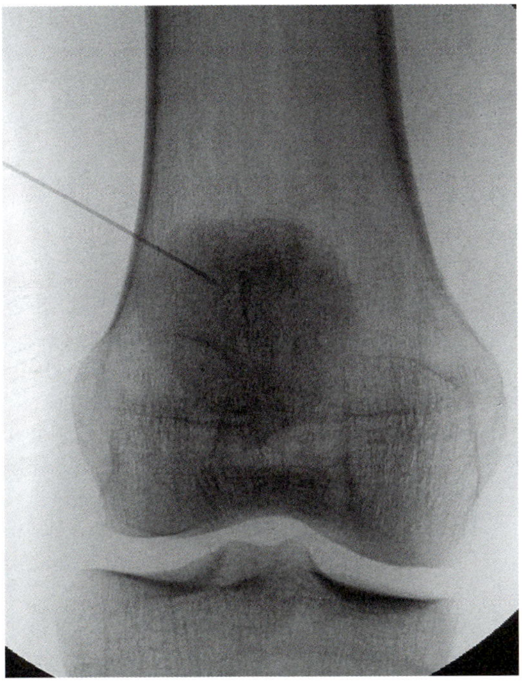

• **Fig. 21.51** Lateral patellar facet injection. AP fluoroscopic view with contrast.

PEARLS AND PITFALLS

- Proceduralist should pull the patella laterally; it can help to open the patellofemoral space to allow for ease of needle entry.
- The medial patellar facet injections are deeper, so the needle angle is different and usually less steep. Sometimes starting a little more superior to the patella will help avoid the middle ridge.
- Inject slowly to allow for possible adhesion of mesenchymal stem cells,

Tibiofibular Joint

KEY POINTS

- An often overlooked cause of lateral knee pain.
- Entire posterolateral corner needs evaluation when assessing for pain in this region.
- There is significant anatomic variability in the angulation of the proximal tibiofibular joint.

Pertinent Anatomy

See Ultrasound section.

Common Pathology

- Degenerative osteoarthritis or direct traumatic injury
- Ganglion cyst, which may or may not compress the common peroneal nerve
- PL corner injury with subsequent instability (requires co-treatment of surrounding injured/lax structures)

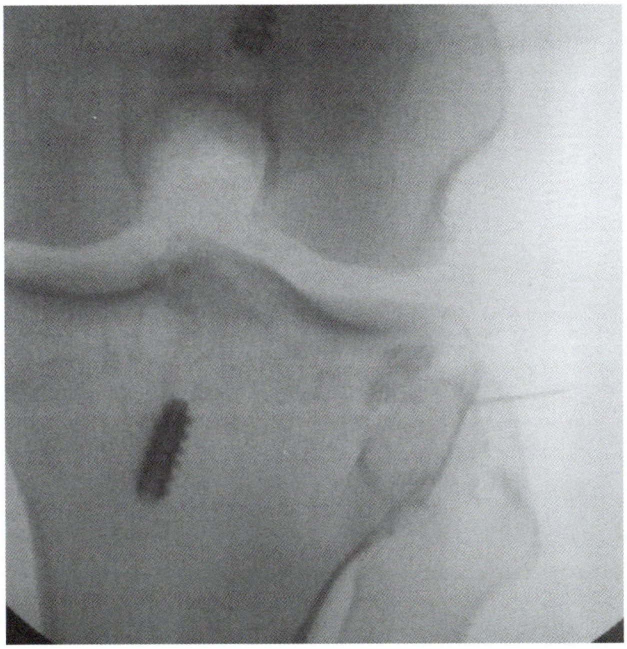

• **Fig. 21.52** Tibiofibular joint injection. AP fluoroscopy with contrast.

Equipment

- C-arm fluoroscopy
- 25 or 27 gauge 2 inch or 1.5 inch needle
- Contrast

Common Injectates

- Local anesthetics for diagnostics, corticosteroids, prolotherapy, orthobiologics (PRP, bone marrow concentrate, etc.).

Injectate Volume

- 2 to 10 mL total

Technique

Patient Position

- Supine with the knee in hook-lying (see Fig. 21.42)

Clinician Position

- Standing on ipsilateral side of the patient

C-Arm Position

- Anterior posterior projection with slight lateral oblique to open the joint
- Lateral view

Needle Position

- Palpate the fibular head. Start needle entry just superior and anterior to the fibular head.
- Aim posteriorly and slightly inferiorly.

Target

- In the AP view, needle should be a third to halfway in the joint space. Contrast should show medial and inferior flow inside the joint (Fig. 21.52).

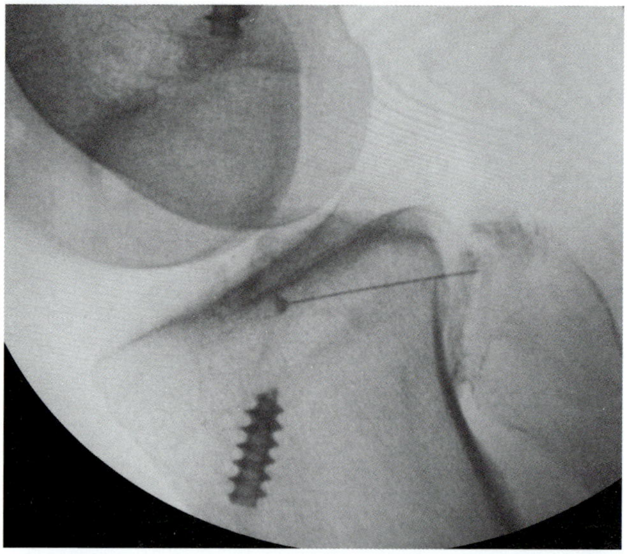

• **Fig. 21.53** Tibiofibular joint injection. Lateral fluoroscopy with contrast.

- In the lateral view, the needle should be halfway in the joint from anterior to posterior. Contrast should show a coin-shaped flow in the joint (Fig. 21.53).

PEARLS AND PITFALLS

- Enter just anterior and superior of the joint to avoid neovasculature.
- Check lateral view to avoid advancing too far posteriorly and to avoid peroneal nerve.
- If contrast is pooling, then adjust the needle to obtain better intra-articular flow.
- It is a small joint, so don't advance the needle more than halfway into the joint to prevent cartilage injury.

Anterior Cruciate Ligament

KEY POINTS

- There is evidence that partial to complete, non-retracted ACL tears can be healed with bone marrow concentrate.[72,73]
- Fluoroscopically guided ACL injection is the preferred technique for partial to complete non-retracted ACL tears.[72,73] It is necessary to treat both bundles, insertion, and origin, as well as mid substance tears if present.
- Ultrasound-guided ACL injections have been shown to reach the insertion, mid substance, and ACL origin[74]; however, fluoroscopy is the preferred method to confirm spread in real time and to readjust needle to achieve full coverage when tears are present.

Pertinent Anatomy

- Two bands of the ACL (Fig. 21.54A to D):
  1. AM bundle:
     - Insertion on medial tibial spine medial and anterior to the PL bundle
     - Origin on the lateral trochlea posterior relative to PL band with the knee in flexion and anterior when in extension in the majority of patients[75]
     - Function: controls AP translation (anterior drawer test/Lachman test)
     - Biomechanics: tight in 45 to 60 degrees of knee flexion
     - Connects with medial meniscal root
  2. PL bundle:
     - Insertion on the medial tibial spine lateral and posterior to the AM bundle
     - Origin on the lateral trochlea slightly posterior and proximal relative to the AM band when the knee is in extension and anterior and slightly distal when in flexion in many patients.[75] In the lateral fluoroscopic view, it is located posterior and distal to the marrow shadow of the femur (see Fig. 21.54D)
     - Function: controls AP translation (anterior drawer/Lachman test) and tibial rotation (pivot shift test, ACL dial)
     - Biomechanics: tight in extension
- ACL sheath: The ACL is surrounded by a synovial sheath shown to provide a protective role, and damage to which is associated with ACL degeneration.[76] The sheath prevents direct contact of synovial fluid with the ligament (Fig. 21.55).[77] The ACL, therefore, lies within the joint capsule, but separated from the synovial membrane.[78]

Common Pathology

- ACL laxity, partial tear, non-retracted full tear, or full tear that is approximated and retracted less than 1 cm.
- Acute ACL tears are more common in women, are associated with cutting sports and valgus stress or hyperextension injury, and are associated with biomechanical imbalance secondary to quadriceps dominance.[79]

Equipment

- C-arm fluoroscopy
- 25 gauge 3,5 inch needle
- Contrast

Common Injectates

- Prolotherapy, orthobiologics (PRP, bone marrow concentrate, etc.).

Injectate Volume

- 1 to 2 mL total

Technique

Patient Position

- Supine hook lying (see Fig. 21.42)

Clinician Position

- Ipsilateral to the side of the patient

C-Arm Position

- True anterior posterior projection where anterior and posterior femur and tibia are aligned.

- Lateral projection where medial and lateral femoral condyles and medial and lateral tibial plateaus are aligned.

Needle Position

- In true AP fluoroscopic view, needle should be centered between the tibial spines.
- Needle will travel through the patella tendon, Hoffa's fat pad, and the anterior joint capsule into the ACL.

Target/Injection Techniques

- Target the ACL insertion, then move on to target origin, and possibly mid portion depending on contrast spread.
- ACL insertion, AM bundle:
  - Palpate the patella. The needle will enter just below the patella.
  - In true AP fluoroscopic view, needle should be centered between the tibial spines.
  - In AP view, advance needle about 1 cm, aiming posterior and inferior, making sure needle is staying in the middle of the tibial spines.
  - Angle should be fairly steep relative to the knee.
  - Advance further in the lateral view to the insertional target.
  - Guide the needle to the tibial plateau just anterior to the medial tibial eminence.
  - Inject a small amount of contrast in the lateral view, which should show flow superior and posterior along the distal to mid ACL fibers. Sometimes flow can go all the way to the proximal portion (Fig. 21.56).

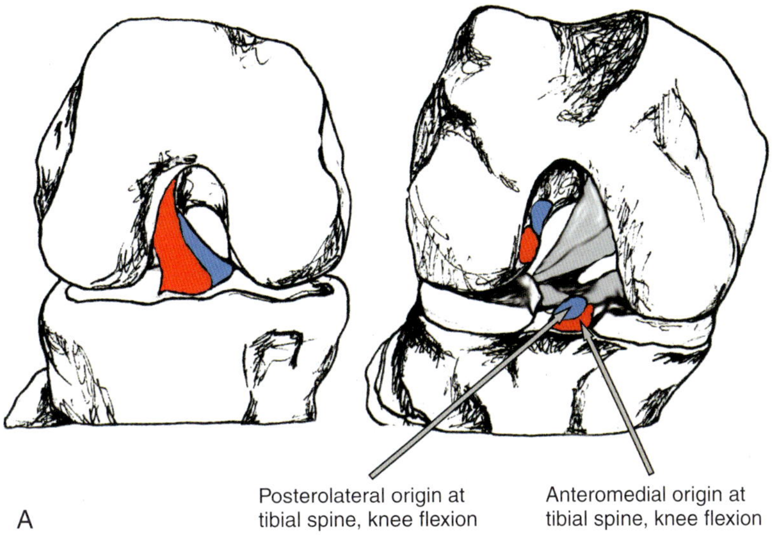

A

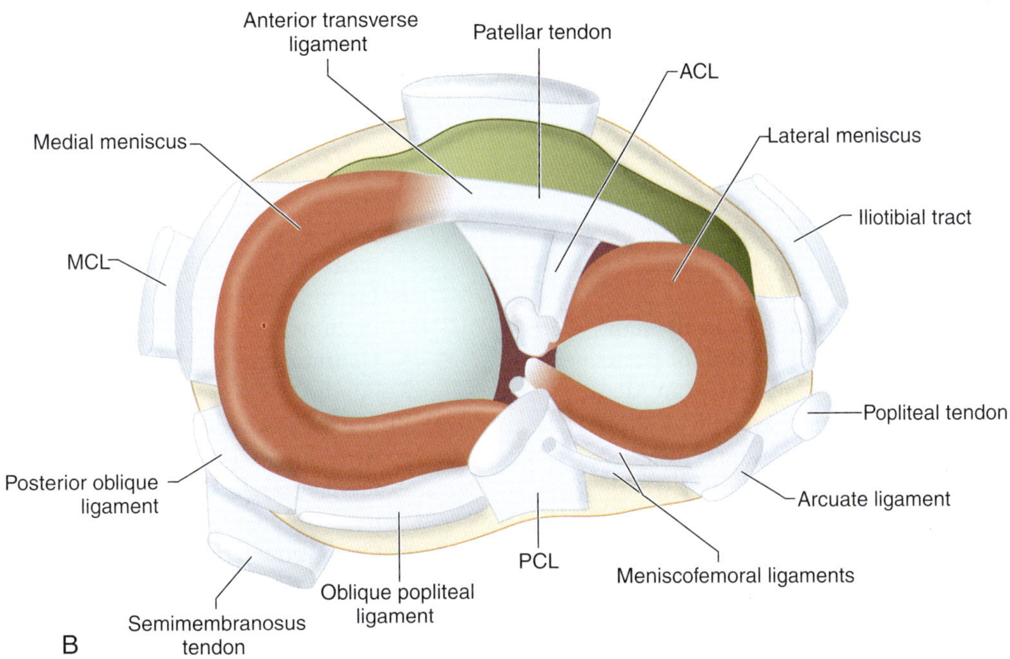

B

• **Fig. 21.54** Anterior Cruciate Ligament Anatomy. (A) ACL coronal. (B) *ACL* insertions transverse. *ACL*, Anterior cruciate ligament; *MCL*, medial collateral ligament; *PCL*, posterior cruciate ligament.

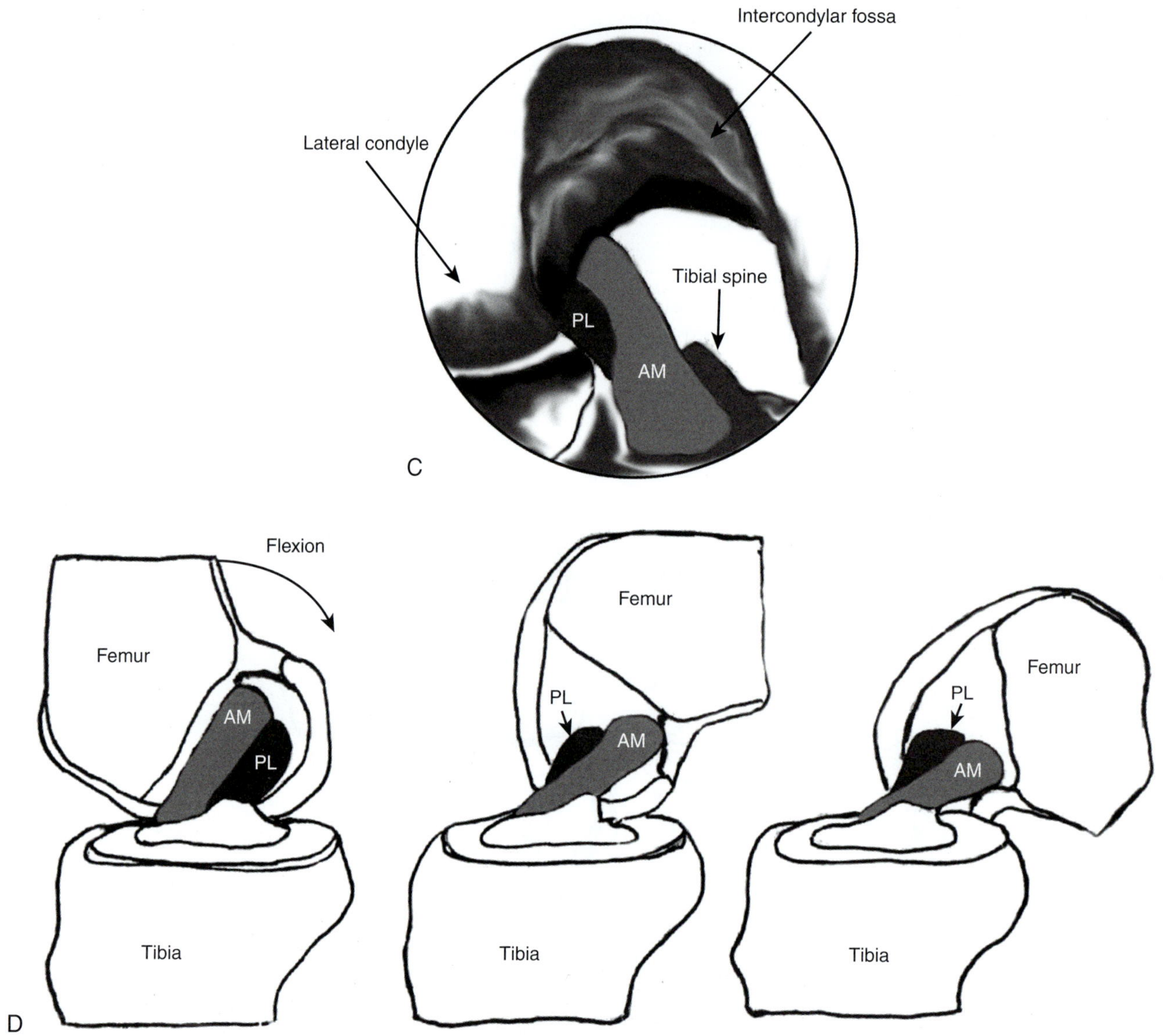

•Fig. 21.54—cont'd (C) ACL bundles from AP with knee in flexion. (D) ACL bundles in extension and flexion, sagittal view. *AM,* Anteromedial bundle, *PL,* posterolateral bundle. (B, From Tafur M, Bencardino JT, et al. *Insall & Scott Surgery of the Knee.* 2018;133–160.e3.)

- If contrast is pooling, then the needle is likely anterior to the ligament, and the needle needs to advance posteriorly.
- If the contrast spreads diffusely in the joint, then the needle is either lateral, medial, or posterior to the ACL. Recheck needle placement in AP.
- Confirm in the AP view as well to show contrast going superior and lateral (Fig. 21.57). Sometimes contrast will additionally flow into the medial > lateral meniscus via connection to the transverse ligament, which can be seen in the AP view.
- Sometimes contrast flow will appear as one large single band; sometimes the bands clearly appear separate.

- AM bundle insertion:
  - With a curved needle tip, turn the needle slightly medially but still just anterior to the tibial spine.
  - Insertion point is slightly anterior and medial to PL bundle.
  - Contrast flow is at a shallower angle than the PL bundle.
- PL bundle insertion:
  - After injecting the AM bundle, turn the curved needle laterally and head slightly posterior (1 to 2 mm) and inject the PL bundle.
  - Contrast flow is at a slightly steeper angle compared to the AM bundle.
- ACL lorigin:
  - Palpate the patella. This time the needle will enter about 1cm below the patella or midway between the patella and the tibia.

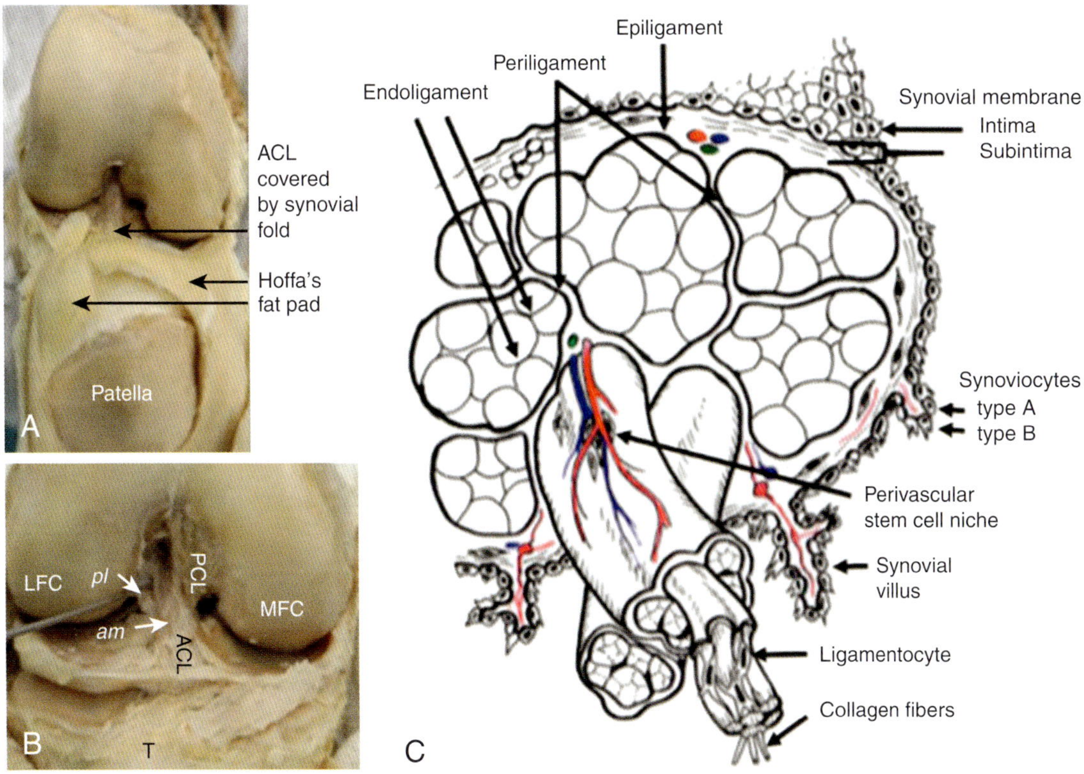

• **Fig. 21.55** ACL Dissection, Sheath, and Blood Supply. (From Schulze-Tanzil G. Intra-articular ligament degeneration is interrelated with cartilage and bone destruction in osteoarthritis. *Cells.* 2019;8:990 with permission.)

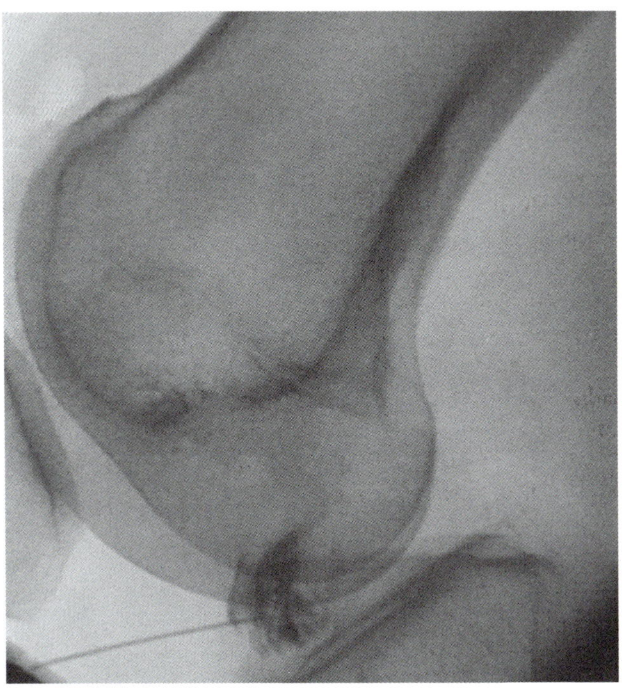

• **Fig. 21.56** Distal ACL Insertion Injection Lateral Fluoroscopy with Contrast Showing Double Bundle Flow.

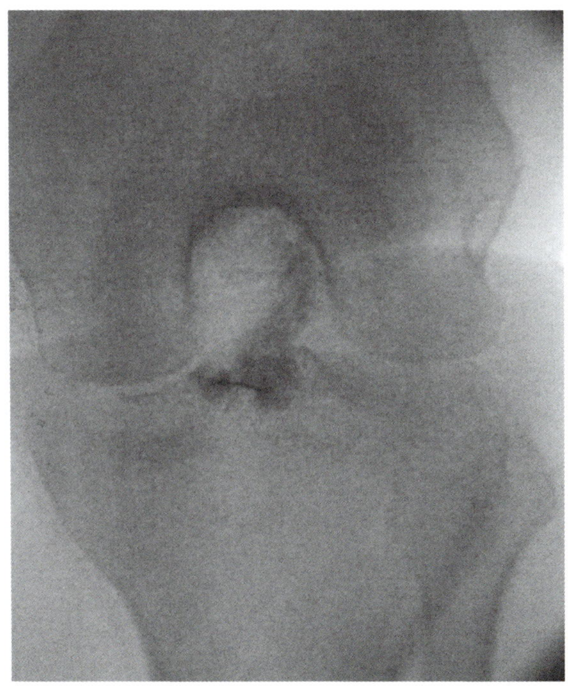

• **Fig. 21.57** Distal ACL Insertion Injection AP Fluoroscopy with Contrast.

- In true AP fluoroscopic view, needle should be centered between the tibial spines.
- In AP view, advance needle about 1 cm, aiming toward the superolateral femoral trochlea.
- Angle will be slightly upwards.
- Advance further in the lateral view gently towards the mid lateral superior trochlear bone.
- The needle should touch down on bone in the anterior half of the medial wall of the lateral femoral condyle.

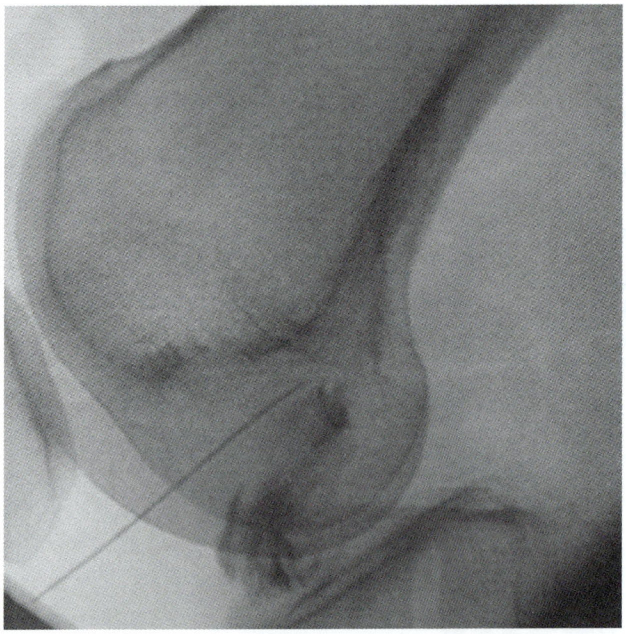

• **Fig. 21.58** Proximal ACL Injection Fluoroscopy Lateral View with Contrast Connecting to Distal ACL.

Then "walk" off the trochlea, aiming posterior to the ACL origin at the posterior superior aspect of the lateral femoral trochlea. Use fluoroscopy to ensure the needle does not advance posterior to the femur. The needle should be at or just 1 mm off the bone.

- Inject a small amount of contrast in the lateral view, which should show flow inferior and anterior along the posterior to mid ACL fibers. The contrast should head toward or connect with contrast flow from insertional injection (Fig. 21.58).
  - If contrast is pooling and not flowing along the ACL fibers or flowing diffusely into the joint, then the needle is likely medial to the ligament, and the needle needs to be adjusted laterally.
- In the AP view, confirm contrast spread inferior, medial, and connecting with contrast flow from insertional injection (Fig. 21.59).
- AM and PL bundles:
  - In the flexed position, the AM bundle is taut, and the origin appears more posterior and inferior on the femur. To target, adjust the curved needle posteriorly in the lateral view.
  - In the flexed position, the PL bundle is lax, and the origin appears more anterior and superior on the femur. To target ,adjust curved needle and direct anteriorly in the lateral view.

- ACL mid portion: target the mid portion of the ACL if there is a specific tear hear on MRI, there is diffuse tearing throughout the ACL, or if contrast flows from the insertion and origin does not completely fill the mid portion of the ACL.
  - In the AP view, start needle entry in the middle of the ACL insertions and origin that should be filled with contrast.
  - Start the needle about ½ to 1 cm below the patella.
  - Advance about 1 cm to make sure the needle is on this trajectory.
  - Should have a less steep angle than the insertion technique.
  - In the lateral view, advance posteriorly to the mid portion of contrast from previous injections at the insertion and origin.
  - Inject a tiny amount of contrast to confirm flow in the mid portion of the ACL in the lateral and confirm in the AP view.
  - Turn and redirect the needle 1 to 2 mm medial, lateral, and superior inferior to make sure to pick up both bands.

PEARLS AND PITFALLS

- Be sure to visualize the patient's ACL on MRI prior to the procedure to notice any anatomic variations and get a better idea of ACL insertion, origin, and mid substance tear characteristics and help predict contrast flow.
- The ACL bundles run parallel to each other in full knee extension where the anteromedial (AM) bundle is lax and the posterolateral (PL) bundle is relatively taut. However, these procedures are done with the knee in 90–120 degrees of flexion. In flexion the mid sections slightly cross as the AM bundle is taut, and the PL bundle is relatively lax. This makes the PL origin appear more anterior and superior, and the AM origin appear more posterior and inferior.
- A slight bend in the needle tip makes it easier to make slight adjustments and redirect the needle tip into multiple areas of the ligament.
- There is a great deal of variation in individual anatomy,[75] so use contrast flow to guide needle placement.
- If you cannot get complete flow from the tibial insertion to femur, then you must also inject the femoral origins.
- Inject both AM and PL bundle for optimal treatment, need to see two-directional flow, otherwise both bundles were not reached.
- In some ACLs with partial healing prior to injection, stump formation can occur. In these cases, needle fenestration of the stump is recommended to encourage fiber growth through the fibrous tissue of the stump.
- Full remodeling of the ACL can take between 6 and 12 months (shorter time periods for younger patients). Repeat MRI at 3-month intervals can show progressing, positive healing. Obtain ACL sagittal and/or coronal oblique views to image better.
- May need to also inject transverse ligament if there is anterior meniscal root instability in association with ACL injury.
- Often can get spread into anterior horns of the lateral and medial menisc; so if also targeting here, watch for contrast flow to add additional injectate.

Anterior Cruciate Graft

KEY POINTS

- Treatment for partial tears only, not complete or retracted. Must have visible intact fibers.
- Similar approach to regular ACL, but look for the graft tunnels to guide needle placement.
- Try to angle inside the tunnel, if possible.

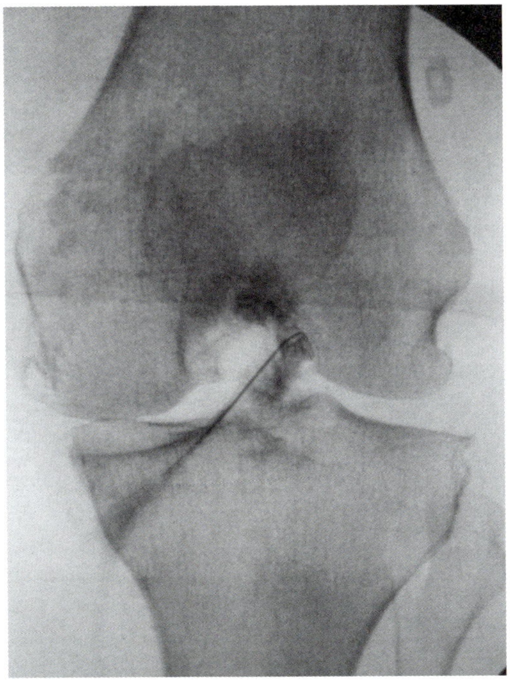

• **Fig. 21.59** Proximal ACL Origin Injection AP Fluoroscopy with Contrast.

Pertinent Anatomy

- Femoral and tibial tunnels with screws to hold them in place.
- Of note, ACL grafts are not contained within a synovial sheath, as is the case with native ACL.

Common Pathology

- Complete or incomplete tears of ACL graft. ACL graft rupture rates range from approximately 2% to 10%.[80]

Equipment

- C-arm fluoroscopy
- 25 gauge 3.5 inch needle
- Contrast

Common Injectates

- Prolotherapy orthobiologics (PRP, bone marrow concentrate, etc.)

Injectate Volume

- 1 to 2 mL total

Technique

Patient Position

- Hook-lying position (see Fig. 21.42)

Clinician Position

- Standing ipsilateral to the side of the patient

Transducer Position or C-Arm Position Fluoro Technique

- Start with AP projection, transition between lateral and AP as needed for needle guidance

Needle Position

- Have a slight bend in the needle tip to make it easier to make slight adjustments injecting multiple areas of the ligament and for redirection.
- Start with targeting the graft tunnel insertion; then target the origin and possible mid portion.
- In true AP fluoroscopic view, needle should be centered (medial/lateral) between the graft tunnel outline.
- Needle will travel through the patella tendon, Hoffa's fat pad, and the anterior joint capsule.

Target

- Follow same step as the ACL with the below adjustments:
- ACL graft orientation, insertion, and origin sites will vary between surgical technique used.
- However, graft tunnels can easily be seen on x-ray to be used as landmarks.
- For the insertional and origin techniques, instead of using set anatomic landmarks, aim directly for the graft tunnel entries on the tibial and femur respectively.
- The majority of grafts are single bundle so no need to consider double bundle techniques.
- Inject the graft thoroughly by redirecting the needle at each site (insertion, origin, mid portion) 1 to 2 mm as able to get full coverage of the graft (Figs. 21.60–21.62).

PEARLS AND PITFALLS

- Use the surgical tunnels as guides for needle placement.
- If possible, try to get needle into the tunnels.
- Redirect needle as much as possible to obtain complete coverage.

Posterior Cruciate Ligament

KEY POINTS

- Biologic injections to treat posterior cruciate ligament (PCL) laxity or tear (partial or complete non-retracted).
- If partial tearing of the PCL, be sure to at least inject origin and insertion. Mid portion if tears there on MRI.

Pertinent Anatomy

- Inserts at posterior tibial plateau with the origin at the anterior wall of the medial femoral trochlea.
- Ligament of Wrisberg (posterior meniscofemoral ligament) attaches to the posterior area of the lateral meniscus and crosses superiorly and medially behind the posterior cruciate ligament to attach to the medial condyle of the femur. This ligament is present in up to 90% of patients and can be confused with the PCL (Fig. 21.63).[81]

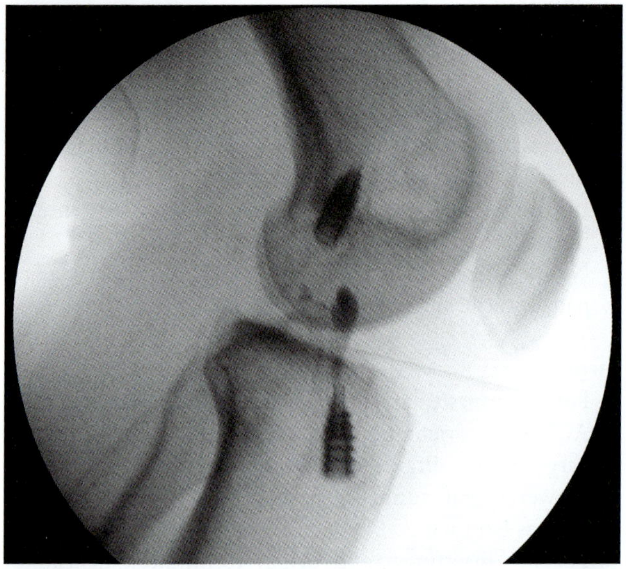

• **Fig. 21.60** Distal ACL Graft Injection Lateral Fluoroscopic View with Contrast.

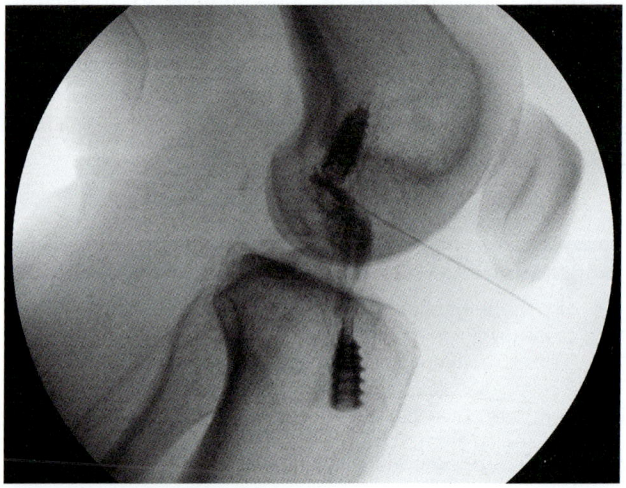

• **Fig. 21.61** Proximal ACL Graft Injection Lateral Fluoroscopic View with Contrast.

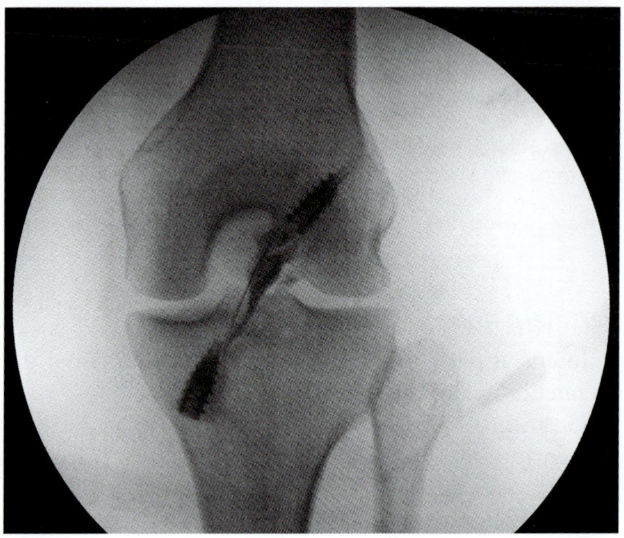

• **Fig. 21.62** Proximal ACL Graft Injection AP Fluoroscopic View with Contrast.

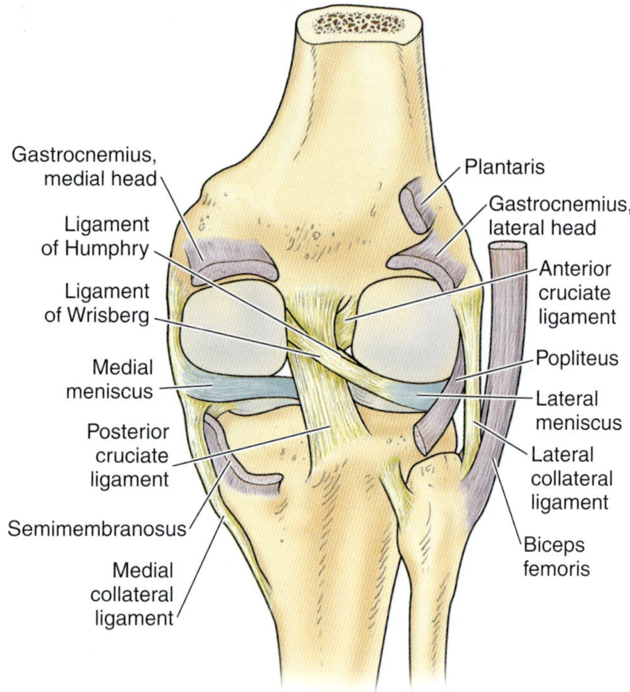

• **Fig 21.63** PCL. (From Clarke HD, Kransdorf MJ, Conley, et al. *Insall & Scott Surgery of the Knee*. 2018;2–49.e3.)

- Two bundles: anterolateral bundle and posteromedial bundle.[82]

Common Pathology

- Lax PCL due to:
  - Trauma, via hyperextension mechanism in sports and most commonly from motor vehicle accidents from direct blow to the tibia with a bent knee.[82]
  - Long-term weakness in the quadriceps with resultant hyperextension to lock the knee.

Equipment

- C-arm fluoroscopy
- 25 gauge 3.5 inch needle
- Contrast

Common Injectates

- Prolotherapy, orthobiologics (PRP, bone marrow concentrate, etc.).

Injectate Volume

- 1 to 2 mL total

Technique

Patient Position

- Supine hook-lying (120 degrees flexion) (see Fig. 21.42).

Clinician Position

- Standing ipsilateral to the side of the patient

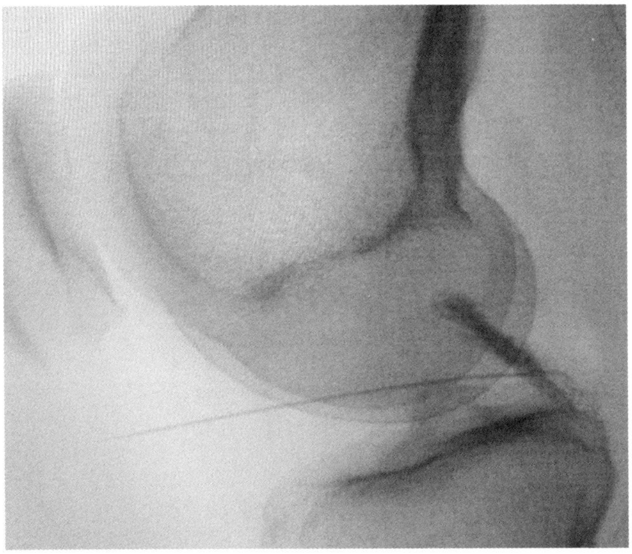

• **Fig. 21.64** Distal PCL Injection Fluoroscopy Lateral View with Contrast.

C-Arm Position

- AP to start and transition to lateral.

Needle Position

- Have a slight bend in the needle tip to make it easier to make slight adjustments when injecting multiple areas of the ligament and for redirection.
- Start with targeting the PCL origin at the posterior tibial plateau; then target insertion on lateral wall of the femoral condyle.
- In true AP fluoroscopic view, needle should be centered between the tibial spines.
- Needle will travel through the patella tendon, Hoffa's fat pad, and the anterior joint capsule.

Target

- PCL origin at tibia:
  - Palpate the patella. The needle will enter just below the patella.
  - In true AP fluoroscopic view, needle should be centered between the tibial spines.
  - In AP view, advance needle about 1 cm, aiming posterior and inferior, making sure needle is staying in the middle of the tibial spines.
  - Angle will be slightly inferior.
  - Advance in the lateral view to the origin of the PCL at posterior tibia about ½ cm anterior to the posterior tibial wall. Be sure not to advance past the femur.
  - Inject a small amount of contrast in the lateral view, which should show flow going superior and anterior (Fig. 21.64). Often flow can go all the way to the proximal portion.
  - If the contrast spreads diffusely in the joint, then the needle is either lateral, medial, or posterior. Recheck needle placement in AP.
  - Confirm in the AP view to show contrast going superior and medial (Fig.21.65).

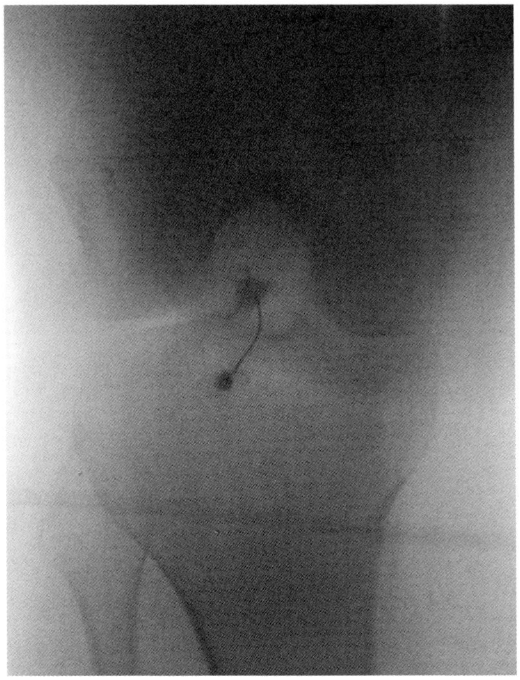

• **Fig. 21.65** Distal PCL Injection Fluoroscopy AP View with contrast.

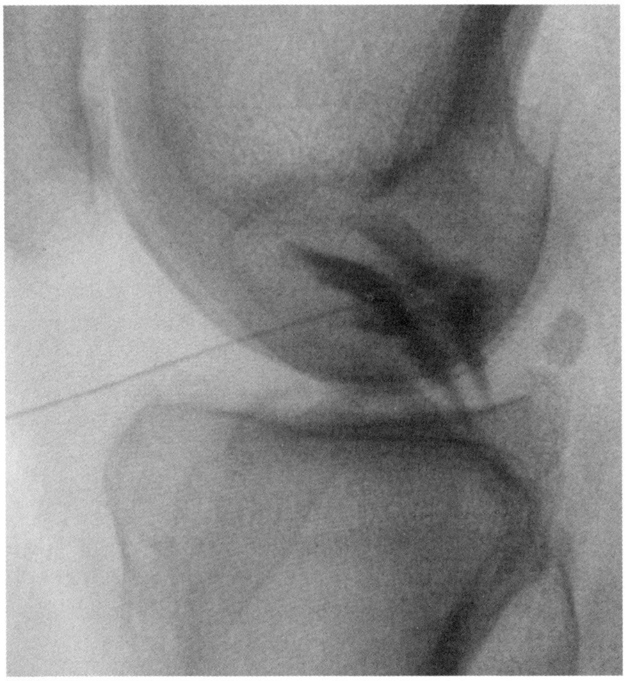

• **Fig. 21.66** PCL Injection Showing Double Bundle Contrast Flow.

  - Rarely you can visualize two bundles in the PCL (Fig. 21.66).
- PCL insertion on the femur:
  - Palpate the patella. This time the needle will enter about 1 cm below the patella or midway between the patella and the tibia.
  - In true AP fluoroscopic view, needle should be centered between the tibial spines.
  - In AP view, advance needle about 1 cm, aiming toward the superior lateral femoral trochlea.

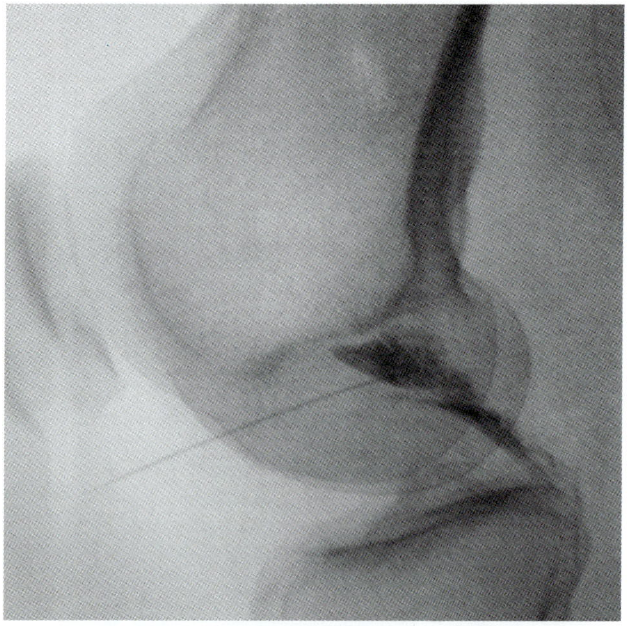

• **Fig. 21.67** Proximal PCL Injection Fluoroscopy Lateral View with Contrast Connecting to Distal Portion.

- Angle will be slightly upwards.
- Advance further in the lateral view slightly toward the anterior, superior medial femur.
- The needle should touch down on the bone in the anterior third of the lateral wall of the medial femoral condyle. Then "walk" off the trochlea, aiming posterior to the PCL origin at the middle superior aspect of the medial femoral trochlea. Needle should be at or just 1 mm off the bone.
- Inject a small amount of contrast in the lateral view, which should show flow going inferior and posterior toward the posterior tibial plateau (Fig. 21.67).
- If contrast is pooling and not flowing along the PCL fibers or flowing diffusely into the joint, then the needle is likely anterior or medial to the ligament.
- Confirm in the AP view to show contrast going inferior and lateral (Fig. 21.68).

• PCL mid portion: target the mid substance of the PCL if there is diffuse tearing throughout the PCL on MRI or if contrast flow does not completely fill the mid substance of the PCL.

- In the AP view, start needle entry in the middle of the tibial spines.
- Start the needle about 1 cm below the patella.
- Advance about 1 cm to make sure the needle is on this trajectory.
- Should have minimal angle on the needle.
- In the lateral view, advance posteriorly to the mid height between the femur and the tibia. Target is posterior one-third of the joint. Should be in mid portion of contrast flow from the origin and insertion.
- Inject a tiny amount of contrast to confirm flow in the mid portion of the PCL in the lateral view and confirm in the AP view.

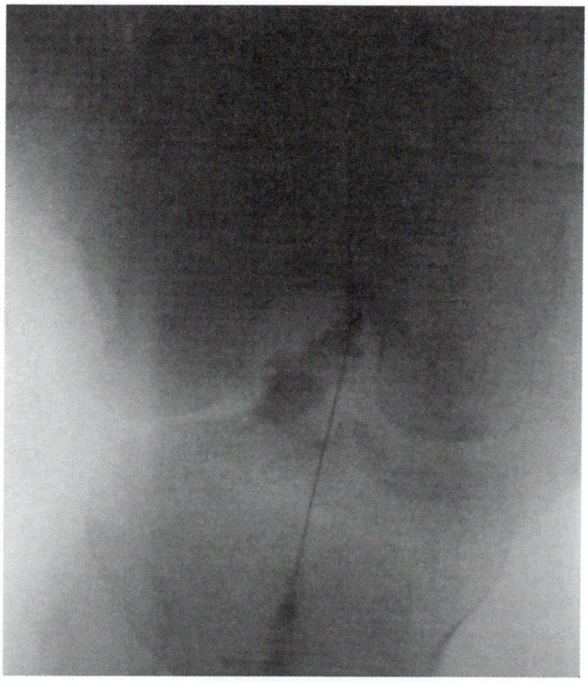

• **Fig. 21.68** Proximal PCL Injection Fluoroscopy AP View with Contrast Connecting to Distal Portion.

PEARLS AND PITFALLS

- Be sure to start the needle trajectory at the true middle of trochlea, not the center of the patella, since patellae are often deviated laterally.

Meniscus

KEY POINTS

- There may be the advantage of going through less meniscal tissue and theoretically less risk of injury.
- Contrast flow can confirm specific targets are injected accurately.
- It may be an easier route to inject micronized adipose tissue to reduce trauma to the meniscus as usually a larger-gauge needle is required.

Pertinent Anatomy

- Medial and lateral.
- Anterior horn, body, and posterior horn.
- Red, red/white, white zones:
  - Red periphery zone rich in vasculature.
  - Inner white zone with no blood supply, nutrition vis diffusion only.
  - Middle red/white zone: transition between vascular and avascular areas.
- Meniscal ligaments (can be variable within patients[21]):
  - Coronary ligaments (meniscotibial),[22] which act to anchor the menisci to the tibia both anteriorly and posteriorly.[23,24]

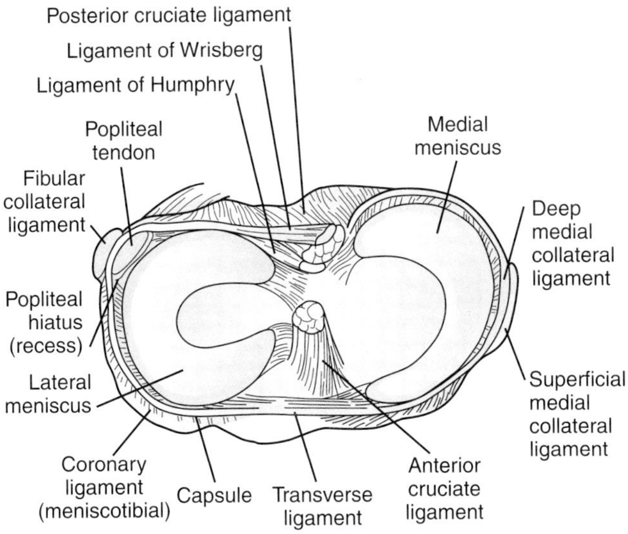

• **Fig. 21.69** Meniscal Ligaments. (From Parvizi J, Kim GK, et al. *High-Yield Orthopaedics*. 2010;292–293.)

- Posterior meniscofemoral ligament (ligament of Wrisberg) connects the posterior horn of the lateral meniscus to the medial femoral condyle and the PCL.[25]
- Anterior meniscofemoral ligament (ligament of Humphry) connects posterior horn of lateral meniscus, but lies anterior to the PCL and inserts at the femoral PCL.[25]
- Anterior intermeniscal ligament, which connects the anterior horns of the medial and lateral menisci (Fig. 21.69)[25]
- Deep MCLs (meniscofemoral and meniscotibial) are deep to the MCL and are with the medial meniscus, connecting it via longitudinal fibers to the femur and the tibia.[83]
- Root attachments:
  - The medial meniscus posterior root attachment is PL to the medial tibial eminence.
  - The lateral meniscus root attachment is posterior and medial to the lateral tibial eminence.
  - The medial meniscus anterior root attachment is AM to the ACL tibial insertion and inserts into the anterior intercondylar crest of the tibia.
  - The lateral meniscus anterior root is anterolateral to the ACL tibial insertion.[26,27]

Common Pathology

- Medial meniscus tears can occur in the anterior portion, body, posterior portion, or root and can have the following types of morphologies: radial (associated with meniscal extrusion), horizontal (parallel to tibial plateau), vertical (perpendicular to tibial plateau), flap (horizontal or oblique fissures with displacement), bucket handle, or complex (combination).[25,28]
- Medial meniscus posterior horn tears are commonly associated with ACL injury,[23] as are lateral meniscus root tears.[27]
- Injury to the posterior medial meniscus coronary ligament is associated with increased tibial internal rotation.[23]
- Horizontal and oblique tears are more commonly asymptomatic. Vertical, complex, radial, and displaced tears have a stronger association with pain and are generally more clinically meaningful.[29]

Equipment

- C-arm fluoroscopy
- 23 to 18 gauge needle depending on injectate, 3 to 3.5 inch length
- Contrast

Common Injectates

- Prolotherapy orthobiologics (PRP, bone marrow concentrate, micronized adipose tissue, etc.)

Injectate Volume

- 1 to 2 mL total

Technique

Patient Position

- Supine hook-lying

Clinician Position

- Standing on ipsilateral side of the patient.

Transducer Position or C-Arm Position Fluoro Technique

- True AP projection, where anterior and posterior femur and tibia are aligned.
- Lateral projection, where medial and lateral femoral condyles and medial and lateral tibial plateaus are aligned.

Needle Position

- MRI imaging should help guide needle starting point. Needle should start over the peripheral edge of the desired tibial plateau using AP projection to identify needle entry point in the sagittal plane.
- Then, in lateral position, start needle entry about 1 cm above the tibial plateau.
- Under intermittent fluoroscopy, advance needle from superior to inferior, anterior to posterior toward the desired area of the meniscus.
- Avoid hitting the femoral condyle articular cartilage.

Target

- Medial meniscus
  - Anterior horn:
    - Aim to gently touch down on the medial meniscus just above the tibial plateau at the depth of the anterior tibial spine on the lateral view.
    - Inject a tiny amount of contrast to confirm.
    - Contrast in lateral should spread anterior and slightly posterior above the tibial surface.
    - In the AP view, be sure the needle is over the tibia and has not traveled too medial outside the joint or too lateral on the tibial plateau.

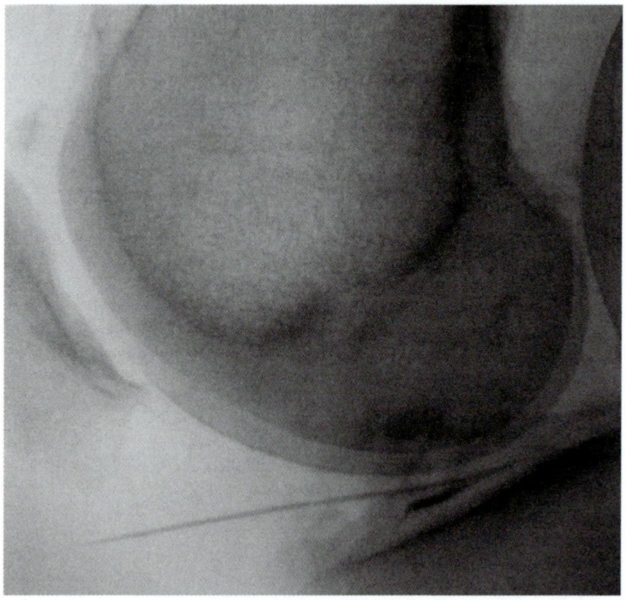

• **Fig. 21.70** Medial Meniscus Body Lateral Fluoroscopy View with Contrast Showing Flow to the Anterior Horn Also.

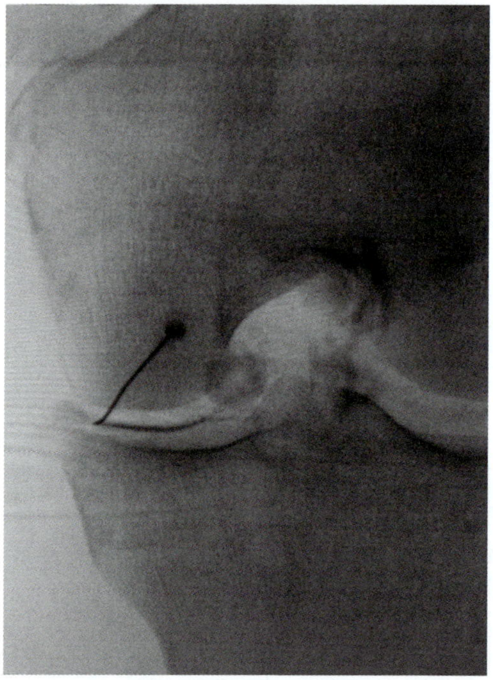

• **Fig. 21.71** Medial Meniscus Body AP Fluoroscopy View with Contrast.

- Contrast in AP should be spread laterally across the anterior horn.
- Body:
  - Aim to gently touch down on the medial meniscus just above the tibial plateau at the depth of the mid portion of the tibial spine on the lateral view.
  - Contrast in lateral should spread slightly anterior and posterior above the tibial surface (see Fig. 21.70).
  - In the AP view, be sure the needle is over the tibia and has not traveled too medially outside the joint or too laterally on the tibial plateau.
  - Contrast in AP should be just over periphery of the tibia. There may be some faint spread to anterior or posterior horn (see Fig. 21.71).
- Posterior horn:
  - Aim to gently touch down on the medial meniscus just above the tibial plateau at the depth of the posterior edge of the tibial spine on the lateral view.
  - You may need to start needle ½ cm lower to get increased depth into the joint.
  - Inject a tiny amount of contrast to confirm.
  - Contrast in lateral should spread anterior and slightly posterior above the tibial surface (Fig. 21.72).
  - In the AP view, be sure the needle is over the tibia and has not traveled too medially outside the joint or too laterally on the tibial plateau (Fig. 21.73).
  - Contrast in AP should be spread laterally across the posterior horn but look similar to anterior horn spread.
- Root:
  - Instead of starting over the medial aspect of the tibial wall, start just medial to the medial tibial spine in the AP view.

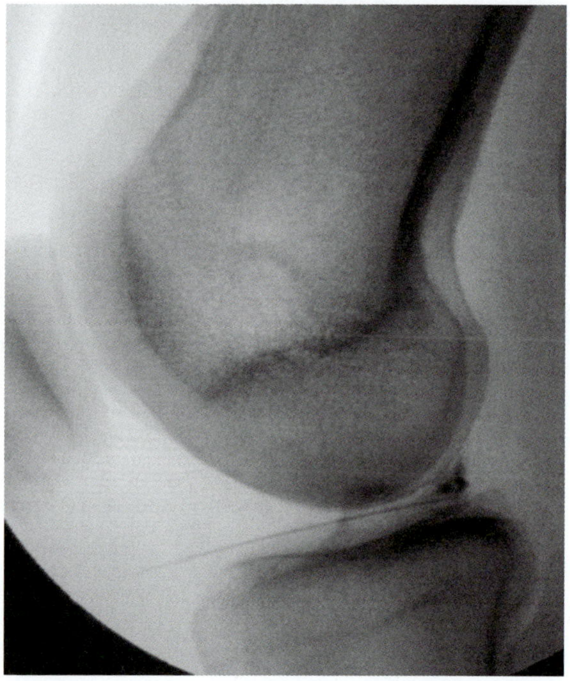

• **Fig. 21.72** Posterior Medial Meniscus Lateral Fluoroscopy View with Contrast.

  - Aim to gently touch down on the medial meniscus root just above the tibial plateau at the depth just posterior to the tibial spine on the lateral view.
  - You may need to start needle ½ cm lower to get increased depth into the joint.
  - Inject a tiny amount of contrast to confirm.

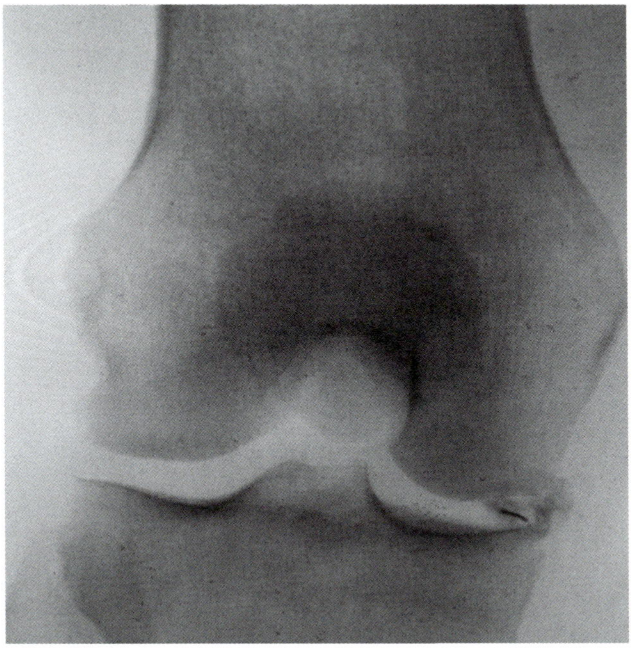

• **Fig. 21.73** Posterior Medial Meniscus AP Fluoroscopy View with Contrast.

        - Contrast in lateral should spread only slightly and stay mostly posteriorly above the tibial surface. Fig. 21.74
        - In the AP view, be sure the needle is just medial to the tibial spines.
        - Contrast in AP should be spread laterally across the posterior horn and root but look similar to anterior horn spread (Figure 21.74).
- Lateral meniscus
    - Anterior horn:
        - Aim to gently touch down on the lateral meniscus just above the tibial plateau at the depth of the anterior tibial spine on the lateral view.
        - Inject a tiny amount of contrast to confirm.
        - Contrast in lateral should spread anterior and slightly posterior above the tibial surface.
        - In the AP view, be sure the needle is over the tibia and has not traveled too laterally outside the joint or too medially on the tibial plateau.
        - Contrast in AP should be spread medially across the anterior horn.
    - Body:
        - Aim to gently touch down on the lateral meniscus just above the tibial plateau at the depth of the mid portion of the tibial spine on the lateral view.
        - Contrast in lateral should spread slightly anterior and posterior above the tibial surface.
        - In the AP view, be sure the needle is over the tibia and has not traveled too laterally outside the joint or too medially on the tibial plateau.
        - Contrast in AP should be just over periphery of the tibia. There may be some faint spread to anterior or posterior horn.
    - Posterior horn:
        - Aim to gently touch down on the lateral meniscus just above the tibial plateau at the depth of the posterior edge tibial spine on the lateral view.
        - May need to start needle ½ cm lower to get increased depth into the joint.
        - Inject a tiny amount of contrast to confirm.
        - Contrast in lateral should spread anterior and slightly posterior above the tibial surface.
        - In the AP view, be sure the needle is over the tibia and has not traveled too laterally outside the joint or too medially on the tibial plateau.
        - Contrast in AP should be spread medially across the posterior horn but look similar to anterior horn spread.
    - Root:
        - Instead of starting over the lateral aspect of the tibial wall, start just lateral to the lateral tibial spine in the AP view.
        - Aim to gently touch down on the lateral meniscus root just above the tibial plateau at the depth just posterior to the tibial spine on the lateral view.
        - You may need to start needle ½ cm lower to get increased depth into the joint.
        - Inject a tiny amount of contrast to confirm.
        - Contrast in lateral should spread only slightly and stay mostly posterior above the tibial surface.
        - In the AP view, be sure the needle is just lateral to the lateral tibial spine.
        - Contrast in AP should be spread medially across the posterior horn and root but look similar to anterior horn spread.

PEARLS AND PITFALLS

- The meniscus is dense; so there can be quite a bit of resistance. Torn areas may be slightly less dense. Using a slightly large needle gauge can help to inject. Slightly pulling back on the needle while injecting can help the flow of injectate.
- Be conscious while advancing in the lateral fluoroscopic view that the needle trajectory is not veering medial or lateral to the joint.
- Be sure to check in both lateral and AP views to ensure needle is in the meniscus and not out of the joint or just over the tibial plateau.
- Be sure to avoid scraping the femoral chondral surface.

Genicular Nerve Radiofrequency Ablation

Radiofrequency Ablation

KEY POINTS

- Radiofrequency (RF) ablation uses a RF current through an electrode tip needle to create a thermal lesion.
- Neurodestructive temperatures range from 65°C to 90°C.
- Traditional monopolar RF ablation probes operate at a constant temperature of 80°C, though temperature reading will not stay perfectly constant at the preset temperature but will go over and under, typically within half a degree, during the ablation. This is due to the probe itself causing the surrounding tissue to oscillate to create heat. The probe then senses the tissue temperature and adjusts to keep the temperature constant. This also limits the size of the "zone of coagulation."
- Cooled RF ablation uses internally cooled RF probes which are able to deliver more energy to surrounding tissues. While internally cooled probes operate at a set temperature of 60°C, temperatures in tissues beyond the probe tip reach 80°C. As a result of the internal cooling of the probe, larger lesions are created, which can help compensate for physiologic variability of nerve location and increase the likelihood of treatment success.
- The RF electrode tip should be placed parallel to the target genicular nerve.

Pertinent Anatomy[84]

- The SMGN course is at the junction of the distal femoral diaphysis and medial femoral epicondyle.
- The SLGN course is at the junction of the distal femoral diaphysis and the lateral femoral epicondyle.
- The IMGN course is at the junction of the medial condyle and diaphysis of the tibia.

Common Pathology

- Utilized for treatment of chronic knee pain due to chronic osteoarthritis that is non-operative or chronic knee pain after total knee arthroplasty.

Equipment

- C-arm fluoroscopy
- 18 to 20 gauge radiofrequency (RF) cannula with 10 mm active tip
- RF generator capable of generating energy for thermal ablation, pulsed radiofrequency ablation, or cooled RF ablation

Common Injectates

- Lidocaine (1%, 2%), bupivacaine (0.25%, 0.5%, 0.75%)
- Corticosteroids

Injectate Volume

- 1 to 2 mL of local anesthetic is typically injected after stimulation and before the ablation to improve the patient's comfort. Practitioners may use lidocaine (1% or 2%), or bupivacaine (0.25%, 0.5%, or 0.75%) with or without corticosteroid in mixture

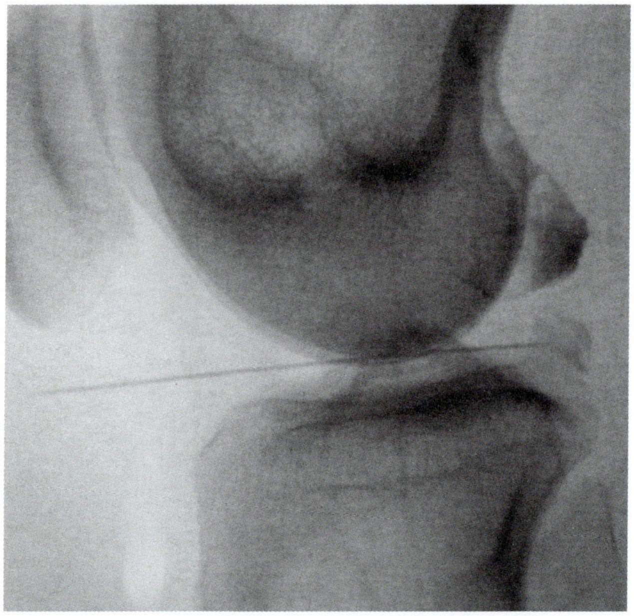

• **Fig. 21.74** Medial Meniscus Root Lateral Fluoroscopy View with Contrast.

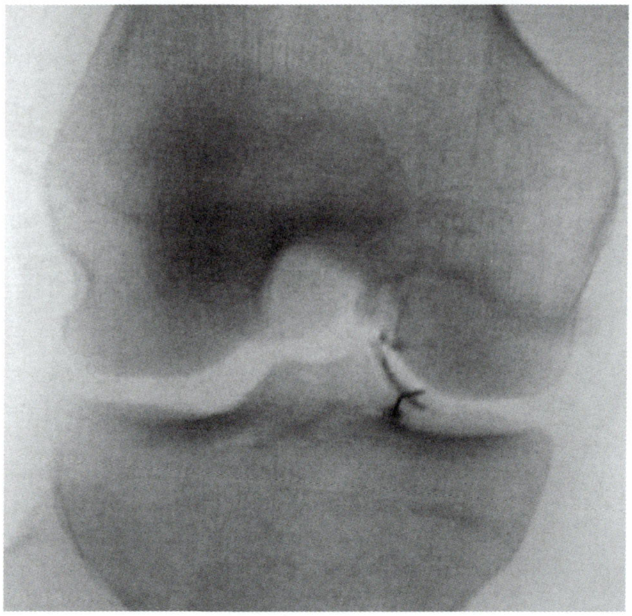

• **Fig. 21.75** Medial Meniscus Root AP Fluoroscopy View with Contrast.

Technique

Patient Position

- Supine with a pillow underneath both knees to provide slight flexion and improve comfort for patient during procedure

C-Arm Position

- Confirm appropriate genicular nerve target zones with an AP view.
- Tilt the C-arm slightly cephalad or caudad to square off the tibial plateau.
- Oblique the C-arm 15 to 20 degrees toward medial aspect of joint to obtain a "down the barrel" view of superomedial and IMGN target zones (Fig. 21.76A).

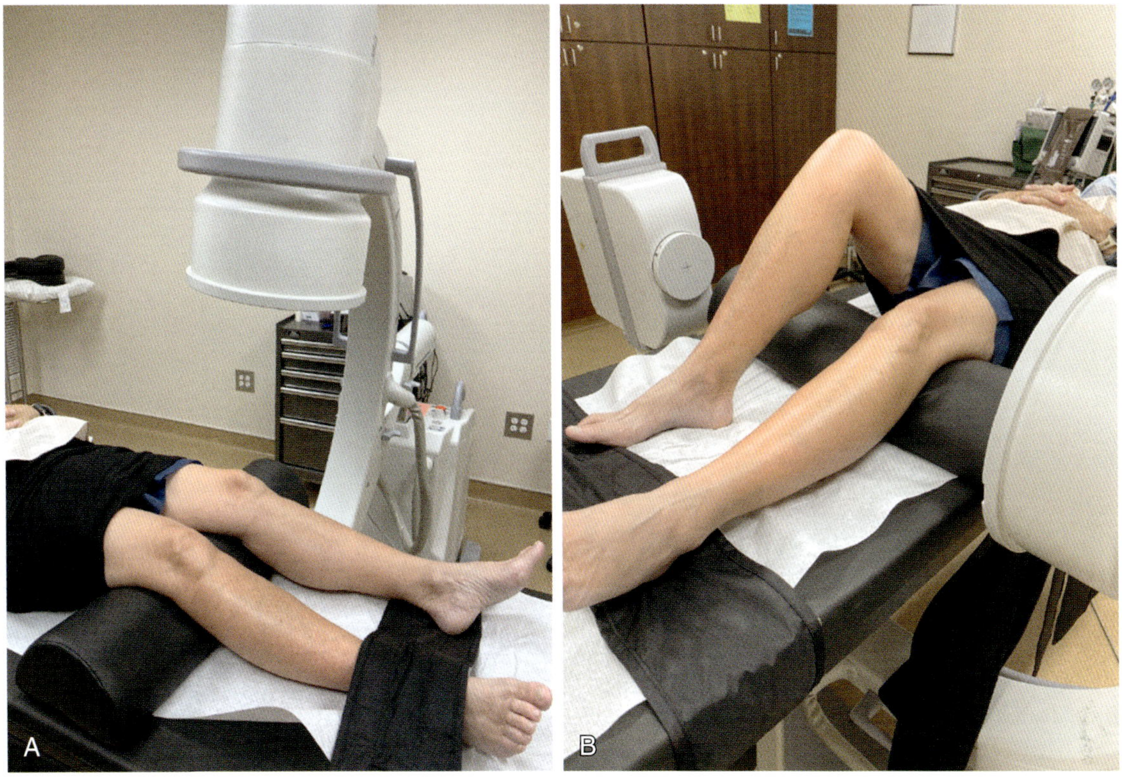

• **Fig. 21.76** (A) Genicular nerves RF C-arm set up. (B) Lateral flouroscopic view set up to ascertain needle depth.

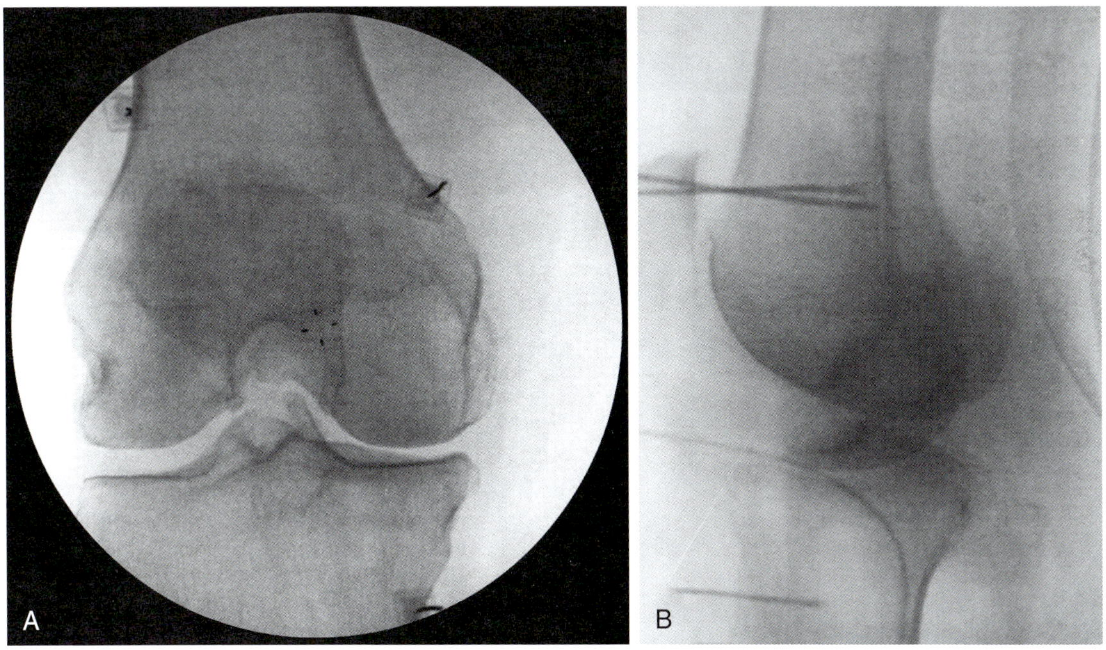

• **Fig. 21.77** Needle placement for SMGN and IMGN RF. (A) AP view; (B) Lateral view.

- Oblique the C-arm 15 to 20 degrees toward lateral aspect of joint to obtain a "down the barrel" view of SLGN target zone (see Fig. 21.76A).
- A lateral view of the C-arm should be obtained to check needle/trocar depth (see Fig. 21.76B).

Needle Position

- Insert the needle coaxially or slightly off plane in order to obtain optimum parallel placement of probes along the course of each nerve on the shaft of each respective bone (femur and tibia) (Fig. 21.77A and B).

Targets

- For the SMGN, needle placement should be at the junction of the distal femoral diaphysis and medial femoral epicondyle (Fig. 21.78A).

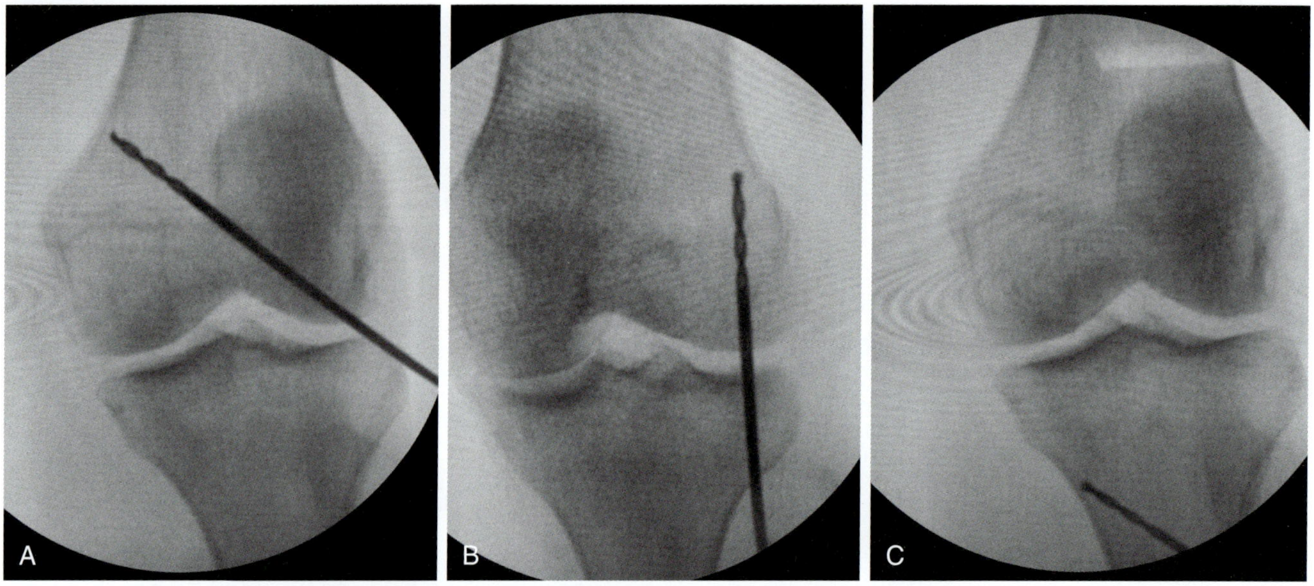

• **Fig. 21.78** RF probe placement for (A) SMGN; (B) SLGN; (C) IMGN.

- For the SLGN, needle placement should be at the junction of the distal femoral diaphysis and the lateral femoral epicondyle (see Fig. 21.78B).
- For the IMGN, needle placement should be at the junction of the medial condyle and diaphysis of the tibia (see Fig. 21.78C).

PEARLS AND PITFALLS[85]

- You want to ensure that the needle is placed at an angle so that there is parallel placement of the tip along the nerve; hence the suggestion to oblique C-arm 15–20 degrees.
- Before the ablation, motor and sensory stimulation should be performed to ensure there are no sensory or motor symptoms from peripheral nerve activation (femoral, saphenous, and/or common peroneal nerves).
- 1–2 mL of local anesthetic is typically injected after stimulation and before the ablation to improve the patient's comfort.
- Practitioners vary in their ablation settings; it can be 70–85 degrees for up to 90 s.
- After the first round of ablation, slightly advance or pull back tip of radiofrequency (RF) cannula a few millimeters before beginning the next round of ablation.
- Practitioners also may rotate the tip of the RF cannula 90–180 degrees to widen the path of RF ablation.
- Due to the variability in genicular nerve anatomy, two or even three rounds of ablation should be performed to account for various possible paths of nerves.
- One method to improve post-ablation pain and reduce discomfort during the ablation is to perform one round of pulsed RF ablation (50 Hz/4 ms at 42°C for 120 s) followed by standard thermal ablation as detailed above.
- Corticosteroid (Kenalog, Depo-Medrol, Decadron) may be injected along with local anesthetic prior to ablating the nerve, if appropriate, for post-procedure analgesia.
- Corticosteroids have not been proven to reduce frequency or severity of post-radiofrequency neuritis.[86]

References

1. Chen B, Lai LP, Putcha N, Stitik TP, Foye PM, et al. Optimal needle placement for ultrasound-guided knee joint injections or aspirations. *J Trauma Treat.* 2014;3:216.
2. Jackson D, Evans N, Thomas B. Accuracy of needle placement into the intra-articular space of the knee. *J Bone Joint Surg Am.* 2002;84:1522–1527.
3. Park Y, Lee SC, Nam HS, Lee J, Nam SH. Comparison of sonographically guided intra-articular injections at 3 different sites of the knee. *J Ultrasound Med.* 2011;30(12):1669–1676.
4. Iizuka M, Yao R, Wainapel S. Saphenous nerve injury following medial knee joint injection: a case report. *Arch Phys Med Rehabil.* 2005;86(10):2062–2065.
5. Lee SY, Gn KK, Chung BJ, Lee SW, Kim TK. Anterolateral portal is less painful than superolateral portal in knee intra-articular injection. *Knee Surg Relat Res.* 2015;27(4):228–232. https://doi.org/10.5792/ksrr.2015.27.4.228.
6. Pierce TP, Elmallah RK, Jauregui JJ, Cherian JJ, Harwin SF, Mont MA. Inferomedial or inferolateral intra-articular injections of the knee to minimize pain intensity. *Orthopedics.* 2016;39(3):e578–e581.
7. Choi JW, Lee JH, Ki M, et al. The comparison of two different intraarticular injections using a sonographic anterolateral approach in patients with osteoarthritic knee. *Korean J Pain.* 2018;31(4):289–295.
8. Koga H, Shimaya M, Muneta T, et al. Local adherent technique for transplanting mesenchymal stem cells as a potential treatment of cartilage defect. *Arthritis Res Ther.* 2008;10(4):R84.
9. Forster BB, Lee JS, Kelly S, et al. Proximal tibiofibular joint: an often-forgotten cause of lateral knee pain. *AJR Am J Roentgenol.* 2007;188(4):W359–W366.
10. Sarma A, Borgohain B, Saikia B. Proximal tibiofibular joint: rendezvous with a forgotten articulation. *Indian J Orthop.* 2015;49(5):489–495.
11. Forster BB, Lee JS, Kelly S, et al. Proximal tibiofibular joint: an often-forgotten cause of lateral knee pain. *AJR Am J Roentgenol.* 2007;188:W359–W366.

12. Wilson TJ, Stone JJ, Howe BM, Rock MG, Spinner RJ. Joint outcomes following surgery for superior tibiofibular joint-associated peroneal intraneural ganglion cysts. *Neurosurgery*. 2019. https://doi.org/10.1093/neuros/nyz205.
13. *Gray's Anatomy. The Anatomical Basis of Clinical Practice*. 41st ed. Elsevier; 2016.
14. Van Den Bergh FR, Vanhoenacker FM, De Smet E, Huysse W, Verstraete KL. Peroneal nerve: normal anatomy and pathologic findings on routine MRI of the knee. *Insights Imaging*. 2013;4(3):287–299.
15. Ward EE, Jacobson JA, Fessell DP, et al. Sonographic detection of Baker's cysts: comparison with MR imaging. *Am J Radiol*. 2001;176:373–380.
16. Mureşan S, Mureşan M, Voidăzan S, Neagoe R. The accuracy of musculoskeletal ultrasound examination for the exploration of meniscus injuries in athletes. *J Sports Med Phys Fitness*. 2017;57(5):589–594.
17. Xia XP, Chen HL, Zhou B. Ultrasonography for meniscal injuries in knee joint: a systematic review and meta-analysis. *J Sports Med Phys Fitness*. 2016;56(10):1179–1187.
18. Timotijevic S, Vukasinovic Z, Bascarevic Z. Correlation of clinical examination, ultrasound sonography, and magnetic resonance imaging findings with arthroscopic findings in relation to acute and chronic lateral meniscus injuries [published correction appears in *J Orthop Sci*. 2014 Mar;19(2):375. Sladjan, Timotijevic [corrected to Timotijevic, Sladjan]; Zoran, Vukasinovic [corrected to Vukasinovic, Zoran]; Zoran, Bascarevic [corrected to Bascarevic, Zoran]] [published correction appears in *J Orthop Sci*. 2014 Mar;19(2):375]. *J Orthop Sci*. 2014;19(1):71–76.
19. Chan PS, Kneeland JB, Gannon FH, Luchetti WT, Herzog RJ. Identification of the vascular and avascular zones of the human meniscus using magnetic resonance imaging: correlation with histology. *Arthroscopy*. 1998;14(8):820–823.
20. Fox AJ, Bedi A, Rodeo SA. The basic science of human knee menisci: structure, composition, and function. *Sports Health*. 2012;4(4):340–351. https://doi.org/10.1177/1941738111429419.
21. Wan AC, Felle P. The menisco-femoral ligaments. *Clin Anat*. 1995;8(5):323–326.
22. Kimura M, Shirakura K, Hasegawa A, Kobayashi Y, Udagawa E. Anatomy and pathophysiology of the popliteal tendon area in the lateral meniscus, 1. Arthroscopic and anatomical investigation. *Arthroscopy: J Arthroscop & Related Surg*. 1992;8(4):419–423.
23. Peltier A, Lording T, Maubisson L, Ballis R, Neyret P, Lustig S. The role of the meniscotibial ligament in posteromedial rotational knee stability. *Knee Surg Sports Traumatol Arthrosc*. 2015;23(10):2967–2973.
24. Seitz A, Kasisari R, Claes L, Ignatius A, Durselen L. Forces acting on the anterior meniscotibial ligaments. *Knee Surg Sports Traumatol Arthrosc*. 2012;20(8):1488–1495.
25. Fox AJS, Wanivenhaus F, Burge AJ, Warren RF, Rodeo SA. The human meniscus: a review of anatomy, function, injury, and advances in treatment. *Clin Anat*. 2015;28(2):269–287.
26. Pache S, Aman ZS, Kennedy M, et al. Meniscal root tears: current concepts review. *Arch Bone Jt Surg*. 2018;6(4):250–259.
27. Koo JH, Choi SH, Lee SA, Wang JH. Comparison of medial and lateral meniscus root tears. *PloS One*. 2015;10(10):e0141021.
28. Jarraya M, Roemer FW, Englund M, et al. Meniscus morphology: does tear type matter? A narrative review with focus on relevance for osteoarthritis research. *Semin Arthritis Rheumatism*. 2017;46(5):552–561.
29. Zanetti M, Pfirrmann CWA, Schmid MR, Romero J, Seifert B, Hodler J. Patients with suspected meniscal tears: prevalence of abnormalities seen on MRI of 100 symptomatic and 100 contralateral asymptomatic knees. *Am J Roentgenol*. 2003;181(3):635–641.
30. MacMahon PJ, Brennan DD, Duke D, Forde S, Eustace SJ. Ultrasound-guided percutaneous drainage of meniscal cysts: preliminary clinical experience. *Clin Radiol*. 2007;62(7):683–687.
31. Niceforo A, Di Giunta AC, Caminiti S, Tirrò S. A rare case of a large lateral meniscal cyst of the knee. *Arthroscopy*. 1998;14(7):759–761.
32. Rutten MJ, Collins JM, van Kampen A, Jager GJ. Meniscal cysts: detection with high-resolution sonography. *AJR Am J Roentgenol*. 1998;171(2):491–496.
33. Tyson LC, Daughters TC, Ryu RK, Crues JV. MRI appearance of meniscal cysts. *Skeletal Radiol*. 1995;24:421–424.
34. Mountney J, Thomas NP. When is a meniscal cyst not a meniscal cyst? *Knee*. 2004;11(2):133–136.
35. Yepes H, et al. "Relationship between hypovascular zones and patterns of ruptures of the quadriceps tendon". *JBJS*. 2008;10(90):2135–2141.
36. Distal patellar tendinosis: an unusual form of jumper's knee. January 2007. *Knee Surg Sports Traumatol Arthrosc*. 15(1):54–57
37. Baumbach SF, Lobo CM, Badyine I, Mutschler W, Kanz KG. Prepatellar and olecranon bursitis: literature review and development of a treatment algorithm. *Arch Orthop Trauma Surg*. 2014;134(3):359–370.
38. Parker CH, Leggit JC. Novel treatment of prepatellar bursitis. *Mil Med*. 2018;183(11–12):e768–e770.
39. Aydingoz U, Oguz B, Aydingoz O, Comert RB, Akgun I. The deep infrapatellar bursa: prevalence and morphology on routine magnetic resonance imaging of the knee. *J Comput Assist Tomogr*. 2004;28(4):557–561.
40. Curtis BR, Huang BK, Pathria MN, Resnick DL, Smitaman E. Pes anserinus: anatomy and pathology of native and harvested tendons. *AJR Am J Roentgenol*. 2019;213(5):1107–1116.
41. Olewnik Ł, Gonera B, Podgórski M, Polguj M, Jezierski H, Topol M. A proposal for a new classification of pes anserinus morphology. *Knee Surg Sports Traumatol Arthrosc*. 2019;27(9):2984–2993.
42. Toktas H, Dundar U, Adar S, Solak O, Ulasli AM. Ultrasonographic assessment of pes anserinus tendon and pes anserinus tendinitis bursitis syndrome in patients with knee osteoarthritis. *Mod Rheumatol*. 2015;25(1):128–133.
43. Alvarez-Nemegyei J. Risk factors for pes anserinus tendinitis/bursitis syndrome: a case control study. *J Clin Rheumatol*. 2007;13(2):63–65.
44. Smith J, Sayeed YA, Finnoff JT, Levy BA, Martinoli C. The bifurcating distal biceps femoris tendon: potential pitfall in musculoskeletal sonography. *J Ultrasound Med*. 2011;30(8):1162–1166.
45. Beltran J, Matityahu A, Hwang K, et al. The distal semimembranosus complex: normal MR anatomy, variants, biomechanics and pathology. *Skeletal Radiol*. 2003;32(8):435–445.
46. Yoon MA, Choi JY, Lim HK, et al. High prevalence of abnormal MR findings of the distal semimembranosus tendon: contributing factors based on demographic, radiographic, and MR features. *AJR Am J Roentgenol*. 2014;202(5):1087–1093.
47. Kim YC, Yoo WK, Chung IH, Seo JS, Tanaka S. Tendinous insertion of semimembranosus muscle into the lateral meniscus. *Surg Radiol Anat*. 1997;19:365–369.
48. Andrews K, Lu A, Mckean L, Ebraheim N. Review: medial collateral ligament injuries. *J Orthop*. 2017;14(4):550–554. https://doi.org/10.1016/j.jor.2017.07.017.

49. Jones L, Bismil Q, Alyas F, Connell D, Bell J. Persistent symptoms following non operative management in low grade MCL injury of the knee—the role of the deep MCL. *Knee.* 2009;16(1):64–68.
50. Galletti L, Ricci V, Andreoli E, Galletti S. Treatment of a calcific bursitis of the medial collateral ligament: a rare cause of painful knee. *J Ultrasound.* 2019;22(4):471–476. https://doi.org/10.1007/s40477-018-0353-y.
51. Del Castillo-González F, Ramos-Álvarez JJ, González-Pérez J, Jiménez-Herranz E, Rodríguez-Fabián G. Ultrasound-guided percutaneous lavage of calcific bursitis of the medial collateral ligament of the knee: a case report and review of the literature. *Skeletal Radiol.* 2016;45(10):1419–1423.
52. Davenport D, Arora A, Edwards MR. Non-operative management of an isolated lateral collateral ligament injury in an adolescent patient and review of the literature. *BMJ Case Rep.* 2018;2018:bcr2017223478. https://doi.org/10.1136/bcr-2017-223478.
53. Keskin D. Fibular collateral ligament-biceps femoris calcific bursitis causing flexion contracture in the knee, external rotation in the leg, and equinus deformity in the ankle. *J Manip Physiol Ther.* 2008;31(3):247–250.
54. Özçakar L, Albarazi NB, Abdulsalam AJ. Ultrasound imaging of the knee showing a fortuitous calcification in the lateral collateral ligament. *Med Ultrason.* 2019;21(2):1954. https://doi.org/10.11152/mu-1954.
55. Bonasia DE, D'Amelio A, Pellegrino P, Rosso F, Rossi R. Anterolateral ligament of the knee: back to the future in anterior cruciate ligament reconstruction. *Orthop Rev (Pavia).* 2015;7(2):5773. https://doi.org/10.4081/or.2015.5773. Published 2015 Jun 11.
56. Claes S, Vereecke E, Maes M, Victor J, Verdonk P, Bellemans J. Anatomy of the anterolateral ligament of the knee. *J Anat.* 2013;223(4):321–328. https://doi.org/10.1111/joa.12087.
57. Getgood, A., Brown, C., Lording, T., Amis, A., Claes, S., Musahl, V. (2018). *The Anterolateral Complex of the Knee: Results from the International ALC Consensus Group Meeting. Knee Surgery, Sports.*
58. Thawait SK, Soldatos T, Thawait GK, Cosgarea AJ, Carrino JA, Chhabra A. High resolution magnetic resonance imaging of the patellar retinaculum: normal anatomy, common injury patterns, and pathologies. *Skeletal Radiol.* 2012;41(2):137–148. https://doi.org/10.1007/s00256-011-1291-3.
59. Tuxoe JI, Teir M, Winge S, Nielsen PL. The medial patellofemoral ligament: a dissection study. *Knee Surg Sports Traumatol Arthrosc.* 2002;10(3):138–140.
60. Garth Jr WP, Connor GS, Futch L, Belarmino H. Patellar subluxation at terminal knee extension: isolated deficiency of the medial patellomeniscal ligament. *J Bone Joint Surg Am.* 2011;93(10):954–962. https://doi.org/10.2106/JBJS.H.00103.
61. Shah KN, DeFroda SF, Ware JK, Koruprolu SC, Owens BD. Lateral patellofemoral ligament: an anatomic study. *Orthop J Sports Med.* 2017;5(12):2325967117741439. https://doi.org/10.1177/2325967117741439. Published 2017 Dec 4.
62. Guerrero P, Li X, Patel K, et al. Medial patellofemoral ligament injury patterns and associated pathology in lateral patella dislocation: an MRI study. *BMC Sports Sci Med Rehabil.* 2009;1:17. https://doi.org/10.1186/1758-2555-1-17.
63. Amis AA, Firer P, Mountney J, Senavongse W, Thomas NP. Anatomy and biomechanics of the medial patellofemoral ligament [published correction appears in *Knee.* 2004 Feb;11(1):73]. *Knee.* 2003;10(3):215–220. http://doi:10.1016/s0968-0160(03)00006-1.
64. Pękala PA, Tomaszewski KA, Henry BM, et al. Risk of iatrogenic injury to the infrapatellar branch of the saphenous nerve during hamstring tendon harvesting: a meta-analysis. *Muscle Nerve.* 2017;56(5):930–937.
65. James NF, Kumar AR, Wilke BK, Shi GG. Incidence of encountering the infrapatellar nerve branch of the saphenous nerve during a midline approach for total knee arthroplasty. *J Am Acad Orthop Surg Glob Res Rev.* 2019;3(12):e19.00160.
66. Yasar E, Kesikburun S, Kılıç C, Güzelküçük Ü, Yazar F, Tan AK. Accuracy of ultrasound-guided genicular nerve block: a cadaveric study. *Pain Physician.* 2015;18(5):E899–E904.
67. Kim D-H, et al. Ultrasound-guided genicular nerve block for knee osteoarthritis: a double-blind, randomized controlled trial of local anesthetic alone or in combination with corticosteroid. *Pain Physician.* 2018;21(1):41–52.
68. Sotelo VG, et al. Ultrasound-guided genicular nerve block for pain control after total knee replacement: preliminary case series and technical note. *Rev Esp Anestesiol Reanim.* 2017;64(10):568–576.
69. Loudon JK. Biomechanics and pathomechanics of the patellofemoral joint. *Int J Sports Phys Ther.* 2016;11(6):820–830.
70. Fox AJ, Wanivenhaus F, Rodeo SA. The basic science of the patella: structure, composition, and function. *J Knee Surg.* 2012;25(2):127–141.
71. Tecklenburg K, Dejour D, Hoser C, Fink C. Bony and cartilaginous anatomy of the patellofemoral joint. *Knee Surg Sports Traumatol Arthrosc.* 2006;14(3):235–240.
72. Centeno C, Markle J, Dodson E, et al. Symptomatic anterior cruciate ligament tears treated with percutaneous injection of autologous bone marrow concentrate and platelet products: a non-controlled registry study. *J Transl Med.* 2018;16(1):246.
73. Centeno CJ, Pitts J, Al-Sayegh H, Freeman MD. Anterior cruciate ligament tears treated with percutaneous injection of autologous bone marrow nucleated cells: a case series. *J Pain Res.* 2015;8:437–447.
74. Smith J, Hackel JG, Khan U, Pawlina W, Sellon JL. Sonographically guided anterior cruciate ligament injection: technique and validation. *PM&R.* 2015;7(7):736–745.
75. Kopf S, Musahl V, Tashman S, Szczodry M, Shen W, Fu FH. A systematic review of the femoral origin and tibial insertion morphology of the ACL. *Knee Surg Sports Traumatol Arthrosc.* 2009;17(3):213–219.
76. Amiel D, Billings E, Harwood FL. Collagenase activity in anterior cruciate ligament: protective role of the synovial sheath. *J Appl Physiol.* 1990;69(3):902–906.
77. Schulze-Tanzil G. Intraarticular ligament degeneration is interrelated with cartilage and bone destruction in osteoarthritis. *Cells.* 2019;8(9):990.
78. Gupta M, Goyal PK, Singh P, Sharma A. Morphology of intra-articular structures and histology of menisci of knee joint. *Int J Appl Basic Med Res.* 2018;8(2):96–99.
79. Hewett TE, Ford KR, Hoogenboom BJ, Myer GD. Understanding and preventing ACL injuries: current biomechanical and epidemiologic considerations—update 2010. *N Am J Sports Phys Ther.* 2010;5(4):234–251.
80. Wright R, Magnussen R, Dunn W, Spindler K. Ipsilateral graft and contralateral ACL rupture at five years or more following ACL reconstruction. A systematic review. *J Bone Joint Surg Am Vol.* 2011;93:1159–1165.
81. Cho JM, Suh JS, Na JB, et al. Variations in meniscofemoral ligaments at anatomical study and MR imaging. *Skeletal Radiol.* 1999;28(4):189–195.

82. Laprade CM, Civitarese DM, Rasmussen MT, Laprade RF. Emerging updates on the posterior cruciate ligament: a review of the current literature. *Am J Sports Med.* 2015;43(12):3077–3092.
83. Masouros SD, Mcdermott ID, Amis AA, Bull AMJ. Biomechanics of the meniscus-meniscal ligament construct of the knee. *Knee Surg Sports Traumatol Arthrosc.* 2008;16(12):1121–1132.
84. Fonkoué L, Behets C, Kouassi JK, et al. Distribution of sensory nerves supplying the knee joint capsule and implications for genicular blockade and radiofrequency ablation: an anatomical study. *Surg Radiol Anat.* 2019;41(12):1461–1471. https://doi.org/10.1007/s00276-019-02291-y.
85. Jamison DE, Cohen SP. Radiofrequency techniques to treat chronic knee pain: a comprehensive review of anatomy, effectiveness, treatment parameters, and patient selection. *J Pain Res.* 2018;11:1879–1888. https://doi.org/10.2147/JPR.S144633.
86. Singh JR, Miccio Jr VF, Modi DJ, Sein MT. The impact of local steroid administration on the incidence of neuritis following lumbar facet radiofrequency neurotomy. *Pain Physician.* 2019;22(1):69–74.

22

Ankle Region Injection Techniques

ALLISON C. BEAN, ALLISON N. SCHROEDER, MATTHEW SHERRIER, ARTHUR JASON DE LUIGI, AND KENTARO ONISHI

Joint Injections

Tibiotalar Joint Injection

KEY POINTS

- Use of a high-frequency small footprint linear ultrasound transducer, like the "hockey stick," is recommended for all ankle region and joint injections.
- Various injection approaches exist, and the choice depends on individual anatomy.

Pertinent Anatomy

- The ankle (also known as tibiocrural or tibiotalar) joint is a hinged synovial articulation between the distal tibia and fibula and the talus.
- The joint also allows primarily ankle plantarflexion and dorsiflexion.

Common Pathology

- Ankle joint pathology often presents with a joint effusion, associated with deep and diffuse pain with restricted range of motion.
- Ankle joint injury can be acute or chronic. Etiologic causes include arthritis, synovitis, fracture, chondral lesion, instability from chronic ligament or tendon pathology, or infection.
- On sonographic examination with the foot in slight plantarflexion and imaging the anterior joint recess, distention of the joint with anechoic fluid is the most sensitive location and position to identify an effusion.[1]
- Of note, 1 to 2 mm of anechoic hyaline cartilage covers the talar dome, and it is important not to mistake this for intra-articular fluid.
- Tibiotalar intra-articular loose bodies are hyperechoic and may migrate to the medial ankle tendon sheaths, as these can communicate with the ankle joint.[2]

Equipment

- High-frequency, small footprint, linear ultrasound transducer.
- 30 to 25 gauge 1 to 2 inch needle.

Common Injectates

- Local anesthetics for diagnostic injections.
- Corticosteroids, hyaluronic acid, prolotherapy, orthobiologics (platelet-rich plasma [PRP], bone marrow concentrate, etc.).

Injectate Volume

- 2 to 4 mL

Patient Position

- Supine or seated on the exam table.
- Knee flexed to approximately 90 degrees and ankle in slight plantarflexion so that the plantar surface of the foot is flat on the exam table.

Clinician Position

- Seated at the foot of the exam table facing the patient and ultrasound machine.

Transducer Orientation

- Preferred approach (Fig. 22.1A):
  - Begin with the transducer in long axis to the distal tibia.
  - Translate the probe distally to identify the joint space.
  - Identify the tibialis anterior tendon in long axis; then translate the probe medial to the tibialis anterior tendon.
- Alternative approach #1:
  - The transducer is rotated 90 degrees from the position described above and is positioned in the transverse plane at the level of the joint.
- Alternative approach #2:
  - The transducer is positioned as described in the preferred approach and translated laterally with the distal

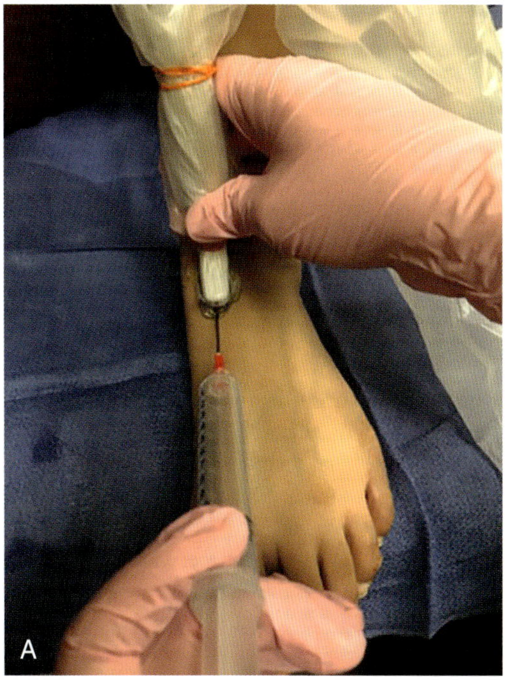

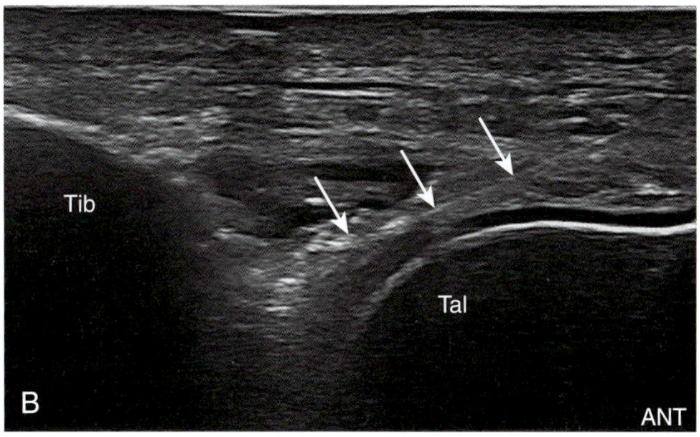

• **Fig. 22.1** (A) Ultrasound-guided tibiotalar joint injection setup for an in-plane, anterior to posterior approach. (B) Intra-articular tibiotalar joint injection using an in-plane, anterior to posterior approach. Arrows point to the needle. *ANT*, Anterior; *Tal*, talus; *Tib*, tibia.

end and slightly rotated medially to view the anterior talofibular ligament (ATFL) in long axis.

Needle Position

- Preferred approach: In-plane, anterior to posterior (Fig. 22.1B). This can also be accomplished using an out-of-plane approach.
- Alternative approach #1: In-plane, medial to lateral or lateral to medial with the needle coursing deep to the overlying tendons.
- Alternative approach #2: In-plane, anterior/distal to posterior/proximal, targeting both the tibiotalar joint and ATFL.

Target

- Anterior joint recess, deep to anterior fat pad, superficial to talar dome cartilage.

PEARLS AND PITFALLS

- There is risk of perforating tendon or neurovascular structures if they lie within the needle trajectory. The preliminary scan is helpful to identify at-risk structures, including the peroneal nerve branches, dorsalis pedis vessels, and anterior ankle tendons.
- Needle contact with the chondral surface should be avoided, since this can result in damage of the cartilage.

Subtalar Joint Injection

KEY POINTS

- Various injection approaches exist, and the choice depends on individual anatomy.
- The posterolateral approach is the preferred method by the authors due to less frequent anatomic variations in this region.[3] This targets the posterior subtalar joint (PSTJ).
- Alternate approaches (anterolateral via sinus tarsi and posteromedial approaches) may be used; however, these approaches require careful consideration to avoid nearby tendons, nerves, and vessels and account for more anatomic variations common to these areas.

Pertinent Anatomy

- The subtalar joint (or talocalcaneal joint) is a multiarticulate joint where the talus articulates with the calcaneus through three facets: anterior, middle, and posterior.
- The joint primarily allows for ankle inversion and eversion.

Common Pathology

- Intra-articular subtalar joint pathology often presents with joint effusion.
- Pain is typically in the hindfoot and worse when walking on uneven surfaces. Joint pain is the most common result of post-traumatic arthritis.
- On sonographic examination of a subtalar joint effusion, anechoic intra-articular fluid can be visualized when the talus and calcaneus are both in view with anterolateral, posterolateral, or posteromedial transducer placement.[3]

Equipment

- High-frequency, small footprint, linear ultrasound transducer.
- 30 to 25 gauge 1 to 2 inch needle.

Common Injectates

- Local anesthetics for diagnostic injections.
- Corticosteroids, hyaluronic acid, prolotherapy, orthobiologics (PRP, bone marrow concentrate, etc.).

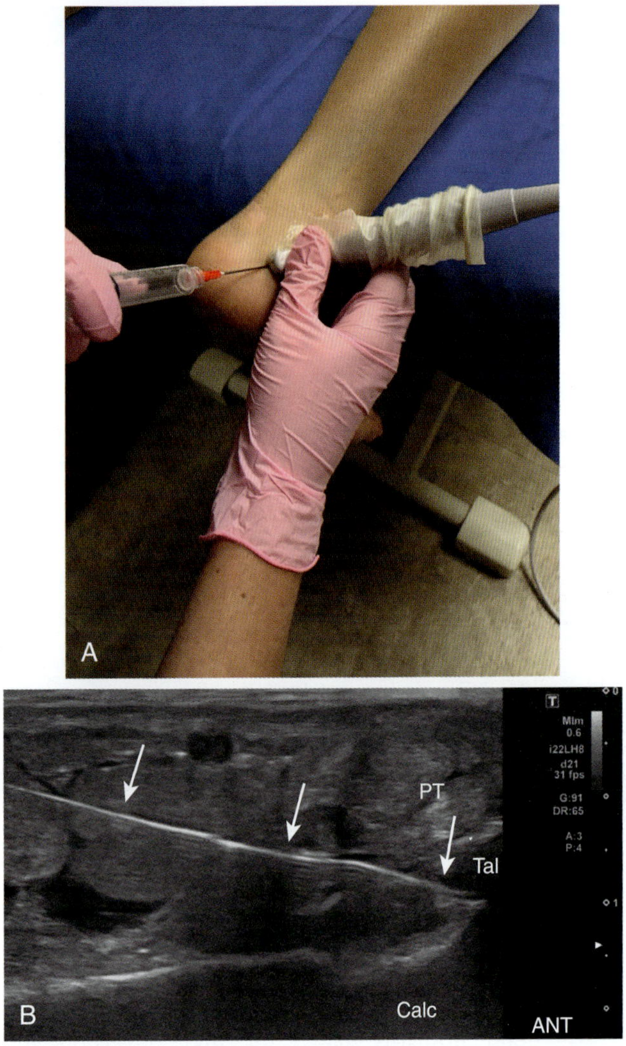

• **Fig. 22.2** (A) Ultrasound-guided subtalar joint injection set-up, for injection into the posterolateral joint. (B) Intra-articular subtalar joint injection using an in-plane, posterior distal to anterior proximal approach. *Arrows* denote the needle. *ANT,* Anterior, *Calc,* calcaneus; *PT,* peroneal tendons; *Tal,* talus.

Injectate Volume

- 1 to 3 mL

Technique

Patient Position

- Prone with the foot hanging off the edge of the exam table and ankle in dorsiflexion.
- Alternative approach: Lateral decubitus with the lateral ankle of the targeted side facing upward.

Clinician Position

- Seated or standing at the foot of the exam table facing the patient and ultrasound machine.
- Proceduralist knee or an assistant can be used to induce ankle dorsiflexion of the patient.

Transducer Orientation

- Preferred approach, posterolateral joint (Fig. 22.2A):
  - Begin with a long-axis view of the Achilles tendon.
  - Translate the transducer laterally while rotating the distal end of the transducer farther laterally. The final transducer position will be in the parasagittal plane.
  - The angle of insonation of the ultrasound beam points toward the medial malleolus and calcaneus.
  - Both the talus and calcaneus should be in view.
  - In case of severe arthritis or difficulty visualizing the posterior joint recess, further anterior translation around the "corner" of the posterolateral calcaneus while maintaining the angle of insonation may allow for improved visualization (with the peroneal tendons in view superficial to the joint).
- Alternative approach, anterolateral through the sinus tarsi. To find sinus tarsi:
  - Begin at the third web space while visualizing third and fourth metatarsal bones in short axis and translate proximally.
  - The first opening you will encounter after the mid-foot bones will be the sinus tarsi.

Needle Position

- Preferred approach: In-plane, distal lateral to proximal medial (Fig. 22.2B).
- Alternative approach: Out-of-plane, anterior to posterior.

Target

- Preferred approach: PSTJ recess.
- Alternative approach: Anterior subtalar joint through the sinus tarsi.

PEARLS AND PITFALLS

- Use of gel stand-off technique over the posterolateral edge of calcaneus will allow for improved needle visualization during the injection.
- Given the steep angle of the needle in this approach, needle localization software may also be helpful to improve needle visualization.
- In the anterolateral approach through the sinus tarsi, the target is also deep and may require the use of a walk-down technique.

Ligament Injections

Anterior Talofibular Ligament

KEY POINTS

- The ATFL is the most commonly injured ligament in the ankle (Figs. 22.3 and 22.4).[4]
- There have not been any high-quality studies on the ideal injectate volume, type of injectate, or clinical outcomes for ATFL injections.

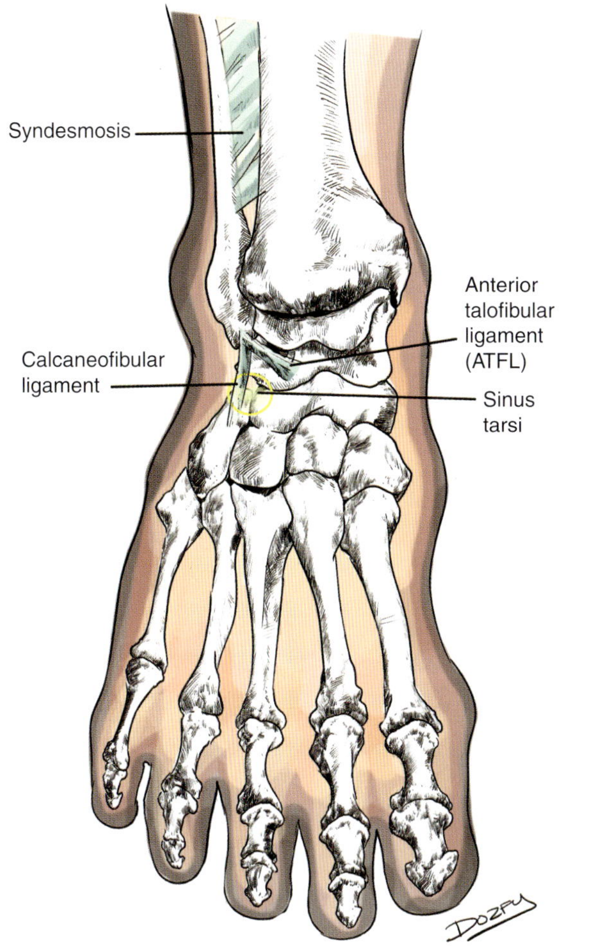

• **Fig. 22.3** Anterior Ankle Bony and Ligamentous Anatomy.

Pertinent Anatomy

- The ATFL extends from approximately the distal 10 mm of the fibula to the neck of the talus, running 45 to 90 degrees anteriorly to the axis of tibia.[5]
- Anatomic variation exists. ATFL may be single-, double-, or triple-bundled in morphology.[6]

Common Pathology

- Injury typically results from inversion of the ankle and should be suspected in patients with tenderness over the ATFL and a positive anterior drawer test.
- On sonographic examination of an injured ATFL, the typically homogeneous hyperechoic ligament that courses obliquely from the anterior distal fibula to the talus will appear relatively hypoechoic or disrupted.[7]
- It is important to note that the ATFL is prone to anisotrophy due to its nonlinear course and this should not be misinterpreted as a tear.[7]
- Dynamic imaging while performing an anterior drawer test can be helpful in equivocal cases.[8]

Equipment

- High-frequency, small footprint, linear ultrasound transducer.
- 30 to 25 gauge 1 to 2 inch needle.

Common Injectates

- Prolotherapy, orthobiologics (PRP, bone marrow concentrate, etc.).
- Avoid intraligamentous corticosteroids.

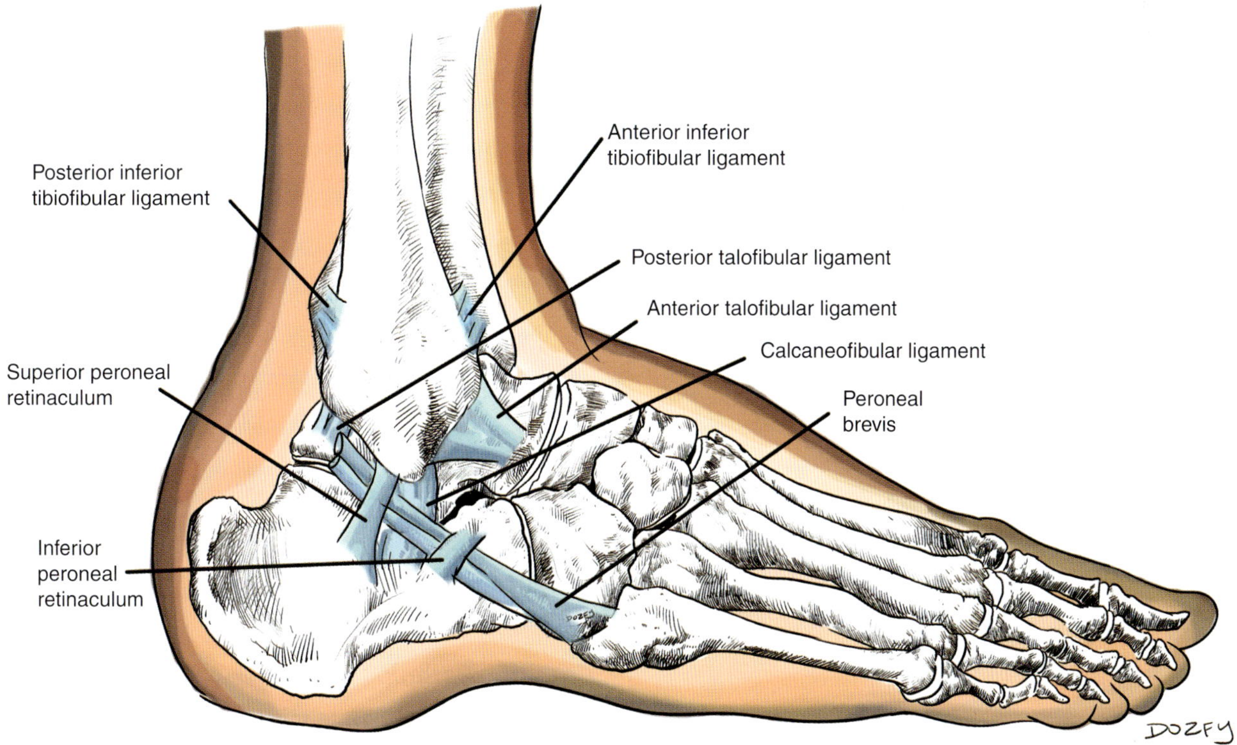

• **Fig. 22.4** Anatomy of the Lateral Ankle Ligaments.

Injectate Volume

- 0.5 to 1 mL

Technique

Patient Position

- Supine or seated on the exam table.
- Knee flexed approximately to 90 degrees and ankle in slight plantarflexion so that the plantar surface of the foot is flat on the exam table.
- Alternatively, the patient can be place in the lateral decubitus position with the lateral aspect of the targeted ankle facing upward.

Clinician Position

- Seated or standing at the foot of the exam table, facing the patient and ultrasound machine.

Transducer Orientation

- The ligament is identified by palpating the distal fibular tip and placing the transducer in the transverse plane at the anterior aspect of the fibula (Fig. 22.5A).
- The medial end of the transducer is distally rotated.
- The ligament is identified in long axis, spanning from the anterior distal fibula to the talus.

Needle Position

- Preferred approach: In-plane, anterior to posterior (Fig. 22.5B).
- Alternate approach: Out-of-plane, distal lateral to proximal medial.

Target

- Areas of hypoechogenicity or interstitial tears in the ATFL and cortical irregularities of the fibula and talus at the ATFL origin and insertion.

PEARLS AND PITFALLS

- Anterior ankle structures, such as the lateral tarsal branch of the inferolateral malleolar artery and intermediate dorsal cutaneous branch of the superficial peroneal nerve, should be identified and avoided during the injection.
- Often the anterior lateral malleolar artery travels adjacent to the mid portion of the ligament. An injured ATFL may have increased vascularization superficial to the ligament. Use color flow Doppler to identify vasculature and avoid it.
- Use of a gentle gel stand-off technique may allow for improved needle visualization during the injection. Aggressive stand-off will result in increased anisotropy of the ATFL.
- The injection can be combined with physical therapy, initially focusing on range of motion, then progressing to strengthening and proprioceptive training. A period of plantarflexion limitation can be considered, as dorsiflexion is the position of tension for ATFL.

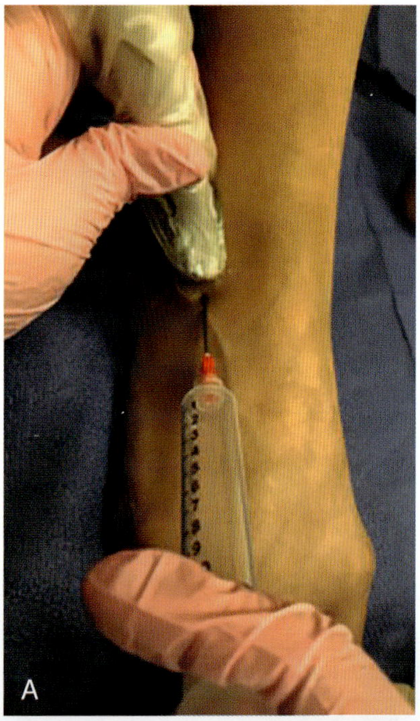

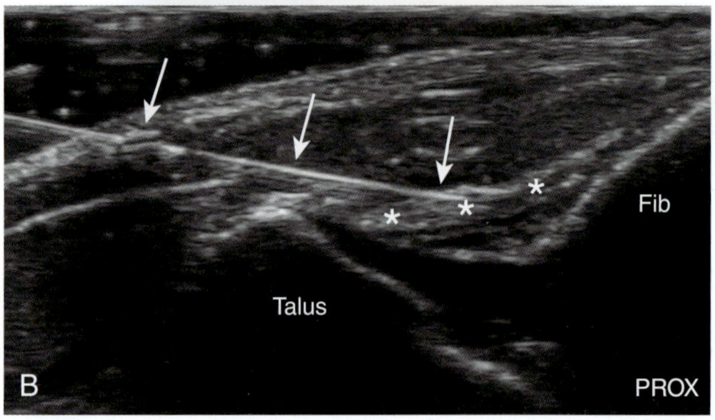

• **Fig. 22.5** (A) Ultrasound-guided ATFL injection setup for an in-plane, anterior to posterior approach. (B) ATFL injection using an in-plane, anterior to posterior approach. ATFL *(asterisk)* is imaged in long axis. *Arrows* point to the needle. *ATFL*, Anterior talofibular ligament; *Fib,* fibula; *PROX,* proximal.

Calcaneofibular Ligament (CFL)

KEY POINTS

- The calcaneofibular ligament (CFL) is commonly injured in combination with the ATFL.

Pertinent Anatomy

- The CFL originates from the tip of the lateral malleolus and inserts on the lateral side of the calcaneus (see Figs. 22.3 and 22.4).[9]
- The CFL restrains inversion of the calcaneus with respect to the fibula.[10]

Common Pathology

- The CFL is commonly injured with moderate to severe sprains of the ATFL with inversion injury.[11]

- Isolated injuries can occur but are infrequent and occur when the ligament is under maximum strain with the foot in dorsiflexion.[11]

Equipment

- High-frequency, small footprint, linear ultrasound transducer.
- 30 to 25 gauge 1 to 2 inch needle.

Common Injectates

- Orthobiologics prolotherapy, orthobiologics (PRP, bone marrow concentrate, etc.).
- Avoid intraligamentous corticosteroids.

Injectate Volume

- 0.5 to 1.5 mL

Technique

Patient Position

- Lateral decubitus position with the lateral aspect of the targeted ankle facing upward.
- Dorsiflexion of the ankle.

Clinician Position

- Seated or standing at the foot of the exam table, facing the patient and ultrasound machine.

Transducer Orientation

- Transducer in oblique coronal plane between the fibular tip and the posterior heel.
- The CFL is visualized under the peroneal tendons (seen in short axis) and appears as a hammock (Fig. 22.6A).
- Long axis to the ligament.

Needle Position

- Out of plane in either direction (Fig. 22.6B).

Target

- Areas of hypoechogenicity or interstitial tears in the CFL.

PEARLS AND PITFALLS

- Use of gel stand-off technique may allow for improved needle visualization during the injection.

Posterior Talofibular Ligament

KEY POINTS

- The PTFL is the strongest and least commonly injured lateral ligament in the ankle, at a rate of 5% to 10%.[12]

Pertinent Anatomy

- The posterior talofibular ligament (PTFL) originates from the malleolar fossa, located on the medial surface of the lateral malleolus, coursing almost horizontally to insert in the posterolateral talus (see Fig. 22.4).[13]

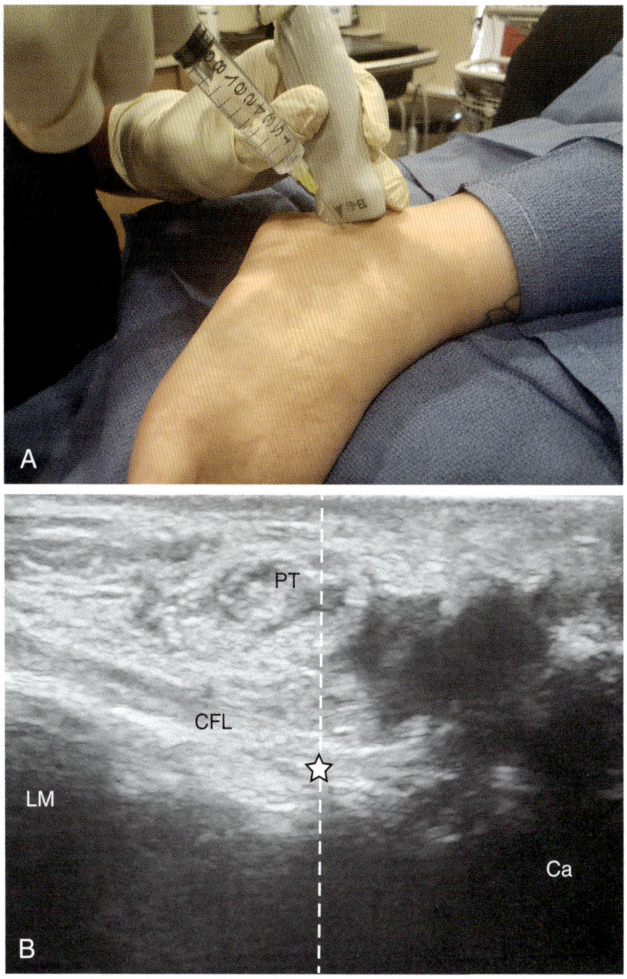

• **Fig. 22.6** (A) Ultrasound-guided CFL out-of-plane injection setup. (B) CFL out-of-plave injection. *Asterisk,* Needle tip; *Ca,* calcaneus; *CFL,* calcaneofibular ligament; *LM,* lateral malleolus; *PT,* peroneal tendons.

- The ligament resists posterior displacement of the talus with respect to the fibula and tibia and is under most tension in dorsiflexion.[14]

Common Pathology

- Isolated PTFL injury is rare and is mostly associated with severe ankle inversion injury resulting in tearing of the ATFL and CFL first.[14]

Equipment

- High-frequency, small footprint, linear ultrasound transducer.
- 30 to 25 gauge 1 to 2 inch needle.

Common Injectates

- Orthobiologics prolotherapy, orthobiologics (PRP, bone marrow concentrate, etc.).
- Avoid intraligamentous corticosteroids.

Injectate Volume

- 0.5 to 1.5 mL

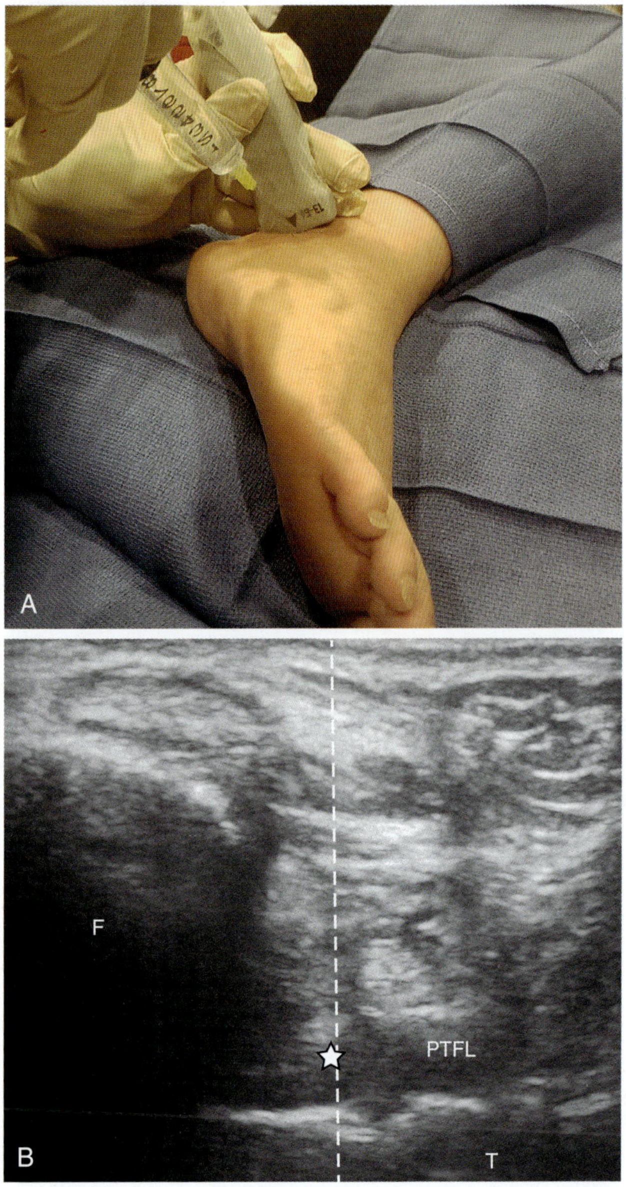

• **Fig. 22.7** (A) Ultrasound-guided PTFL injection setup. (B) PTFL injection out-of-plane ultrasound injection. *Asterisk,* Needle tip; *F,* fibular head; *PTFL,* posterior talofibular ligament; *T,* talus.

Technique

Patient Position

- Lateral decubitus position with the lateral aspect of the targeted ankle facing upward.

Clinician Position

- Seated or standing at the foot of the exam table facing the patient and ultrasound machine.

Transducer Orientation

- Long axis to the ligament (Fig. 22.7A).

Needle Position

- Out of plane in either direction (Fig. 22.7B).

Target

- Areas of hypoechogenicity or interstitial tears in the PTFL and cortical irregularities of the fibula and talus at the PTFL origin and insertion.

PEARLS AND PITFALLS

- Use of gel stand-off technique may allow for improved needle visualization during the injection.

Inferior Tibiofibular Ligaments Injection

KEY POINTS

- This injection can be performed using an in-plane or out-of-plane technique.
- Deltoid ligament injury can be associated with the same mechanism of anterior inferior tibiofibular ligament (AITFL) injury as well, so often both need to be evaluated and possibly treated.

Pertinent Anatomy

- The inferior tibiofibular joint is a syndesmotic articulation between the distal tibia and fibula and is stabilized by the AITFL and posterior inferior tibiofibular ligament (PITFL) (see Fig. 22.4).
- The interosseous tibiofibular ligament provides additional stabilization to the distal tibiofibular joint and extends between the crest of the fibula medially and proximally to the crest of the tibia, with its most distal portion approximately 1 cm proximal to the tibiotalar joint.[15]
- Variability exists in the number of bundles or fascicles of the AITFL.[16,17] The AITFL is a flat ligament that courses superior and medial from the distal fibula to the distal tibia. An accessory AITFL (Bassett's ligament) may also be identified as a discrete bundle distal to the AITFL, spanning a greater distance between the tibia and fibula in a slightly more horizontal orientation than the AITFL.[18]
- The PITFL courses superior and medial from the posterior aspect of the distal fibula to the distal tibia and is analogous to AITFL. The deep portion of this ligament is referred to as the inferior transverse ligament and is identifiable in 70% of ankles.[19]

Common Pathology

- The AITFL and distal tibiofibular joint are commonly injured by forced external rotation and dorsiflexion at the ankle.[15]
- Isolated injuries to the AITFL can lead to external rotary instability, even with an intact PITFL.[20]
- AITFL injuries can be evaluated with the dorsiflexion external rotation stress test, which causes joint widening.[21]

- On sonographic examination of an injured AITFL, the typical homogeneously hyperechoic structure spanning between the anterior distal tibia and fibula will appear disrupted. Dynamic imaging with dorsiflexion and external rotation stress testing will show widening between the distal tibia and fibula in a grade 3 AITFL tear.[22]

Equipment

- High-frequency, small footprint, linear ultrasound transducer.
- 30 to 25 gauge 1 to 2 inch needle.

Common Injectates

- Prolotherapy, orthobiologics (PRP, bone marrow concentrate, etc.).
- Avoid intraligamentous corticosteroids.

Injectate Volume

- 0.5 to 1 mL

Technique

Patient Position

- Lateral decubitus with the lateral ankle of the targeted side facing upward.

Clinician Position

- Seated or standing at the foot of the exam table, facing the posterior ankle and ultrasound machine.

Transducer Orientation

- The transducer is placed in short axis across the distal tibia and fibula.
- Identify the most distal aspect of the tibia. The lateral aspect of the transducer is rotated inferiorly on the distal fibula (anterior for AITFL or posterior for PITFL).
- The transducer will be long axis to the AITFL or PITFL (Figs. 22.8A and 22.9A)

Needle Position

- In-plane, lateral to medial (Fig. 22.8B).
- Alternatively, it can be out of plane in either direction (Fig. 22.9B).

Target

- Areas of hypoechogenicity within the ligament and/or area of maximum tenderness on sonopalpation.

PEARLS AND PITFALLS

- Use of a gel stand-off may allow for improved needle visualization during the injection.
- The superficial peroneal nerve courses superficial to the AITFL and this should be avoided. Out-of-plane injection risks injury to the peroneal nerve branches and is not recommended.
- Injection can be combined with physical therapy focused on range of motion and progressing to strengthening and proprioceptive training.

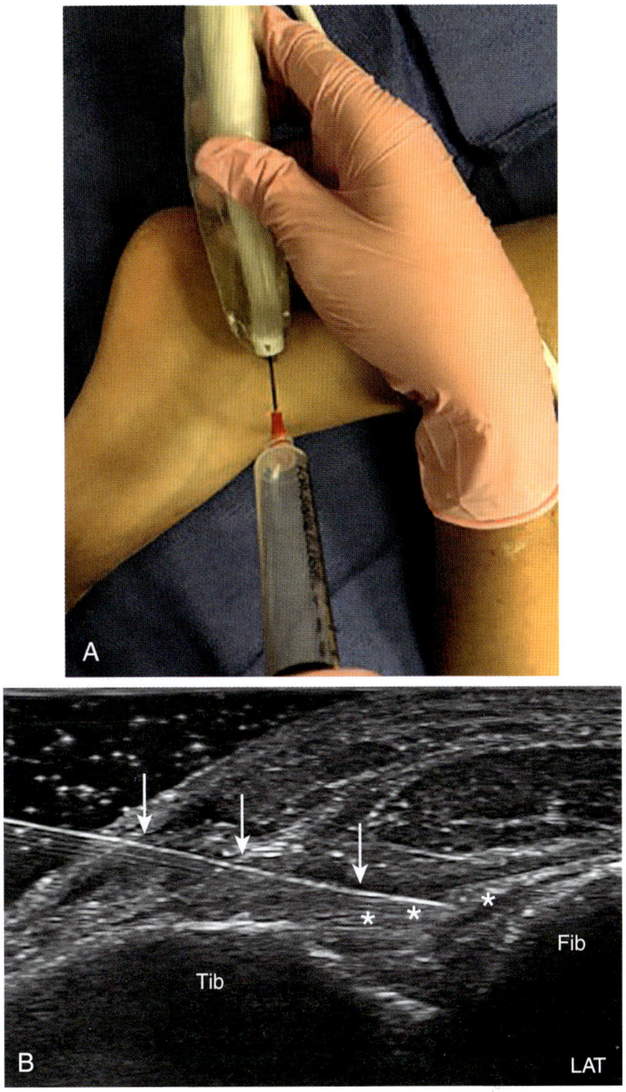

• **Fig. 22.8** (A) Ultrasound-guided AITFL injection setup for an in-plane, lateral to medial approach. (B) AITFL injection using an in-plane, lateral to medial approach. AITFL *(asterisks)* is imaged in long axis. *Arrows* point to the needle. *AITFL*, Anterior inferior tibiofibular ligament; *Fib*, fibula; *LAT*, lateral; *Tib*, tibia.

Deltoid Ligament Complex Injection

KEY POINTS

- The deltoid ligament consists of up to six bands, each of which can be targeted for injection using a slightly different transducer position and approach.

Pertinent Anatomy

- The deltoid ligament consists of superficial and deep components with up to six bands: (1) tibionavicular; (2) tibiospring, also called the plantar calcaneonavicular ligament; (3) tibiocalcaneal; (4) superficial posterior

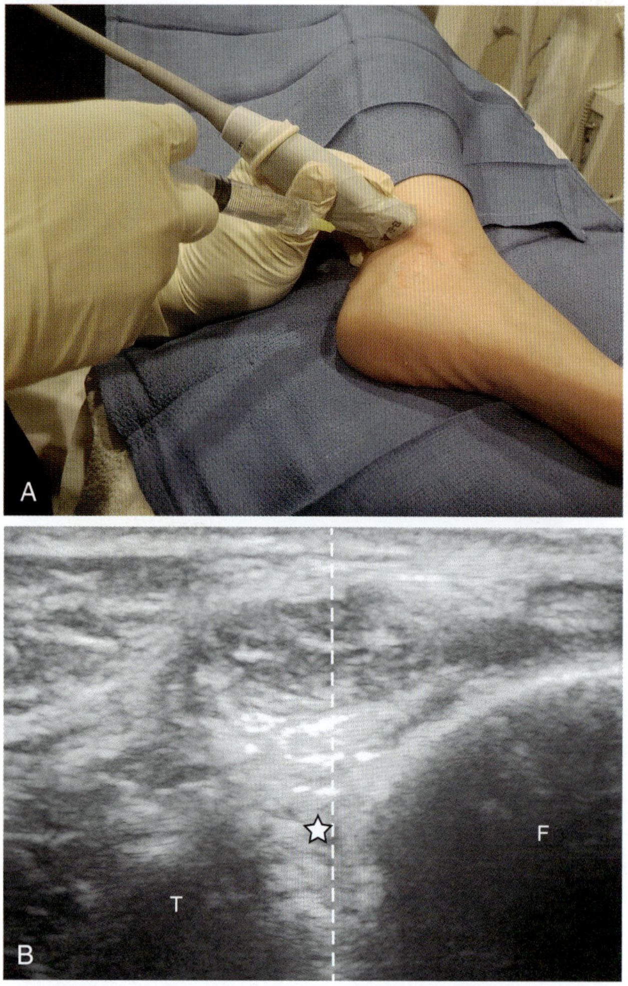

• **Fig. 22.9** (A) PITFL injection setup. (B) PITFL out-of-plane injection. *Asterisk,* Needle tip in PITFL; *F,* fibular; posterior inferior tibiofibular ligament; *T,* tibia.

tibiotalar, (5) deep posterior tibiotalar; and (6) deep anterior tibiotalar (Fig. 22.10).[23]

- It attaches the tibia to the talus, navicular, and calcaneus and resists ankle eversion.[23]
- The spring ligament has two main components: superomedial calcaneonavicular ligament (SMCNL) and inferior calcaneonavicular ligament (ICNL). Some anatomic variants also have a third band, referred to as the medioplantar oblique ligament. The SMCNL originates from the anterior middle facet of the subtalar joint and attaches medial side of the navicular articular margin. The ICNL originates between the anterior and medial subtalar facets and inserts on the lateral navicular break. The third band can originate between the first two and attaches to the navicular tuberosity.[24]
- The SMCNL is intimately connected to the tibialis posterior tendon and superficial component of the deltoid ligament, adding medial stability for the ankle and hindfoot.[25]
- The spring ligament helps to maintain arch height and stability and resists forefoot abduction.[25]

Common Pathology

- Injuries to the deltoid ligament are less common than lateral ankle injuries. They occur with forced ankle eversion combined with external rotation.
- Injuries to the spring ligament accur most often in the SMCNL and are mostly correlated with posterior tibialis injury. One study found that 92% of patients with posterior tibialis dysfunction had damage to the SMCNL.[26]
- Isolated spring ligament injury is rare but has been reported and is associated with loss of the foot arch.[27]

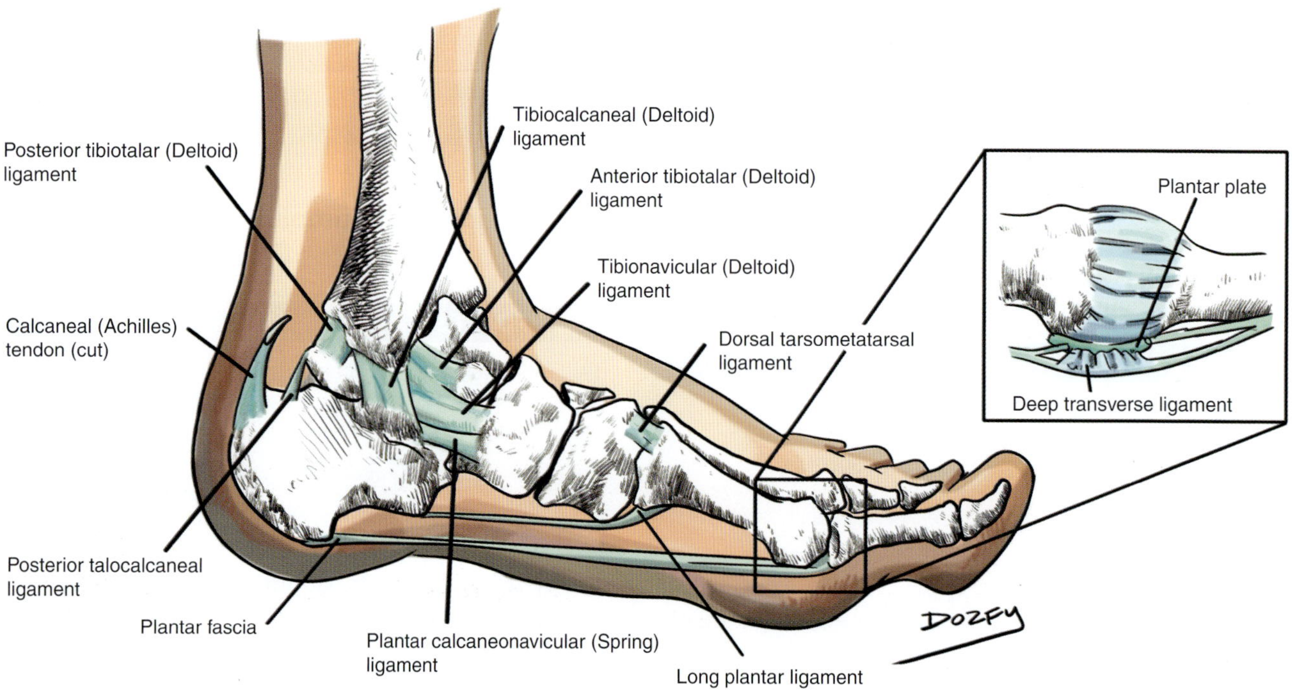

• **Fig. 22.10** Anatomy of the Medial Ankle Ligaments.

- On sonographic evaluation, injury may be identified by disruption of the normal fibrillar pattern, diffuse hypoechoic enlargement, or discontinuity of the ligament with possible hyperechoic avulsion fracture fragments.[22,28]

Equipment

- High-frequency, small footprint, linear ultrasound transducer.
- 30 to 25 gauge 1 to 2 inch needle.

Common Injectates

- Prolotherapy, orthobiologics (PRP, bone marrow concentrate, etc.).
- Avoid intraligamentous corticosteroids.

Injectate Volume

- 0.5 to 1.5 mL per ligament.

Technique

Patient Position

- Lateral decubitus with the medial ankle of the targeted side facing upward.

Clinician Position

- Seated or standing at the foot of the exam table, facing the patient and ultrasound machine.

Transducer Orientation

- Each component of the deltoid ligament (listed above) can be visualized spanning between the respective bones it connects (Figs. 22.11A and 22.12A).
- The transducer is oriented in long axis to the target ligament component.

Needle Position

- In-plane, distal to proximal (Fig. 22.11B).
- Alternatively, inject the ligaments out of plane (Fig. 22.12B).

Target

- Areas of hypoechogenicity within the ligament and/or area of greatest tenderness on sonopalpation.

PEARLS AND PITFALLS

- Evaluate each component of the deltoid ligament and pathologic-appearing bands.
- Care should be taken to identify and avoid the tibialis posterior, extensor digitorum longus (EDL) tendons, and tibial neurovascular bundle, as these structures course around the medial malleolus and run superficial to the posterior components of the deltoid ligament.
- Gel stand-off technique may allow for improved needle visualization during the injection.

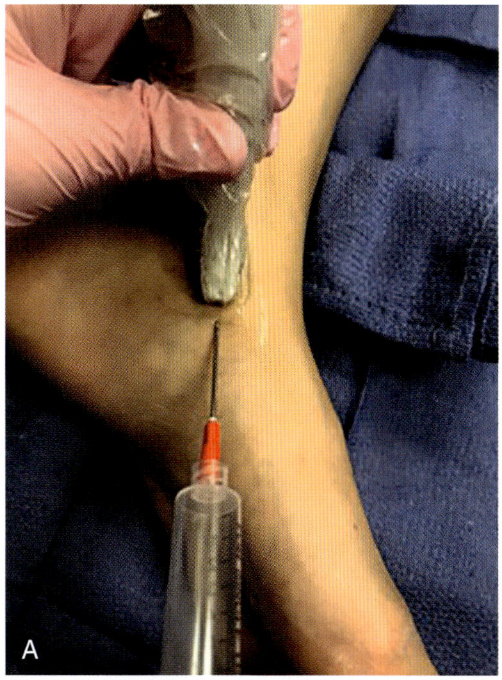

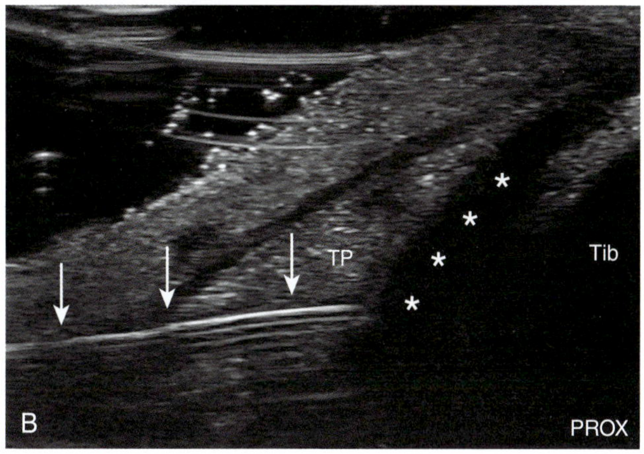

• **Fig. 22.11** (A) Ultrasound-guided deltoid ligament injection setup for the deep anterior tibiotalar portion of the deltoid ligament. (B) Deltoid ligament injection using and in-plane, distal to proximal approach. Deep anterior tibiotalar portion of the deltoid ligament *(asterisks)* is imaged in long axis deep to tibialis posterior *(TP)* tendon. *Arrows* point to the needle. *PROX,* proximal; *Tib,* tibia.

Tendon Injections

Achilles Tendon or Paratenon Injection

KEY POINTS

- Intratendinous or peritendinous injections may be performed.
- Intratendinous injections are typically performed if there is a clear tendon defect, using an orthobiologic.
- If tendinosis or pathologic thickening without obvious tear is present for injection of orthobiologcs, needle passages (needle tenotomy/fenestration) might be needed in order to create space to inject.

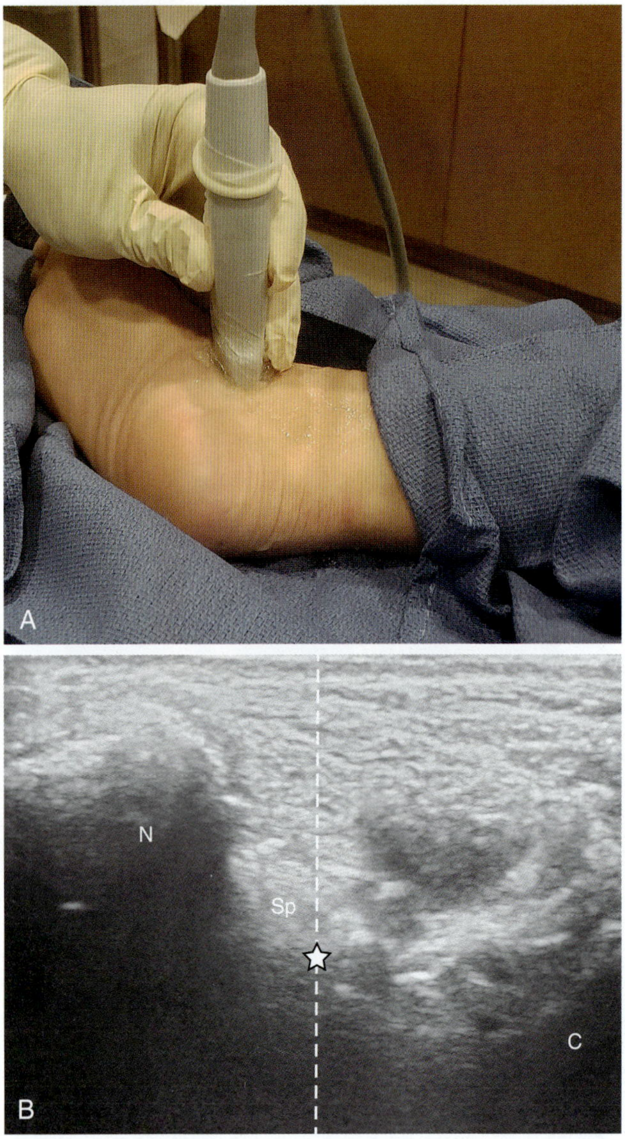

• **Fig. 22.12** (A) Plantar calcaneal navicular ligament (spring ligament) setup. (B) Plantar calcaneal navicular ligament spring ligament injection. *Asterisk,* Needle tip; *C,* calcaneus; *N,* navicular bone; *Sp,* spring ligament.

Pertinent Anatomy

- The Achilles tendon is the longest, thickest, and strongest tendon in the body.[29]
- It connects the gastrocnemius and soleus muscles to the calcaneus.

Common Pathology

- Tendinopathy or rupture of the Achilles commonly occurs 2 to 6 cm proximal to its insertion at the calcaneus, as this region is relatively hypovascular.[30]
- On sonographic evaluation, tendinosis appears as a hypoechoic fusiform enlargement of the Achilles tendon without significant disruption of the tendon fibers. Increased neovascularity or hyperemia visualized on color or power Doppler is suggestive of tendinopathy and has been found to correlate with patient symptoms; vascularity should be evaluated with light transducer pressure and the foot in a neutral position so as to reduce the tissue tension.[31,32]
- Partial-thickness Achilles tendon tears may initially appear as a more defined hypoechoic or anechoic area or cleft within the tendon.[33]
- Tendinopathy associated with retrocalcaneal bursitis and Haglund's deformity may occur at the Achilles tendon insertion.
- Haglund's deformity is an enlargement of the posterior superior aspect of the calcaneus and, when present, has a more guarded prognosis in Achilles tendinopathy.[34]
- On sonographic evaluation, findings may include (1) a hypoechoic region or thickened tendon size that may represent general tendinopathy; (2) an anechoic region within the tendon that may represent a tear; and/or (3) hyperechoic region that is likely due to calcification; finally, (4) calcaneal cortical irregularities representing enthesophyte may be seen.
- Care must be taken to ensure that anisotropy is not mistaken for pathology.[35]

Equipment

- High-frequency linear ultrasound transducer.
- 30 to 25 gauge 1 to 2 inch needle.

Common Injectates

- Prolotherapy, orthobiologics (PRP, bone marrow concentrate, etc.).
- Local anesthetic (diagnostic) or corticosteroid (therapeutic) can be used in peritendinous injections.
- Avoid intratendinous corticosteroids.

Injectate Volume

- 1 to 3 mL intratendinous, or as much as can be injected without significant resistance.
- 1 to 3 mL peritendinous.

Technique of Mid-Portion Achilles Tendon Injection

Patient Position

- Prone with the foot hanging off the edge of the exam table and ankle positioned in slight passive dorsiflexion applied by the clinician.

Clinician Position

- Seated at the foot of the exam table, facing the affected lateral ankle and ultrasound machine.

Transducer Orientation

- The mid-portion Achilles tendon is easily palpable. The Achilles tendon is visualized in short axis by placing the transducer in the anatomic transverse plane and in long axis by placing the transducer in the anatomic longitudinal plane (Fig. 22.13A).
- The injection can be performed in short axis or long axis to the tendon, whichever minimizes damage to surrounding healthy tissues.

Needle Position

- Preferred approach: In-plane, lateral to medial (Fig. 22.13B).
- Alternate approach: Out-of-plane, lateral to medial.

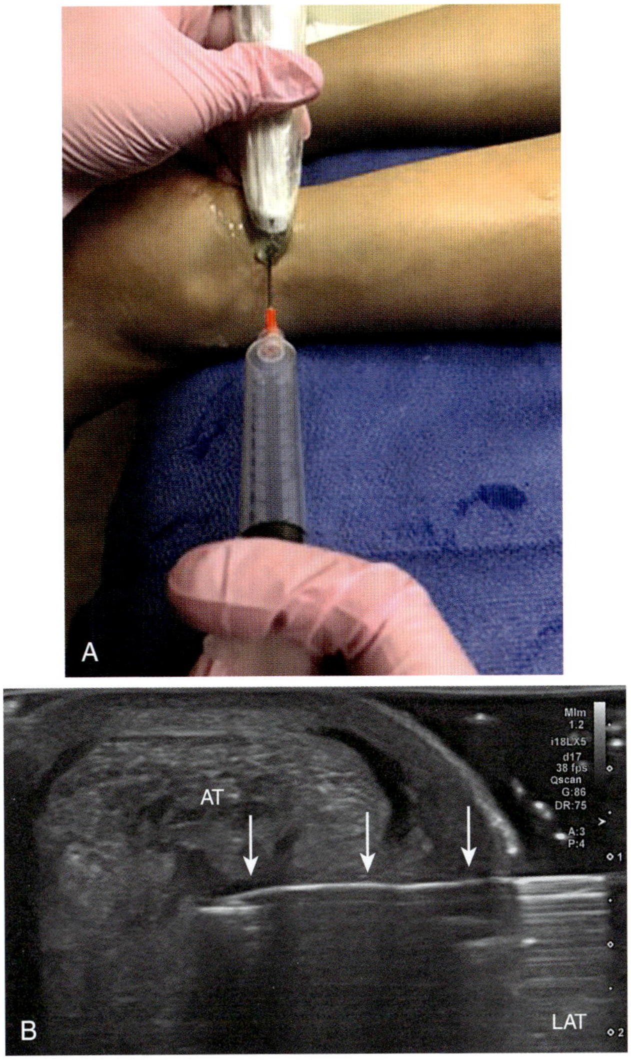

• **Fig. 22.13** (A) Ultrasound-guided mid-portion Achilles tendon injection setup of an in-plane, lateral to medial approach targeting deep to the Achilles tendon. (B) Mid-portion Achilles tendon injection using an in-plane lateral to medial approach. The Achilles tendon *(AT)* is visualized in short axis. *Arrows* point to the needle. *LAT,* lateral.

Target

- Intratendinous or peritendinous in regions of tendon hypoechogenicity, thickening, tears, hyperemia, or sonopalpation tenderness.

PEARLS AND PITFALLS

- When approaching the tendon laterally, care must be taken to avoid the sural nerve and small saphenous vein, which lie lateral to the Achilles.[36]
- Color Doppler can be used to identify areas of neovascularization, a surrogate marker for neonerves, which are thought to contribute to pain in Achilles tendinopathy.
- Orthobiologic injections can be combined with an ultrasound-guided tendon scraping procedure which mechanically separates the deep surface of the Achilles tendon from Kager's fat pad (as described later in this chapter).[37]
- Procedures are often combined with an eccentric or heavy slow resistance exercise protocol.[38]

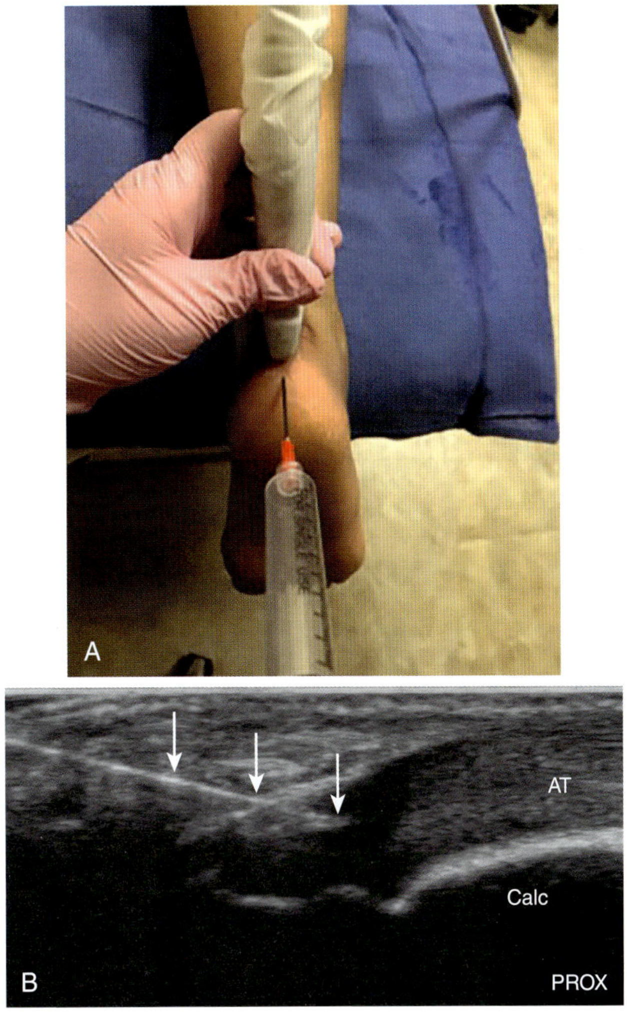

• **Fig. 22.14** (A) Ultrasound-guided insertional Achilles tendon injection setup for a distal to proximal approach. (B) Insertional Achilles tendon injection using an in-plane, distal to proximal approach. The Achilles tendon *(AT)* is visualized in long axis. *Arrows* point to the needle. *Calc,* Calcaneus; *PROX,* proximal.

Technique of Insertional Achilles Tendon Injection

Patient Position

- Prone with the foot hanging off the edge of the exam table and ankle positioned in slightly passive dorsiflexion applied by the clinician.

Clinician Position

- Seated at the foot of the exam table, facing the plantar aspect of the foot and ultrasound machine.

Transducer Orientation

- The insertional Achilles tendon is visualized in the anatomic longitudinal view by placing the transducer over the posterior aspect of calcaneus (Fig. 22.14A).
- Can visualize some of the fibers in the transverse view as well.

Needle Position

- In-plane, distal to proximal (Fig. 22.14B).
- For the transverse view can also inject in-plane lateral to medial.

Target

- Areas of tendon hypoechogenicity, calcification/enthesopathy, and cortical irregularities.

PEARLS AND PITFALLS

- Evaluate for anisotropy, particularly at the calcaneal insertion of the Achilles, to avoid misidentifying a tear.
- Target tendon enthesis as well and excoriate, if desired, if insertional tendinosis is present.
- Percutaneous needle tenotomy/fenestration can also be performed until a change in tissue texture is achieved.[78]

Tibialis Anterior Tendon/Tendon Sheath Injection

KEY POINTS

- Injury to the tibialis anterior tendon is less common than injury to other tendons about the ankle.[39]

Pertinent Anatomy

- The tibialis anterior originates from the upper two-thirds of the lateral surface of the tibia. The tendinous portion passes beneath the inferomedial band of the extensor retinaculum to insert on the medial surface of the medial cuneiform and the base of the first metatarsal (Fig. 22.15).
- The distal tibialis anterior tendon may have a longitudinal split near its insertion, which is a normal variant.[40]

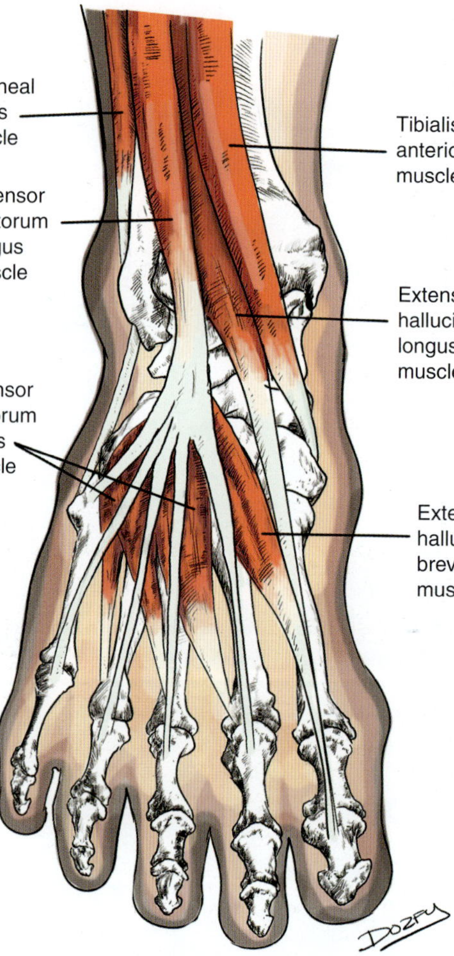

• **Fig. 22.15** Anterior Ankle and Mid Foot Musculature.

Common Pathology

- Injuries most commonly occur within 3.5 cm of the insertion.[40]
- On sonographic evaluation, tendinopathy can be identified by loss of the typical hyperechoic and fibrillar echotexture of the tibialis anterior tendon. Anechoic fluid may also be present within the tendon sheath.[41]

Equipment

- High-frequency, small footprint, linear ultrasound transducer.
- 30 to 25 gauge 1 to 2 inch needle.

Common Injectates

- Prolotherapy, orthobiologics (PRP, bone marrow concentrate, etc.).
- Local anesthetic (diagnostic) or corticosteroid (therapeutic) can be used in peritendinous injections.
- Avoid intratendinous corticosteroids.

Injectate Volume

- 1 to 3 mL intratendinous, or as much as can be injected without significant resistance.
- 1 to 3 cc peritendinous.

Technique

Patient Position

- Supine or seated on the exam table.
- Knee flexed to approximately 90 degrees and ankle in slight plantarflexion so that the plantar surface of the foot is flat on the exam table.

Clinician Position

- Seated or standing at the foot of the exam table, facing the affected medial ankle and ultrasound machine.

Transducer Orientation

- The tibialis anterior tendon is visualized in short axis as the most medially located anterior ankle tendon when placing the transducer in the anatomic transverse plane anterior to the ankle joint (Fig. 22.16A).

Needle Position

- In-plane, medial to lateral (Fig. 22.16).

Target

- Tibialis anterior tendon or tendon sheath at site of tendon hypoechogenicity, enlargement, intra-sheath fluid, or sonopalpation tenderness.

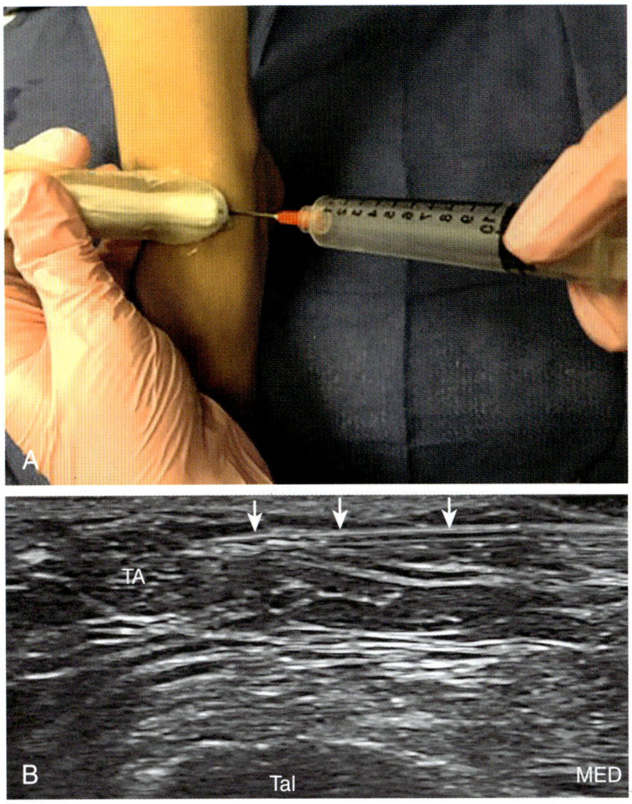

• **Fig. 22.16** (A) Ultrasound-guided tibialis anterior peritendon injection setup for an in-plane, medial to lateral approach. (B) Tibialis anterior injection using an in-plane, medial to lateral approach. The tibialis anterior *(TA)* is visualized in short axis, superficial to the talus *(Tal)*. *Arrows* point to the needle. *MED,* Medial.

PEARLS AND PITFALLS

- Identify and avoid the dorsalis pedis artery and deep fibular nerve which run laterally to the tendon.
- A longitudinal split of the distal tendon may be a normal variant and should not be mistaken for a split tear.[42]

Extensor Digitorum Tendon/Tendon Sheath Injection

KEY POINTS

- Injection can be performed anywhere along the tendon from the ankle joint to the distal insertions at the phalanges.

Pertinent Anatomy

- The EDL muscle originates on the anterior tibia, runs down the front of the tibia anterior to the ankle joint and deep to the extensor retinaculum. It inserts on the middle and distal phalanges of digits 2 to 5 (see Fig. 22.15).
- The extensor digitorum brevis (EDB) muscle originates from the proximal lateral calcaneus, the interosseous talocalcaneal ligament, and the inferior extensor retinaculum and passes medially over the foot to insert on the lateral side of the EDL on digits 2 to 4.

Common Pathology

- The extensor tendons may become irritated as they course over the dorsal aspect of the foot.
- Tendinopathy of the EDL and EDB is commonly caused by shoes tied too tightly, resulting in compression of the tendons, or due to overuse, such as with running uphill for prolonged periods.
- On sonographic evaluation, each slip of the EDL and EDB can be visualized and evaluated for loss of the normal fibrillar tendon pattern or fluid within the tendon sheath.[41]

Equipment

- High-frequency, small footprint, linear ultrasound transducer.
- 30 to 25 gauge 1 to 2 inch needle.

Common Injectates

- Prolotherapy, orthobiologics (PRP, bone marrow concentrate, etc.).
- Local anesthetic (diagnostic) or corticosteroid (therapeutic) can be used in peritendinous injections.
- Avoid intratendinous corticosteroids.

Injectate Volume

- 1 to 3 mL intratendinous, or as much as can be injected without significant resistance.
- 1 to 3 mL peritendinous.

Technique

Patient Position

- Supine or seated on the exam table.
- Knee flexed approximately to 90 degrees and ankle in slight plantarflexion so that the plantar surface of the foot is flat on the exam table.

Clinician Position

- Seated or standing at the foot of the exam table, facing the affected lateral ankle and ultrasound machine.

Transducer Orientation

- The EDL tendon is visualized in short axis by placing the transducer in the axial plane over the anterior ankle (Fig. 22.17A).
- When visualized over the talus, it lies just lateral to the tibialis anterior tendon.
- Identification of the EDL can be confirmed by following it distally into the foot and visualizing its branches to the phalanges.
- Injection is performed with the tendon visualized in short axis.

Needle Position

- In-plane, lateral to medial (Fig. 22.17B).

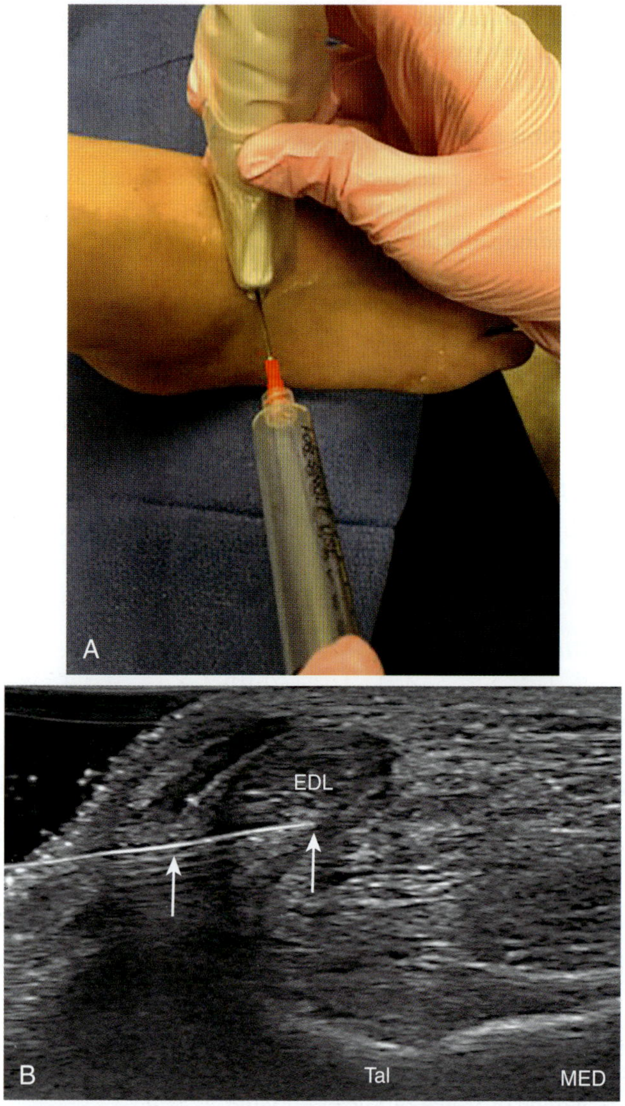

• **Fig. 22.17** (A) Ultrasound guided extensor digitorum longus *(EDL)* tendon sheath injection setup for an in-plane, lateral to medial approach. (B) EDL tendon sheath injection using an in-plane, lateral to medial approach. EDL is visualized in short axis. Note the use of gel stand-off technique. *Arrows* point to the needle. *MED,* Medial; *Tal,* talus.

Target

- Areas of tendon hypoechogenicity, intra-sheath fluid, or sonopalpation tenderness of the EDB or EDL tendon/tendon sheath.

PEARLS AND PITFALLS

- Each individual tendon of the EDL or EDB can be targeted at the location of sonopalpation tenderness.
- Identify and avoid the dorsalis pedis artery, common digital arteries, deep peroneal nerve, and digital nerves during injection.
- A unilocular, anechoic, compressible fluid collection identified deep to the EDL and superficial to the talus is the Gruberi bursa. This should be distinguished from anechoic fluid within the EDL tendon sheath or ganglion cysts, which are typically non-compressible and multilocular, and can be a target for injection.[43]

Retromalleolar Peroneus Brevis and/or Longus Tendon/Tendon Sheath Injection

KEY POINTS

- Non-traumatic subluxation of the tendons in the retromalleolar region can contribute to tendon inflammation that can be targeted during injection.

Pertinent Anatomy

- The peroneus (fibularis) longus and brevis tendons course posterior to the lateral malleolus with the peroneus brevis lying medially in the supramalleolar region. The tendons course through the osteofibrous tunnel formed by the bony retromalleolar groove and the fibrous superior peroneal retinaculum. The superior peroneal retinaculum is a band of deep fascia that extends from the posterior aspect of the lateral malleolus to the lateral surface of the calcaneus.[44]
- The peroneus brevis tendon inserts on the base of the fifth metatarsal. The peroneus longus courses across the plantar aspect of the foot and inserts on the first metatarsal and medial cuneiform.

Common Pathology

- Tendon injury may occur due to forceful contraction of the peroneal muscles in attempts to correct for sudden abnormal plantarflexion and inversion, the typical mechanism for a lateral ankle sprain.
- Non-traumatic subluxation or tendon irritation may occur in individuals with ligamentous laxity, a shallow retromalleolar groove, hypertrophied peroneal tubercle, low-lying peroneus brevis muscle, or with disruption of the superior peroneal retinaculum.
- On sonographic evaluation, tendinosis of the peroneus longus or brevis will appear as hypoechoic enlargement without well-defined tendon defects, whereas a tear will have a distinct cleft in the tendon. Visualization of two hemitendons is indicative of a longitudinal split tear.[45]
- Dynamic sonographic evaluation with dorsiflexion and eversion of the ankle may be helpful for identifying subluxation (Rankin type A = subluxation of tendons over one another; Rankin type B = subluxation of the peroneus longus tendon through a longitudinal split tear in the peroneus brevis) or dislocation of the peroneal tendons.[45-47]
- The superior peroneal retinaculum can also be evaluated sonographically and disruptions can be classified into four anatomic types based on the Oden classification.[48]

Equipment

- High-frequency, small footprint, linear ultrasound transducer.
- 30 to 25 gauge 1 to 2 inch needle.

Common Injectates

- Prolotherapy, orthobiologics (PRP, bone marrow concentrate, etc.).

- Local anesthetic (diagnostic) or corticosteroid (therapeutic) can be used in peritendinous injections.
- Avoid intratendinous corticosteroids.

Injectate Volume

- 1 to 3 mL intratendinous, or as much as can be injected without significant resistance.
- 1 to 3 mL peritendinous.

Technique

Patient Position

- Lateral decubitus with the lateral ankle of the targeted side facing upward. A towel roll may be placed under the medial ankle to position the ankle in relative inversion and plantarflexion.

Clinician Position

- Seated at the foot of the exam table, facing the affected anterior ankle and ultrasound machine.

Transducer Orientation

- Preferred approach:
  - The peroneal tendons are identified in the retromalleolar groove by placing the transducer in the axial plane, just posterior to the fibula. The peroneus brevis can be identified lying closer to the lateral malleolus (Fig. 22.18A).
  - The tendons can be scanned in short axis by translating the transducer distally and proximally along the course of the tendons.
- Alternate approach:
  - For visualization of the tendons in long axis, the transducer is placed over the posterior aspect of the distal fibula in the oblique-sagittal plane in the supramalleolar region. This allows for visualization of the peroneus brevis and longus tendons in one imaging plane.

Needle Position

- Preferred approach: In-plane, anterior to posterior (Fig. 22.18B).
- Alternate approach: In-plane, proximal to distal or distal to proximal.

Target

- Common peroneal tendons/tendon sheath in the retromalleolar groove.

PEARLS AND PITFALLS

- Dynamic ultrasound evaluation with eversion and dorsiflexion or circumduction of the foot may reveal tendon subluxation or superior retinaculum disruption.
- Fluid within the tendon sheath (tenosynovitis) should be distinguished from extratendinous fluid related to injury of the calcaneofibular ligament located distally and deep to the peroneus longus and brevis.
- A peroneus quartus is an anatomic variant (6%) that should not be confused with a split tear of the peroneus brevis.[49]

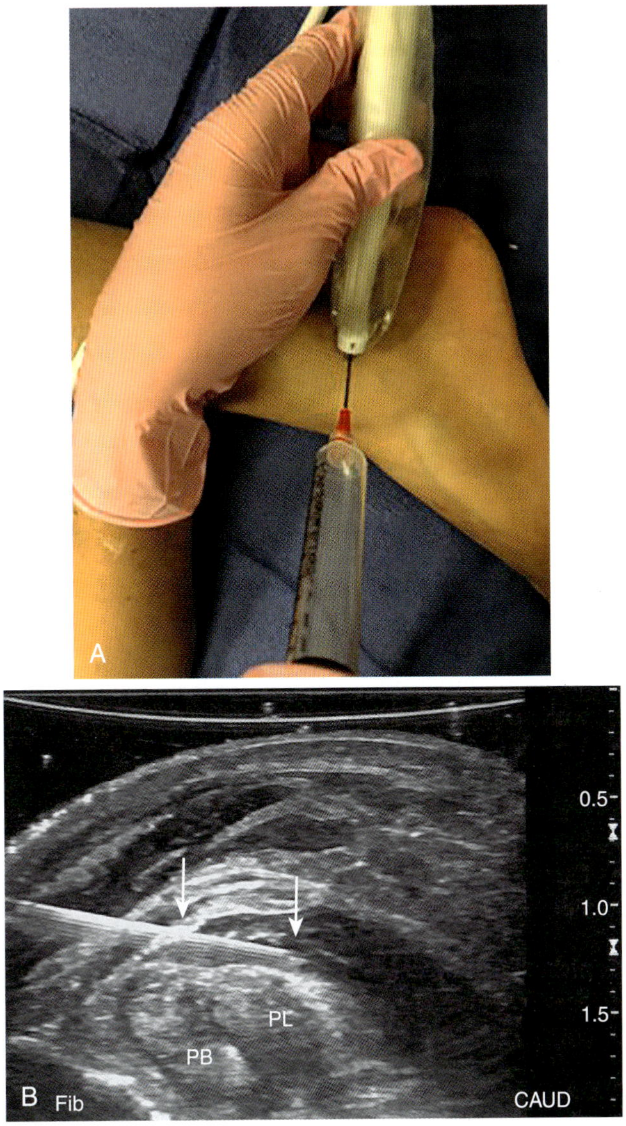

• **Fig. 22.18** (A) Ultrasound-guided peroneus longus/brevis tendon sheath injection setup at the level of the lateral malleolus, using anterior to posterior approach. (B) Peroneus longus/brevis tendon sheath injection using an in-plane, anterior to posterior approach. Peroneus longus *(PL)* and peroneus brevis *(PB)* are visualized in short axis. *Arrows* point to the needle. Note the use of gel stand-off technique. *CAUD,* Caudal; *Fib,* fibula.

Insertional Peroneus Brevis Tendon/Tendon Sheath Injection

KEY POINTS

- When scanning with ultrasound, the peroneus "B"revis is the tendon closest to the "B"one (lateral malleolus).

Pertinent Anatomy

- The peroneus brevis tendon inserts on the base of the fifth metatarsal.

Common Pathology

- Insertional peroneus brevis tendinopathy is uncommon, but may occur with repetitive eversion or in the setting of a traumatic inversion injury as the muscle forcefully contracts in response.[50]
- On sonographic evaluation, cortical irregularity at the base of the fifth metatarsal with microcalcification and/or a hypoechoic tendon structure may be visualized.[51]

Equipment

- High-frequency, small footprint, linear ultrasound transducer.
- 30 to 25 gauge 1 to 1.5 inch needle.

Common Injectates

- Prolotherapy, orthobiologics (PRP, bone marrow concentrate, etc.).
- Local anesthetic (diagnostic) or corticosteroid (therapeutic) can be used in peritendinous injections.
- Avoid intratendinous corticosteroids.

Injectate Volume

- 1 to 3 mL intratendinous, or as much as can be injected without significant resistance.
- 1 to 3 mL peritendinous.

Technique

Patient Position

- Lateral decubitus with the lateral ankle of the targeted side facing upward.

Clinician Position

- Seated or standing at the foot of the exam table, facing the anterior ankle and ultrasound machine.

Transducer Orientation

- The peroneus brevis can be identified by following it distally from the retromalleolar groove to the base of the fifth metatarsal in short axis and then rotating the transducer 90 degrees to visualize it in long axis (Fig. 22.19A).
- Alternatively, the peroneus brevis can be identified by placing the transducer parallel to the plantar aspect of the foot with the distal aspect of the transducer over the base of the fifth metatarsal.
- Injection is performed with the transducer in long axis to the tendon.

Needle Position

- In-plane, distal to proximal or proximal to distal (Fig. 22.19B).

Target

- Peroneus brevis insertion/enthesopathy.

PEARLS AND PITFALLS

- Use of a gel standoff technique may allow for improved needle visualization during the injection.
- If calcifications are present in the tendon insertional fibers, needle tenotomy/fenestration can also be performed.

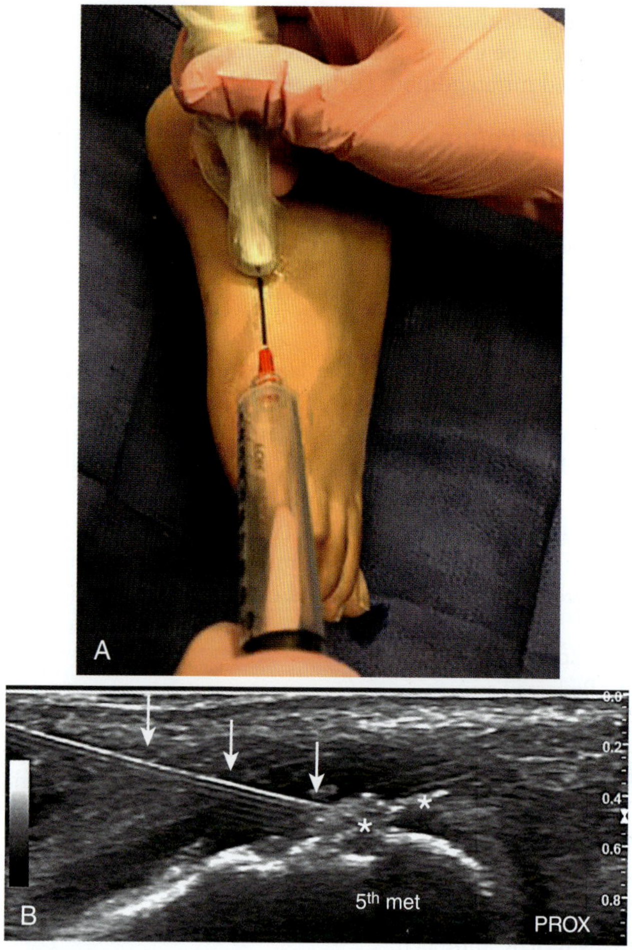

• **Fig. 22.19** (A) Ultrasound-guided peroneus brevis insertional tendon injection setup for an in-plane, distal to proximal approach. (B) Peroneus brevis insertional tendon injection using an in-plane, distal to proximal approach. The peroneus brevis is visualized in long axis and is calcific *(asterisk)*. *Arrows* point to the needle. *5th met,* Base of fifth metatarsal; *PROX,* proximal.

Tibialis Posterior Tendon/Tendon Sheath Injection

KEY POINTS

- Injection should target the area of pathology.

Pertinent Anatomy

- The tibialis posterior tendon emerges distally from tibialis posterior muscle that originates in the deep compartment of the lower leg, running posterior to the medial malleolus and under the flexor retinaculum. This tendon, along with the spring ligament, supports the medial longitudinal arch through its broad and complex attachment (navicular, cuboid, cuneiforms, metatarsals 2 to 4).[52]

Common Pathology

- Tendinopathic changes occur most commonly in the retromalleolar region or distally at the navicular insertion.[53]

- Injuries often occur insidiously without discrete injury and are usually secondary to overuse or repetitive microtrauma, resulting in degeneration or a longitudinal split thickness tear in the retromalleolar region.[54]
- On sonographic evaluation, tendon sheath distention greater than 5.8 mm with anechoic fluid, hypoechoic and hypertrophied tendon (after accounting for anisotropy), or areas of discrete anechoic clefts with disruption of the fibrillar pattern can indicate pathology.[55]
- A longitudinal split tear may be associated with abnormal tendon dislocation or subluxation, which may be apparent only during ankle movement.[56]
- Of note, it is normal to see up to 4 mm of fluid in the tendon sheath of the tibialis posterior tendon just beyond the medial malleolus, but this should not be present at the navicular where the tendon sheath is absent.[57]

Equipment

- High-frequency, small footprint, linear ultrasound transducer.
- 30 to 25 gauge 1 to 1.5 inch needle.

Common Injectates

- Prolotherapy, orthobiologics (PRP, bone marrow concentrate, etc.).
- Local anesthetic (diagnostic) or corticosteroid (therapeutic) can be used in peritendinous injections.
- Avoid intratendinous corticosteroids.

Injectate Volume

- 1 to 3 mL intratendinous, or as much as can be injected without significant resistance.
- 1 to 5 mL peritendinous.

Technique

Patient Position

- Lateral decubitus with the medial ankle of the targeted side facing upward.
- Unaffected leg will be positioned away from the injection site.

Clinician Position

- Seated or standing at the foot of the exam table, facing the patient and ultrasound machine.

Transducer Orientation

- If targeting the retromalleolar region, the transducer is placed in short axis to the tendon in the anatomic axial plane just posterior to the medial malleolus (Fig. 22.20A).
- If targeting the tendon insertion, the transducer is placed in long axis to the distal tendon at the navicular insertion (Fig. 22.21A).

Needle Position

- Proximal, retromalleolar region: In-plane, anterior to posterior (Fig. 22.20B).
- Distal, navicular region: In-plane, distal to proximal (Fig. 22.21B).

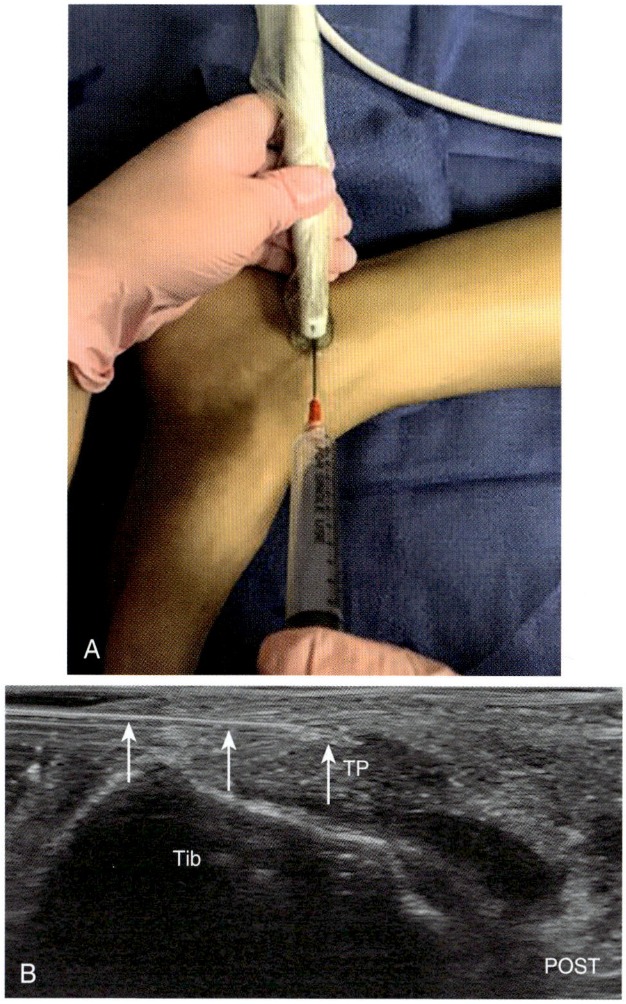

• **Fig. 22.20** (A) Ultrasound-guided retromalleolar tibialis posterior injection setup for an in-plane, anterior to posterior approach. (B) Retromalleolar tibialis posterior injection using an in-plane, anterior to posterior approach. The tibialis posterior tendon *(TP)* is visualized in short axis. *Arrows* point to the needle. Note use of gel stand-off technique. *POST,* Posterior; *Tib,* tibia.

Target

- Tendon or tendon sheath in region(s) of hypoechogenicity, thickening, interstitial tearing, sonopalpation tenderness.

PEARLS AND PITFALLS

- Identify and avoid the tibial neurovascular bundle.
- Injections are commonly targeted to just within the tendon sheath to avoid disrupting the tendon structure. Orthobiologic injections can target areas of hypoechogenicity as well as fill interstitial tears with injectate. You can target the enthesopathy and insertion at the navicular if pathologic.
- When injecting near the retromalleolar groove, an anterior to posterior approach is preferred to avoid neurovascular structures.

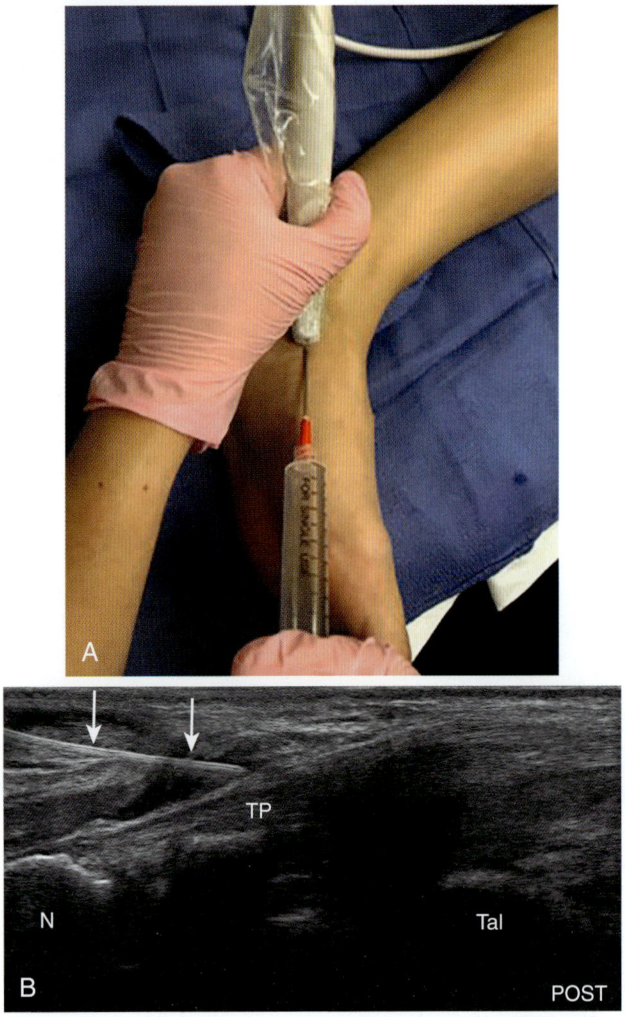

• **Fig. 22.21** (A) Ultrasound-guided distal tibialis posterior injection setup for an in-plane, distal to proximal approach. (B) Distal tibialis posterior injection using an in-plane, distal to proximal approach. The tibialis posterior tendon *(TP)* is visualized in long axis as it nears its insertion on the navicular *(N)*. *Arrows* point to the needle. *POST,* Posterior; *Tal,* talus.

Flexor Digitorum Longus Tendon/Tendon Sheath Injection

KEY POINTS

- The injection can be performed at the retromalleolar groove, near the sustentaculum tali, or at the knot of Henry, depending on the area of pathology.

Pertinent Anatomy

- The flexor digitorum longus (FDL) muscle originates on the posterior tibia, medial to the tibialis posterior. The FDL and tibialis posterior tendons cross just proximal to the medial malleolus and the FDL tendon continues distally posterior to the medial malleolus and tibialis posterior tendon.
- The FDL then courses around the sustentaculum tali, crosses over the flexor hallucis longus (FHL) tendon at the level of the navicular at the knot of Henry, joins the quadratus plantae in the sole of the foot, and finally splits into four separate tendons that insert on the plantar aspect of the distal phalanges of digits 4 to 5.
- The flexor digitorum accessory longus (FDAL) is the most common accessory muscle in the foot and ankle region, present in 6% to 12% of individuals. It has a variable origin and insertion, and commonly runs through the tarsal tunnel posterior to the FHL.[58,59]

Common Pathology

- The FDL is prone to tendinopathy where it courses around the sustentaculum tali and crosses the FHL at the knot of Henry; the FDL and FHL interact closely, with fibrous interconnections at the knot of Henry where it is prone to friction.[60,61]
- Tendinopathy of the FDL often occurs after walking barefoot on uneven or sandy surfaces where the toes are not fully able to grip the surface.
- On sonographic evaluation, tendon sheath distention with anechoic fluid, hypoechoic and hypertrophied tendon (after accounting for anisotropy), or areas of discrete anechoic clefts with disruption of the fibrillar pattern are suggestive of tendon injury.[62]

Equipment

- High-frequency, small footprint, linear ultrasound transducer.
- 30 to 25 gauge 1 to 2 inch needle.

Common Injectates

- Prolotherapy, orthobiologics (PRP, bone marrow concentrate, etc.).
- Local anesthetic (diagnostic) or corticosteroid (therapeutic) can be used in peritendinous injections.
- Avoid intratendinous corticosteroids.

Injectate Volume

- 1 to 3 mL intratendinous, or as much as can be injected without significant resistance.
- 1 to 3 mL peritendinous.

Technique

Patient Position

- Lateral decubitus with the medial ankle of the targeted side facing upward.

Clinician Position

- Seated or standing at the foot of the exam table, facing toward the anterior ankle and ultrasound machine.

Transducer Orientation

- Preferred approach: The FDL tendon is visualized in short axis just posterior to the tibialis posterior tendon

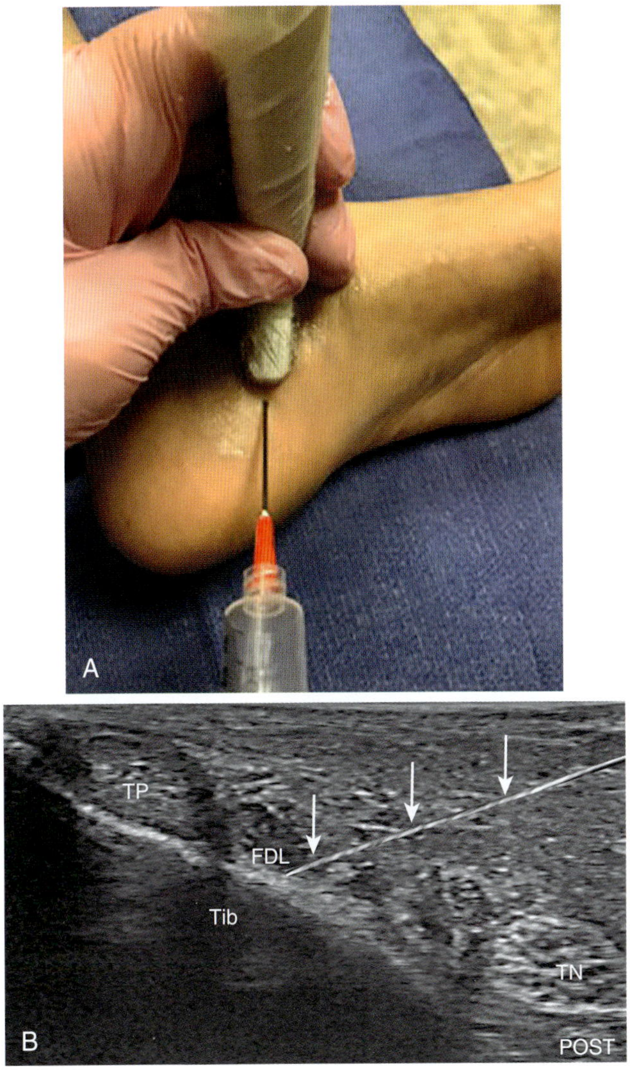

• **Fig. 22.22** (A) Ultrasound-guided flexor digitorum longus *(FDL)* injection setup for an in-plane, posterior to anterior approach. (B) FDL injection using an in-plane, posterior to anterior approach. The FDL is visualized in short axis. *Arrows* point to the needle. *POST,* Posterior; *Tib,* tibia; *TN,* tibial nerve; *TP,* tibialis posterior.

with the transducer placed posterior to the medial malleolus in the transverse plane (Fig. 22.22A).

- Alternate approach: The transducer is rotated 90 degrees to visualize the tendons in short axis.

Needle Position

- Preferred approach: In-plane, posterior to anterior (Fig. 22.22B).
- Alternate approach: In-plane, proximal to distal.

Target

- Tendon in region(s) of hypoechogenicity, thickening, interstitial tearing, sonopalpation tenderness, or tendon sheath.
- FDL tendon/tendon sheath.

PEARLS & PITFALLS

- The tibial neurovasculature is located in close proximity to the FDL and must be identified prior to the injection and avoided.
- Use of a gel stand-off technique may allow for improved visualization during the injection.

Flexor Hallucis Longus Tendon/Tendon Sheath Injection in the Tarsal Tunnel

KEY POINTS

- During the injection, care must be taken to avoid injury to the tibial neurovasculature, which is located in close proximity to the tendon.

Pertinent Anatomy

- The FHL muscle is located deep in the posterior compartment. The FHL tendon courses posterior to the medial malleolus over the posterior talus between the lateral and medial posterior tubercles and under the sustentaculum tali. It crosses under the FDL at the knot of Henry, continuing into the sole of the foot to run between the hallux sesamoid bones, inserting onto the plantar aspect of the distal phalanx.

Common Pathology

- Tenosynovitis of the FHL in the tarsal tunnel at the level of the posterior talus and os trigonum is the most common seen pathology; however, tendinopathy may also occur more distally at the knot of Henry or at the level of the sesamoids.
- On sonographic evaluation, tendinosis is characterized by hypoechoic enlargement of the involved tendon and anechoic fluid may be seen surrounding the tendon at sites of irritation in tenosynovitis.[62] Of note, the FHL tendon sheath communicates with the ankle joint, so additional sonographic evaluation of the anterior joint recess must be performed to rule out intra-articular cause to intra-sheath fluid.
- Dynamic sonographic evaluation can reveal great toe triggering and confirm the diagnosis of hallux saltans.[63]

Equipment

- High-frequency, small footprint, linear ultrasound transducer.
- 30 to 25 gauge 1 to 2 inch needle.

Common Injectates

- Prolotherapy, orthobiologics (PRP, bone marrow concentrate, etc.).

- Local anesthetic (diagnostic) or corticosteroid (therapeutic) can be used in peritendinous injections.
- Avoid intratendinous corticosteroids.

Injectate Volume

- 1 to 3 mL intratendinous, or as much as can be injected without significant resistance.
- 1 to 3 mL peritendinous.

Technique

Patient Position

- Lateral decubitus with the medial ankle of the targeted side facing upward skyward or prone.

Clinician Position

- Seated or standing at the foot of the exam table, facing the posterior ankle and ultrasound machine.

Transducer Orientation

- The FHL tendon is visualized in short axis just posterior and deep to the tibial neurovasculature with transducer in transverse plane (Fig. 22.23A).

Needle Position

- In-plane, posterior to anterior (Fig. 22.23B).

Target

- Tendon or tendon sheath in region(s) of hypoechogenicity, thickening, interstitial tearing, sonopalpation tenderness.

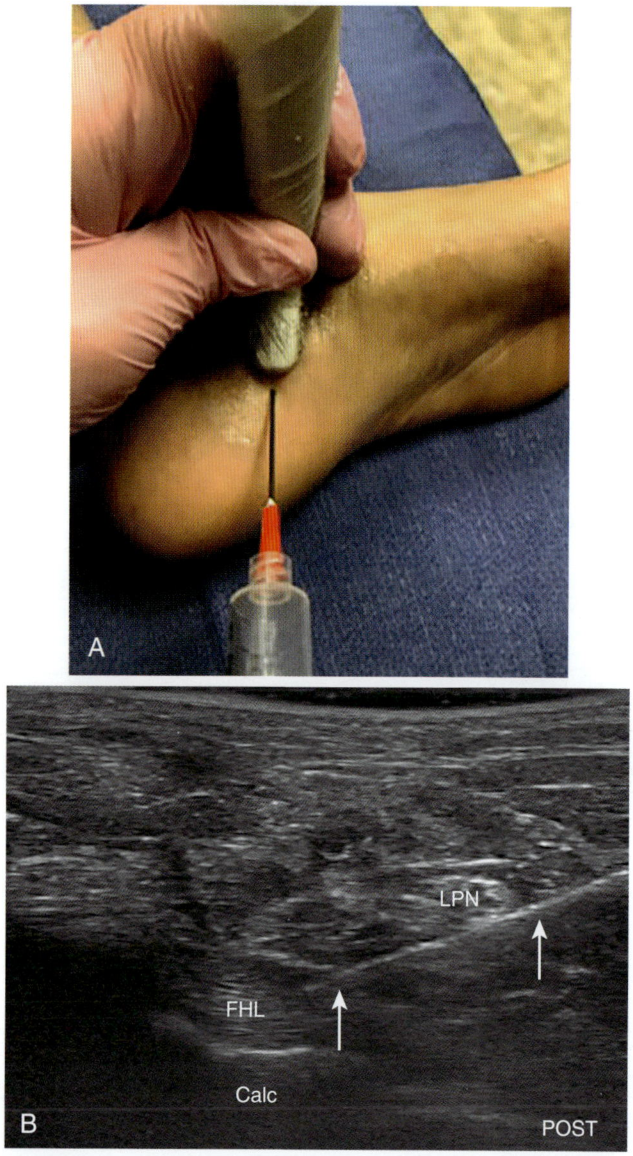

• **Fig. 22.23** (A) Ultrasound-guided flexor hallucis longus *(FHL)* injection setup for an in-plane, posterior to anterior approach. (B) FHL injection using an in-plane, posterior to anterior approach. FHL is visualized in short axis. *Arrows* point to the needle. *Calc,* Calcaneus; *LPN,* lateral plantar nerve; *POST,* posterior.

PEARLS AND PITFALLS

- The tibial neurovasculature and branches vary but are most commonly located anterior to the FHL and should be identified and avoided during injection.[64]
- Use of a gel stand-off technique may allow for improved visualization during the injection.
- Injection may also be performed by entering on the lateral aspect of the ankle and advancing the needle medially anterior to the Achilles tendon to reach the medial aspect of the FHL tendon sheath.
- Tendinopathy of the FDL can occur with FHL tendinopathy at the knot of Henry and can also be a target for intervention.

Perineural Injections

KEY POINTS

- Injections can be performed along the course of the nerve, targeting regions of clinical symptoms, focal nerve enlargement, or sonopalpation tenderness.
- Diagnostic perineural injections can be used to confirm that symptoms are resulting from nerve injury.
- Therapeutic hydrodissection/hydrorelease of the nerve can be performed to free the nerve from surrounding adhesions. Indications for therapeutic injections have not been well studied in the literature but are likely effective for compressive neuropathy. To date, there have been no studies examining the specificity, sensitivity, or accuracy of the use of ultrasound-guided hydrodissection/release in mononeuropathies of the superficial peroneal nerve, deep peroneal nerve, or tibial nerve and its branches.
- On sonographic evaluation, the nerve may appear larger and hypoechoic proximal to the level of entrapment, with loss of the normal fascicular architecture.[62] Sonopalpation tenderness can assist in localizing the region of nerve injury. The nerve is targeted at this location during a hydrodissection/hydrorelease procedure.
- Neuromas appear as focal, hypoechoic masses with poor internal fascicular definition, and are continuous with the nerve. These can be the target of perineural injections.

Superficial Peroneal Nerve

Pertinent Anatomy

- The superficial peroneal (fibular) nerve generally carries fascicles from the L4-S1 root levels.
- The common peroneal nerve branches from the sciatic nerve in the posterior distal thigh and courses around the fibular neck before dividing into superficial and deep peroneal nerves at the anterolateral aspect of the proximal fibula.
- Although great variability has been described, the superficial peroneal nerve typically descends in the lateral compartment of the lower leg between the peroneal muscles and the lateral aspect of the EDL.[65]
- When it reaches the lower third of the leg, it pierces the deep crural fascia to course superficially and terminates to divide into the medial and intermediate dorsal cutaneous nerves.[65]
- The superficial peroneal nerve supplies motor function to peroneus longus and brevis and provides sensory function to the anterolateral leg and dorsum of the foot.

Common Pathology

- Due to its superficial location, the superficial peroneal nerve is prone to injury from direct trauma, lacerations, ankle sprains, etc.
- The nerve is commonly compressed or stretched at the fibular neck or compressed where it pierces the deep crural fascia at the lower third of the leg. This neural strain may trigger a cascade of inflammation and scarring to the surrounding soft tissue, which can result in chronic neuropathic pain.

Equipment

- High-frequency linear ultrasound transducer.
- 30 to 25 gauge 1 to 2 inch needle.

Common Injectates

- For nerve block: Local anesthetic with or without corticosteroid.
- For hydrodissection/hydrorelease Mixture of normal saline and local anesthetic solution, 5% dextrose solution, or platelet lysate solutions.

Injectate Volume

- For nerve block: 5 to 10 mL.
- For hydrodissection/hydrorelease: 5 to 15 mL along the course of the nerve.

Technique

Patient Position

- Supine with the affected leg internally rotated or lateral decubitus with the lateral ankle of the targeted side facing upward.

Clinician Position

- Seated at the foot of the exam table, facing the posterior ankle and ultrasound machine.

Transducer Orientation

- The superficial peroneal nerve is most commonly identified in short axis at the distal third of the leg where it exits the crural fascia with the transducer in the axial plane (Figs. 22.24A and 22.25A).
- The transducer can be translated distally and proximally along the course of the superficial peroneal nerve to identify the area of pathology.
- Injection is performed with the transducer positioned to view the nerve in short axis, unless long-axis view is indicated to cover a longer segment of the nerve.
- Injection can be performed anywhere along the course of the nerve.

Needle Position

- In-plane, posterolateral to anteromedial (Fig. 22.24B and Fig. 22.25B).

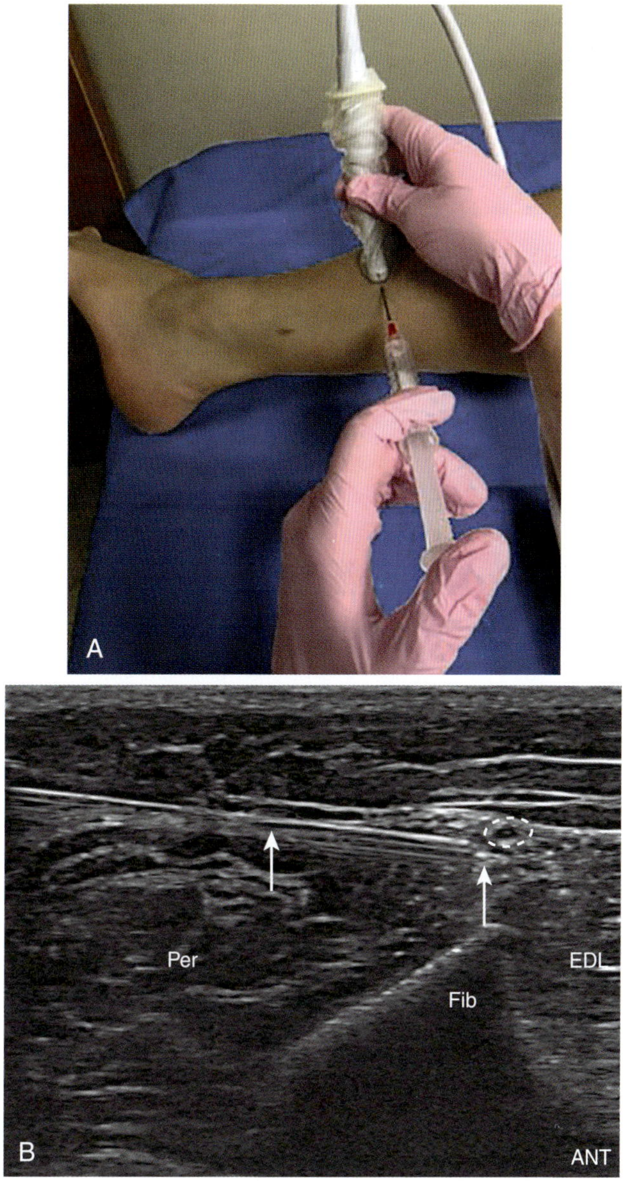

• **Fig. 22.24** (A) Ultrasound-guided superficial peroneal perineural injection setup for an in-plane, posterolateral to anteromedial injection at the distal third of the leg. (B) Superficial peroneal perineural injection at the distal third of the lower leg using an in-plane, posterolateral to anteromedial approach. Superficial peroneal nerve *(circled)* is visualized in short axis near where it exits the crural fascia and is commonly entrapped. *Arrows* point to the needle. *ANT,* Anterior; *EDL,* extensor digitorum longus muscle; *Fib,* fibula; *Per,* peroneal musculature.

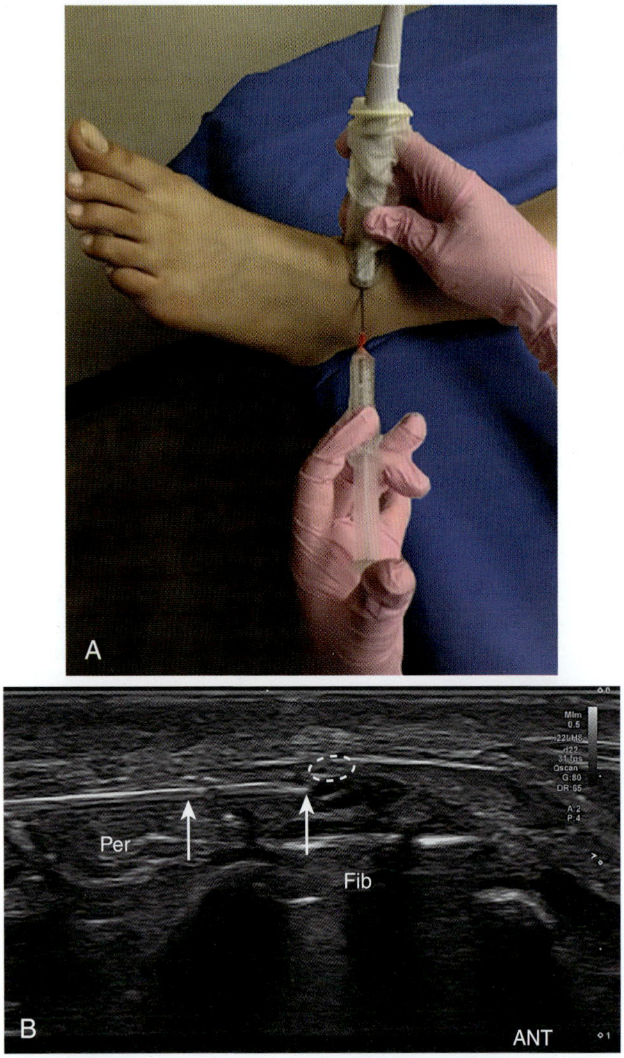

• **Fig. 22.25** (A) Ultrasound-guided superficial peroneal perineural injection setup for an in-plane, posterolateral to anteromedial injection at the mid-fibula level. (B) Superficial peroneal perineural injection using an in-plane, posterolateral to anteromedial approach. Superficial peroneal nerve *(circled)* is visualized in short axis where it courses over the ankle joint. *Arrows* point to the needle. *ANT,* Anterior; *Fib,* fibula; *Per,* peroneal musculature.

Target

- Mesoneurium in regions of focal flattening, proximal enlargement, or sonopalpation tenderness along the nerve.

PEARLS AND PITFALLS

- The nerve is most commonly targeted where it pierces the crural fascia since this is a common site of pathology.
- The procedure should be planned so that one can minimize damage to the nerve and nearby muscle, tendons, and vasculature.
- Begin injecting while approaching the mesoneurium and advance the needle while injecting slowly to gently push the nerve away, reducing the risk of intraneural injection.
- With proper release, accompanying vessels have been observed to appear to have a stronger pulse, although the significance of this phenomenon is unknown.

Deep Peroneal Nerve

Pertinent Anatomy

- The deep peroneal (fibular) nerve generally carries fascicles from the L4-S1 root levels.
- The common peroneal nerve branches from the sciatic nerve in the posterior distal thigh and courses around the fibular head before dividing into the superficial and deep peroneal nerves.
- The deep peroneal nerve runs inferomedially, deep to the EDL along the anterior surface of the interosseous membrane, where it runs with the anterior tibial artery in the middle of the leg. It descends with the artery anterior to the tibiotalar joint, where it divides into the lateral and medial terminal branches.
- The medial terminal branch runs with the dorsalis pedis artery to the first interosseous space. The lateral terminal branch passes beneath the EDB.
- It provides motor function to the muscles of the anterior compartment of the leg, the EDB, and the extensor hallucis brevis. It provides sensory innervation to the first dorsal webspace.

Common Pathology

- The nerve is commonly compressed or stretched at the fibular neck.
- Injury to the deep peroneal nerve in the distal lower leg is rare and is typically a result of an ankle sprain, ganglion cyst,[66,67] or iatrogenic injury.[68]

Equipment

- High-frequency, small footprint, linear ultrasound transducer.
- 30 to 25 gauge 1 to 2 inch needle.

Common Injectates

- For nerve block: Local anesthetic with or without corticosteroid
- For hydrodissection/hydrorelease: Mixture of normal saline and local anesthetic solution or 5% dextrose solution, or platelet lysate solution have been used.

Injectate Volume

- For nerve block: 2 to 5 mL.
- For hydrodissection/hydrorelease: 5 to 15 mL along the course of the nerve.

Technique

Patient Position

- Supine or seated on the exam table.
- Knee extended and ankle in slight plantarflexion.

Clinician Position

- Seated or standing at the foot of the exam table, facing toward the patient and ultrasound machine.

Transducer Orientation

- The deep peroneal nerve is visualized in short axis over the anterior talus deep to the extensor hallucis longus (EHL) and lateral to the dorsalis pedis artery (Fig. 22.26A).

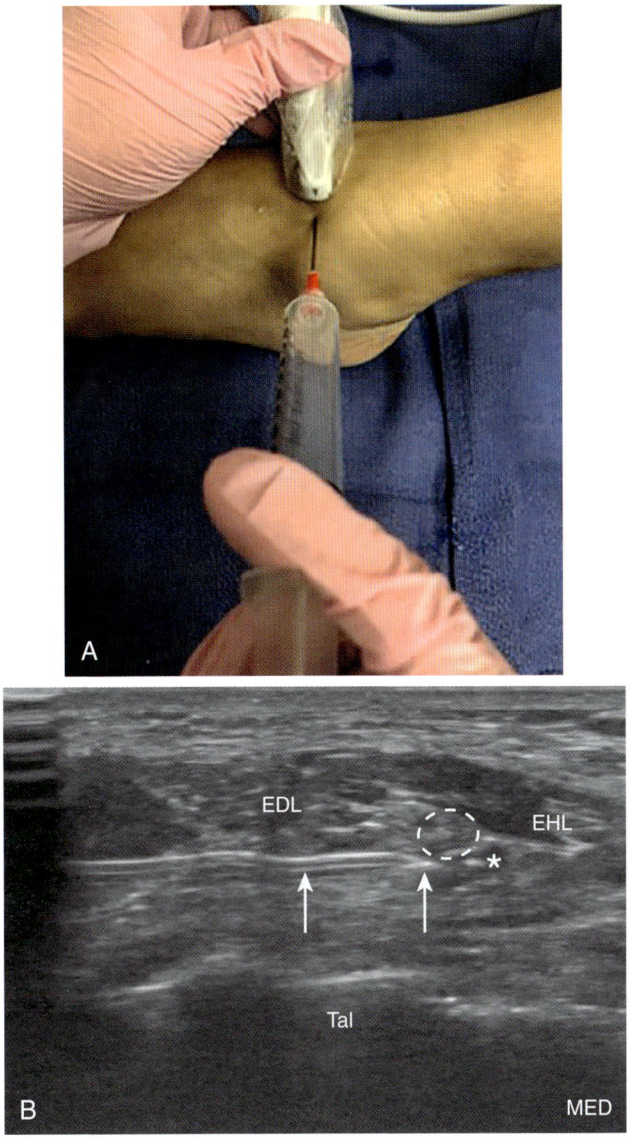

• **Fig. 22.26** (A) Ultrasound-guided deep peroneal perineural injection setup for an in-plane, lateral to medial approach. (B) Deep peroneal perineural injection using an in-plane, lateral to medial approach. Deep peroneal nerve *(circled)* is visualized in short axis near the dorsalis pedis artery *(asterisk)*. *Arrows* point to the needle. *EDL*, Extensor digitorum longus tendon; *EHL*, extensor hallucis longus muscle/tendon; *MED*, medial; *Tal,* talus.

- The transducer can be translated distally and proximally along the course of the deep peroneal nerve to identify the area of pathology.
- Injection is performed with the transducer positioned to view the nerve in short axis, unless long-axis view is indicated to cover a longer segment of the nerve.

Needle Position

- In-plane, lateral to medial or medial to lateral, depending on the location of the dorsalis pedis artery (Fig. 22.26B).

Target

- Mesoneurium in regions of focal flattening, proximal enlargement, or sonopalpation tenderness along the nerve.

PEARLS AND PITFALLS

- Perineural injections of the deep peroneal nerve are mostly performed anterior to the ankle joint.
- Take care to avoid injury to the nerve and nearby tendons and vasculature. Color Doppler should be used to identify the dorsalis pedis artery prior to injection and an appropriate approach should be taken to avoid injury to the artery.
- Begin injecting while approaching the mesoneurium and advance the needle while injecting slowly to gently push the nerve away, reducing the risk of intraneural injection.
- With proper release, accompanying vessels are observed to have a stronger pulse, although the significance of this phenomenon is unknown.

Tibial Nerve

Pertinent Anatomy

- The tibial nerve generally carries fascicles from the L5-S2 root levels. It branches from the sciatic nerve in the posterior distal thigh and courses down the posterior calf and into the medial ankle, where it enters the tarsal tunnel after dividing into the medial and lateral plantar nerves.
- The tarsal tunnel is located at the medial ankle posterior to the medial malleolus and is divided into an upper compartment (bound superficially by the deep aponeurosis) and lower ("classic") compartment (bound superficially by the flexor retinaculum, also called the laciniate ligament).

Common Pathology

- Tarsal tunnel syndrome typically involves entrapment of the tibial nerve or its branches, causing pain or paresthesias in the plantar aspect of the foot.
- Baxter's neuritis is characterized by chronic heel pain from entrapment of the first branch of the lateral plantar nerve by the deep fascia of the abductor hallucis muscle and/or beneath the medial edge of the quadratus plantae fascia.
- Jogger's foot refers to medial plantar nerve compression, often seen with hyperpronation with running.

Equipment

- High-frequency, small footprint, linear ultrasound transducer.
- 30 to 25 gauge 1 to 2 inch needle.

Common Injectates

- For nerve block: Local anesthetic with or without corticosteroid.
- For hydrodissection/hydrorelease: Mixture of normal saline and local anesthetic solution or 5% dextrose solution, or platelet lysate solution may be used.

Injectate Volume

- For nerve block: 5 to 10 mL.
- For hydrodissection/hydrorelease: 10 to 15 mL along the course of the nerve.

Technique

Patient Position

- Prone or lateral decubitus with the medial ankle of the targeted side facing upward.

Clinician Position

- Seated or standing at the foot of the exam table, facing the posterior ankle and ultrasound machine.

Transducer Orientation

- The tibial nerve is visualized in short axis posterior to the FDL tendon with the transducer placed in the axial plane just posterior to the proximal medial malleolus (Fig. 22.27A).
- The transducer can be translated distally and proximally along the course of the tibial nerve to identify its branches and the area of pathology.
- Injection is performed with the transducer positioned to view the nerve in short axis, unless long-axis view is indicated to cover a longer segment of the nerve.

Needle Position

- In-plane, posterior to anterior (Fig. 22.27B).

Target

- Mesoneurium in regions of focal flattening, proximal enlargement, or sonopalpation tenderness along the nerve.

PEARLS AND PITFALLS

- Take care to avoid injury to the nerve and nearby tendons and vasculature. Color Doppler should be used to identify the posterior tibial artery and veins prior to injection.
- Begin injecting while approaching the mesoneurium and advance the needle while injecting slowly to gently push the nerve away, reducing the risk of intraneural injection.
- With proper release, accompanying vessels are observed to have a stronger pulse, although the significance of this phenomenon is unknown.
- Branches of the tibial nerve in the foot, including Baxter's nerve and the medial plantar nerve, can also be targeted.

Saphenous Nerve

Pertinent Anatomy

- The saphenous nerve is the sensory terminal branch of the femoral nerve, arising in the femoral triangle, coursing deep to Hunter's canal, before becoming subcutaneous by piercing the fascia lata between the gracilis and sartorius tendons in the thigh. In the lower leg, it runs distally behind the medial border of the tibia with the great saphenous vein and divides into two branches in the distal third of the lower leg.
- One branch continues along the margin of the tibia and terminates at the ankle while the other branch travels

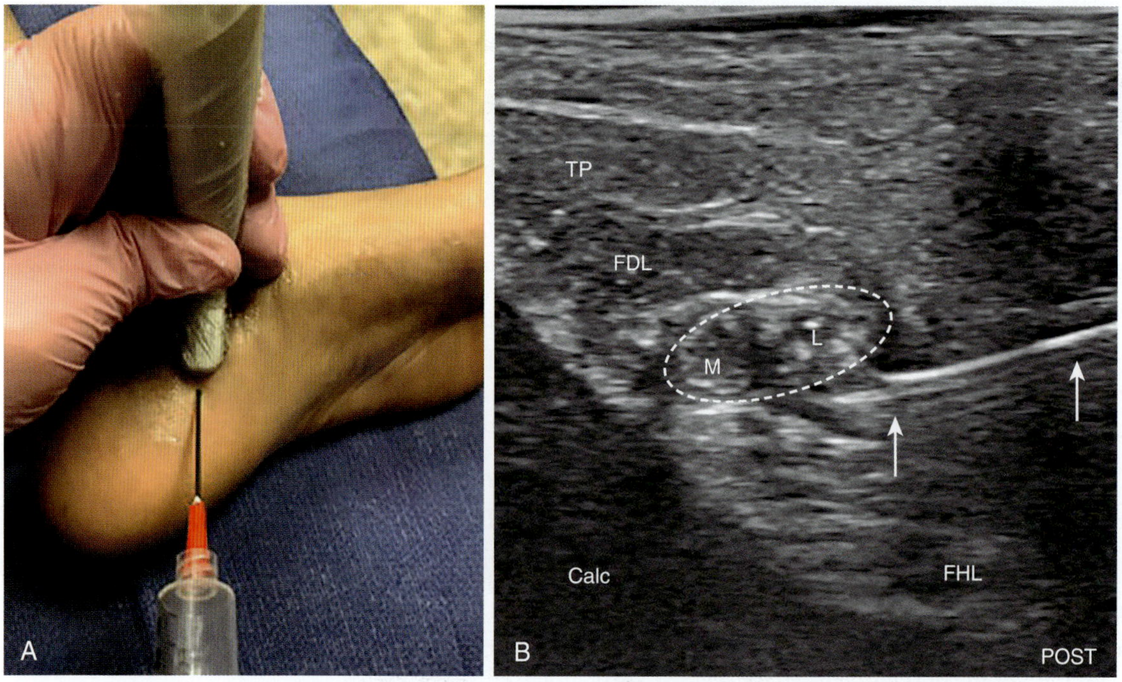

• **Fig. 22.27** (A) Ultrasound-guided tibial perineural injection setup for an in-plane, posterior to anterior approach. (B) Tibial perineural injection using an in-plane, posterior to anterior approach. The tibial nerve *(circled)* has split into the medial plantar nerve *(M)* and lateral plantar nerve *(L)*. *Arrows* point to the needle. *Calc,* Calcaneus; *FDL,* flexor digitorum longus; *FHL,* flexor hallucis longus; *POST,* posterior; *TP,* tibialis posterior.

with the great saphenous vein anterior to the medial malleolus and into the foot.[69]

- The branch of the saphenous nerve at the ankle supplies the medial side of the foot.

Common Pathology

- The saphenous nerve is susceptible to injury anywhere along its pathway. Injury may occur from direct trauma, stretching (such as ankle dislocation), or compression to anterior thigh, medial knee and shin, or over medial ankle.

Equipment

- High-frequency, small footprint, linear ultrasound transducer.
- 30 to 25 gauge 1 to 2 inch needle.

Common Injectates

- For nerve block: Local anesthetic with or without corticosteroid.
- For hydrodissection/hydrorelease: Mixture of normal saline and local anesthetic solution or 5% dextrose solution, or platelet lysate solution may be used.

Injectate Volume

- For nerve block: 2 to 5 mL.
- For hydrodissection/hydrorelease: 5 to 15 mL along the course of the nerve, per expert opinion.

Technique

Patient Position

- Lateral decubitus with the medial ankle of the targeted side facing upward.

Clinician Position

- Seated at the foot of the exam table, facing toward the patient and ultrasound machine.

Transducer Orientation

- The saphenous nerve can be visualized in short axis lateral and proximal to the medial malleolus with the transducer in the anatomic axial plane (Fig. 22.28A).
- The transducer can be translated distally and proximally along the course of the saphenous nerve to identify its branches and the area of pathology.
- Injection is performed with the transducer positioned to view the nerve in short axis, unless long-axis view is indicated to cover a longer segment of the nerve.

Needle Position

- In-plane, posteromedial to anterolateral, or anteromedial to posterolateral (Fig. 22.28B).

Target

- Mesoneurium in regions of focal flattening, proximal enlargement, or sonopalpation tenderness along the nerve.

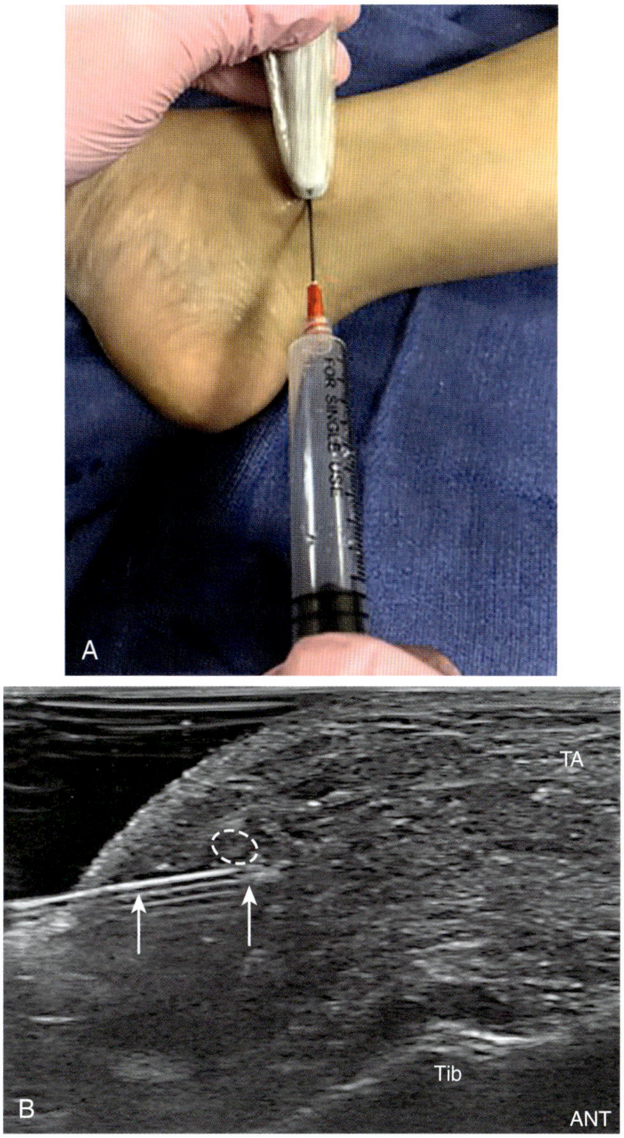

• **Fig. 22.28** (A) Ultrasound-guided saphenous perineural injection setup for an in-plane, posteromedial to anterolateral approach. (B) Saphenous injection using an in-plane, posteromedial to anterolateral approach. The saphenous nerve *(circled)* is visualized in short axis. *Arrows* point to the needle. *ANT,* Anterior; *TA,* tibialis anterior; *Tib,* tibia.

PEARLS AND PITFALLS

- Care should be taken to avoid injury to the saphenous nerve or greater saphenous vein.
- If a nerve block is being performed and the distal saphenous nerve branches above the level of the block due to anatomic variation, and an additional block more proximally may be necessary.
- The saphenous nerve can be difficult to identify. Localization may be facilitated by first identifying the greater saphenous vein followed by the adjacent nerve.
- Begin injecting while approaching the mesoneurium and advance the needle while injecting slowly to gently push the nerve away, reducing the risk of intraneural injection.
- With proper release, accompanying vessels are observed to have a stronger pulse, although the significance of this phenomenon is unknown.

Sural Nerve

Pertinent Anatomy

- The sural nerve is formed by contributions of the tibial and common fibular nerves.
- It travels in the posterior calf with the small (lesser) saphenous vein along the lateral border of the Achilles, continuing posterior to the lateral malleolus and deep to the peroneal tendon sheath. It extends to the fifth metatarsal base, branching into lateral and medial terminal branches.
- The sural nerve provides sensation to the posterolateral lower leg, lateral malleolus, lateral heel, and lateral foot to the base of the fifth toe.

Common Pathology

- The sural nerve can be compromised as a result of traumatic injuries such as ankle sprains, fractures of the fifth metatarsal or os peroneum, in addition to compression by ganglion cysts, bony osteophytes, tenosynovitis, or hypertrophic muscles.

Equipment

- High-frequency, small footprint, linear ultrasound transducer.
- 30 to 25 gauge 1 to 2 inch needle.

Common Injectates

- For nerve block: Local anesthetic with or without corticosteroid.
- For hydrodissection/hydrorelease: Mixture of normal saline and local anesthetic solution or 5% dextrose solution, or platelet lysate solution may be used.

Injectate Volume

- For nerve block: 2 to 5 c.
- For hydrodissection/hydrorelease: 5 to 15 mL along the course of the nerve, per expert opinion.

Technique

Patient Position

- Prone or lateral decubitus with the lateral ankle of the targeted side facing upward.

Clinician Position

- Seated or standing at the foot of the exam table, facing the anterior ankle and ultrasound machine.

Transducer Orientation

- The sural nerve can be visualized in short axis halfway between the Achilles tendon and the lateral malleolus with the transducer in the axial plane (Fig. 22.29A).
- The transducer can be translated distally and proximally along the course of the sural nerve to identify the area of pathology.
- Injection is performed with the transducer positioned to view the nerve in short axis, unless long-axis view is indicated to cover a longer segment of the nerve.

Needle Position

- In-plane, posteromedial to anterolateral, or anterolateral to posteromedial (Fig. 22.29B).

Target

- Mesoneurium in regions of focal flattening, proximal enlargement, or sonopalpation tenderness along the nerve.

PEARLS AND PITFALLS

- Pre-procedural scanning should be performed to identify the small saphenous vein to avoid intravenous injection.
- Begin injecting while approaching the mesoneurium and advance the needle while injecting slowly to gently push the nerve away, reducing the risk of intraneural injection.
- With proper release, accompanying vessels are observed to have a stronger pulse, although the significance of this phenomenon is unknown.

Bursa Injections

Retrocalcaneal Bursa Injection

KEY POINTS

- Retrocalcaneal bursitis often coexists with Achilles tendinopathy and Haglund's deformity.

Pertinent Anatomy

- The retrocalcaneal bursa lies in the posterior ankle between the posterior calcaneus and distal Achilles tendon.
- Retrocalcaneal bursa has an anterior to posterior diameter less than 1.5 to 3 mm and changes shape with ankle plantarflexion and dorsiflexion.[70]

Common Pathology

- When inflamed and enlarged, the bursa will appear as a comma-shaped anechoic or hypoechoic structure between the distal Achilles tendon and the calcaneus on sonographic evaluation.
- Retrocalcaneal bursitis may be associated with Haglund's deformity and Achilles tendinopathy with neovascularization.

Equipment

- High-frequency linear ultrasound transducer.
- 30 to 27 gauge 1 to 1.5 inch needle.

Common Injectates

- Anesthetic and corticosteroid.
- Dextrose solution for sclerosis.

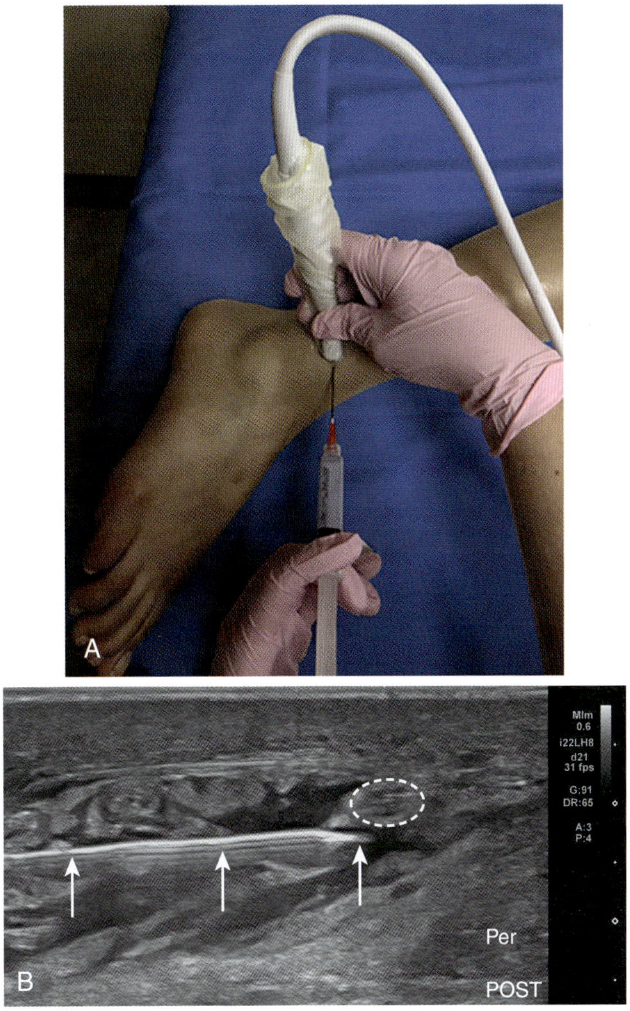

• **Fig. 22.29** (A) Ultrasound-guided sural perineural injection setup for an in-plane, anterior to posterior approach. (B) Sural perineural injection using an in-plane, anterior to posterior approach. The sural nerve *(circled)* is visualized in short axis *Arrows* point to the needle. *Per,* Peroneal musculature; *POST,* posterior.

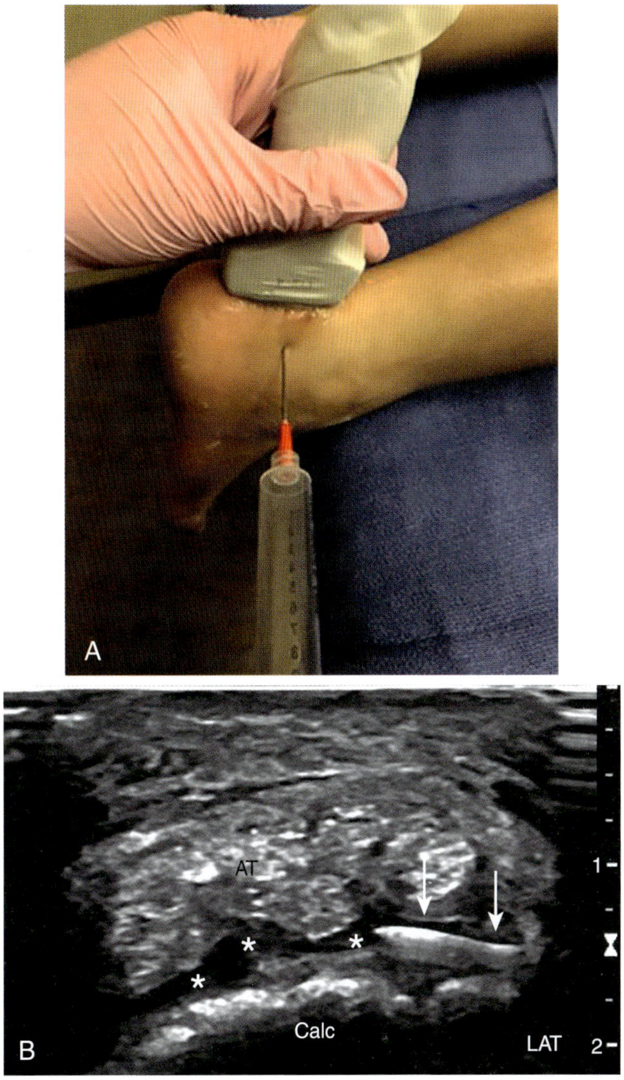

• **Fig. 22.30** (A) Ultrasound-guided retrocalcaneal bursa injection setup for an in-plane, lateral to medial approach. (B) Retrocalcaneal bursa injection using an in-plane, lateral to medial approach. The retrocalcaneal bursa *(asterisks)* is seen deep to the Achilles tendon *(AT)*. Arrows point to the needle. *Calc,* Calcaneus; *LAT,* lateral.

Injectate Volume

- 1 to 3 mL.

Technique

Patient Position

- Prone with the foot hanging off the edge of the exam table.

Clinician Position

- Seated or standing at the foot of the exam table, facing the affected lateral ankle and ultrasound machine.

Transducer Orientation

- The Achilles tendon is located in long or short axis as described above.
- The retrocalcaneal bursa can be visualized deep to the Achilles tendon (Fig. 22.30A).
- Injection is performed with the transducer oriented in short axis to the Achilles tendon.

Needle Position

- In-plane, lateral to medial (Fig. 22.30B).

Target

- Hypoechoic distended bursae between the Achilles tendon and the calcaneus.

PEARLS AND PITFALLS

- When approaching the bursa laterally, care must be taken to avoid the sural nerve.

Retroachilles Bursa Injection

KEY POINTS

- When imaging the retroachilles bursa, a thick layer of gel and light transducer pressure must be used or compression of tissues may cause displacement of fluid, making it difficult to identify bursitis.

Pertinent Anatomy

- The retroachilles bursa lies superficial to the distal Achilles tendon insertion on the calcaneus and is not typically visualized with ultrasound in the absence of pathology.

Common Pathology

- Retroachilles bursitis is typically a result of local mechanical irritation from footwear or Haglund's deformity.
- On sonographic evaluation, bursitis will appear as an anechoic or hypoechoic fluid collection between the subcutaneous tissue and Achilles tendon. Hypervascularity may also be seen.

Equipment

- High-frequency linear ultrasound transducer.
- 30 to 27 gauge 1 to 1.5 inch needle.

Common Injectates

- Anesthetic and corticosteroid.
- Dextrose solution for sclerosis.

Injectate Volume

- 1 to 3 mL.

Technique

Patient Position

- Prone with the foot hanging off the edge of the exam table.

Clinician Position

- Seated at the foot of the exam table, facing the affected lateral ankle and ultrasound machine.

Transducer Orientation

- The distal Achilles tendon is located in long or short axis as described above.
- Light transducer pressure with a gel stand-off is used to visualize fluid in the retroachilles bursa (Fig. 22.31A).
- Injection is performed with the transducer oriented in oblique long axis to the Achilles tendon.

Needle position

- In-plane, distal lateral to proximal medial (Fig. 22.31B).

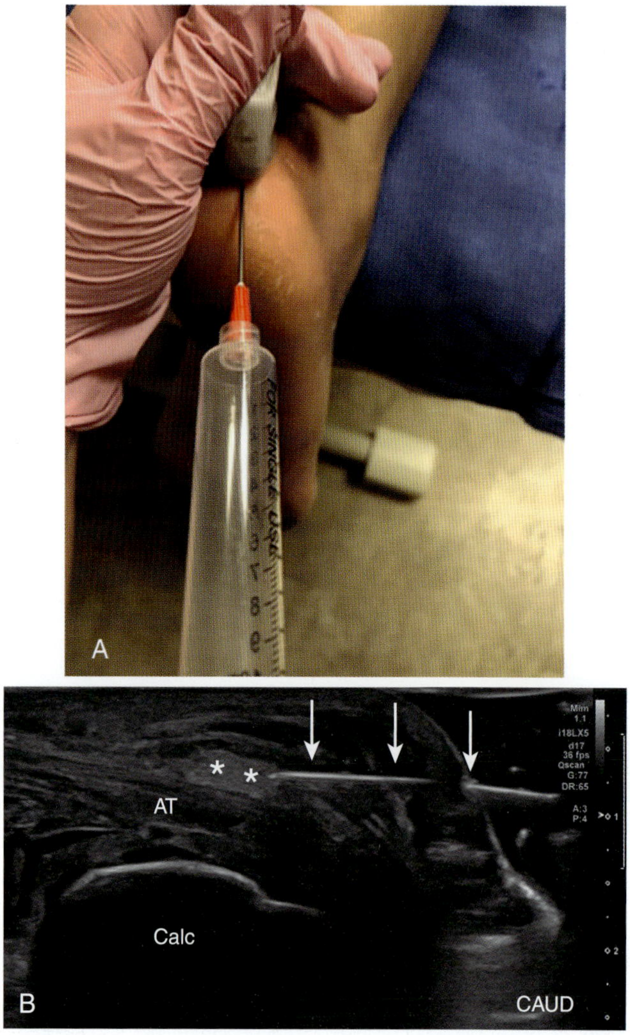

• **Fig. 22.31** (A) Ultrasound-guided retroachilles bursa injection setup for an in-plane, distal lateral to proximal medial approach. (B) Retroachilles bursa injection using an in-plane, distal lateral to proximal medial approach. The retroachilles bursa *(asterisks)* is superficial to the Achilles tendon *(AT)*. *Arrows* point to the needle. *Calc*, Calcaneus; *CAUD*, caudal.

Target

- Bursa superficial to the Achilles tendon near the tendon insertion on the calcaneus.

PEARLS AND PITFALLS

- Using light transducer pressure with a thick layer of gel is important to avoid compression and displacement of fluid in the Achilles bursa if only a small amount of fluid is present.
- When approaching the bursa laterally, care must be taken to avoid the sural nerve.
- Avoid injection into the Achilles tendon.

Other Injections

Achilles Tendon Scraping/High-Volume Image-Guided Injection

KEY POINTS

- Use of a high-frequency linear ultrasound transducer is recommended.
- In Achilles tendinopathy, neovessels and neonerves can be a source of pain and tendon scraping and high-volume image-guided injection (HVIGI) aims to separate neonerves away from the tendon using mechanical blunt force and fluid pressure, respectively.

Pertinent Anatomy

- The Achilles tendon is the longest, thickest, and strongest tendon in the body and connects the gastrocnemius and soleus muscles to the calcaneus.
- Kager's fat pad is located directly anterior to the Achilles tendon and posterior to the ankle joint.

Common Pathology

- In mid-portion Achilles tendinopathy, it is thought that neovessels and neonerves extend from Kager's fat pad to the Achilles tendon.
- On sonographic evaluation, neovessels can be visualized with color or power Doppler and serve as a surrogate marker for neonerves, which are thought to contribute to pain in Achilles tendinopathy.[37]

Equipment

- Needle size: 27 to 30 gauge 1 to 1.5-inch needle for local anesthetic.
- #11 blade scalpel.
- 18 gauge needle or meniscotome for scraping procedure. This is not needed if the goal is just to perform HVIGI.
- High-frequency linear ultrasound transducer.
- Syringes, probe cover, sterile gel, gauze, bandage, local anesthetic.

Technique

Patient Position

- Prone with the foot hanging off the edge of the exam table and ankle positioned in slight passive dorsiflexion applied by the clinician.

Clinician Position

- Seated at the foot of the exam table, facing the affected lateral ankle and ultrasound machine.

Transducer Orientation

- Short axis to the Achilles tendon (Fig. 22.32A).

Needle Entry

- In-plane, lateral to medial (Fig. 22.32B).

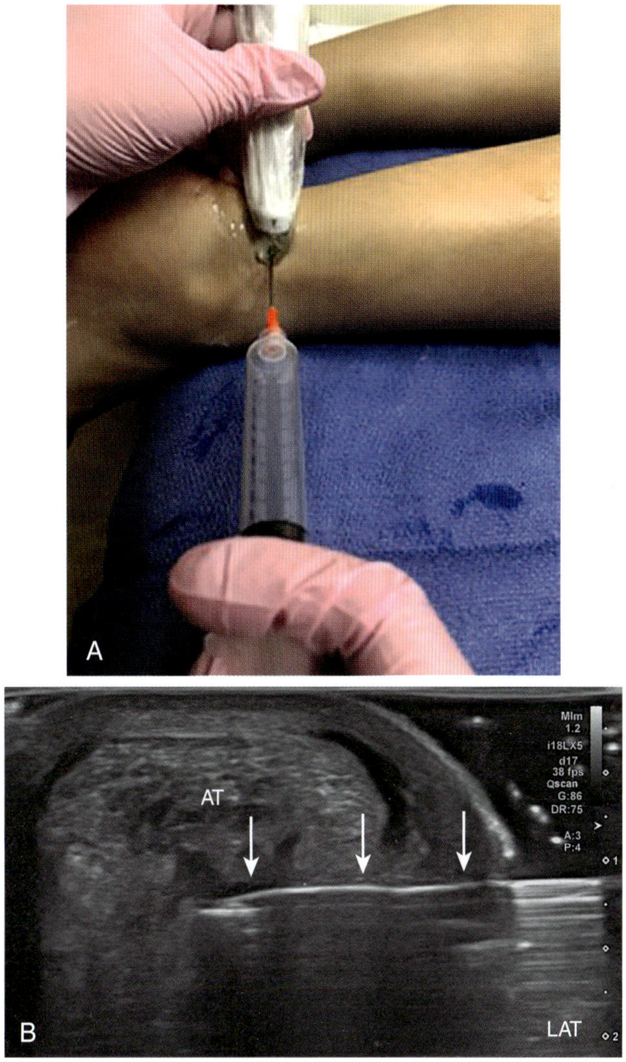

• **Fig. 22.32** (A) Ultrasound-guided Achilles tendon scraping setup. (B) Kager's fat pad hydrorelease using an in-plane, lateral to medial approach. The Achilles tendon *(AT)* is visualized in short axis. *Arrows* point to the needle. *LAT,* Lateral.

Target

- Areas of vascularity extending from Kager's fat pad to the deep surface of the Achilles tendon should be targeted.

Injectate Volume

- 5 to 40 mL (use more volume if HVIGI is combined with tendon scraping).
- Common injectates: Anesthetic, sterile water, normal saline, dextrose.

Additional Procedure Details

- Following administration of local anesthetic, a stab incision is made on the skin with an #11 blade.
- An 18 gauge needle or meniscotome is then inserted under ultrasound guidance, deep to the Achilles tendon at the site of neovascularization identified on Doppler.
- The needle or meniscotome is moved in a cephalo-caudad direction in a swiping motion to disrupt neovessels and neonerves. Use of a meniscotome allows for a single

swipe rather than a needle, which might require a few repetitions.

PEARLS AND PITFALLS

- Tendon scraping and HVIGI can be performed alone, or in combination to separate the Achilles tendon from Kager's fat pad.
- Anecdotally, high-volume injection may result in more post-injection discomfort, likely due to tissue stretching.
- Identify the sural nerve and avoid when approaching from the lateral side.
- Color Doppler should be used to identify areas of neovascularization, a surrogate marker for neonerves.
- As both tendon scraping and HVIGI are extratendinous procedures, clinicians may feel more comfortable returning patients to normal loading activity more quickly compared to other intratendinous procedures that may result in compromised tendon integrity and a heightened risk for a tendon rupture/tear for a period of time following the procedure.
- Procedures are often combined with an eccentric or heavy slow resistance exercise protocol.[38]

Fluoroscopy-guided ankle injections.

Tibiotalar Joint

KEY POINTS

- The joint can be injected from either anterior or posterior.

Pertinent Anatomy[71–73]

- The tibiotalar joint is the space between the distal tibia and the talus.
- The anterior tibiotalar joint is the most pertinent location for injections.
- There are several structures that are superficial to the joint, including the tibialis anterior tendon, FHL tendon, EDL tendon, and the neurovascular bundle containing the dorsalis pedis and the deep peroneal nerve.
- The posterior tibiotalar joint can also be accessed for injections.
- The posterior joint is narrow and traversed by a groove that runs obliquely downward and inward.

Common Pathology

- The tibiotalar joint commonly sustains traumatic injury, which can produce fractures, osteochondral lesions, synovitis, effusion, and hemarthrosis.
- It is also a common site for arthropathies, including osteoarthritis and inflammatory arthropathies such as rheumatoid arthritis.
- It is less commonly affected by pigmented villonodular synovitis (PVNS).
- Infection is another rare pathology of the joint.

Equipment

- Needle size: 27 to 22 gauge 1.5 to 3 inch needle.
- Sterile preparation.
- Fluoroscopy C-arm.

Common Injectates

- Local anesthetics for diagnostics, corticosteroids.
- Biologics (PRP, bone marrow concentrate, etc.)

Injectate Volume

- 1 to 3 mL.

Technique 1: Anterior

Patient Position

- Patient is seated supine with the foot on a flat surface and joint slightly plantarflexed.

Clinician Position

- Standing on the side of the patient.

C-Arm Position.

- True lateral view.

Needle Position

- Palpate the dorsalis pedis pulse and option to mark.
- Start the needle just lateral or medial to the dorsalis pulse.
- Identify the joint space with lateral fluoroscopy and start the needle just below the joint line (Fig. 22.33).

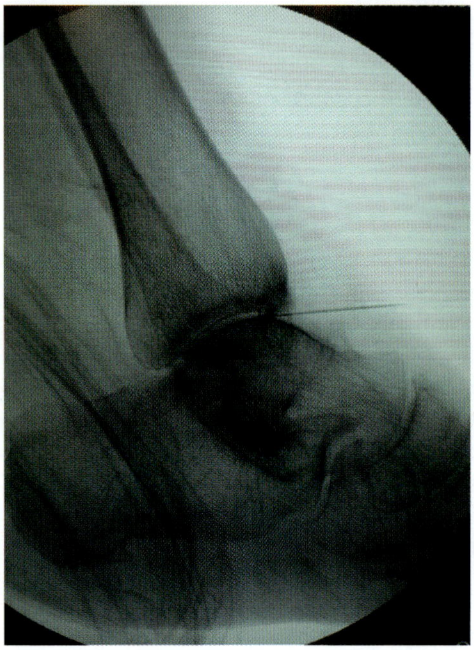

• **Fig. 22.33B** Ankle Fluoro Tibiotalar Joint Intra-Articular Anteior Approach.

Target

- Anterior third of the joint space.
- Inject a small amount of contrast to confirm arthrogram.

PEARLS AND PITFALLS

- There is risk of neurovascular (dorsalis pedis, superficial peroneal nerve) or anterior tibialis tendon injury.
- Palpation of the dorsalis pedis is recommended prior to needle entry to avoid injury to the artery.
- Going medial to the artery risks the tendon injury, going too far lateral can injure the nerve.

Technique 2: Posterior

Patient Position

- Patient is prone with foot elevated on a pillow or wedge or hanging over the edge of table (Fig. 22.34A).

Clinician Position

- Standing on the side of the patient.

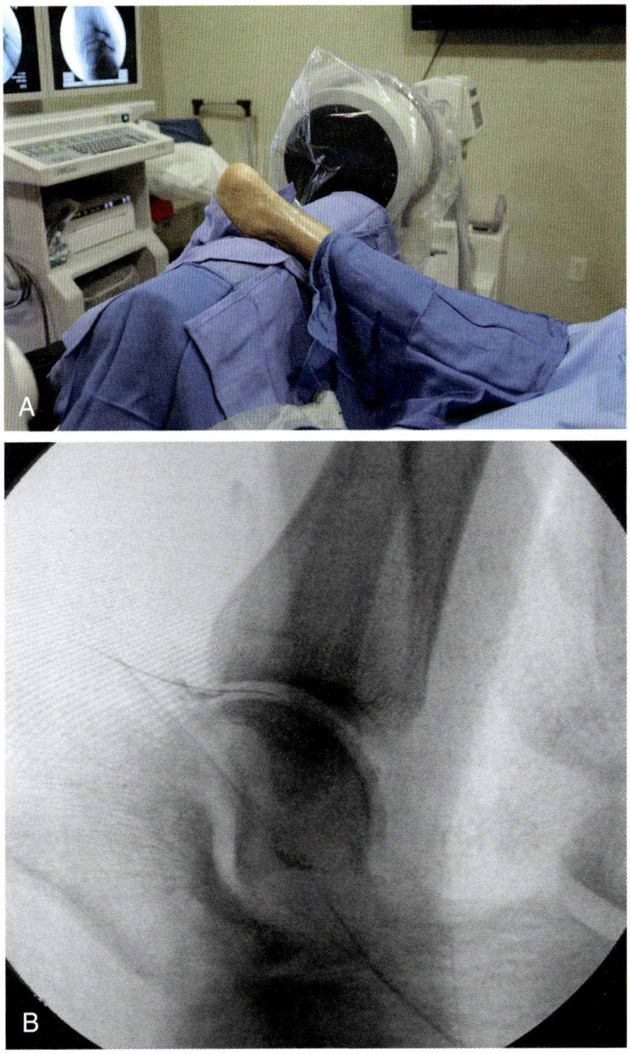

• **Fig. 22.34** (A) Setup. (B) Ankle fluoro IA posterior lateral view.

C-Arm Position

- True lateral view.
- May use AP view if needle to confirm medial to lateral orientation.

Needle Position

- Identify the joint with lateral fluoroscopy and start the needle 1cm below the joint line.
- Needle entry should be just lateral to the Achilles tendon.
- Aim the needle slight superior and medially.

Target

- Posterior third of the joint space (Fig. 22.34B).
- Inject a small amount of contrast to confirm arthrogram.

PEARLS AND PITFALLS

- A slight bend in the needle helps navigation.
- Be aware of needle trajectory not to venture too lateral or media: you can use the AP view to confirm.
- Taking a medial to Achilles approach increases the risk of tibial neurovascular injury.

Subtalar Joint: Posterior Approach

KEY POINTS

- Most injections will be performed with fluoroscopy, with the patient prone and foot elevated on a pillow or wedge or hanging over the edge of the table.

Pertinent Anatomy[71-73]

- The subtalar (talocalcaneal) joint is the space between the calcaneus and the talus. It is composed of three facets (posterior, middle, and anterior). The posterior facet is the largest and the most common target for injections. Although the motion at the subtalar joint is small, it primary allows inversion-eversion of the ankle and hindfoot.

Common Pathology

- The subtalar joint commonly sustains traumatic injury, which can produce sprains, fractures, chondral lesions, synovitis, effusion, and hemarthrosis.
- A severe inversion injury, leading to rupture of the calcaneofibular ligament, can lead to instability.
- It is also a common site for arthropathies, including osteoarthritis and inflammatory arthropathies such as rheumatoid arthritis, reactive (Reiter's) arthritis, and gout.

Equipment

- Needle size: 25 to 22 gauge 2 to 3-inch needle.
- C-arm fluoroscopy.
- Contrast.

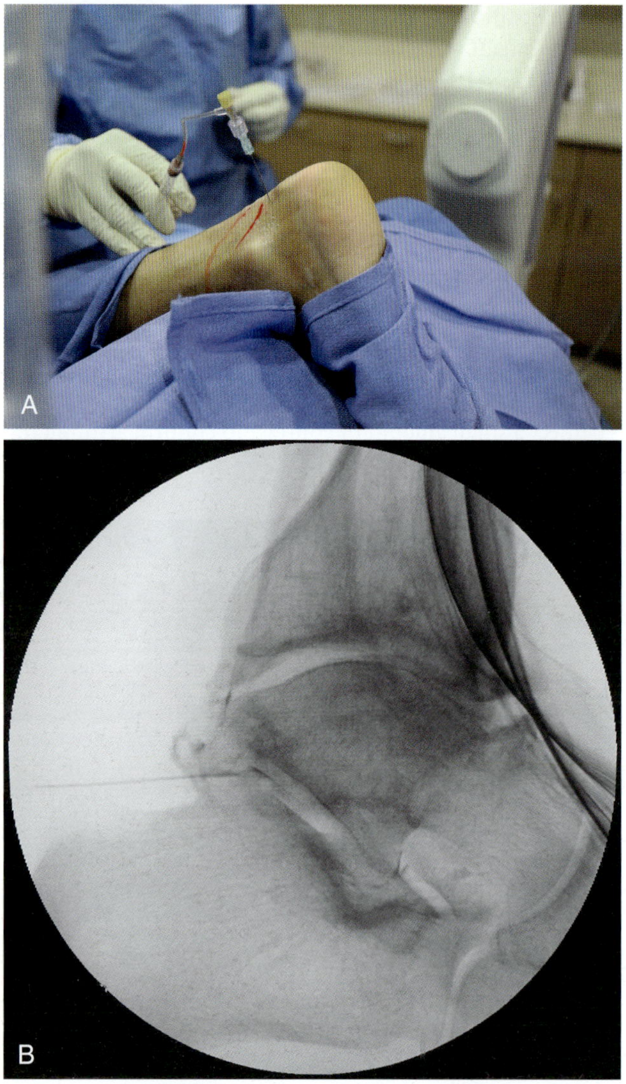

• **Fig. 22.35** Ankle Fluoro Subtalar Joint IA.

Common Injectates

- Local anesthetics for diagnostics, corticosteroids.
- Biologics (PRP, bone marrow concentrate, etc.).

Injectate Volume

- 1 to 2 mL.

Technique

Patient Position

- Patient is lying prone with foot elevated on a pillow or wedge or hanging over the edge of the table (Fig. 22.35A).

Clinician Position

- Clinician standing on the side of the patient.

C-Arm Position

- True lateral view.
- May use AP view if needle to confirm medial to lateral orientation.

Needle Position

- Identify the joint with lateral fluoroscopy and start the needle 0.5 cm below the joint line.
- Needle entry should be just lateral to the Achilles tendon.
- Aim the needle slightly superior and medially.

Target

- Posterior third of the joint space (Fig. 22.35B).
- Inject a small amount of contrast to confirm arthrogram.

PEARLS AND PITFALLS

- Put the ankle in dorsiflexion to open the joint more.
- A slight bend in the needle helps navigation.
- Be aware of needle trajectory not to venture too lateral or medial; you can use the AP view to confirm.
- The posteromedial approach requires passage of the needle in close proximity to the tibial neurovascular bundle.
- When there is a significant subtalar joint effusion present, an aspiration can be performed prior to injection. Laboratory analysis of the joint fluid may be beneficial in assessing for crystalline or inflammatory arthropathy.
- In 14% of population there may be communication between the ankle and subtalar joint.[74]

Subtalar Joint (Sinus Tarsi): Anterior Approach

KEY POINTS

- Most injections will be performed with fluoroscopy, with the patient side-lying and foot elevated on a pillow or wedge.

Pertinent Anatomy[72,73]

- The sinus tarsi, also known as the tarsal sinus, serves as a boundary between the anterior and posterior aspects of the joint.
- It contains five ligamentous structures, comprising the medial, intermediate, and lateral roots of the extensor retinaculum, the cervical ligament, and the ligament of the tarsal canal.
- The sinus tarsi also contains an arterial anastomosis, nerve endings, fat, and the joint capsule.
- The sinus tarsi is bordered posteriorly by the PSTJ, and can be separated from the PSTJ in 95% of cases by the anterior capsular ligament.[75]

Common Pathology

- The subtalar joint commonly sustains traumatic injury, which can produce sprains, fractures, chondral lesions, synovitis, effusion, and hemarthrosis.
- A severe inversion injury, leading to rupture of the calcaneofibular ligament, can lead to instability.
- It is also a common site for arthropathies, including osteoarthritis, ankylosing spondylitis, inflammatory

arthropathies such as rheumatoid arthritis, and crystalline arthropathies such as gout.
- Ganglion cysts may also occur in this area.

Equipment

- Needle size: 25 to 22 gauge 2 to 3 inch needle.
- Contrast fluoroscopy C-arm.

Common Injectates

- Local anesthetics for diagnostics, corticosteroids.
- Biologics (PRP, bone marrow concentrate, etc.).

Injectate Volume

- 1 to 2 mL.

Technique

Patient Position

- Patient is side-lying with foot elevated on a pillow or wedge.
- Alternatively, the patient can be supine with the knee flexed and foot flat on the table.
- The opposite leg will need to be positioned out of the C-arm view (Fig. 22.33A).

Clinician Position

- Clinician is standing on the opposite side of the C-arm.

C-Arm Position

- True lateral view with the anterior subtalar joint clearly open.
- May use true AP view to confirm medial lateral needle placement.

Needle Position

- Start directly over the joint space anterior-inferior to the lateral malleolus and just above the calcaneus.
- The entry point is marked with a metallic wand prior to sterile preparation or with a sterile sheathed needle after sterile preparation.
- The needle is advanced slightly anterior-posterior from lateral to medial.

Target

- Mid portion of the anterior subtalar joint/sinus tarsi (Fig. 22.36).
- Can check an AP view to ensure the needle is in the mid portion of the joint.
- Inject a small amount of contrast to confirm intra-articular spread.

PEARLS AND PITFALLS

- When there is a significant subtalar joint effusion present, an aspiration can be performed prior to injection. Laboratory analysis of the joint fluid may be beneficial in assessing for crystalline or inflammatory arthropathy.
- Optimize joint visualization with the C-arm.
- Avoid going too deep through the joint; the AP view can confirm needle depth.
- Option to also inject the joint from medial to lateral if patient in the hook-lying position.

Talonavicular Joint

KEY POINTS

- Most injections will be performed with fluoroscopy, with the patient side-lying with the lateral aspect of the affected foot on the table, exposing the medial aspect and the talonavicular joint.

Pertinent Anatomy[72,73]

- The talonavicular joint is the space between the distal talus and navicular. It is a ball and socket joint and has an incomplete fibrous capsule. There are ligamentous structures that overlie the joint with the spring ligament along the medial inferior portion and the deltoid ligament covering the medial joint line.
- There are several structures that are superficial to the joint. These include the tibialis posterior tendon, extensor hallucis longus tendon, and the saphenous nerve and vein along the medial aspect. The tibialis anterior, superficial peroneal nerve, and the medial tarsal arteries are located over the dorsomedial joint. The deep peroneal nerve and lateral tarsal artery are superficial to the dorsolateral aspect of the joint. The dorsalis pedis artery and deep peroneal nerve pass under the extensor retinaculum on the dorsal aspect of the joint with dorsal digital nerves passing superficially.

Common Pathology

- The talonavicular joint commonly sustains traumatic injury, which can produce fractures, chondral lesions, synovitis, effusion, and hemarthrosis. It is also a common site for arthropathies, including osteoarthritis, posttraumatic arthritis, tarsal coalition, diabetic neuropathic arthropathy, and congenital deformities (club foot).

Equipment

- Needle size: 27 to 22 gauge 1.5 to 2 inch needle.
- C-arm fluoroscopy.

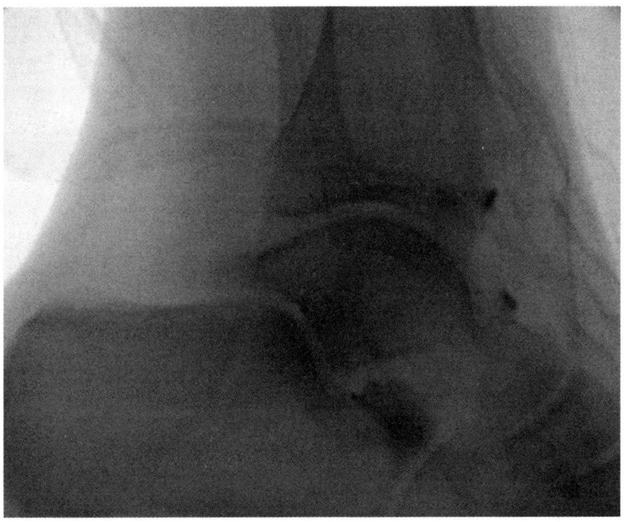

• **Fig. 22.36** Ankle Fluoro Sinus Tarsi.

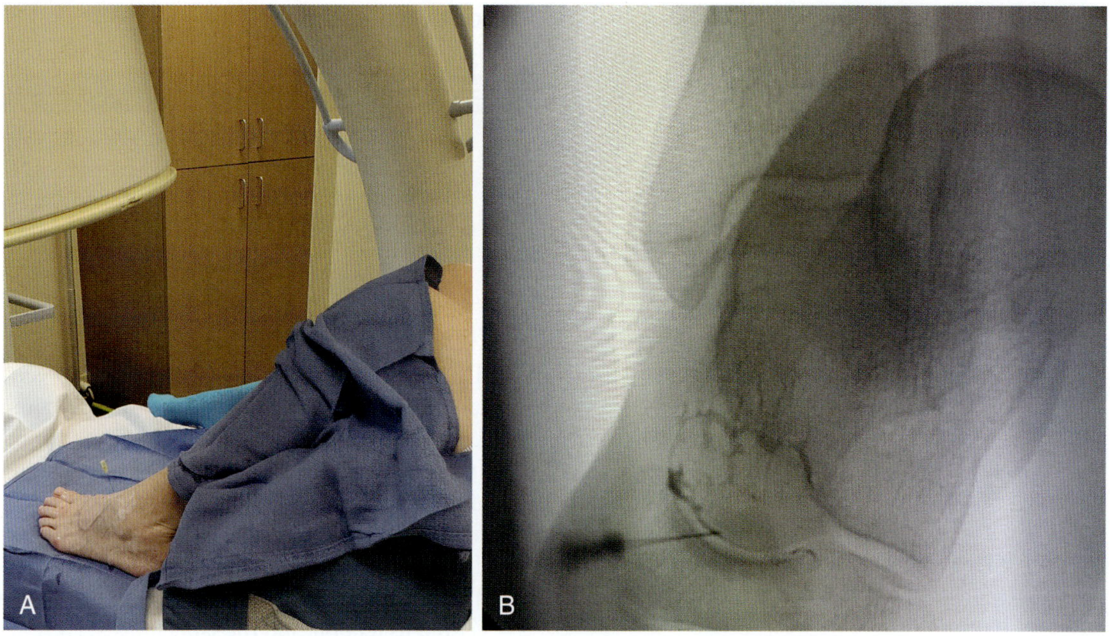

• **Fig. 22.37** (A) Set up. (B) Ankle Fluoro Talonavicular intraarticular.

Common Injectates

- Local anesthetics for diagnostics, corticosteroids.
- Biologics (PRP, bone marrow concentrate, etc.).

Injectate Volume

- 1 to 2 mL.

Technique

Patient Position

- Patient is side-lying with the lateral aspect of the affected foot on the table, exposing the medial aspect and the talonavicular joint (Fig. 22.37A).

Clinician Position

- Clinician is sterile and standing on the opposite side of the table as the C-arm, with clear visualization of the fluoroscopy screen.

C-Arm Position

- True AP view of the joint.
- Option to confirm in a lateral view as well.

Needle Position

- The entry point is marked with a sheathed needle or a metallic wand.
- Start the needle directly over the joint line in the AP view.

Target

- Talonavicular joint (Fig. 22.37B).
- Inject a small amount of contrast to confirm arthrogram.

PEARLS AND PITFALLS

- There is risk of neurovascular or tendon injury. Palpation of the dorsalis pedis is recommended prior to needle entry to avoid insertion of the needle into the artery.
- Damage to small sensory branches adjacent to the joint has been associated with neuropathic pain.[76,77]

References

1. Jacobson JA, et al. Detection of ankle effusions: comparison study in cadavers using radiography, sonography, and MR imaging. *AJR Am J Roentgenol.* 1998;170(5):1231–1238.
2. Na JB, et al. The flexor hallucis longus: tenographic technique and correlation of imaging findings with surgery in 39 ankles. *Radiology.* 2005;236(3):974–982.
3. Smith J, et al. Accuracy of sonographically guided posterior subtalar joint injections: comparison of 3 techniques. *J Ultrasound Med.* 2009;28(11):1549–1557.
4. Woods C, et al. The Football Association Medical Research Programme: an audit of injuries in professional football: an analysis of ankle sprains. *Br J Sports Med.* 2003;37(3):233–238.
5. Burks RT, Morgan J. Anatomy of the lateral ankle ligaments. *Am J Sports Med.* 1994;22(1):72–77.
6. Edama M, et al. Morphological features of the anterior talofibular ligament by the number of fiber bundles. 216:69–74.
7. Oae K, et al. Evaluation of anterior talofibular ligament injury with stress radiography, ultrasonography and MR imaging. *Skeletal Radiol.* 2010;39(1):41–47.
8. Campbell DG, Menz A, Isaacs J. Dynamic ankle ultrasonography. A new imaging technique for acute ankle ligament injuries. *Am J Sports Med.* 1994;22(6):855–858.
9. Drez DJ, Kaveney MF. Ankle ligament injuries. Practical guidelines for examination and treatment. *J Musculoskel Med.* 1989;6:21–36.

10. Makhani JS. Lacerations of the lateral ligament of the ankle. An experimental appraisal. *J Int Coll Surg*. 1962;38:454–466.
11. Renström, Per AFH, Lynch SA. Ankle ligament injuries. *Rev Bras Med do Esporte*. 1998;4(3):71–80. https://doi.org/10.1590/S1517-86921998000300002.
12. Haraguchi N, Toga H, Shiba N, Kato F. Avulsion fracture of the lateral ankle ligament complex in severe inversion injury: incidence and clinical outcome. *Am J Sports Med*. 2007;35(7):1144–1152.
13. Golanó P, Vega J, de Leeuw PA, et al. Anatomy of the ankle ligaments: a pictorial essay. *Knee Surg Sports Traumatol Arthrosc*. 2016;24(4):944–956. https://doi.org/10.1007/s00167-016-4059-4.
14. Mollon B, Wasserstein D, Murphy GM, White LM, Theodoropoulos J. High ankle sprains in professional ice hockey players: prognosis and correlation between magnetic resonance imaging patterns of injury and return to play. *Orthop J Sports Med*. 2019;7(9). https://doi.org/10.1177/2325967119871578. 2325967119871578.
15. Hermans JJ, et al. Anatomy of the distal tibiofibular syndesmosis in adults: a pictorial essay with a multimodality approach. *J Anat*. 2010;217(6):633–645.
16. Boonthathip M, et al. Tibiofibular syndesmotic ligaments: MR arthrography in cadavers with anatomic correlation. *Radiology*. 2010;254(3):827–836.
17. van den Bekerom MP, Raven EE. The distal fascicle of the anterior inferior tibiofibular ligament as a cause of tibiotalar impingement syndrome: a current concepts review. *Knee Surg Sports Traumatol Arthrosc*. 2007;15(4):465–471.
18. Subhas N, et al. MRI appearance of surgically proven abnormal accessory anterior-inferior tibiofibular ligament (Bassett's ligament). *Skeletal Radiol*. 2008;37(1):27–33.
19. Lilyquist M, et al. Cadaveric analysis of the distal tibiofibular syndesmosis. *Foot Ankle Int*. 2016;37(8):882–890.
20. Clanton TO, et al. Biomechanical analysis of the individual ligament contributions to syndesmotic stability. *Foot Ankle Int*. 2017;38(1):66–75.
21. Cha SW, et al. Reliable measurements of physiologic ankle syndesmosis widening using dynamic 3D ultrasonography: a preliminary study. *Ultrasonography*. 2019;38(3):236–245.
22. Mei-Dan O, et al. A dynamic ultrasound examination for the diagnosis of ankle syndesmotic injury in professional athletes: a preliminary study. *Am J Sports Med*. 2009;37(5):1009–1016.
23. Campbell KJ, et al. The ligament anatomy of the deltoid complex of the ankle: a qualitative and quantitative anatomical study. *J Bone Joint Surg Am*. 2014;96(8):e62.
24. Domzalski M, Kwapisz A, Król A, Jedrzejewski K. The role of plantar calcaneonavicular ligament complex in the development of the adult flat foot—anatomical study. *Chir Narzadow Ruchu Ortop Pol*. 2007;72(4):265–268.
25. Ribbans WJ, Garde A. Tibialis posterior tendon and deltoid and spring ligament injuries in the elite athlete. *Foot Ankle Clin*. 2013;18(2):255–291. https://doi.org/10.1016/j.fcl.2013.02.006.
26. Balen PE, Helms CA. Association of posterior tibial tendon injury with spring ligament injury, sinus tarsi abnormality and plantar fasciitis on MR imaging. *AJR Am J Roentgenol*. 2001;176(5):1137–1143.
27. Orr JD, Nunley 2nd JA. Isolated spring ligament failure as a cause of adult-acquired flatfoot deformity. *Foot Ankle Int*. 2013;34(6):818–823. https://doi.org/10.1177/1071100713483099.
28. Chen PY, Wang TG, Wang CL. Ultrasonographic examination of the deltoid ligament in bimalleolar equivalent fractures. *Foot Ankle Int*. 2008;29(9):883–886.
29. O'Brien M. The anatomy of the Achilles tendon. *Foot Ankle Clin*. 2005;10(2):225–238.
30. Carr AJ, Norris SH. The blood supply of the calcaneal tendon. *J Bone Joint Surg Br*. 1989;71(1):100–101.
31. Sunding K, et al. Evaluation of Achilles and patellar tendinopathy with greyscale ultrasound and colour Doppler: using a four-grade scale. *Knee Surg Sports Traumatol Arthrosc*. 2016;24(6):1988–1996.
32. Richards PJ, Win T, Jones PW. The distribution of microvascular response in Achilles tendonopathy assessed by colour and power Doppler. *Skeletal Radiol*. 2005;34(6):336–342.
33. Astrom M, et al. Imaging in chronic Achilles tendinopathy: a comparison of ultrasonography, magnetic resonance imaging and surgical findings in 27 histologically verified cases. *Skeletal Radiol*. 1996;25(7):615–620.
34. Ahn KS, et al. Ultrasound elastography of lateral epicondylosis: clinical feasibility of quantitative elastographic measurements. *AJR Am J Roentgenol*. 2014;202(5):1094–1099.
35. Bianchi S, Becciolini M, Urigo C. Ultrasound imaging of disorders of small nerves of the extremities: less recognized locations. *J Ultrasound Med*. 2019;38(11):2821–2842.
36. Kammar H, et al. Anatomy of the sural nerve and its relation to the Achilles tendon by ultrasound examination. *Orthopedics*. 2014;37(3):e298–e301.
37. Alfredson H. Ultrasound and Doppler-guided mini-surgery to treat midportion Achilles tendinosis: results of a large material and a randomised study comparing two scraping techniques. *Br J Sports Med*. 2011;45(5):407–410.
38. Wilson F, et al. Exercise, orthoses and splinting for treating Achilles tendinopathy: a systematic review with meta-analysis. *Br J Sports Med*. 2018;52(24):1564–1574.
39. Beischer AD, et al. Distal tendinosis of the tibialis anterior tendon. *Foot Ankle Int*. 2009;30(11):1053–1059.
40. Mengiardi B, et al. Anterior tibial tendon abnormalities: MR imaging findings. *Radiology*. 2005;235(3):977–984.
41. Ng JM, et al. US and MR imaging of the extensor compartment of the ankle. *Radiographics*. 2013;33(7):2047–2064.
42. Olewnik L, et al. A cadaveric and sonographic study of the morphology of the tibialis anterior tendon—a proposal for a new classification. *J Foot Ankle Res*. 2019;12:9.
43. Gaetke-Udager K, et al. Ultrasound of the Gruberi bursa with cadaveric and MRI correlation. *AJR Am J Roentgenol*. 2016;207(2):386–391.
44. Davis WH, et al. The superior peroneal retinaculum: an anatomic study. *Foot Ankle Int*. 1994;15(5):271–275.
45. Lee SJ, et al. Ultrasound and MRI of the peroneal tendons and associated pathology. *Skeletal Radiol*. 2013;42(9):1191–1200.
46. Raikin SM, Elias I, Nazarian LN. Intrasheath subluxation of the peroneal tendons. *J Bone Joint Surg Am*. 2008;90(5):992–999.
47. Draghi F, et al. Intrasheath instability of the peroneal tendons: dynamic ultrasound imaging. *J Ultrasound Med*. 2018;37(12):2753–2758.
48. Oden RR. Tendon injuries about the ankle resulting from skiing. *Clin Orthop Relat Res*. 1987;(216):63–69.
49. Zammit J, Singh D. The peroneus quartus muscle. Anatomy and clinical relevance. *J Bone Joint Surg Br*. 2003;85(8):1134–1137.
50. Brodsky JW, Zide JR, Kane JM. Acute peroneal injury. *Foot Ankle Clin*. 2017;22(4):833–841.
51. Sussman WI, Hofmann K. Treatment of insertional peroneus brevis tendinopathy by ultrasound-guided percutaneous ultrasonic

needle tenotomy: a case report. *J Foot Ankle Surg.* 2019;58(6): 1285–1287.
52. Lhoste-Trouilloud A. The tibialis posterior tendon. *J Ultrasound.* 2012;15(1):2–6.
53. Schweitzer ME, Karasick D. MR imaging of disorders of the posterior tibialis tendon. *AJR Am J Roentgenol.* 2000;175(3):627–635.
54. Manske MC, et al. Arterial anatomy of the tibialis posterior tendon. *Foot Ankle Int.* 2015;36(4):436–443.
55. Bianchi S, et al. Ultrasound appearance of tendon tears. Part 2: lower extremity and myotendinous tears. *Skeletal Radiol.* 2006;35(2):63–77.
56. Prato N, et al. Sonography of posterior tibialis tendon dislocation. *J Ultrasound Med.* 2004;23(5):701–705.
57. Nazarian LN, et al. Synovial fluid in the hindfoot and ankle: detection of amount and distribution with US. *Radiology.* 1995;197(1):275–278.
58. Bowers CA, et al. The flexor digitorum accessorius longus—a cadaveric study. *J Foot Ankle Surg.* 2009;48(2):111–115.
59. Deleu PA, et al. Anatomical characteristics of the flexor digitorum accessorius longus muscle and their relevance to tarsal tunnel syndrome a systematic review. *J Am Podiatr Med Assoc.* 2015;105(4):344–355.
60. Zhao XY, et al. Anatomical study of the compositions and internal connections of the chiasma plantare (master knot of Henry): exploring its possible clinical impact. *J Foot Ankle Surg.* 2019;58(6):1235–1244.
61. Lui TH, Chow FY. "Intersection syndrome" of the foot: treated by endoscopic release of master knot of Henry. *Knee Surg Sports Traumatol Arthrosc.* 2011;19(5):850–852.
62. Jacobson JA. *Fundamentals of Musculoskeletal Ultrasound E-Book.* Elsevier Health Sciences; 2017.
63. Martinez-Salazar EL, et al. Hallux saltans due to stenosing tenosynovitis of flexor hallucis longus: dynamic sonography and arthroscopic findings. *Skeletal Radiol.* 2018;47(5):747–750.
64. Mehdizade A, Adler RS. Sonographically guided flexor hallucis longus tendon sheath injection. *J Ultrasound Med.* 2007;26(2): 233–237.
65. Solomon LB, et al. Surgical anatomy of the sural and superficial fibular nerves with an emphasis on the approach to the lateral malleolus. *J Anat.* 2001;199(Pt 6):717–723.
66. Nikolopoulos D, et al. Deep peroneal nerve palsy caused by an extraneural ganglion cyst: a rare case. *Case Rep Orthop.* 2015;2015:861697.
67. Brestas P, Protopsaltis I, Drossos C. Role of sonography in the diagnosis and treatment of a ganglion cyst compressing the lateral branch of deep peroneal nerve. *J Clin Ultrasound.* 2017;45(2): 108–111.
68. Lui TH, Chan LK. Deep peroneal nerve injury following external fixation of the ankle: case report and anatomic study. *Foot Ankle Int.* 2011;32(5):S550–S555.
69. Mercer D, et al. The course of the distal saphenous nerve: a cadaveric investigation and clinical implications. *Iowa Orthop J.* 2011;31:231–235.
70. Hamada M, et al. Width of the retrocalcaneal bursa is not altered by the ankle motion or flexor hallucis longus contraction. *J Functional Morphol Kinesiol.* 2016;1(4):378–381.
71. Gray H. The tibia. Articulations. In: Gray H, ed. *Gray's Anatomy.* 1st ed. Philadelphia, PA: Courage Books; 1901:195–196.
72. Gray H. The tarsus. The astralgus. In: Gray H, ed. *Gray's Anatomy.* 1st ed. Philadelphia, PA: Courage Books; 1901:203–204.
73. Gray H. Articulations of the tarsus. In: Gray H, ed. *Gray's Anatomy.* 1st ed. Philadelphia, PA: Courage Books; 1901:287–288.
74. Carmont MR, et al. Variability of joint communications in the foot and ankle demonstrated by contrast-enhanced diagnostic injections. *Foot Ankle Int.* 2009;30:439–442.
75. Jotoku T, Kinoshita M, Okuda R, Abe M. Anatomy of ligamentous structures of the tarsal sinus and canal. *Foot Ankle Int.* 2006;27:533–538.
76. Lui T, Chan LK. Safety and efficacy of talonavicular arthroscopy in arthroscopic triple arthrodesis. A cadaveric study. *Knee Surg Sports Trauma Arthrosc.* 2010;8(5):607–611.
77. Hammond AW, Phisitkul P, Femino J, Amendola A. Arthroscopic debridement of the talonavicular joint using dorsomedial and dorsolateral portals: a cadaveric study of safety and access. *Arthroscopay.* 2011;27(2):228–234.
78. Chimenti RL, et al. Percutaneous ultrasonic tenotomy reduces insertional Achilles tendinopathy pain with high patient satisfaction and a low complication rate. *J Ultrasound Med.* 2019;38(6):1629–1635.

23 Foot Injection Techniques

DOUGLAS HOFFMAN, JACOB JONES, PIERRE D'HEMECOURT, JOHN PITTS, AND ARTHUR JASON DE LUIGI

Foot Ultrasound Introduction

Ultrasound (US) has emerged as a valuable imaging modality for addressing many foot disorders and allows a more precise approach to intra-articular and soft tissue injections. US-guided injection techniques involving the plantar fascia, medial and inferior calcaneal nerves, the intersection of flexor hallucis longus (FHL) and flexor digitorum longus (FDL), midfoot joints, metatarsophalangeal (MTP) joints, sesamoids, plantar plate, and Morton's neuromas are reviewed in this chapter. This chapter does not contain an exhaustive list of all foot injections, but rather, serves as an outline for the different approaches to common foot injections.

Plantar Fascia

KEY POINTS

- Disorders of the central cord of the plantar fascia are the most common cause of heel pain in the adult population.[1] Enthesopathy of the lateral cord of the plantar fascia is an often overlooked cause of lateral foot pain and can coexist with plantar fasciopathy.[2]
- Corticosteroid injections are controversial in the setting of degenerative plantar fasciopathy, particularly when used repetitively. However, they are occasionally utilized for pain control during the rehabilitative process and while addressing underlying biomechanical factors.
- There is no strong evidence for a preference of placing a corticosteroid injection deep, superficial, or directly within the central cord of the plantar fascia. In theory, a corticosteroid injection superficial to the central cord may cause fat pad atrophy. Alternatively, an injection within the central cord may propagate undersurface partial-thickness tears, which are common with plantar fasciopathy.

Pertinent Anatomy (Fig. 23.1)

- The plantar fascia is composed of three components: the central, medial, and lateral cords. The central and lateral cords are the most clinically relevant.
- The central cord originates from the plantar aspect of the medial tubercle of the calcaneus and has a complex insertion distally onto the MTP joint and plantar fat pad. The lateral cord originates on the lateral aspect of the medial tubercle of the calcaneus and inserts onto the base of the fifth metatarsal lateral to the insertion of the peroneus brevis.

Pathology

- Undersurface partial-thickness tears are often present adjacent to a calcaneal enthesophyte.
- Enthesopathy of the lateral cord of the plantar fascia (LCPF) at its insertion onto the base of the fifth metatarsal can occur in isolation or coexist with plantar fasciopathy.

Equipment

- 27–22 gauge, 1.5–2 inch needle for fascia injection
- 25–18 gauge, 1.5–2 inch needle for tenotomy
- High- or medium-frequency linear array transducer

Common Injectates

- Local anesthetics for diagnostics, corticosteroids
- Prolotherapy
- Orthobiologics

Injectate Volume

- 1–3 mL

TECHNIQUE: Approach for injection of the central cord of the plantar fascia

Patient Position

- Prone with knee fully extended and ankle resting on a towel or over the edge of the table.
- Alternatively, patient lying supine, knee fully extended with the ankle on a towel and/or hanging over edge of table.

Clinician Position

- Seated at end of table

Transducer Position

- Short axis (SAX) to plantar fascia near its origin on the calcaneus (in-plane approach) (Fig. 23.2A and B)

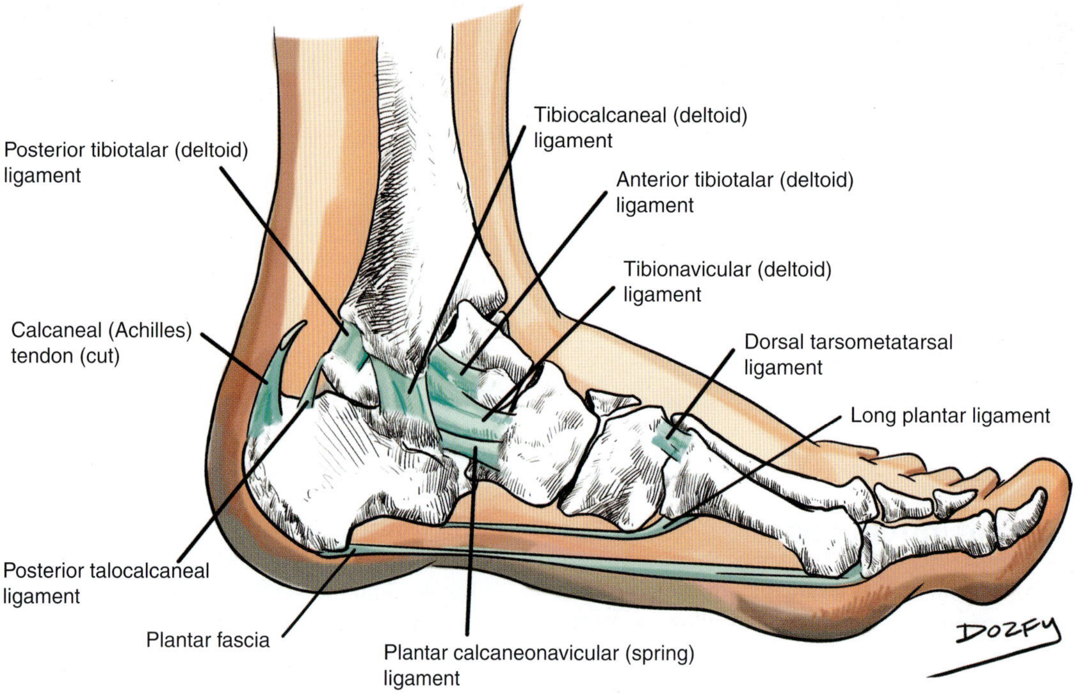

• **Fig. 23.1** Anatomy of The Medial Ankle Ligaments and Plantar Fascia.

- Long axis (LAX) to the plantar fascia (in-plane approach) (Fig. 23.3A)

Needle Position
- SAX in-plane approach directed medial to lateral (see Fig. 23.2C)
- LAX in-plane approach directed either proximal to distal or distal to proximal (see Fig. 23.3B)

Target
- Pathogenic areas of the tendon if using orthobiologics or needle tenotomy
- Peritendinous if using corticosteroids

PEARLS AND PITFALLS
- Avoid placing injectate directly into the plantar fat pad when utilizing a corticosteroid.
- A tibial nerve block may minimize the need for local anesthetic when using an orthobiologic or needle tenotomy.
- The principle of needle fenestration is to pass the needle repeatedly through the tendinopathic areas of the central cord. The number of fenestrations can vary widely, depending on the severity and extent of the central cord involvement.
- Alternating SAX and LAX imaging during the fenestration assures that the full extent of the tendinopathic portion of the tendon is addressed.

Technique: Approach for injection or fenestration of the lateral cord of the plantar fascia

Patient Position
- Side-lying with the lateral aspect of the affected foot facing up. Towel under the ankle for comfort (Fig. 23.4A)

Clinician Position
- Seated at end of table

Transducer Position

- LAX to the LCPF (in-plane approach) (see Fig. 23.4A)
- SAX to the LCPF (in-plane approach) (Fig. 23.5A)

Needle Position

- LAX in-plane approach directed proximal to distal or distal to proximal (see Fig. 23.4B)
- SAX in-plane approach directed dorsal to plantar (see Fig. 23.5B)

Target
- Pathogenic areas of the lateral cord if using orthobiologics or needle tenotomy
- Peritendinous if using corticosteroids

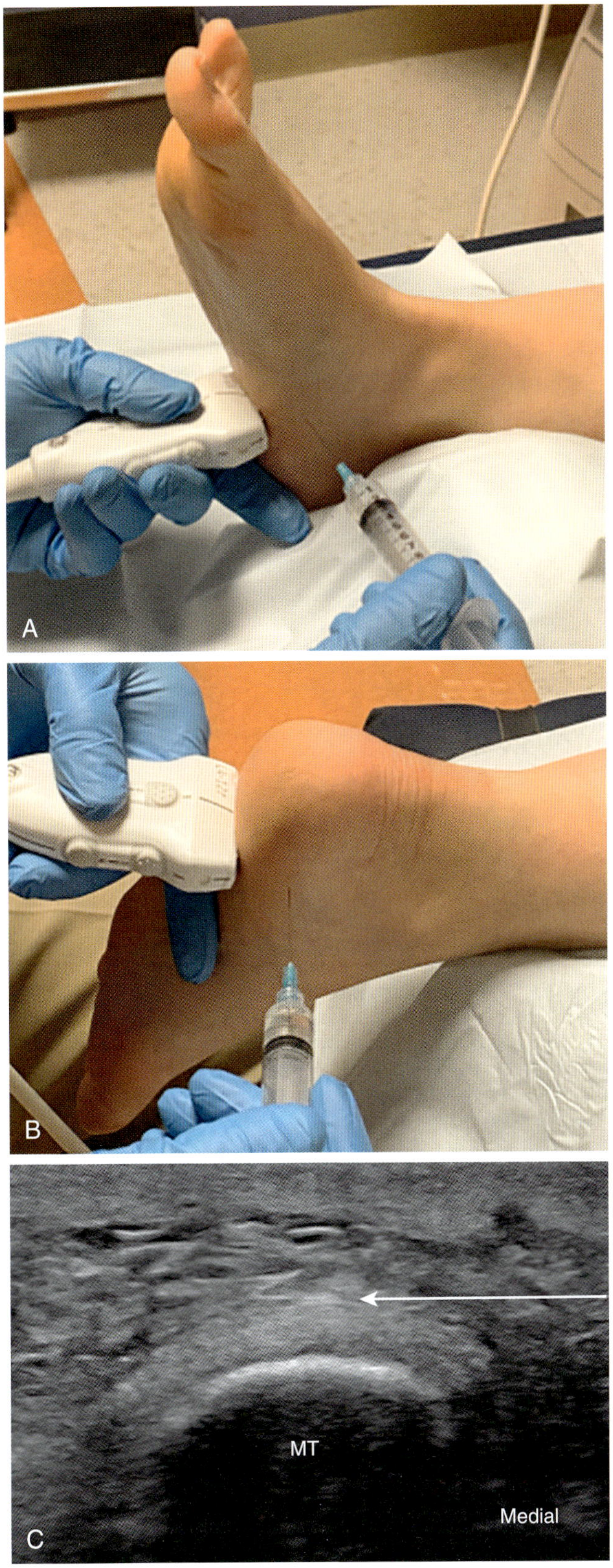

• **Fig 23.2** Sax In-Plane Approach for Injection of The Proximal Central Cord of The Plantar Fascia. (A) Patient and needle position for medial to lateral SAX in-plane approach (patient supine). (B) Patient and needle position for medial to lateral SAX in-plane approach (patient prone). (C) Ultrasound image and needle position (*arrow*) for medial to lateral SAX in-plane approach, corresponding to the images shown in A and B. *MT*, Medial tubercle of the calcaneus.

PEARLS AND PITFALLS

- If utilizing a corticosteroid, consider placing the injectate along the superficial border of the LCPF to minimize the risk of tearing.
- Fenestration and/or orthobiologic injection may take months for full recovery.

Medial Calcaneal Nerve and Inferior Calcaneal Nerve (Baxter's Nerve)

KEY POINTS

- Neuropathic pain is not an uncommon cause of heel pain.
- Selectively blocking the medial calcaneal nerve (MCN) or inferior calcaneal nerve (ICN) can help decipher heel pain arising from nerve entrapment versus plantar fasciopathy. However, pain from an entrapment neuropathy can coexist with symptomatic proximal plantar fasciopathy.
- Both the ICN and MCN are approached similarly with a posterior to anterior SAX in-plane approach.

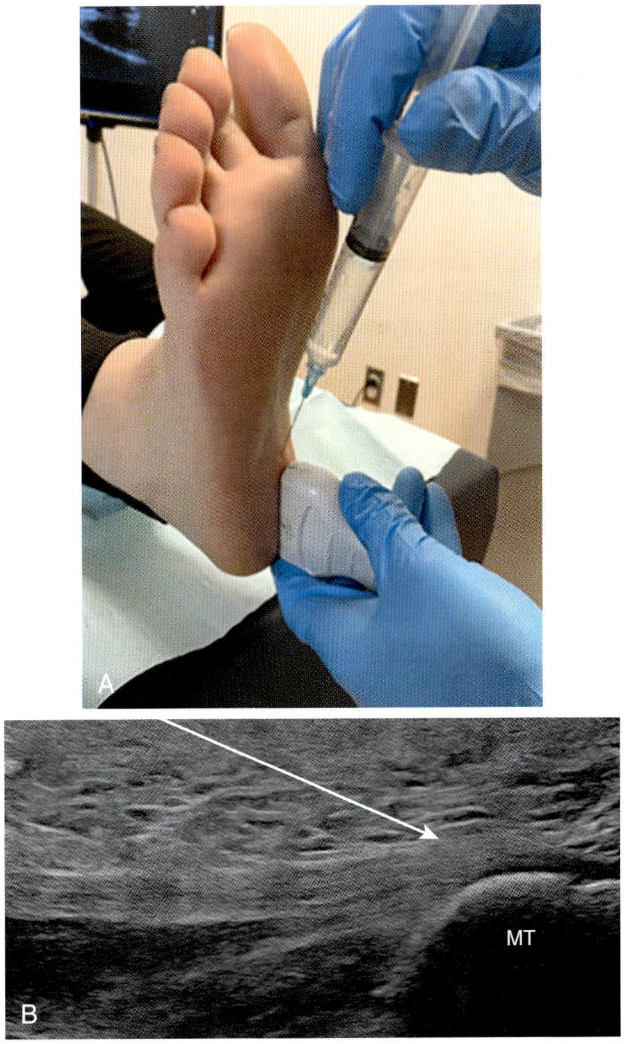

• **Fig. 23.3** LAX in-Plane Approach for Injection of the Proximal Central Cord of the Plantar Fascia. (A) Patient and needle position for distal to proximal LAX in-plane approach. (B) Ultrasound image and needle position (*arrow*) for distal to proximal LAX in-plane approach corresponding to image A. *MT*, Medial tubercle of the calcaneus.

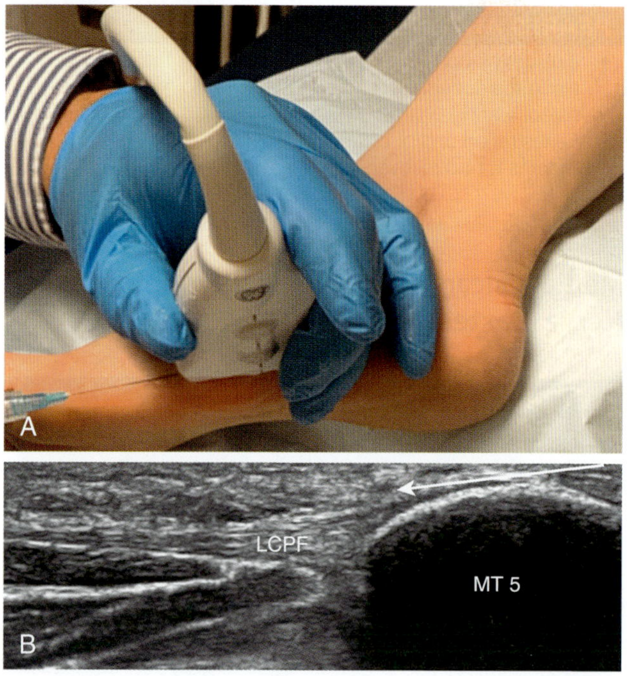

• **Fig 23.4** LAx In-Plane Approach for Injection of The LCPF. (A) Patient and transducer position for distal to proximal LAX in-plane approach. (B) Corresponding US image and needle position (*arrow*) for distal to proximal LAX in-plane approach. May also approach this injection from proximal to distal. *LCPF*, Lateral cord of the plantar fascia; *MT 5*, fifth metatarsal.

Pertinent Anatomy (see Fig. 23.6)

- The MCN most commonly comes directly off the tibial nerve and remains in the superficial subcutaneous tissue as it traverses towards the posteromedial calcaneal region.
- The ICN is typically the first branch of the lateral plantar nerve (LPN). It travels posteriorly from its take-off point before turning inferiorly between the abductor hallucis (AH) and the quadratus plantae (QP) muscles. It then courses between the flexor digitorum brevis (FDB) and the QP, deep to the calcaneal osteophyte (if present), before terminating at the abductor digiti minimi (ADM) muscle.
- There is some variability in the take-off of the ICN and may divide above the tarsal tunnel in 12% of cases.[3]
- The ICN is motor to the ADM muscle.

Common Pathology

- Neuropathies involving both the MCN and ICN can lead to heel pain and mimic plantar fasciopathy. An entrapment neuropathy of the ICN can occur in isolation or in conjunction with plantar fasciopathy. Up to 20% of cases of heel pain have been attributed to ICN entrapment.[4] Entrapment of the ICN typically occurs as it traverses between the QP and AH muscles, or more distally between the FDB and QP muscles adjacent to the calcaneal osteophyte.

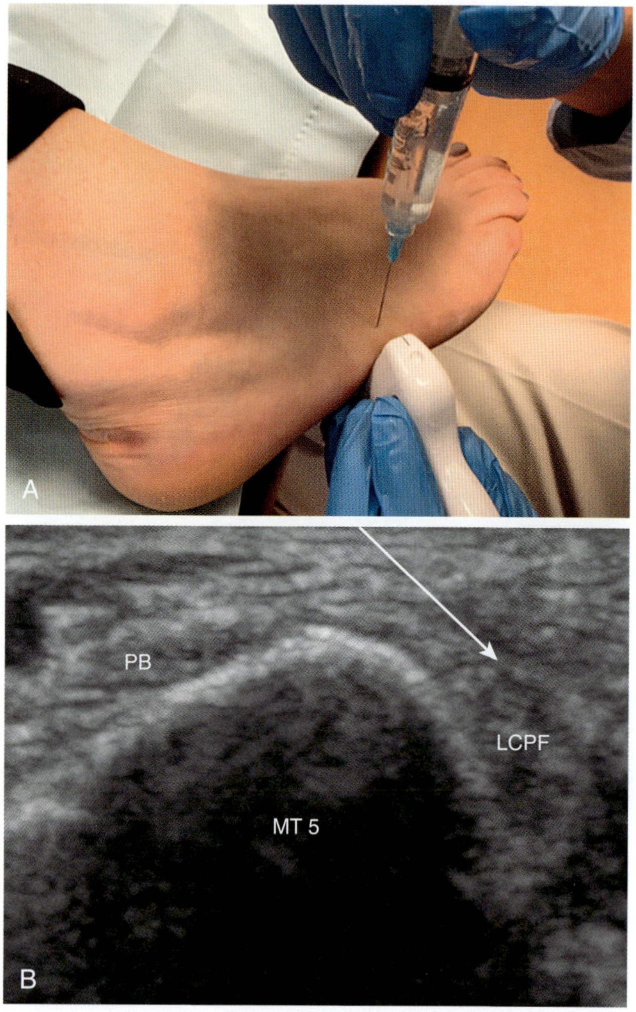

• **Fig 23.5** SAX in-plane approach for injection of the LCPF. (A) Patient and transducer position for dorsal to plantar SAX in-plane approach. (B) Corresponding US image and needle position (*arrow*) for a dorsal to plantar SAX in-plane approach. *LCPF*, Lateral cord of the plantar fascia; *MT 5*, fifth metatarsal; *PB*, peroneus brevis. The top of the image is dorsal. To the left is medial.

- Atrophy and fatty replacement of the ADM muscle is a clue to entrapment of the ICN.

Equipment

- High-frequency linear or hockeystick ultrasound transducer
- 27–22 gauge, 1.25–1.5 inch needle for perineural injection

Common Injectates

- Local anesthetics, corticosteroids

Injectate Volume

- Local anesthetic 0.5–2mL

Technique

Patient Position

- Supine

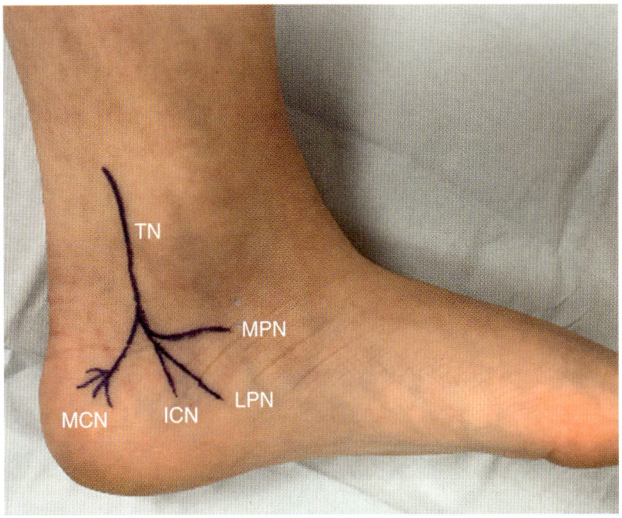

• **Fig 23.6** MCN and ICN. The MCN typically branches off the tibial nerve before the bifurcation of the medial plantar nerve (*MPN*) and lateral plantar nerve (*LPN*). Note that the MCN travels posterior to the ICN. *ICN,* Inferior calcaneal nerve; *MCN,* medial calcaneal nerve; *TN*, tibial nerve.

- Affected leg is externally rotated to expose the medial ankle. The lateral ankle rests comfortably on a towel or over the side of the examination table (Fig. 23.6).
- Alternatively, patient is prone with ankle over the side of the examination table.

Clinician Position

- Seated directly distal to the foot being injected.

Transducer Position

- SAX to the targeted nerve (see Fig. 23.7A)

Needle Position

- SAX in-plane approach from posterior to anterior (see Fig. 23.7B and C).

Target

- Perineural

PEARLS AND PITFALLS

- Identify the MCN by tracing in SAX as it separates from the tibial nerve and traverses inferiorly and posteriorly. It remains fairly superficial, which helps distinguish it from the ICN, which will dive between the AH and QP muscles.
- An isolated local block of the MCN will often differentiate it from ICN entrapment. In such a case, an MCN block will anesthetize the medial calcaneal region but should not affect plantar heel pain if the pain arises from ICN entrapment.
- The ICN is identified by tracing the LPN until a small single fascicle branches posteriorly toward the AH and QP interval. Occasionally, the ICN branches from the tibial nerve proximal to its bifurcation into the medial and lateral plantar nerves.
- Lighten the probe pressure to assure that adjacent venous structures are not compressed and properly identified in planning the needle approach.

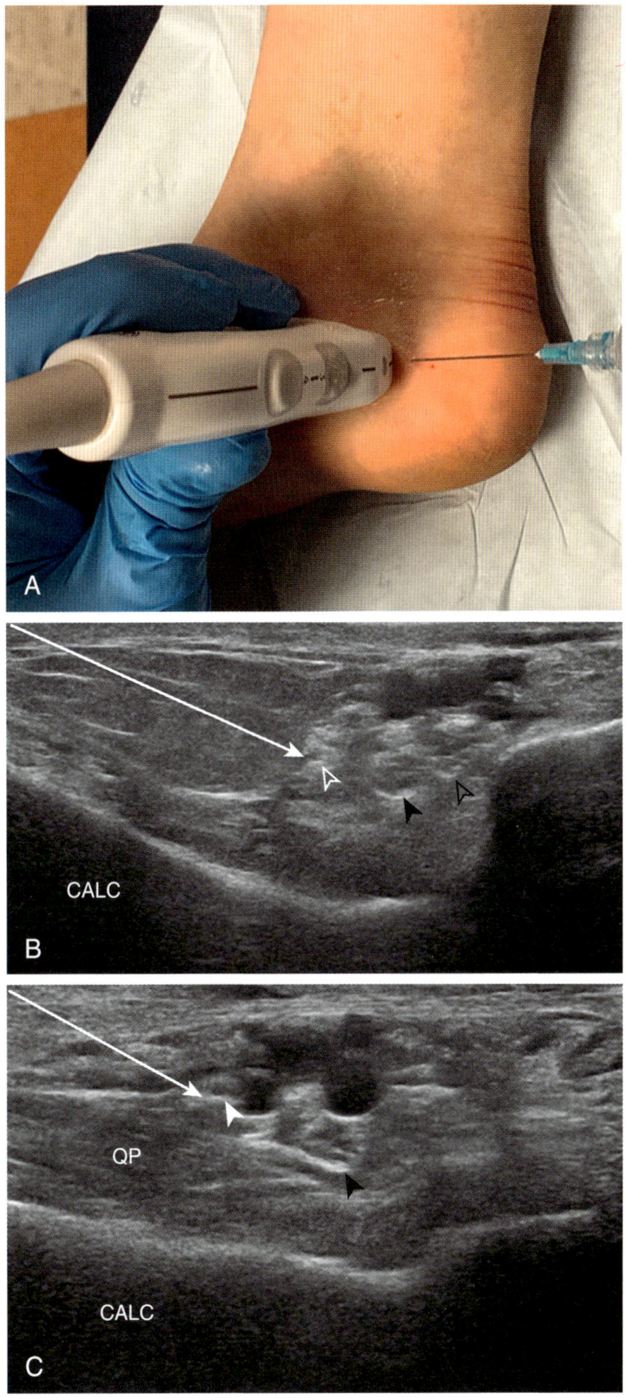

• **Fig 23.7** Approach to Injection of the Medial Calcaneal Nerve (MCN) and Inferior Calcaneal Nerve (ICN). (A) Patient and transducer position for a posterior to anterior SAX in-plane approach for injection of either the MCN or ICN. (B) Corresponding image and needle position (*arrow*) for injection of the MCN (*open white arrowhead*), which appears as a single hypoechoic fascicle traversing posteriorly into the subcutaneous tissue superficial to the calcaneus (*CALC*). *Black arrowhead* = lateral plantar nerve; *open black arrowhead* = medial plantar nerve. (C) Corresponding image and needle position (*arrow*) for injection of the ICN (*white arrowhead*), which appears as a single hypoechoic fascicle branching posteriorly from the lateral plantar nerve (*black arrowhead*) and is located adjacent to the quadratus plantae (*QP*) muscle before it enters the interval between the QP and AH muscles.

Intersection Syndrome

KEY POINTS

- This represents a friction syndrome between the flexor digitorum longus (FDL) and flexor hallucis longus (FHL) tendons as they cross distal to the medial tarsal tunnel (master knot of Henry).
- The differential diagnosis of medial ankle and/or midfoot pain is broad, and an injection into the knot of Henry can be both diagnostic and potentially therapeutic.

Pertinent Anatomy

- The FHL and the FDL are viewed in proximity to each other at the sustentaculum tali (ST) in short axis. The FDL is visualized just superficial to the ST while the FHL is located slightly distal and posterior. Scanning distal to the ST in short axis, the two tendons will intersect. The point of intersection, or the knot of Henry, is the common location of pathology.
- The medial plantar neurovascular bundle is most often medial to the tendons at their intersection point.

Common Pathology

- Tendinosis or tenosynovitis
- Adhesions between the two tendons

Equipment

- High- or medium-frequency linear array ultrasound transducer
- 30–25 gauge. 1.25–1.5 inch needle

Common Injectates

- Local anesthetics for diagnostics, corticosteroids
- Saline for hydrodissection
- Orthobiologics

Injectate Volume

- 1-2 mL
- 5-10 mL for hydrodissection

Technique

Patient Position

- Supine or seated
- Affected leg externally rotated to expose the medial ankle. Lateral ankle resting comfortably on a towel or over the side of the examination table (Figs. 23.8A and 23.9A)

Clinician Position

- Seated directly distal to the foot being injected

Transducer Position

- SAX to the crossover of the FDL and FHL (in-plane approach) (see Fig. 23.8A)
- LAX to the crossover of the FDL and FHL (in-plane approach) (see Fig. 23.9A)

Needle Position

- SAX in-plane approach directed dorsal to plantar (see Fig. 23.8B)
- LAX in-plane approach from distal to proximal (see Fig. 23.9B)

Target

- Between the FDL and FHL at the knot of Henry

PEARLS AND PITFALLS

- Identify and carefully map the medial plantar neurovascular bundle as they traverse adjacent to the knot of Henry.
- Lighten the probe pressure to avoid compression of the medial plantar vein during pre-injection planning.

Midfoot Joints

KEY POINTS

- US-guided midfoot injections can provide both diagnostic and therapeutic benefits.
- Osteoarthrosis (OA) is the most common midfoot joint disorder in the adult population.
- View radiographs as part of injection planning to become familiar with the bony anatomy.
- Patients often have multiple joints involved with midfoot OA. Careful scanning with correlative sono-palpatory pain can help guide providers with information regarding which joint(s) to inject.

Pertinent Anatomy

- The midfoot joints include the talonavicular, calcaneocuboid, naviculo-cuneiform, and tarsometatarsal joints.
- Synovial compartments of the midfoot involve joint complexes rather than separate compartments for each individual joint (Fig. 23.10).
- Abnormal communication between joint compartments is likely to occur in the setting of osteoarthrosis or inflammatory arthropathy.
- At-risk structures include the dorsalis pedis artery and vein, branches of the superficial and deep fibular nerves, and extensor tendons.

Common Pathology

- Osteoarthrosis
- Inflammatory arthropathy

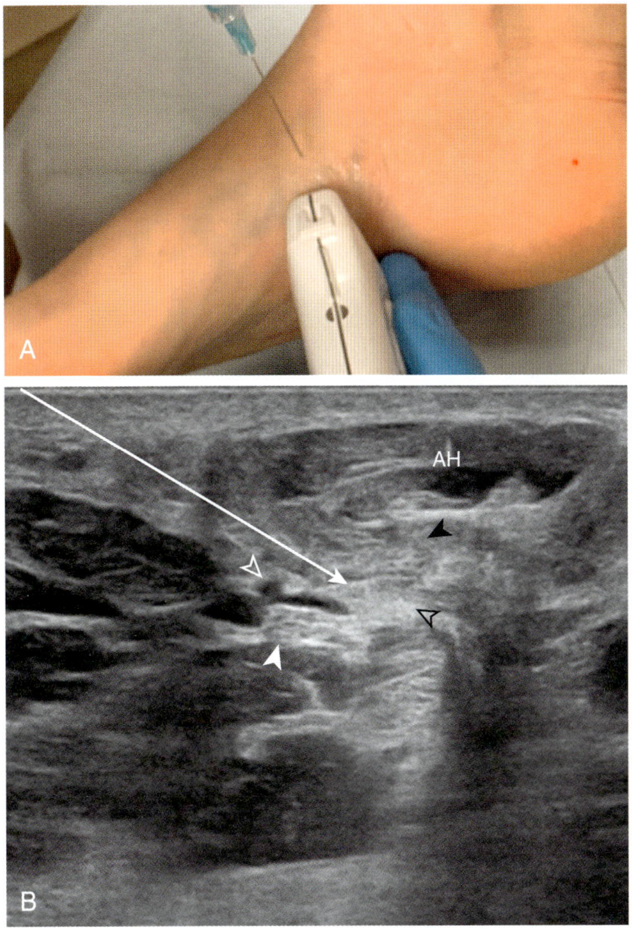

• **Fig 23.8** Intersection Syndrome Injection. SAX in-plane approach to injection of the intersection of the FDP and flexor halluceis longus (FHL) at the knot of Henry: (A) Patient and transducer position for a dorsal to plantar SAX in-plane approach. (B) Corresponding US image and needle position (*arrow*) for the dorsal to plantar SAX in-plane approach. The MPN (*white arrowhead*) and medial plantar artery and vein (*open white arrowhead*) are typically adjacent to the fexor digitorum profundus (FDP) and flexor hallucis longus (FHL) tendons. *Black arrowhead*, FDP; *open black arrowhead*, FHL; *AH*, abductor hallucis.

Equipment
- High-frequency linear or hockeystick ultrasound transducer
- 30–27 gauge, 1.0–1.25 inch if using local anesthetic before injection; 27–22 gauge, 1.0–1.5 inch for injectate

Common Injectates
- Local anesthetics for diagnostics, corticosteroids
- Prolotherapy
- Orthobiologics

Injectate Volume
- 0.5–1.5 mL

Technique
Patient Position
- Supine with posterior ankle on towel or hanging over the edge of the table
- Alternatively, knee flexed with foot on table (Figs. 23.11A and 23.12A)

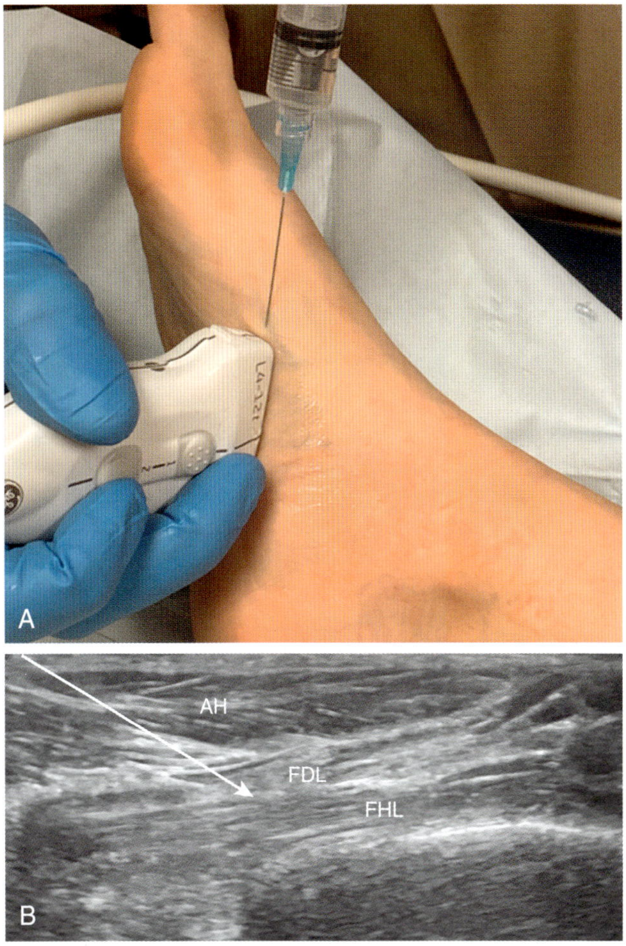

• **Fig 23.9** Intersection Syndrome Injection. LAX in-plane approach to injection of the intersection of the FDP and FHL at the knot of Henry: (A) Patient and transducer position for a distal to proximal long-axis (LAX) in-plane approach. (B) Corresponding US image and needle position (*arrow*) for the distal to proximal LAX in-plane approach. *AH,* Abductor hallucis; *FDL*, flexor digitorum longus; *FHL,* flexor hallucis longus.

Clinician Position
- Seated at the end of the table

Transducer Position
- LAX to the joint (out-of-plane approach) (see Fig. 23.11A)
- SAX to the joint (in-plane approach) (see Fig. 23.12A)

Needle Position
- Dorsal medial to lateral or lateral to medial (depending on location of at-risk structures) LAX out-of- plane approach (see Fig. 23.11B)
- Dorsal medial to lateral or lateral to medial (depending on location of at-risk structures) SAX in-plane approach (see Fig. 23.12B)

Target
- Directly between the bones into the joint.
- Can also inject the overlying joint capsule with prolotherapy or orthobiologics.

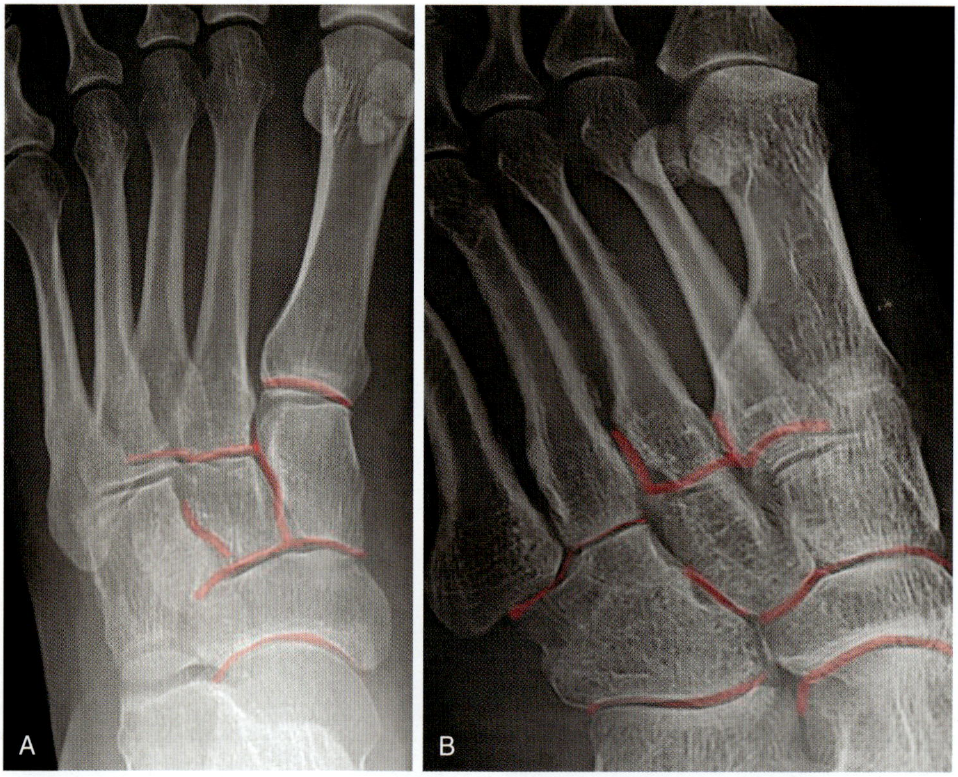

• **Fig 23.10** Anteroposterior (AP) and Oblique Radiographs of The Foot Demonstrating The Midfoot Joint Complexes (*red lines*). (A) AP radiograph of the foot showing the medial column joint complexes. Note that the medial tarsometatarsal joints communicate with the naviculocuneiform joints. (B) Oblique radiograph of the foot showing the lateral midfoot joint complexes.

PEARLS AND PITFALLS

- In advanced talonavicular joint arthrosis, dorsal overhanging of bony hypertrophic changes may obscure the joint line. In this case, scan distal to proximal to definitively identify the metatarsals, cuneiforms, and navicular bones. A more medial or lateral approach may also allow better visualization of the joint space and access to the intra-articular joint space.
- Apply light transducer pressure in pre-injection images to avoid compression of vascular structures.
- Assess overlying extensor tendons for attritional changes. In the setting of OA, the joint space may communicate with the overlying tendons due to capsular attrition. Thus, the injectate that contains a corticosteroid may leak into the tendon sheath and predispose to rupture.

Approach to Injection of the Lisfranc Joint

Injections Key Points

- The Lisfranc joint complex often remains symptomatic after injury due to instability or post-traumatic osteoarthrosis.
- An injection into the joint complex may provide diagnostic value for surgical planning or for management of pain.
- View radiographs as part of injection planning to become familiar with bony anatomy. Normal bony articulations may be altered after injury.

Pertinent Anatomy

- The Lisfranc joint is the articulation between the medial cuneiform and medial base of the second metatarsal.
- The Lisfranc ligament complex lies in an oblique plane between the medial cuneiform and second metatarsal base. It is composed of a dorsal, interosseous, and plantar component. The dorsal component is visible on ultrasound.
- At-risk structures include the medial branch of the deep fibular nerve, which most commonly travels directly over the Lisfranc joint.
- Scan SAX on the first and second metatarsals from distal to proximal until the first metatarsal disappears and the medial cuneiform appears (Fig. 23.13A and B).

Common Pathology

- Ligamentous injury with or without associated fracture
- Post-traumatic osteoarthrosis

Equipment

- High-frequency linear or hockeystick ultrasound transducer
- 30–27 gauge, 1.0–1.25 inch if using local anesthetic before injection; 30–22 gauge, 1.0–1.5 inch for injectate

Common Injectates

- Local anesthetics for diagnostics, corticosteroids
- Prolotherapy
- Orthobiologics

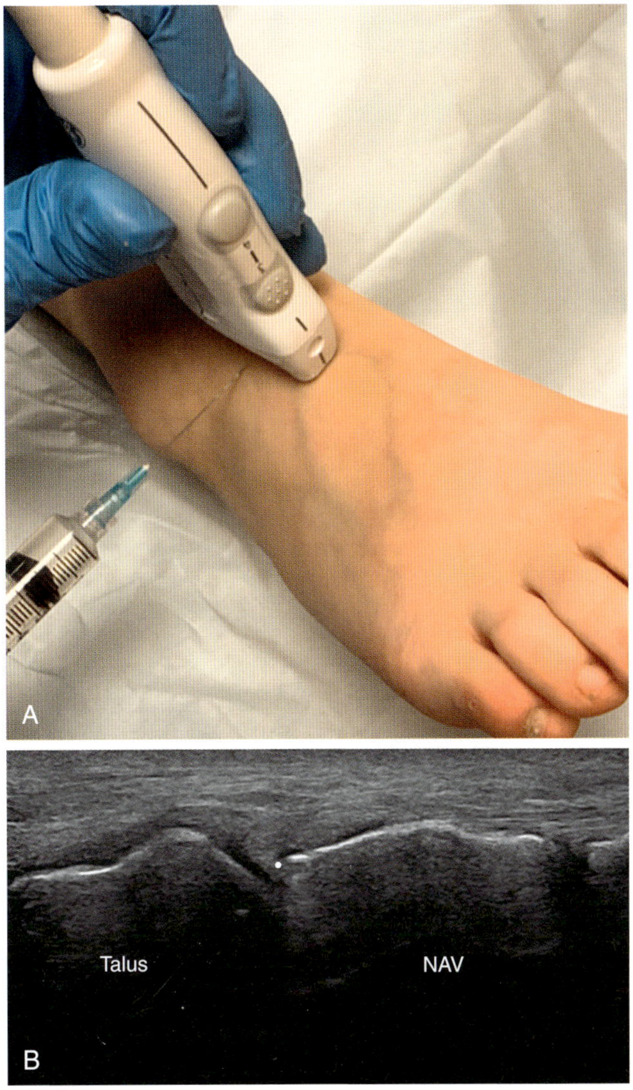

• **Fig 23.11** Midfoot Joint Injection. Long-Axis (LAX) out-of-Plane Approach. (A) Transducer and needle position for a lateral to medial LAX out-of-plane approach for an injection into the talonavicular joint. The approach may be medial to lateral or lateral to medial, depending on the location of at-risk structures. A similar approach is applied for injections involving the naviculocuneiform and tarsometatarsal joints. (B) Corresponding ultrasound image and needle position (*white dot*) for the LAX out-of-plane approach. *NAV*, Navicular bone.

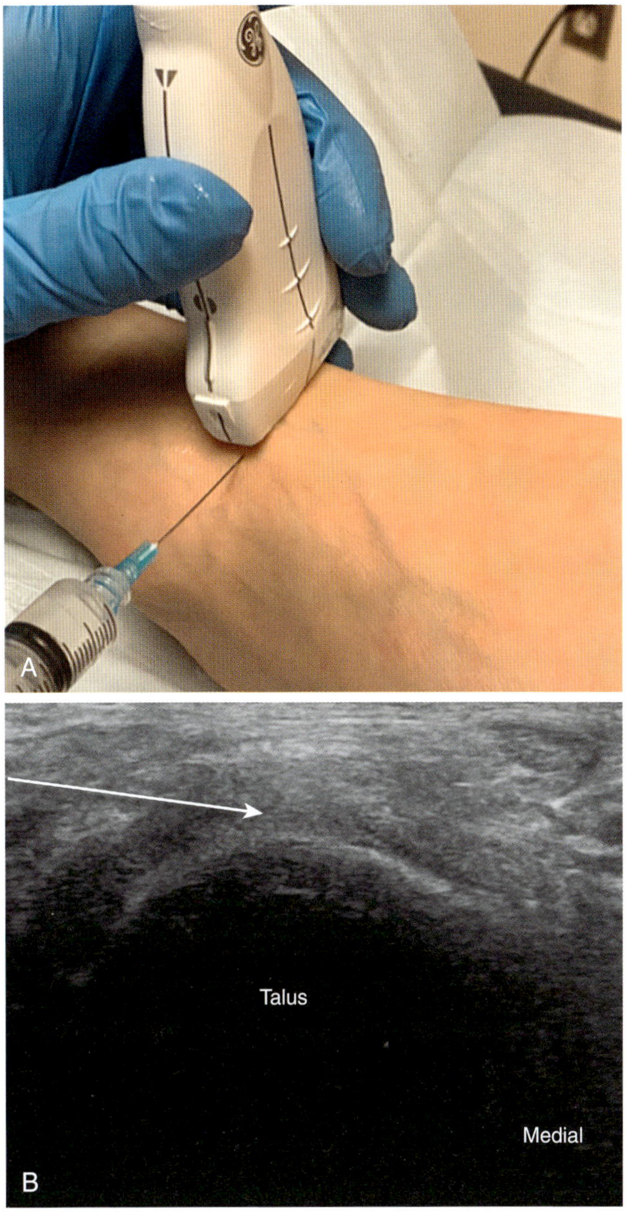

• **Fig 23.12** Midfoot Joint Injection. SAX in-Plane Approach. (A) Transducer and needle position for a lateral to medial SAX in-plane approach for an injection into the talonavicular joint. The approach may be medial to lateral or lateral to medial, depending on the location of at-risk structures. A similar approach is applied for injections involving the naviculocuneiform and tarsometatarsal joints. (B) Corresponding ultrasound image and needle position (*arrow*) for the SAX in-plane approach.

Injectate Volume

- 1–2 mL

Technique

Patient Position

- Supine with posterior ankle on towel or hanging over the edge of the table (Fig. 23.14A and B; see also Fig. 23.13A and B)
- Alternatively, knee flexed with foot on table

Clinician Position

- Seated at the end of the table

Transducer Position

- Transverse at the mid-substance of the first and second MT and translate the probe proximately until the first metatarsal disappears and the medial cuneiform appears adjacent to the second metatarsal (see Fig. 23.13).

Needle Position

- Joint injections, LAX distal to proximal out-of-plane approach, beginning at the proximal first metatarsal interspace
- Alternately, SAX view of second metatarsal middle cuneiform joint
- For biologic injections, LAX out-of-plane approach to Lisfranc ligament complex

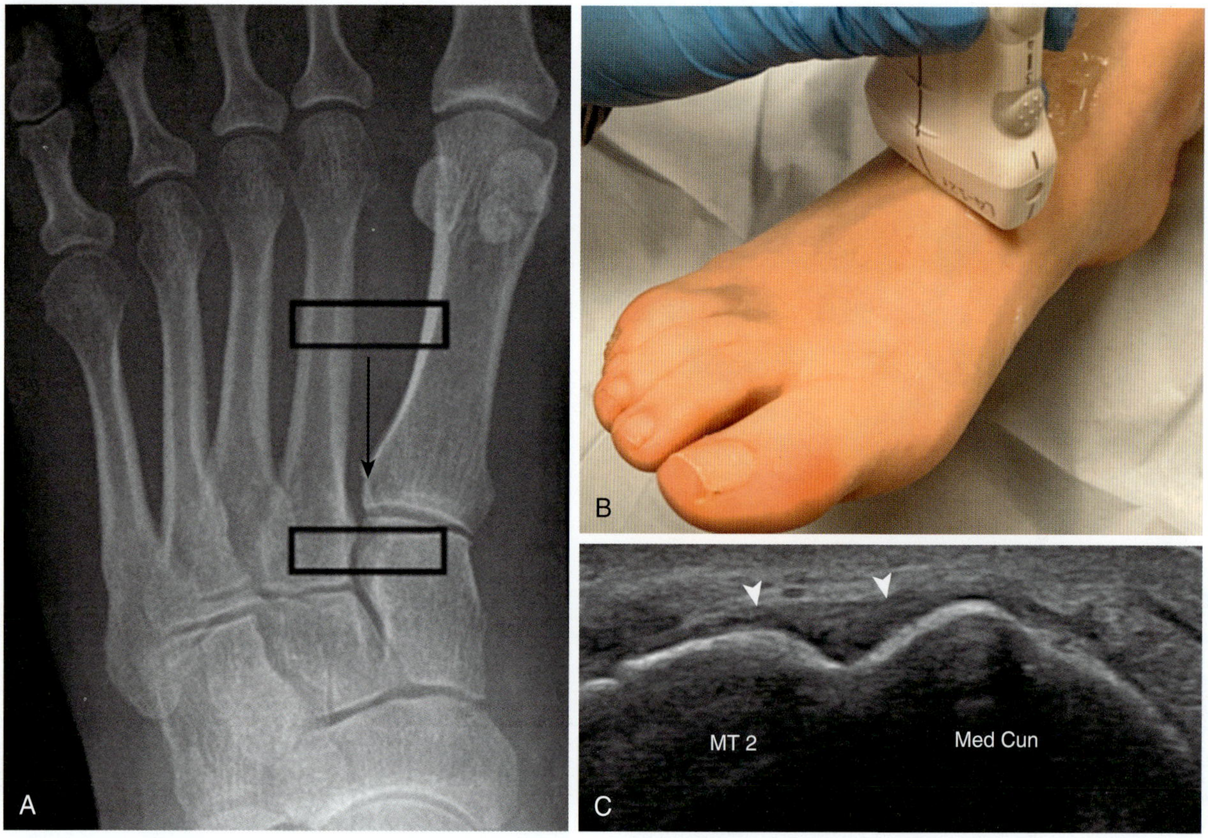

• **Fig 23.13** Sonographic Localization of Lisfranc Joint. (A) AP radiograph of the foot showing the transducer position for localizing the Lisfranc joint. Beginning anatomic coronal at the mid-metatarsal level between the first and second metatarsals (more distal probe position), translate the probe proximally until the first metatarsal disappears and the medial cuneiform (*Med Cun*) is visualized adjacent to the second metatarsal (proximal probe position). (B) Ultrasound transducer position to visualize Lisfranc joint corresponding to the more proximal transducer position in A. (C) Corresponding ultrasound image of Lisfranc joint. Note the overlying dorsal Lisfranc ligament (*arrowheads*). *Med Cun*, Medial metatarsal; *MT 2*, second metatarsal.

Target

- Lisfranc ligament superficial to the second metatarsal and medial cuneiform

PEARLS AND PITFALLS

- Identify the dorsalis pedis artery and vein(s) and medial branch of deep fibular nerve.
- If one has difficulty injecting the Lisfranc joint, one can inject the middle cuneiform second metatarsal joint since it often communicates with the Lisfranc joint.

First Metatarsophalangeal Joint and Lesser Metatarsophalangeal Joints

KEY POINTS

- Assess for presence of effusion if considering aspiration.
- Assess for signs of urate deposition disease if clinically pertinent.
- Hyperechoic aggregates or punctate echogenic debris (snowstorm appearance), often with hypervascularity, in dorsal synovial recess.
- Subcutaneous edema and vascularity in acute gout attack.
- Double contour sign (two echogenic lines) involving the articular cartilage of metatarsal head.

Pertinent Anatomy

- Extensor tendons traverse dorsal to the MTP joint

Common Pathology

- Osteoarthrosis
- Urate deposition disease
- Inflammatory arthropathy

Equipment

- High-frequency linear or hockeystick ultrasound transducer
- 22–20 gauge, 1–1.5 inch needle for aspiration
- 27–22 gauge, 1.0–1.5 inch needle for injection

Common Injectates

- Local anesthetics for diagnostics, corticosteroids
- Prolotherapy
- Orthobiologics

Injectate Volume

- 0.5–1 mL

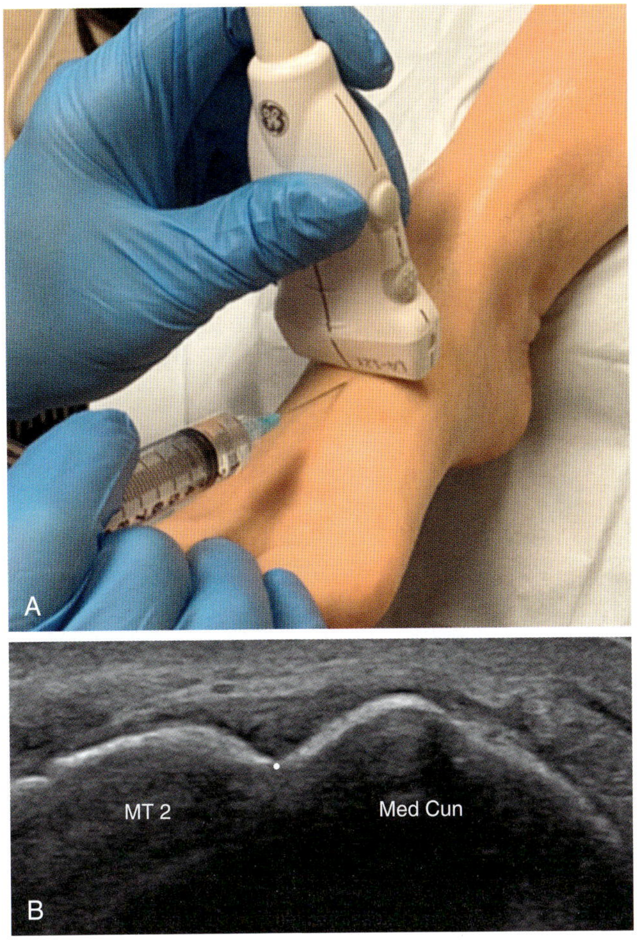

• **Fig 23.14** Lisfranc Joint Injection. (A) Transducer and needle position for a LAX (transverse) distal to proximal out-of-plane approach to injecting the Lisfranc joint. (B) Corresponding ultrasound image and needle target (*white dot*) for Lisfranc joint injection. *Med Cun*, Medial metatarsal; *MT 2*, second metatarsal.

Technique

Patient Position

- Supine with posterior ankle on towel or hanging over the edge of the table (Figs. 23.15A and 23.16A)
- Alternatively, knee flexed with foot on table

Clinician Position

- Seated directly distal to the foot being injected

Transducer Position

- LAX to the joint (out-of-plane approach) (see Fig. 23.15A)
- SAX to the joint (in-plane approach) (see Fig. 23.16A)

Needle Position

- Dorsal medial to lateral or lateral to medial LAX out-of-plane approach (see Fig. 23.15B)
- Dorsal medial to lateral or lateral to medial SAX in-plane approach (preferred approach for aspiration) (see Fig. 23.16B)

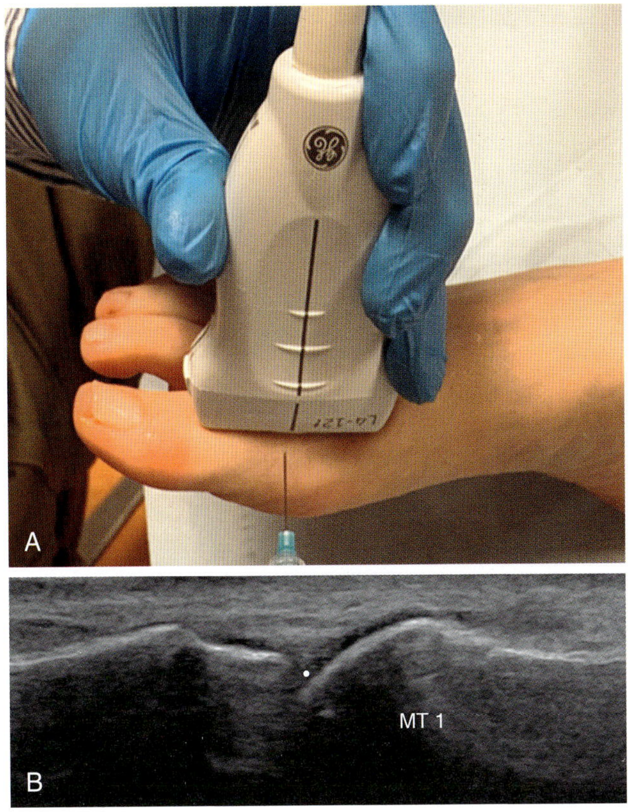

• **Fig 23.15** First Metatarsophalangeal (MTP) Joint Injection. LAX Out-of-Plane Approach. (A) Transducer and needle position for a LAX out-of-plane injection of the first MTP joint. The approach can be medial to lateral or lateral to medial. (B) Corresponding ultrasound image and needle location (*white dot*) for a LAX out-of-plane approach. A similar approach is utilized for injections of the lesser MTP joints. *MT 1*, First metatarsal.

PEARLS AND PITFALLS

- Avoid going through the extensor tendon to reach the joint.
- Traction to phalange or/or slight plantar flexion often opens up the joint space.

Great Toe Sesamoid Bones

KEY POINTS

- Both the tibial and fibular sesamoid articulations may be reached with an intra-articular first MTP joint injection.

Pertinent Anatomy

- Medial (tibial) and lateral (fibular) hallux sesamoids
- Intersesamoid ligament between the two sesamoid bones
- FHL tendon runs between the two sesamoid bones plantar to the intersesamoid ligament
- The joint between the sesamoid bones and first metatarsal communicates with the first MTP joint.[5]
- The tibial sesamoid bone is more prone to multiple ossification centers, and therefore more likely to have a bipartite or multipartite morphology.[6]

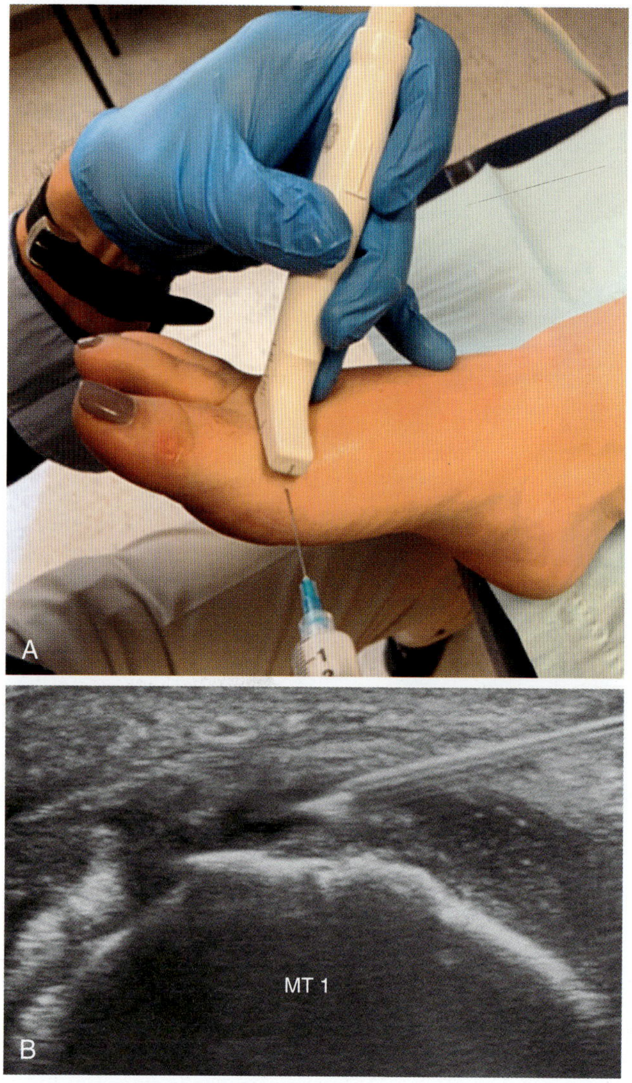

• **Fig 23.16** First Metatarsophalangeal (MTP) Joint Injection or Aspiration. SAX In-Plane Approach. (A) Transducer and needle position for a SAX in-plane injection or aspiration of the first MTP joint. The approach can be medial to lateral or lateral to medial. (B) Ultrasound image of a SAX in-plane aspiration of the first MTP joint. *MT 1*, First metatarsal.

Common Pathology

- Chronic sesamoid pain may be due to insertional tendinosis of the flexor hallucis brevis (FHB) tendons, stress fracture, avascular necrosis (AVN), and/or degenerative changes of the sesamoid articulation with the metatarsal head.[7]
- Stress fractures occur secondary to repetitive overuse trauma most commonly seen in dancers and runners.[8] This may overlap with secondary degenerative changes as the sesamoids form a true joint articulation with the metatarsal head.

Equipment

- High-frequency linear or hockeystick ultrasound transducer
- 30–27 gauge, 1.0–1.25 inch if using local anesthetic before injection; 25–22 gauge, 1.0-1.5 inch for injectate

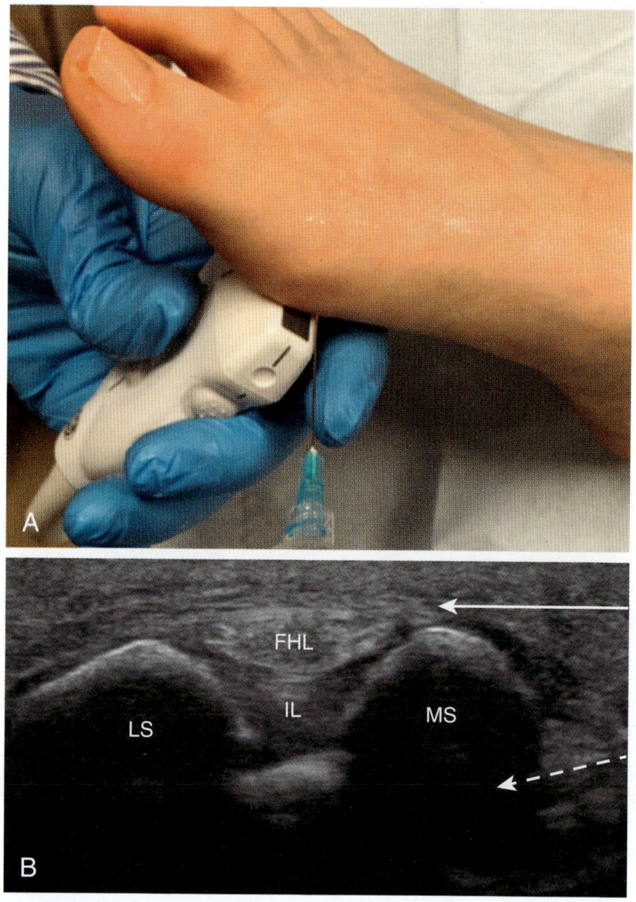

• **Fig 23.17** Great Toe Sesamoid Injection. Sax Axis In-Plane Approach. (A) Transducer and needle position for a medial to lateral SAX in-plane injection for a medial sesamoid injection. A lateral to medial approach can be utilized for a lateral sesamoid injection. (B) Corresponding ultrasound image and needle pathways showing the SAX in-plane approach for injecting either the superficial border of the sesamoid (*solid arrow*) or the deeper sesamoid-metatarsal articulation (*dotted arrow*). *FHL*, Flexor hallucis longus tendon; *LS*, lateral sesamoid; *MS*, medial sesamoid; *IL*, intersesamoid ligament.

Common Injectates

- Local anesthetics for diagnostics, corticosteroids
- Prolotherapy
- Orthobiologics

Injectate Volume

- 0.5–1 mL

Technique

Patient Position

- Supine with knee fully extended and ankle plantar flexed and resting on the table (Fig. 23.17A)

Clinician Position

- Seated directly below the foot being injected

Transducer Position

- SAX to the sesamoid-metatarsal articulation (in-plane approach) (see Fig. 23.17A)

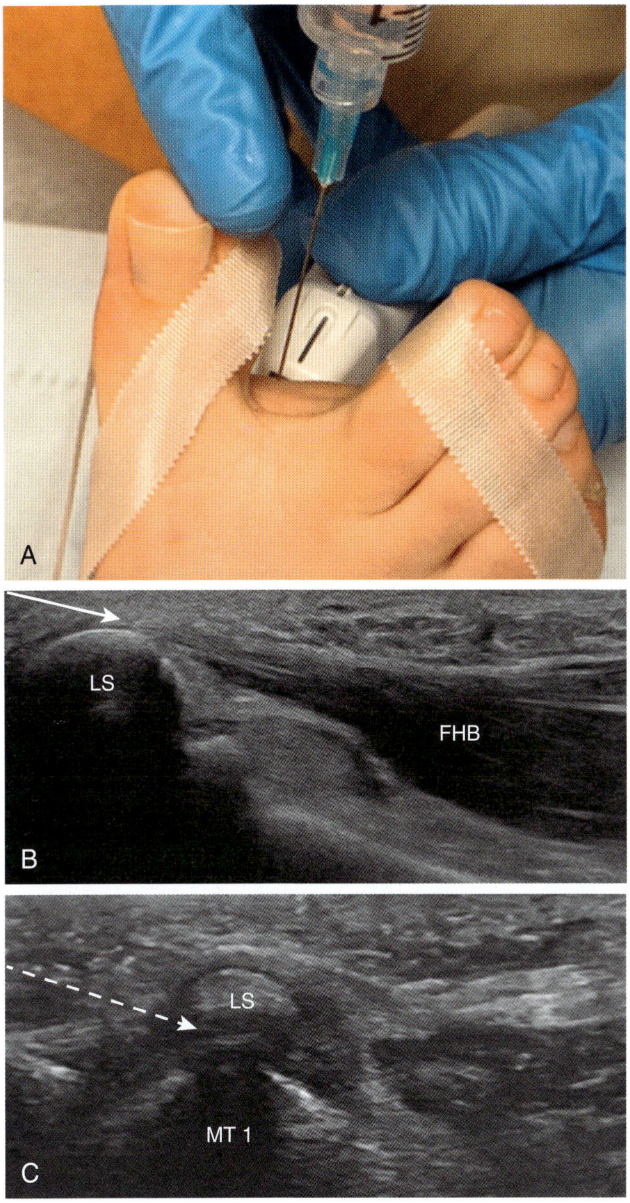

• **Fig 23.18** Great Toe Sesamoid Injection. Distal to Proximal Lax Approach. (A) Transducer and needle position for a LAX in-plane injection of the lateral sesamoid. A similar approach can be used for a medial sesamoid injection. Taping the toes apart may allow easier access for lateral sesamoid injections. (B) Corresponding ultrasound image and needle pathway (*solid arrow*) showing the distal to proximal LAX in-plane approach for injecting the superficial border of the lateral sesamoid. (C) Corresponding ultrasound image and needle pathway (*dotted arrow*) showing the distal to proximal LAX in-plane approach for injecting the lateral sesamoid/first metatarsal articulation. *FHB,* flexor hallucis brevis; *LS,* Lateral sesamoid; *MT 1*, first metatarsal.

- LAX to the sesamoid-metatarsal articulation (in-plane approach) (Fig. 23.18A)

Needle Position

- SAX in-plane to the sesamoid articulation with the needle approaching medial to lateral (see Fig. 23.17B)
- LAX in-plane to the sesamoid articulation from distal to proximal (see Fig. 23.18B and C)

PEARLS AND PITFALLS

- The fibular sesamoid is best approached with an LAX in-plane approach.
- Avoid the interdigital nerve and artery with the fibular sesamoid.

Interdigital (Morton's) Neuroma

Injections Key Points

- High-frequency linear or hockeystick ultrasound probe.
- Corticosteroids may result in temporary relief and provide diagnostic information when more than multiple pathologies are present (i.e., plantar plate or fat pad abnormalities).
- Serial alcohol injections, cryoablation, or radiofrequency ablation may provide more long-term relief in selected patients.

Pertinent Anatomy

- The interdigital nerve runs plantar to the dorsal intermetatarsal ligament.
- The intermetatarsal bursa is located dorsal to the dorsal intermetatarsal ligament.

Common Pathology

- Neuroma is somewhat of a misnomer, in that it is a fibrous thickening of the interdigital nerve associated with edema of the endoneurium. The intermetatarsal bursopathy accompanies the abnormal digital nerve. Thus, an interdigital neuroma should be thought of as a neuroma-bursal complex.[9]
- Most common location is within the third metatarsal interspace.[10]
- Post-surgical complications include fibrous adhesions around nerve, symptomatic stump neuroma, or intermetatarsal bursopathy.[11]
- Symptomatic interdigital neuroma often coexists with plantar plate and plantar fat pad abnormalities.

Equipment

- High-frequency linear or hockeystick ultrasound transducer
- 30–27 gauge, 1.0–1.25 inch if using local anesthetic before injection; 25–22 gauge, 1.0–1.5 inch for injectate

Common Injectates

- Local anesthetics for diagnostics, corticosteroids
- 98% alcohol for neurolysis[12]
- Neuroprolotherapy (5% dextrose)
- Radiofrequency ablation or cryoa[13,14]

Injectate Volume

- Corticosteroid—0.5-1mL
- Alcohol—various volumes reported in the literature (authors use 40–60% solution when combined with a local anesthetic)[15]
- 3–5 mL for hydrodissection for post-surgical scar tissue

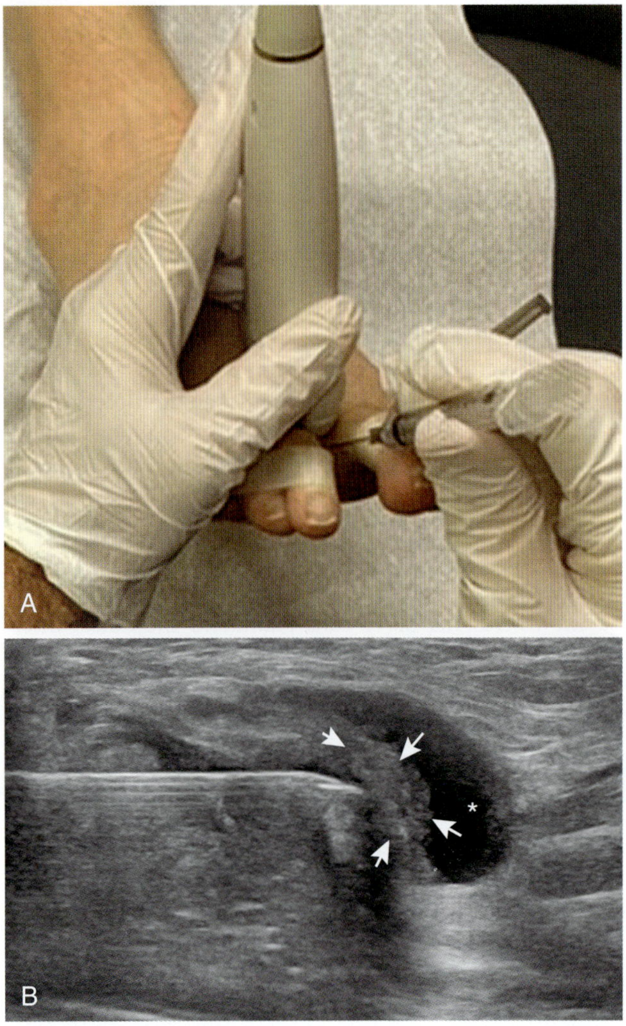

• **Fig 23.19** Neuroma-Bursal Complex (Morton's Neuroma) Injection. Long-Axis In-Plane Approach. (A) Transducer and needle position for a distal to proximal LAX in-plane approach, entering through the webspace. (B) Corresponding ultrasound image of a distal to proximal LAX in-plane neuroma-bursal complex injection. Note the extension of the neuroma-bursal complex (*white arrowheads*) and fluid from the injection within the intermetatarsal bursa (*asterisk*).

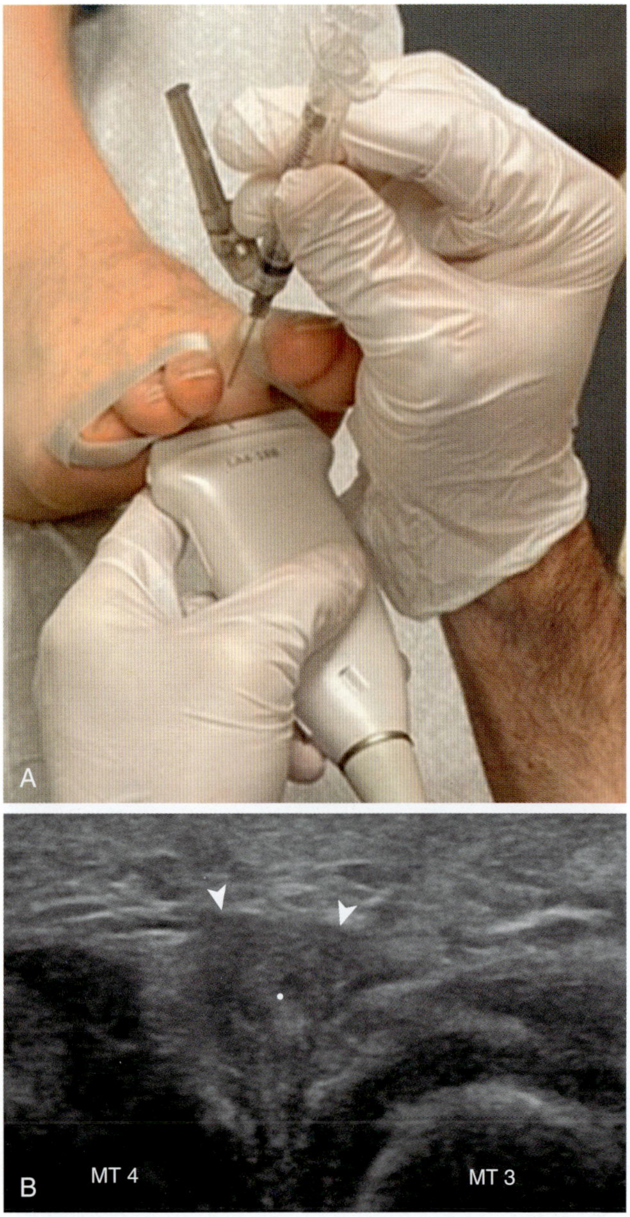

• **Fig 23.20** Neuroma-Bursal Complex Injection. Sax Out-of-Plane Approach. (A) Transducer and needle position for a distal to proximal SAX out-of-plane approach, entering through the plantar aspect of the webspace. (B) Corresponding ultrasound image and needle placement (*white dot*) of a distal to proximal SAX out-of-plane neuroma-bursal complex injection (*white arrowheads*). *MT 3*, Third metatarsal; *MT 4*, fourth metatarsal.

Technique

Patient Position

- Supine
- The patient has knees extended with feet hanging off the edge of the table or rolled towel, allowing the provider to push up under the neuroma (Fig. 23.19A)
- Consider taping the toes apart if the toes are anatomically malpositioned and obstructing the view (see Fig. 23.19A)

Clinician Position

- Seated or standing directly below the foot being injected

Transducer Position

- For dorsal approach—LAX (in-plane approach) (Fig. 23.19A)
- For plantar approach—SAX (out-of-plane approach) or LAX (in-plane approach) (Fig. 23.20A)

Needle Position

- For dorsal approach—LAX, in-plane to the transducer, distal to proximal (see Fig. 23.19B and 23.21) or proximal to distal
- For plantar approach—SAX, out-of-plane distal to proximal (Fig. 23.20B) or LAX, in-plane distal to proximal

Target

- Needle directed toward the neuroma-bursal complex

PEARLS AND PITFALLS

- Smaller MNs may be asymptomatic. Correlate the MN with either sono-palpatory pain or a diagnostic injection.[16]
- If plantar plate injury is present, then one would consider treating that as well with prolotherapy or orthobiologics.

Plantar Plates

KEY POINTS

- Consider prolotherapy or orthobiologics in the presence of a plantar plate tear with associate instability. Cortisone is usually not indicated.
- Plantar plate tears most often occur at their insertion onto the proximal phalanx, and can become more conspicuous on ultrasound with dynamic dorsiflexion of the MTP joint.

Pertinent Anatomy

- The plantar plate represents a fibrocartilaginous structure along the plantar aspect of the MTP joints.[17] It plays a crucial role in the stability of the MTP joint.[18]
- The plantar plate of the first MTP joint has a central component from the metatarsal to proximal phalanx, and medial and lateral components from the sesamoids to proximal phalanx.
- Flexor tendons traverse plantar to the plantar plate.

Common Pathology

- Capsuloligamentous complex (turf toe) injuries involving the first MTP joint most commonly involve injury to the plantar plate. More advanced injuries may also include other structures of the capsuloligamentous complex and the FHL tendon.
- Attritional-type tears at the insertion of the plantar plate onto the proximal phalanx are the most common abnormality involving the plantar plates of the lesser MTP joints.

Equipment

- High- or medium-frequency linear array ultrasound transducer
- 27–22 gauge, 1–1.5 inch needle

Common Injectates

- Prolotherapy
- Orthobiologics for plantar plate tear

Injectate Volume

- 0.5–2 mL

Technique

Patient Position

- Prone with knee fully extended and ankle plantar flexed over a rolled towel

Clinician Position

- Seated directly below the foot being injected

Transducer Position

- LAX to the plantar plate in the sagittal plane (Fig. 23.22A)

Needle Position

- LAX in plane from distal to proximal (Fig. 23.22B)

Target

- Directly into the plantar plate tear

PEARLS AND PITFALLS

- Use a small-gauge needle through the flexor tendon. It is important to avoid injecting into the flexor tendons.
- Foot deformity, such as a hammer toe, may necessitate a proximal to distal approach to the plantar plate.

Foot Fluoroscopy Injection Techniques

Joints

KEY POINTS

- Joint position can vary between patients, especially if deformities or a history of foot or ankle surgery. Adjust the C-arm to optimize joint visualization.
- If using prolotherapy or orthobiologics, one can inject the capsule of the joints as well if instability is present.

Calcaneocuboid Joint

Pertinent Anatomy

- The anterior process of the calcaneus articulates with posterior portion of the cuboid, forming the calcaneocuboid (CC) joint
- Intermediate dorsal cutaneous nerve can travel over the dorsum of the joint
- The calcaneocuboid has a relatively prominent inferior joint recess
- Peroneal longus tendon traverses under the lateral and plantar aspect of the joint
- The CC joint is intrinsically stable due to the congruency of the articular surfaces, and is reinforced by ligaments and tendon attachments[19–21]

Common Pathology

- Osteoarthrosis
- Traumatic injury
- Cuboid syndrome (dropped or subluxed cuboid), disrupting CC joint congruity

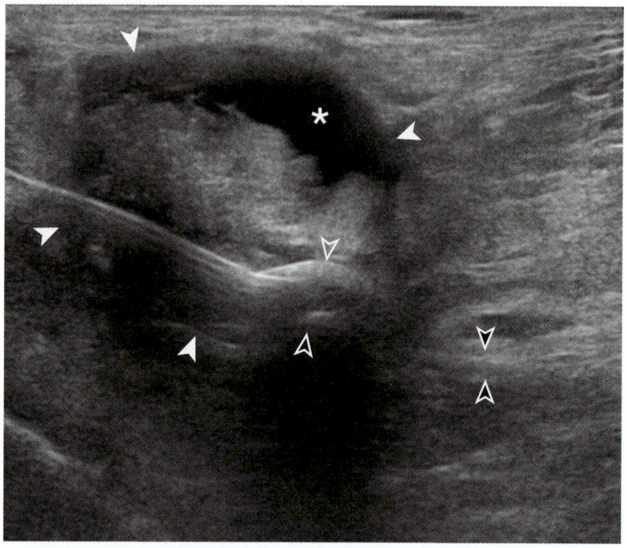

• **Fig 23.21** Cryoablation of A Neuroma-Bursal Complex (Morton's Neuroma). Long-axis in-plane approach similar to Fig. 23.19. The target of the ice ball (*open arrowheads*) is the interdigital nerve (*black arrowheads*) at or proximal to the neuroma-bursal complex. A similar location is utilized for a radiofrequency ablation. The *white arrowheads* outline the extent of the neuroma-bursal complex. The fluid within the neuroma-bursal complex (*asterisk*) is from local anesthesia infiltration prior to the ablation.

Equipment

- C-arm fluoroscopy
- 27–22 gauge, 1–2 inch needle
- Contrast

Common Injectates

- Local anesthetics for diagnostics, corticosteroids
- Prolotherapy
- Orthobiologics

Injectate Volume

- 1–2 mL

Technique

Patient Position

- Supine with the knee bent so that the foot is flat on the table (Fig. 23.23)
- Can place pillows or a bolster under the knee for comfort

Clinician Position

- Standing ipsilateral side of the patient

C-Arm Position Fluoro Technique

- Start in anteroposterior (AP) projection, then oblique laterally to view the lateral aspect of the calcaneal cuboid joint
- C-arm aligned so joint space is "opened up," resulting in increased lucency

Needle Position

- Start directly over the lateral joint line, directing needle from superior to inferior

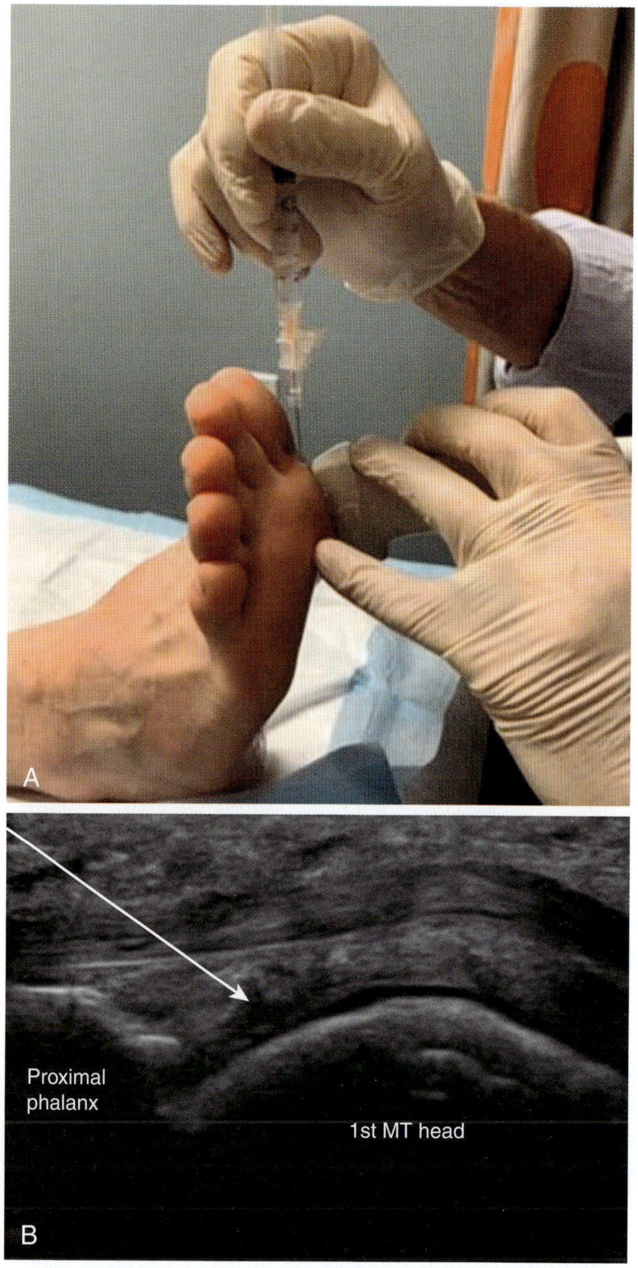

• **Fig 23.22** First Metatarsophalangeal (MTP) Plantar Plate Injection. A similar approach is utilized for injection of the plantar plates of the lesser MTP joints. LAX in-plane approach. (A) Transducer and needle position for a distal to proximal LAX in-plane injection to the plantar plate. (B) Corresponding ultrasound image and needle pathways showing LAX in-plane approach to the plantar plate (*arrow*). *1st MT*, First metatarsal.

Target

- Advance and inject a small amount of contrast to confirm intra-articular placement (Fig. 23.24)

PEARLS AND PITFALLS

- Entering the joint laterally avoids the intermediate dorsal cutaneous nerve.
- Internal rotation of the foot can help open the joint.

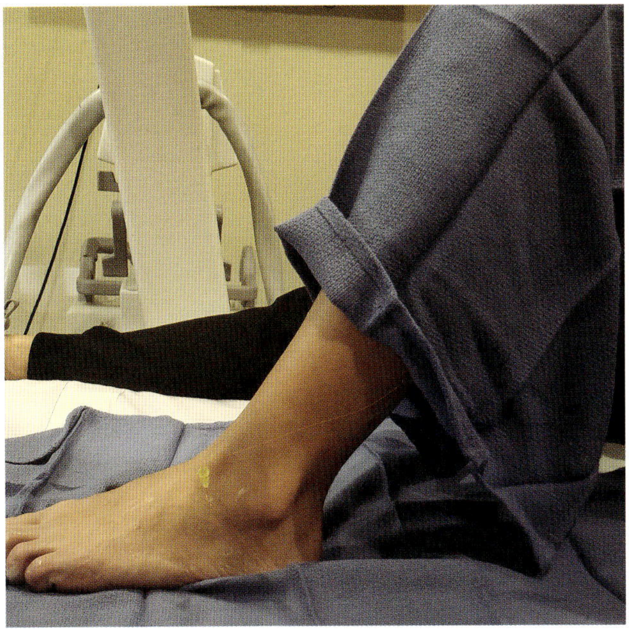

• **Fig 23.23** Calcanocuboidal Joint Injection with Fluoroscopy Setup.

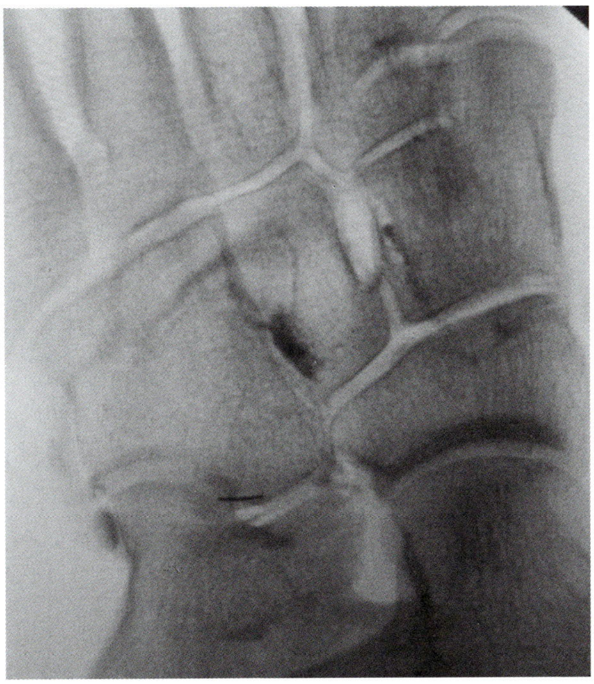

• **Fig 23.24** Calcanocuboidal Joint Injection AP Fluoroscopic View, with Contrast Showing Communication with Intercuneiform Joints.

Naviculocuboid (Cuboideonavicular) Joint

Pertinent Anatomy

- Intermediate dorsal cutaneous nerve from the superficial peroneal nerve travels dorsal and lateral to the joint

Common Pathology

- Joint arthritis
- Traumatic injury

Equipment

- C-arm fluoroscopy
- 27–22 gauge, 1–2 inch needle
- Contrast

Common Injectates

- Local anesthetics for diagnostics, corticosteroids
- Prolotherapy
- Orthobiologics

Injectate Volume

- 1–2 mL

Technique

Patient Position

- Supine with the knee bent and the foot flat on the table
- Can place pillows or a bolster under the knee

Clinician Position

- Standing ipsilateral side of the patient

C-Arm Position

- Start in AP projection, then oblique laterally 20-35 degrees to bring the navicular cuboid joint into view.
- C-arm aligned so joint space is "opened up," resulting in increased lucency

Needle Position

- Start directly over the inferior aspect of the joint line

Target

- Advance needle until gently touching the inferior lateral navicular.
- Then "walk off" into the joint and inject a small amount of contrast to confirm intra-articular positioning (Fig. 23.25).

PEARLS AND PITFALLS

- If the patient feels radiating sensation during the injection, redirect the needle dorsal medial to avoid the intermediate dorsal cutaneous nerve. C-arm rotation may have to be adjusted as well.
- The naviculocuboid joint is a deeper joint. To obtain good intra-articular flow, the needle may have to be advanced further into the joint.
- There is variable communication in midfoot joints. Contrast may communicate with the adjacent joints (anteriosubtalar, cubocuneiform, navicular cuneiform).

Intercuneiform Joints

Pertinent Anatomy

- Intercuneiform joints are articulations among the three cuneiform bones (lateral-intermediate cuneiform joint

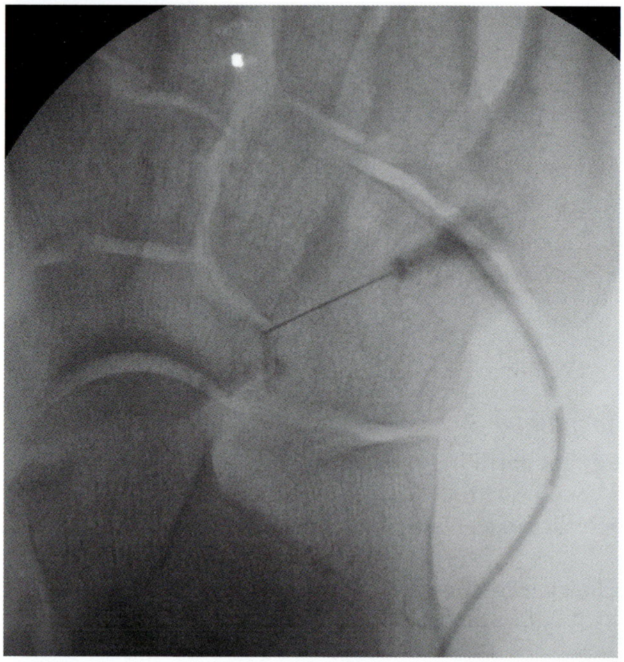

• **Fig 23.25** Naviculocuboid Joint Injection AP Fluoroscopic View, with Contrast.

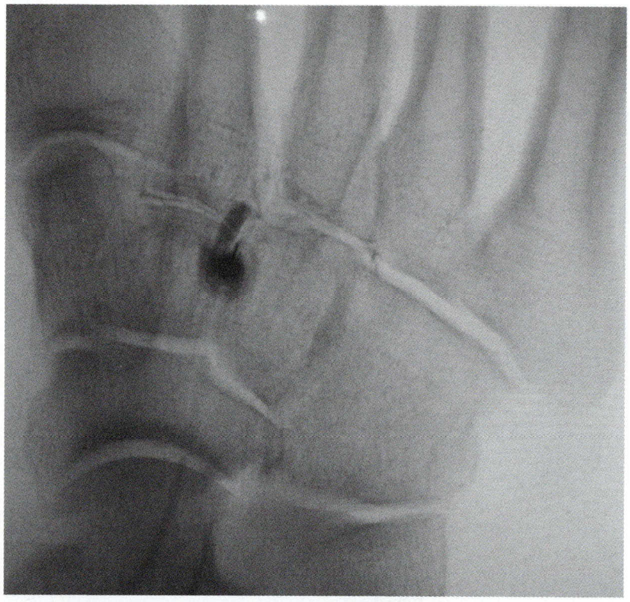

• **Fig 23.26** Intercuneiform Joint Injection with AP Fluoroscopic View, with Contrast also Showing Communication with Medial Tarsometatarsal Joints.

and medial-intermediate cuneiform joint). The cuneocuboid joint describes the joint between the cuboid and lateral cuneiform.

- Intercuneiform joints
- Lateral-intermediate cuneiform joint
- Medial-intermediate cuneiform joint
- The intermediate dorsal cutaneous nerve from the superficial peroneal nerve travels dorsal and lateral to the cubocuneiform joint

Common Pathology

- Joint arthritis
- Traumatic injury

Equipment

- C-arm fluoroscopy
- 27–22 gauge, 1–2 inch needle
- Contrast

Common Injectates

- Local anesthetics for diagnostics, corticosteroids
- Prolotherapy
- Orthobiologics

Injectate Volume

- 1–2 mL

Technique

Patient Position

- Supine with the knee bent so that the foot is flat on the table
- Can place pillows or a bolster under the knee

Clinician Position

- Standing ipsilateral side of the patient

C-Arm Position

- Obtain view to most "open up" the desired joint, resulting in increased joint lucency
- Cubocuneiform
  - Start in AP projection, then oblique laterally 25–40 degrees to visualize the joint clearly
- Lateral-intermediate cuneiform joint
  - AP view requiring lateral oblique 15–25 degrees to visualize the joint clearly
- Medial-intermediate cuneiform joint
  - Cuneiform and first AP view requiring medial oblique 5–15 degrees to visualize the joint clearly

Needle Position

- Start directly over the mid portion of the desired joint line

Target

- Advance and inject a small amount of contrast to confirm intra-articular placement (Fig. 23.26).

PEARLS AND PITFALLS

- Needle trajectory risks penetration of the intermediate dorsal cutaneous nerve.
- If the patient feels radiating sensation during the injection, redirect needle more dorsal medial to avoid the nerve. C-arm rotation may have to be adjusted as well.

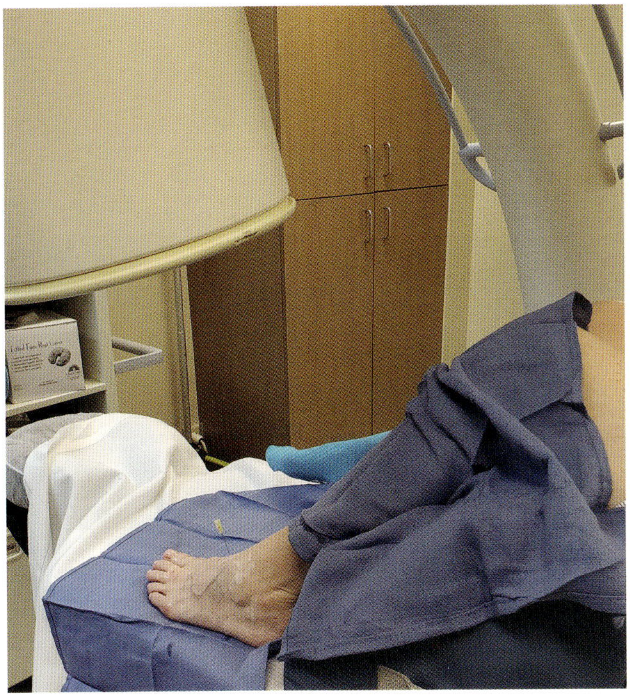

• **Fig 23.27** Naviculocuneiform Joint Injection with Fluoroscopy Setup.

Naviculocuneiform Joints

Pertinent Anatomy

- The distal aspect of the navicular has three facets, one for each cuneiform (medial, intermediate, and lateral).
- There is one joint capsule for all three articulations.
- The naviculocuneiform (NC) joint also communicates with the second and third tarsometatarsal joint via the medial and intermediate cuneiform intercuneiform joint.
- The dorsalis pedis artery traverses dorsally over the navicular, and the medial and lateral tarsal branches off the dorsalis pedis can course over the NC joints.[22,23]

Common Pathology

- Joint arthritis
- Traumatic injury

Equipment

- C-arm fluoroscopy
- 27–22 gauge, 1–2 inch needle
- Contrast

Common Injectates

- Local anesthetics for diagnostics, corticosteroids
- Prolotherapy
- Orthobiologics

Injectate Volume

- 1–2 mL

Technique

Patient Position

- Supine with the knee bent so that the foot is flat on the table (Fig. 23.27)
- Can place pillows or a bolster under the knee

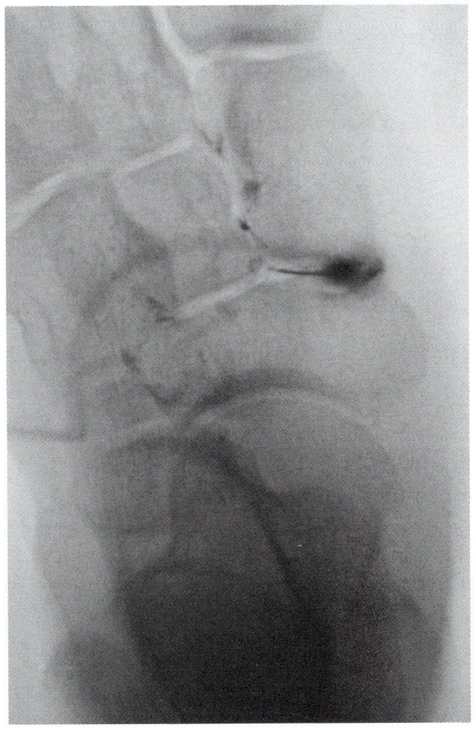

• **Fig 23.28** Naviculocuneiform Joint Injection AP Fluoroscopic View with Contrast.

Clinician Position

- Standing ipsilateral side of the patient

C-Arm Position

- Obtain view to most "open up" the desired joint, resulting in increased joint lucency
- Navicular-medial cuneiform
  - AP view of the joint requiring medial oblique of 15–20 degrees to visualize the joint clearly
- Navicular-intermediate cuneiform or navicular-medial cuneiform-intermediate cuneiform
  - Direct AP view; may require 5–10 degree medial oblique to visualize the joint clearly
- Navicular lateral cuneiform or navicular-intermediate cuneiform-lateral cuneiform joints
  - AP view of the joint requiring lateral oblique of 10–20 degrees to visualize the joint clearly

Needle Position

- Palpate the dorsalis pedis pulse and position needle to avoid damaging the artery
- Start directly over the mid portion of the desired joint line
- Alternatively, can start at Y intersection of the navicular and medial and intermediate cuneiforms

Target

- Advance and inject a small amount of contrast to confirm intra-articular placement (Fig. 23.28)

PEARLS AND PITFALLS

- Needle trajectory risks penetration of the medial dorsal cutaneous nerve or dorsalis pedis artery.
- If the patient feels radiating sensation during the injection, redirect needle more dorsal medial to avoid the nerve. The C-arm rotation may have to be adjusted as well.

Tarsometarsal Joints

Pertinent Anatomy

- The Lisfranc joint is composed of the five tarsometatarsal (TMT) joints, and represents the junction between the midfoot and forefoot.
- The joint encompasses articulations between the three cuneiforms and the cuboid proximally, and the base of the five metatarsal heads distally. The TMT joints have three separate joint capsules:
  - Medial cuneiform and first metatarsal base
  - Intermediate and lateral cuneiforms and second and third metatarsal bases
  - Cuboid and fourth and fifth metatarsal bases
- TMT joints may communicate with the intercuneiform joints.
- The second and third TMT joints communicate with the naviculocuneiform joint.
- Intermediate and medial dorsal cutaneous nerves travel dorsally to the joints.
- The dorsalis pedis artery travels dorsally and usually between the first and second tarsals and metatarsals.
- The lateral tarsal artery branches form the dorsalis pedis, usually at the level of the navicular bone over the lateral cuneiform and between fourth and fifth tarsals and metatarsals.
- The arcuate artery usually traverses just distal to the proximal metatarsal heads over the second, third, and fourth metatarsals.[24-26]

Common Pathology

- Joint arthritis
- Traumatic injury
- Lisfranc ligament injury[27]

Equipment

- C-arm fluoroscopy
- 27–22 gauge, 1–2 inch needle
- Contrast

Common Injectates

- Local anesthetics for diagnostics, corticosteroids
- Prolotherapy
- Orthobiologics

Injectate Volume

- 1–2 mL

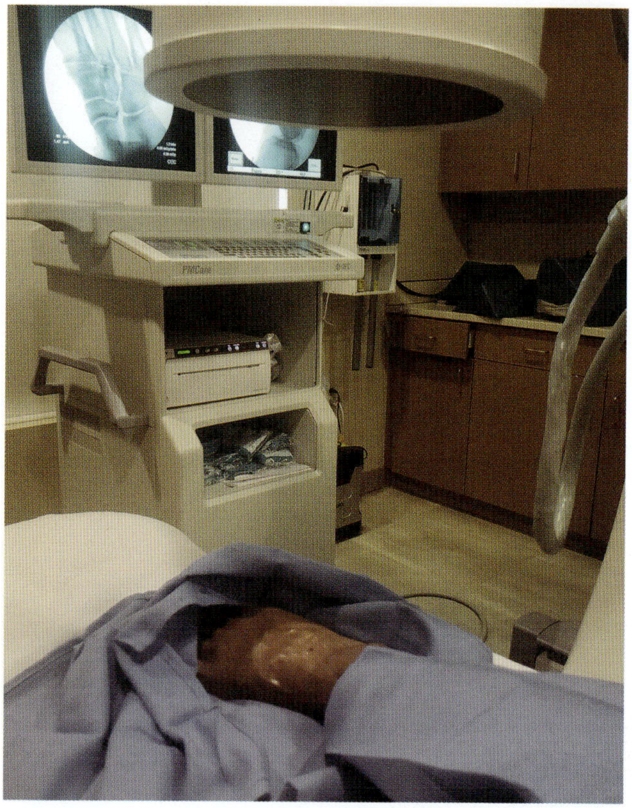

• **Fig 23.29** Fourth and Fifth Tarsometatarsal Joint Injection Setup Lateral Decubitus.

Technique

Patient Position

- Supine with the knee bent so that the foot is flat on the table
- Can place pillows or a bolster under the knee
- Optional for the fourth and fifth metatarsal joints to have patient in the lateral decubitus position (Fig. 23.29)

Clinician Position

- Standing ipsilateral side of the patient

C-Arm Position

- Obtain view to most "open up" the desired joint, resulting in increased joint lucency
- Medial cuneiform and first metatarsal base:
  - Direct AP view
- Intermediate and lateral cuneiforms and second and third metatarsal bases:
  - AP view may require 5–10 degrees of lateral oblique
- Cuboid and fourth and fifth metatarsal bases:
  - AP view may require 10–20 degrees of lateral oblique

Needle Position

- First three TMT joints: aim directly over desired joint, palpating and avoiding the dorsalis pedis pulse prior to placing needle

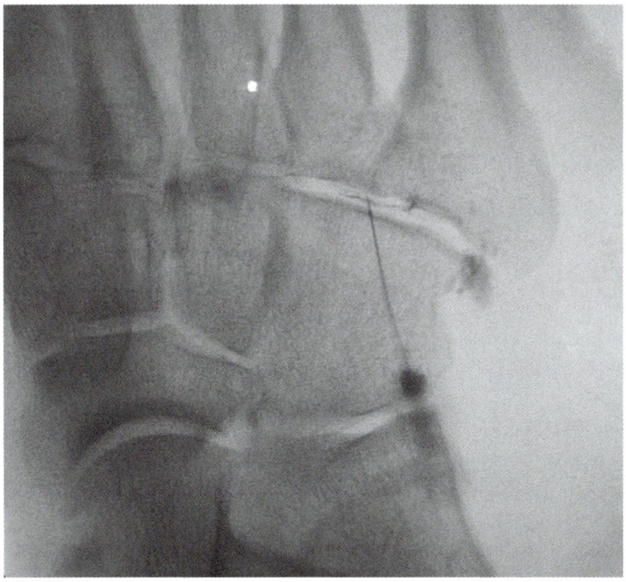

• **Fig 23.30** Lateral Tarsometatarsal Joint Injection AP View, with Contrast.

- Fourth and fifth TMT joints: aim at T-shaped intersections of the cuboid and fourth and fifth metatarsal heads

Target

- Advance and inject a small amount of contrast to confirm intra-articular placement (Fig. 23.30)

Metatarsophalangeal Joints

Pertinent Anatomy

- The metatarsophalangeal (MTP) joints have a ball-and-socket articulation. The proximal phalanx has a prominent dorsal lip.
- The first MTP joint has distinct anatomy, including paired sesamoids with their own articulations at the crista or plantar aspect of the metatarsal head.
- The first MTP joint communicates with the sesamoid articulations and has small dorsal and plantar recesses.
- The second through fifth, or lesser MTP joints, have small dorsal and larger plantar capsular recesses, which extend from the metatarsal necks to the bases of the proximal phalanges.
- The extensor tendons travel over the midline of the joints.
- The dorsal digital nerves and arteries travel medial and lateral to the bones/joints.[20,21]

Common Pathology

- Joint arthritis
- First MTP joint is the most common site for gout[28]

Equipment

- C-arm fluoroscopy
- 27–22 gauge, 1–2 inch needle
- Contrast

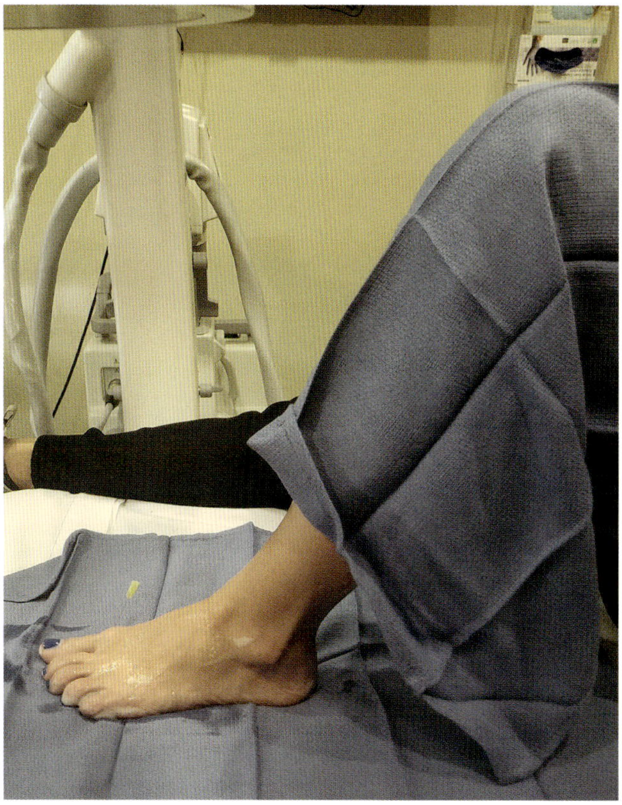

• **Fig 23.31** First Metatarsal Phalangeal Joint Injection with Fluoroscopy Setup.

Common Injectates

- Local anesthetics for diagnostics, corticosteroids
- Prolotherapy
- Orthobiologics

Injectate Volume

- 1–2 mL

Technique

Patient Position

- Supine with the knee bent so that the foot is flat on the table (Fig. 23.31)
- Can place pillows or a bolster under the knee

Clinician Position

- Standing ipsilateral side of the patient

C-Arm Position Fluoro Technique

- Direct AP view of the joint with the most joint line lucency

Needle Position

- Start needle just off the mid-line and proximal to the joint over the metatarsal head to avoid the dorsal lip of the proximal phalanx or osteophytes

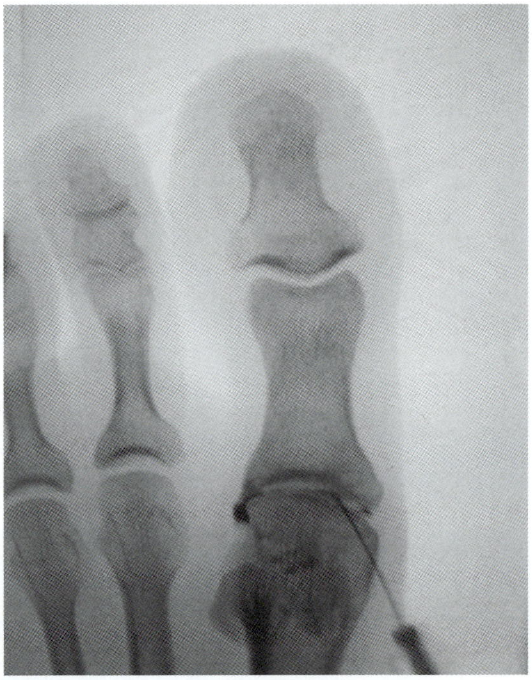

• **Fig 23.32** First Metatarsal Phalangeal Joint Injection AP Fluoroscopic View, with Contrast.

Target

- Touch down on metatarsal head and walk off 1 mm distal from the joint
- Inject a small amount of contrast to confirm intra-articular flow (Fig. 23.32)

PEARLS AND PITFALLS

- Start over the metatarsal head to avoid the dorsal lip of the proximal phalanx. The joint capsule extends from the metatarsal necks to the bases of the proximal phalanges. Guiding the needle and targeting the metatarsal head will result in intra-articular placement.
- Rule out gout flare for first MTP joint pain and swelling before injecting any orthobiologics.
- If suspected gout, use local anesthetic, then use 22-20 gauge needle to aspirate.

Interphalangeal

Pertinent Anatomy

- The interphalangeal (IP) joints are hinge joints between the phalanges.
- Dorsal digital nerves and arteries travel medial and lateral to the bones/joints.[20-21]

Common Pathology

- Joint arthritis
- Traumatic injury

Equipment

- C-arm fluoroscopy
- 27–22 gauge, 1–2 inch needle
- Contrast

Common Injectates

- Local anesthetics for diagnostics, corticosteroids
- Prolotherapy
- Orthobiologics

Injectate Volume

- 0.5–1 mL

Technique

Patient Position

- Supine with the knee bent so that the foot is flat on the table
- Can place pillows or a bolster under the knee

Clinician Position

- Standing ipsilateral side of the patient

C-Arm Position

- Direct AP view of the joint with the most joint line lucency

Needle Position

- Start needle just off the mid-line and proximal to the joint over the head of the phalanx to avoid the dorsal lip of the middle or distal base of the phalanx

Target

- Touch down on head of the phalanx (Fig. 23.33).
- Option to inject a very small amount of contrast to confirm intra-articular flow. If no intra-articular flow, ensure the needle is not on the dorsal lip and then reposition to direct needle distally until it drops into the joint.

PEARLS AND PITFALLS

- Can slightly flex the toe to open up the joint more.
- These are small joints, so keep injectate volume low.

Metatarsosesamoid

Pertinent Anatomy

- The two sesamoid bones of the first MTP joint are contained within the tendons of the FHB and form a part of the plantar plate.
- They articulate with the plantar facets of the metatarsal head.
- A crista, or intersesamoid ridge, separates the medial and lateral metatarsal facets.
- They function to distribute weight of the first ray, with the tibial or medial sesamoid assuming most of the weight-bearing forces.

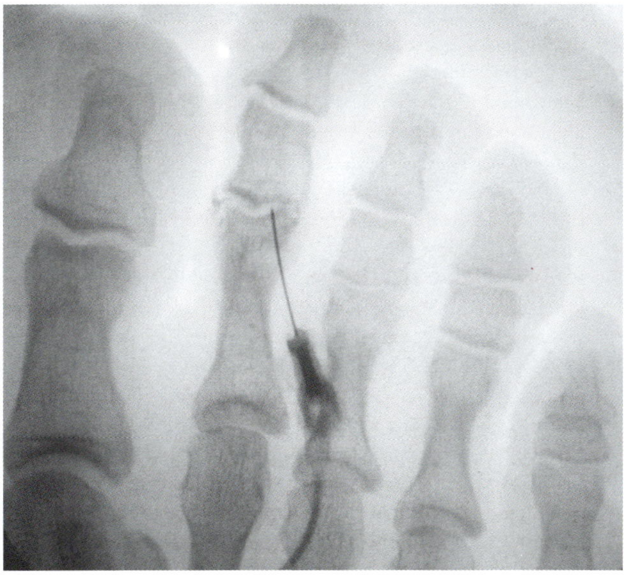

• **Fig 23.33** Interphalangeal Joint Injection AP Fluoroscopic View, with Contrast.

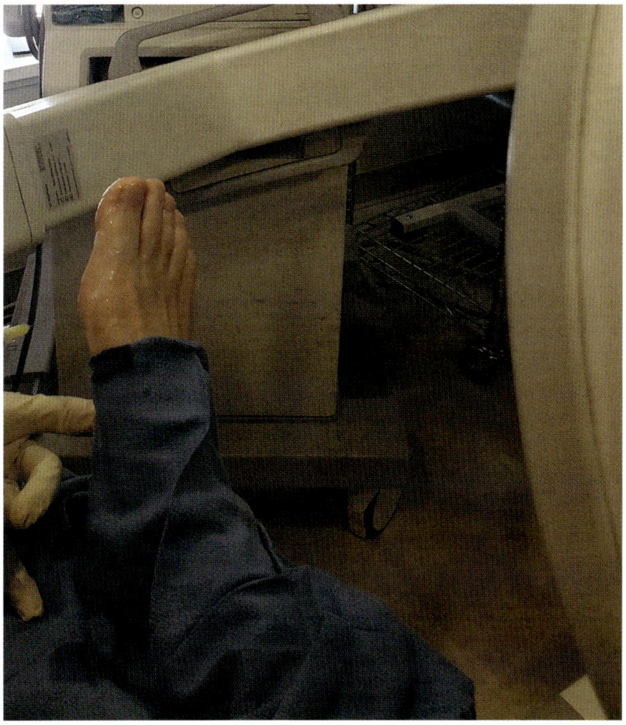

• **Fig. 23.34** Metatarsosesamoid with Fluoroscopy Injection Setup.

- They have a tenuous blood supply, so injury can lead to delayed healing.
- Bipartite sesamoids are a normal anatomic variant, with an incidence of 7% to 30%.

Common Pathology

- Intractable plantar keratosis can develop under the metatarsal heads
- Bursitis
- Arthritis secondary to trauma, chondromalacia, or sesamoiditis
- Fracture[29]

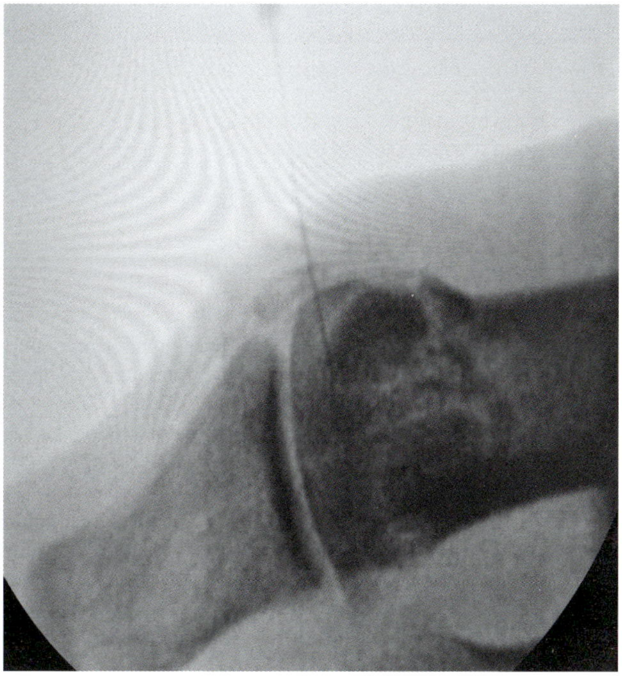

• **Fig 23.35** Metatarsosesamoid Injection with Fluoroscopy.

Equipment

- C-arm fluoroscopy
- 27–22 gauge, 1–2 inch needle
- Contrast

Common Injectates

- Local anesthetics for diagnostics, corticosteroids
- Prolotherapy
- Orthobiologics

Injectate Volume

- 0.5–1 mL

Technique

Patient Position

- Supine

Clinician Position

- Same side as affected limb

C-Arm Position

- AP view where the MTP joint and sesamoids can be visualized clearly

Needle Position

- Start medially (Fig. 23.34)

Target

- Aim for the space between tibial sesamoid and plantar aspect of the metatarsal head
- Inject a small amount of contrast to ensure flow in the joint (Fig. 23.35)

PEARLS AND PITFALLS

- Can be a painful injection, so use local anesthetic prior to injection.
- Hold the toe steady during injection as this is a sensitive area and prone for patient movement.

References

1. Draghi F, Gitto S, Bortolotto C, et al. Imaging of plantar fascia disorders: findings on plain radiography, ultrasound and magnetic resonance imaging. *Insights Imaging*. 2017;8:69–78.
2. Hoffman DF, Nazarian LN, Smith J. Enthesopathy of the lateral cord of the plantar fascia. *J Ultrasound Med*. 2014;33:1711–1716.
3. Presley J, Maida E, Pawlina W, et al. Sonographic visualization of the first branch of the lateral plantar nerve (Baxter nerve). *J Ultrasound Med*. 2013;32:1643–1652.
4. Alshami AM, Souvlis T, Coppieters MW. A review of plantar heel pain of neural origin: differential diagnosis and management. *Man Ther*. 2008;13:103–111.
5. Wempe M, Sellon J, Sayeed Y, et al. Feasibility of the first metatarsophangeal joint injections for sesmoid disorders: a cadaveric investigation. *Pharm Manag PM R*. 2012;4(8):556–560.
6. Taylor J, Sartoris D, Huang G, et al. Painful conditions affecting the first metatarsal bones. *Radiographics*. 1993;13:817–830.
7. Miller TT. Painful accessory bones of the foot. *Semin Musculoskelet Radiol*. 2002;6:153–161.
8. Potter HG, Pavlov H, Abrahams TG. The hallux sesamoids revisited. *Skeletal Radiol*. 1992;21:437–444.
9. Cohen SL, Miller TT, Ellis SJ, et al. Sonography of Morton neuromas: what are we really looking at? *J Ultrasound Med*. 2016;35:2191–2195.
10. Gomez D, Jha K, Jepson. Ultrasound scan for the diagnosis of interdigital neuroma. *Foot Ankle Surg*. 2005;11(3):175–177.
11. Beard N, Gouse R. Current ultrasound application in the foot and ankle. *Orthop Clin N Am*. 2018;49:109–121.
12. Hughes R, Ali K, Jones H, et al. Treatment of Morton's neuroma with alcohol injection under sonographic guidance: follow-up of 101 cases. *AJR Am J Roentgenol*. 2007;188:1535–1539.
13. Masala S, Cuzzolino A, Morini M, et al. Ultrasound-guided percutaneous radiofrequency for the treatment of Morton's neuroma. *Cardiovasc Intervent Radiol*. 2018;41:137–144.
14. Cazzato RL, Garnon J, Ramamurthy N, et al. Percutaneous MR-guided cryoablation of Morton's neuroma: rationale and technical details after the first 20 patients. *Cardiovasc Intervent Radiol*. 2016;39(10):1491–1498.
15. Pabinger C, Malaj I, Lothaller H, et al. Improved injection technique of ethanol of Morton's neuroma. *Foot Ankle Int*. 2020;41(5):590–595.
16. Symeonidis PD, Iselin LD, Simmons N, et al. Prevalence of interdigital nerve enlargements in an asymptomatic population. *Foot Ankle Int*. 2012;33(7):543–547.
17. Deland JT, Lee KT Sobel M, et al. Anatomy of the plantar plate and its attachments in the lesser metatarsal phalangeal joint. *Foot Ankle Int*. 1995;16:480–548.
18. Ford LA, Collins KB, Christensen JC. Stabilization of the subluxed second metatarsophalangeal joint: flexor tendon transfer versus primary repair of the plantar plate. *J Foot Ankle Surg*. 1998;37:217–222.
19. Standring S. In: *Gray's Anatomy: The Anatomical Basis of Clinical Practice*. 41st ed. New York: Elsevier; 2016:1339–1340.
20. Kelikian AS. *Sarrafian's Anatomy of the Foot and Ankle: Descriptive, Topographic, Functional*. 3rd ed. Philadelphia: Wolters Kluwer/Lippincott Williams & Wilkins; 2011:550–552.
21. Manaster BJ. *Imaging Anatomy. Knee, Ankle, Foot*. 2nd ed. Philadelphia: Elsevier; 2017:438–439.
22. Hansford BG, Mills MK, Stilwill SE, McGow AK, Hanrahan CJ. Naviculocuneiform and second and third tarsometatarsal articulations: underappreciated normal anatomy and how it may affect fluoroscopy-guided injections. *AJR Am J Roentgenol*. 2019;212:874–882.
23. RennerK, McAlister JE, GalliMM, Hyer CF. Anatomic description of the naviculocuneiform articulation. *J Foot Ankle Surg*. 2017;56:19–21.
24. Desmond EA, Chou LB. Current concepts review: Lisfranc injuries. *Foot Ankle Int*. 2006;27:653–660.
25. Siddiqui NA, Galizia MS, Almusa E, Omar IM. Evaluation of the tarsometatarsal joint using conventional radiography, CT, and MR imaging. *Radiographics*. 2014;34:514–531.
26. Preidler KW, Wang YC, Brossman J, Trudell D, Daenen B, Resnick D. Tarsometatarsal joint: anatomic details on MRI images. *Radiology*. 1996;199:733–773.
27. Wynter S, Grigg C. Lisfranc injuries. *Australian Family Physician*. 2017;46(3):116–119.
28. Stewart S, Dalbeth N, Vandal AC, Rome K. The first metatarsophalangeal joint in gout: a systematic review and meta-analysis. *BMC Musculoskelet Disord*. 2016;17:69.
29. Sims AL, Kurup HV. Painful sesamoid of the great toe. *World J Orthop*. 2014;5(2):146–150. https://doi.org/10.5312/wjo.v5.i2.146.

24 Calcific Tendonitis Barbotage/Lavage

JASON IAN BLAICHMAN AND KENNETH S. LEE

KEY POINTS

- Calcific tendonitis, or more appropriately tendinosis, of the rotator cuff is a relatively common cause of shoulder pain. Calcifications are usually self-limiting but can also be recurrent, progressive, and debilitating.
- Calcific deposits can develop in any rotator cuff tendon, but the vast majority occur in the supraspinatus tendon, followed by the infraspinatus and the subscapularis tendons.
- Calcific tendonitis is usually the most symptomatic during the resorptive phase, when there is an acute inflammatory reaction to the calcification.
- Radiographs of the shoulder are essential to confirm the diagnosis of calcific tendonitis, exclude other potential causes of shoulder pain, and allow planning for intervention.
- Conservative treatment, including nonsteroidal antiinflammatory drugs (NSAIDs), subacromial-subdeltoid (SASD) bursa corticosteroid injections and physiotherapy, should be the first line of therapy for calcific tendonitis.
- When conservative treatment fails, ultrasound (US)-guided barbotage/lavage is a safe, quick, and effective way to provide immediate and long-term relief of symptoms.
- A SASD bursa corticosteroid injection should be performed immediately following barbotage to prevent a calcific bursitis flare up due to some retrograde passage of calcium into the bursa during the procedure.
- Although the shoulder is the most common site for calcific tendinitis, other tendons can be affected, including at the elbow, knee (quadriceps and patella), gluteal tendons, Achilles, etc. The techniques described in this chapter can be adapted and applied to other areas.

Clinically Relevant Anatomy

The rotator cuff is composed of four muscles arising from the scapula that attach to the humeral head. The supraspinatus, infraspinatus, and teres minor tendons attach to the superior, middle, and inferior facets of the greater humeral tuberosity, respectively. The subscapularis tendon attaches to the lesser humeral tuberosity.

Pathophysiology

Calcific tendonitis is the result of hydroxyapatite crystal deposition in an otherwise healthy tendon. The exact etiology remains uncertain, with several proposed theories.[1,2] The multiphasic disease model posited by Uhthoff and Loehr is one of the most accepted and divides the cycle of calcific tendonitis into three stages[2–6]:

1. **Precalcific stage:** an unknown trigger, postulated to be a decrease in oxygen tension, induces fibrocartilaginous metaplasia of tenocytes into chondrocytes with formation of intracellular calcifications. This stage is asymptomatic.
2. **Calcific stage:** this stage is further subdivided into three phases.
   - 2.1. *Formative phase:* hydroxyapatite crystals rupture into the extracellular space and coalesce, taking on a chalklike consistency.
   - 2.2. *Resting phase*: the calcific deposits are walled-off and quiescent. This phase is of variable length and usually asymptomatic, unless there is rotator cuff impingement caused by mass effect of large calcific deposits.
   - 2.3. *Resorptive phase*: an unknown trigger induces angiogenesis, inflammation, and resorption of the calcific deposit, which becomes liquefied, taking on a toothpaste-like consistency. Increased internal pressure in the deposit due to increased volume from liquefaction may cause decompression of the calcification into the subacromial-subdeltoid (SASD) bursa, inciting bursitis. This phase corresponds to the most painful and symptomatic clinical stage, often characterized by sudden onset of severe pain.
3. **Postcalcific stage:** fibroblasts migrate into the tendon defect and form a scar, with the tendon returning to a

relatively normal appearance. This stage is again usually asymptomatic.

Several of the phases may occur concurrently within a calcific deposit, and the sequence of the stages may not always be regular.[5]

Calcific tendonitis can occur in any rotator cuff tendon, but the vast majority (≈80%) of deposits are located in the supraspinatus tendon, usually in the so-called critical zone 1.5 to 2.0 cm from its insertion onto the greater tuberosity.[5] The infraspinatus tendon is involved 15% of the time, followed by the subscapularis tendon in approximately 5% of cases.[5] The teres minor tendon is rarely involved.[1,4]

Clinical Presentation and Epidemiology

Calcific tendonitis is a common disease with reported incidence rates ranging from 2.7% to 54%, accounting for 7% of cases of shoulder pain.[3,7,8] It is usually symptomatic between the ages of 40 and 60 years and is more common in women and diabetic patients.[1,2,4,5] Calcific deposits in the rotator cuff are present on radiographs in 7.5% to 20% of asymptomatic individuals and in 6.8% of symptomatic individuals.[9,10] Deposits are bilateral in 10% to 20% of patients and become symptomatic in 50% of patients.[4,7,10] Rotator cuff tears are generally not associated with calcific tendinitis.[5]

Clinical symptoms vary significantly depending on the stage and location of calcific deposits.[5] Sudden and excruciating pain often occurs during the resorptive phase.[5] Pain is usually referred to the deltoid region, and limitation in range of motion and function can clinically mimic adhesive capsulitis or a rotator cuff tear.[2,5] If the calcific deposit decompresses into the SASD bursa during the resorptive phase, the resultant crystal-induced SASD bursitis will usually dominate the clinical picture.[5] During more quiescent stages of calcific tendonitis, larger calcific deposits can cause symptoms of impingement.[5]

Imaging and Sonographic Evaluation

Given the multiple clinical presentations of calcific tendonitis, and the aforementioned overlap of symptoms with those of other shoulder pathologies, a differential diagnosis should always be considered clinically; however, calcific tendonitis can usually be readily distinguished from the other diagnostic considerations based on a combination of appropriate history, physical exam, and correlative imaging.

Confirming the clinical suspicion of calcific tendonitis requires imaging of the shoulder. Radiographs (Fig. 24.1A) can help to confirm the presence of calcific deposits.[1] Dystrophic insertional calcifications, or enthesophytes, should not be confused with calcific tendonitis. Enthesophytes are usually significantly smaller in size, linear in morphology, and located directly above, or in contact with, the greater humeral tuberosity, whereas calcific tendonitis is generally located 1 to 2 cm away from the greater humeral tuberosity with no osseous contact and is typically ovoid in morphology.[5] Further cross-sectional imaging of the shoulder with either magnetic resonance imaging (MRI) or ultrasound (US) (see Fig. 24.1B and C) is recommended to assess the integrity of the rotator cuff and exclude other possible etiologies for shoulder pain.[1]

US can also help to confirm and localize the calcifications.[1] The sonographic appearance of a calcific deposit correlates with its consistency.[5] In the formative and quiescent phases, calcific deposits have a high density of hydroxyapatite crystals, which cause strong reflection of sound waves.[5] This results in the calcific deposits appearing solid and echogenic with pronounced posterior acoustic shadowing, making them easy to delineate from the surrounding tendon.[5] As liquefaction proceeds in the resorptive phase, the calcific deposit becomes progressively less echogenic with diminished posterior shadowing.[5]

Treatment Options

Symptomatic calcific tendonitis can be highly debilitating, limiting activities of daily living and resulting in a significant economic impact due to missed work.[7,11] Calcific tendonitis is often described as a self-limiting entity, which usually resolves spontaneously[4,7,10]; however, a significant portion of patients will continue to remain symptomatic for an extended period or may experience a cyclic clinical course, with repeated episodes of acute, disabling pain and progressive loss of function.[4,10]

There is general agreement that conservative management should be the first line of treatment in the acute phase of calcific tendonitis.[4,5,7,8,11] Conservative management usually involves a combination of nonsteroidal antiinflammatory drugs (NSAIDs) and corticosteroid injections into the SASD bursa for symptom relief, and occasionally physiotherapy to prevent loss of joint mobility. Conservative therapy can be effective, but residual significant symptoms persist in approximately 30% to 50% of patients.[5] Many authors suggest a trial of conservative therapy for a period of at least 3 to 6 months; however, this could vary on an individual basis depending on the severity of pain and the patient's ability to tolerate a conservative approach.[5]

Several researchers have investigated risk factors for predicting poor outcomes from conservative management of calcific tendonitis, although results have been mixed. In general, female gender, dominant arm involvement, bilateral disease, longer duration of symptoms at presentation, and larger number of calcifications were found to be negative prognostic factors.[8] In contrast, the significance of common radiographic parameters, such as size, morphologic features (based on the Gartner classification[11]), and location of the calcific deposits, have been more inconsistent in the literature.[8,12,13]

Given the often self-limiting nature of calcific tendonitis, an ideal intervention should not only be effective at removing the culprit calcification and improving the patient's symptoms but should also be as minimally invasive and of as short a duration as possible; relatively comfortable for

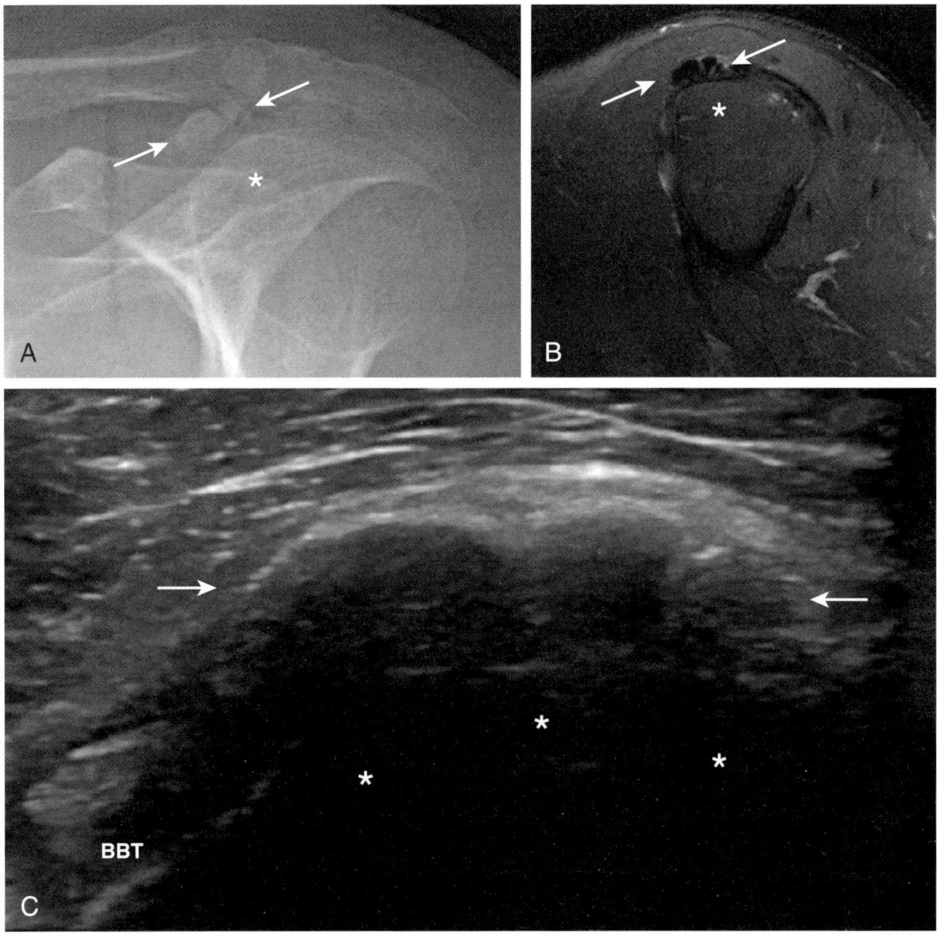

• **Fig. 24.1** Imaging of Calcific Tendonitis. A large cluster of calcifications *(white arrows)* in the supraspinatus tendon is demonstrated on (A) a transscapular radiograph, (B) a double oblique sagittal T2 fat-saturation magnetic resonance image, and (C) a transverse sonographic image. The greater tuberosity *(white asterisks)* serves as a landmark. Note the lack of surrounding edema and overlying bursitis. Large deposits can result in mild chronic pain and may cause limitations in motion due to mechanical obstruction. *BBT*, Biceps tendon.

the patient; have minimal associated complications; and be cost-effective.[1,7,14] Several treatments have been investigated and employed when conservative management of calcific tendonitis fails. Acetic acid iontophoresis is one potential treatment shown to be no more effective than physical therapy or placebo.[15] The efficacy of other treatments has been demonstrated, although they are not without their own drawbacks. They include the following procedures.

Shockwave Lithotripsy

Shockwave lithotripsy, or extracorporeal shock wave therapy (ESWT) uses shock waves to dissolve the calcifications. This treatment has been demonstrated to be effective at resolving calcific deposits and significantly improving clinical symptoms.[5,7,14] However, the utility of ESWT is limited due to several factors, including: a protracted treatment course requiring at least three sessions separated by 2 to 4 weeks, during which the patient often remains symptomatic; significant pain often experienced by patients during the procedure; and the need for specialized equipment, which increases the cost of offering this treatment.[1,7,14]

Open or Arthroscopic Surgical Excision of Calcifications

Surgical excision of calcifications can provide significant clinical improvement, but prospective randomized controlled trials are limited. Surgical resection has been shown to be more effective than ESWT in reducing pain and radiographic resolution of calcifications, but studies are inconclusive as to whether this difference is significant by 2 years post treatment.[16,17] No study has compared surgical outcomes with US-guided barbotage. Although surgery is an effective treatment for calcific tendonitis, controversy remains over the optimal surgical management, with ongoing debate regarding repairing the resultant tendon defect.[16,17] Surgery has significant potential drawbacks, including higher risk of complications such as infection, adhesive capsulitis, reflex sympathetic dystrophy, protracted recovery and rehabilitation period, and significantly increased costs.[1,7,11] For these reasons, surgery is currently considered the option of last resort, to be used only when other less-invasive methods have failed.[7]

Barbotage/Lavage

Two-needle barbotage under fluoroscopic guidance was first described by Comfort and Arafiles in 1978,[17] and Farin et al. first demonstrated the feasibility of US-guided barbotage in 1995.[18,19,20] These studies described a barbotage technique with fenestration, which involves puncturing the calcific deposit with a needle multiple times. Citing concern regarding the potential risk of tendon injury caused by fenestration, Aina et al. first described a modified US-guided single-needle technique in 2001.[28] No high-quality studies have compared the efficacy of lavage with simple fenestration, but subsequent double-needle approaches have also largely forgone fenestration.[21,22] More recent randomized controlled studies have demonstrated no significant difference in clinical outcomes up to 1 year between the single- and double-needle lavage technique, with the main difference being a slightly shorter procedure time treating denser calcifications using the double-needle technique.[23,24]

Clinical trials have generally shown significant pain relief and improvement of symptoms with US-guided barbotage both in the short term and at 1 year post treatment.[7,14,25] Barbotage also results in a statistically significant decrease in the size of calcific deposits versus conservative therapy at 1 year post treatment.[25] The self-limiting natural history of calcific tendonitis becomes more relevant during a more protracted time frame, and longer-term follow-up studies have shown that clinical outcomes of patients who were treated with barbotage are not significantly different from patients treated conservatively at 5 and 10 years post treatment.[14,26]

Equipment

- High-frequency (>10 MHz) linear US
- 18- to 20-gauge 1.5-inch needle for lavage
- 25-gauge 1.5-inch needle for initial anesthetic
- Optional: 30-gauge 0.5-inch needle for initial skin anesthetic
- 10-mL syringes with 50:50 mixture of anesthetic and bacteriostatic sterile saline for lavage
- 10-mL syringe for initial anesthetic
- 5-mL syringe for corticosteroid

Common Injectates

- *Anesthetic: 1% lidocaine for barbotage, 0.5% ropivacaine for SASD bursa injection*
- *For SASD bursa injection: corticosteroid (40 mg triamcinolone acetonide or methylprednisolone acetate) and local anesthetic*

  Author's Preferred Technique:
- Both single- and double-needle techniques have been described. We use the single-needle technique at our institution (Fig. 24.2), which is described in detail later, followed by a SASD bursa corticosteroid injection.[27] The double-needle technique is subsequently described for completeness.[22,23]

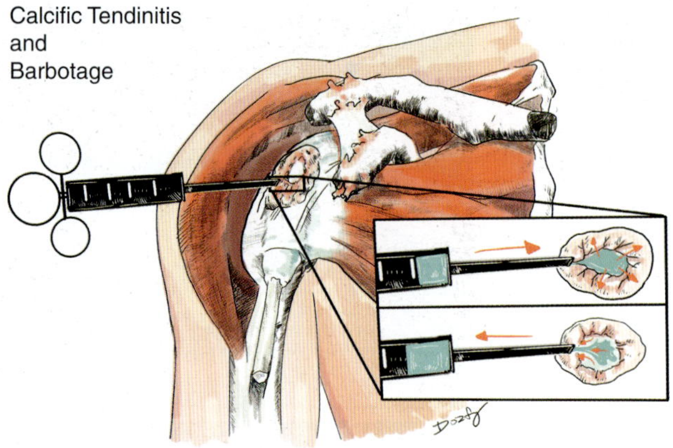

• **Fig. 24.2** Barbotage Technique. Under ultrasound guidance, the 18-gauge needle is advanced into the calcific deposit along the axis of the tendon fibers, and directed cranially to allow gravity to assist with aspiration of the calcific debris. *(Inset, top)* Once the needle tip is positioned within the calcific deposit, continuous small pumps of the syringe plumber are applied, causing breakdown of the calcification due to dissolution and pressure waves from the injected fluid. *(Inset, bottom)* Between each pump, the buildup of backpressure pushes fluid and calcific debris back into the syringe without the operator needing to actively aspirate. It is important to avoid fenestrating the calcific deposit because doing so might allow the injected fluid to decompress through the resultant holes and prevent backpressure from building up.

- The single-needle technique relies on the buildup of backpressure within the calcific deposit to dissolve and carry calcific debris in a retrograde fashion back into the syringe.
- The double-needle technique creates a lavage circuit, with one needle used to push fluid into the calcific deposit to dissolve it and the second needle serving as an outflow tract for the injected fluid and calcific debris to egress. This technique generally uses larger, 16-gauge needles.

Patient Position

- The patient is placed in a semireclined supine position.
- The ipsilateral arm is ideally placed behind the patient's back with palm toward the stretcher, which results in anterior rotation of the greater tuberosity of the humeral head along with the distal supraspinatus tendon, uncovering it from the overlying acromion.
- If the calcification is located in a different tendon, slight alterations in patient positioning may be necessary. The goal is to be able to visualize the entire calcification under US.

Clinician Position

- The clinician is positioned in a comfortable standing or seated fashion adjacent to the targeted shoulder.

Transducer Position

- The US transducer is positioned over the site of calcific tendonitis and oriented along the long axis of the rotator cuff fibers.

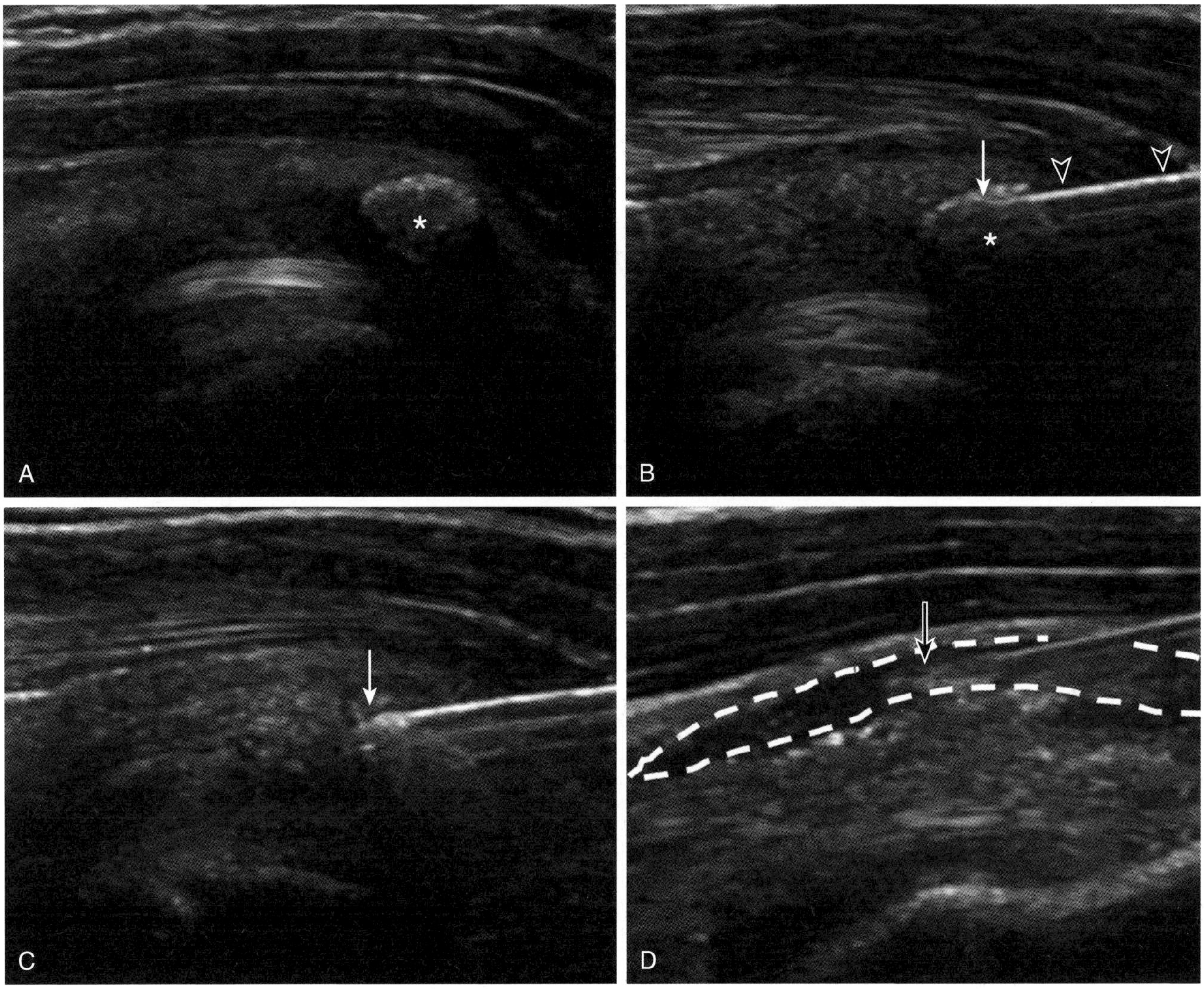

• **Fig. 24.3** Ultrasound-Guided Barbotage Example. (A) A calcific deposit *(white asterisk)* is identified in the anterior supraspinatus tendon. (B) An 18-gauge needle *(black arrowheads)* has been advanced into the calcification in a single pass with the needle tip *(white arrow)* located in the center of the deposit *(white asterisk)*. (C) Following barbotage *(white arrow)*, the calcification has essentially completely resolved and is no longer seen. (D) The needle is pulled back slightly and repositioned so that its tip *(black arrow)* is located in the subacromial bursa. A mixture of corticosteroid and local anesthetic is then injected into the bursa, which will become mildly distended *(white dashed line)*.

Single-Needle Technique

Needle Position

- After local anesthetic is administered, the 18-gauge needle should be advanced in plane with the US probe, and along the long axis of the rotator cuff tendon fibers, to minimize potential injury to the tendon.

Target

- The largest calcific deposit should be targeted first with the goal of advancing the needle tip into the center of the deposit in a single pass without interruption of the medial wall or fenestration of the calcification (Fig. 24.3A and B).
- Maintaining integrity of the wall of the deposit is key to ensure buildup of backpressure within the calcification, which is essential for barbotage. Fenestration will allow the injectate to decompress through the resultant holes in the deposit.

Lavage

- Once the 18-gauge needle is positioned with its tip in the calcific deposit, the first syringe containing a 50:50 mixture of local anesthetic and saline is connected directly to the needle, and the syringe is oriented with the needle tip directed cranially, to allow gravity to assist with calcium aspiration (see Fig. 24.2).
- At this point, the clinician begins applying repeated intermittent small pumps on the syringe plunger, lavaging the center of the calcification with small volumes of injectate, which causes breakdown of the calcification

from the inside due to dissolution and pressure waves (see Fig. 24.2, *inset top*).

- Between each pump, the buildup of backpressure pushes fluid and calcific debris back into the syringe without requiring active aspiration from the operator (see Fig. 24.2, *inset bottom*).
- The clinician should periodically check the syringe for calcific debris and switch to the next prepared syringe if there is significant buildup of calcium debris within.
- This process is continued until as much calcium as possible is removed and the syringe remains relatively clear (see Fig. 24.3C).
- If there are multiple significant deposits, the needle should be repositioned and the process should be repeated. US evaluation of the deposits during lavage is helpful to ensure all areas of the deposits are being treated.
- Once all of the calcium deposits have been treated, the needle tip is pulled back and repositioned in the SASD bursa, and the syringe containing the corticosteroid mixture is attached and injected into the bursa (see Fig. 24.3D).
- The average needle-in to needle-out time is approximately 10 minutes.

Double-Needle Technique

Needle Position

- After anesthetic is administered, two 16-gauge needles are advanced in plane with the US probe, and along the long axis of the rotator cuff tendon fibers, to minimize potential injury to the tendon.

Target

- The largest calcific deposit should be targeted first. The first needle is inserted into the lower portion of the calcium deposit with the bevel turned upward to face the probe.[22,23] The second needle is then inserted parallel and superficial to the first needle with the bevel turned downward, so that both needle bevels face one another.[22,23] Ideally the needle tips should be located within 2 to 3 mm of each other.[22,23]

Lavage

- Once the 16-gauge needles are positioned with tips in the calcific deposit, a syringe containing a 50:50 mixture of anesthetic and saline is connected directly to one of the needles.
- At this point, the clinician begins applying repeated intermittent small pumps on the syringe plunger, lavaging the center of the calcification with small volumes of injectate, which causes breakdown of the calcification from the inside due to dissolution and pressure waves.
- As the calcification dissolves, the injectate and calcium debris will egress from the deposit via the free needle.
- This process is continued until as much calcium as possible is removed and the fluid draining out of the free needle becomes relatively clear.
- If there is difficulty dissolving dense calcifications, the needles can be gently rotated and laterally displaced while still inside the calcification to increase fragmentation.[22]
- Once all of the calcium deposits have been treated, the free needle is removed and the other needle tip is pulled back and repositioned in the SASD bursa, and the syringe containing the corticosteroid mixture is attached and injected into the bursa.

Complications

Barbotage is generally very well tolerated with most studies reporting minimal immediate complications, usually consisting of mild vasovagal reactions.[7,14] Transient worsening of symptoms may occur in the 48 hours following the procedure due to SASD bursitis.[7] Frozen shoulder and septic bursitis have also been documented, although they are uncommon.[14,28] Temporary recurrence of symptoms approximately 15 weeks after treatment has been described in at least one study but was found to be generally less intense than prebarbotage symptoms and controlled adequately with NSAIDs.[7]

Postprocedure Care and Follow-Up

The patient should be advised to rest the shoulder for 48 hours following the procedure and to avoid heavy lifting for 2 weeks. NSAIDs medication can be used for pain relief as needed and physiotherapy can be resumed after 1 week. Patients should also be warned that their symptoms may become worse for the first few days until the corticosteroid injection takes effect. Follow-up shoulder radiographs can be obtained several weeks following the procedure to ensure a decreased burden of rotator cuff calcification.

PEARLS AND PITFALLS

- It is not necessary to remove all of the calcification, as lavage often incites a reaction by the body that usually leads to removal of most, if not all, of the residual calcifications.[1]
- If the needle becomes blocked, first try switching the syringe. If this fails to resolve the blockage, a smaller-gauge needle can be threaded through the 18-gauge needle to attempt to unblock it. If this also fails, switching to a new needle may be necessary, but this is uncommon.
- If the calcification is too firm to break up with lavage, fenestration can be used as a last-ditch effort. Although this precludes aspiration of debris, the mechanical disruption of the calcific deposit will usually elicit a reaction from the body that will result in resorption of at least some of the calcium.
- Barbotage leading to a tendon tear is a theoretical risk but is very uncommon when proper technique is use, including ensuring a needle approach along the long axis of the tendon.
- Barbotage should be followed immediately by a subacromial-subdeltoid (SASD) bursa injection, as the procedure itself, and release of some of the calcific debris into the bursa during the procedure, will likely irritate the bursa.

References

1. Saboeiro GR. Sonography in the treatment of calcific tendinitis of the rotator cuff. *J Ultrasound Med*. 2012;31(10):1513–1518.
2. De Carli A, Pulcinelli F, Rose GD, Pitino D, Ferretti A. Calcific tendinitis of the shoulder. *Joints*. 2014;2(3):130–136.
3. Kachewar SG, Kulkarni DS. Calcific tendinitis of the rotator cuff: a review. *J Clin Diagn Res*. 2013;7(7):1482–1485.
4. Merolla G, Singh S, Paladini P, Porcellini G. Calcific tendinitis of the rotator cuff: state of the art in diagnosis and treatment. *J Orthop Traumatol*. 2016;17(1):7–14.
5. Diehl P, Gerdesmeyer L, Gollwitzer H, Sauer W, Tischer T. Calcific tendinitis of the shoulder. *Orthopä*. 2011;40(8):733–746.
6. Uhthoff HK, Loehr JW. Calcific tendinopathy of the rotator cuff: pathogenesis, diagnosis, and management. *J Am Acad Orthop Surg*. 1997;5(4):183–191.
7. Del Cura JL, Torre I, Zabala R, Legorburu A. Sonographically guided percutaneous needle lavage in calcific tendinitis of the shoulder: short- and long-term results. *AJR Am J Roentgenol*. 2007;189(3):W128–W134.
8. De Witte PB, van Adrichem RA, Selten JW, Nagels J, Reijnierse M, Nelissen RGHH. Radiological and clinical predictors of long-term outcome in rotator cuff calcific tendinitis. *Eur Radiol*. 2016;26(10):3401–3411.
9. Burke CJ, Adler RS. Ultrasound-guided percutaneous tendon treatments. *AJR Am J Roentgenol*. 2016;207(3):495–506.
10. Lin JT, Adler RS, Bracilovic A, Cooper G, Sofka C, Lutz GE. Clinical outcomes of ultrasound-guided aspiration and lavage in calcific tendinosis of the shoulder. *HSS J*. 2007;3(1):99–105.
11. Gartner J, Heyer A. Calcific tendinitis of the shoulder. *Orthopä*. 1995;24(3):284–302.
12. Ogon P, Suedkamp NP, Jager M, Izadpanah K, Koestler W, Maier D. Prognostic factors in nonoperative therapy for chronic symptomatic calcific tendinitis of the shoulder. *Arthritis Rheum*. 2009;60(10):2978–2984.
13. Serafini G, Sconfienza LM, Lacelli F, Silvestri E, Aliprandi A, Sardanelli F. Rotator cuff calcific tendonitis: short-term and 10-year outcomes after two-needle US-guided percutaneous treatment--nonrandomized controlled trial. *Radiology*. 2009;252(1):157–164.
14. Leduc BE, Caya J, Tremblay S, Bureau NJ, Dumont M. Treatment of calcifying tendinitis of the shoulder by acetic acid iontophoresis: a double-blind randomized controlled trial. *Arch Phys Med Rehabil*. 2003;84(10):1523–1527.
15. Rompe JD, Zoellner J, Nafe B. Shock wave therapy versus conventional surgery in the treatment of calcifying tendinitis of the shoulder. *Clin Orthop Relat Res*. 2001;(387):72–82.
16. Rebuzzi E, Coletti N, Schiavetti S, Giusto F. Arthroscopy surgery versus shock wave therapy for chronic calcifying tendinitis of the shoulder. *J Orthop Traumatol*. 2008;9(4):179–185.
17. Comfort TH, Arafiles R. Barbotage of the shoulder with image-intensified fluoroscopic control of needle placement for calcific tendinosis. *Clin Orthop Relat Res*. 1978;135:171–178.
18. Farin PU, Jaroma H, Soimakallio S. Rotator cuff calcifications: treatment with US-guided technique. *Radiology*. 1995;195(3):841–843.
19. Farin PU, Rasanen H, Jaroma H, Harju A. Rotator cuff calcifications: treatment with ultrasound-guided percutaneous needle aspiration and lavage. *Skeletal Radiol*. 1996;25(6):551–554.
20. Vignesh KN, McDowall A, Simunovic N, Bhandari M, Choudur HN. Efficacy of ultrasound-guided percutaneous needle treatment of calcific tendinitis. *AJR Am J Roentgenol*. 2015;204(1):148–152.
21. Sconfienza LM, Vigano S, Martini C, et al. Double-needle ultrasound guided percutaneous treatment of rotator cuff calcific tendinitis: tips & tricks. *Skeletal Radiol*. 2013;42(1):19–24.
22. Ferrero G, Fabbro E, Orlandi D, et al. Ultrasound-guided percutaneous treatment of rotator cuff calcific tendinitis: randomized comparison between one- and two-needle procedure. Presented at European Congress of Radiology, Vienna, 2014.
23. Orlandi D, Mauri G, Lacelli F, et al. Rotator cuff calcific tendinopathy: randomized comparison of US-guided percutaneous treatments by one or two needles. *Radiology*. 2017;285(2):518–527.
24. De Witte PB, Selten JW, Navas A, et al. Calcific tendinitis of the rotator cuff: a randomized controlled trial of ultrasound-guided needling and lavage versus subacromial corticosteroids. *Am J Sports Med*. 2013;41(7):1665–1673.
25. De Witte PB, Kolk A, Overes F, Nelissen RGHH, Reijnierse M. Rotator cuff calcific tendinitis: ultrasound-guided needling and lavage versus subacromial corticosteroids: five-year outcomes of a randomized controlled trial. *Am J Sports Med*. 2017;45(14):3305–3314.
26. Lee KS, Rosas HG. Musculoskeletal ultrasound: how to treat calcific tendinitis of the rotator cuff by ultrasound-guided single-needle lavage technique. *AJR Am J Roentgenol*. 2010;195(3):638.
27. Oudelaar BW, Schepers-Bok R, Ooms EM, Huis In `t Veld R, Vochteloo AJ. Needle aspiration of calcific deposits (NACD) for calcific tendinitis is safe and effective: six months follow-up of clinical results and complications in a series of 431 patients. *Eur Radiol*. 2016;85(4):689–694.
28. Aina R, Cardinal E, Bureau NJ, Aubin B, Brassard P. Calcific shoulder tendinitis: treatment with modified US-guided fine-needle technique. *Radiology*. 2001;221(2):455–461.

25

High-Volume Ultrasound-Guided Capsular Distention for Adhesive Capsulitis

ALYSSA NEPH SPECIALE AND BRIAN DAVIS

KEY POINTS

- Adhesive capsulitis occurs due to thickening and fibrosis of the coracohumeral ligament (CHL), glenohumeral ligament, rotator interval (RI), and axillary joint recess.
- The condition is more common in middle-aged females with a history of diabetes mellitus but is also linked to collagen vascular disease, thyroid disease, rheumatologic disorders, trauma, and surgery.[1–3]
- Course is reportedly self-limiting but may persist for up to 18 to 24 months or longer.[4–6]
- If conservative measures fail, hydrodistention may be considered as a treatment option. Hydrodistention has been found to be superior to manipulation under anesthesia (MUA) in one study[7] and superior during earlier stages of disease and treatment course.[8]
- Recommend using high-volume saline and anesthetic rather than corticosteroid for distention due to risk of chondrotoxicity, hyperglycemia in diabetes mellitus, labile hypertension, and lack of superior benefit with addition of steroids.
- Use a 20- to 25-gauge 3.5-inch or 10-cm needle for an out-of-plane approach to the glenohumeral joint (GHJ) during injection (authors' preferred method due to decreased tissue disruption).
- Perform preprocedure and postprocedure shoulder joint range of motion testing.
- Perform proprioceptive neuromuscular facilitation (PNF) and active release therapy (ART) immediately following the procedure and start physical therapy (PT) within 2 to 4 hours after procedure for maximal sustained benefit of capsular distention.

Anatomy

The glenohumeral joint (GHJ) is a diarthrodal joint, stabilized by the capsule, glenohumeral and coracohumeral ligaments (CHLs), glenoid labrum, and rotator cuff musculature. The rotator interval (RI) is a tendinous triangular gap covered exclusively by capsular tissue. It is bordered by the supraspinatus tendon superiorly, subscapularis tendon inferiorly, and coracoid process medially. The RI contains the long head of the biceps tendon. The joint capsule is reinforced by the CHL and superior glenohumeral ligament (SGHL) in this location, forming the "biceps pulley."[9] The RI contributes to stabilization of the joint and the biceps tendon. The inferior portion of the GHJ capsule is termed the "axillary recess" and lies between the anterior and posterior bands of the inferior glenohumeral ligament (IGHL) (Fig. 25.1A).[10]

Common Pathology

Adhesive capsulitis (AC), or "frozen shoulder," can be a debilitating condition, affecting 2% to 5% of the population, middle-aged females more than males. Risk factors include diabetes mellitus (13.4% prevalence of AC),[2] thyroid disease, rheumatologic disorders, collagen vascular disease, and Parkinson disease.[1–3] Secondary AC often results from surgery or trauma. The course of AC is typically self-limiting but may persist upward of 18 to 24 months or longer for full resolution through the three characteristic phases: freezing stage, frozen stage, and thawing phase.[4–6] In addition, it has been suggested that there is a higher incidence of contralateral AC in the future in younger patients (<50 years old) and those with diabetes.[11]

Arthroscopic findings in AC include replacement of the subscapularis recess with scar tissue, tightened axillary recess, reduced joint fluid volume, and contracture of RI and CHL. Histopathologic appearance demonstrates tissue similar to that found in Dupuytren contracture, consisting of dense type III collagen, fibroblasts, contractile myofibroblasts, and neovascularization.[12] Clinically, external rotation is typically affected first and progresses to include limitations in flexion, abduction, and internal rotation.

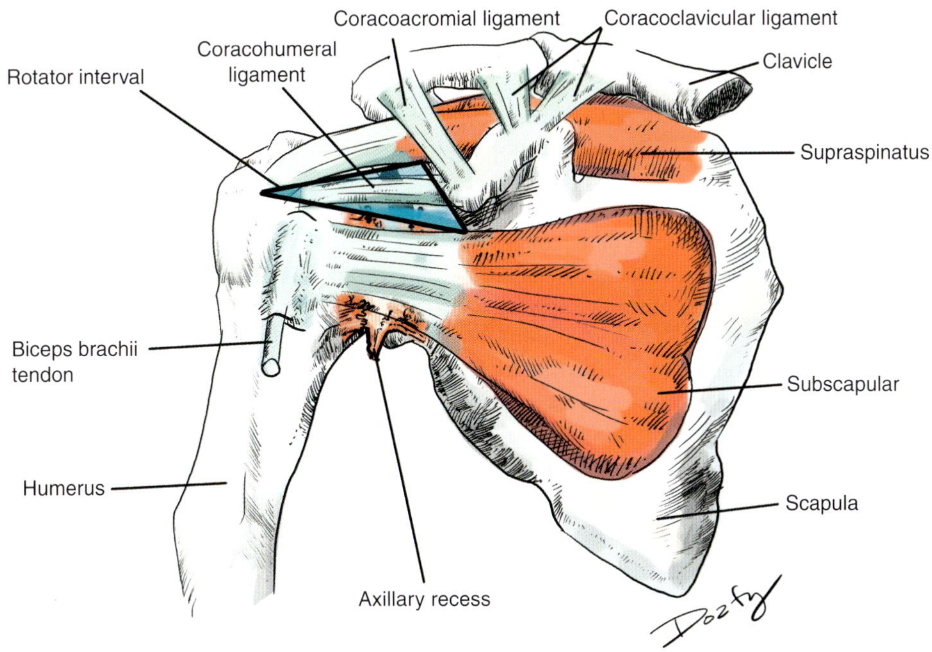

• **Fig. 25.1** Normal shoulder anatomy demonstrating glenohumeral and coracohumeral ligaments, and the rotator interval with the long head of the biceps tendon.

Imaging

Magnetic resonance imaging (MRI) or ultrasound (US) imaging is preferred over x-ray to rule out significant rotator cuff tear or other pathology prior to interventional treatment. MRI and MR arthrography (MRA) can demonstrate thickening of the CHL, thickening and reduction in the size of the axillary recess or RI, and obliteration of the subcoracoid fat triangle.[13] Similar pathologic thickening may be seen on US (higher sensitivity with US arthrography than US alone) as well as hypoechoic soft tissue and hypervascular synovium on power Doppler within the RI.[14,15]

Treatment Options

Typically, the first-line treatment for AC is physical therapy (PT), including strengthening, stretching, mobilization, US, and medications such as nonsteroidal antiinflammatory drugs (NSAIDs) or oral steroids.[16,17] The authors recommend pursuing injection therapy after at least 6 weeks of conservative measures and advanced imaging. Although hydrodistention has shown improved efficacy in the earlier stages of treatment, it may not be approved by insurance prior to a course of conservative treatment.[8] RI, subacromial, and intra-articular steroid injections can also be performed.[18,19] There is no proven difference in outcome after subacromial versus intra-articular injection.[18,20]

Capsular hydrodistention under pressure has long been regarded as an effective treatment option to rapidly improve range of motion (ROM) in AC by stretching or rupturing the contracted joint capsule.[21] There is no consensus on the inclusion of corticosteroid within the injectate. In some studies, hydrodilation with cortisone has been shown to have better outcomes in pain and ROM compared with intra-articular or subacromial steroid injections or hydrodilation alone.[22] However, the study that found dilation to be inferior to intra-articular corticosteroid only used a volume of 9 mL for dilation, which is inadequate to cause capsular distention.[23–25] Although the use of corticosteroid may aid in reducing inflammation due to capsular stretch during hydrodistention and reduce risk of recontracture of the capsule,[22,26] the authors have had very successful results with use of anesthetic and saline alone and prefer to avoid the chondrotoxic effects of steroid when possible.[27,28] In addition, avoiding steroid is essential in the setting of poorly controlled diabetics, labile hypertension, and steroid sensitivity. Dilation of the joint capsule with the goal of capsular rupture is controversial because there is no evidence that rupture is required for desired outcome. Some studies have even shown that capsular preservation may actually result in increased ROM and decreased pain in the short term.[29,30] The volume used for hydrodilation has widely ranged from 10 to 90 mL, most commonly in the 25- to 50-mL range.[7,22,25,31–33] The authors recommend avoiding intentional capsular rupture by monitoring for backflow of injectate in the syringe and patient's tolerance to pressure during injection. Another described hydrodilation approach is via the rotator cuff interval. One study by Yoong et al. showed good results in the treatment of AC with rotator cuff interval hydrodilation with 21 mL of combination of local anesthetic and steroid; however, the authors have not had clinic experience with this technique.[34] Orthobiologic treatments such as platelet-rich plasma (PRP), platelet lysate, and platelet-poor plasma (PPP) can also be considered as dilation solutions due to antiinflammatory and chrondroprotective cytokines, and one study showed that intra-articular PRP injection had better results for AC compared with steroid injection.[35,36] Although there is a paucity of data for use in AC, the editors have had good success using platelet lysate and PPP to replace saline for dilation solution in practice.

Another option if conservative measures fail is manipulation under anesthesia (MUA), which has been found to be inferior to hydrodistention in regards to pain and ROM in one study.[7,37] MUA should be avoided in elderly osteoporotic patients due to the risk of fracture. If MUA fails, arthroscopic capsular release of the CHL, anterior capsule, and subscapularis bursa can be pursued.[38] This technique may be challenging with tighter capsular contracture due to difficulty inserting the arthroscope.[39] Although arthroscopic capsular release has been shown to have slightly better outcomes than hydrodistention, both arthroscopy and MUA require general anesthesia, increasing the risk of adverse outcomes in certain populations.

Indications for High-Volume Ultrasound-Guided Injection for Adhesive Capsulitis

Patient Selection

Candidates for capsular hydrodistention or high-volume ultrasound-guided injection (HVUGI) are those with AC who fail at least 6 weeks of conservative PT, modalities, and medication management, unless conservative measures are contraindicated or there are severe functional limitations. Hydrodistention has been found to have improved efficacy in the early stages[8] and in those with less severe limitations in ROM at the time of procedure ("freezing" rather than "frozen" stage) but may not be approved by insurance prior to a trial of conservative treatment.[40] Long-term outcomes with HVUGI may be less favorable in diabetic patients.[41]

Authors' preferred diagnostic criteria for AC include greater than 25% reduction of passive ROM in two or more of the four cardinal shoulder motions (internal rotation, external rotation, abduction, and extension) without another explanation for the loss of motion, such as GHJ osteoarthritis or impingement. Preprocedurally, we test and record the degree of shoulder motion in abduction, external rotation, internal rotation, and extension, as well as the Apley scratch test. We perform GHJ ROM testing with the scapula fixed and shoulder in 90 degrees of abduction (or at end range if patient cannot achieve 90 degrees) and elbow in 90 degrees of flexion. Normal ROM in this position is at least 45 degrees of internal rotation, 90 degrees of external rotation, 90 to 110 degrees of abduction (isolated GHJ), and 45 to 60 degrees of extension.[42]

Equipment

- Musculoskeletal US machine with a high-frequency linear or curvilinear array transducer (10 to 18 MHz preferred)
- Sterile probe cover and sterile US gel (entirely sterile procedure recommended)
- Sterile gloves
- ChloraPrep cleansing solution sticks × 2
- Two extension tubing sets
- Syringes: 10 mL, 20 mL, 60 mL
- Needles: 18-gauge 1.5-inch needle (to draw medications); 25-gauge 1.5-inch needle (for local anesthesia); 20- to 25-gauge 3.5-inch or 20-gauge 10-cm Chiba (Cook Medical, Bloomington, IN) or 2- to 3.5 inch spinal needle (for injectate)
- Injectate:
  - Up to 12 mL of local anesthetic for the skin and extra-articular soft tissue such as 1% lidocaine without epinephrine.
  - 10 mL of preferred intra-articular anesthetic
    - Recommend use of ropivacaine 0.5% over bupivacaine and especially lidocaine due to risk of chondrotoxicity with intra-articular injection.[43]
  - 50 mL of preservative-free 0.9% normal saline solution or preferred dilation solution (connected to tubing and primed, Fig. 25.2B)[24]
  - Option to use platelet lysate, PRP, and/or PPP as part of dilation solution.

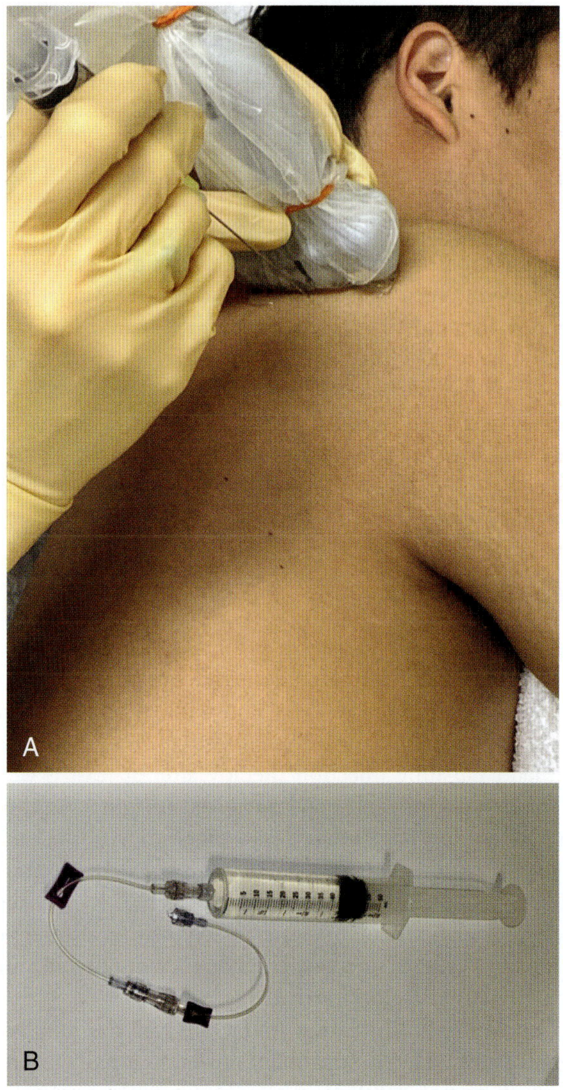

• **Fig. 25.2** (A) Patient position, transducer position, and needle position for the out-of-plane approach for glenohumeral capsular distention. (B) Setup of intravenous tubing connected end to end and attached to 60-mL syringe to allow for easier injection of saline under pressure.

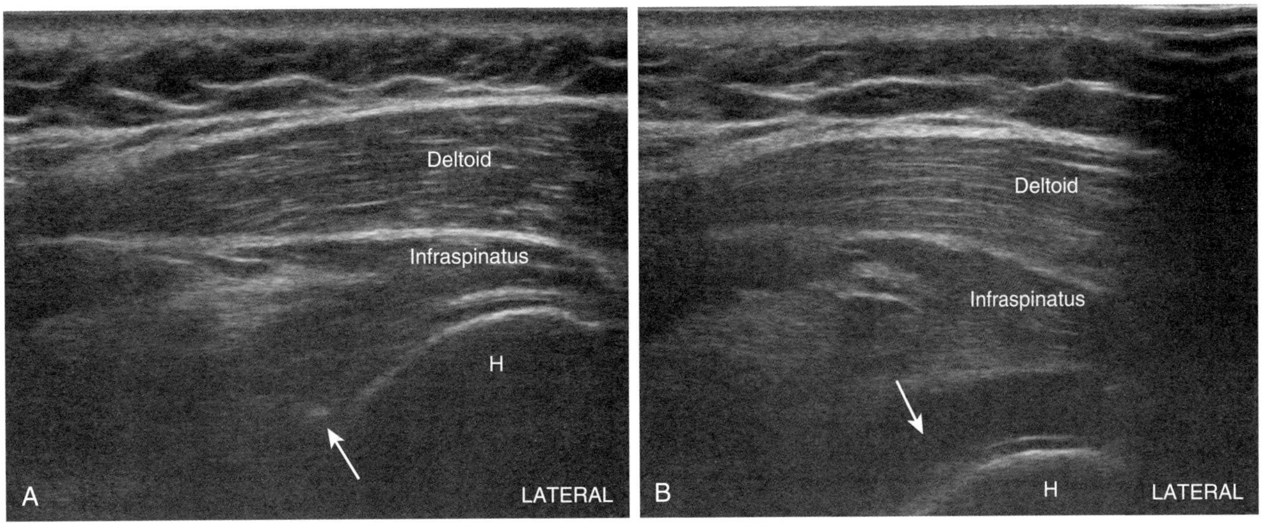

• **Fig. 25.3** (A) Out-of-plane injection approach from distal to proximal. *White arrow* shows needle tip. (B) Distended joint recess as shown by *white arrow* after saline distention. *H,* Humerus.

Author's Preferred Technique

Patient Position

- Lateral recumbent with affected side up.
- Arm bent at patient's side; may have bolster under arm for comfort.
- Prep entire forequarter region of posterior and anterior shoulder with two ChloraPrep cleansing solution sticks, and apply sterile probe cover and gel to transducer.

Clinician Position

- Sitting or standing behind patient with US machine in visual line, across from clinician.

Transducer Orientation

- Over the posterior aspect of the GHJ, parallel with infraspinatus fibers (see Fig. 25.2A).

Needle Orientation and Technique

- Procedure can be performed with the needle out of plane (Fig. 25.3A) or in plane (Fig. 25.4) to the transducer.
- Suprascapular or interscalene nerve block prior to the procedure may be considered for anesthesia. Oral anxiolytics may be considered in some patients, but intravenous (IV) anxiolytics or narcotics are typically not required or recommended due to increased risk of adverse effects and necessity for monitoring. In the current opioid crisis, judicious use of postprocedure narcotics is optional.
- Skin wheal and local anesthesia with 1% lidocaine using 25-gauge 1.5- to 2-inch needle, walking down toward the humeral head and glenoid labrum.
- Monitor for nearby vascular structures to avoid intravascular injection.
- HVUGI performed with 20- to 25-gauge, 2- to 3.5-inch spinal needle or 10-cm Chiba needle. Insert needle along same trajectory, anesthetizing deeper tissues and extracapsular area with local anesthetic. Then penetrate the capsule.

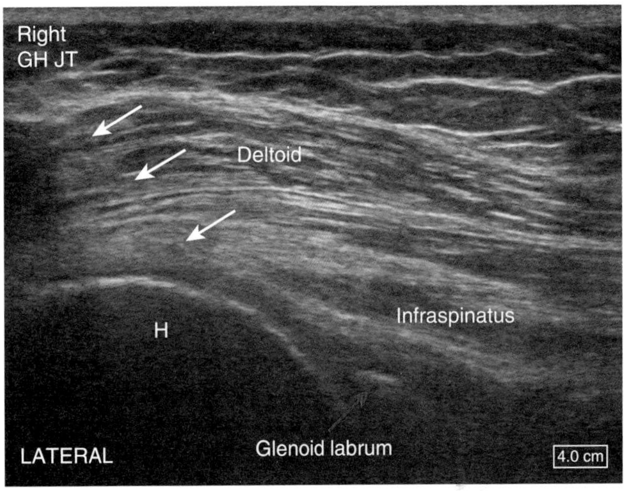

• **Fig. 25.4** In-plane injection approach from lateral to medial. *White arrow* shows shaft of the needle entering posterior capsule and joint recess. *H,* Humerus. *GH JT,* Glenohumeral Joint.

- Leave the needle in place, switch the syringe, and inject 10 mL preferred anesthetic into the joint, ensuring adequate capsular distention (see Fig. 25.3A and B).
- Leave the needle in place and then attach IV tubing (see Fig. 25.2B) primed and connected to a 50-mL syringe of dilating solution (tubing allows for easier injection under pressure).
- Slowly inject dilation solution, monitoring the patient's comfort and ensuring that the joint capsule continues to expand. Small aliquots and occasional release of pressure is preferred to maintain patient comfort.
- Inject volume until there is backflow of injectate in the syringe, extracapsular leak of fluid, or the patient in unable to tolerate the pressure any longer. In the authors' experience, total injectate volume can range from 20 to 70 mL with the most common volume between 35 and 50 mL.

- Wrap sterile gauze around the base of needle and remove needle while applying pressure to site of entry. Apply bandage.

Postprocedure Protocol

The physician should perform 5 to 10 minutes of proprioceptive neuromuscular facilitation (PNF) and active release therapy (ART) along with passive stretching and deep breathing following the procedure once the local anesthetic has taken effect. All cardinal movements should be addressed to stretch out the capsular fibers. Retest and record the ROM after PNF or ART in abduction, external rotation, internal rotation, extension, and the Apley scratch test for comparison with pretest values. These can also be compared with posttherapy values. Recommend scheduling a PT session within 2 to 4 hours after the procedure for additional stretching and to maintain beneficial capsular stretch from distention.[44] Instruct patient in use of shoulder pulley exercises 4 to 5 times daily after procedure.

Postprocedure Complications

Although rare, complications can include bleeding, infection, temporary muscle weakness, paresthesia, and capsular rupture. Transient muscle weakness may occur due to anesthetization of a branch of the suprascapular nerve, leading to temporary external rotation weakness. Weakness will be more severe if direct suprascapular or interscalene nerve block is performed. If a proper stretching program is not performed post procedure, stiffness may worsen or persist due to inflammatory effect of capsular distention and disease process. Most commonly, patients may have sensation of fullness or aching due to volume of injectate, but this should dissipate over the course of a few hours to days. Postprocedure fullness in the chest wall may be more prominent with capsular rupture.

PEARLS AND PITFALLS

- Can consider performing a suprascapular or interscalene nerve block prior to distention to improve patient comfort during the procedure, although many patients can tolerate the procedure with local anesthetization and anesthetization of the glenohumeral joint. Give adequate time (10 to 15 minutes) to allow the intra-articular anesthetic to take effect before performing postprocedural stretching.
- For the in-plane approach, the needle bevel should be facing the articular surface of the humerus to avoid damaging the cartilage surface.
- Solution should be visualized expanding the joint capsule/space. If expansion is not seen or fluid is seen accumulating in one place, reposition the needle tip to insure intra-articular placement. Power Doppler can be used to confirm intra-articular injection. May assess anterior shoulder with ultrasound for fluid accumulation; hence need for anterior shoulder sterilization.
- Take short breaks during infusion of the saline under pressure to improve patient comfort.
- If you feel sudden loss of resistance during saline injection, the capsule may have ruptured. Fluid will be observed extracapsular, and additional injection of dilation solution is likely unnecessary.
- Remember to provide proprioceptive neuromuscular facilitation, active release therapy, and passive stretch post procedure (once anesthetic has taken full effect) and start physical therapy within 2 to 4 hours to reduce loss of beneficial capsular stretch secondary to the distention.
- Commonly, during the postprocedural stretching, the provider will feel or hear "pops" that indicate breaking of adhesions followed by immediate improvement in range of motion.
- Performing shoulder pulley exercises and self-stretching is critical for successful outcome.

References

1. Milgrom C, Novack V, Weil Y, Jaber S, Radeva-Petrova DR, Finestone A. Risk factors for idiopathic frozen shoulder. *Isr Med Assoc J*. 2008;10:361–364.
2. Zreik NH, Malik RA, Charalambous CP. Adhesive capsulitis of the shoulder and diabetes: a meta-analysis of prevalence. *Muscles Ligaments Tendons J*. 2016;6:26–34.
3. Dias R, Cutts S, Massoud S. Frozen shoulder. *BMJ*. 2005;331:1453–1456.
4. Reeves B. The natural history of the frozen shoulder syndrome. *Scand J Rheumatol*. 1975;4:193–196.
5. Vastamaki H, Kettunen J, Vastamaki M. The natural history of idiopathic frozen shoulder: a 2- to 27-year followup study. *Clin Orthop Relat Res*. 2012;470:1133–1143.
6. Diercks RL, Stevens M. Gentle thawing of the frozen shoulder: a prospective study of supervised neglect versus intensive physical therapy in seventy-seven patients with frozen shoulder syndrome followed up for two years. *J Shoulder Elbow Surg*. 2004;13:499–502.
7. Quraishi NA, Johnston P, Bayer J, Crowe M, Chakrabarti AJ. Thawing the frozen shoulder. A randomised trial comparing manipulation under anaesthesia with hydrodilatation. *J Bone Joint Surg Br*. 2007;89:1197–1200.
8. Lin MT, Hsiao MY, Tu YK, Wang TG. Comparative efficacy of intra-articular steroid injection and distension in patients with frozen shoulder: a systematic review and network meta-analysis. *Arch Phys Med Rehabil*. 2018;99:1383–1394.e1386.
9. Woertler K. Rotator interval. *Semin Musculoskelet Radiol*. 2015;19:243–253.
10. Fields BKK, Skalski MR, Patel DB, et al. Adhesive capsulitis: review of imaging findings, pathophysiology, clinical presentation, and treatment options. *Skeletal Radiol*. 2019;48:1171–1184.
11. Lamplot JD, Lillegraven O, Brophy RH. Outcomes from conservative treatment of shoulder idiopathic adhesive capsulitis and factors associated with developing contralateral disease. *Orthop J Sports Med*. 2018;6:2325967118785169.
12. Bunker TD. Frozen shoulder: unravelling the enigma. *Ann R Coll Surg Engl*. 1997;79:210–213.
13. Sofka CM, Ciavarra GA, Hannafin JA, Cordasco FA, Potter HG. Magnetic resonance imaging of adhesive capsulitis: correlation with clinical staging. *HSS J*. 2008;4:164–169.
14. Cheng X, Zhang Z, Xuanyan G, et al. Adhesive capsulitis of the shoulder: evaluation with US-arthrography using a sonographic contrast agent. *Sci Rep*. 2017;7:5551.

15. Lee JC, Sykes C, Saifuddin A, Connell D. Adhesive capsulitis: sonographic changes in the rotator cuff interval with arthroscopic correlation. *Skeletal Radiol.* 2005;34:522–527.
16. Levine WN, Kashyap CP, Bak SF, Ahmad CS, Blaine TA, LU B. Nonoperative management of idiopathic adhesive capsulitis. *J Shoulder Elbow Surg.* 2007;16:569–573.
17. Buchbinder R, Hoving JL, Green S, Hall S, Forbes A, Nash P. Short course prednisolone for adhesive capsulitis (frozen shoulder or stiff painful shoulder): a randomised, double blind, placebo controlled trial. *Ann Rheum Dis.* 2004;63:1460–1469.
18. Oh JH, Oh CH, Choi JA, Kim SH, Kim JH, Yoon JP. Comparison of glenohumeral and subacromial steroid injection in primary frozen shoulder: a prospective, randomized short-term comparison study. *J Shoulder Elbow Surg.* 2011;20:1034–1040.
19. Cho CH, Kim du H, Bae KC, Lee D, Kim K. Proper site of corticosteroid injection for the treatment of idiopathic frozen shoulder: results from a randomized trial. *Joint Bone Spine.* 2016;83:324–329.
20. Goyal T, Singh A, Negi P, Kharkwal B. Comparative functional outcomes of patients with adhesive capsulitis receiving intra-articular versus sub-acromial steroid injections: case-control study. *Musculoskelet Surg.* 2019;103:31–35.
21. Rizk TE, Gavant ML, Pinals RS. Treatment of adhesive capsulitis (frozen shoulder) with arthrographic capsular distension and rupture. *Arch Phys Med Rehabil.* 1994;75:803–807.
22. Yoon JP, Chung SW, Kim JE, et al. Intra-articular injection, subacromial injection, and hydrodilatation for primary frozen shoulder: a randomized clinical trial. *J Shoulder Elbow Surg.* 2016;25:376–383.
23. Jacobs LG, Barton MA, Wallace WA, Ferrousis J, Dunn NA, Bossingham DH. Intra-articular distension and steroids in the management of capsulitis of the shoulder. *BMJ.* 1991;302:1498–1501.
24. Haughton DN, Barton S, Meenan E, et al. Can we improve the outcome of hydrodilatation for adhesive capsulitis? *Shoulder Elbow.* 2018;10:93–98.
25. Wu WT, Chang KV, Han DS, Chang CH, Yang FS, Lin CP. Effectiveness of glenohumeral joint dilatation for treatment of frozen shoulder: a systematic review and meta-analysis of randomized controlled trials. *Sci Rep.* 2017;7:10507.
26. Tveita EK, Tariq R, Sesseng S, Juel NG, Bautz-Holter E. Hydrodilatation, corticosteroids and adhesive capsulitis: a randomized controlled trial. *BMC Musculoskelet Disord.* 2008;9:53.
27. Braun HJ, Wilcox-Fogel N, Kim HJ, Pouliot MA, Harris AH, Dragoo JL. The effect of local anesthetic and corticosteroid combinations on chondrocyte viability. *Knee Surg Sports Traumatol Arthrosc.* 2012;20:1689–1695.
28. Wernecke C, Braun HJ, Dragoo JL. The effect of intra-articular corticosteroids on articular cartilage: a systematic review. *Orthop J Sports Med.* 2015;3:2325967115581163.
29. Rymaruk S, Peach C. Indications for hydrodilatation for frozen shoulder. *EFORT Open Rev.* 2017;2:462–468.
30. Kim K, Lee KJ, Kim HC, Lee KJ, Kim DK, Chung SG. Capsule preservation improves short-term outcome of hydraulic distension in painful stiff shoulder. *J Orthop Res.* 2011;29:1688–1694.
31. Buchbinder R, Green S. Effect of arthrographic shoulder joint distension with saline and corticosteroid for adhesive capsulitis. *Br J Sports Med.* 2004;38:384–385.
32. Lee DH, Yoon SH, Lee MY, Kwack KS, Rah UW. Capsule-preserving hydrodilatation with corticosteroid versus corticosteroid injection alone in refractory adhesive capsulitis of shoulder: a randomized controlled trial. *Arch Phys Med Rehabil.* 2017;98:815–821.
33. Mun SW, Baek CH. Clinical efficacy of hydrodistention with joint manipulation under interscalene block compared with intra-articular corticosteroid injection for frozen shoulder: a prospective randomized controlled study. *J Shoulder Elbow Surg.* 2016;25:1937–1943.
34. Yoong P, Duffy S, McKean D, Hujairi NP, Mansour R, Teh JL. Targeted ultrasound-guided hydrodilatation via the rotator interval for adhesive capsulitis. *Skeletal Radiol.* 2015;44(5):703–708. https://doi.org/10.1007/s00256-014-2047-7.
35. Barman A, Mukherjee S, Sahoo J, et al. Single intra-articular platelet-rich plasma versus corticosteroid injections in the treatment of adhesive capsulitis of the shoulder: a cohort study. *Am J Phys Med Rehabil.* 2019;98:549–557.
36. Yan L, Zhou L, Xie D, et al. Chondroprotective effects of platelet lysate towards monoiodoacetate-induced arthritis by suppression of TNF-alpha-induced activation of NF-κB pathway in chondrocytes. *Aging (Albany NY).* 2019;11:2797–2811.
37. Kivimaki J, Pohjolainen T. Manipulation under anesthesia for frozen shoulder with and without steroid injection. *Arch Phys Med Rehabil.* 2001;82:1188–1190.
38. Gallacher S, Beazley JC, Evans J, et al. A randomized controlled trial of arthroscopic capsular release versus hydrodilatation in the treatment of primary frozen shoulder. *J Shoulder Elbow Surg.* 2018;27:1401–1406.
39. Robinson CM, Seah KT, Chee YH, Hindle P, Murray IR. Frozen shoulder. *J Bone Joint Surg Br.* 2012;94:1–9.
40. Vad VB, Sakalkale D, Warren RF. The role of capsular distention in adhesive capsulitis. *Arch Phys Med Rehabil.* 2003;84:1290–1292.
41. Bell S, Coghlan J, Richardson M. Hydrodilatation in the management of shoulder capsulitis. *Australas Radiol.* 2003;47:247–251.
42. Vairo GL, Duffey ML, Owens BD, Cameron KL. Clinical descriptive measures of shoulder range of motion for a healthy, young and physically active cohort. *Sports Med Arthrosc Rehabil Ther Technol.* 2012;4:33.
43. Jayaram P, Kennedy DJ, Yeh P, Dragoo J. Chondrotoxic effects of local anesthetics on human knee articular cartilage: a systematic review. *Pharm Manag PM R.* 2019;11:379–400.
44. Jellad A, May W, Zrig A, et al. Intra-articular distension preceded by physical therapy versus intra-articular distension followed by physical therapy for treating adhesive capsulitis of the shoulder. *J Back Musculoskelet Rehabil.* 2020;33(3):443–450.

26

Ultrasound-Guided Needle Tenotomy and Ultrasound-Guided Tenotomy and Debridement With Tenex Health TX System

RYAN C. KRUSE AND MEDERIC M. HALL

KEY POINTS

- A subset of tendinopathy appears to become chronic and nonresponsive to conservative treatments such as activity modification and exercise-based rehabilitation.
- Ultrasound-guided needle tenotomy is a simple office-based procedure that has been shown effective at multiple tendon locations throughout the body.
- Ultrasound-guided tenotomy and debridement with the Tenex Health TX System provides a less-invasive and cost-effective option for chronic tendinopathy compared to traditional surgical management.
- An in-depth understanding of the regional anatomy and the ability to obtain optimal ultrasound images of the region are essential prerequisites of either procedure.

Introduction

Tendinopathy is a clinical condition characterized by pain and dysfunction related to mechanical loading of a tendon. While often self-limited and responsive to conservative measures, such as activity modification and exercised-based rehabilitation, a subset of patients goes on to develop chronic and recalcitrant symptoms. While the optimal treatment for this group remains poorly defined in the literature, minimally invasive ultrasound-guided mechanical treatments have shown favorable results. In this chapter we review ultrasound-guided needle tenotomy and ultrasound-guided tenotomy and debridement with the Tenex Health TX System. Procedural technique, post-procedure care and rehabilitation, and patient selection are discussed.

Pathology

The term "tendinopathy" includes a wide array of potential histopathology involving the tendon and its paratenon or sheath. Chronic tendon pain is felt to predominately represent a condition characterized histologically as mucoid collagen degeneration with other variable features such as collagen disorganization, fibrocartilaginous metaplasia, calcification, and neovascularity. These changes are often referred to as tendinosis. Although primarily an overuse and degenerative process with an absence of acute inflammatory infiltrate, inflammatory mediators are present.[1] Clinically, tendinopathy is characterized by pain and dysfunction with mechanical loading of a tendon and can lead to significant time loss from sport and work.[2] While the optimal treatment for this group remains poorly defined in the literature, minimally invasive ultrasound-guided mechanical treatments have shown favorable results.[3–8]

Treatment Options

Ultrasound-guided percutaneous needle tenotomy was first described in the early 1980s as a nonsurgical treatment option for common extensor tendinopathy.[9] Subsequent studies have reported favorable outcomes across multiple tendon locations.[10–13] The basic principle of the procedure is to stimulate a healing response within a region of disorganized nonhealing tendon tissue *via local acute trauma produced by multiple needle fenestrations.*[14,15]

Despite early encouraging outcomes with simple needle fenestration, there are inherent limitations with this technique. The Tenex Health TX system (Tenex Health, Lake Forest, CA) is an ultrasonic cutting instrument designed to focally debride and remove pathologic tissue from tendons allowing for both a true tenotomy and debridement.[16] The rationale is that when the pathologic tissue is removed, a chronic degenerative process is converted to an acute process, introducing inflammatory growth factors and promoting tendon healing.[17] Recent advances in the technology now allow for removal of hard calcifications and bone. Early clinical experience has been favorable, even for challenging locations such as the Achilles insertion.[6] The procedure is safely performed in a clinical setting under local anesthesia, which reduces cost significantly compared to an open or endoscopic tenotomy. Furthermore, the minimally invasive nature allows for less post-procedure pain and faster recovery than traditional surgical approaches.[4]

Techniques

A pre-procedural ultrasound should be performed to confirm pathology amendable to treatment and to identify local structures at risk such as nerves and blood vessels. Ergonomics for both patient and physician should be considered. Nuances in treatment of each individual tendon location are outside the scope of this chapter. An in-depth understanding of the regional anatomy and the ability to obtain optimal ultrasound images of the region are essential prerequisites of either procedure.

While there may be variance in clinical practice, we have found that ultrasound-guided needle tenotomy and ultrasound-guided tenotomy and debridement are safely and effectively performed in an outpatient setting under local or regional anesthesia. We recommend a sterile technique including a sterile ultrasound transducer cover and sterile acoustic coupling gel. Our local anesthetic preference is a 50:50 mixture of 1% lidocaine without epinephrine and 0.5% ropivacaine. Between 4 and 10 mL should provide adequate anesthesia in most cases. This can be titrated to patient comfort using the lowest effective dose.

Ultrasound-Guided Needle Tenotomy/ Fenestration

After anesthesia is obtained, a large-gauge needle (typically 18 to 20 G) is advanced with live ultrasound guidance to the area of pathology, and multiple fenestrations are made through the pathologic tissue. Whenever possible, fenestrations should be made parallel to tendon fibers in order to avoid unnecessary trauma to surrounding normal tissue. While determining the necessary amount of tissue fenestration is subjective, a change in tissue resistance to the needle will be appreciated as adequate fenestration is achieved.[13]

Ultrasound-Guided Tenotomy and Debridement With the TX System

Once anesthesia is achieved, a #11 blade is used to make a 5-mm skin incision and create a tract to the tendon or fascia

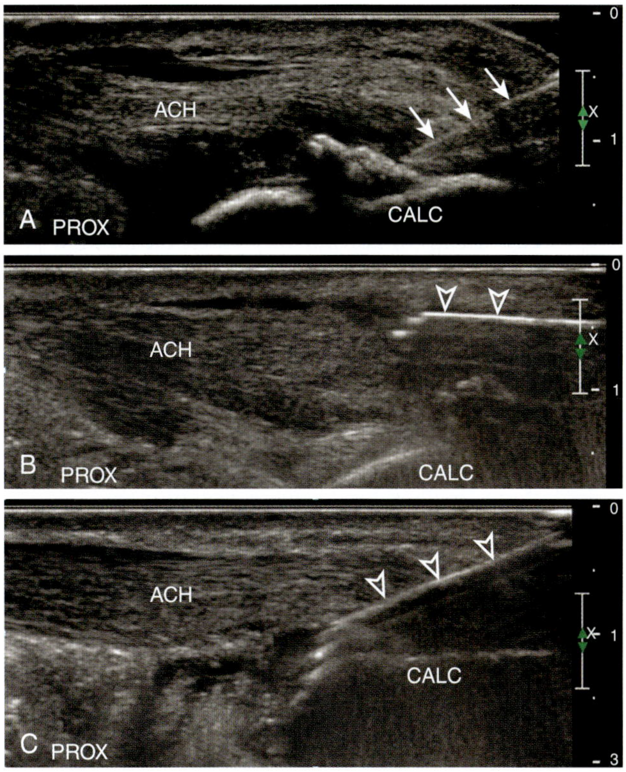

• **Fig. 26.1** **Ultrasound-Guided Tenotomy and the Debridement Procedural Technique.** Long-axis image of Achilles tendon demonstrating procedural technique. (A) After obtaining local anesthesia, a #11 blade *(arrows)* is used to make an incision down to the tendon. (B) The TX MicroTip *(open arrowheads)* is then introduced superficial/posterior to the tendon and the hypertrophied paratenon and connective tissue are debrided from the tendon. (C) The MicroTip is then guided into the tendon and the regions of tendinosis are debrided. In this example, there was concomitant retrocalcaneal bursitis and a limited bursectomy was performed. *ACH*, Achilles tendon; *CALC*, calcaneus; *PROX*, proximal.

being treated (Fig. 26.1A). We prefer to perform the incision under live ultrasound guidance to maximize safety. The incision should always be performed in line with the tendon or fascia to avoid iatrogenic horizontal fiber laceration. Occasionally, more than one incision/entry site is required to effectively address the full extent of the pathologic tissue.

The TX MicroTip is then guided into the region of pathologic tissue (see Fig. 26.1B and C). The cutting energy is activated via a foot pedal and a gentle oscillating motion should be used to allow for debridement and aspiration of tissue. The tip of the device should stay within the tendon while the foot pedal is activated, if possible, to avoid excess leakage of irrigation fluid into the local muscle and subcutaneous tissues. Care should be taken to only move the device in a linear direction to avoid torque at the hub, which can lead to device failure. With improper technique, the internal needle may fracture at the hub. This will be accompanied by an auditory change to a higher pitch. The internal needle may also be visualized extending farther beyond the external needle. If there is any concern for device failure, the procedure should be terminated immediately, and the device carefully removed from the patient for inspection. When removing the MicroTip one should ensure not to leave a fractured internal needle in the procedure site. As the pathologic tissue is removed there will be a tactile change in resistance at the tip of the device and the debrided region will often demonstrate hyperechoic microbubbles from the irrigation fluid. Calcifications will lose posterior acoustic shadowing artifact and should visibly decrease in size as the MicroTip moves freely through the debrided tissue region (Fig. 26.2). Energy times will vary based on location and extent of pathology, with as little as 30 seconds for focal regions in small tendons and up to 10 minutes in large regions of calcified tissue when using the TX1 or TX2 system. Cumulative energy time (both hard and soft tissue) may be extended to 15 minutes when using the TX-Bone, but hard tissue applications should generally not exceed 10 minutes. Energy should always be administered in a pulsatile fashion to allow for adequate aspiration and cooling of the device. The recommended duty cycle is 15 seconds on, 45 seconds off, on HIGH cutting power. This is of particular importance with the TX-Bone as continuous energy administration may result in superficial burns at the skin surrounding the entry site. The device will provide an auditory signal if aspiration slows and has a safety mechanism to shut off the cutting energy if the device becomes clogged and aspiration stops.

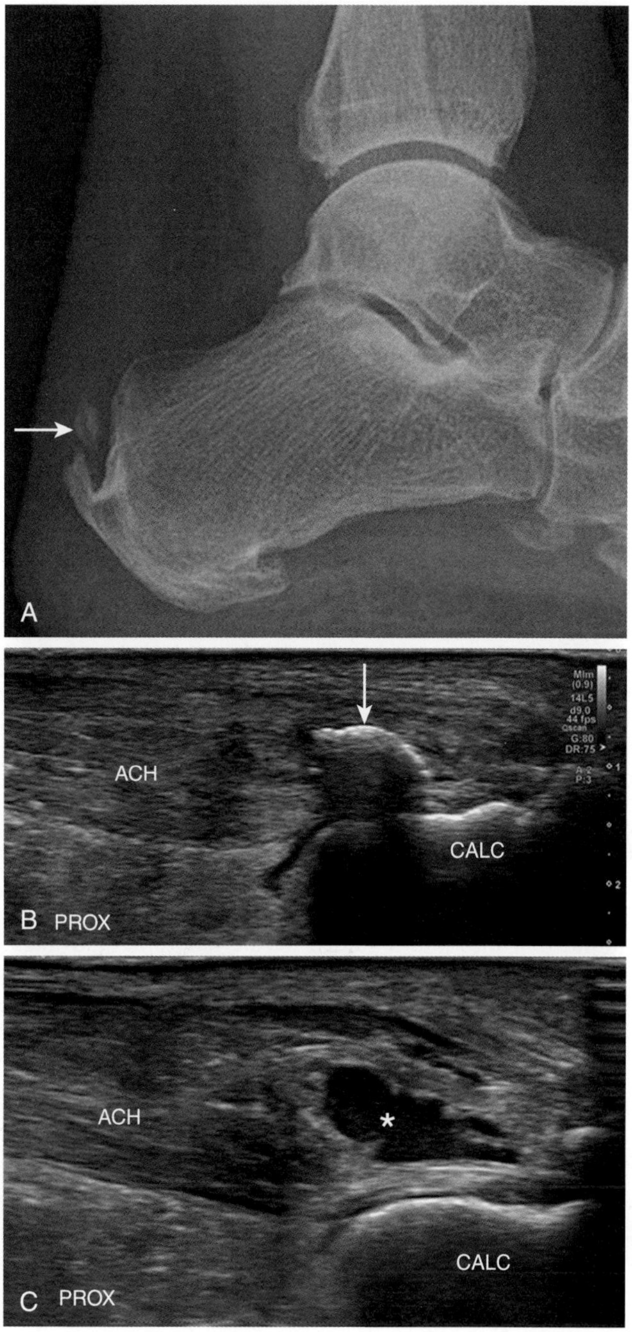

• **Fig. 26.2** Achilles Calcification Treated With the Tenex System. Pre- and post-procedure images of an Achilles insertional calcification treated with the TX-Bone MicroTip. (A) Lateral X-ray demonstrates a large calcification *(arrow)* within the Achilles tendon insertion. (B) Long-axis ultrasound image prior to procedure shows the same calcification *(arrow)* represented as a hyperechoic linear structure with posterior acoustic shadowing. (C) Post-procedure image confirms complete debridement of the calcification with anechoic fluid–filled defect at site of prior calcification *(asterisk)*. *ACH*, Achilles tendon; *CALC*, calcaneus; *PROX*, proximal.

Post-Procedure Care and Rehabilitation

Upon completion of the procedure, either a small adhesive bandage is applied to the needle entry site or the skin incision is closed with a single adhesive wound closure strip followed by gauze and a transparent film dressing. A compression sleeve is recommended if possible. We recommend avoiding submersion of the procedure site for 72 hours after needle tenotomy and for 2 weeks after tenotomy and debridement with the TX system. Post-procedure rehabilitation will vary slightly by the site, the degree of pathology, and the functional demands of the patient. We currently use a criterion-based rehabilitation protocol, which commonly takes between 6 and 12 weeks for return to activities.

Patient Selection and Rationale

Regardless of the technique chosen, optimal outcomes begin with appropriate patient selection. In our experience, patients most likely to respond to tenotomy have clinical features of focal tendon pain with loading and correlative findings on diagnostic ultrasound or magnetic resonance imaging. Patients should have chronic symptoms (>3 months) and fail appropriate initial conservative treatment, which should include activity modification/load management and an exercise-based rehabilitation program. Although further research is needed to identify negative prognosticating factors, we recommend careful evaluation for significant tendon tearing (>50% of cross-sectional area), associated ligament instability (e.g., radial collateral ligament laxity of the lateral elbow in association with common extensor tendinosis), and bony impingement (e.g., Haglund deformity at the Achilles insertion), which may require a more traditional surgical approach or consideration of the TX-Bone. Other factors, such as history of local corticosteroid injections, non-loading pain, and diffuse widespread pain, also should be considered.

The decision to proceed with ultrasound-guided needle fenestration versus ultrasound-guided tenotomy and debridement with the TX system is largely one of available resources and clinician preference at this point, with no studies directly comparing the two treatment options. However, we have found that tenotomy and debridement with the TX system often results in much less post-procedure pain and allows for the introduction of earlier rehabilitation. In fact, we only prescribe over-the-counter analgesics post-procedure. We hypothesize this is because the TX system allows for focal removal of the pathologic tissue and local aspiration/irrigation of nociceptive mediators with much less trauma to the surrounding healthy tissue. In contradistinction, the primary goal of needle fenestration is to create a traumatic injury to stimulate a healing response. There are certain clinical scenarios in which ultrasound-guided tenotomy and debridement with the TX system offers a clear advantage, including addressing calcifications within tendons, associated hypertrophic and inflamed bursal tissue, and local bony impingement. A clear limitation of the TX system is length of the MicroTip. The longest MicroTip currently available (TX 2) is approximately 2 inches in length. Deep targets in large patients (such as gluteal tendons) may not be possible; needle fenestration offers a good alternative in these cases.

References

1. Dean BJF, Dakin SG, Millar NL, Carr AJ. Review: emerging concepts in the pathogenesis of tendinopathy. *Surgeon*. 2017;15(6):349–354. https://doi.org/10.1016/j.surge.2017.05.005.
2. Neph A, Onishi K, Wang JH. Myths and facts of in-office regenerative procedures for tendinopathy. *Am J Phys Med Rehabil*. 2019;98(6):500–511.
3. Morrey BF. A new safe and effective treatment for chronic refractory tendinopathy. *Ortho Rheum Open Access J*. 2018;11(5).
4. Barnes DE, Beckley JM, Smith J. Percutaneous ultrasonic tenotomy for chronic elbow tendinosis: a prospective study. *J Shoulder Elbow Surg*. 2015;24(1):67–73.
5. Battista CT, et al. Ultrasonic percutaneous tenotomy of common extensor tendons for recalcitrant lateral epicondylitis. *Tech Hand Up Extrem Surg*. 2018;22(1):15–18.
6. Chimenti RL, et al. Percutaneous ultrasonic tenotomy reduces insertional Achilles tendinopathy pain with high patient satisfaction and a low complication rate. *J Ultrasound Med*. 2019;38(6):1629–1635.
7. Elattrache NS, Morrey BF. Percutaneous ultrasonic tenotomy as a treatment for chronic patellar tendinopathy—jumper's knee. *Operat Tech Orthopaed*. 2013;23(2):98–103.
8. Stover D, et al. Ultrasound-guided tenotomy improves physical function and decreases pain for tendinopathies of the elbow: a retrospective review. *J Shoulder Elbow Surg*. 2019;28(12):2386–2393.
9. Yerger B, Turner T. Percutaneous extensor tenotomy for chronic tennis elbow: an office procedure. *Orthopedics*. 1985;8(10):1261–1263.
10. Housner JA, Jacobson JA, Misko R. Sonographically guided percutaneous needle tenotomy for the treatment of chronic tendinosis. *J Ultrasound Med*. 2009;28(9):1187–1192.
11. Mattie R, et al. Percutaneous needle tenotomy for the treatment of lateral epicondylitis: a systematic review of the literature. *PM R*. 2017;9(6):603–611.
12. McShane JM, Nazarian LN, Harwood MI. Sonographically guided percutaneous needle tenotomy for treatment of common extensor tendinosis in the elbow. *J Ultrasound Med*. 2006;25(10):1281–1289.
13. Peck E, Jelsing E, Onishi K. Advanced ultrasound-guided interventions for tendinopathy. *Phys Med Rehabil Clin N Am*. 2016;27(3):733–748.
14. Finnoff JT, et al. Treatment of chronic tendinopathy with ultrasound-guided needle tenotomy and platelet-rich plasma injection. *PM R*. 2011;3(10):900–911.
15. Krey D, Borchers J, McCamey K. Tendon needling for treatment of tendinopathy: a systematic review. *Phys Sportsmed*. 2015;43(1):80–86.
16. Barnes DE. Ultrasonic energy in tendon treatment. *Operat Techniq Orthopaed*. 2013;23(2):78–83.
17. Khan KM, Cook JL, Bonar F, Harcourt P, Astrom M. Histopathology of common tendinopathies: update and implications for clinical management. *Sports Med*. 1999;27(6):393–408.

27

High-Volume Image-Guided Injections

MARIA-CRISTINA ZIELINSKI, NICOLA MAFFULLI, OTTO CHAN, AND ROMAIN HAYM

KEY POINTS

Features of the high-volume image-guided injection technique:

- It is designed to improve pain, function, and to reduce tendon thickness.
- It enables patients follow a specific tendon loading program by reducing pain.
- Ultrasound imaging is crucial to ensure correct needle placement at the interface between the paratenon and peritendinous structures.
- The injection is extra-tendinous, eliminating the risks associated with intratendinous corticosteroid injection.

Pathology

Tendinopathies can be acute or chronic and can affect athletic and sedentary patients, leading to long periods of sport cessation and interfering with the activities of daily living.[1,2] Intrinsic (age, gender, body composition, tendon temperature, systemic diseases, muscle strength, flexibility, previous injuries, anatomic variants, genetic predisposition and blood supply) and extrinsic factors (overloading, underloading, training loading error, drugs), alone or in combination, can cause tendinopathy.[3] Pathologic tendons become increasingly painful in response to loading. Clinically, they appear swollen and thickened, and are painful on palpation.

The diagnosis of tendinopathy is based on careful history and detailed clinical examination.[4] High-resolution real-time ultrasonography is frequently used to image tendon disorders and confirm the diagnosis.[5] Ultrasonography is an operator-dependent technique that can influence the image obtained, depending on transducer handling and machine settings. Consequently, the interobserver reliability of ultrasonographic assessment of tendon structures can be problematic, and changes over time may make it difficult to evaluate the progression or the improvement of the tendinopathy.[5]

Ultrasound Imaging Findings

Sonographic features of tendinopathy include abnormal tendon size (thickness), shape (bulging), changes in echogenicity, altered fibrillar appearance, the presence of fluid, sheath thickening, and neovascularization in the tendon or its sheath. Neovessels are associated with abnormal nerves ingrowth, which are thought to contribute to tendinopathic pain.[6,7] Color Doppler and power Doppler ultrasonography are established methods to detect increased blood flow associated with neovascularization within the tendons.[8] Neovascularization in the absence of pain may not be pathologic, and can just indicate a physiologic response to recent physical activity; however, neovascularization within the tendinopathic area is generally present in patients with chronic painful tendinopathy.[9,10]

Treatment Options

Conservative treatment of tendinopathy can be disappointing, and 25% to 45% of patients may require surgery.[1,11] Surgery used to be indicated after a 6-month period of nonoperative management,[12] but is now advocated only as a last resort.

Platelet-rich plasma (PRP) injections have become popular in clinical practice for chronic tendinopathy, as it is hypothesized that a variety of growth factors may promote a healing response in the tissue.[13–16] However, the results of randomized controlled trials (RCTs) have been mixed, and at present there is insufficient evidence for the effectiveness of PRP for tendinopathy of the main body of the Achilles tendon.[17]

There is no accepted standard regimen for the management of tendinopathies, but the inclusion of progressive tendon loading through heavy load concentric and/or eccentric exercise as part of the management plan is crucial.[18,19] Loading exerts beneficial effects on tenocyte homeostasis and promotes tendon collagen synthesis, and can result in decreased pain and increased performance.[20–22] If the clinical symptoms of tendinopathy do not resolve, other nonoperative treatments are available, including extracorporeal shockwave therapy or nitric oxide patches. Injections at the interface between the tendon and peritendinous tissues should also be considered if physiotherapy and shockwave therapy are unsuccessful in reducing pain and facilitate tendon loading.[12]

The rationale behind high-volume image-guided injections (HVIGIs) for the management of tendinopathy is to use a large quantity of fluid to mechanically sever the neovessels and the accompanying nerve ingrowth, either by direct mechanical trauma or through pressure-mediated secondary ischemia.[23–25] In addition, the local anesthetic used in the HVIGI contributes to reducing nociception by producing a short-term local block of the neonerves, and through longer-term neonerve neurotoxicity. Local anesthetics produce a variable neurotoxic effect.[26] The use of corticosteroids likely counteracts the mechanically induced reaction to the injection of the large volume of fluid; it may also contribute to slowing down the re-formation of adhesions between the tendon and peritendinous tissues.[27,28]

HVIGI may be more effective than PRP in improving outcomes of chronic tendinopathies in the short term and similar results long term,[29] with numerous studies confirming the value of HVIGI in tendinopathies.[28,30,31] In patients with chronic tendinopathies, HVIGI significantly reduces pain and stiffness, reduces tendon thickness and intratendinous vascularity on ultrasonographic imaging, and improves function at both the short-term follow-up (2 weeks) and up to an average of 30.3 weeks.[10,32–36] The success rate of HVIGI in returning patients to the desired level of sport is up to 68%.[10]

Corticosteroids are an adjunct to the high-volume injection (very diluted with 0.25 mL in 50 mL of local anesthetics + saline), and are injected at the interface between the Achilles Tendon and Kager's fat to minimize the risk of tendon rupture or other adverse events associated with intratendinous injections.[28] Some authors believed that HVIGI without corticosteroids yielded similar effects on pain reduction and functional improvement in comparison to HVIGI with corticosteroids.[27] However, a recent level 1 RCT found HVIGI with corticosteroids had better outcomes in pain reduction, improved function, and reduced tendon thickness.[28,37]

The clinical diagnosis and management of tendinopathies are not straightforward. Hence, patients should understand that symptoms may recur with either conservative or surgical approaches.[27] Below we describe the technique for the Achilles tendon in detail but see Table 27.1 for general instructions for other areas.

PATIENT SELECTION

- Patients who failed conservative treatment in the past
- Patients unable to tolerate tendon loading
- Patients in whom conservative treatment aggravates symptoms
- Patients unable to have surgery because of comorbidities
- Patients who do not want surgery

Equipment (e.g., Achilles Tendon) *see Fig. 27.1*

- Luer Lock syringes (5 × 10 mL)
- High-pressure Luer Lock connecting tube
- Green needle (21 G × 40 mm)
- Sterile gloves
- Aseptic solution (Hydrex Pink Chlorhexidine Gluconate 0.5% w/v and 70% denatured alcohol [DEB])
- Cotton wool gauze and skin plaster
- High frequency linear ultrasound transducer

Technique (Achilles Mid-portion Tendinopathy HVIGI)

Common Injectates

- Local anesthetic, typically: Bupivacaine 0.5%
- Corticosteroid, typically: Depo-Medrone
- Normal saline

Injectate Volume

- 10 mL of local anesthetics mixed with
- 0.25 mL of corticosteroid (= 10 mg)
- followed by 40 mL of normal saline

Patient Position

- Supine, with the affected leg externally rotated to expose the medial ankle. The lateral ankle rests comfortably on a towel or over the side of the examination table
- Alternatively, the patient can be placed prone with a pillow or bolster under the shin

Clinician Position

- Seated directly distal to the foot being injected

Transducer Ultrasound

- Short axis to Achilles tendon

Needle Orientation

- 21 G × 40 mm needle is inserted from a medial approach in-line with the transducer

Target

- Interface between the anterior surface of the Achilles tendon and Kager's fat pad, with the bevel facing away from

TABLE 27.1 Local Anesthetic and Corticosteroid Dosages, Saline Volumes, Needle Approach and Injection Site, Ultrasound Transducer Placement, and Equipment Needed for the High-Volume Image-Guided Injection (HVIGI) of Different Pathologies.

HVIGI	Local Anesthetic	Corticosteroid Dosage	Saline Volume	Needle Approach and Injection Site (US Imaging Plane)	Equipment
Achilles tendinopathy	Bupivacaine 0.5% 10 mL	Depo-Medrone 0.25 mL (=10 mg)	4 × 10 mL	Medial approach, interface between Achilles tendon and Kager's fat pad (US transverse plane)	5 × 10 mL Luer Lock syringes Long connecting tube Green needle (21 G × 40 mm)
Patellar tendinopathy	Bupivacaine 0.5% 10 mL	Depo-Medrone 0.25 mL (=10 mg)	3 × 10 mL	Medial or lateral approach, interface between patellar tendon and Hoffa's fat pad (US transverse plane)	4 × 10 mL Luer Lock syringes Long connecting tube Green needle (21 G × 40 mm)
Shoulder subacromial impingement (rotator cuff tendinopathy, SASD bursitis)	Bupivacaine 0.5% 20–30 mL	Depo-Medrone 40 mg	—	Lateral approach into the SASD bursa (US transverse plane)	2–3 × 10 mL Luer Lock syringes Long connecting tube Green needle (21 G × 40 mm)
Sinus tarsi syndrome	Bupivacaine 0.5% 10 mL	Triamcinolone 40 mg	—	Anterolateral approach perpendicular to skin, deep at the apex of the sinus tarsi.	1 × 10 mL Luer Lock syringe Long connecting tube Green needle (21 G × 40 mm)
Elbow lateral epicondyle tendinopathy ("tennis elbow")	Bupivacaine 0.5% 10 mL	Depo-Medrone 40 mg	—	Distal approach until needle is in contact with bone, at common extensor tendon enthesis (US longitudinal plane)	3 × 3 mL Luer Lock syringes Long connecting tube Orange needle (25 G × 25 mm)
Plantar fasciopathy	Bupivacaine 0.5% 10 mL	Depo-Medrone 40 mg	—	Medial approach, at plantar fascia insertion onto calcaneus (US transverse plane)	1 × 10 mL Luer Lock syringe Long connecting tube Green needle (21 G × 40 mm)
Greater trochanteric pain syndrome (gluteal tendinopathy)	Bupivacaine 0.5% 20 mL	Depo-Medrone 40 mg	—	Lateral approach until needle is in contact with bone, at lateral facet of greater trochanter	2 × 10 mL Luer Lock syringes Long connecting tube 22 G spinal needle
Small tendons tendinopathy/ tenosynovitis (tibialis posterior, finger flexor, etc.)	Bupivacaine 0.5% 10–20 mL	Depo-Medrone 40 mg	—	Transverse or longitudinal approach, interface between tendon and tendon sheath (US TS or LS plane)	1–2 × 10 mL Luer Lock syringe Short connecting tube Orange needle (25 G × 25 mm)
Morton's neuroma	Bupivacaine 0.5% 10 mL	Depo-Medrone 40 mg	—	Approach from dorsum via intermetatarsal space, directly into the fibrotic capsule of the neuroma (US on plantar aspect, transverse across metatarsal heads)	1 × 10 mL Luer Lock syringe Long connecting tube Green needle (21 G × 40 mm)

SASD, Subacromial-subdeltoid; *US*, ultrasound.

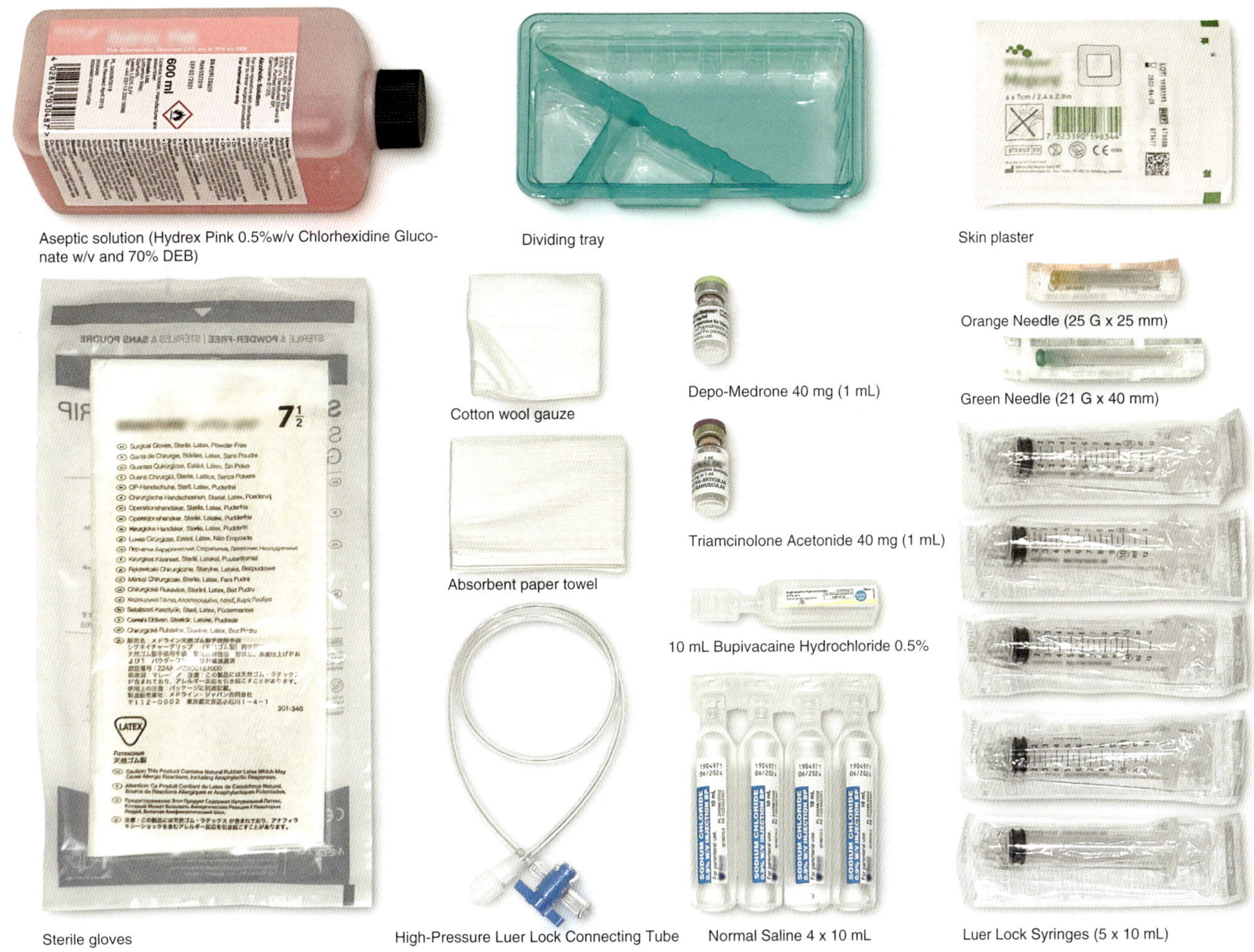

• **Fig. 27.1** Equipment for the High-Volume Image-Guided Injection. *DEB*, Denatured alcohol.

the tendon. Care is taken to avoid placing the needle into the tendon itself. The needle tip is repositioned in real time after each syringe to be as close as possible to the anterior surface of the Achilles tendon.

Please see Table 27.1 for details on dosages, volumes, needle placement and equipment for different pathologies, and Figs. 27.2 and 27.3 for injection sites and ultrasound views.

Post-Injection Management, Physiotherapy, Return-to-Sport

Patients are advised to rest the injected limb for 3 days, and are made aware of a possible steroid flare reaction.[32] Immediately after the procedure, patients are referred to a specialist physiotherapist for initial post-injection management, and tendon loading program.[38] On day 4, the progressive tendon loading program is selected and specifically adapted[38] to each patient taking previous history, current symptoms, tendon's tolerance to loading, and short- and long-term goals into consideration. The 12–16 weeks program includes concentric-eccentric Heavy Slow Resistance,[39] eccentrics[18] if previously well tolerated, concentric-eccentric-plyometrics combined loading,[40] progressing to sport-specific high-intensity and high-speed plyometrics.[41] If the tendon pain was severe and the tendon was irritable up until the injection, isometric exercises are initially performed.[42] Care is also given to initially avoid compressive loads onto the affected tendons (for example: ankle dorsiflexion in insertional Achilles tendinopathy, etc.), and are eventually reintroduced at a later stage.[43,44] Patients are also educated to monitor tendon pain and adjust the loading progression if pain increases past a 5/10 on the Numerical Pain Rating Scale (NPRS) during loading, increased stiffness the following morning, or worsening over time.[45–47]

By day 10, patients are advised to start a course of supervised physiotherapy to improve any relevant biomechanical and functional issues, and progress the tendon loading program; plyometrics or stretch-shortening cycle training is introduced as soon as tolerated, aiming to transition to sport-specific training to match the physical requirements (speed, duration, intensity) and technical skills of the target activity/sport at pre-tendinopathy levels.

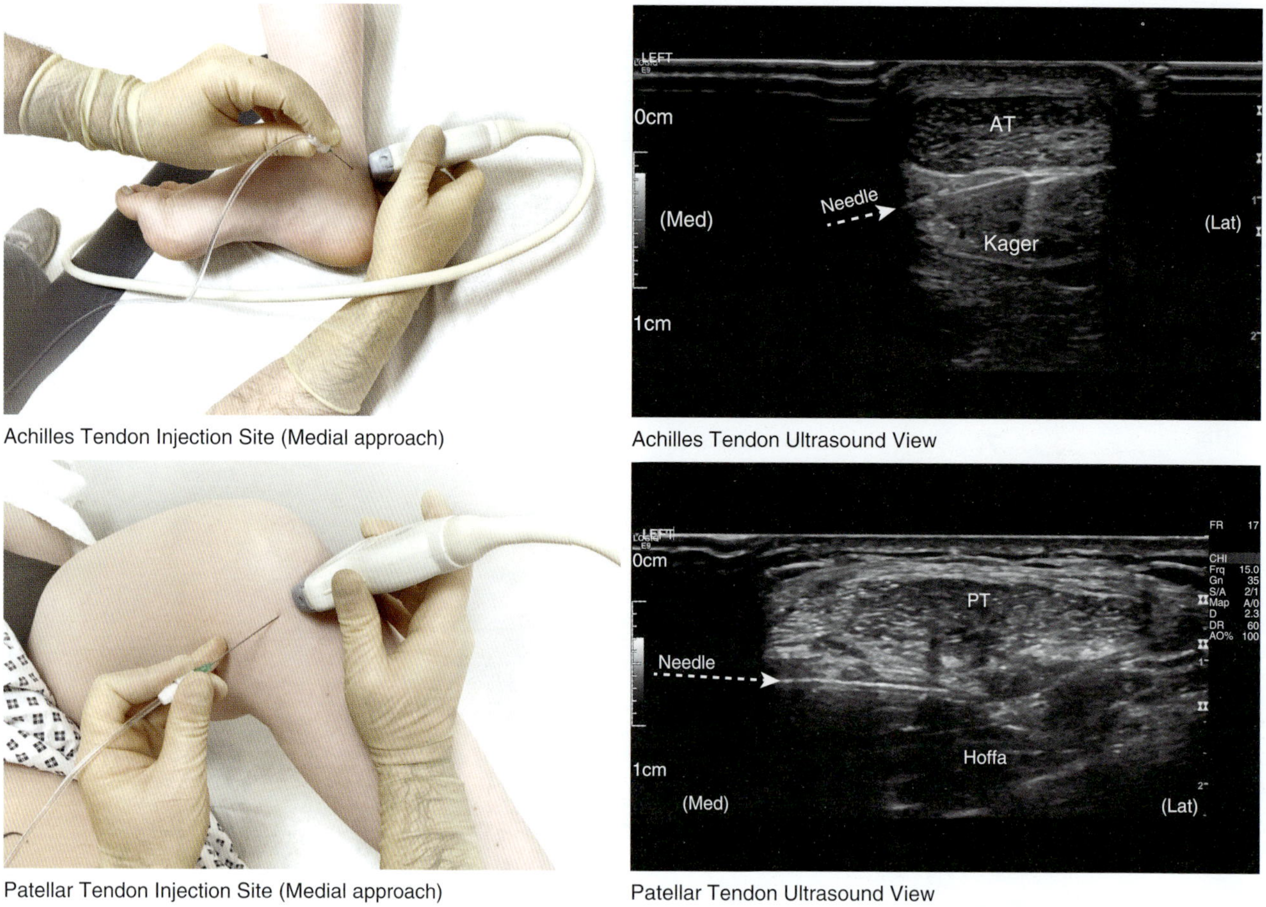

• **Fig. 27.2** Needle approach, transducer positioning, and ultrasound view of the high-volume image-guided injection of Achilles tendon and patellar tendon.

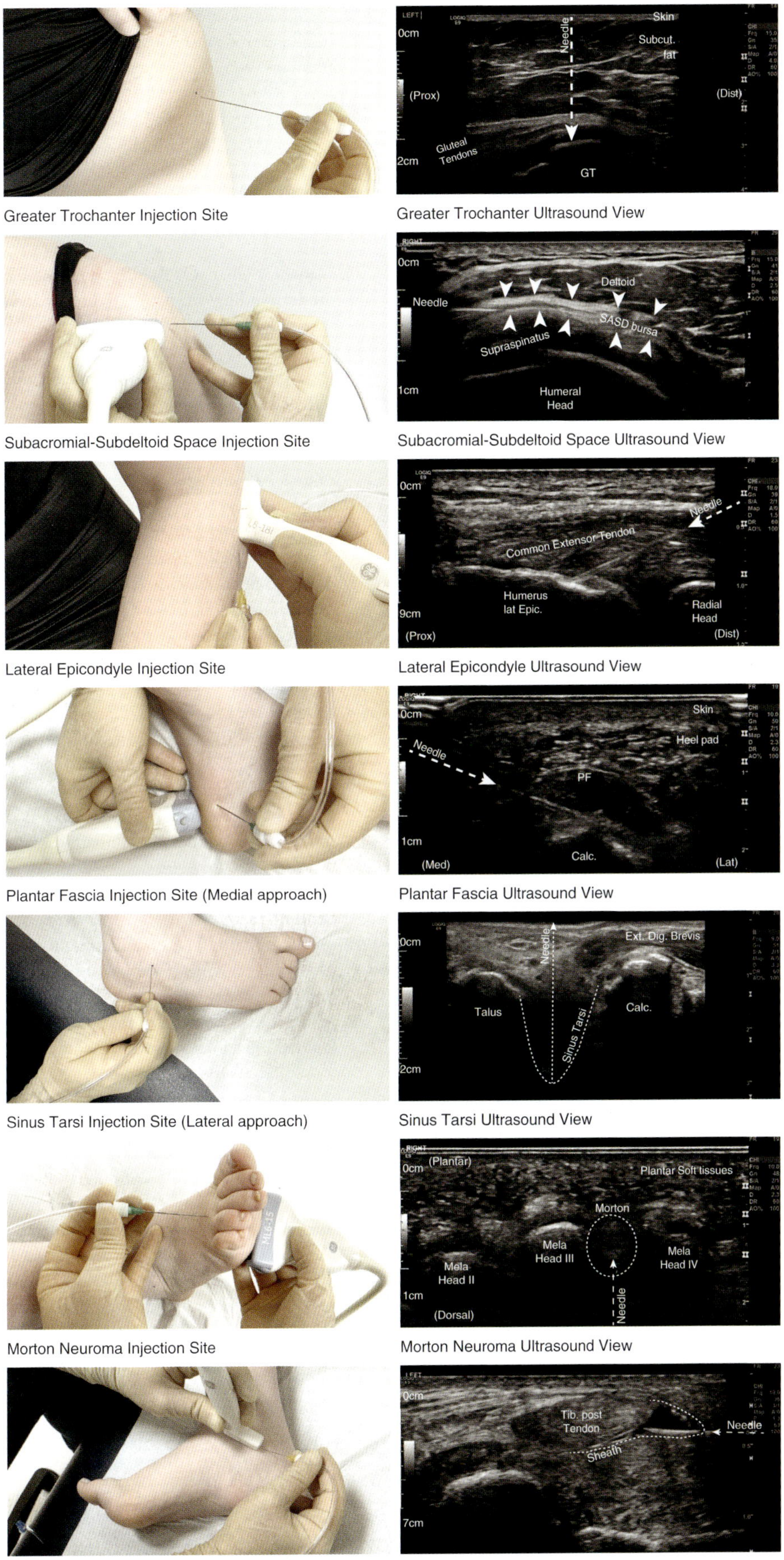

• **Fig. 27.3** Needle approach, transducer positioning, and ultrasound view of the high-volume image-guided injection for subacromial-subdeltoid space, sinus tarsi, and lateral epicondyle.

References

1. Maffulli N, Sharma P, Luscombe KL. Achilles tendinopathy: aetiology and management. *J Royal Society Med.* 2004;97:472–476.
2. Rompe JD, Furia JP, Maffulli N. Mid-portion Achilles tendinopathy—current options for treatment. *Disability Rehabil.* 2008;30:1666–1676.
3. Magnan B, Bondi M, Pierantoni S, et al. The pathogenesis of Achilles tendinopathy: a systematic review. *Foot Ankle Surg.* 2014;20:154–159.
4. Longo UG, Ronga M, Maffulli N. Achilles tendinopathy. *Sports Med Arthrosc Rev.* 2018;26:16–30. 2018/01/05. https://doi.org/10.1097/jsa.0000000000000185.
5. Van Schie H, De Vos R, De Jonge S, et al. Ultrasonographic tissue characterisation of human Achilles tendons: quantification of tendon structure through a novel non-invasive approach. *Brit J Sports Med.* 2010;44:1153–1159.
6. Maffulli N. Tendon problems: a basic science primer. *J Sports Traumatol Related Res.* 1999;21:3–10.
7. Longo UG, Ronga M, Maffulli N. Achilles tendinopathy. *Sports Med Arthroscopy Rev.* 2009;17:112–126.
8. Öhberg L, Lorentzon R, Alfredson H. Neovascularisation in Achilles tendons with painful tendinosis but not in normal tendons: an ultrasonographic investigation. *Knee Surg Sports Traumatol Arthroscop.* 2001;9:233–238.
9. Longo UG, Rittweger J, Garau G, et al. No influence of age, gender, weight, height, and impact profile in Achilles tendinopathy in masters track and field athletes. *Am J Sports Med.* 2009;37:1400–1405.
10. Maffulli N, Spiezia F, Longo UG, et al. High volume image guided injections for the management of chronic tendinopathy of the main body of the Achilles tendon. *Physical Therap Sport.* 2013;14:163–167.
11. Alfredson H. Chronic midportion Achilles tendinopathy: an update on research and treatment. *Clin Sports Med.* 2003;22:727–741.
12. Maffulli N, Longo UG, Kadakia A, et al. Achilles tendinopathy. *J Foot Ankle Surg.* 2019 2019/04/30. https://DOI: 10.1016/j.fas.2019.03.009.
13. De Vos RJ, Weir A, van Schie HT, et al. Platelet-rich plasma injection for chronic Achilles tendinopathy: a randomized controlled trial. *JAMA.* 2010;303:144–149.
14. Hansen M, Boesen A, Holm L, et al. Local administration of insulin–like growth factor–I (IGF–I) stimulates tendon collagen synthesis in humans. *Scandinavian J Med Sci Sports.* 2013;23:614–619.
15. Khan K, Forster B, Robinson J, et al. Are ultrasound and magnetic resonance imaging of value in assessment of Achilles tendon disorders? A two year prospective study. *Brit J Sports Med.* 2003;37:149–153.
16. Olesen JL, Heinemeier KM, Langberg H, et al. Expression, content, and localization of insulin-like growth factor I in human achilles tendon. *Connect Tissue Res.* 2006;47:200–206.
17. Andia I, Martin JI, Maffulli N. Advances with platelet rich plasma therapies for tendon regeneration. *Expert Opin Biol Therap.* 2018;18:389–398.
18. Alfredson H, Pietilä T, Jonsson P, et al. Heavy-load eccentric calf muscle training for the treatment of chronic Achilles tendinosis. *Am J Sports Med.* 1998;26:360–366.
19. Loppini M, Maffulli N. Conservative management of tendinopathy: an evidence-based approach. *Muscles Ligaments Tendons J.* 2011;1:134.
20. Langberg H, Ellingsgaard H, Madsen T, et al. Eccentric rehabilitation exercise increases peritendinous type I collagen synthesis in humans with Achilles tendinosis. *Scandinavian J Med Sci Sports.* 2007;17:61–66.
21. Rees JD, Maffulli N, Cook J. Management of tendinopathy. *Am J Sports Med.* 2009;37:1855–1867.
22. Kjær M, Langberg H, Heinemeier K, et al. From mechanical loading to collagen synthesis, structural changes and function in human tendon. *Scandinavian J Med Sci Sports.* 2009;19:500–510.
23. Tan SC, Chan O. Achilles and patellar tendinopathy: current understanding of pathophysiology and management. *Disabil Rehabil.* 2008;30:1608–1615.
24. Wheeler PC, Mahadevan D, Bhatt R, et al. A comparison of two different high-volume image-guided injection procedures for patients with chronic noninsertional Achilles tendinopathy: a pragmatic retrospective cohort study. 2016;55:976–979.
25. Wheeler PC, Tattersall CJCjosmojotCAoSM. *Novel Interventions for Recalcitrant Achilles Tendinopathy: Benefits Seen Following High-Volume Image-Guided Injection or Extracorporeal Shockwave Therapy-A Prospective Cohort Study*; 2018.
26. Verlinde M, Hollmann MW, Stevens MF, et al. Local anesthetic-induced neurotoxicity. *Intl J Mol Sci.* 2016;17:339.
27. Abdulhussein H, Chan O, Morton S, et al. High volume image guided injections with or without steroid for mid-portion Achilles tendinopathy: a pilot study. *Clin Res Foot Ankle.* 2017; 5:249.
28. Boesen AP, Langberg H, Hansen R, et al. High volume injection with and without corticosteroid in chronic midportion Achilles tendinopathy. *Scandinavian J Med Sci Sports.* 2019.
29. Boesen AP, Hansen R, Boesen MI, et al. Effect of high-volume injection, platelet-rich plasma, and sham treatment in chronic midportion Achilles tendinopathy: a randomized double-blinded prospective study. *Am J Sports Med.* 2017;45:2034–2043.
30. Andia I, Maffulli N. Platelet-rich plasma for muscle injury and tendinopathy. *Sports Med Arthroscopy Rev.* 2013;21:191–198.
31. Andia I, Maffulli N. A contemporary view of platelet-rich plasma therapies: moving toward refined clinical protocols and precise indications. *Regenerat Med.* 2018;13:717–728.
32. Chan O, O'Dowd D, Padhiar N, et al. High volume image guided injections in chronic Achilles tendinopathy. *Disabil Rehabil.* 2008;30:1697–1708.
33. Crisp T, Khan F, Padhiar N, et al. High volume ultrasound guided injections at the interface between the patellar tendon and Hoffa's body are effective in chronic patellar tendinopathy: a pilot study. *Disabil Rehabil.* 2008;30:1625–1634.
34. Humphrey J, Chan O, Crisp T, et al. The short-term effects of high volume image guided injections in resistant non-insertional Achilles tendinopathy. *J Sci Med Sport.* 2010;13:295–298.
35. Maffulli N, Del Buono A, Oliva F, et al. High-volume image-guided injection for recalcitrant patellar tendinopathy in athletes. *Clin J Sport Med.* 2016;26:12–16.
36. Morton S, Chan O, King J, et al. High volume image-guided injections for patellar tendinopathy: a combined retrospective and prospective case series. *Muscles Ligaments Tendons J.* 2014;4:214.
37. Wheeler PC, Mahadevan D, Bhatt R, Bhatia M. A comparison of two different high-volume image-guided injection procedures for patients with chronic noninsertional Achilles tendinopathy: a pragmatic retrospective cohort study. *J Foot Ankle Surg.* 2016;55(5):976–979. https://doi.org/10.1053/j.jfas.2016.04.017.

38. Scott A, Docking S, Vicenzino B, et al. Sports and exercise-related tendinopathies: a review of selected topical issues by participants of the Second International Scientific Tendinopathy Symposium (ISTS), Vancouver, 2012. 2013;47:536–544.
39. Beyer R, Kongsgaard M, Hougs Kjær B, et al. Heavy slow resistance versus eccentric training as treatment for Achilles tendinopathy: a randomized controlled trial. 2015;43:1704–1711.
40. GrävareSilbernagel K, Crossley KMJjoo, therapy sp. A proposed return-to-sport program for patients with midportion Achilles tendinopathy: rationale and implementation. 2015;45:876–886.
41. Silbernagel KG, Thomeé R, Eriksson BI, et al. Continued sports activity, using a pain-monitoring model, during rehabilitation in patients with Achilles tendinopathy: a randomized controlled study. 2007;35:897–906.
42. Rio E, Kidgell D, Purdam C, et al. Isometric exercise induces analgesia and reduces inhibition in patellar tendinopathy. 2015;49:1277–1283.
43. Cook J, Purdam C. Is compressive load a factor in the development of tendinopathy? *Brit J Sports Med.* 2012;46:163–168.
44. Docking S, Samiric T, Scase E, et al. Relationship between compressive loading and ECM changes in tendons. 2013;3:7.
45. GrävareSilbernagel K, Thomee R, Thomee P, et al. Eccentric overload training for patients with chronic Achilles tendon pain—a randomised controlled study with reliability testing of the evaluation methods. 2001;11:197–206.
46. Kongsgaard M, Kovanen V, Aagaard P, et al. Corticosteroid injections, eccentric decline squat training and heavy slow resistance training in patellar tendinopathy. 2009;19:790–802.
47. Malliaras P, Barton CJ, Reeves ND, et al. Achilles and patellar tendinopathy loading programmes. *Sports Med.* 2013;43:267–286.

28

Ultrasound-Guided Release of Trigger Finger and de Quervain Tenosynovitis

RICARDO E. COLBERG AND JAVIER A. JURADO

Ultrasound-Guided Trigger Finger Release at the First Annular (A1) Pulley

KEY POINTS

- Compared to open surgery, releasing the A1 pulley under ultrasound guidance has a better safety profile with a lower risk of complications and a quicker return to work.[1]
- Percutaneous release is performed through a small puncture incision that does not require sutures.
- Ultrasound image guidance allows the physician to visualize the neurovascular bundle before making the incision as well as during the procedure, which diminishes the risk of neurovascular injury.[2–5]
- Return to basic daily activities and resuming full duties at work is quicker since the wound heals more quickly.[1,6,7]
- This procedure should be avoided in patients that present with evidence of Dupuytren contracture.
- The Colberg criteria help confirm a complete release of the A1 pulley.[8]

Anatomy

The flexor tendons in the finger lay palmar (volar) to the metacarpal bones with the flexor digitorum profundus (FDP) closer to the metacarpal bone and the flexor digitorum superficialis (FDS) farthest from the metacarpal bone. The FDP and FDS tendons are surrounded by a common synovial tendon sheath. There are five annular ligaments, referred to as "A pulleys," which are superficial to the tendon sheath that hold the tendons close to the bone. The A1 pulley is the most proximal and clinically significant ligament.[9,10] The length of the A1 pulley can be estimated by measuring the distance between the palmar creases of the metacarpophalangeal (MCP) and proximal interphalangeal (PIP) joints. The A1 pulley is found at the level of the metacarpal head and MCP joint, and this measurement is roughly equivalent to the distance between the proximal edge of the A1 pulley and the MCP crease (Fig. 28.1).[11] There is a neurovascular bundle at both the radial and ulnar side of the tendon.[11] The digital arteries originate from the superficial palmar arch (artery), which is roughly 1 inch proximal to the MCP joint.

Common Pathology

Stenosing tenosynovitis of the finger flexor tendons, more commonly referred to as "trigger finger," can lead to pain and loss of mechanical hand function. In the acute phase, inflammation of the tendon and the synovial lining of the tendon sheath causes severe pain with finger bending. The inflammation eventually can cause mechanical catching or locking of the tendon at the A1 pulley as the tendon gets so swollen that it does not glide well under the pulley with finger flexion and extension.[12] The friction created from the catching leads to chronic thickening of the A1 pulley, which may lead to a permanently locked finger.[13] The severity of the trigger finger is graded based on the Quinnell grading system[14]:

- Grade 1—pain with flexion at the A1 pulley with no mechanical symptoms
- Grade 2—painful catching at the A1 pulley with active release with the same finger extension
- Grade 3—painful locking that requires passive release with the other hand
- Grade 4—permanently locked finger

Ultrasound Imaging Findings

Ultrasound is used to evaluate the A1 pulley, flexor tendons, and neurovascular structures, as well as to diagnose mechanical catching of the tendon (Fig. 28.2). In the

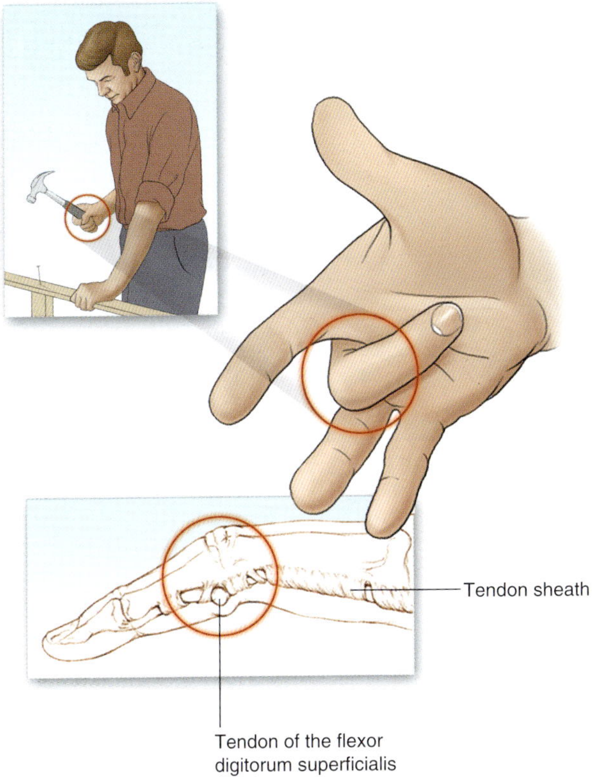

• **Fig. 28.1** Anatomy of the Flexor Tendons and Pulleys. (From Waldman S. *Atlas of Common Pain Syndromes*. 4th ed. Elsevier, Philadelphia, PA; 2019.)

cross-sectional view, the A1 pulley is at the level of the metacarpal head superficial to the tendon sheath. The neurovascular structures are seen radial and ulnar (i.e., lateral and medial) to the tendons (see Fig. 28.2A). The A1 pulley can be further evaluated in the longitudinal view for any evidence of tendinopathy such as hypoechoic thickening of the tendon and/or hyperemia in the tendon sheath or A1 pulley on power Doppler imaging.[15,16] Hypertrophy of the A1 pulley and a swollen nodule in the tendon with a mechanical catching at the A1 pulley (see Fig. 28.2C) during dynamic ultrasound examination confirms the diagnosis of trigger finger.[15]

Treatment Options

Patients are generally first treated with nonsteroidal anti-inflammatory drugs (NSAIDs), finger night splints, cortisone injection, and/or physical therapy.[17] Injecting the trigger finger using ultrasound guidance improves accuracy of the placement of the needle, avoiding neurovascular structures.[18,19] Cortisone injection and splinting have been shown to provide significant relief in 50% to 56% of patients.[20–24] However, more than 30% of cases do not resolve, especially if the treatment did not start before the onset of mechanical symptoms.[23,24] These cases require a release of the A1 pulley by either open surgery, palpation guided, or ultrasound-guided release of the A1 pulley.[1,8,25–29]

Equipment

- Needles: 25-gauge, 1.5-inch needle/18-gauge, 1.5-inch needle with a blade at the tip (Nokor Admix, Becton, Dickinson and Company, Franklin Lakes, NJ) (Fig. 28.3). Other instruments such as the hook knife have also been reported and shown to be effective.[2]
- Musculoskeletal ultrasound machine with a high-frequency linear array transducer.

Technique

Patient Position

- Seated with the palmar side of the hand facing up and the hand resting at the edge of the table in order to allow hyperextension of the MCP joint. The palmar side is cleansed in a sterile fashion from mid-palm down to the distal interphalangeal joint, creating a sterile field (Fig. 28.4A).
- For patients with risk of vasovagal syncope, we recommend having them lay down supine with the hand facing up, resting at their side at the edge of the table.

Clinician Position

- Seated distal to the trigger finger.

Transducer Orientation

- Short axis to the metacarpal bone and flexor tendon to identify the neurovascular structures.
- Long axis to the flexor tendon over the A1 pulley and the MCP joint to perform the release.

Needle Orientation

- In-plane with the transducer with a distal to proximal approach toward the A1 pulley.

Target

- Inject local anesthesia with a 25-gauge, 1.5-inch needle from distal to proximal over the A1 pulley and inside the tendon sheath (see Fig. 28.4B)
- Create a puncture incision in the skin using the 18-gauge Nokor needle and advance towards the A1 pulley and flexor tendons.
- Make an incision through the A1 pulley and the tendon sheath from distal to proximal (see Fig. 28.4A). Irrigate the tendon with normal saline solution to ensure a complete release.

Injectate Volume

- Local anesthesia: 1 to 3 mL of local anesthetic
- Author prefers 1% lidocaine with epinephrine (1:100,000)
- Irrigation: 3 mL normal saline solution

Pearls and Pitfalls

- Avoid puncturing the neurovascular structures and blood vessels by keeping the Nokor needle tip (blade) in the visual field at all times.

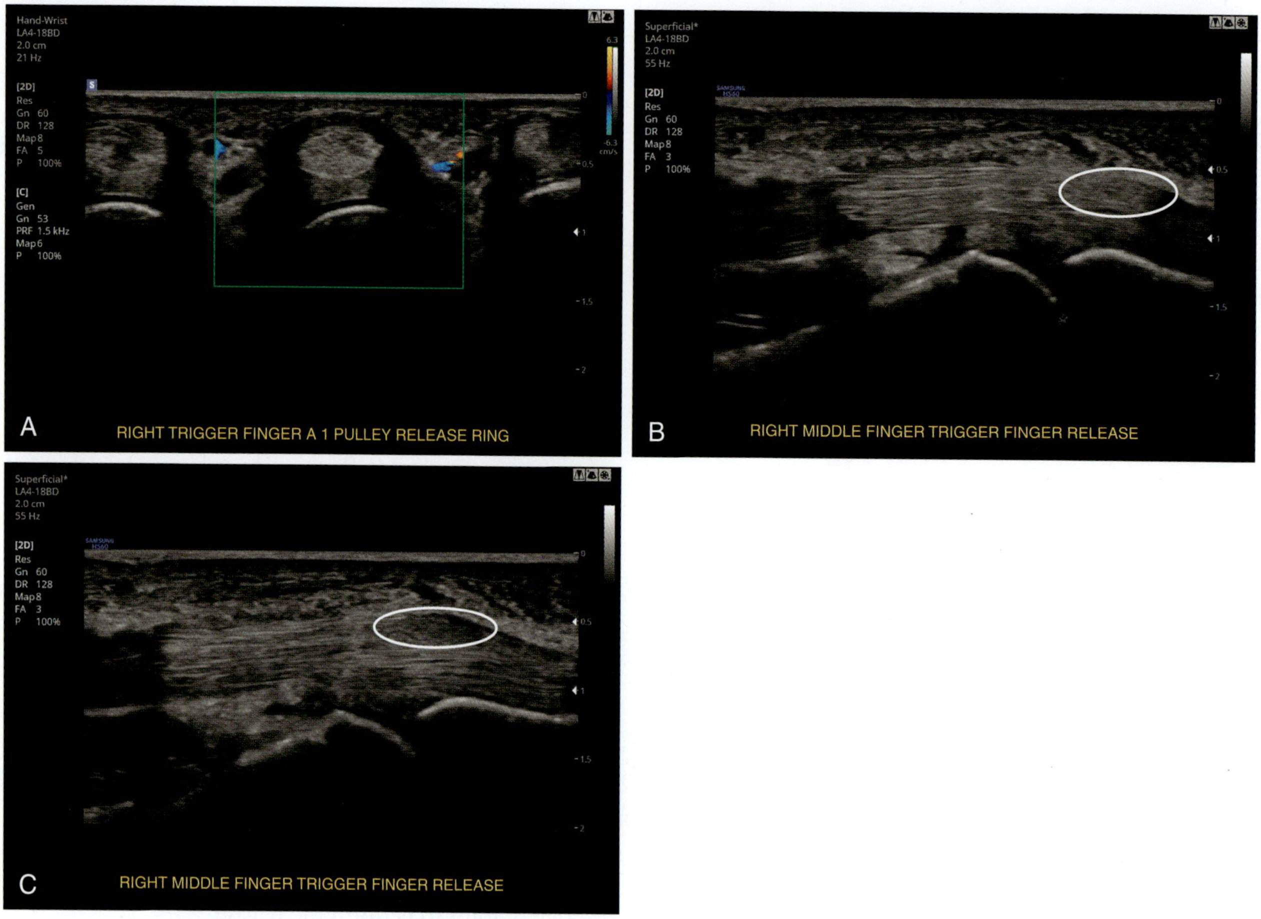

• **Fig. 28.2** Flexor digitorum superficialis and profundus at the metacarpophalangeal joint (oval: A1 pulley). (A) Short-axis view of the tendons and surrounding neurovascular structures. (B) Finger in full extension with the nodule (oval) away from the A1 pulley. (C) Finger in flexion with the nodule (oval) catching at the A1 pulley.

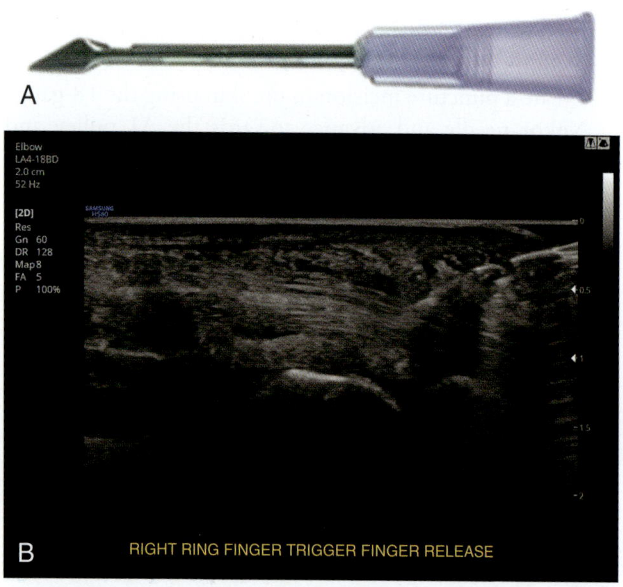

• **Fig. 28.3** Nokor Admix 18-gauge, 1.5-inch hypodermic needle (A) with blade at the tip and ultrasound image of the needle (B).

- Despite popular belief, epinephrine is safe to use near fingers, even for digital nerve blocks, and it greatly reduces the amount of bleeding that occurs with the procedure, minimizing complications.[30]
- This procedure should be avoided in patients that have widespread hand pain, complex regional pain syndrome, or evidence of Dupuytren contracture.
- Complete release of the A1 pulley can be confirmed after the procedure using the Colberg criteria (Fig. 28.5B–D)[8]:
  1. Irrigate the tendon and the area where the A1 pulley was released in order to visualize an anechoic defect between the two ends of the severed A1 pulley (see Fig. 28.5B and D).
  2. Perform a dynamic ultrasound evaluation of the tendon by doing active and passive range of motion in order to visualize the tendon gliding smoothly without any mechanical catching/locking (see Fig. 28.5E and F).
  3. Have the patient make a fist 10 times by doing full active range of motion of the hand/fingers, closing and opening all of the fingers to make sure there is no residual mechanical catching/locking of the tendon.

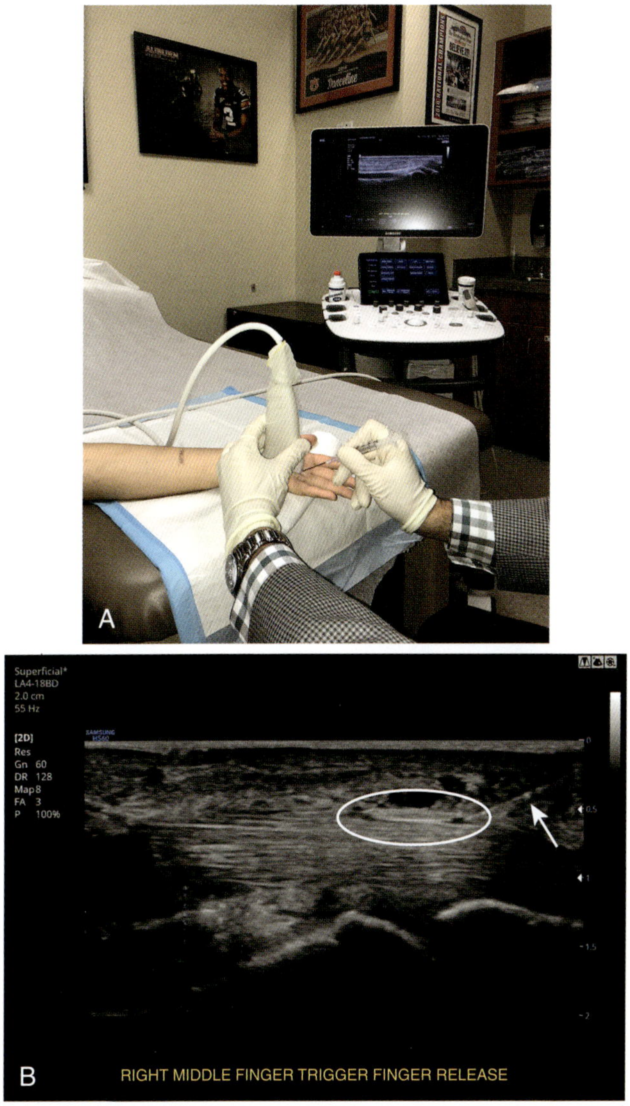

• **Fig. 28.4** (A) Position of patient, clinician, transducer, needle, and ultrasound machine. (B) Flexor digitorum superficialis and profundus at the metacarpophalangeal joint. *Oval*: A1 pulley. *Arrow*: 25-gauge, 1.5-inch hypodermic needle distal to the A1 pulley inside the tendon sheath. The fluid was injected from distal to proximal inside the tendon sheath. It can be seen spreading through the superficial and deep aspect of the tendon sheath proximal to the A1 pulley.

- If a patient does not pass any of the three tests, residual A1 pulley fibers may be present and the incision should be extended proximal or distal according to where the residual catching is identified. The Colberg criteria should be performed again to ensure complete release of the A1 pulley.
- If done correctly, patients should not feel any residual catching/locking after the procedure and rate of recurrence is less than 1%.[8]
- Avoid immobilizing after the procedure in order to minimize scar tissue formation around the tendon that may lead to flexion contracture.
- Preexisting PIP joint flexion contracture is a risk factor for residual pain at the PIP joint after releasing the trigger finger because the finger range of motion increases from eliminating the mechanical catching of the trigger finger.[8,31]

Post-Procedure

Once the A1 pulley has been released, an adhesive bandage is placed over the puncture incision and it may be removed 24 hours post-procedure. Patients are instructed to avoid heavy lifting or gripping for 2 weeks. Patients can perform all basic activities of daily living and light duties as tolerated 24 hours post-procedure. If there is pain, patients can ice the treated area and take acetaminophen or an over-the-counter NSAID as needed. Patients may have mild residual soft tissue swelling after the release that will resolve within the first 4 weeks post-procedure.

Complications Post-Procedure

Possible complications after the procedure, although extremely rare, include residual pain, infection, flexor tendon laceration, neurovascular injury, and incomplete release of the A1 pulley.[32] The thumb presents two additional challenges to the procedure: (1) the thumb digital nerve can cross over the A1 pulley and is at risk of laceration; and (2) the thumb frequently has a sesamoid bone within the adductor pollicis and abductor pollicis brevis tendons, which may displace the tendon and make it difficult to navigate the needle into the A1 pulley without lacerating the tendon.[5,33] These are similar to complications that may be seen with open surgery and palpation-guided percutaneous release.[12] Open surgeries carry a risk rate of 12% to 28%, ranging from nerve injury, vascular injury, wound infection to wound dehiscence and scar hypertrophy.[34–36] Ultrasound minimizes the risks associated with palpation-guided percutaneous release, especially the risk of an incomplete release, tendon laceration and neurovascular injury.[5] PIP joint flexion contracture and diabetes are risk factors for residual pain at the PIP joint after releasing the trigger finger.[37]

Ultrasound-Guided Release of De Quervain Tenosynovitis

KEY POINTS

- Compared to open surgery, an ultrasound-guided first compartment release has a better safety profile with a lower risk of complications.[38]
- It is performed through a small puncture incision that does not require sutures.[39]
- Ultrasound image guidance allows the physician to visualize the neurovascular bundle before making the incision, as well as during the procedure, which diminishes the risk of neurovascular injury.[38]
- Return to basic daily activities and resuming full duties at work is quicker since the wound heals more quickly.
- This procedure should be avoided in patients with a history of first dorsal compartment release and recurrence.

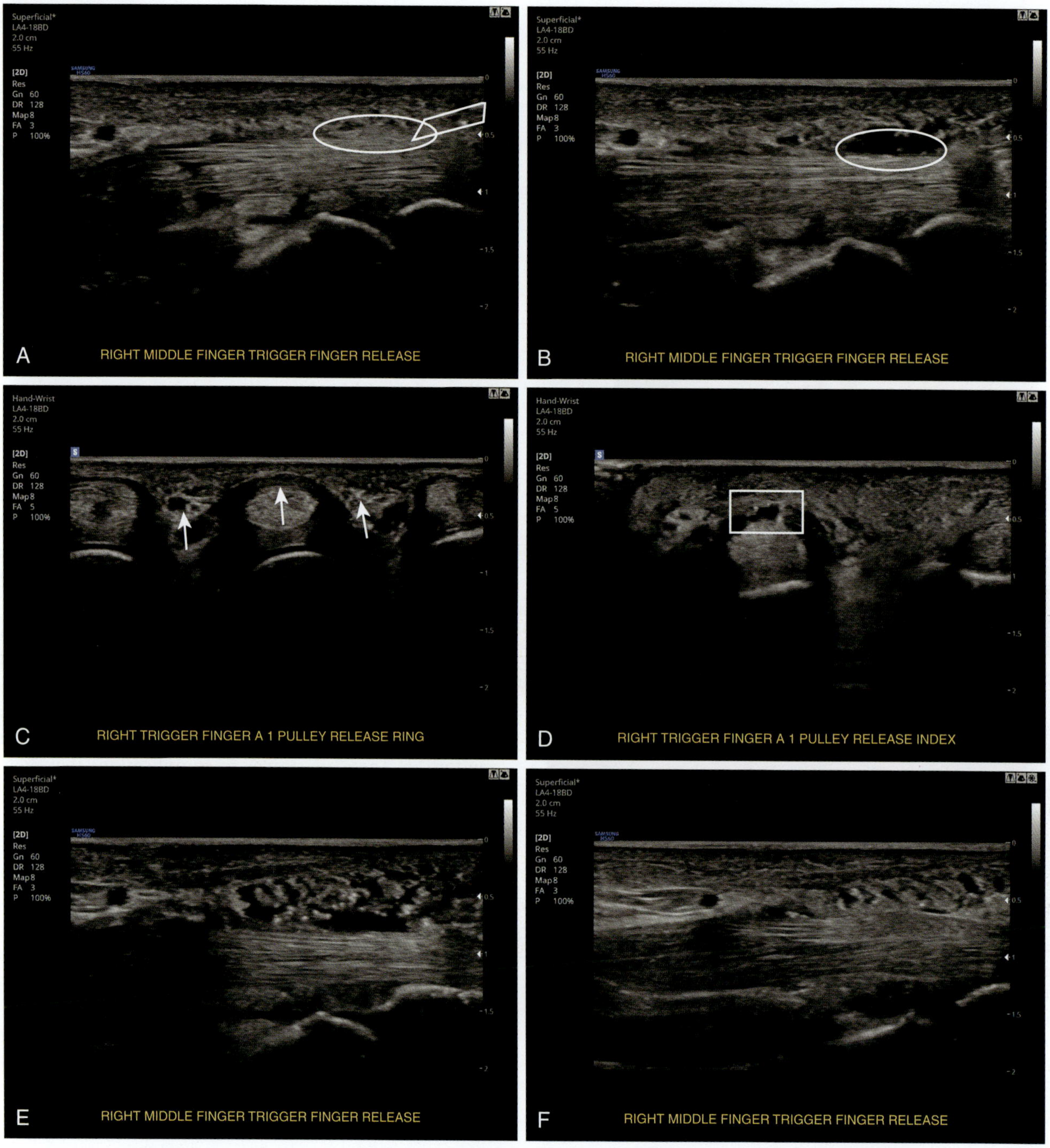

• **Fig. 28.5** Flexor digitorum superficialis and profundus at the metacarpophalangeal joint before and after A1 pulley release. (*Oval*: A1 pulley). (A) Longitudinal view of tendons showing intact A1 pulley before release. *truncated rectangle*: 18-gauge Nokor needle. The needle was advanced from distal to proximal. (B) Longitudinal view of tendons post-release showing an empty space where the A1 pulley used to be. (C) Cross-sectional view of the tendons showing intact A1 pulley and neurovascular bundles *(arrows)*. (D) Cross-sectional view of the tendons showing a transected A1 pulley (empty space inside the rectangle between (the two ends of the A1 pulley after release). (E) Finger in full extension with the nodule away from the area of the A1 pulley. (F) Finger in full flexion with the nodule gliding smoothly through the area where the A1 pulley used to be not catching anymore.

Anatomy

The extensor retinaculum is a bandlike structure that extends over the dorsal wrist at the level of the distal radius. It holds the abductor and extensor tendons of the wrist and fingers in place (Fig. 28.6). These tendons cross the wrist joint under the extensor retinaculum within six dorsal compartments. The abductor pollicis longus and extensor pollicis brevis tendons are found in the first compartment. In some cases, the two cross the compartment in a common tendon sheath, while in other cases they travel through the compartment separated by

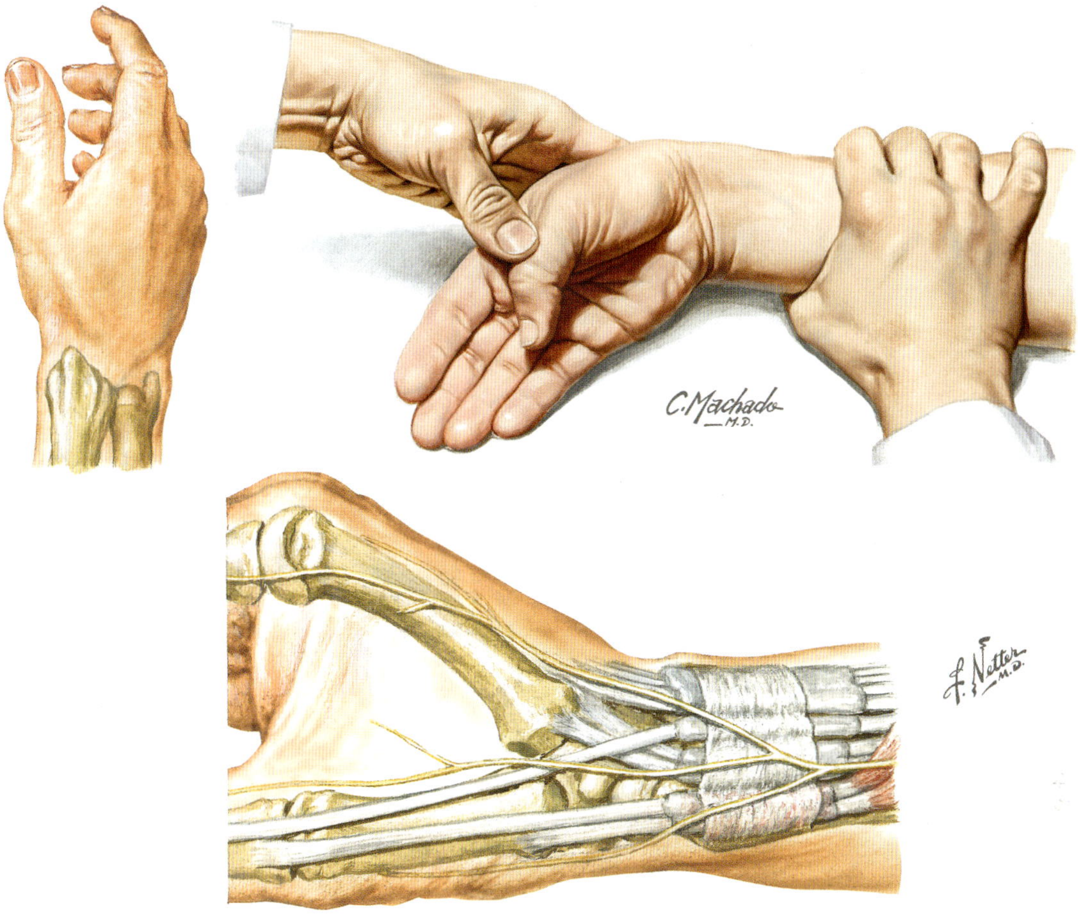

• **Fig. 28.6** Anatomy of the Extensor Retinaculum and First Dorsal Compartment. (From Greene W. *Netter's Orthopaedics*. Saunders, Philadelphia, PA; 2006. Used with permission of Elsevier. All rights reserved.)

a septum.[40] The radial artery and vein as well as the superficial radial nerve are adjacent to the first dorsal compartment.

Common Pathology

de Quervain tenosynovitis, one of the most common tenosynovitis, occurs at the first dorsal compartment and involves the abductor pollicis longus and extensor pollicis brevis tendons. Inflammation and swelling cause mechanical catching/locking and tenderness at the extensor retinaculum.[41–43] The Finkelstein test can be performed to confirm the diagnosis (pain reproduced with flexing the thumb into the palm of the hand, forming a fist around the thumb and ulnar deviating the wrist).[42]

Ultrasound Imaging Findings

Ultrasound can be used to visualize pathology in the extensor retinaculum, abductor pollicis longus (APL) and extensor pollicis brevis (EPB) tendons, and neurovascular structures.[39] The extensor retinaculum can be identified in the longitudinal view above both tendons over the distal radius (Fig. 28.7A).[39] Fig. 28.5B shows the extensor retinaculum in short-axis view covering the radial styloid and the APL and EPB tendons. In the axial view, the radial artery is found volar to the first dorsal compartment and the superficial radial artery dorsally, with small branches covering the area.[39] In over 60% of patients with de Quervain tenosynovitis, an intra-compartment septum can be identified, separating the APL and EPB tendons in the axial view.[40]

Treatment Options

Patients are generally first encouraged to rest, avoid painful activities, and wear a thumb spica wrist splint. Additionally, patients may be treated with NSAIDs, a cortisone injection, and physical therapy.[41–45] Injecting the first dorsal compartment with ultrasound guidance ensures accurately placing the needle inside the tendon sheath while avoiding the neurovascular structures.[46] However, many cases do not resolve, especially if the treatment did not start before the osnet of the mechanical symptoms. These cases require a release of the extensor retinaculum and incision of the tendon sheath by either open surgical release or an ultrasound guided release.[38]

Equipment

- Needles: 25-gauge, 1.5-inch needle/18-gauge, 1.5-inch needle with a blade at the tip (Nokor Admix, Becton, Dickinson and Company, Franklin Lakes, NJ) (see Fig. 28.2)/20-gauge, 1.5-inch needle. A release using

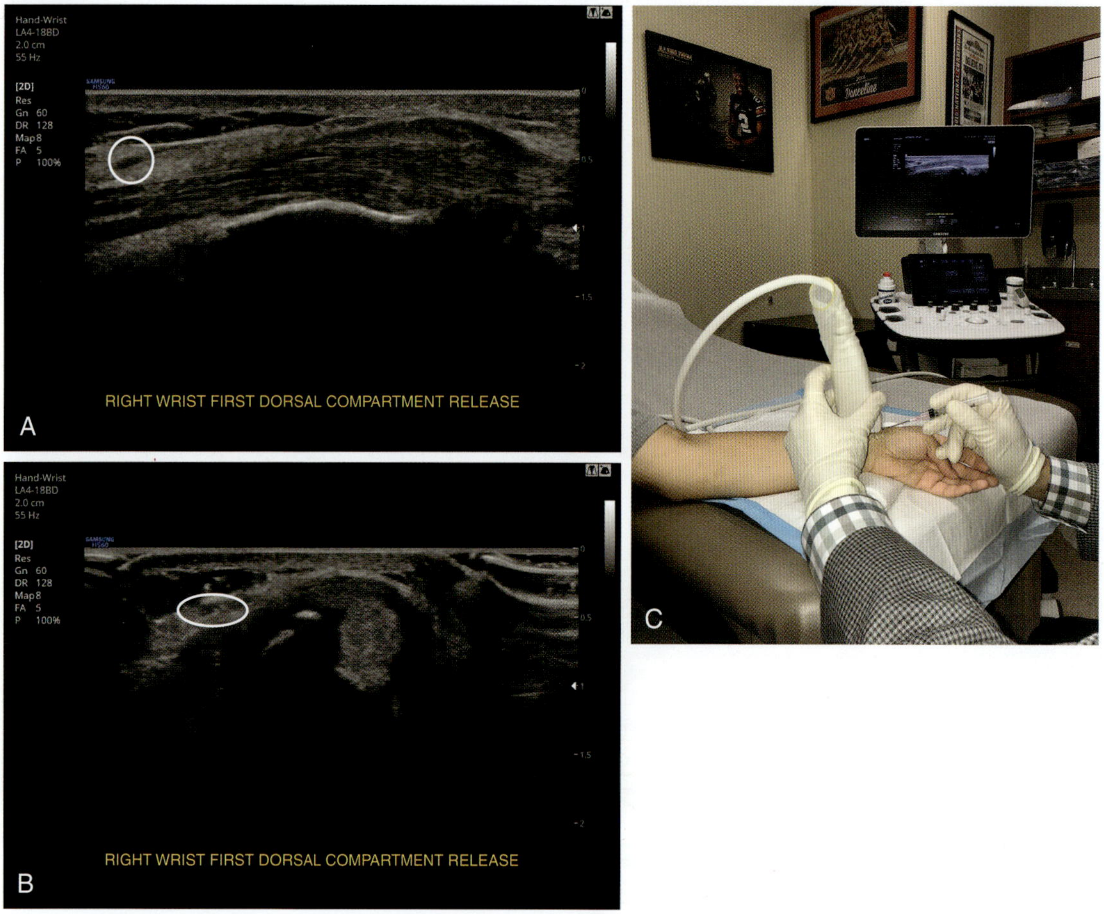

• **Fig. 28.7** Ultrasound images of abductor pollicis longus and extensor pollicis brevis at the end of the radius and patient position. (A) Longitudinal view of tendons showing intact extensor retinaculum with the finger in full extension. (*Circle:* small cutaneous branch from superficial radial nerve.) (B) Cross-sectional view of the tendons showing intact extensor retinaculum. (*Oval:* superficial radial nerve.) (C) Position of patient, clinician, transducer, needle, and ultrasound machine.

a regular hypodermic needle (20 or 21 gauge) has also been described in the literature.[38]

- Ultrasound machine with a high-frequency linear array transducer.

Technique

Patient Position

- Seated or supine with the wrist in neutral between pronation and supination (thumb up). The radial side of the distal forearm and wrist is cleansed in sterile fashion in order to create a sterile field (see Fig. 28.7C).

Clinician Position

- Seated distal and volar to the thumb.

Transducer Orientation

- Short axis to identify the neurovascular structure and perform the nerve block.
- Longitudinal axis over the tendons of the first dorsal compartment of the wrist for the release.

Nerve Block

Needle Orientation

- In-plane with the transducer in short axis to the superficial radial nerve about 3 inches proximal to the first dorsal compartment of the wrist.

Target

- Inject using the 25-gauge, 1.5-inch needle to create a superficial radial nerve block.
- Then inject additional local anesthesia from distal to proximal in longitudinal axis over the first dorsal compartment, injecting into the soft tissue and tendon sheath.

de Quervain Release

Needle Orientation

- In-plane with the transducer, with a distal to proximal approach toward the first dorsal compartment of the wrist.

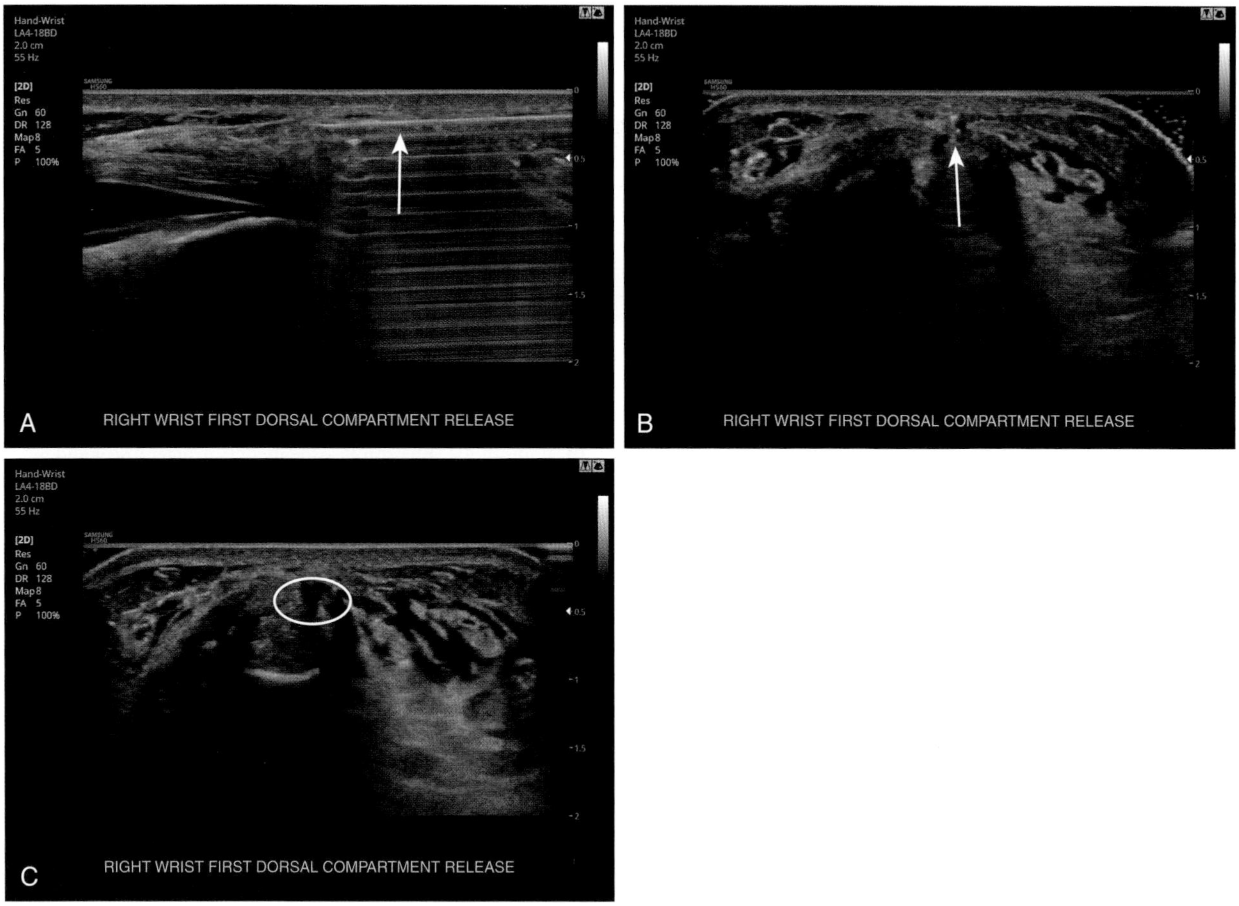

• **Fig. 28.8** The extensor retinaculum during the procedure and after the incision made. *Arrow*: location of the 18-gauge, 1.5-inch needle with a blade at the tip. (A) Longitudinal view of the needle cutting the extensor retinaculum. (B) Short-axis view of the needle cutting the extensor retinaculum. (C) Short-axis view of the extensor retinaculum post-procedure with the incision created. (*Oval*: incision through the extensor retinaculum.)

Target

- Create a puncture incision in the skin using the 18-gauge Nokor needle and advance toward the extensor retinaculum and first dorsal compartment.
- Make an incision through the extensor retinaculum and tendon sheath from distal to proximal (Fig. 28.8A–C). Irrigate the tendon with normal saline solution to ensure a complete release.

Injectate Volume

- Local anesthesia: 3 mL 1% lidocaine plain for the superficial radial nerve block
- 1 mL to 3 mL of local anesthetic; Author prefers 1% lidocaine with epinephrine (1:100,000)
- Irrigation: 3 mL normal saline solution

Pearls and Pitfalls

- Avoid puncturing the neurovascular structures and blood vessels by keeping the Nokor needle tip (blade) in the visual field at all times.
- Complete release of the first dorsal compartment may be confirmed after the procedure applying the Colberg criteria mentioned above.
- Complete incision of the extensor retinaculum can be seen in Fig. 28.8C.
- Patients can perform all basic activities of daily living and light duties as tolerated 24 hours post-procedure. A thumb spica brace may be offered for severe cases to be worn for 1 week in order to avoid instability of the tendon.
- Patients may have mild residual soft tissue swelling after the release that will resolve within the first 4 weeks post-procedure.
- If done correctly, patients should not feel any residual catching/locking after the procedure.
- Avoid immobilizing for more than 1 week after the procedure in order to minimize scar tissue formation around the tendon that may lead to extension contracture.
- This procedure should be avoided in patients that previously had a surgery in the first dorsal compartment of the wrist, have widespread hand pain, or complex regional pain syndrome.

Post-Procedure

An adhesive bandage is placed over the puncture incision and it may be removed 24 hours post-procedure. Patients are given a thumb spica brace to wear during the night for 1 week and are instructed to avoid heavy lifting or gripping for 2 weeks. Patients can perform all basic activities of daily living and light duties as tolerated 24 hours post-procedure. If there is pain, patients can ice the treated area and take acetaminophen or an over-the-counter NSAID as needed. Patients may have mild residual soft tissue swelling after the release that typically resolve within the first 4 weeks post-procedure.

Complications Post-Procedure

Complications are rare and include residual pain, infection, bruising, tendon laceration, neurovascular injury, incomplete release, and instability of the tendons leading to subluxation.[38,40,47] These complications are similar to the ones seen with an open surgical release.[48,49] Open surgery carries a risk of adverse events of up to 42%, including pain, nerve injury, wound complications, and tendon subluxation.[48] Ultrasound minimizes the risks associated with open surgery, especially the risk of neurovascular injury since the nerves and blood vessels can be visualized at all times.[5,50] Tendon subluxation is a rare complication, but if present may require surgery to repair the retinaculum. Immobilization with the thumb spica splint attempts to reduce the risk of subluxation.[51] In addition, given the anatomic variability of the superficial radial nerve and its branches, there is also risk of injuring this nerve or one of the branches and they should be identified with ultrasound imaging prior to initiating the procedure.[52,53] Given this, a palpation-guided release is not recommended for de Quervain tenosynovitis due to the high risk of neurovascular injury. Ultrasound guidance should always be used.

References

1. Nikolaou VS, Malahias MA, Kaseta MK, Sourlas I, Babis GC. Comparative clinical study of ultrasound-guided A1 pulley release vs open surgical intervention in the treatment of trigger finger. *World J Orthop*. 2017;8(2):163.
2. Smith J, Rizzo M, Lai JK. Sonographically guided percutaneous first annular pulley release. *J Ultrasound Med*. 2010;29(11):1531–1542.
3. Weiss ND, Richter MB. Percutaneous release of trigger digits. *Am J Orthop (Belle Mead, NJ)*. 2017;46(4):E263–E267.
4. Werthel JD, Cortez M, Elhassan BT. Modified percutaneous trigger finger release. *Hand Surg Rehabil*. 2016;35(3):179–182.
5. Zhao JG, Kan SL, Zhao L, et al. Percutaneous first annular pulley release for trigger digits: a systematic review and meta-analysis of current evidence. *J Hand Surg*. 2014;39(11):2192–2202.
6. Gilberts EC, Beekman WH, Stevens HJ, Wereldsma JC. Prospective randomized trial of open versus percutaneous surgery for trigger digits. *J Hand Surg*. 2001;26(3):497–500.
7. Dierks U, Hoffmann R, Meek MF. Open versus percutaneous release of the A1-pulley for stenosing tendovaginitis: a prospective randomized trial. *Tech Hand Extrem Surg*. 2008;12(3):183–187.
8. Colberg R, Fleisig G, Drogosz M, Pantuosco J. A novel U/S-guided trigger finger release and diagnostic testing techniques. Oral poster session presented at: 2019 AMSSM Annual Meeting. 28th Annual Meeting for the American Medical Society for Sports Medicine; April 12–17, 2019; Orlando, FL.
9. Fiorini HJ, Santos JBG, Hirakawa CK, Sato ES, Faloppa F, Albertoni WM. Anatomical study of the A1 pulley: length and location by means of cutaneous landmarks on the palmar surface. *J Hand Surg*. 2011;36A:464–468.
10. Wilhelmi BJ, Snyder NIV, Verbesey JE, Ganchi PA, Lee WP. Trigger finger release with hand surface landmark ratios: an anatomic and clinical study. *Plast Reconstr Surg*. 2001;108:908–915.
11. Kaplan 3rd SJ, FW. Anatomical study of the A1 pulley: length and location by means of cutaneous landmarks on the palmar surface. *J Hand Surg*. 2011;36(6):1114.
12. Langer D, Maeir A, Michailevich M, Luria S. Evaluating hand function in clients with trigger finger. *Occupation Therap Intl*. 2017;2017.
13. Lundin AC, Eliasson P, Aspenberg P. Trigger finger and tendinosis. *J Hand Surg (European Volume)*. 2012;37(3):233–236.
14. Quinnell RC. Conservative management of trigger finger. *The Practitioner*. 1980;224:187–190.
15. Guerini H, Pessis E, Theumann N, et al. Sonographic appearance of trigger fingers. *J Ultrasound Med*. 2008;27(10):1407–1413.
16. Sato J, Ishii Y, Noguchi H, Takeda M. Sonographic appearance of the flexor tendon, volar plate, and A1 pulley with respect to the severity of trigger finger. *J Hand Surg*. 2012;37(10).
17. Amirfeyz R, McNinch R, Watts A, et al. Evidence-based management of adult trigger digits. *J Hand Surg*. 2017;42(5):473–480.
18. Lee DH, Han SB, Park JW, et al. Sonographically guided tendon sheath injections: implications for trigger finger treatment. *J Ultrasound Med*. 2011;30(2):197–203.
19. Mardani-Kivi M, Karimi-Mobarakeh M, Babaei Jandaghi A, Keyhani S, Saheb-Ekhtiari K, Hashemi-Motlagh K. Intra-sheath versus extra-sheath ultrasound guided corticosteroid injection for trigger finger: a triple blinded randomized clinical trial. *Physician Sportsmed*. 2017:1–5.
20. Patel MR, Bassini L. Trigger fingers and the thumb: when to splint, inject or operate. *J Hand Surg Am*. 1992;17(1):110–113.
21. Rodgers JA, McCarthy JA, Tiedeman JJ. Trigger fingers and themb: when to splint, inject and operatre. *Orthopedics*. 1998;21(3): discussion 309–310.
22. Benan DA, Nakhdjevani A, Lloyd MA, Schreuder FB. The efficacy of steroid injection in the treatment of trigger finger. *Clin Orthop Surg*. 2012;4(4):263–268.
23. Rozental TD, Zurakowsky D, Blazer PE. Trigger finger prognostic indicator of recurrence following corticosteroid injection. *J Bone Joint Surg Am*. 2008;90(8):1665–1672.
24. Benson LS, Ptaszek AJ. Injection versus surgery in the treatment of trigger finger. *J Hand Surg Am*. 1997;22(1):138–144.
25. Kuo LC, Su FC, Tung WL, Lai KY, Jou IM. Kinematical and functional improvements of trigger digits after sonographically assisted percutaneous release of the A1 pulley. *J Orthop Res*. 2009;27(7):891–896.
26. Marij Z, Aurangzeb Q, Rizwan HR, Haroon R, Pervaiz MH. Outpatient percutaneous release of trigger finger: a cost effective and safe procedure. *Malaysian Orthop J*. 2017;11(1):52.
27. Mishra SR, Gaur AK, Choudhary MM, Ramesh J. Percutaneous A1 pulley release by the tip of a 20G hypodermic needle before open surgical procedure in trigger finger management. *Techniques Hand Upper Extremity Surg*. 2013;17(2):112–115.
28. Rojo-Manaute JM, Rodríguez-Maruri G, Capa-Grasa A, Chana-Rodríguez F, Soto MD, Martín JV. Sonographically guided intrasheath percutaneous release of the first annular pulley for trigger digits, Part 1. *J Ultrasound Med*. 2012;31(3):417–424.

29. Jou IM, Chern TC. Sonographically assisted percutaneous release of the A1 pulley: a new surgical technique for treating trigger digit. *J Hand Surg*. 2006;31(2):191–199.
30. Ilicki J. Safety of epinephrine in digital nerve blocks: a literature review. *J Emerg Med*. 2015;49(5):799–809.
31. Salim N, Abdullah S, Sapuan J, Haflah NH. Outcome of corticosteroid injection versus physiotherapy in the treatment of mild trigger fingers. *J Hand Surg Eur Vol*. 2012;37(1):27–34.
32. Paulius KL, Maguina P. Ultrasound-assisted percutaneous trigger finger release: is it safe? *Hand*. 2009;4(1):35–37.
33. Cebesoy O, Karakurum G, Kose KC, Baltaci ET, Isik M. Percutaneous release of the trigger thumb: is it safe, cheap and effective? *Int Orthopaedic*. 2007;31(3):345–349.
34. Everding NG, Bishop GB, Belyea CM, Soong MC. Risk factors for complications of open trigger finger release. *Hand*. 2015;10(2):297–300.
35. Finsen V, Hagen S. Surgery for trigger finger. *Hand Surg*. 2003;8(2):201–203.
36. Will R, Lubahn J. Complications of open trigger finger release. *J Hand Surg Am*. 2010;34(4):594–596.
37. Siddiqui AA, Rajput IM, Adeel M. Outcome of percutaneous release for trigger digits in diabetic and non-diabetic patients. *Cureus*. 2019;11(5):e4585.
38. Lapègue F, André A, Pasquier Bernachot E, et al. US-guided percutaneous release of the first extensor tendon compartment using a 21-gauge needle in de Quervain's disease: a prospective study of 35 cases. *Eur Radiol*. 2018.
39. Colberg RE, Henderson RG. Ultrasound-guided first dorsal compartment release for refractory de Quervain tenosynovitis: a case report. *PM R*. 2019;11(6):665.
40. Sato J, Ishii Y, Noguchi H. Ultrasonographic evaluation of the prevalence of an intracompartmental septum in patients with de Quervain's disease. *Orthopedics*. 2016;39(2):112–116.
41. Peck E, Ely E. Successful treatment of de Quervain tenosynovitis with ultrasound-guided percutaneous needle tenotomy and platelet-rich plasma injection: a case presentation. *PM R*. 2013;5(5):438–441.
42. Som A, Singh P. *Finkelstein Sign*. StatPearls Publishing. 2019.
43. Roh YH, Noh JH, Gong HS, Baek GH. Effects of metabolic syndrome on the functional outcomes of corticosteroid injection for de Quervain tenosynovitis. *J Hand Surg Euro Vol*. 2017;42(5):481.
44. Huisstede BM, Gladdines S, Randsdorp MS, Koes BW. Effectiveness of conservative, surgical, and post-surgical interventions for trigger finger, Dupuytren's disease, and de Quervain's disease. A systematic review. *Archives Physical Med Rehabil*. 2017.
45. Cavaleri R, Schabrun SM, Te M, Chipchase LS. Hand therapy versus corticosteroid injections in the treatment of de Quervain's disease: a systematic review and meta-analysis. *J Hand Therap*. 2016;29(1):3–11.
46. Kutsikovich J, Merrell G. Accuracy of injection into the first dorsal compartment: a cadaveric ultrasound study. *J Hand Surg*. 2018;43(8): 777–e1.
47. Güleç A, Türkmen F, Toker S, Acar MA. Percutaneous release of the first dorsal extensor compartment: a cadaver study. *Plastic Reconstru Surg Global Open*. 2016;4(10).
48. Rogozinski B, Lourie GM. Dissatisfaction after first dorsal compartment release for de Quervain tendinopathy. *J Hand Surg Am*. 2016;41(1):117–119.
49. Bruijnzeel H, Neuhaus V, Fostvedt S, Jupiter JB, Mudgal CS, Ring DC. Adverse events of open A1 pulley release for idiopathic trigger finger. *J Hand Surg Am*. 2012;37(8):1650–1656.
50. Danda RS, Kamath J, Jayasheelan N, Kumar P. Role of ultrasound in the treatment of de Quervain tenosynovitis by local steroid infiltration. *J Hand Microsurg*. 2016;8(1):34–37.
51. Horn BJ, Zondervan R, Hornbach E. Prevention of tendon subluxation in de Quervain's tenosynovitis release using retinacular repair. *Spartan Med Res J*. 2016;1(1):4705.
52. Abrams RA, Brown RA, Botte MJ. The superficial branch of the radial nerve: an anatomic study with surgical implications. *J Hand Surg*. 1992;17(6):1037–1041.
53. Robson AJ, See MS, Ellis H. Applied anatomy of the superficial branch of the radial nerve. *Clin Anat*. 2008;21(1):38–45.

29 Compartment Pressure Testing

JONATHAN T. FINNOFF AND JACOB REISNER

KEY POINTS

- Chronic exertional compartment syndrome (CECS) is a painful condition characterized by an increase in intracompartmental pressure (ICP) with exercise.[1]
- This is seen most commonly in the four muscular compartments of the leg but has also been described in the foot, the four compartments of the arm, and the hand.[1,2] This chapter focuses on compartment pressure testing for the leg, but the principles can be applied to the other locations.
- Preexercise and postexercise ICP is the "gold standard" test to diagnose CECS.
- Compartment pressures are obtained by inserting an ICP monitor with palpation guidance into the four compartments of the leg.
- ICPs are obtained prior to exercise and at 1 minute and 5 minutes post exercise.
- CECS is confirmed using the Pedowitz criteria[3] if the preexercise ICP greater than 15 mm Hg, 1-minute postexercise ICP greater than 30 mm Hg, or 5-minute postexercise ICP greater than 20 mm Hg.

Pertinent Anatomy

The leg contains four distinct compartments: anterior, lateral, superficial posterior, and deep posterior.[2] The anterior compartment contains the tibialis anterior muscle, extensor hallicus longus muscle, extensor digitorum longus muscle, peroneus tertius muscle, deep peroneal nerve, and the anterior tibial artery and vein.[2] The lateral compartment contains the peroneus longus muscle, peroneus brevis muscle, and superficial peroneal nerve (which exits through the fascia of the lateral compartment in the distal third of the leg).[2] The superficial posterior compartment contains the plantaris muscle, gastrocnemius muscle, soleus muscle, sural nerve, and branches of tibial artery and vein.[2] The deep posterior compartment contains the flexor digitorum longus muscle, tibialis posterior muscle, flexor hallucis longus muscle, popliteus muscle, tibial nerve, posterior tibial artery and vein, and the peroneal artery and vein.[2] The tibialis posterior muscle is contained in its own fascia and is sometimes referred to as the fifth compartment of the leg.[2]

Common Pathology

Chronic exertional compartment syndrome (CECS) most commonly affects the anterior (40% to 60%) and deep posterior compartments (32% to 60%), followed by the lateral (12% to 35%) and superficial posterior compartments (2% to 20%).[2] Thickened and less-compliant compartment fascia, reduced microcapillary capacity, and venous congestion have all been postulated to contribute to the development of CECS, but the pathophysiology is still debated.[2]

In normal muscle physiology, there is a 20% increase in muscle volume during exercise and, as a result, intracompartmental pressure (ICP) increases.[4] In CECS, increased compartment pressure during exercise may also lead to transient neuropraxia manifesting as transient changes in sensation and strength. The neurologic symptoms are related to the nerve contained in the effected compartment. CECS involving the anterior compartment may present with deep peroneal neuropraxia with foot drop and first web space numbness that progressively develops with activity.[2] CECS of the lateral compartment may present with activity-related progressive ankle eversion weakness and dorsal foot numbness.[2] CECS involving the superficial and/or deep posterior compartment may present with activity-related progressive plantar foot paresthesias and ankle plantar flexion weakness.[2]

The differential diagnosis for CECS includes medial tibial stress syndromes, stress fracture, fascial defects or herniations, popliteal artery entrapment syndrome, claudication, peripheral nerve entrapment syndromes, and lumbosacral radiculopathy. Clinical suspicion will guide the work-up, but ICP testing is the "gold standard" test to confirm the diagnosis of CECS.[2–4] Normally, increases in compartment pressures return to normal within 3 to 5 minutes after exercise.[4] A delay in normalizing pressures or pre-exercise pressure measurements greater than 15 mm Hg are suggestive of CECS.[4] The Pedowitz criteria (Table 29.1) are the established gold standard for diagnosing CECS.

Equipment

- STIC ICP Monitor System (C2Dx, Schoolcraft, MI); or Compass ICP Monitor System (Centurion Medical Products, Williamston, MI).
- ChloraPrep skin applicator (Becton Dickenson, Franklin Lakes, NJ)
- Needle size: 27 gauge, 1.25 inch for local anesthesia and 18-gauge 2.5-inch ICP monitor needle
- Local anesthesia: 1% lidocaine
- Sterile gauze
- Tubular elastic retention netting
- Bandages

Technique

Patient Position

- Supine with bolsters supporting both ankles.

TABLE 29.1 Pedowitz Criteria for the Diagnosis of Chronic Exertional Compartment Syndrome by Intracompartmental Pressure.[3]

Time	Pressure measurement
Pre exercise	>15 mm Hg
1-min post exercise	>30 mm Hg
5-min post exercise	>20 mm Hg

Clinician Position

- Standing next to patient.

Needle Position

- Anterior compartment (Fig. 29.1A): four fingerbreadths below the tibial tuberosity and one fingerbreadth lateral to the tibial crest directed in an anterior to posterior direction.[5]
- Lateral compartment (see Fig. 29.1B): three fingerbreadths below the fibular head directed in a lateral to medial direction toward the fibula.[5]
- Superficial posterior compartment (see Fig. 29.1C): one handbreadth below the popliteal crease over the medial mass of the calf directed to toward the medial head of the gastrocnemius.[5]
- Deep posterior compartment (see Fig. 29.1D): one handbreadth distal to the tibial tuberosity and one fingerbreadth posterior the medial edge of the tibia. The needle is directed in a medial to lateral direction through the soleus into the deep posterior compartment. This occurs at a depth of approximately 4 cm.[5]

Protocol

- The needle entry site is marked with a skin marker.
- The skin at the needle entry site is cleansed using ChloraPrep skin applicator.
- The skin and subcutaneous tissue at the needle entry site are anesthetized using approximately 1 mL of 1% lidocaine. Care is taken not to inject local anesthetic into the muscles of the compartment.

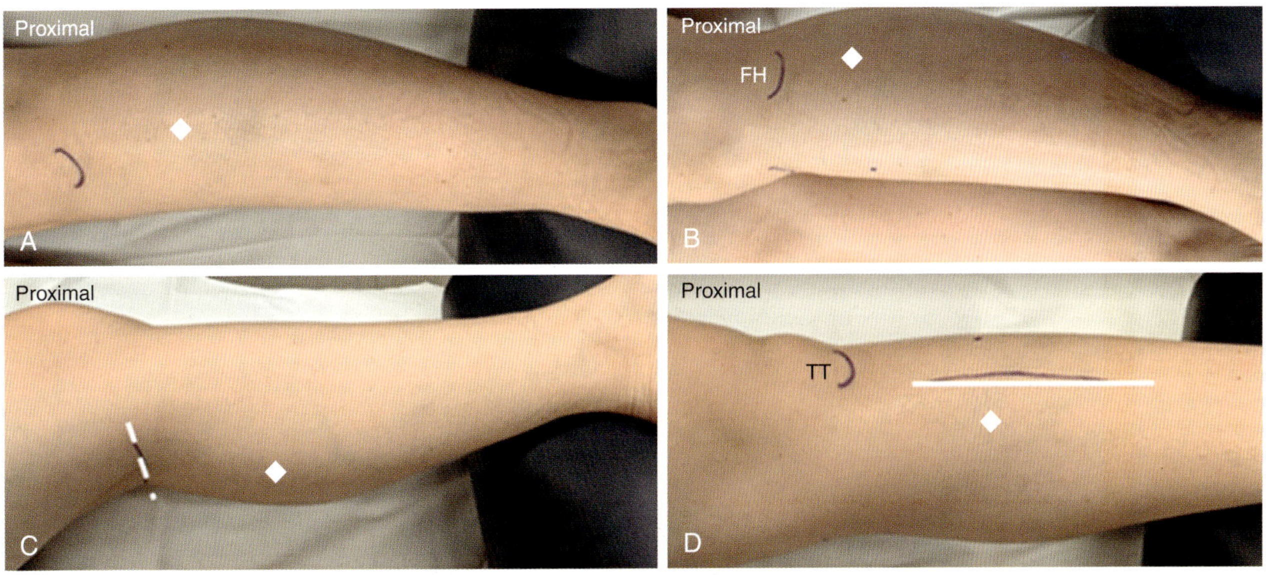

• **Fig. 29.1** Needle Entry Sites for Intracompartmental Pressure Testing of the Four Leg Compartments. (A) Anterior compartment. (B) Lateral compartment. (C) Superficial posterior compartment. (D) Deep posterior compartment. *Diamond*, needle entry site; *dashed line*, popliteal crease; *FH*, fibular head; *solid line*, medial edge of tibia; *TT*, tibial tubercle.

- The ICP monitor is assembled as directed by the manufacturer.
- The ICP monitor is turned on and aligned in the position of needle insertion.
- The ICP monitor is zeroed while holding the pressure monitor in the same plane/position that it will be inserted into the compartment.
- A small amount of saline is injected into the compartment to create a continuous fluid cylinder into the compartment.
- The compartment pressure monitor is held in position until the compartment pressure stabilizes, at which time the compartment pressure is recorded.

PEARLS AND PITFALLS

- Based on the study by Peck et al.,[6] ultrasound-guided needle placement was not shown to be superior to palpation-guided needle placement based on surface landmarks described by Perotta et al.[5]
- A bolster is used to "float" the calf musculature to eliminate the theoretical risk of spuriously elevating compartment pressures due to direct pressure to the compartments by the examination table.
- Care should be taken to only anesthetize the skin and subcutaneous tissues at the needle entry sites to eliminate introducing fluid into the compartment which may theoretically elevate the compartment pressure.
- Patients should be encouraged to exercise until their leg pain is maximal. Ideally, the activity that provokes their symptoms should be used for the exercise portion of the test.
- The normal saline used for the intracompartmental pressure monitor can be replaced with 1% lidocaine, thereby reducing pain during compartment pressure testing.

- The ICP monitor needle is withdrawn from the compartment
- Sterile gauze is applied over the needle entry site.
- Tubular elastic retention netting is donned to secure gauze in place.
- The patient follows a graded exercise protocol until maximal symptoms are achieved.
- Patients discontinue exercising and are immediately taken to the examination room.
- They are placed in a supine position with their ankles on a bolster.
- The tubular elastic retention netting is cut off and the compartment(s) in question are retested at 1 and 5 minutes post exercise.
- The needle entry site is covered by a simple dressing.

References

1. Liu B, Barrazueta G, Ruchelsman DE. Chronic exertional compartment syndrome in athletes. *J Hand Surg Am*. 2017;42(11):917–923.
2. Rajasekaran S, Finnoff JT. Exertional leg pain. *Phys Med Rehabil Clin N Am*. 2016;27(1):91–119.
3. Pedowitz RA, Hargens AR, Mubarak SJ, Gershuni DH. Modified criteria for the objective diagnosis of chronic compartment syndrome of the leg. *Am J Sports Med*. 1990;18(1):35–40.
4. Brennan Jr FH, Kane SF. Diagnosis, treatment options, and rehabilitation of chronic lower leg exertional compartment syndrome. *Curr Sports Med Rep*. 2003;2(5):247–250.
5. Perotto A. *Anatomical Guide for the Electromyographer*, 5th ed. Springfield, IL: Thomas Books; 2011.
6. Peck E, Finnoff JT, Smith J, Curtiss H, Muir J, Hollman JH. Accuracy of palpation-guided and ultrasound-guided needle tip placement into the deep and superficial posterior leg compartments. *Am J Sports Med*. 2011;39(9):1968–1974.
7. Peck E, Finnoff JT, Smith J. Neuropathies in runners. *Clin Sports Med*. 2010;29(3):437–457.

30 Ultrasound-Guided Anterior and Lateral Compartment Fasciotomies for Chronic Exertional Compartment Syndrome

JONATHAN T. FINNOFF AND JACOB REISNER

KEY POINTS

- Chronic exertional compartment syndrome (CECS) is characterized by pain and increased intracompartmental pressure with exertion.[1]
- Ultrasound-guided (USG) fasciotomies have been described for the treatment of anterior and lateral leg compartment CECS.[2]
- USG fasciotomies are performed through a 3-mm skin incision, reducing tissue trauma, and potentially reducing complications, and facilitating more rapid return to activity.[2]

Pertinent Anatomy and Common Pathology

For more information refer to Chapter 29 (Compartment Pressure Testing).

Traditional Treatment Options

There are several nonsurgical treatment options for chronic exertional compartment syndrome (CECS). Activity modification is one option in cases where a specific activity (i.e., cycling or running) provokes symptoms.[1] In runners with anterior compartment symptoms and a heel strike pattern, gait re-training and adopting a forefoot running pattern may assist in treating CECS.[1,2] Intramuscular botulinum toxin A injections have also been used in the treatment of CECS.[4–6] However, their duration of action is limited and anterior compartment injections can cause temporary weakness, resulting in foot drop. Ultrasound-guided (USG) needle fenestration of the anterior and lateral compartments was reported as a treatment in the case of a collegiate lacrosse player with CECS, who returned to full activity after 10 days and had resolution of symptoms at the 18-month follow-up.[7]

Open surgical fasciotomy is the traditional and best-described definitive treatment for CECS.[1,7] Waterman et al.[7] reviewed 754 fasciotomy procedures performed for CECS in a military population. In this population 77% of cases involved a release of both the anterior and lateral compartments. They reported a complication rate of 15.7%, with infection being the most common followed by neurologic injury. The recurrence rate was 44.7%, and 5.9% went on to surgical revision.[8] More recently, endoscopic procedures involving a balloon catheter dilation have been described.[9] Ultrasound-assisted surgical procedures also have been reported in a recent case series. This procedure utilized Metzenbaum scissors but required initial nonguided blunt dissection to the fascial plane.[10]

USG fasciotomy using a V-shaped meniscotome for the anterior and lateral compartments was first described in a cadaveric model by Lueders et al. in 2017.[2] Since then it has been translated into clinical practice and was recently described in a case report of a 41-year-old female runner who underwent anterior compartment USG fasciotomy without complications; she returned to full activity 7 days after the procedure.[11] Recently, a retrospective review of

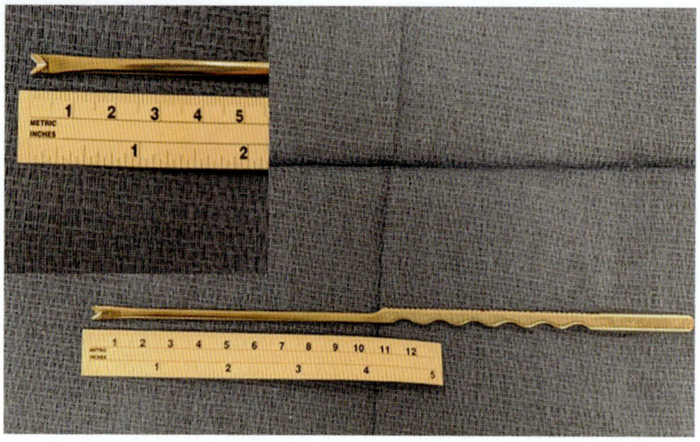

• **Fig. 30.1** Three-millimeter V-shaped meniscotome.

50 USG fasciotomies showed a single complication, "sharp nerve pain," that resolved without treatment in 2 weeks, and an average return to full activity of 10 days.[12]

Equipment

- High-resolution ultrasound machine with a high-frequency linear array transducer.
- Indelible marker.
- Needle size: 25-guage, 2-inch and 22-gauge, 3.5-inch needles.
- Local anesthetic: a mixture of 4 mL 1% lidocaine, 4 mL 0.5% lidocaine with epinephrine, 4 mL of 0.2% ropivacaine, and 8 mL of sterile saline per compartment.
- Number 11-blade scalpel.
- A 3.00-mm V-shaped meniscotome (Smith and Nephew, Inc., Andover, MA) (Fig. 30.1).
- Skin closure: Dermabond (Ethicon, LLC, San Lorenzo, Puerto Rico), benzoin tincture (3M, Maplewood, MN), and three ¼ × 1.5-inch Steri-Strips (3M, Maplewood, MN).

Technique

Pre-Procedure Planning—Anterior Compartment

- The anterior compartment borders are identified with ultrasound.
- The common peroneal nerve (CPN), superficial peroneal nerve (SPN), and deep peroneal nerve (DPN) are identified and their course is marked on the skin.
- The start (3 cm distal to tibial tuberosity) and finish (10 cm proximal to the inferior aspect of the lateral malleolus) locations for the procedure are marked on the skin.
- The optimal course of the fasciotomy from proximal to distal is determined with ultrasound and marked on the skin.

Pre-Procedure Planning—Lateral Compartment

- The lateral compartment borders are identified with ultrasound.
- The CPN and SPN are identified and their course is marked on the skin.
- The start (3 cm distal to the fibular head) and finish (10 cm proximal to the inferior aspect of the lateral malleolus) locations for the procedure are marked on the skin.
- The optimal course of the fasciotomy from proximal to distal is determined with ultrasound and marked on the skin.

Patient Position

- Supine.
- Legs extended in neutral rotation.

Clinician Position

- Seated next to the patient.

Local Anesthesia

Transducer Position

- Alternating between the long- and short-axis views relative to the needle/meniscotome trajectory.

Needle Position

- Alternating between a 25-gauge, 2-inch needle and 22-guage, 3.5-inch needle, guided in-plane relative to the ultrasound transducer, the skin surface at the proximal incision site, adjacent subcutaneous tissues, and the fascia along the pre-marked course of the fasciotomy are anesthetized.
- Multiple needle entry sites, spaced approximately 3 inches apart, are required to anesthetize the entire length of the fascia.

Injectate Volume

- 10 to 20 mL per compartment.
- Recommended injectate: a mixture of 4 mL of 1% lidocaine, 4 mL of 0.5% lidocaine with epinephrine, 4 mL of 0.2% ropivacaine, and 8 mL of sterile saline.

Target

- Superficial to the fascia and deep to the subcutaneous tissue layer.
- The injection will create a plane, separating the subcutaneous tissue from fascia.

Fasciotomy

Transducer Position

- Alternate between long-short-axis views relative to the meniscotome.

Meniscotome Position

- A No.11-blade scalpel is used to make a 3-mm skin incision at the proximal fasciotomy start site for each respective compartment (Fig. 30.2).
- The V-shaped meniscotome is introduced through the skin incision in a proximal to distal direction.
- The deep portion of the meniscotome is pushed through the fascia while maintaining the superficial portion of the meniscotome above the fascia, such that the fascia is captured in the cleft of the V-shaped cutting blade.

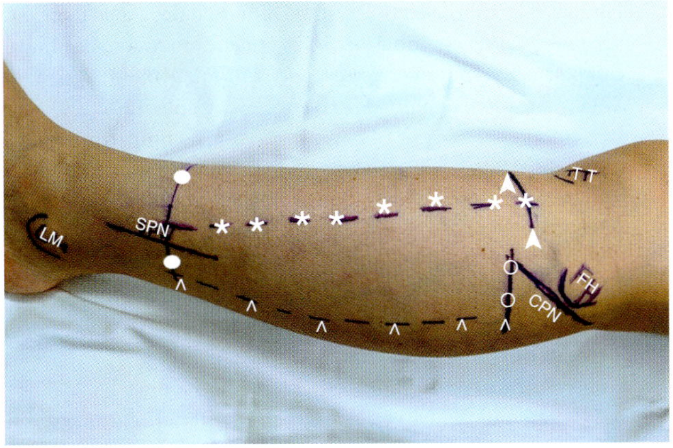

• **Fig. 30.2** Anatomy Pre-Scan Markings. Anterior compartment fasciotomy course (*asterisk*). Lateral compartment fasciotomy course (*open arrows*). Proximal border of anterior compartment fasciotomy (*arrowheads*) and lateral compartment fasciotomy border (*open circles*). Distal border of anterior and lateral compartment fasciotomies (*closed circles*). *CPN*, Common peroneal nerve; *FH*, fibular head; *LM*, lateral malleolus; *SPN*, superficial peroneal nerve; *TT*, tibial tubercle.

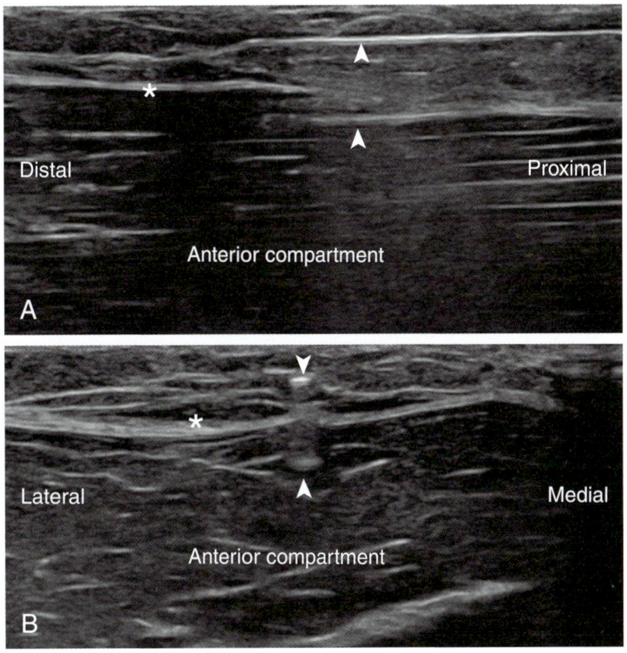

• **Fig. 30.3** (A) Long-axis view of V-shaped meniscotome cutting through fascia of anterior compartment with superficial blade seen superficial to fascia and deep blade seen deep to the fascia. (B) Short-axis view of the V-shaped meniscotome cutting the fascia of the anterior compartment with the tip of the superficial blade seen superficial to the fascia and the tip of the deep blade seen deep to the fascia. *, Anterior compartment fascia; *arrowhead*, V-shaped meniscotome.

- The V-shaped meniscotome is advanced distally along the predetermined fasciotomy course, maintaining visualization on the meniscotome cutting blade with ultrasound.
- Care is taken to ensure the fascia remains in the cleft of the V-shaped cutting blade to ensure the fascia is transected as the meniscotome is advanced (Fig. 30.3).

Target

- The fascia is transected by the meniscotome along the predetermined fasciotomy course from the start to finish locations to ensure adequate transection of the fascia.

Skin Closure

- Dermabond is used to approximate the skin margins.
- Two inches of benzoin tincture is applied circumferentially around the incision site and allowed to dry.
- Three ¼ × 1.5-inch Steri-Strips are applied across the incision site to re-enforce the Dermabond closure.
- Compressive sleeves or stockings are placed over the leg.

Post-Procedure Instructions

Ice the area three to four times per day for 15 minutes for 7 days. Elevate the legs for a minimum of 15 minutes several times a day for 7 days. Ambulate as tolerated after the procedure. Increase activity as tolerated after 7 days. Wear compressive sleeves or stockings for 3 to 4 weeks. Perform self-massage/tissue mobilization for 3 to 4 weeks.

Potential Complications

Potential complications include injury to the CPN or SPN. Care should be taken to identify and mark each nerve's course in relation to the planned fasciotomy (see Fig. 30.2). Pain and swelling at the incision site and along the fasciotomy course may be observed. This may be mitigated with post-procedure compression. Finally, with the skin incision, local infection is a potential complication. Although the procedure is performed in an office-based setting, sterile technique is utilized at all times and the patient is advised not to submerge the incision for 48 hours.

Pearls and Pitfalls

- Oral analgesics may be considered prior to and immediately after the procedure for patient comfort.
- A 22-gauge, 3.5-inch needle can be placed under the ultrasound probe on the patient's skin to assist in marking the course of relevant structures (e.g., CPN, DPN, and SPN).
- Frequently alternate between long- and short-axis views to ensure the fascia remains in the cleft of the V-shaped meniscotome tip throughout the procedure (see Fig. 30.3).
- Keeping the deep portion of the V-shaped meniscotome just deep to the fascia may reduce muscle tissue damage and pain during the procedure.
- Frequently alternate between long- and short-axis views to ensure the meniscotome is advanced under direct ultrasound visualization while monitoring relevant adjacent tissues/structures (e.g., neurovascular structures, tendons, etc.), and ensuring the meniscotome remains on the pre-planned fasciotomy course.
- Additional local anesthetic may be administered during the fasciotomy for patient comfort. This may be injected in a distal to proximal direction to allow the meniscotome to remain in place.

- Post-procedure, ice, compression, and elevation will reduce swelling.

References

1. Diebal AR, Gregory R, Alitz C, Gerber JP. Effects of forefoot running on chronic exertional compartment syndrome: a case series. *Int J Sports Phys Ther.* 2011;6(4):312–321.
2. Rajasekaran S, Finnoff JT. Exertional leg pain. *Phys Med Rehabil Clin N Am.* 2016;27(1):91–119.
3. Lueders DR, Sellon JL, Smith J, Finnoff JT. Ultrasound-guided fasciotomy for chronic exertional compartment syndrome: a cadaveric investigation. *PM R.* 2017;9(7):683–690.
4. Isner-Horobeti ME, Dufour SP, Blaes C, Lecocq J. Intramuscular pressure before and after botulinum toxin in chronic exertional compartment syndrome of the leg: a preliminary study. *Am J Sports Med.* 2013;41(11):2558–2566.
5. Hutto WM, Schroeder PB, Leggit JC. Botulinum toxin as a novel treatment for chronic exertional compartment syndrome in the U.S. military. *Mil Med.* 2019;184(5-6):e458–e461.
6. Baria MR, Sellon JL. Botulinum toxin for chronic exertional compartment syndrome: a case report with 14 month follow-up. *Clin J Sport Med.* 2016;26(6):e111–e113.
7. Finnoff JT, Rajasekaran S. Ultrasound-guided, percutaneous needle fascial fenestration for the treatment of chronic exertional compartment syndrome: a case report. *PM R.* 2016;8(3):286–290.
8. Waterman BR, Laughlin M, Kilcoyne K, Cameron KL, Owens BD. Surgical treatment of chronic exertional compartment syndrome of the leg: failure rates and postoperative disability in an active patient population. *J Bone Joint Surg Am.* 2013;95(7):592–596.
9. Wittstein J, Moorman 3rd CT, Levin LS. Endoscopic compartment release for chronic exertional compartment syndrome: surgical technique and results. *Am J Sports Med.* 2010;38(8):1661–1666.
10. Balius R, Bong DA, Ardevol J, Pedret C, Codina D, Dalmau A. Ultrasound-guided fasciotomy for anterior chronic exertional compartment syndrome of the leg. *J Ultrasound Med.* 2016;35(4):823–829.
11. Finnoff J, Johnson W. Ultrasound-guided fasciotomy for chronic exertional compartment syndrome: a case report. *Clin J Sport Med.* 2020;30(6):e231–e233.
12. Reisner J, Johnson W, Hollman J, Sellon J, Finnoff J. Safety and feasibility of ultrasound-guided fasciotomy for chronic exertional compartment syndrome. In: AMSSM 29th Annual Meeting; 2020.

31 Principles of Perineural Injections

JEFFREY A. STRAKOWSKI

Ultrasound-Guided Perineural Injections

KEY POINTS

- In-plane injections should be used for peripheral nerves because of the relative vulnerability of the target.
- The image should be optimized for maximum conspicuity of the nerve and to reliably identify the border of the outer epineurium.
- The nerve should be scanned proximally and distally to the injection field in both the short- and long-axis views prior to the procedure.
- Applying a small amount of hypoechoic injectate adjacent to the nerve will increase the nerve's conspicuity.
- The flow of the injectate should be observed carefully to ensure that it is not intraneural.

Peripheral Nerve Anatomy and Image Optimization

Anatomy

Peripheral nerves have a characteristic fascicular pattern that is readily distinguished from the fibrillar pattern of tendons (Fig. 31.1).[1] The hypoechoic fascicles are seen among the intervening hyperechoic inner epineurium. In the short-axis view, the contrast of this tissue creates the appearance of a honeycomb. The fascicles reflect the bundle of nerve fibers surrounding by perineurium. The inner epineurium consists of connective tissue and intraneural vascular structures. The highly reflective outer border is the outer epineurium.[2]

Scanning and Image Optimization

Peripheral nerves should initially be scanned in the short-axis view for identification and recognition of the surrounding anatomy. The long-axis view also should be included for a complete perspective (Fig. 31.2). When the nerve is surrounded by relatively isoechoic tissue, such as tendons, and is difficult to identify, scanning should be done to follow the nerve to a more conspicuous location such as surrounding hypoechoic muscle. Once reliably identified, the nerve can be followed back to the preferred location. Increasing the speed of scanning of the nerve in the short-axis view can also improve its conspicuity.[3]

The peripheral nerve image can be optimized by toggling the transducer to create an orthogonal position of the nerve and minimize anisotropic artifact.[4] Typically, the highest-frequency transducer that can adequately penetrate to the desired depth should be used. The depth should be set so that the nerve takes up a large portion of the image rather than a small area at the surface. The focal zone should be placed at the level of the nerve, and the gray-scale gain should be set to create the greatest contrast between the outer epineurium and surrounding tissue.

Common Pathology

The most consistent abnormal finding with focal neuropathies is enlargement of the nerve.[5] The mechanism of this is complex but can include: blocking of axoplasmic flow, endoneurial edema, distal axonal degeneration, perineural and endoneurial inflammation, perineural fibrosis, axons sprouting, remyelination, and thickening of the perineurium and epineurium.[6] Assessment of the cross-sectional area at the area of maximal nerve swelling is the most commonly used parameter to distinguish nerve abnormality. This is performed by tracing the inner border of the outer epineurium and the calculation is performed by most ultrasound machines. Techniques that help distinguish pathologic enlargement include comparison to unaffected areas of the same nerve and, when needed, comparison to the opposite limb. Sufficient inspection should be performed to determine whether the enlargement is focal, which is typical of entrapment neuropathies, or more diffuse, as seen with stretch injuries. The internal echotexture of the nerve also should be assessed. Enlargement or distortion of the internal fascicles often suggests more severe injury. The effect of surrounding tissue, such as scarring, should also be identified.[7] In the context of trauma, careful inspection should be performed to establish that the nerve is in continuity.

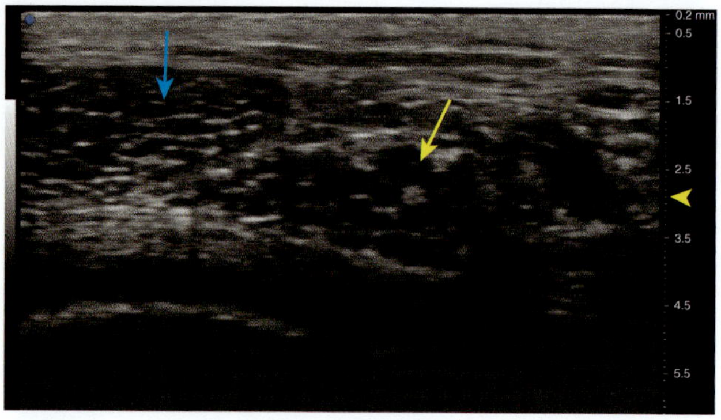

• **Fig. 31.1** Ultra-high frequency (70 MHz) sonogram demonstrating the fascicular pattern of the ulnar nerve *(yellow arrow)* at the distal forearm in the short-axis view. Note the contrast of the fibrillar pattern of the neighboring flexor carpi ulnaris tendon *(blue arrow)*.

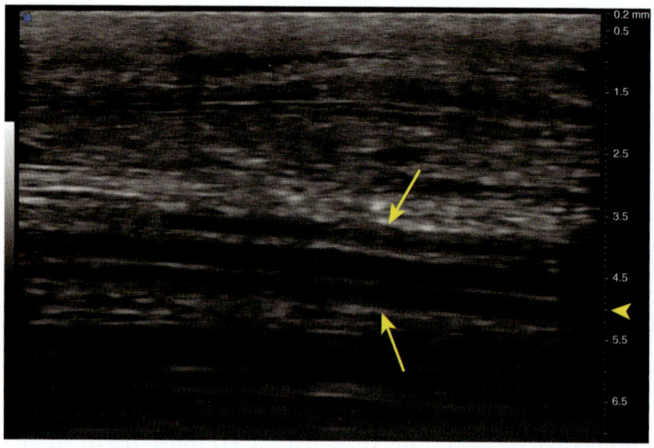

• **Fig. 31.2** Ultra high frequency (70MHz) sonogram demonstrating the fascicular pattern of the medial plantar branch of the tibial nerve *(yellow arrows)* in long axis.

Identification of a complete neurotmesis leads to the consideration of surgical treatment for repair.

Indications for Peripheral Nerve Injections

Ultrasound-guided peripheral nerve injections are performed for anesthetic blocks for pain management during surgery or other procedures, diagnostic blocks to help determine the source of pain, and therapeutic treatment of a known peripheral nerve injury.[8–10] The nature of the injectate and relative volume is based on the indication and type of procedure.[11] Ultrasound guidance has changed the nature of anesthetic and therapeutic injections by allowing direct visualization of the nerve, enabling the clinician to change the needle position and target multiple nerves from the same external landmark.[12,13] Diagnostic blocks are performed by injecting a small amount of local anesthetic around the nerve, instead of wide infiltration into the surrounding tissue, in an effort to help determine the pain generator. Ultrasound guidance provides greater precision of diagnostic injections over nonguided injections.[14] Procedures performed for therapeutic effect can consist of any combination of local anesthetic, steroid, saline, and dextrose. The purpose is to provide direct therapeutic effect from the injectate and, when appropriate, use the injected volume to alleviate compression and encroaching scar by hydrodissecting the nerve.[15,16]

Peripheral Nerve Injection Technique

Equipment

- Needles:
  - 27-gauge, 1.0-inch needle to anesthetize the skin
  - 25-gauge, 1.5-inch needle for most superficial injections
  - 25-gauge, 3.5-inch needle for deeper injections
- Injectate options:
  - Local anesthetic (e.g., 1% lidocaine, 0.25% bupivacaine)
  - Normal saline solution
  - 5% dextrose
  - Steroid (e.g., dexamethasone 4 mg/mL, triamcinolone acetonide (Kenalog) 40 mg/mL)
  - Platelet products: platelet-rich plasma (PRP) or platelet lysate
- Ultrasound machine with a high-frequency (10 to 15 MHz) linear array transducer
- Sterile conduction gel
- Sterile gloves

Peripheral Nerve Injection Principles

- There should be complete knowledge of the function of the peripheral nerve prior to the procedure.
- The nerve and surrounding tissue should be thoroughly pre-scanned in both short- and long-axis views. This includes both cranially and caudally to the injection field.
- The field should be scanned with varying transducer pressure to assess for neighboring vessels that could be potentially collapsed.
- Doppler imaging should also be used, with pre-scanning to further assess for vascular structures.
- The image should be optimized so the margins of outer epineurium are adequately visualized.
- The injections should be performed with an in-plane view of the needle and a short-axis view of the nerve.
- Aseptic technique should be used with all injections.
- Anoblique stand-off of sterile conduction gel can help with needle visualization prior to insertion. This is particularly beneficial with superficial targets.[17]
- It is helpful to slowly introduce a small amount of the hypoechoic injectate to increase the conspicuity of the outer epineurium (Fig. 31.3), then proceed with the remainder of the injection.
- The flow of the injectate should be carefully observed during the procedure to avoid intraneural injection and potential injury.[18]
- Doppler imaging can be used during the procedure to highlight the flowing of the injectate.
- When using higher volumes of injectate, it is often useful to alternate between short- and long-axis views to confirm injectate flow along the nerve sheath.

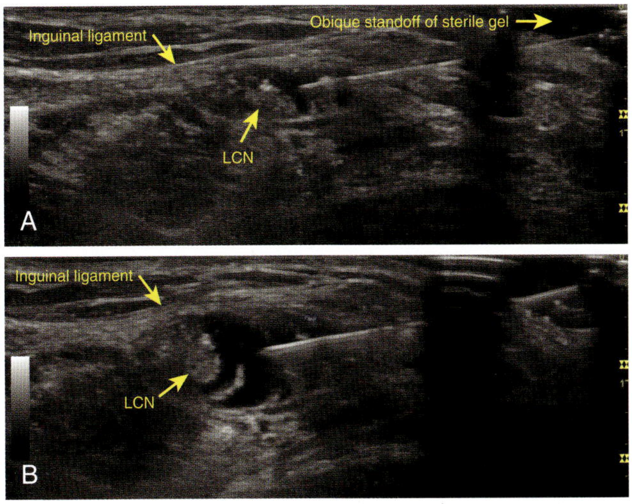

• **Fig. 31.3** Sonograms demonstrating a perineural injection of the lateral cutaneous nerve *(LCN)* of the thigh. The injection is performed with an in-plane view to the transducer and the nerve is seen in the short-axis view. The inguinal ligament and hypoechoic oblique standoff of sterile gel is also seen. (A) A small amount of injectate is placed between the nerve and inguinal ligament as the needle is slowly withdrawn to increase conspicuity of the small nerve. (B) After a clear halo is created with the initial slow injection and the outer epineurium is more conspicuous, the remainder of the injectate is introduced.

- Local anesthetics are used for anesthetic blocks and to anesthetize the skin for other injections. There is potential neurotoxicity and they are therefore minimized with therapeutic injections, particularly repeated hydrodissections.
- Generally, higher volumes of injectate are used for hydrodissections. This can be in the range of 4 to 15 mL. There is not complete consensus regarding the composition of the injectate, but it can involve any combination of local anesthetic, injectable steroid, normal saline solution, PRP, and 5% dextrose.[19] There are anecdotal reports and some initial studies of the therapeutic effect of 5% dextrose around peripheral nerve injures; however, further studies are needed.[20]
- The use of PRP and platelet lysate are also advocated by some for enhancing recovery of peripheral nerve injuries. Further studies are also needed to demonstrate efficacy for this purpose.[21–23]

Post-Procedure

- Post-injection scanning should be considered, particularly after higher-volume injections, to assess the injectate placement. Dynamic ultrasound to assess nerve mobility after hydrodissection can also provide insight into the effect of the injection.
- The patient should be able to resume nonstressful activities immediately after the injection.
- Ice and over-the-counter analgesic medications can be used if there is a temporary increase in discomfort after the injection.
- The patient is generally scheduled for follow-up evaluation 2 to 6 weeks after the procedure to assess the response to treatment.

References

1. Martinoli C, Bianchi S, Dahmane M, Pugliese F, Bianchi-Zamorani MP, Valle M. Ultrasound of tendons and nerves. *Eur Radiol.* 2002;12(1):44–55.
2. Strakowski JA. *Introduction to Musculoskeletal Ultrasound: Getting Started.* New York: Demos Medical; 2015.
3. Strakowski JA. *Ultrasound Evaluation of Focal Neuropathies. Correlation with Electrodiagnosis.* New York: Demos Medical; 2014.
4. Kremkau FW. *Diagnostic Ultrasound: Principles and Ultrasound.* St. Louis: Sauders; 2002.
5. Walker FO, Cartwright MS, Wiesler ER, Caress J. Ultrasound of nerve and muscle. *Clin Neurophysiol.* 2004;115(3):495–507.
6. Rempel D, Dahlin L, Lundborg G. Pathophysiology of nerve compression syndromes: response of peripheral nerves to loading. *J Bone Joint Surg Am.* 1999;81(11):1600–1610.
7. Martinoli C, Bianchi S, Pugliese F, et al. Sonography of entrapment neuropathies in the upper limb (wrist excluded). *J Clin Ultrasound.* 2004;32(9):438–450.
8. Markovic M, Crichton K, Read JW, Lam P, Slater HK. Effectiveness of ultrasound-guided corticosteroid injection in the treatment of Morton's neuroma. *Foot Ankle Int.* 2008;29(5):483–487.
9. Tagliafico A, Serafini G, Lacelli F, Perrone N, Valsania V, Martinoli C. Ultrasound-guided treatment of meralgia paresthetica (lateral femoral cutaneous neuropathy): technical description and results of treatment in 20 consecutive patients. *J Ultrasound Med.* 2011;30(10):1341–1346.
10. Pasquali C, Vulcano E, Novario R, Varotto D, Montoli C, Volpe A. Ultrasound-guided alcohol injection for Morton's neuroma. *Foot Ankle Int.* 2015;36(1):55–59.
11. Strakowski JA. Ultrasound-guided peripheral nerve procedures. *Phys Med Rehabil Clin N Am.* 2016;27(3):687–715.
12. Yamamoto H, Sakura S, Wada M, Shido A. A prospective, randomized comparison between single- and multiple-injection techniques for ultrasound-guided subgluteal sciatic nerve block.
13. Re M, Blanco J, Gómez de Segura IA. Ultrasound-guided nerve block anesthesia. *Vet Clin North Am Food Anim Pract.* 2016;32(1):133–147.
14. Lento PH, Strakowski JA. The use of ultrasound in guiding musculoskeletal interventional procedures. *Phys Med Rehabil Clin N Am.* 2010;21(3):559–583.
15. Cass SP. Ultrasound-guided nerve hydrodissection: what is it? A review of the literature. *Curr Sports Med Rep.* 2016;15(1):20–22.
16. Dettori N, Choudur H, Chhabra A. Ultrasound-guided treatment of peripheral nerve pathology. *Semin Musculoskelet Radiol.* 2018;22(3):364–374.
17. Smith J, Finnoff JT. Diagnostic and interventional musculoskeletal ultrasound: part 1. Fundamentals. *PM R.* 2009;1(1):64–75.
18. Choquet O, Morau D, Biboulet P, Capdevila X. Where should the tip of the needle be located in ultrasound-guided peripheral nerve blocks? *Curr Opin Anaesthesiol.* 2012;25(5):596–602.
19. Lam SKH, Reeves KD, Cheng AL. Transition from deep regional blocks toward deep nerve hydrodissection in the upper body and torso: method description and results from a retrospective chart review of the analgesic effect of 5% dextrose water as the primary hydrodissection injectate to enhance safety. *Biomed Res Int.* 2017;2017:7920438.

20. Dufour E, Cymerman A, Nourry G, Balland N, Couturier C, Liu N, et al. An ultrasonographic assessment of nerve stimulation-guided median nerve block at the elbow: a local anesthetic spread, nerve size, and clinical efficacy study. *Anesth Analg.* 2010;111(2):561–567.
21. Kuffler DP. Platelet-rich plasma and the elimination of neuropathic pain. *Mol Neurobiol.* 2013;48(2):315–332.
22. Malahias MA, Chytas D, Babis GC, Nikolaou VS. Platelet-rich plasma guided injections: clinical application in peripheral neuropathies. *Front Surg.* 2014;1:41.
23. Kuffler DP. Platelet-rich plasma promotes axon regeneration, wound healing, and pain reduction: fact or fiction. *Mol Neurobiol.* 2015;52(2):990–1014.

32

Ultrasound-Guided Release of the Transverse Carpal Ligament (Carpal Tunnel)

ADAM M. POURCHO, PHILLIP HENNING, AND JAY SMITH

ABBREVIATIONS

CSA cross-sectional area
CTR carpal tunnel release
CTS carpal tunnel syndrome
TCL transverse carpal ligament
TSZ transverse safe zone
LAX long-axis view
US ultrasound
USCTR ultrasound-guided carpal tunnel release
USG ultrasound guidance
SAX short axis

KEY POINTS

- Ultrasound-guided carpal tunnel release (USCTR) has the advantage of a smaller incision size, as well as the advantage of being performed in an office/procedure room setting using only local anesthesia, potentially lowering cost.
- Ultrasound guidance (USG) allows the ability to directly visualize all carpal tunnel structures and control the transverse safe zone (TSZ).
- USCTR has documented faster recovery and less post-procedure pain medication use when compared to mini-open carpal tunnel release (MOCTR).
- Pre-scanning protocol and knowledge of the anatomy of the carpal tunnel with special attention to potential anatomic variants of the median nerve is recommended prior to performing any carpal tunnel release (CTR) procedures.

Ultrasound-Guided Transverse Carpal Ligament Release

Pertinent Anatomy

The carpal tunnel (CT) is a fibro-osseous canal on the volar side of the wrist, formed by the carpal bones (floor) and transverse carpal ligament (TCL) (roof) (Figs. 32.1 and 32.2B and C). The TCL is approximately 1.5 to 4 mm thick on average.[1–3] The proximal TCL inserts on the scaphoid bone and traverses medially to the pisiform, while the distal TCL inserts on the trapezium and traverses medial to the hook of the hamate (see Fig. 32.2B and C). The proximal portion of the TCL is the distal continuation of the antebrachial fascia, with transverse instead of longitudinally oriented fibers.[1,2,4,5] The radial side of the TCL divides into two layers, a superficial layer and a deep layer, to accommodate the tendon of the flexor carpi radialis (FCR).[1,2,4]

The carpal canal contains the median nerve and nine tendons: the flexor pollicis longus (FPL), the four flexor digitorum superficialis (FDS), and the four flexor digitorum profundus (FDP) (see Fig. 32.1). The FPL has its own synovial sheath, while the FDS and FDP have a common synovial sheath. The FCR, flexor carpi ulnaris, ulnar nerve, and palmaris tendons are external to the CT.[3] The abductor pollicis brevis (APB) and flexor pollicis brevis (FPB) have anatomic connections on the radial side of the TCL, while ulnarly, the flexor digiti minimi brevis (FDMb) originates from the TCL.[2–4]

The median nerve is anatomically located in the forearm between the FDS and FDP muscles. As the nerve travels distally, it becomes more superficial just proximal to the TCL by looping radially around the FDS muscles and tendons in the distal forearm.[1,2,4,6] The palmar cutaneous branch arises off the radial side of the median nerve, most commonly between the FCR and palmaris longus (if present), providing sensation to the palmar surface of the thumb (see Fig. 32.1).[7] From here, the median nerve travels superficially between the tendons of the FPL and FDS to the index and middle fingers. The median nerve normally travels in the CT as a single nerve, prior to dividing into radial and ulnar branches at the distal border of the TCL.

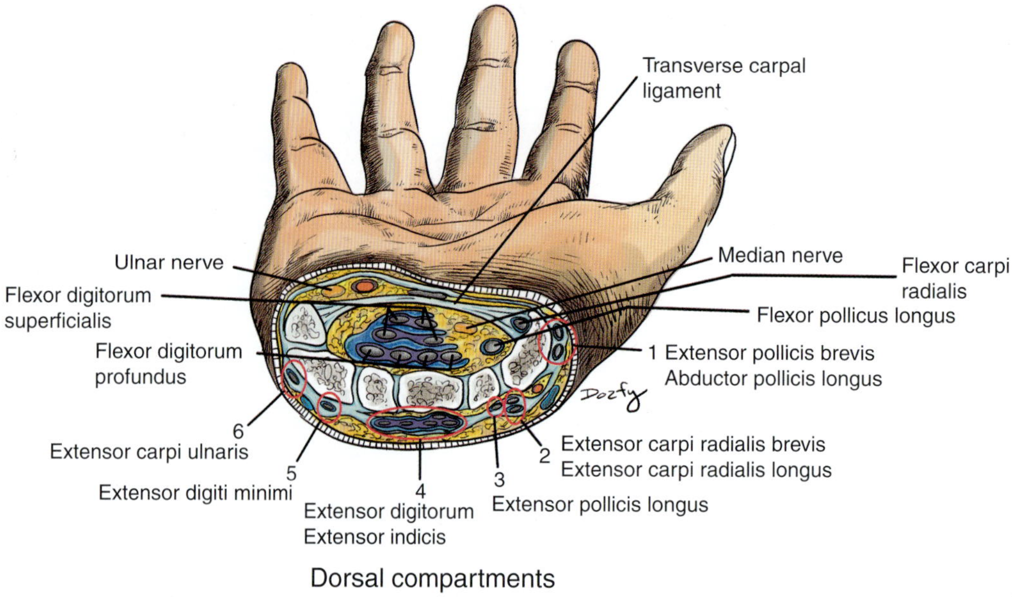

• **Fig. 32.1** Anatomy. Anatomic view of the carpal tunnel.

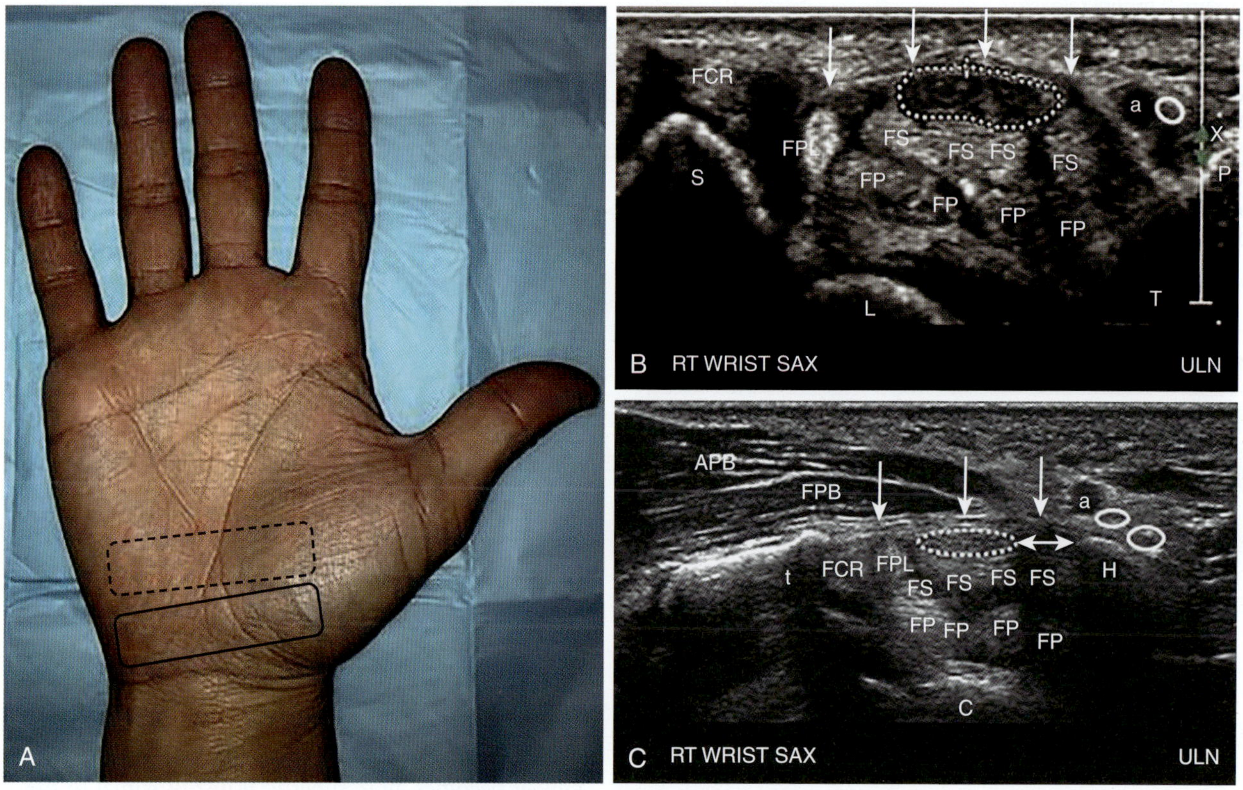

• **Fig. 32.2** Ultrasound of the Carpal Tunnel With Anatomic Correlates. (A) Transducer positioning for sonographic short-axis (SAX) view of the proximal *(solid rectangle)* and distal *(dotted rectangle)* carpal tunnel (CT). (B) US SAX correlate, with transducer positioned as shown in Fig. 32.2A, of the proximal CT with ulnar *(ULN)* to the right. Note the bony landmarks of the scaphoid *(S)* radially and the pisiform *(P)* ulnarly. The median nerve *(dotted circle)* is situated superficial within the CT. (C) US SAX correlate, with transducer positioned as shown in Fig. 32.2A, of the distal CT with ULN to the right. Note the transverse safe zone (TSZ) *(double arrow)*, in this patient bordered on the ULN side by the hook of the hamate (H). *a*, Ulnar artery; *APB*, abductor pollicis brevis; *C*, capitate; *FCR*, flexor carpi ulnaris; *FP*, flexor digitorum profundus; *FPB*, flexor pollicis brevis; *FPL*, flexor pollicis longus; *FS*, flexor digitorum superficialis; *L*, lunate; *solid circles*, ulnar nerve; *t*, trapezoid; *T*, triquetrum.

The thenar motor branch (TMB) (also referred to as the recurrent motor branch of the median nerve) typically originates from the antero-ulnar aspect of the radial division at the distal TCL and travels vertically in a palmar direction around the distal TCL to innervate the thenar musculature (see Fig. 32.1).[8–26] The TMB is a critically important structure within the CT region because it is the primary motor innervation to the thenar muscles in most people.[8–26] A detailed knowledge of anatomic variations of the TMB (mentioned later in this chapter) is recommended prior to performing procedures on or about the CT.

In the palm, the median nerve supplies sensation to the palmar surface of the thumb, index and middle finger, and radial palmar surface of the ring finger, while also providing motor innervation of the thenar eminence as well as the first and second lumbricals via the TMB.[4,7,26]

Anatomic Variants

There are many reported anatomic variants of the wrist, involving vessels, nerves, tendons, and muscle; some of these have significant clinical relevance when it comes to USCTR.[8–12,15,18,26–28] The operator should be aware that the presence of one anatomic variant should alert to the presence of potential additional anatomic variants.

The most common variant of the median nerve itself is a bifid median nerve with or without a persistent median artery (PMA).[2,27] A PMA, which is present in 12% to 23% of the population, arises from the ulnar artery and travels distally along the ulnar side of the median nerve and may contribute to symptoms of carpal tunnel syndrome (CTS).[8–12,15,18,26–28] The superficial location of the PMA in the CT puts the artery at risk for injury during USCTR, and its presence should be noted prior to attempting release. Furthermore, a PMA is often associated with a bifid or trifid median nerve. The use of color Doppler can help to identify this variant.[2,27]

PMA with bifid median nerve can also often be associated with an anomalous FDS muscle belly that can be seen dynamically with flexion and extension of the fingers.[1,2,8,15,25,29,30] Another variant is proximal bifurcation of the median nerve, which can be seen in 1% to 3% of the population. Early division of the terminal branches is even less common.[1,2,8,15,25,29,30]

Anatomic variants of the TMB are common and present in 46% to 90% of the population. There are four main anatomic variants of the TMB: the distal ligamentous (most common); the subligamentous branch (33%); the transligamentous branch (8% to 12%); and the ulnar division take off (rare).[8,10–17,20,24–26,31] Hypertrophy of the thenar muscles has been associated with transligamentous TMB.[8] A firm understanding of normal and anatomic variants of the TMB and identification of the TMB and possible variants with ultrasound (US) prior to any USG procedures about the TCL is highly recommended.[32]

There are two main variants of the palmar cutaneous nerve described in the literature. The first variant arises on the radial side of the median nerve, and the second, on the ulnar side of the median nerve. The latter crosses the nerve prior to going through the fibro-osseous tunnel before becoming subcutaneous.[7,27] Damage to this nerve during surgery has been shown to cause the development of a neuroma, and therefore, demands consideration when performing USCTR.[33]

There is one anatomic variation of the ulnar nerve that warrants mention. In 1% to 3% of the population, the nerve travels in an osseo-fibrous canal (different from Guyon's canal) situated on the anteromedial portion of the TCL, extending approximately 4 cm from the pisiform to the hook of the hamate bifurcation.[1,2]

The palmaris longus (PL) muscle has the greatest number of possible variants in the human body.[34,35] Two variants are particularly important when considering USCTR and must be identified before surgery. The first variant involves the PL traversing the CT, possibly contributing to symptomatology. The second, referred to as a reverse PL, involves the muscle belly in a distal rather than proximal position. In the case of a reverse PL, the muscle belly may extend into the CT, possibly increasing or contributing to compression.[30,34] The low-lying FDS muscle bellies, as well as more proximally located lumbrical muscle bellies, may also dynamically impinge on the median nerve with dynamic testing. There are also reports at the wrist of other anatomic variants to the tendons, including accessory FDS to the index finger and the palmar surface.[2,30,34,35]

The CT can also be compromised by any number of cystic or mass-like structures.[36] If discovered, care should be taken to note these structures and make appropriate referrals for either diagnosis or treatment.

The sonographer should always report the presence of anatomic variants of the nerves, ligaments, and tendons about the TCL, which might otherwise be damaged or require additional treatment during any surgical release of the TCL.

Pathophysiology/Diagnosis

Median nerve entrapment at the TCL, leading to CTS, is the most common peripheral entrapment neuropathy, with an incidence of 3.5% to 6.2%.[37–39] Approximately 450,000 surgical releases are performed annually in the United States, with a total cost of over 2 billion dollars.[37–39] More than 90% of patients report clinical improvement following release.[37–40]

The diagnosis of CTS is primarily clinical, with most patients complaining of numbness and tingling in the lateral three digits of the hand with or without associated weakness. Patients may have a positive Tinel's sign over the median nerve at the TCL or a positive Phalen's test. Electrodiagnostic (EDX) testing may be obtained to assess the severity of injury to the median nerve and differentiate CTS from competing diagnoses, such as peripheral neuropathy or cervical radiculopathy.[41,42] Isolated or predominant TMB involvement has been implicated in some patients with CTS who present with disproportionate thenar atrophy or weakness, particularly in the setting of a relatively normal-appearing median nerve.[8,11,17,19,20,22,23,26,43]

Sonographic Evaluation/Findings

Recently, the use of musculoskeletal US has increasingly been used to evaluate and manage patients with CTS.[1,2,24,32,42,44–49] The most commonly reported findings on US in the setting of CTS are that of median nerve enlargement, focal median nerve constriction, reduced median nerve gliding (dynamically), TCL bowing, flexor tenosynovitis, or space-occupying lesions (e.g., ganglia, tumors, thrombosed or anomalous arteries, abnormal muscle slips, or supernumerary muscles or tendons).[2,6,36,42,45–48,50] Other studies have indicated cross-sectional area (CSA) at the proximal TCL may provide more conventional diagnostic parameters.[6,51] The normal CSA can vary from 6.5 to 12 mm^2, depending on the study.[6,51] Enlargement of the median nerve CSA (with contralateral comparison) in conjunction with EDX testing and clinical examination should lead to an accurate diagnosis. In postoperative evaluation, US may identify incomplete TCL transection, TCL regrowth, scarring and adhesions, improvement of CSA, and injury to the median nerve or its palmar cutaneous or TMB in patients with continued symptoms.[42,49,52–56]

Sonographic evaluation of the CT typically begins in the anatomic axial plane and eventually in the anatomic sagittal plane. In the axial view, the nerve has a "honeycomb" appearance, with individual hypoechoic fascicles separated by echogenic septa representing the interfascicular perineurium (see Fig. 32.2B and C). The nerve bundles are less susceptible to anisotropy, unlike other structures, such as muscles and ligaments. Differential anisotropy with toggling of the transducer can be used to make the nerve more conspicuous for identification. The nerve is followed from the pronator quadratus in the forearm through the proximal and eventually distal CT. Dynamic maneuvers, with flexion and extension of the fingers, is recommended to identify possible muscle variants. Color Doppler should be used to identify vascular anatomy. Sagittal plane (longitudinal images) is useful in cases of focal compression, showing the compressed portion of the median nerve as well as the proximal and/or distal swollen portion of the nerve ("notch sign").[1,44,45] Special care is taken to note the aforementioned anatomic variants as they pertain to the TCL.

It is suggested that the following structures are viewed as part of a pre-screening protocol:[32,57–59]

- The median nerve:
  - With CSA measurements at the distal border pronator quadratus, the proximal TCL, and the distal TCL
- The palmar cutaneous branch of the median nerve
- The TMB of the median nerve
- The ulnar nerve and artery:
  - Location of the superficial palmar arch to the hook of the hamate
  - Location of the ulnar nerve to the hook of the hamate
- The vasculature and presence of anatomic variants, including persistent median artery (if present)
- Measurement of length of the TCL in sagittal plane
- The native transverse safe zone
  - Distance between the median nerve and ulnar artery or hamate
- The FCR, FDS, FDP, flexor carpi ulnaris (FCU), and FPL tendons
- Superficial palmar artery and palmar fat pad
- The bony acoustic landmarks of scaphoid, pisiform, trapezium, and hook of hamate

Contraindications to USCTRS

- Inability to adequately visualize at-risk structures:
  - TMB/recurrent motor branch of the median nerve
  - Palmar cutaneous branch of the median nerve
  - Ulnar vessels
  - Superficial palmar arterial arch
  - Median and ulnar palmar digital nerves
- Variant anatomy that would preclude establishment of a safe transverse safe zone
- Presence of mass lesion or other process that requires treatment beyond CTR

Treatment Options

Conservative treatment options for CTS typically include activity modification, occupational therapy, bracing, steroid injections, and alternative medicine (i.e., acupuncture, low-level laser, yoga, and static magnetic field therapy). For patients who fail conservative treatment, surgical release is considered the definitive treatment. Although historically performed via a large (3 to 5 cm) palmar incision, CTR techniques have evolved to reduce trauma with less-invasive treatments.[49,60–62] The goal of less-invasive treatments is improving cosmesis, reducing postoperative pain, and promoting faster recovery.[49,52,57,58,63] The currently available CTR techniques include mini-open CTR (mOCTR) via a single 1 to 3 cm palmar incision, endoscopic CTR (ECTR) via one (wrist) or two (wrist and palm) 1 to 2 cm incisions, and more recently, ultrasound-guided CTR (USCTR) via a single less than 1 cm wrist or palmar incision.[49,57,59,64–75]

Ultrasound-Guided Release

The primary goal of CTR is to transect the TCL while avoiding injury to the neurovascular structures.[59–61,76,77] Although ECTR may promote a faster recovery than mOCTR, there is a concern that limited visualization of the surrounding structures during ECTR may increase complications.[60,61,66,76] USCTR combines a single or dual incision (Manos procedure) with direct

US visualization of at-risk structures.[52,53,57,58,67,70,72–75,78–84] Despite many different devices being used to perform USCTR, review of the current publications on USCTR report a greater than 98% clinical success rate without any documented neurovascular injuries.[49,52,57,58,67–71,73,74,78,81,83–85] Rojo-Maudate et al published their randomized clinical trial comparing mOCTR versus USCTR, demonstrating a five times faster functional recovery, pain reduction, and pain medication discontinuation with USCTR.[68]

ECTR techniques and most USCTR techniques place the surgical device within the TSZ. The TSZ is defined as a region bordered radially by the median nerve and ulnarly by the hook of the hamate or ulnar vessels, whichever lies more radial (see Fig. 32.2C).[32,84] The TSZ has been shown to vary from approximately 4.4 to 12.4 mm, and was statistically larger in men when compared to women, but exhibits significant inter-individual variability. In some cases, a 0 mm TSZ has been documented.[32,52,57,58,81,84] It can be therefore technically challenging to establish a consistent TSZ while performing CTR. During ECTR, the size of the TSZ is determined by the size of the introducer and endoscopic device.[44,61,66,76,86] This is contrasted to USCTR, in which the cutting instrument is smaller, requiring a small incision, but also presenting the same challenge of establishing a TSZ.[67,68,70–75,83–85]

More recently, the SX-One MicroKnife (Sonex Health LLC, Rochester, MN), a disposable device with ability to protect the TSZ, has become available. A cadaveric investigation using the SX-One device to perform USCTR on cadaveric specimens documented a 100% rate of TCL release and no neurovascular injury.[87] Initial studies on this device have shown promising results, with faster recovery and return to normal function with no reported neurovascular injuries to date.[49,52,57,58,81]

Equipment

- High-frequency linear transducer (e.g., 12 to 5 MHz)
- Arm board
- Surgical drapes
- Lidocaine ~8 to 10 mL
- Dilator
- 21-gauge, 2-inch needle
- A #15 blade
- Skin glue vs 4-0 sutures for closure
- Steri-strips
- Sterile towels and gauze
- Sterile saline (10 mL)
- Cutting device (SX-One MicroKnife by Sonex, hook knife, Gou wire)

Authors' Preferred Technique

Patient Position

- Supine or lateral recumbent, with the arm on an arm board and a pillow between the patient's knees (Fig. 32.3B)

Clinician Position

- Clinician is seated either between patient's underarm and body or between patients arm and head, per clinician preference (see Fig. 32.3B).
- US display located directly in front of clinician's line of vision.

Transducer Orientation

- A combination of orthogonal anatomic axial and sagittal views are used for the procedure (Fig. 32.4A–C).

Technique

- Using USG, the surgical limb is marked with pre-surgical skin markings. The superficial palmar arch, hook of hamate, pisiform, median nerve, ulnar nerve and artery, scaphoid, and trapezium are marked prior to start of procedure. The proximal wrist crease (starting point) is also marked (Fig. 32.3A and B).
- The SX-One MicroKnife is first primed via the manufacturer's recommendations with sterile saline.
- Following aseptic preparation, an USG in-plane proximal-to-distal anesthetic of ~8 mL of 1% lidocaine without epinephrine is injected into the superficial palmar fascia and deep to the TCL with a 21-gauge, 50 mm needle.
- This needle is withdrawn, and using USG, a second 21-gauge, 2 inch needle is used to hydrodissect the median nerve away from the flexor tendons and TCL using 10 mL of sterile 0.9% normal saline, making the TCL more conspicuous.
- Following adequate anesthesia, a #15 blade scalpel with the blade positioned upward is used to make a vertical stab incision through the antebrachial fascia, at the proximal wrist crease.
- USG is then used to accurately place the device into the CT, ulnar to the median nerve within the TSZ. The distal end of the device is advanced until 1 cm distal to the hook of the hamate, taking care to note the location of the SPA (see Fig. 32.4A). A ureteral dilator can be inserted through the track first to help accommodate the device more easily.
- US evaluation in two orthogonal planes is utilized to ensure proper positioning of the device within the TSZ (see Fig. 32.4A).
- Once proper positioning is sonographically confirmed, the handle on the device is depressed and locked, filling the balloons with sterile saline and expanding the TSZ (see Fig. 32.4B).
- The device can then be adjusted ulnarly or radially to create an optimal cutting position away from the path of the median nerve and ulnar neurovascular structures.
- Following confirmation of adequate placement of the device and cutting angle, the blade is then deployed from a distal to proximal direction, cutting the TCL (see Fig. 32.4C).
- After release, the blade is left recessed in the proximal location.

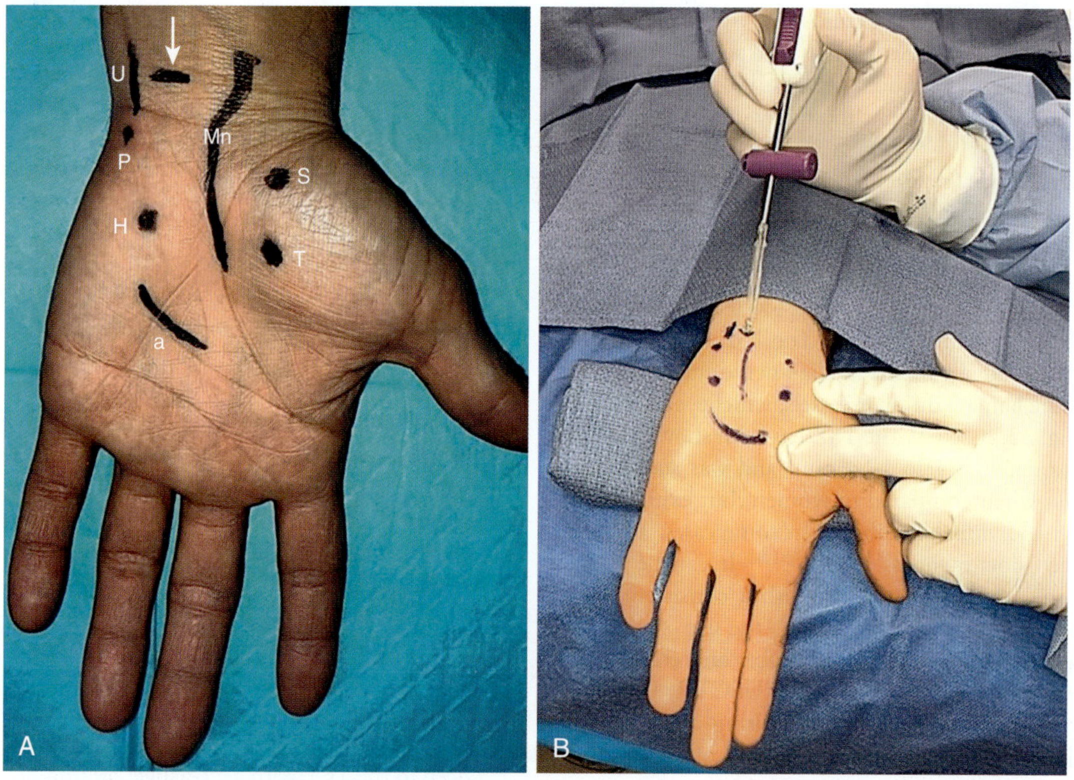

• **Fig. 32.3** Pre-Surgical Markings and Patient Position. (A) Picture of incision placement at the proximal wrist crease along the distal forearm and device direction of insertion *(arrow). Black skin markings* represent pre-surgical marking scanning protocol to assist with safe procedure. (B) With the patient positioned supine (or lateral recumbent) and arm outstretched on an arm board, the device is inserted as demonstrated in the photo. *a*, Superficial palmar arch; *H*, hook of hamate; *Mn*, median nerve; *P*, pisiform; *S*, scaphoid; *T*, trapezoid; *U*, ulnar nerve.

Confirmation of Complete Release

Following release, the balloons are deflated, and the device is used to probe the TCL to ensure complete release. The device should be superficial to the hook of the hamate and the TCL ligament through the probing process. If complete release is not obtained, the device can be reused by re-inflating the balloons and resetting the blade to the distal retracted position. Following the above steps, a repeat pass can be made.

On confirmation of complete release, the device can be removed from the incision so excess fluid and blood can be expressed through the wound. The incision is closed with skin glue and steri-strips, or suture if preferred. A sterile gauze and occlusive dressing are applied to the wound.

Post-procedure neurologic and physical exam are recommended to ensure no neurologic or tendon injuries have occurred. The published average total time of the procedure is approximately 7 minutes, with an average incision length of less than 5 mm.[49,52,57,58,81]

Post-Procedure Management

Following the procedure, patients are instructed to keep the incision covered with bio-occlusive dressing until the wound heals (5 to 7 days). Patients are allowed to return to usual activities as tolerated, letting pain be their guide. Indeed, some patients with comorbid functional limitations, such as those in wheelchairs, are allowed to immediately resume ambulation.[58,81] Recommended follow-up screening surveys are the Boston Carpal Tunnel Questionnaire and the Quick Disabilities of the Arm, Shoulder, and Hand.[88,89]

Complications

Pillar pain, or pain over the prominences of the trapezial ridge, scaphoid tubercle, pisiform, or the hook of the hamate, is present in as many as 60% of individuals following CT release.[31,39,56,61,62,76,86,90,91] This can be debilitating, causing a decrease in strength and delayed return to work/recreational activities. Early data on USCTR show an early return to prior level of function with faster decrease in peroperative and operative pillar pain when compared to mini-open technique.

Iatrogenic injury to any of the aforementioned nervous structures is a potential complication of any CTR procedure. Perhaps the most-feared complication of CT release is injury to the TMB; the theoretical risk increases dramatically in the setting of anatomic variations in the origin or

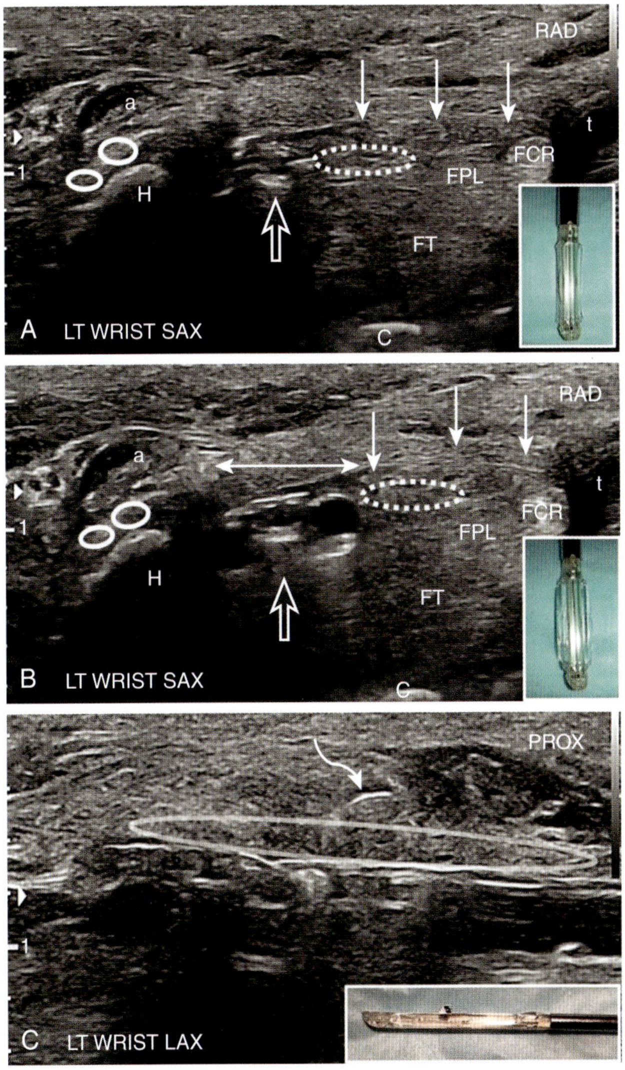

• **Fig. 32.4** Ultrasound-Guided Carpal Tunnel Release. (A) Out-of-plane sonographic SAX view of the device *(open arrow)* within the TSZ in a left wrist at the level of the distal CT *(solid arrows)*, with transducer positioned as shown *(dotted ellipse)*. Note the balloons are deflated, as seen in the insert. (B) SAX US of the device *(open arrow)* at the same level with the balloons now inflated (as in insert), expanding the TSZ to 8 mm *(double arrow)* (C) In-plane view of the device engaged (as in insert) with the blade *(curved arrow)* cutting the TCL *(solid ellipse)*. a, Ulnar artery; *APB*, abductor pollicis brevis; *C*, capitate; *FCR*, flexor carpi ulnaris; *FPB*, flexor pollicis brevis; *FPL*, flexor pollicis longus; *FT*, flexor tendons; *H*, hook of hamate; *PROX*, proximal; *RAD*, radial; *solid circles*, ulnar nerve; *solid ellipse*, ulnar nerve; *t*, trapezoid.)

course of the TMB.[j] Even in the absence of injury, the TMB may be a source of persistent symptoms following USCTR. A thorough sonographic preoperative screening should help identify these patients so that appropriate referral for traditional release with neurolysis can be made.

To date, USCTR has reported a greater than 98% clinical success rate, with no reported neurologic injuries, indicating this procedure can be safely performed by a trained sonographer, with careful protection of neurologic structures.[49,52,57,58,81]

[j]References 8, 10, 12, 21, 25, 28, 31, 60–62, 76, 86, 90–92.

References

1. Jayaraman S, Naidich TP. The carpal tunnel: ultrasound display of normal imaging anatomy and pathology. *Neuroimaging Clin N Am*. 2004;14(1):103–113. viii.
2. Presazzi A, Bortolotto C, Zacchino M, Madonia L, Draghi F. Carpal tunnel: normal anatomy, anatomical variants and ultrasound technique. *J Ultrasound*. 2011;14(1):40–46.
3. Pacek CA, Chakan M, Goitz RJ, Kaufmann RA, Li ZM. Morphological analysis of the transverse carpal ligament. *Hand (N Y)*. 2010;5(2):135–140.
4. Cobb TK, Dalley BK, Posteraro RH, Lewis RC. Anatomy of the flexor retinaculum. *J Hand Surg Am*. 1993;18(1):91–99.
5. Deak N, Bordoni B. *Anatomy, Shoulder and Upper Limb, Wrist Flexor Retinaculum*. Treasure Island (FL): StatPearls; 2019.
6. Klauser AS, Halpern EJ, De Zordo T, et al. Carpal tunnel syndrome assessment with US: value of additional cross-sectional area measurements of the median nerve in patients versus healthy volunteers. *Radiology*. 2009;250(1):171–177.
7. Tagliafico A, Pugliese F, Bianchi S, et al. High-resolution sonography of the palmar cutaneous branch of the median nerve. *AJR Am J Roentgenol*. 2008;191(1):107–114.
8. Al-Qattan MM. Variations in the course of the thenar motor branch of the median nerve and their relationship to the hypertrophic muscle overlying the transverse carpal ligament. *J Hand Surg Am*. 2010;35(11):1820–1824.
9. Wolfswinkel EM, Hoang D, Kulber DA. Anatomic variations of the median nerve identified during endoscopic carpal tunnel release with STRATOS. *Plast Reconstr Surg Glob Open*. 2017;5(9):e1458.
10. Beris AE, Lykissas MG, Kontogeorgakos VA, Vekris MD, Korompilias AV. Anatomic variations of the median nerve in carpal tunnel release. *Clin Anat*. 2008;21(6):514–518.
11. Hurwitz PJ. Variations in the course of the thenar motor branch of the median nerve. *J Hand Surg Br*. 1996;21(3):344–346.
12. Lanz U. Anatomical variations of the median nerve in the carpal tunnel. *J Hand Surg Am*. 1977;2(1):44–53.
13. Mizia E, Tomaszewski K, Depukat P, et al. Median nerve (anatomical variations) and carpal tunel syndrome—revisited. *Folia Med Cracov*. 2013;53(4):37–46.
14. Mizia E, Tomaszewski KA, Goncerz G, Kurzydlo W, Walocha J. Median nerve thenar motor branch anatomical variations. *Folia Morphol (Warsz)*. 2012;71(3):183–186.
15. Tountas CP, Bihrle DM, MacDonald CJ, Bergman RA. Variations of the median nerve in the carpal canal. *J Hand Surg Am*. 1987;12(5 Pt 1):708–712.
16. Ahn DS, Yoon ES, Koo SH, Park SH. A prospective study of the anatomic variations of the median nerve in the carpal tunnel in Asians. *Ann Plast Surg*. 2000;44(3):282–287.
17. Johnson RK, Shrewsbury MM. Anatomical course of the thenar branch of the median nerve—usually in a separate tunnel through the transverse carpal ligament. *J Bone Joint Surg Am*. 1970;52(2):269–273.
18. Lindley SG, Kleinert JM. Prevalence of anatomic variations encountered in elective carpal tunnel release. *J Hand Surg Am*. 2003;28(5):849–855.
19. Mannerfelt L, Hybbinette CH. Important anomaly of the thenar motor branch of the median nerve. A clinical and anatomical report. *Bull Hosp Joint Dis*. 1972;33(1):15–21.
20. Mumford J, Morecraft R, Blair WF. Anatomy of the thenar branch of the median nerve. *J Hand Surg Am*. 1987;12(3):361–365.

21. Jegal M, Woo S, Lee H, Shim J, Shin J, Park M. Anatomical relationships between muscles overlying distal transverse carpal ligament and thenar motor branch of the median nerve. *Clin Orthop Surg.* 2018;10(1):89–93.
22. Yamanaka K, Horiuchi Y, Yabe Y. Compression neuropathy of the motor branch of the median nerve due to an anomalous thenar muscle. *J Hand Surg Br.* 1994;19(6):711–712.
23. Alp M, Marur T, Akkin SM, Yalcin L, Demirci S. Ramification pattern of the thenar branch of the median nerve entering the thenar fascia and the distribution of the terminal branches in the thenar musculature: anatomic cadaver study in 144 hands. *Clin Anat.* 2005;18(3):195–199.
24. Smith J, Barnes DE, Barnes KJ, et al. Sonographic visualization of thenar motor branch of the median nerve: a cadaveric validation study. *Pharm Manag PM R.* 2017;9(2):159–169.
25. Al-Qattan MM, Al-Zahrani K. An unusual pre-ligamentous thenar motor branch of the median nerve. *Eur J Plast Surg.* 2017;40(3):259–262.
26. Ajmani ML. Variations in the motor nerve supply of the thenar and hypothenar muscles of the hand. *J Anat.* 1996;189(Pt 1):145–150.
27. Mitchell R, Chesney A, Seal S, McKnight L, Thoma A. Anatomical variations of the carpal tunnel structures. *Can J Plast Surg.* 2009;17(3):e3–e7.
28. Lutsky KF, Jones CM, Kim N, Medina J, Matzon JL, Beredjiklian PK. Frequency of incidental median thenar motor nerve branch visualization during mini-open and endoscopic carpal tunnel release. *Hand (N Y).* 2017;12(1):60–63.
29. Hong JT, Lee SW, Han SH, et al. Anatomy of neurovascular structures around the carpal tunnel during dynamic wrist motion for endoscopic carpal tunnel release. *Neurosurgery.* 2006;58(suppl 1): ONS127–133; discussion ONS127–133.
30. Sookur PA, Naraghi AM, Bleakney RR, Jalan R, Chan O, White LM. Accessory muscles: anatomy, symptoms, and radiologic evaluation. *Radiographics.* 2008;28(2):481–499.
31. Wolf AW, Packard S, Chow JC. Transligamentous motor branch of the median nerve discovered during endoscopically assisted carpal tunnel release. *Arthroscopy.* 1993;9(2):222–223.
32. Sytsma T, Ryan H, Lachman N, Kakar S, Smith J. Anatomic relationship between the hook of the hamate and the distal transverse carpal ligament: implications for ultrasound-guided carpal tunnel release. *Am J Phys Med Rehabil.* 2018;97(7):482–487.
33. Evans GR, Dellon AL. Implantation of the palmar cutaneous branch of the median nerve into the pronator quadratus for treatment of painful neuroma. *J Hand Surg Am.* 1994;19(2):203–206.
34. Olewnik L, Wysiadecki G, Polguj M, Podgorski M, Jezierski H, Topol M. Anatomical variations of the palmaris longus muscle including its relation to the median nerve—a proposal for a new classification. *BMC Musculoskelet Disord.* 2017;18(1):539.
35. Ioannis D, Anastasios K, Konstantinos N, Lazaros K, Georgios N. Palmaris longus muscle's prevalence in different nations and interesting anatomical variations: review of the literature. *J Clin Med Res.* 2015;7(11):825–830.
36. Chen CH, Wu T, Sun JS, Lin WH, Chen CY. Unusual causes of carpal tunnel syndrome: space occupying lesions. *J Hand Surg Eur Vol.* 2012;37(1):14–19.
37. Nordstrom DL, DeStefano F, Vierkant RA, Layde PM. Incidence of diagnosed carpal tunnel syndrome in a general population. *Epidemiology.* 1998;9(3):342–345.
38. Atroshi I, Englund M, Turkiewicz A, Tagil M, Petersson IF. Incidence of physician-diagnosed carpal tunnel syndrome in the general population. *Arch Intern Med.* 2011;171(10):943–944.
39. Palmer DH, Hanrahan LP. Social and economic costs of carpal tunnel surgery. *Instr Course Lect.* 1995;44:167–172.
40. Fajardo M, Kim SH, Szabo RM. Incidence of carpal tunnel release: trends and implications within the United States ambulatory care setting. *J Hand Surg Am.* 2012;37(8):1599–1605.
41. Keith MW, Masear V, Chung KC, et al. American Academy of Orthopaedic Surgeons Clinical Practice Guideline on diagnosis of carpal tunnel syndrome. *J Bone Joint Surg Am.* 2009;91(10):2478–2479.
42. Cartwright MS, Hobson-Webb LD, Boon AJ, et al. Evidence-based guideline: neuromuscular ultrasound for the diagnosis of carpal tunnel syndrome. *Muscle Nerve.* 2012;46(2):287–293.
43. Olave E, Prates JC, Del Sol M, Sarmento A, Gabrielli C. Distribution patterns of the muscular branch of the median nerve in the thenar region. *J Anat.* 1995;186(Pt 2):441–446.
44. Abicalaf CA, de Barros N, Sernik RA, et al. Ultrasound evaluation of patients with carpal tunnel syndrome before and after endoscopic release of the transverse carpal ligament. *Clin Radiol.* 2007;62(9):891–894; discussion 895–896.
45. Al-Hashel JY, Rashad HM, Nouh MR, et al. Sonography in carpal tunnel syndrome with normal nerve conduction studies. *Muscle Nerve.* 2015;51(4):592–597.
46. McDonagh C, Alexander M, Kane D. The role of ultrasound in the diagnosis and management of carpal tunnel syndrome: a new paradigm. *Rheumatology (Oxford).* 2015;54(1):9–19.
47. Fowler JR, Cipolli W, Hanson T. A comparison of three diagnostic tests for carpal tunnel syndrome using latent class analysis. *J Bone Joint Surg Am.* 2015;97(23):1958–1961.
48. Sernik RA, Abicalaf CA, Pimentel BF, Braga-Baiak A, Braga L, Cerri GG. Ultrasound features of carpal tunnel syndrome: a prospective case-control study. *Skeletal Radiol.* 2008;37(1):49–53.
49. Chappell CD, Beckman JP, Baird BC, Takke AV. Ultrasound (US) changes in the median nerve cross-sectional area after microinvasive US-guided carpal tunnel release. *J Ultrasound Med.* 2019.
50. Fumiere E, Dugardeyn C, Roquet ME, Delcour C. US demonstration of a thrombosed persistent median artery in carpal tunnel syndrome. *J Belg Radiol.* 2002;85(1):1–3.
51. Klauser AS, Abd Ellah MM, Halpern EJ, et al. Sonographic cross-sectional area measurement in carpal tunnel syndrome patients: can delta and ratio calculations predict severity compared to nerve conduction studies? *Eur Radiol.* 2015;25(8):2419–2427.
52. Latzka EW, Henning PT, Pourcho AM. Sonographic changes after ultrasound-guided release of the transverse carpal ligament: a case report. *Pharm Manag PM R.* 2018;10(10):1125–1129.
53. Aydin K, Cokluk C, Piskin A, Kocabicak E. Ultrasonographically checking the sectioning of the transverse carpal ligament during carpal tunnel surgery with limited uni skin incisions. *Turk Neurosurg.* 2007;17(3):219–223.
54. Mondelli M, Filippou G, Aretini A, Frediani B, Reale F. Ultrasonography before and after surgery in carpal tunnel syndrome and relationship with clinical and electrophysiological findings. A new outcome predictor? *Scand J Rheumatol.* 2008;37(3):219–224.
55. Lee CH, Kim TK, Yoon ES, Dhong ES. Postoperative morphologic analysis of carpal tunnel syndrome using high-resolution ultrasonography. *Ann Plast Surg.* 2005;54(2):143–146.
56. Karabay N, Toros T, Cetinkol E, Ada S. Correlations between ultrasonography findings and surgical findings in patients with refractory symptoms after primary surgical release for carpal tunnel syndrome. *Acta Orthop Traumatol Turc.* 2015;49(2): 126–132.

57. Joseph AE, Leiby BM, Beckman JP. Clinical results of ultrasound-guided carpal tunnel release performed by a primary care sports medicine physician. *J Ultrasound Med.* 2020 Mar;39(3):441-452.
58. Henning PT, Yang L, Awan T, Lueders D, Pourcho AM. Minimally invasive ultrasound-guided carpal tunnel release: preliminary clinical results. *J Ultrasound Med.* 2018;37(11): 2699–2706.
59. Chern TC, Wu KC, Huang LW, et al. A cadaveric and preliminary clinical study of ultrasonographically assisted percutaneous carpal tunnel release. *Ultrasound Med Biol.* 2014;40(8):1819–1826.
60. Williamson ERC, Vasquez Montes D, Melamed E. Multistate comparison of cost, trends, and complications in open versus endoscopic carpal tunnel release. *Hand (N Y).* 2019. 1558944719837020.
61. Devana SK, Jensen AR, Yamaguchi KT, et al. Trends and complications in open versus endoscopic carpal tunnel release in private payer and Medicare patient populations. *Hand (N Y).* 2019;14(4):455–461.
62. Cunningham DJ, Baumgartner RE, Federer AE, Richard MJ, Mithani SK. Elevated preoperative hemoglobin A1c associated with increased wound complications in diabetic patients undergoing primary, open carpal tunnel release. *Plast Reconstr Surg.* 2019;144(4):632e–638e.
63. Rojo-Manaute JM, Capa-Grasa A, Chana-Rodriguez F, et al. Ultra-minimally invasive ultrasound guided carpal tunnel release: a randomized controlled trial. *J Ultrasound Med.* 2016;35(6):1149–1157.
64. Kim PT, Lee HJ, Kim TG, Jeon IH. Current approaches for carpal tunnel syndrome. *Clin Orthop Surg.* 2014;6(3):253–257.
65. Papatheodorou LK, Sotereanos DG. Treatment recommendations for carpal tunnel syndrome and peripheral nerve repair. 64:273–280.
66. Hansen TB, Majeed HG. Endoscopic carpal tunnel release. *Hand Clinics.* 2013;30(1):47–53.
67. Capa-Grasa A, Rojo-Manaute JM, Rodriguez FC, Martin JV. Ultra-minimally invasive sonographically guided carpal tunnel release: an external pilot study. *Orthop Traumatol Surg Res.* 2014;100(3):287–292.
68. Rojo-Manaute J, Capa-Grasa A, Chana-Rodriguez F, et al. Ultra-minimally invasive ultrasound guided carpal tunnel release: a randomized controlled trial. *J Ultrasound Med.* 2016;35:1149–1157.
69. Rojo-Manaute JM, Capa-Grasa A, Rodriguez-Maruri GE, Moran LM, Martinez MV, Martin JV. Ultra-minimally invasive sonographically guided carpal tunnel release: anatomic study of a new technique. *J Ultrasound Med.* 2013;32(1):131–142.
70. Wang PH, Li CL, Shao CJ, Wu KC, Chern TC, Jou IM. Ultrasound-guided percutaneous carpal tunnel release in patients on hemodialysis: early experiences and clinical outcomes. *Ther Clin Risk Manag.* 2019;15:711–717.
71. Burnham RS, Loh EY, Rambaransingh B, Roberts SL, Agur AM, Playfair LD. A controlled trial evaluating the safety and effectiveness of ultrasound-guided looped thread carpal tunnel release. *Hand (N Y).* 2019. 1558944719842199.
72. Mittal N, Sangha H, Flannery J, Robinson LR, Agur A. Ultrasound-guided incisionless carpal tunnel release using a hook knife: a cadaveric study. *Pharm Manag PM R.* 2019;11(10): 1101–1106.
73. Petrover D, Silvera J, De Baere T, Vigan M, Hakime A. Percutaneous ultrasound-guided carpal tunnel release: study upon clinical efficacy and safety. *Cardiovasc Intervent Radiol.* 2017;40(4): 568–575.
74. Markison RE. Percutaneous ultrasound-guided MANOS carpal tunnel release technique. *Hand.* 2013;8(4):445–449.
75. de la Fuente J, Miguel-Perez MI, Balius R, Guerrero V, Michaud J, Bong D. Minimally invasive ultrasound-guided carpal tunnel release: a cadaver study. *J Clin Ultrasound.* 2013;41(2):101–107.
76. Benson LS, Bare AA, Nagle DJ, Harder VS, Williams CS, Visotsky JL. Complications of endoscopic and open carpal tunnel release. *Arthroscopy.* 2006;22(9):919–924. 924 e911-912.
77. Lecoq B, Hanouz N, Morello R, et al. Ultrasound-assisted surgical release of carpal tunnel syndrome: results of a pilot, open-label uncontrolled trial conducted outside of the operating room. *Joint Bone Spine.* 2015;82:442–445.
78. Buncke G, McCormack B, Bodor M. Ultrasound-guided carpal tunnel release using the manos CTR system. *Microsurgery.* 2013;33(5):362–366.
79. Dekimpe C, Andreani O, Camuzard O, et al. Ultrasound-guided percutaneous release of the carpal tunnel: comparison of the learning curves of a senior versus a junior operator. A cadaveric study. *Skeletal Radiol.* 2019;48(11):1803–1809.
80. Hebbard PD, Hebbard AIT, Tomka J, Appleyard R. Ultrasound-guided microinvasive carpal tunnel release using a novel retractable needle-mounted blade: a cadaveric study. *J Ultrasound Med.* 2018;37(8):2075–2081.
81. Henning T, Lueders D, Chang K, Yang L. Ultrasound-guided carpal tunnel release using dynamic expansion of the transverse safe zone in a patient with postpolio syndrome: a case report. *Pharm Manag PM R.* 2018;10(10):1115–1118.
82. Rowe NM, Michaels J, Soltanian H, Dobryansky M, Peimer CA, Gurtner GC. Sonographically guided percutaneous carpal tunnel release: an anatomic and cadaveric study. *Ann Plast Surg.* 2005;55(1):52–56; discussion 56.
83. Nakamichi K, Tachibana S, Yamamoto S, Ida M. Percutaneous carpal tunnel release compared with mini-open release using ultrasonographic guidance for both techniques. *J Hand Surg.* 2010;35(3):437–445.
84. Nakamichi KTS. Ultrasonographically assisted carpal tunnel release. *J Hand Surg.* 1997:853–862.
85. McShane JM, Slaff S, Gold JE, Nazarian LN. Sonographically guided percutaneous needle release of the carpal tunnel for treatment of carpal tunnel syndrome: preliminary report. *J Ultrasound Med.* 2012;31(9):1341–1349.
86. Boeckstyns ME, Sorensen AI. Does endoscopic carpal tunnel release have a higher rate of complications than open carpal tunnel release? An analysis of published series. *J Hand Surg Br.* 1999;24(1):9–15.
87. Presley J, Smith J, Barnes D, Lachman N, Kakar S, Sellon J. Ultrasound-guided carpal tunnel release (USCTR) using dynamic safe zone expansion: a cadaveric validation study [abstract]. *Clin J Sport.* 2017;27(suppl):221.
88. Levine DW, Simmons BP, Koris MJ, et al. A self-administered questionnaire for the assessment of severity of symptoms and functional status in carpal tunnel syndrome. *J Bone Joint Surg Am.* 1993;75(11):1585–1592.
89. Hudak PL, Amadio PC, Bombardier C. Development of an upper extremity outcome measure: the DASH (disabilities of the arm, shoulder and hand) [corrected]. The Upper Extremity Collaborative Group (UECG). *Am J Ind Med.* 1996;29(6):602–608.
90. Kuschner SH, Brien WW, Johnson D, Gellman H. Complications associated with carpal tunnel release. *Orthop Rev.* 1991;20(4):346–352.
91. Palmer AK, Toivonen DA. Complications of endoscopic and open carpal tunnel release. *J Hand Surg Am.* 1999;24(3):561–565.
92. Vasiliadis HS, Tokis AV, Andrikoula SI, et al. Microsurgical dissection of the carpal tunnel with respect to neurovascular structures at risk during endoscopic carpal tunnel release. *Arthroscopy.* 2006;22(8):807–812.

33

Ultrasound-Guided Percutaneous Bone Spur Excision and Cheilectomy

BRIAN J. SHIPLE

KEY POINTS

- Bone spurs that form along joints are known as osteophytes, and bone spurs that form at the attachment of tendons to bones are called enthesophytes.
- Bone spurs may cause pain by causing joint impingement, nerve irritation, and direct mechanical irritation to soft tissue.
- Not all bone spurs cause pain. Many bone spurs that are identified may be asymptomatic, and the osteophyte or enthesophyte a sign of the underlying degenerative or inflammatory pathology or instability.
- A cheilectomy is the removal of bony irregularities, or osteophytes, at the osteochondral margin of a joint that limit joint range of motion. Classically this applies to a hallux rigidus patient from the dorsal surface of the great toe, but this term may be applied to any joint where there is an impinging bone spur.
- Minimally invasive percutaneous bone spur or intratendinous calcification removal using a cannula or Tenex TX-Bone tool is a novel way to remove impinging bone spurs along joint surfaces or enthesophytes at tendon attachments.
- Patient selection should be based on careful examination, diagnostic blocks, and diagnostic imaging (e.g., ultrasound, x-ray, and magnetic resonance imaging [MRI]/computed tomography [CT]).

Anatomy and Pathology

Bony exostosis, or bone spurs, is thought to develop in response to inflammatory or mechanical stimuli.[1] There are three main types of bony proliferation: (1) chondro-osteophyte or osteophyte at the synovium-articular cartilage junction along the joint margins; (2) traction spur or enthesophyte at the insertion of a tendon or ligament; and (3) syndesmophytes within the vertebral column along the annulus fibrosus or spinal ligament and associated with inflammatory spondyloarthropathies such as ankylosing spondylitis.[2,3]

Osteophytes and enthesophytes have similar developmental process and composition.[3,4] Osteophytes are typically lateral outgrowths of bone at the joint line and are features of degenerative and inflammatory joint diseases or mechanical stress from joint instability.[2,5] The degree of spurring can vary considerably, and there is some evidence that small spurs can be unrelated to associated joint pathology.[6,7]

Enthesophytes are also common and form in the direction of tension of the involved ligament or tendon.[3] Enthesophytes can form at any tendon or ligament enthesis and are associate with microtears or in response to inflammatory pathology, and risk factors include spondyloarthritis and age.[8,9] One radiographic survey found heel spurs at the Achilles tendon or plantar fascia in 25% of the population.[10] Similar to osteophytes, enthesophytes do not always indicate pain or disease.[8,11–15]

Imaging and Ultrasound Findings

Conventional radiographs are the standard imaging modality for the assessment of osteoarthritis, and osteophytes are a common radiographic feature. Radiographic grading of osteophytes or enthesophytes is often subjective. Different semiquantitative scoring systems have been described.[16–18] Few studies have examined the reliability of these scales or if there is a clinical correlation, and there is an no established universal or standardized grading method for osteophytes or enthesophytes.[19]

Radiographs are in imperfect way of assessing osteophyte formation and enthesophyte changes.[20] In some studies, ultrasound has been shown to be more sensitive than conventional radiography in detecting osteophytes in the hand and knee.[21–25] Sonographic findings of bone spurs, whether an osteophyte or enthesophyte, include a hyperechoic cortical protrusion with acoustic shadowing. Different grading systems have been described, but few studies have examined the reliability of these scales and clinical correlation, and a review of these scales is beyond the scope of this chapter.[17–19] Dynamic ultrasound can also be used to visualize impingement due to osteophytes.[26]

Ultrasound evaluation can also be used for preprocedural planning, and the osteophyte or enthesophyte should be assessed for its size (length, width, and depth) in long and short axis. Examination of surrounding neurovascular structures is necessary to assess a treatment pathway (e.g., place an instrument safely down to the bone spur for possible removal).

Treatment Options

Asymptomatic osteophytes or enthesophytes do not need treatment, and conservative management includes medications, changing footwear, or adding padding. Ultrasound-guided fenestration and cortisone injection have been reported to be an effective way to manage anterior ankle impingement. In a retrospective case series of 49 patients with anterior ankle impingement, Nazarian et al. showed 4/79.6% of patients were able to avoid surgical treatment of their painful anterior ankle impingement at follow-up (average 27 months).[27]

Symptomatic spurs that fail conservative management may need to be removed. Open or arthroscopic/endoscopic surgery is the standard of care for painful osteophytes that limit motion or cause impingement,[28–30] and painful enthesophytes within a tendon.[31,32] Using a cheilectomy to remove painful dorsal osteophytes for hallux rigidus has been well described in the literature, with open, arthroscopic, and percutaneous approaches being described.[33] The literature on percutaneous approaches is limited. Percutaneous minimally invasive techniques for dorsal cheilectomy have been reported with a wedge burr (Wright Medical, Memphis, TN) and have similar complications to an open cheilectomy.[33–36] One limitation may be a higher reoperation rate with the percutaneous palpation-guided approach. One publication comparing open versus minimally invasive cheilectomy with a wedge burr had a higher reoperation rate with the minimally invasive approach (12.8% compared with 2.6% with open surgery).[36]

Minimally invasive arthroscopic and endoscopic resection of bone spurs and exostosis have also been reported at varying locations. Anterior ankle impingement[37,38] has also been managed with arthroscopic removal of bone spurs, effectively treating pain and loss of motion. Successful arthroscopic and endoscopic resection of olecranon spur[39–41] and endoscopic management of chronic Osgood-Schlatter disease[42] have also been described in a case series. Compared with open procedures, arthroscopic procedures have shorter recovery time and quicker resumption of sport.[43,44] Endoscopic calcaneoplasty of Haglund deformity has been shown to be superior to open techniques, with less morbidity and fewer complications.[45,46] Osteophytes can occur at other locations, but the literature on percutaneous and arthroscopic/endoscopic spur excision is limited.

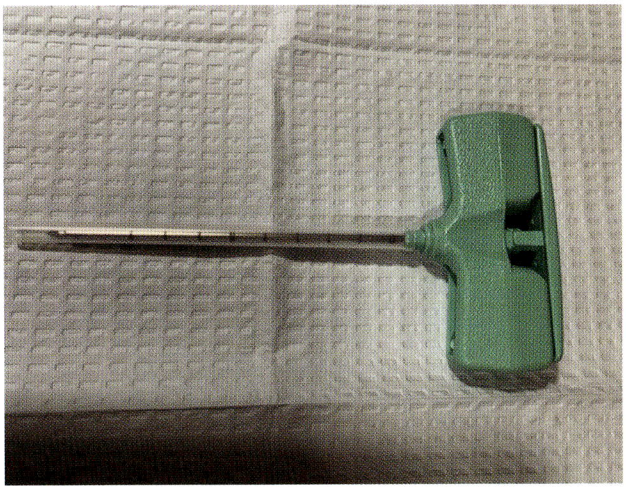

• **Fig. 33.1** The Jamshidi 11-gauge × 4.5-inch trocar and cannula used to remove bone spurs and enthesophytes.

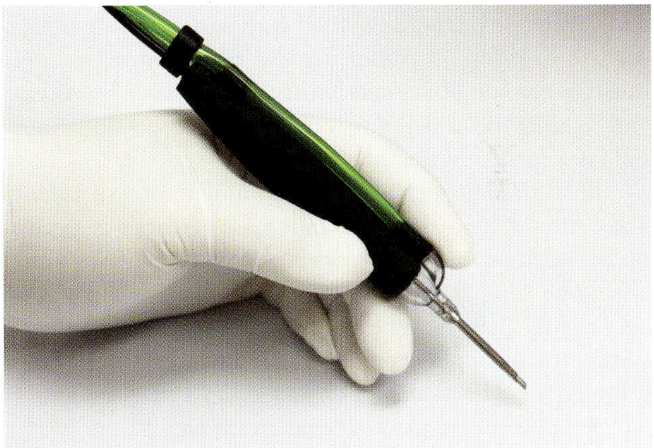

• **Fig. 33.2** TX-Bone (TXB) Micro Tip. Tenex Health TX-Bone (TXB) Micro Tip device designed for bone removal. The Tenex TX-Bone tool is a 14-gauge needle to facilitate debriding bone spurs and enthesophytes.

Ultrasound-guided percutaneous spur excision has not been widely described in the literature. Excision of a painful osteophyte or enthesophyte can be performed with an 11-gauge × 4.5-inch Jamshidi trocar and cannula (Fig. 33.1) or an OnControl trocar and cannula or more recently with the aid of the Tenex TXB Micro Tip bone tool (Fig. 33.2).

Patient Selection

Any patient with a painful osteophyte or enthesophyte that is safely accessible may be a candidate for a bone spur excision, cheilectomy, or tendon enthesophyte excision. Whether a bone spur needs to be addressed as part of a patient's treatment plan can be assessed by a process of exclusion and the use of carefully targeted diagnostic blocks. Many bone spurs that are identified may be asymptomatic, and the osteophyte or enthesophyte may be a sign of the underlying degenerative or inflammatory pathology.

In cases of calcaneal heel spur, radiographic and histologic findings suggest that changes within the fascia rather than the spur are primarily responsible for pain.[47] In one study of subjects who underwent an endoscopic plantar fasciopathy, 53.8% of the patients had a calcaneal spur. The spur was never resected in these subjects, and the outcomes of the plantar fasciopathy remained the same whether the patients had an associated spur or not.[48] Other studies have also shown good results with treating the plantar fascia alone, again showing that, although calcaneal spurs may be present, there are many other causes of heel pain (e.g., plantar fasciitis, tears in the plantar fascia, fat pad atrophy, calcaneal fractures).[49–51]

The challenge of localizing the source of pain extends to other locations of osteophytosis or enthesophytes. Image-guided diagnostic blocks can be very helpful in confirming whether the bone spur is a cause of pain or not. Use a minimal amount of 1% lidocaine around the bone spur to increase the diagnostic accuracy of the block and assess whether good anesthesia is achieved within a few minutes of the injection. Commonly, osteophytes are associated with degenerative or inflammatory joint disease or instability, and enthesophytes are associated with partial tearing of ligament on tendon. The spur may be asymptomatic or only one of a number of factors contributing to pain. Identifying and treating the underlying source of pain is possibly essential for a successful treatment plan.

The ultrasonic percutaneous treatment of osteophytes and enthesophytes is early, and more research is needed on patient outcomes and possible adverse events. Caution should be taken in patient selection. Joint pain, night pain, and resting pain may be negative prognostic factors, and symptoms of impingement or osteophyte rubbing against footwear may be positive prognostic signs that the patient will respond well to percutaneous treatment.

Equipment

- Sterile procedure tray with nonfenestrated sterile tray cover
  - Fenestrated drape or sterile cloth or paper towels to create a sterile field
  - Sterile prep applicators (e.g., ChloraPrep or Betadine) with manufacturer-required drying time to establish a dry sterile barrier prior to the procedure
  - 4 × 4 gauze sponges
  - Sterile surgical marking pen
  - Introducer with an 18-gauge needle or an 11-blade disposable scalpel
  - Sterile 3- to 10-cc syringe for skin to target local anesthesia
  - 27-gauge needle for skin wheel anesthesia
  - 25- to 22-gauge needle for anesthetizing the soft tissue pathway to the target
  - Steri-Strips for wound closure
  - Tincture of benzoin for sterile adhesive to hold Steri-Strip in place
  - 2 × 2 gauze for hemostasis under waterproof wound dressing
  - Tegaderm for waterproof sterile wound barrier
  - Diagnostic ultrasound machine with a high-frequency linear array transducer or a low-frequency curvilinear transducer for deeper approaches
  - Sterile probe cover and sterile gel
  - Percutaneous cutting tool: Jamshidi 11-gauge × 4.5-in trocar and cannula, Tenex TX-Bone Micro Tip Bone tool kit, or 11- to 15-gauge OnControl trocar and cannula

Injectates

- Lidocaine 1% or 2% with and/or without epinephrine and normal saline for skin wheel and local anesthesia and irrigation as needed. If 11-blade is planned as the introducer to puncture the skin, consider using epinephrine for the skin wheel.
- Ropivacaine 0.2% to 0.5% and lidocaine 1% or 2% to help provide longer-term anesthesia from the procedure.
- Optional: an orthobiologic injectate to help facilitate healing of any damaged tissue after the bone spur removal (e.g., dextrose prolotherapy, platelet-rich plasma [PRP] amniotic membrane graft, bone marrow concentrate).

Injectate Volume

- Local anesthesia:
  - Skin wheel 2 to 5 mL of lidocaine 1% with or without epinephrine
  - 3 to 10 mL of mixture of 1 lidocaine 1 or 2% with or without epinephrine mixed with an equal part of ropivacaine 0.2% to 0.5%

Ultrasound-Guided Bone Spur Resection (Author's Preferred Technique)

Patient and Clinician Position

- Patient position will vary depending on the target osteophyte or enthesophyte.
- The physician should preferably be seated across from the ultrasound screen and the patient's limb between the physician and the ultrasound screen for good ergonomics.

Transducer Orientation

- Short- and long-axis views over the bone spur to identify neurovascular structures and plan how much bone needs to be removed to address the soft tissue impingement or restricted joint range of motion. Power Doppler imaging can be used to help localize neurovascular structures.
- The pathway to access the bone spur needs to be planned to minimize risk of iatrogenic injury to the neurovascular structures.
- Detailed knowledge of the neurovascular anatomy will help to ensure a safe pathway to place the cheilectomy tool. Always use Doppler settings (e.g., Doppler perfusion index [DPI] or color Doppler) prior to starting the procedure to make sure no significant blood vessels or nerves are in the way of the cheilectomy tool placement.

- Once the pathway for the needle has been chosen, the entry point should be marked on the skin with a sterile surgical marking pen.

Needle Orientation

- The needle should be placed in-plane to ensure visualization of the needle tip and cutting device. This may necessitate a distal to proximal or medial to lateral approach, etc., depending on the patient's target bone spur location.
- A smaller-gauge anesthetic needle can be used to confirm the pathway for the cutting device to safely access the spur, keeping in mind the neurovascular anatomy and musculoskeletal tissues in the pathway and adjacent to the spur.
    - Anesthetic should be injected around the spur/periosteum, ensuring to cover the three-dimensional location of the spur. Local anesthesia with a 27- to 25-gauge, 1.25-inch needle to make a skin wheel and a 25- to 22-gauge, 1.5- to 4-inch needle to anesthetize a pathway for the cutting tool to the bone spur.
    - In enthesophytes, note any soft tissue defects adjacent to the bone spur that "open up" when injecting the anesthetic. These can represent interstitial tears or delaminating tears and may also need to be addressed (e.g., with an orthobiologic injection) in addition to removing the bone spur.

Target

- Ensure adequate anesthesia of the bone spur and adjacent soft tissue to facilitate a painless procedure. When possible, an adjacent nerve block should be considered to help with pain during the procedure (e.g., tibial and sural nerve block for Achilles spur or Haglund resection).
- An 18-gauge, 1- or 1.5-inch hypodermic needle or an 11-blade disposable scalpel is used as an introducer to puncture the patient's skin to facilitate entry of the larger-bore cutting tools.
- The cutting tool is placed through the introducer hole under, and advanced under, ultrasound guidance to the surface of the bone spur using in-plane views. Orthogonal out-of-plane views are obtained to confirm needle placement. Alternate probe positions will ensure the three dimensions of the bone spur are addressed during the procedure.

Consideration if Using the Jamshidi Trocar

- If using the Jamshidi trocar and cannula, the trocar is removed from the cannula. A 3- to 5-cc syringe with lidocaine with epinephrine is placed on the open Luer-Lock port after removing the trocar in the event the patient needs more anesthesia. This also covers the Luer port opening and helps maintain sterility. Blood backing into the cannula alerts the physician for the need for more hemostasis, and lidocaine with epinephrine is injected through the cannula.

LT ISCHIAL BONE SPUR

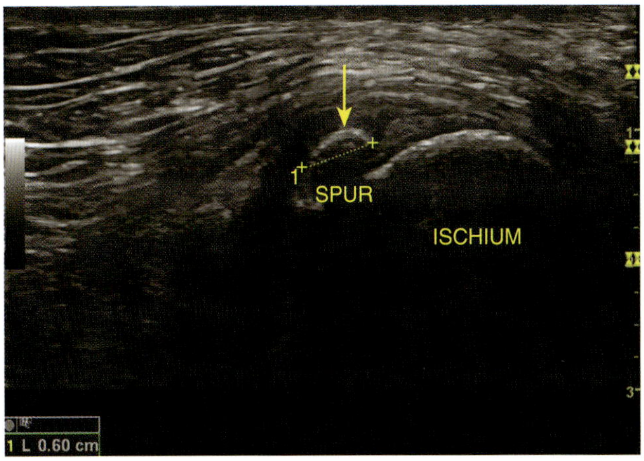

• **Fig. 33.3** Left ischial bone spur at origin of conjoined hamstring tendon in an avid hiker and mountain climber with a history of chronic hamstring origin tendinopathy.

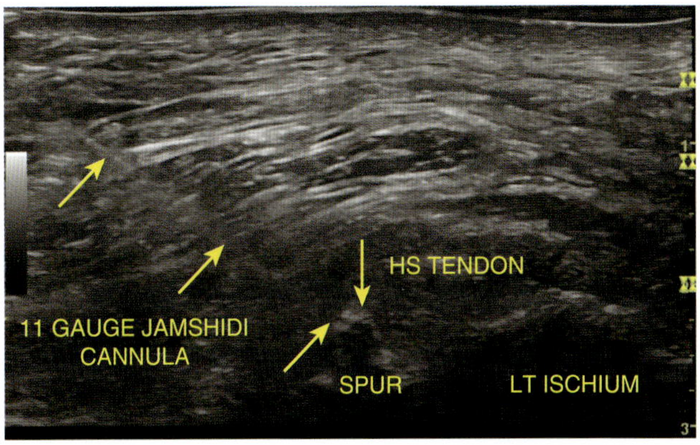

• **Fig. 33.4** Left ischial bone spur with Jamshidi cannula placed in-plane against the bone spur from a lateral to medial approach and ready for the cheilectomy procedure.

- The cannula is then twisted clockwise and counterclockwise and advanced through the bone spur like a leather punch or kitchen apple core tool until the cannula is seen to be all the way through the bone spur on ultrasound imaging. The bone spur is now inside the cannula (Figs. 33.3–33.5).
- An additional pass can be attempted to remove more of the spur. In the author's experience, two passes through a 3-mm bone spur will fill the cannula up approximately 2 cm into the cannula. Removing more bone may be difficult and may increase the risk of leaving a loose body in the surgery site.
- If more of the spur needs to be removed a second Jamshidi trocar and cannula can be placed back through the surgical opening and the procedure repeated

Consideration if Using the Tenex Bone Needle

- In May 2019, the Tenex TXB Micro Tip tool became commercially available. The Tenex TXB cutting tool uses a foot pedal to activate the needle and begin the bone spur removal.

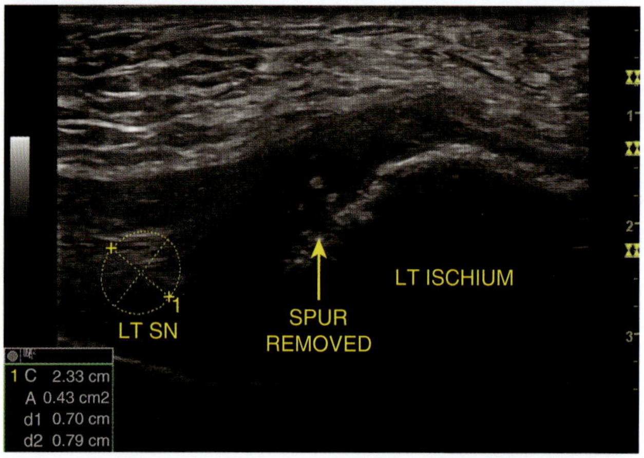

• **Fig. 33.5** The left ischium 8 weeks later showing the bone spur has been removed with some minor specs of bone left in the soft tissue area. Note the proximity of the sciatic nerve to the bone spur removal site.

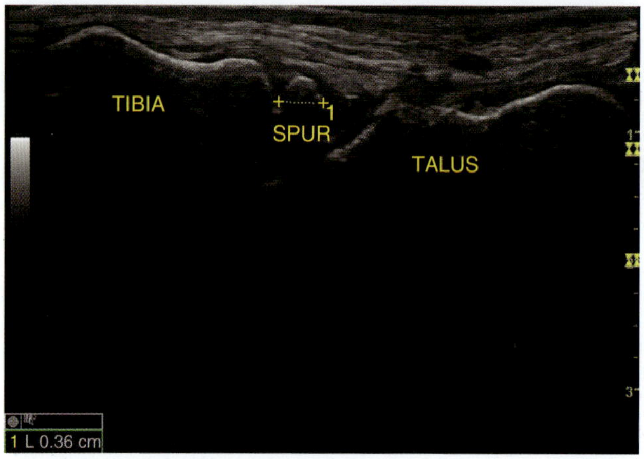

• **Fig. 33.6** A tibial bone spur causing left anterior ankle impingement in a triathlete with a history of pseudogout and keloid scar former.

- The cutting tool removes bone tissue using ultrasonic cavitation and irrigation.
- Ultrasound guidance with alternating in-plane and out-of-plane views should be used to make sure the bone spur has been fully removed.
- The TXB Micro Tip should start along the superficial aspect of the spur and remove bone in layers, moving deeper until the desired amount of bone is removed (Figs. 33.6–33.9). Most enthesophytes or bone spurs are removed with 1 to 3 minutes of cutting time with the TXB tool.

Post Procedure

Once the bone spur is removed, diagnostic ultrasound can confirm if there is adequate removal. The spur site should be studied in short and long axis. If the spur was causing joint impingement, dynamic ultrasound with passive joint range of motion should be used to confirm the impingement has been resolved. If a portion of the spur or enthesophyte in a

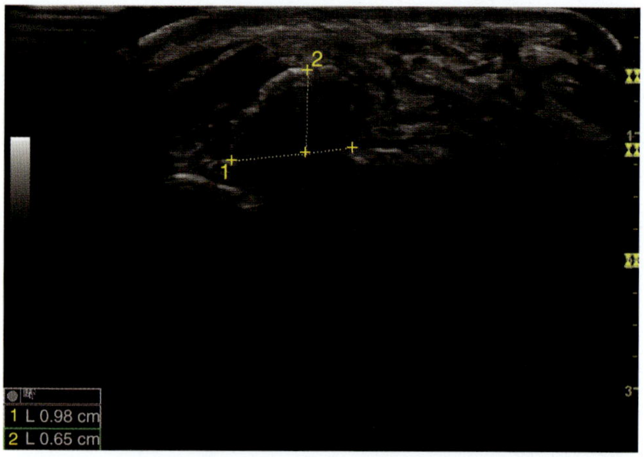

• **Fig. 33.7** Short-axis view of an anterior medial ankle tibial bone spur causing anterior impingement in a triathlete.

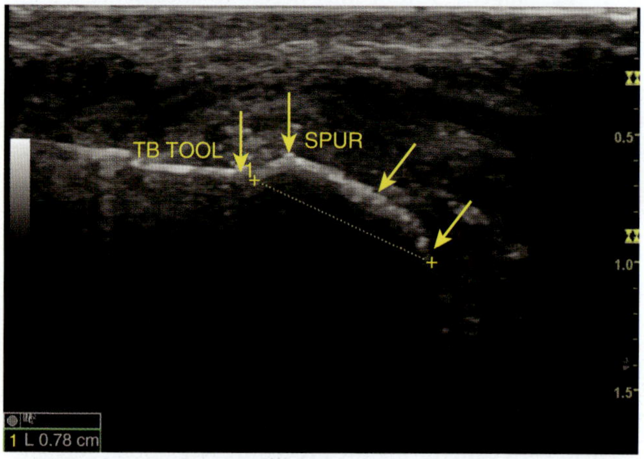

• **Fig. 33.8** Tenex TX-Bone Micro Tip tool placed against the bone spur and ready for the cheilectomy procedure.

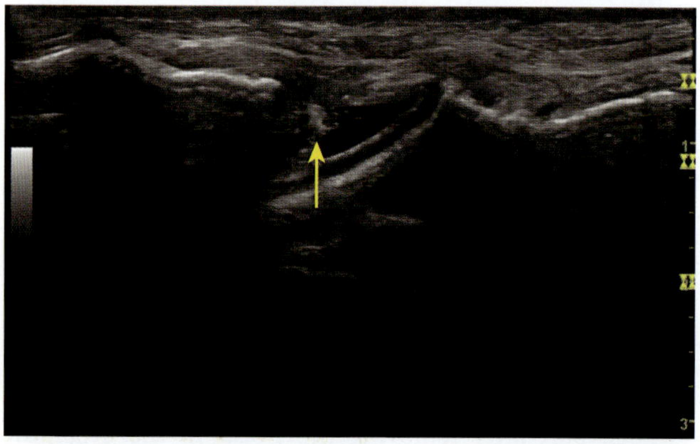

• **Fig. 33.9** Eight weeks post cheilectomy showing some small bony debris left in the soft tissue where the bone spur used to be as well as scant joint fluid in the tibial talar joint and some thickening of the synovial tissue just superficial to the ankle joint. At 3-month follow-up the patient's impingement pain and ankle dorsiflexion had returned to normal.

tendon was not adequately removed, a decision to repeat the procedure should be made. The goal is to remove all or most of the bone spur or enthesophyte.

Once the decision is made that the bone spur resection is adequate, the decision should be made to address any soft tissue defect, such as a tendon tear, ligament tear, or joint capsule tear. The possibility of needing to address an associated soft tissue lesion should be made even before the procedure and reflected in the consent, if the physician decides to do the treatment at the time of the bone spur resection. Associated soft tissue pathology can be treated with an orthobiologic injection at the time of the treatment (e.g., PRP, prolotherapy, etc.). Some physicians will decide to do this treatment at the time of the bone spur resection, and others may decide to delay this treatment until 4 to 8 weeks after the bone spur resection procedure. The author prefers to use an orthobiologic at the time of the bone spur resection using a different needle entry site.

After bone spur removal, compression with sterile gauze can be used for up to 4 to 10 minutes and will usually achieve hemostasis. Bone spurs have a blood supply and, if hemostasis is slow or incomplete, a simple suture closure with Nylon suture material may also be used depending on the depth of the procedure. Once hemostasis has been achieved, tincture of benzoin with Steri-Strips can be used to close the incision site and the Steri-Strips covered by a 2 × 2 sterile gauze and Tegaderm.

The patient is instructed to keep the waterproof dressing on until postoperative day 5. If needed, the dressing can be replaced with a simple adhesive bandage to keep the wound clean and dry. Steri-Strips may be removed between 6 and 7 days. If a suture was placed, it should be removed in 7 to 10 days.

For lower extremity spur excisions, the patient should be non–weight bearing for 1 to 4 days to ensure hemostasis is maintained and allow the postprocedure pain to subside. The goal of non–weight bearing is to allow the early inflammatory phase to pass. For enthesophyte removal in a weight-bearing limb a walking boot is recommended to support the debrided tendon after the non–weight-bearing period and for a total of 2 weeks to allow for early healing of the tendon.

Protected weight bearing as tolerated can resume on day 2 to 5, and range of motion exercises should be started on day 3. The patient may work on range of motion outside of the boot 3 to 5 times a day, keeping the Visual Analog Scale (VAS) pain score no higher than a 3 out of 10. Resistance training should start once the VAS pain score is at 3 out of 10 or less and should not be allowed to go over 3 out of 10 as healing progresses. This may take up to 2 to 4 weeks to achieve that level of pain control. After the initial 2-week healing period, the boot may be weaned and used for longer weight-bearing periods to keep the VAS pain score less than a 3 out of 10.

Patients with painful impinging bone spurs usually notice early pain relief within days to a week or two, but full healing may require 2 to 4 months. The patient may be brought back for a wound check at 1 week, 4 weeks for progression to full rehabilitation, and 8 to 12 weeks to determine if a regenerative injection treatment is needed or the procedure needs to be repeated. During the postprocedure follow-up evaluation, the physician should examine the patient for improvement in symptoms. Diagnostic ultrasound and/or radiographs should be obtained to confirm successful removal of the bone spur or enthesophyte.

Patients with advanced osteoarthritis that have an impinging bone spur are at higher risk of being a nonresponder, but in the author's hands the results have been successful at restoring joint motion and pain relief, especially when combined with an advanced orthobiologic medicine procedure, such as a bone marrow concentrate injection to help treat the arthritic joint.

Complications Post Procedure

Complications are similar to those of open or arthroscopic/endoscopic bone spur removal, including infection, bleeding, and continued or worsening pain. Failure to adhere to sterile technique could result in a wound infection and in cases of bone spur removal from a joint could result in a septic joint. In the author's 10 years of experience, he has not experienced an infection with this procedure and he has not used preprocedure antibiotics or placed any patient on postprocedure antibiotics. Therefore the author does not recommend routinely using antibiotics to help prevent infection but would not view a physician's decision to use antibiotics in this case as improper.

Hemostasis is the most common challenge a physician will encounter on larger bone spurs. Apart from having to use a suture or two, the author has not encountered a patient he was not able to achieve hemostasis. Although rare, the physician should be prepared for a case of uncontrolled bleeding. Other options available to the in-office physician could include silver nitrate sticks, a battery-operated surgical Bovie, or Gelfoam.

Iatrogenic neurologic injury can occur, and in the surgical literature complications of hallux valgus surgery include injury to the dorsomedial cutaneous nerves.[52–54] A decision to remove a spur on or near a nerve is precision work and can cause a minor temporary nerve injury that will recover in days to weeks and rarely months.[55] However, an inadvertent nerve transection can occur without advanced knowledge of the neuroanatomy, and this risk should be discussed with the patient and noted on the signed informed consent. In the author's experience he has not encountered a permanent nerve injury.

Bony debris may remain in the soft tissue using either technique described earlier. Manipulation and compression of the soft tissue toward the incision site, and irrigation of the tissue can be used to try and remove the remaining bony debris. Small pieces of bone left behind in a tendon or ligament again is common and is not of any consequence. Usually on long-term follow-up, the remaining small pieces of bone are adsorbed as the soft tissue continues to remodel and heal (Figs. 33.10 and 33.11). Leaving a loose body in a joint has not occurred in the author's experience and the risk of occurring should be very low risk, but not zero.

In some uncommon situations, the enthesophyte or bone spur may grow back, especially if the joint stability is not addressed as part of the treatment plan. Spur reoccurrence can occur with or without recurrent symptoms.[31,56] All area pathology should be addressed prior to deciding if repeat bone excision is needed to restore tendon function or to try to help the patient's joint movement. No studies have examined recurrence rates after a percutaneous approach. In one study of open versus minimally invasive cheilectomy with a wedge burr for hallux rigidus, the open group did not require further surgery for impingement, while the minimally invasive group 4% required repeat surgery for dorsal impingement pain.[41] In symptomatic cases, a decision to repeat the procedure may be made and may still be successful.

In addition, tendon rupture is a potential risk of enthesophyte resection. Enthesophytes can occupy a larger percentage of the cross-sectional area of a tendon and resection could cause the tendon to be substantially weakened until it is healed. The tendon should be supported (e.g., taping, shoe inserts/heel wedges, prescription orthotics, a boot, and/or bracing) and weight bearing limited for the first 2 weeks after the treatment. Strong consideration should be given to addressing associated tendon pathology, with an advanced orthobiologic injection in the tendon defect left behind to guard against this rare complication and stimulate early healing.

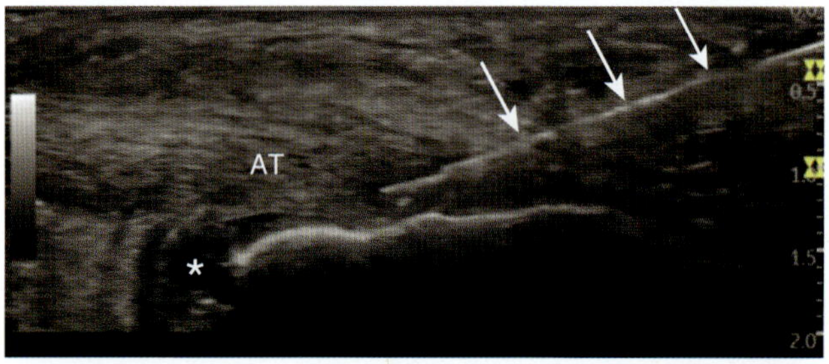

• **Fig. 33.10** Ultrasound of TX-Bone needle *(arrows)* approaching Haglund deformity. The needle track is through the Achilles tendon and the Haglund deformity is removed in layers from superficial to deep. *Asterisks*, Retrocalcaneal bursa; *AT*, Achilles tendon.

PEARLS AND PITFALLS

- Percutaneous osteophyte and enthesophyte resection require real-time ultrasound guidance and precise needle placement.
- The goal of the procedure is to remove painful bony exostosis and restore or improve joint motion; however, the procedure may not work and could leave a loose body behind or make the patient's pain worse.
- Informed consent must be obtained bearing out these facts as well as the lack of controlled studies with efficacy and adverse event data.
- The Tenex 1 and 2 tools have been used to remove very small enthesophytes and bone spurs but often fail to do an adequate job of removing bone from larger lesions of over 1 to 2 mm in size. The Tenex TX-Bone Micro Tip was designed to remove bone. In the author's experience, it is proving to be an efficient way to remove impinging osteophytes and tendon enthesophytes. One limitation is the TX-Bone Micro Tip is 1.3-inch long, and preprocedural planning should take into account whether the tip can reach the pathologic site.
- A Jamshidi trocar and cannula has been used by the author successfully for 10 years to safely remove intratendinous enthesophytes and impinging bone spurs.
- Using the techniques described in this chapter a bone spur approximately 0.5 × 0.5 cm to 1 × 1 cm in size can be safely removed.

References

1. Venne G, Tse MY, Pang SC, Ellis RE. Mechanically-induced osteophyte in the rat knee. *Osteoarthritis Cartilage.* 2020;28(6):853–864.
2. van der Kraan PM, van den Berg WB. Osteophytes: relevance and biology. *Osteoarthritis Cartilage.* 2007;15(3):237–244.

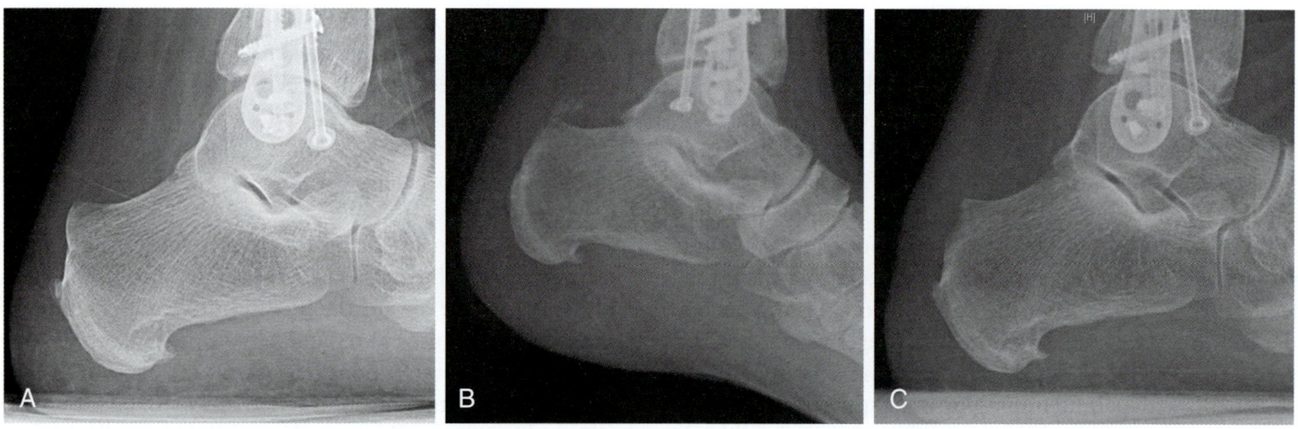

• **Fig. 33.11** Preprocedure radiograph (A) and postprocedure radiographs immediately after the TX-Bone (B) and at 3 months (C) demonstrating the removal of the Haglund deformity. The bony debris visible immediately following the procedure in the retrocalcaneal bursa (B) is resorbed at the 3-month follow-up (C).

3. Rogers J, Shepstone L, Dieppe P. Bone formers: osteophyte and enthesophyte formation are positively associated. *Ann Rheum Dis*. 1997;56(2):85–90.
4. Benjamin M, Rufai A, Ralphs JR. The mechanism of formation of bony spurs (enthesophytes) in the Achilles tendon. *Arthritis Rheum*. 2000;43(3):576–583.
5. Cannon LB, Hackney RG. Anterior tibiotalar impingement associated with chronic ankle instability. *J Foot Ankle Surg*. 2000;39(6):383–386.
6. Felson DT. Developments in the clinical understanding of osteoarthritis. *Arthritis Res Ther*. 2009;11:203e13.
7. Roemer FW, Jarraya M, Niu J, Silva J-R, Frobell R, Guermazi A. Increased risk for radiographic osteoarthritis features in young active athletes: a cross-sectional matched case control study. *Osteoarthritis Cartilage*. 2015;23:239e43.
8. Kamo K, Yahiro K. Incidence and risk factors of calcaneal enthesophytes in spondyloarthritis and trauma patients. *Mod Rheumatol*. 2016;26(4):598–600.
9. Niepel GA, Sit'aj S. Enthesopathy. *Clin Rheum Dis*. 1979;5:857–872.
10. Resnick D, Feingold ML, Curd J, Niwayama G, Goergen TG. Calcaneal abnormalities in articular disorders: rheumatoid arthritis, ankylosing spondylitis, psoriatic arthritis, and Reiter's syndrome. *Radiology*. 1977;125:355–366.
11. Menz HB, Zammit GV, Landorf KB, Munteanu SE. Plantar calcaneal spurs in older people: longitudinal traction or vertical compression? *J Foot Ankle Res*. 2008;1(1):7.
12. Toumi H, Davies R, Mazor M, et al. Changes in prevalence of calcaneal spurs in men and women: a random population from a trauma clinic. *BMC Musculoskelet Disord*. 2014;15:87.
13. Rubin G, Whitten M. Plantar calcaneal spurs. *Am J Orthop*. 1963;5:38.
14. Shama SS, Kominsky SJ, Lemont H. Prevalence of nonpainful heel spurs & its relation to postural foot position. *J Am Podiatr Med Assoc*. 1983;73:122–123.
15. Tanz SS. Heel pain. *CORR*. 1963;28:169–177.
16. Kettler A, Wilke H-J. Review of existing grading systems for cervical or lumbar disc and facet joint degeneration. *Euro Spine J*. 2005;15(6):705–718.
17. Wright RW, MARS Group. Osteoarthritis classification scales: interobserver reliability and arthroscopic correlation. *J Bone Joint Surg Am*. 2014;96(14):1145–1151. https://doi.org/10.2106/JBJS.M.00929.
18. Kijowski R, Blankenbaker D, Stanton P, Fine J, De Smet A. Arthroscopic validation of radiographic grading scales of osteoarthritis of the tibiofemoral joint. *AJR Am J Roentgenol*. 2006;187(3):794–799.
19. Guermazi A, Hunter DJ, Li L, et al. Different thresholds for detecting osteophytes and joint space narrowing exist between the site investigators and the centralized reader in a multicenter knee osteoarthritis study—data from the Osteoarthritis Initiative. *Skeletal Radiol*. 2012;41(2):179–186. https://doi.org/10.1007/s00256-011-1142-2.
20. Rogers J, Watt I, Dieppe P. Comparison of visual and radiographic detection of bony changes at the knee joint. *BMJ*. 1990;300:367–368.
21. Mathiessen A, Haugen IK, Slatkowsky-Christensen B, et al. Ultrasonographic assessment of osteophytes in 127 patients with hand osteoarthritis: exploring reliability and associations with MRI, radiographs and clinical joint findings. *Ann Rheum Dis*. 2013;72:51–56. https://doi.org/10.1136/annrheumdis-2011-201195.
22. Koski JM, Kamel A, Waris P, et al. Atlas-based knee osteophyte assessment with ultrasonography and radiography: relationship to arthroscopic degeneration of articular cartilage. *Scand J Rheumatol*. 2016;45:158–164.
23. Podlipská J, Guermazi A, Lehenkari P, et al. Comparison of diagnostic performance of semi-quantitative knee ultrasound and knee radiography with MRI: Oulu Knee Osteoarthritis Study. *Sci Rep*. 2016;6:22365. https://doi.org/10.1038/srep22365.
24. Slimani S, Haddouche A, Bencharif I, Ladjouze-Rezig A. Superiority of knee ultrasound over radiographs in osteophyte detection in knee osteoarthritis. *Osteoarthritis Cartilage*. 21:31–63. [Abstract].
25. Mortada M, Zeid A, Al-Toukhy MA, Ezzeldin N, Elgawish M. Reliability of a proposed ultrasonographic grading scale for severity of primary knee osteoarthritis. *Clin Med Insights Arthritis Musculoskelet Disord*. 2016;9:161–166. https://doi.org/10.4137/CMAMD.S38141.
26. Shetty M, Fessell DP, Femino JE, Jacobson JA, Lin J, Jamadar D. Sonography of ankle tendon impingement with surgical correlation. *AJR Am J Roentgenol*. 2002;179(4):949–953.
27. Nazarian L, Gulvartian N, Freeland E, Chao W. Ultrasound-guided percutaneous needle fenestration and corticosteroid injection for anterior and anterolateral ankle impingement. *Foot Ankle Specialist*. 2017;11(1):61–66.
28. Yang Q, Zhou Y, Xu Y. Arthroscopic debridement of anterior ankle impingement in patients with chronic lateral ankle instability. *BMC Musculoskelet Disord*. 2018;19(1):239.
29. Razik A, Sott AH. Cheilectomy for hallux rigidus. *Foot Ankle Clin*. 2016;21(3):451–457.
30. Tol JL, van Dijk CN. Anterior ankle impingement. *Foot Ankle Clin*. 2006;11(2):297 (vi.).
31. Alvi HM, Kalainov DM, Biswas D, Soneru AP, Cohen MS. Surgical management of symptomatic olecranon traction spurs. *Orthop J Sports Med*. 2014;2(7):2325967114542775. https://doi.org/10.1177/2325967114542775.
32. McBeth ZL, Galvin JW, Robbins J. Proximal to distal exostectomy for the treatment of insertional Achilles tendinopathy. *Foot Ankle Spec*. 2018;11(4):362–364.
33. Redfern D, Vernois J, Legre BP. Percutaneous surgery of the forefoot. *Clin Podiatr Med Surg*. 2015;32(3):291–332.
34. Teoh KH, Tan WT, Atiyah Z, Ahmad A, Tanaka H, Hariharan K. Clinical outcomes following minimally invasive dorsal cheilectomy for hallux rigidus. *Foot Ankle Int*. 2019;40(2):195–201.
35. Walter R, Perera A. Open, arthroscopic, and percutaneous cheilectomy for hallux rigidus. *Foot Ankle Clin*. 2015;20(3):421–431. https://doi.org/10.1016/j.fcl.2015.04.005.
36. Stevens R, Bursnall M, Chadwick C, et al. Comparison of complication and reoperation rates for minimally invasive versus open cheilectomy of the first metatarsophalangeal joint. *Foot Ankle Int*. 2020;41(1):31–36.
37. Ogilvie-Harris DJ1, Mahomed N, Demazière A. Anterior impingement of the ankle treated by arthroscopic removal of bony spurs. *J Bone Joint Surg Br*. 1993;75(3):437–440.
38. Bauer T, Breda R, Hardy P. Anterior ankle bony impingement with joint motion loss: the arthroscopic resection option. *Orthop Traumatol Surg Res*. 2010;96:462–468.
39. Valkering KP, van der Hoeven H, Pijnenburg BC. Posterolateral elbow impingement in professional boxers. *Am J Sports Med*. 2008;36(2):328–332.
40. Matsuura T, Iwame T, Suzue N, et al. Clinical outcome of arthroscopic treatment for posteromedial elbow impingement in adolescent baseball players. *Arthroscopy*. 2018;34(1):105–110.

41. Singh VR, Bain GI. Endoscopic extrabursal excision of olecranon spur. *Arthrosc Tech*. 2018;7(9):e893–e898.
42. Lui TH. Endoscopic management of Osgood-Schlatter disease. *Arthrosc Tech*. 2016;5(1):e121–e125. https://doi.org/10.1016/j.eats.2015.10.023.
43. van Dijk CN. Anterior and posterior ankle impingement. *Foot Ankle Clin N Am*. 2006;11:663–683.
44. Tol JL, van Dijk CN. Etiology of the anterior ankle impingement syndrome: a descriptive anatomical study. *Foot Ankle Int*. 2004;25(6):382–386. https://doi.org/10.1177/107110070402500603.
45. Jerosch J. Endoscopic calcaneoplasty. *Foot Ankle Clin*. 2015;20(1):149–165.
46. Jerosch J, Sokkar S, Dücker M, Donner A. [Endoscopic calcaneoplasty (ECP) in Haglund's syndrome. Indication, surgical technique, surgical findings and results]. *Z Orthop Unfall*. 2012;150(3):250–256.
47. Tountas AA, Fornasier VL. Operative treatment of subcalcaneal pain. *Clin Orthop Relat Res*. 1996;332:170–178.
48. Nery C, Raduan F, Mansur N, Baunfeld D, Del Buono A, Maffulli N. Endoscopic approach for plantar fasciopathy: a long-term retrospective study. *Int Orthop*. 2013;37(6):1151–1156.
49. Snider MP, Clancy WF, McBeath A. Plantar fascial release for chronic plantar fasciitis in runners. *AJSpMed*. 1983;11:215.
50. Kinley S, Frascone S, et al. Endoscopic plantar fasciotomy versus traditional heel surgery—a prospective study. *JFAS*. 1993;32:595–603.
51. Tomczak RL, Haverstock BD. A retrospective comparison of endoscopic plantar fasciotomy to open plantar fasciotomy with heel spur resection for chronic plantar fasciitis/heel spur syndrome. *JFAS*. 1995;34:305–311. 26.
52. Campbell DA. Sensory nerve damage during surgery on the hallux. *J R Coll Surg Edinb*. 1992;37:422–444.
53. Meier PJ, Kenzora JE. The risks and benefits of distal first metatarsal osteotomies. *Foot Ankle*. 1985;6:7–17.
54. Teoh KH, Haanaes EK, Alshalawi S, Tanaka H, Hariharan K. Minimally invasive dorsal cheilectomy of the first metatarsal: a cadaveric study. *Foot Ankle Int*. 2018;39(12):1497–1501.
55. Teoh KH, Haanaes EK, Alshalawi S, Tanaka H, Hariharan K. Minimally invasive dorsal cheilectomy of the first metatarsal: a cadaveric study. *Foot Ankle Int*. 2018;39(12):1497–1501.
56. Miyamoto K, Sugiyama S, Hosoe H, Iinuma N, Suzuki Y, Shimizu K. Postsurgical recurrence of osteophytes causing dysphagia in patients with diffuse idiopathic skeletal hyperostosis. *Eur Spine J*. 2009;18(11):1652–1658. https://doi.org/10.1007/s00586-009-1133-3.

34 Intraosseous Injections

STEVEN SAMPSON, HUNTER VINCENT, AND SONALI LAL

KEY POINTS

Knee osteoarthritis treatment summary:
- Intra-articular (IA) arthrocentesis (if needed)
- 3 to 8 mL IA (if needed)
- 5 to 10 mL tibial plateau intraosseous (IO)
- 5 to 10 mL femoral condyle IO

Patellofemoral osteoarthritis treatment summary:
- IA arthrocentesis (if needed)
- 3 to 8 mL IA (if needed)
- 5 to 10 mL femoral trochlear IO
- 2 to 3 mL patella IO

Hip osteoarthritis treatment summary:
- IA arthrocentesis (if needed)
- 3 to 8 mL IA (if needed)
- 5 to 8 mL acetabular IO
- 5 to 10 mL femoral head IO

Pertinent Anatomy

To understand the role of intraosseous (IO) injections in the treatment of advanced osteoarthritis with experienced practitioners, it is important to understand the functional anatomy of subchondral bone. Subchondral bone is located beneath the calcified cartilage line forming what is known as the osteochondral unit. The structure consists of a plate of cortical bone, where the bone marrow and trabecular bone areas emerge. Despite the calcified cartilage layer and the cortical plate being nonporous, it is well known that communication between the articular cartilage and subchondral bone does exist (Fig. 34.1).[1] The intercommunication between these layers has been identified to play a more significant role in osteoarthritis (OA) progression than previously thought.[2]

Pathophysiology

Although the pathophysiology of joint osteoarthritis has long been attributed to wear and tear of articular cartilage over time, a growing volume of evidence suggests that joint osteoarthritis may be the result of a multidimensional change in the whole joint inflammatory environment. It is proposed that the inflammatory state of other structures such as synovium and subchondral bone can contribute to the overlying health of the joint.[3] Significant research has identified subchondral bone as a primary starting place for such pathologic changes and is illustrated through objective findings such bone marrow edema. Because of the cross-talk between subchondral bone and articular cartilage, lesions in the subchondral tissue can ultimately affect the overall health of articular cartilage and lead to degeneration, if not properly treated.[1] This chapter provides instruction on targeting subchondral bone in the treatment of joint pain, particularly for hip and knee osteoarthritis. Other less common anatomic locations such as the ankle, hand, foot, shoulder, and clavicle will also be demonstrated.

Treatment Options and Published Studies

Treatment options for bone marrow lesions include bisphosphonates, extracorporeal shock wave therapy, arthroplasty, subchondroplasty with bone cement (calcium phosphate or polymethyl methacrylate), platelet-rich plasma (PRP), bone marrow concentrate (BMC), and mesenchymal stem cells.[4,5] Astur et al. performed a review of subchondroplasty with calcium phosphate that showed, in 164 subjects, significant improvement in the International Knee Documentation Committee (IKDC) score or Knee injury and Osteoarthritis Outcome Score (KOOS) and 70% reduction in total knee arthroplasty at 2 years. Side effects were one deep venous thrombosis and two cases of extravasation of cement into the joint, and 25% still had complaints of pain.[6]

Sanchez et al. conducted a study (n = 30) of case-matched IO and intra-articular (IA) PRP versus IA alone in patients with severe medial or patella femoral OA. They used leukocyte-poor PRP, low concentration (1.5 to 2.5×) with 5 mL injected into the medial tibia plateau (MTP) and medial femoral condyle (MFC) 2 cm above the chondral surface (i.e., 10 mL injected into subchondral bone of each knee). The IO and IA group had significant improvements in KOOS, Western Ontario and McMaster Universities Osteoarthritis Index (WOMAC), and visual analog scale (VAS) score in comparison with the IA alone group at the 6- and 12-month follow-up intervals. They reported that 53% and 46.7% reached the minimum clinically important difference (MCID) for pain reduction at 6 and 12 months, respectively, versus 26.7% and 16.7% for the IA only group.[7] Fiz et al. treated 40 patients with severe hip OA who failed IA PRP with IA 8 mL and IO (5 mL each in acetabulum and femur), placing the PRP 1 cm above the bone. There was significant improvement in WOMAC and Hip disability and

Osteoarthritis Outcome Score (HOOS), 40% met MCID at 12 months, and there were no adverse events.[4]

Hernigou recently published outcomes on long-term follow-up (mean 12 years) for young patients with bilateral knee steroid - induced osteonecrosis. One knee was randomized to receive total knee arthroplasty, and the other knee received autologous BMAC. There were 30 patients and 60 knees injected with 10 mL into each of the medial and lateral tibial and femoral compartments of the knee (i.e., 40 mL injected into the subchondral bone of each treated knee). Both groups had similar knee scores, with 21 of 30 preferring the BMAC-treated knee. There were no serious adverse events in the BMAC-treated knee; the surgery knees had one infection, five had thrombophlebitis, nine required transfusions, and six required revision surgery, whereas only three patients in the BMAC group received a total knee arthroplasty (TKA) at 6, 8, and 12 years later.[8] Another study published by Davidson et al. presented outcomes for 49 patients (age 10 to 17 years old) with osteochondritis dissecans who were treated using high-volume subchondral BMAC, and 76.9% had healing on postprocedural imaging and no serious side effects.[9] Kasik et al. treated 20 patients with knee arthritis and bone marrow edema with a subchondral injection of BMAC and demineralized bone matrix in addition to arthroscopic surgery, with a mean of 14.5-month follow-up. VAS decreased from 7 to 1.3, IKDC scores increased from 29.2 to 66.1, and three of the four patients who had postprocedure imaging showed improvement.[10]

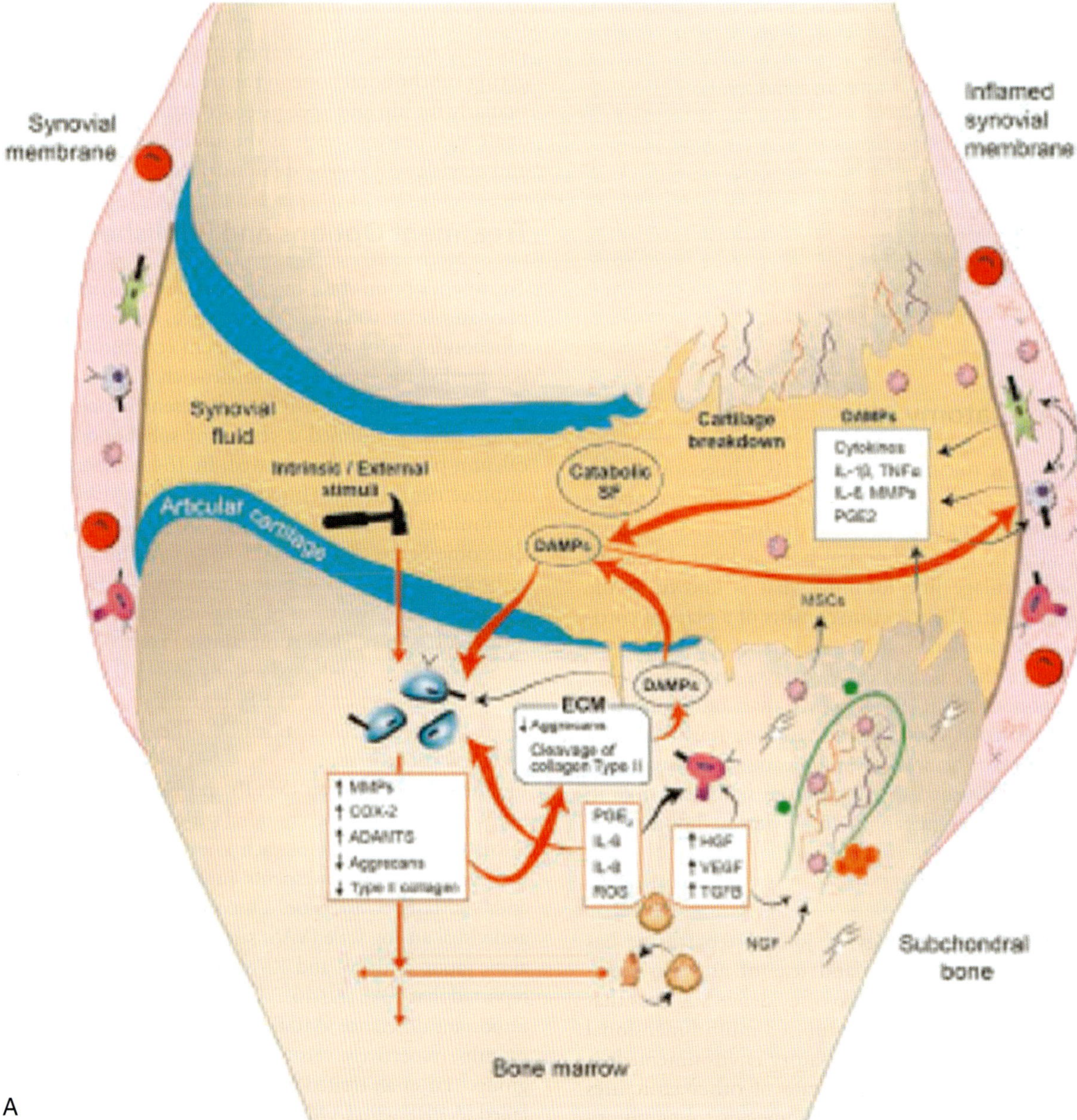

A

• **Fig. 34.1** The Complex Yet Important Role of Subchondral Bone on Joint Homeostasis. (Courtesy of Mikel Sanchez and Nico Fiz.)

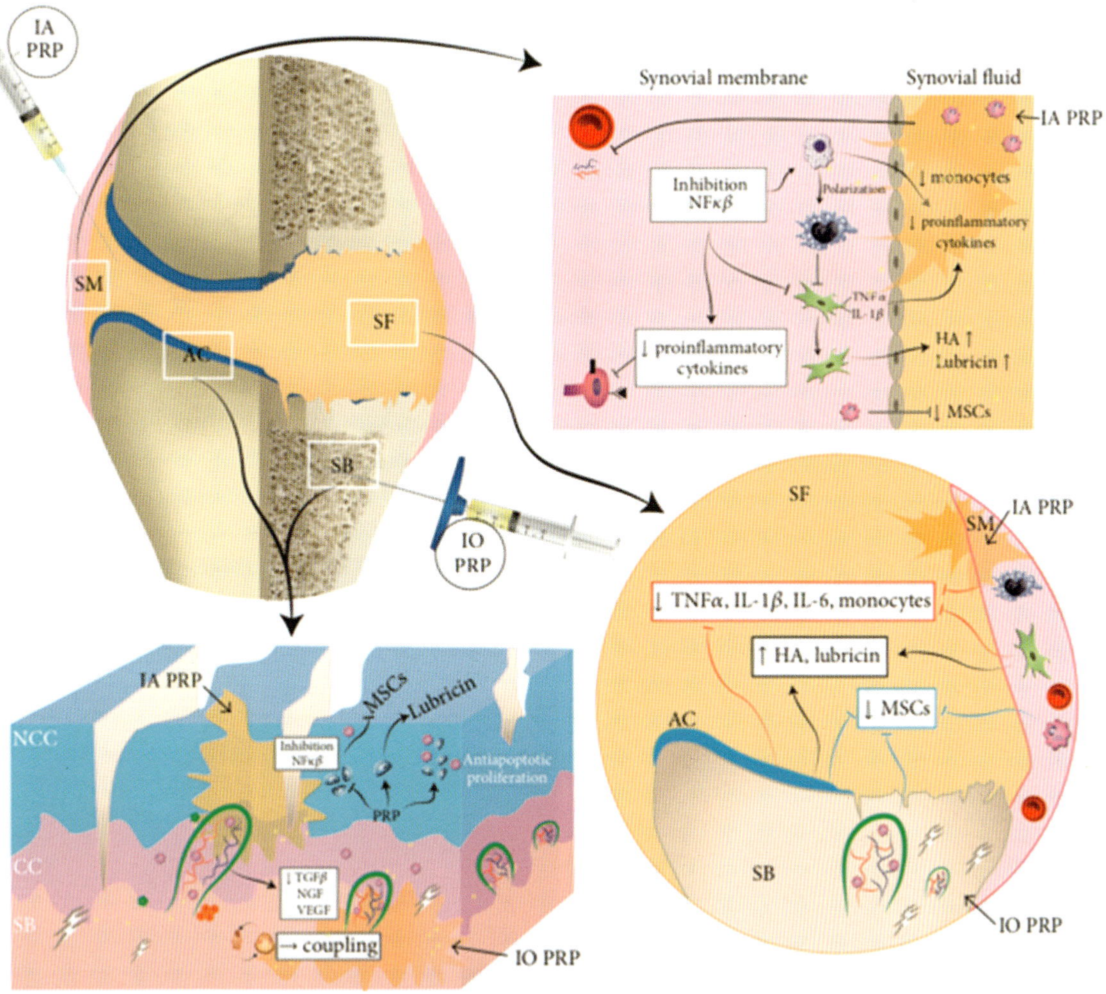

B

• **Fig. 34.1—cont'd**

Lastly, Kyle et al. reported on two cases of knee subchondral edema treated with IO BMAC, and both had symptom and imaging improvements.[11]

An additional study published in 2018 by Hernigou et al. with 30-year follow-up looked at outcomes for the treatment of stage I or II hip osteonecrosis (Fig. 34.2) with cellular therapy versus core decompression. The study enrolled 125 patients (i.e., 250 hips) with bilateral hip osteonecrosis from 1988 to 1998; the hip with the larger-sized osteonecrotic lesion on magnetic resonance imaging (MRI) was treated with percutaneous cellular therapy (i.e., BMAC) and the hip with the contralateral smaller lesion was treated with core decompression. At the most recent follow-up (average of 25 years post treatment), 24% (i.e., 30 hips) in the cellular therapy group versus 76% (i.e., 95 hips) in the core decompression group had undergone total hip arthroplasty. In addition, only 28% versus 72% also had progression to collapse on repeat MRI at the follow-up, cellular therapy versus core decompression, respectively.[12] Several additional studies have also been published on the topic of cellular therapy for the treatment of hip osteonecrosis,[13–19] with the goal of developing best practices for treatment.

The current published research demonstrates very promising results for the use of BMAC to treat bone marrow lesions of the knee and osteonecrotic lesions of the knee and hip. There is some reported positive benefit of IO PRP for subchondral lesions in OA but not as robust.

Technique

Fluoroscopic Guidance: Knee Osteoarthritis

Patient position: Supine, knee in extension. Alternatively, can place the knee in hook lying with a bolster under the knee for support.
Clinician position: Contralateral side as the treatment limb.
Setup: Sedation or MAC optimal, Completely sterile field,

Equipment Needed

25- to 22-gauge needle
18- to 15-gauge bone trocar 1-inch to 2.7-inch length
Automated power driver and/or mallet
Syringes as necessary for volume

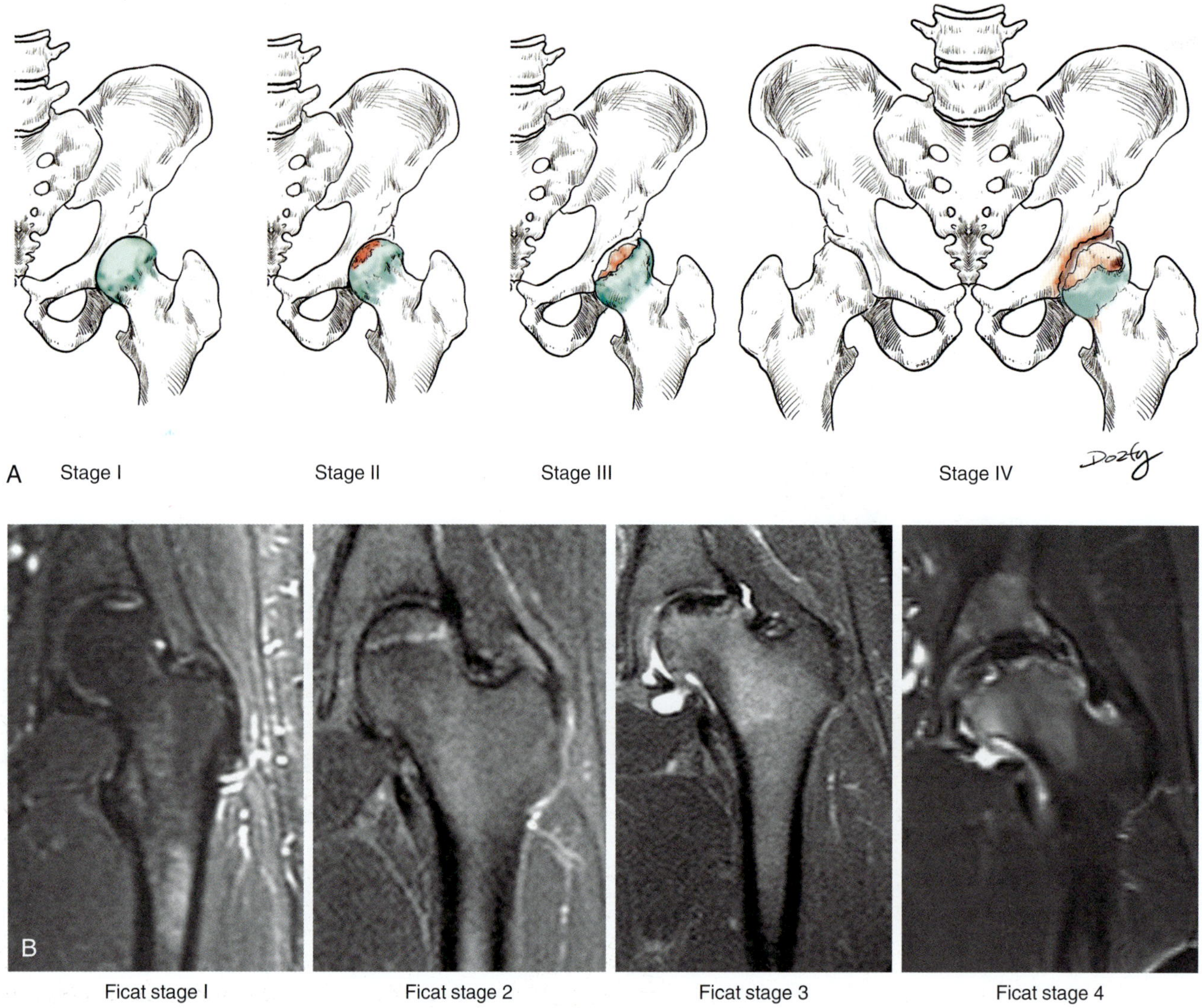

• **Fig. 34.2** Avascular Necrosis. Stage 1: MRI with signs of boney edema, and often presented as groin pain in patient. Stage 2: associated with pain and stiffness, MRI shows geographic defect. Stage 3: Pain and stiffness with occasional radiation to knee, MRI shows increased edema, and eventual cortical collapse. Stage 4: end stage degenerative changes with evidence of cortical collapse.

Procedural Steps

1. Tibial Plateau IO Infiltration:
   a. Using fluoroscopic guidance, the medial joint line is identified in the anteroposterior (AP) and lateral views. Ensure the medial and lateral tibial plateau are aligned in the lateral view and the anterior and posterior plateaus are aligned in AP. Mark the skin approximately 2 cm distal to the joint line and centered in the midline sagittal plane (Fig. 34.3).
   b. If available, linear ultrasound should be used to identify vasculature that could course in the needle trajectory. Use color flow Doppler to identify smaller vessels. Adjust needle entry/skin mark to avoid vasculature.
   c. Optional to add a small amount of local anesthetic, with 0.25% ropivacaine being the preferred choice.
   d. An 18- to 15-gauge trocar used for bone biopsy is introduced into the skin and advanced down to the periosteum (Fig. 34.4).
   e. Under fluoroscopic guidance, the trocar is advanced approximately 1.5 to 2.0 cm, directed in a parallel trajectory toward the articular surface, into the medial portion of subchondral bone in the tibial plateau (Fig. 34.5).
   f. Once the trocar is correctly placed, it is optional to inject contrast to view the spread of injectate through the bone and observe if there is excess vascular uptake.
   g. Approximately 5 to 8 mL of injectate is infiltrated through the trocar.
2. MFC IO Infiltration:
   a. Using fluoroscopic guidance, the medial joint line is identified in the AP and lateral views. Ensure the medial and lateral femoral condyles are aligned in the lateral view and the anterior and posterior plateaus are aligned in AP. Mark the skin approximately 2 cm proximal to the joint line and centered in the midline sagittal plane (Fig. 34.6).

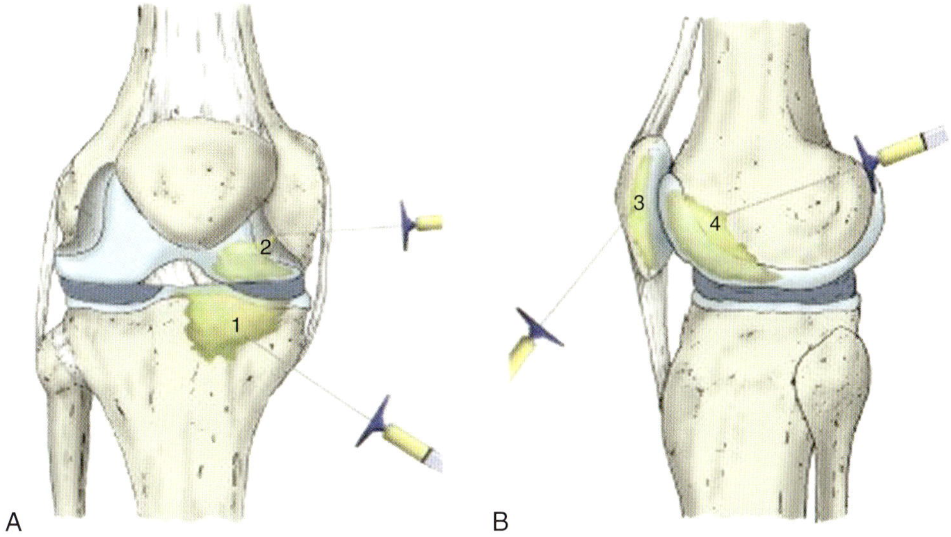

• **Fig. 34.3** Subchondral bone injections for joint osteoarthritis. (A) Subchondral bone injections for Tibial plateau (1) and Medial Femoral Condyle (2). (B) Subchondral bone injections for Patella (3) and femoral condyle (4). (Courtesy of Mikel Sanchez.)

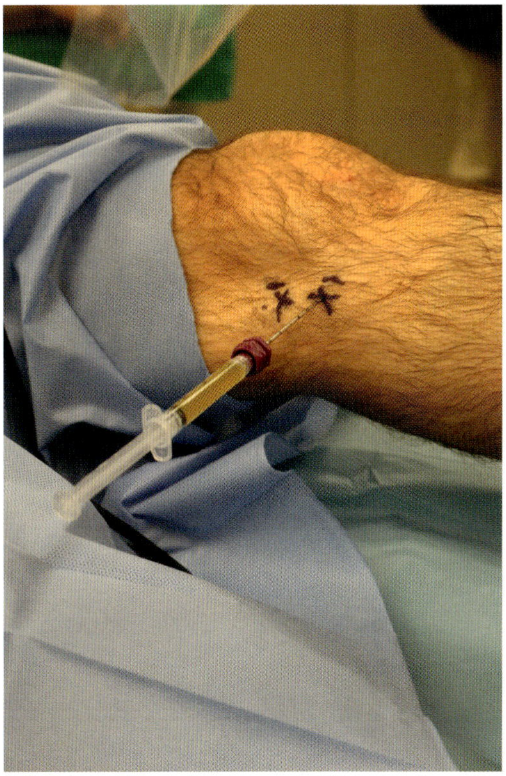

• **Fig. 34.4** Bone trocar advanced into subchondral bone of tibial plateau with injectate ready for infiltration.

b. If available, use ultrasound to identify vasculature that could course in the needle trajectory. Use color flow Doppler to identify smaller vessels. Adjust needle entry/skin mark to avoid vasculature.

c. Optional to add a small amount of local anesthetic, with 0.25% ropivacaine being the preferred choice.

d. The trocar is advanced to the level of the periosteum and again advanced 1.5 to 2 cm toward the medial portion of the femoral condyle, in a parallel trajectory to the articular surface (Fig. 34.7).

e. Once the trocar is in the desired position, it is optional to inject contrast to view the spread of injectate through the bone and observe if there is excess vascular uptake.

f. Five to 8 mL of injectate is infiltrated into the subchondral bone.

3. Lateral Femoral Condyle: The same landmarks and technique are used for the lateral femoral condyle, except using the lateral joint line as a starting point. See Fig. 34.8 as a reference for the placement of the bone trocar in the middle portion of subchondral bone in the lateral femoral condyle.
4. Patellar IO Infiltration: If a patient has significant patellofemoral degeneration, IO infiltration can also be used in treating the patella.
   a. Under fluoroscopic guidance, the midlateral or medial portion of the patella is identified in lateral and AP views.
   b. The bone trocar is advanced to the level of periosteum and advanced approximately 1 to 2 cm toward the middle portion of the patella (Fig. 34.9).
   c. Once proper trocar placement is achieved, it is optional to inject contrast to view the spread of injectate through the bone and observe if there is excess vascular uptake.
   d. Two to 4 mL of injectate can be infiltrated into the patella.

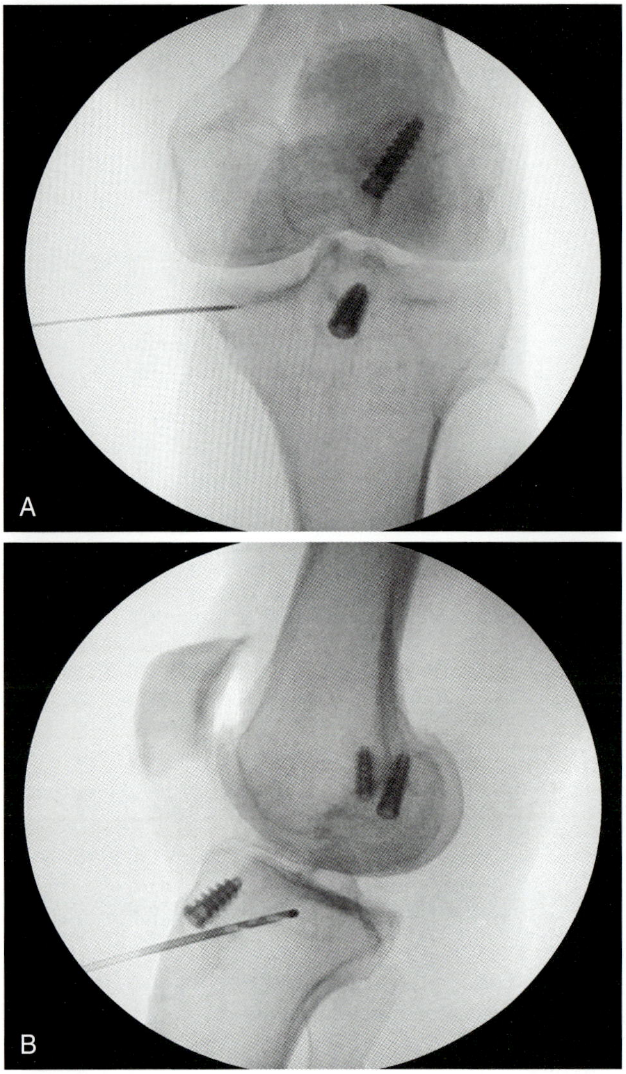

• **Fig. 34.5** (A) Anteroposterior and (B) lateral fluoroscopy views of bone trocar in subchondral bone.

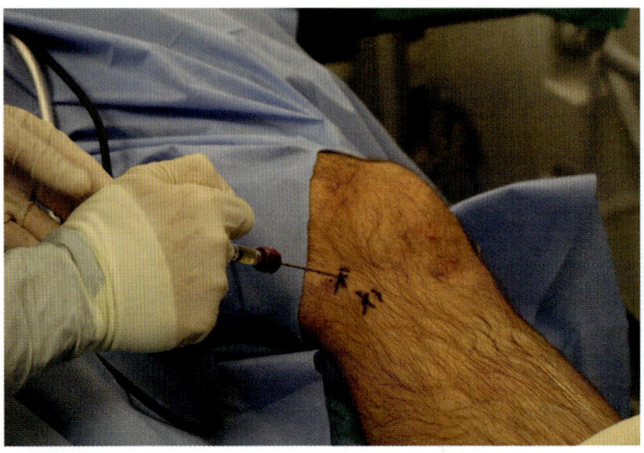

• **Fig. 34.6** Bone trocar is advanced into subchondral bone, approximately 2 cm proximal to the joint line.

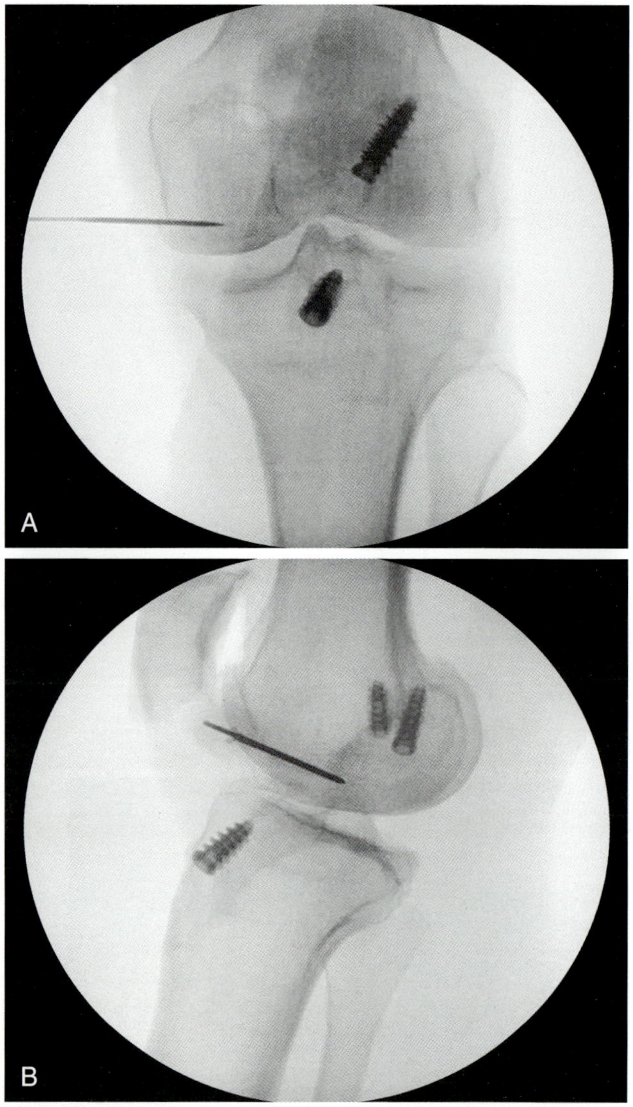

• **Fig. 34.7** (A) Anteroposterior and (B) lateral fluoroscopic views of bone trocar in the subchondral bone in medial femoral condyle.

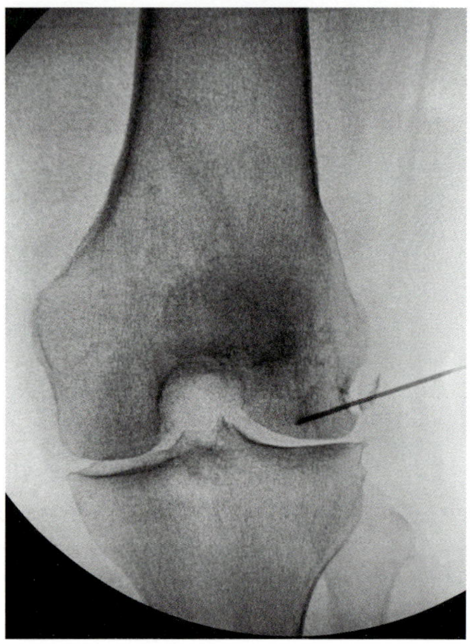

• **Fig. 34.8** Anteroposterior fluoroscopic view of bone trocar advanced into subchondral bone of lateral femoral condyle. (Courtesy of Chris Williams.)

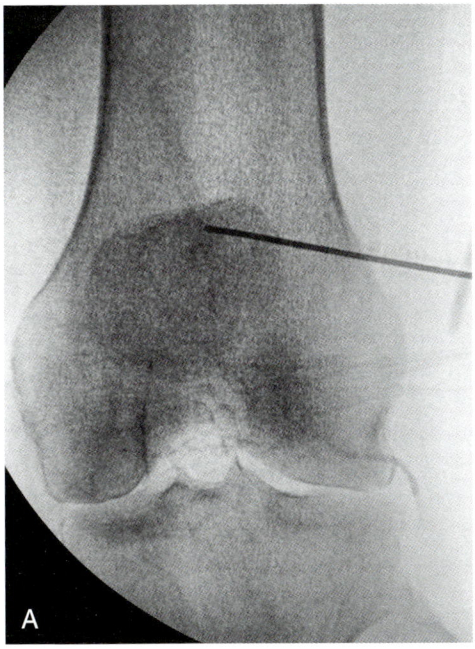

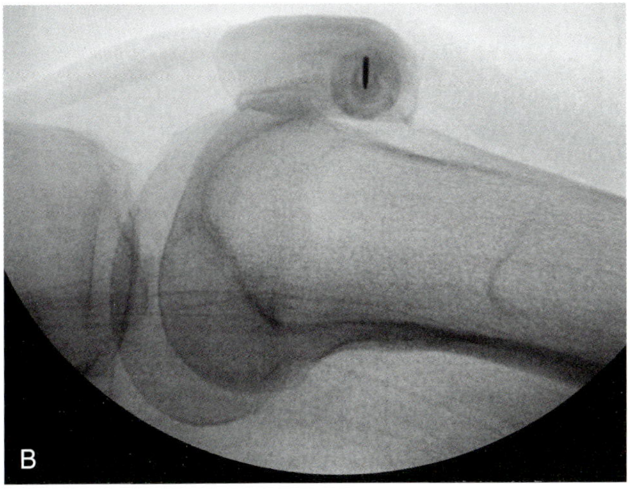

• **Fig. 34.9** (A) Anteroposterior and (B) lateral fluoroscopic views of bone trocar placement into the patella. (Courtesy of Chris Williams.)

Alternative Techniques

For femoral condyle and tibial plateau IO injections, one can also directly target a specific bone marrow lesion as seen on MRI. Technique would be similar, except instead of targeting 2 cm above or below the joint line and injecting subchondral 1.5 to 2 cm into the bone, vary needle position to match specific lesion (Fig. 34.10).

Fluoroscopic Guidance: Hip Osteoarthritis and Avascular Necrosis

Patient position: Supine, hip in 30 degrees of flexion.
Clinician position: Same side as the treatment limb.
Setup: Sedation or MAC optimal, completely sterile field.

PEARLS AND PITFALLS

- Remember, it is important not to advance the trocar beyond the articular cartilage, as this could create a new cartilaginous lesion. Furthermore, in cases of osteoporosis, severe OA, or articular cartilage damage, it is expected to experience less resistance as injectate flows from subchondral bone to intra-articular (IA).
- Patients may experience more postprocedural pain with intraosseous (IO) infiltration versus standard IA orthobiologic injection in the first 48 to 72 hours. This can be due to changes in pressure within the bone.
- Infection secondary to IO infiltration can be more serious than standard IA injection and should be treated as so.

Equipment Needed

18-gauge needle
15-gauge bone trocar
Automated power driver and/or mallet
Syringes, as needed, for volume

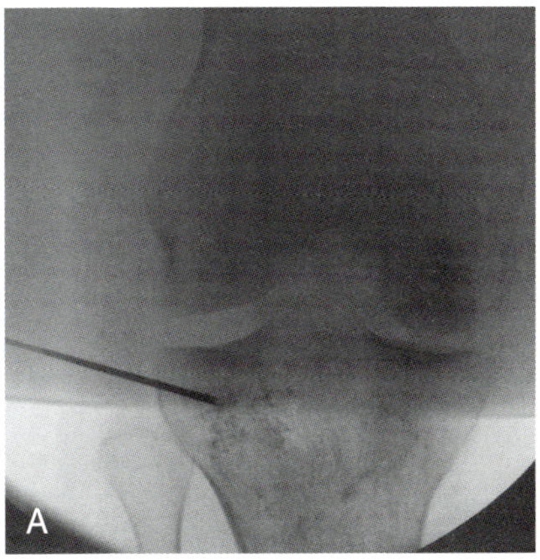

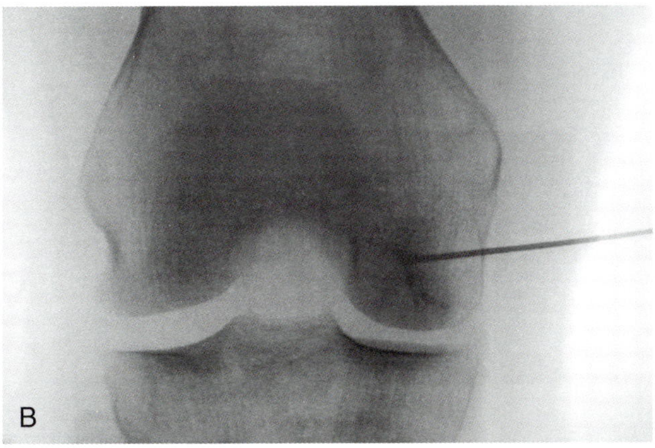

• **Fig. 34.10** Injecting specific lesions for both femoral and tibial plateau lesions for intraosseous patella injections, one can alternatively inject from the anterior aspect of the patella instead of lateral (see Figs. 34.11 and 34.12). (A) Injecting lateral femoral condyle under fluoroscopic guidance (B) Injecting medial femoral condyle undergo fluoroscopic guidance.

Procedural Steps

1. Femoral Head IO Infiltration:
   a. Obtain a true AP projection of the hip joint and proximal femur.
   b. With the proper anatomy identified under fluoroscopic guidance, the skin is marked approximately 1 cm lateral to the sartorius muscle, directly superficial to the femoral neck.
   c. The bone trocar is advanced down to the periosteum of the femoral neck at a 45-degree angle, in line with the anatomic angle of the femoral neck. The trocar should be advanced to within approximately 1 cm of the articular surface (Figs. 34.13–34.15).
   d. Once the trocar is correctly placed, it is optional to inject contrast to see the flow of injectate and make sure there is not excessive vascular uptake.
   e. Approximately 5 to 10 mL of injectate is infiltrated through the trocar.
2. Femoral Head IO Technique 2
   a. Patient positioned in the lateral decubitus position. A 30-degree bend in the target hip with the contralateral hip at 15 degrees to identify the correct femur on fluoroscopy. Pillows and inflated bean bag are helpful to maintain the patient position while under MAC (Fig. 34.16).
   b. Using AP and lateral fluoroscopic views triangulate a needle trajectory starting below the greater trochanter headed toward the middle superior femoral head and mark the skin.
   c. Insert an 11-gauge 6-inch trocar into the periosteum 1 to 2 cm below the greater trochanter, aiming for the superior and middle portion of the femoral head.
   d. Attach the power drill and guide the needle using intermittent fluoroscopy, alternating between the AP and lateral views. Ensure the needle traverses through the middle of the femoral neck.
   e. Once the trocar is correctly placed, it is optional to inject contrast to see flow of injectate and make sure there is not excessive vascular uptake.

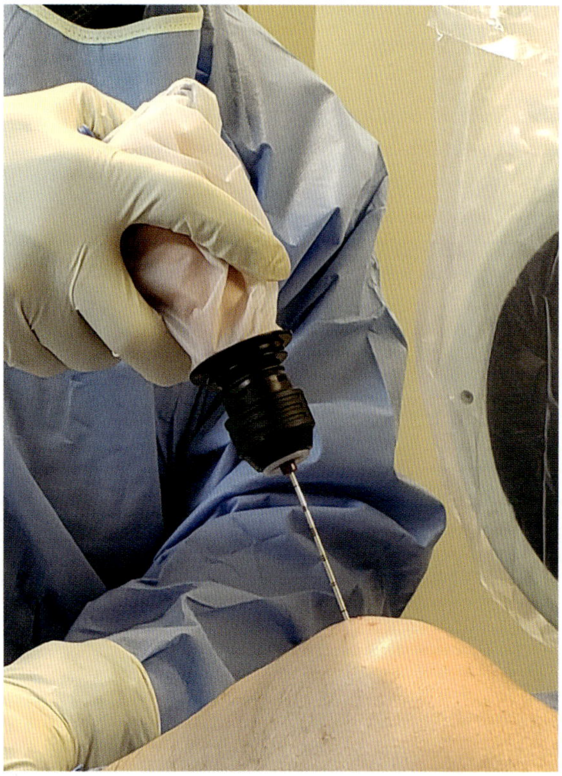

• **Fig. 34.11** Anterior Approach to Intraosseous Patellar Injection.

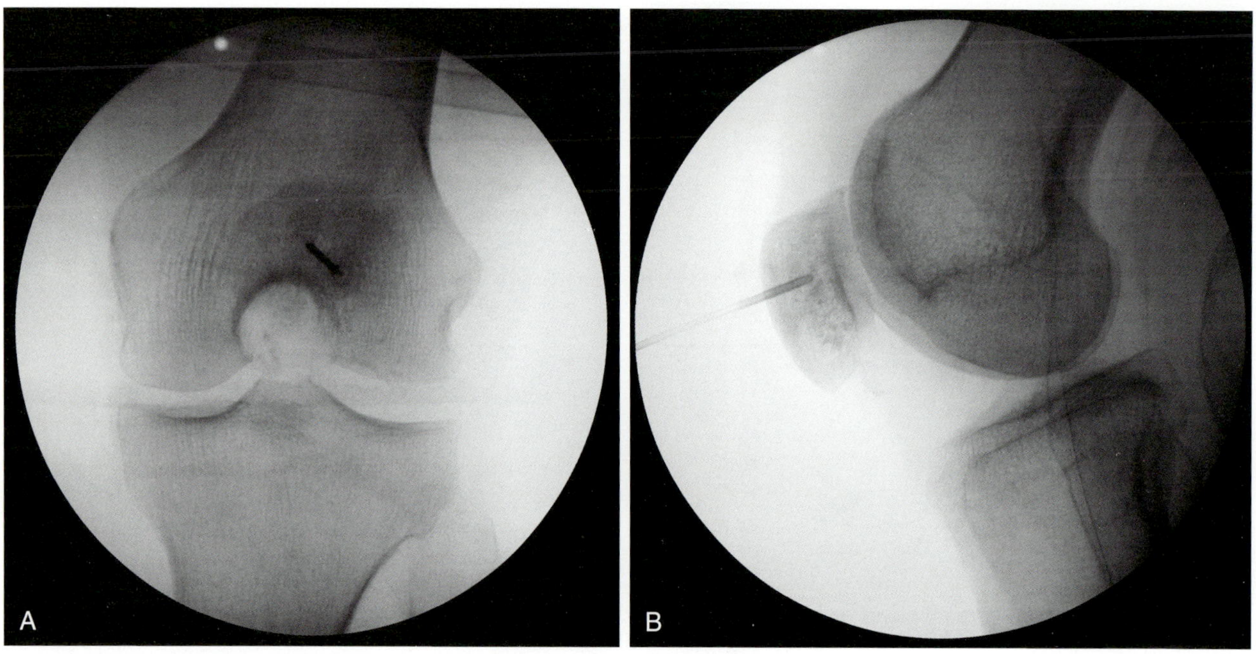

• **Fig. 34.12** (A) Anteroposterior and (B) lateral fluoroscopic images for anterior approach to intraosseous patella injection.

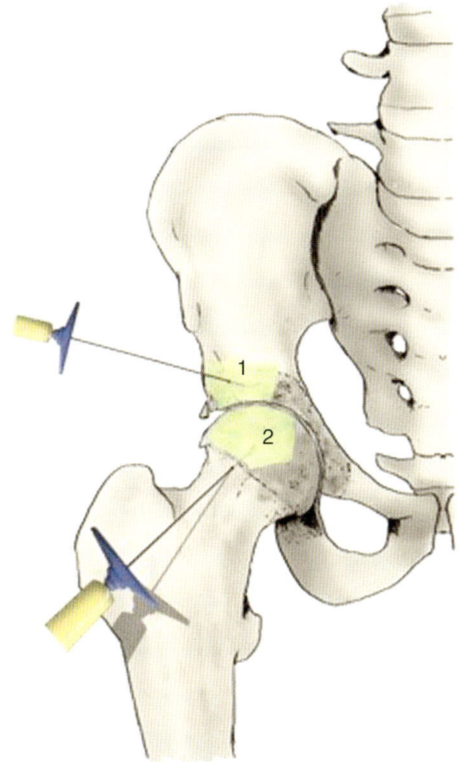

• **Fig. 34.13** Subchondral bone injection locations for hip osteoarthritis, including the acetabulum and femoral head. (1) acetabulum subchondral bone injections. (2) femoral head subchondral. bone injection. (Courtesy of Mikel Sanchez and Nicolas Fiz.)

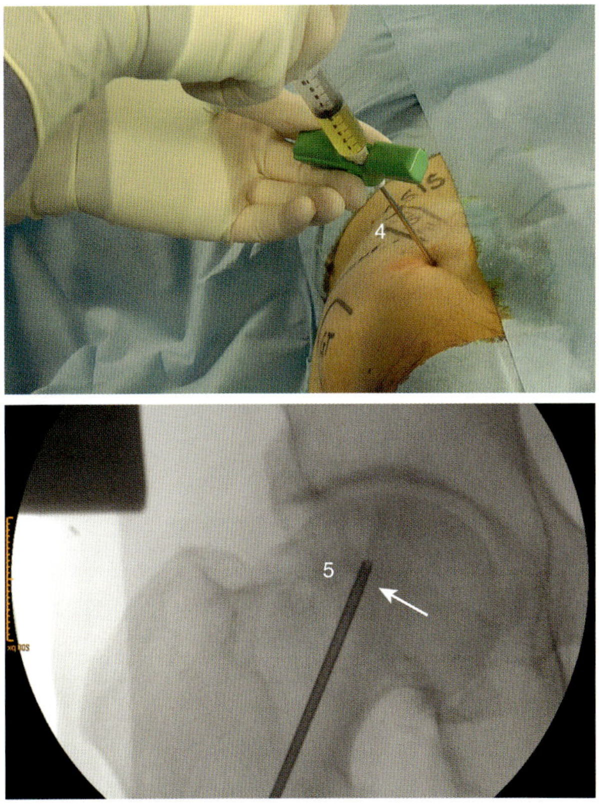

• **Fig. 34.14** *(Top)* Bone trocar alignment and trajectory shown with injectate attached. *(Bottom)* Anteroposterior fluoroscopic view of bone trocar (arrow) within subchondral bone and close to articular surface of femoral head. (Courtesy of Nicolas Fiz.)

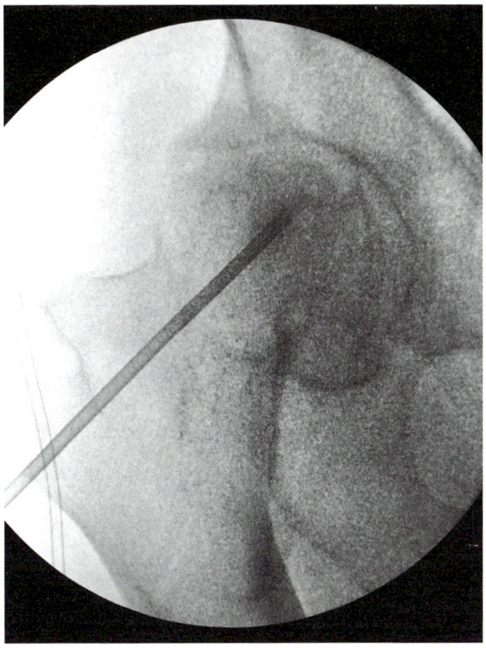

• **Fig. 34.15** Anteroposterior fluoroscopic view of bone trocar within subchondral bone and close to articular surface of femoral head. (Courtesy of Chris Williams.)

   f. Approximately 5 to 10 mL of injectate is infiltrated through the trocar.
   g. Use the power drill to remove the trocar.
3. Acetabulum IO Infiltration:
   a. Using fluoroscopic guidance, a standard AP hip x-ray image is obtained and the femoroacetabular joint line is identified.
   b. The skin is marked approximately 3 cm proximal to the joint line and centered in the midline sagittal plane, just superior to the greater trochanter.
   c. A 15-gauge trocar is introduced into the skin and advanced down to the acetabular periosteum. Under fluoroscopic guidance, the trocar is advanced at a 20-degree cranial-caudal angle, directed parallel to the horizontal plane.
   d. The trocar is advanced to within approximately 1 cm of the articular surface (Figs. 34.17 and 34.18).
   e. Once the trocar is correctly placed, it is optional to inject contrast to see flow of injectate and to make sure there is not excessive vascular uptake.
   f. Approximately 5 to 8 mL of injectate is infiltrated through the trocar.

PEARLS AND PITFALLS

- During femoral intraosseous (IO) infiltration, penetrating the skin lateral to the sartorius muscle minimizes the risk of injury to the lateral femoral cutaneous nerve.
- Infection secondary to IO infiltration can be more serious than standard intra-articular (IA) injections and should be treated as so.

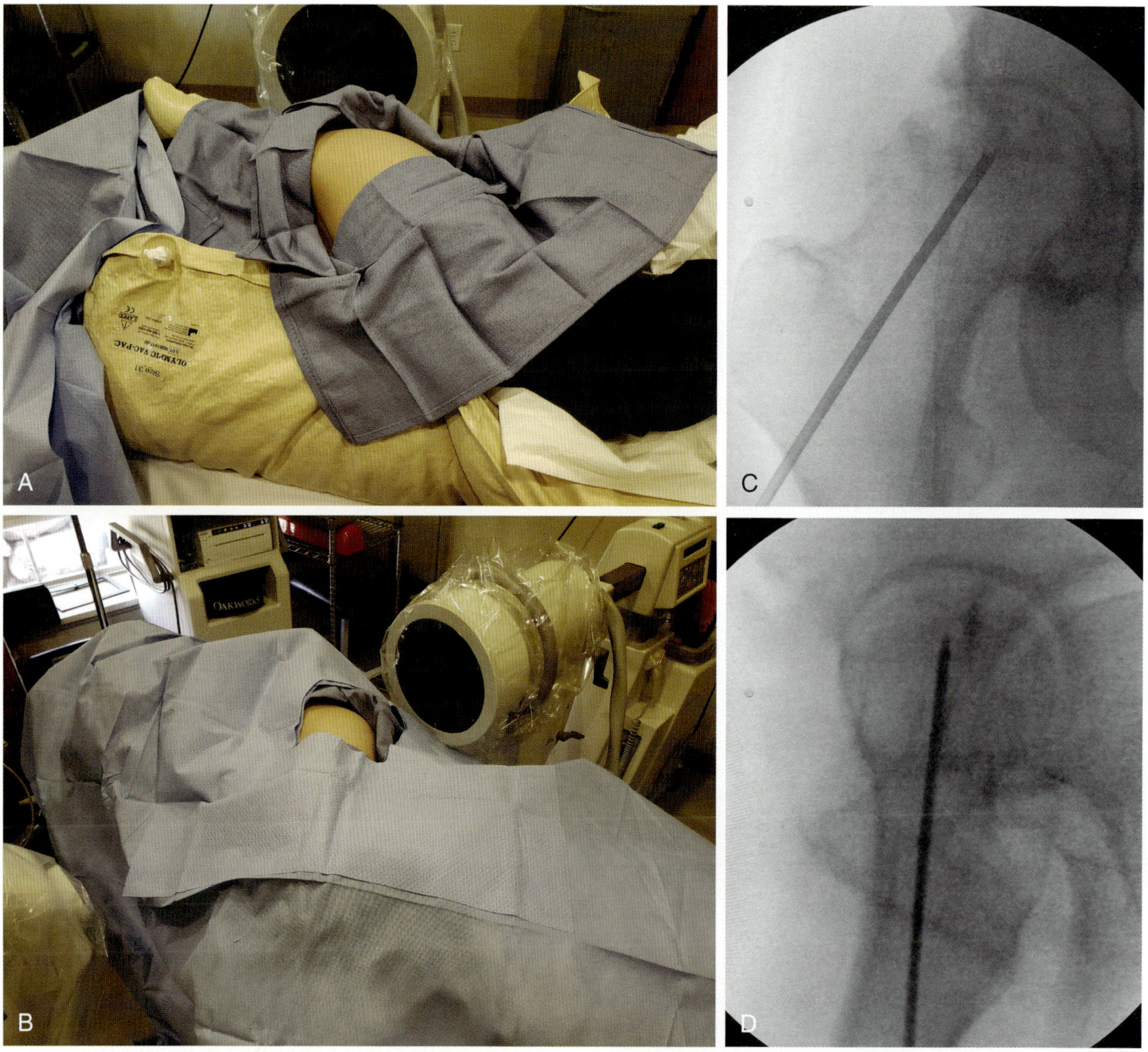

• **Fig. 34.16** Fluoroscopic view of trocar in ideal position for femoral head infiltration. (A and B) Patient positioned in the lateral decubitus position with notable wedge or inflatable bag placed anterior and posterior around patient to secure position while sedated. (C) C-arm placed in the anteroposterior (AP) fluoroscopic view. (D) AP and lateral fluoroscopic view of femur with 11-gauge trocar advanced into the femoral head from a lateral to medial trajectory.

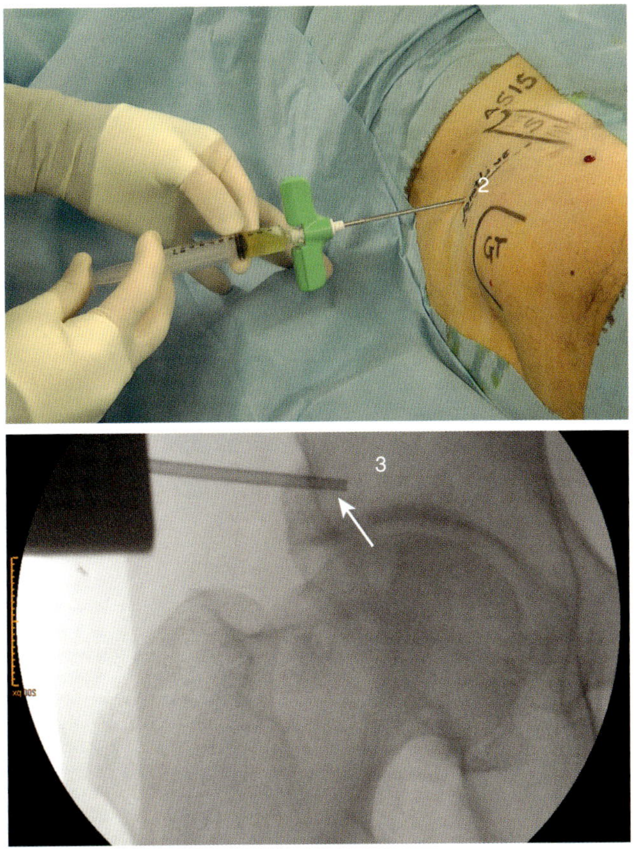

• **Fig. 34.17** *(Top)* Bone trocar alignment and trajectory for acetabulum intraosseous injection. *(Bottom)* Anteroposterior fluoroscopic view for acetabulum subchondral bone injection. (2) trajectory of injection into acetabulum with correlating fluoroscopic image. (3) Arrow shows tip of the boney trocar under fluoroscopic guidance (Courtesy of Nicolas Fiz.)

Ultrasound Guidance: Knee Osteoarthritis

Patient position: Supine with approximately 30 to 40 degrees of knee flexion.
Clinician position: Same side as the treatment limb.
Setup: Sedation or MAC optimal, completely sterile field.

Equipment Needed

18- or 22-gauge needle
15-gauge bone trocar
Automated power driver and/or mallet
Syringes, as needed, for volume

Procedural Steps

1. Preparing for IO Infiltration
   a. Under ultrasound guidance, identify the medial joint line and the medial meniscus.
   b. Using a 25-gauge needle or surgical marker, mark the anatomic midpoint of the medial meniscus. The red arrow in Fig. 34.19 shows the location of the needle at the midpoint of the meniscus.
   c. With the needle acting as the anatomic midpoint, measure 2 cm proximal along the femur and 2 cm distal along the tibia (Fig. 34.20).
2. Tibial Plateau IO Infiltration:
   a. Using a 15-gauge bone access trocar, pierce the skin and advance the trocar down the level of the periosteum. Ensuring a firm position on the tibia, add a small amount of caudal tilt to the trocar (≈10 to 15 degrees) and angle the trocar tip toward the joint line.
   b. Using a mallet, lightly seed the trocar into the periosteum, ensuring the same trajectory (Fig. 34.21).

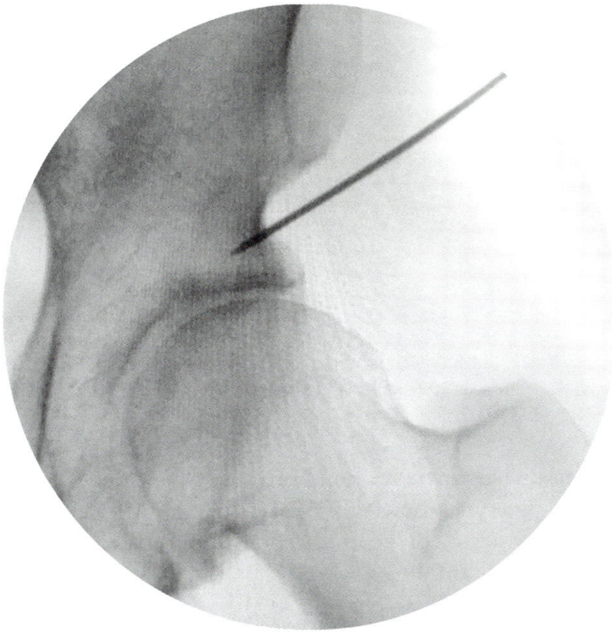

• **Fig. 34.18** Anteroposterior Fluoroscopic View of Acetabulum Subchondral Bone Injection.

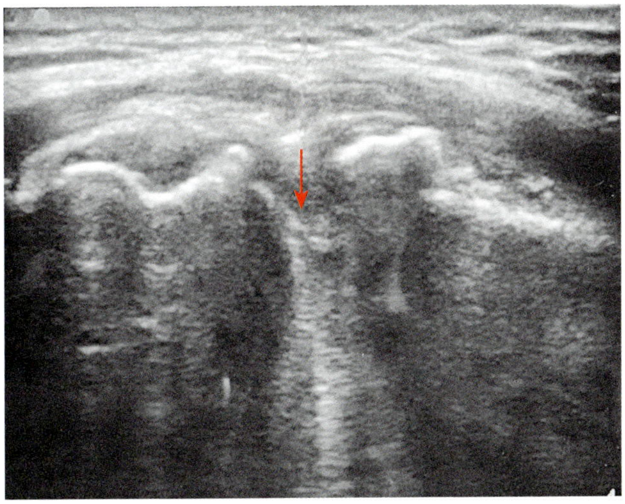

• **Fig. 34.19** Ultrasound image showing the medial joint line with the *red arrow* aligning with medial meniscus. This image is used to create a starting point for accurate measuring.

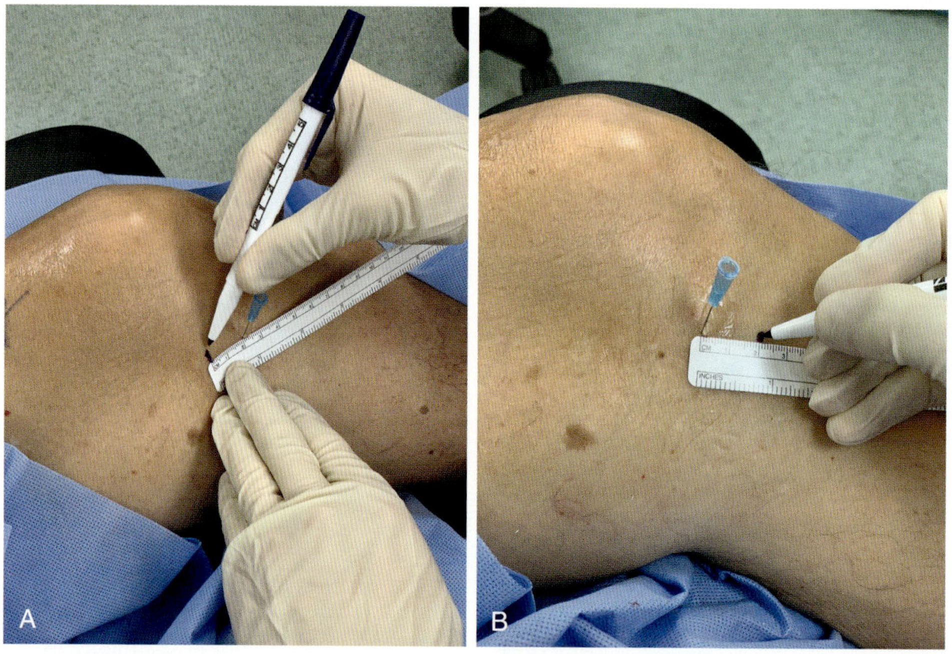

• **Fig. 34.20** With the needle confirmed in the medial meniscus, it acts as a midpoint to accurately measure 2 cm proximal (A) and distal (B) for intraosseous infiltration.

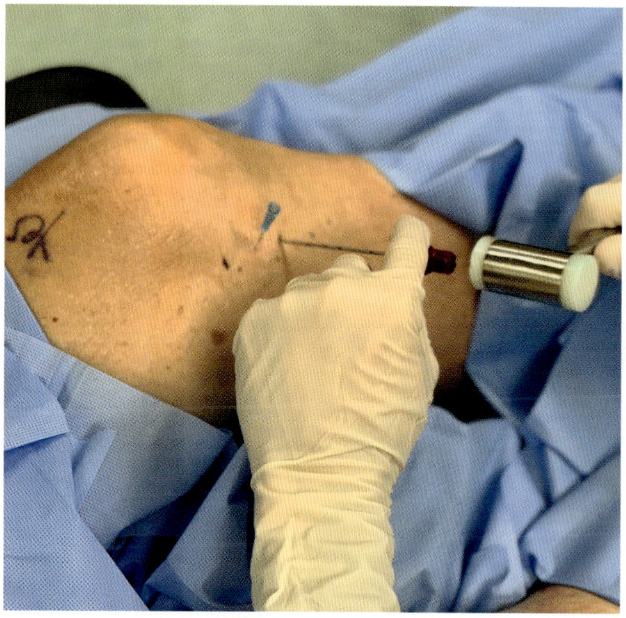

• **Fig. 34.21** Mallet being used to lightly seed the trocar into the periosteum.

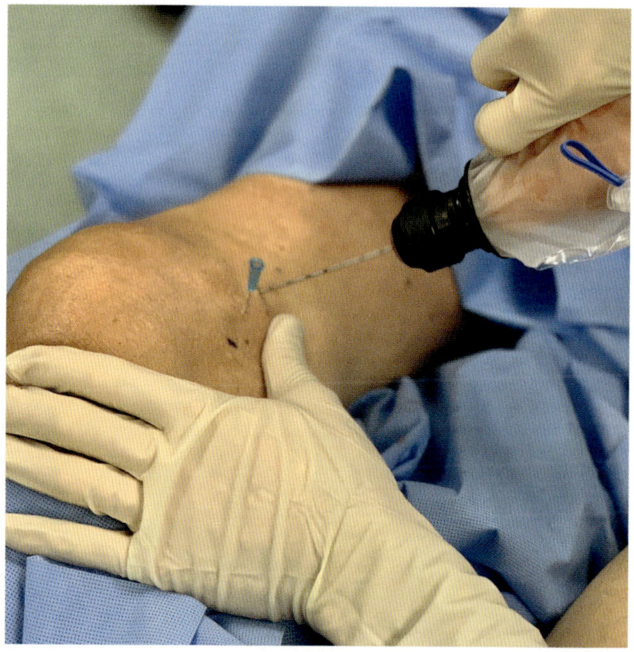

• **Fig. 34.22** Automated power driver used to advance the trocar approximately 1 to 1.5 cm in the same trajectory.

c. Attach the automated power driver to the trocar and advance approximately 1 to 1.5 cm (Fig. 34.22). Alternatively, this can be performed with manual advancement.
d. Attach injectate to the trocar and infiltrate 5 to 10 mL of orthobiologic (Fig. 34.23).
e. The trocar can be removed manually or with assistance from the power driver.

3. Femoral Condyle IO Infiltration:
   a. Using a 15-gauge bone access trocar, pierce the skin and advance the trocar down to the level of the periosteum.
   b. Ensuring a firm position on the femoral condyle, add a small amount of cranial tilt to the trocar (≈10 to 15 degrees) and angle the trocar tip toward the joint line.

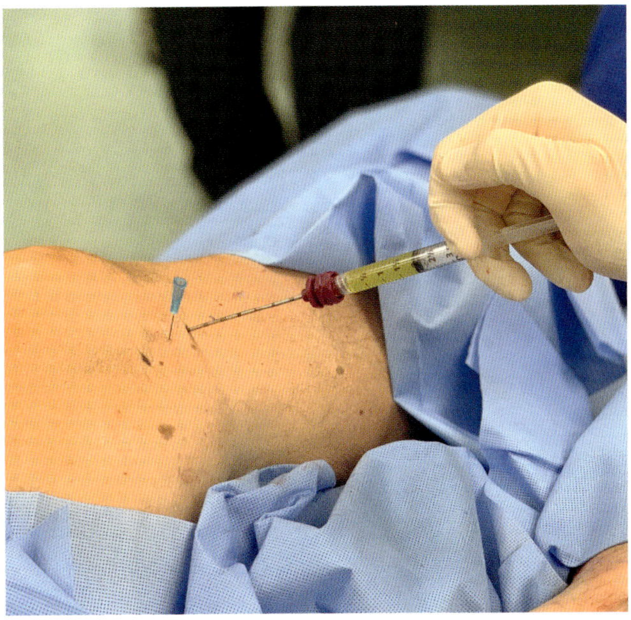

• **Fig. 34.23** Intraosseous Infiltration of Injectate Into Tibial Plateau.

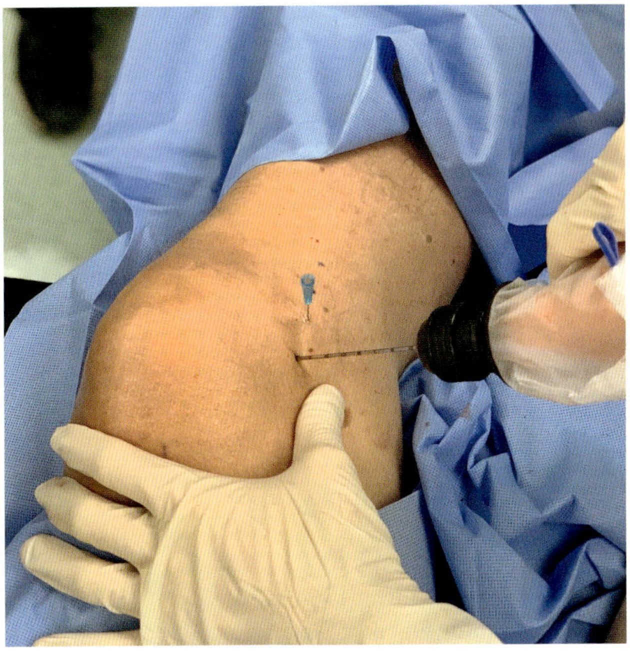

• **Fig. 34.24** Automated power driver being used to advance bone trocar into medial femoral condyle.

c. Using a mallet, lightly seed the trocar into the periosteum, ensuring the same trajectory.
d. Attach the automated power driver to the trocar and advance approximately 1 to 1.5 cm (Fig. 34.24).
e. Attach injectate to the trocar and infiltrate 5 to 10 mL of orthobiologic (Fig. 34.25).

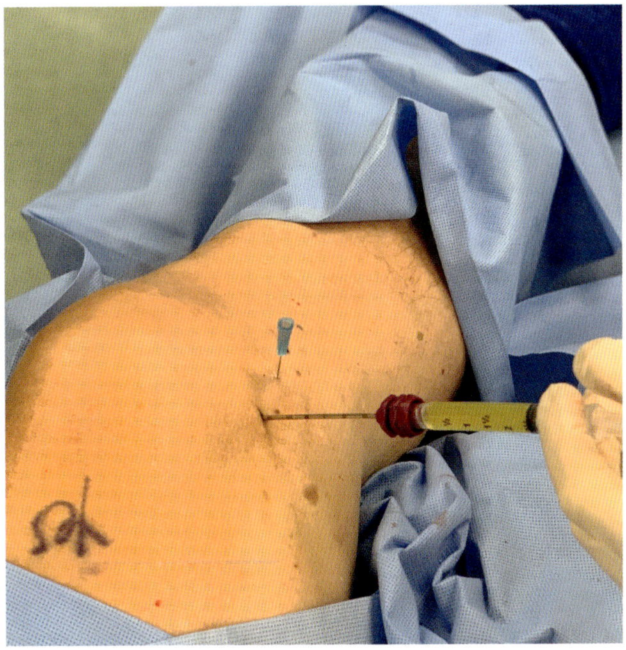

• **Fig. 34.25** Injectate Being Infiltrated Into Medial Femoral Condyle.

Ultrasound Guidance: Hip Osteoarthritis

Patient position: Supine.
Clinician position: Same side as the treatment limb.
Setup: Sedation or MAC optimal, completely sterile field.

Equipment Needed

18/22-gauge needle
15-gauge bone trocar
Automated power driver and/or mallet
Syringe volumes, as needed. for injectate

Procedural Steps

1. Femoral Head IO Infiltration:
   a. Isolate the femoral head using the sagittal oblique view under ultrasound guidance, ensuring a clear view of the femoral head-neck junction.
   b. Maintaining approximately a 45-degree angle, guide the 15-gauge bone access trocar toward the junction of the surgical neck of the femur and femoral head (Fig. 34.26).
   c. Advance the trocar down to the level of the bone, and attach the automated power driver to the trocar.
   d. Advance the trocar into the femoral head approximately 1 to 2 cm, until the trocar is firmly set.
   e. Remove the automated power driver, and infiltrate 5 to 10 mL of injectate.

Ultrasound guidance is used to identify the femoral head-neck junction *(FH)* and guide the bone trocar down to the level of the femoral head *(arrow)*. Note the 45-degree insertional angle of the trocar in the sagittal oblique ultrasound view.

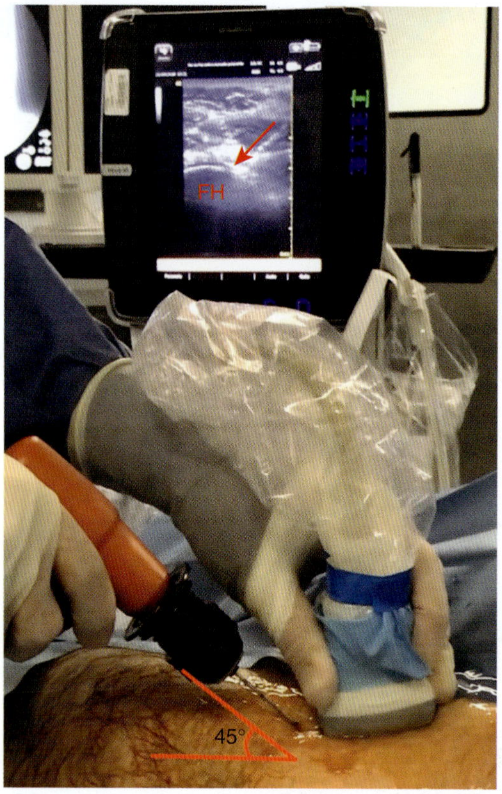

• **Fig. 34.26** Ultrasound-Guided Intraosseous Femoral Head Infiltration. Ultrasound guidance used to identify the femoral head-neck junction (see FH) and guide the bone trocar down to the level of the femoral head (*arrow*). Note the 45-degree insertional angle of the trocar in the sagittal oblique ultrasound view.

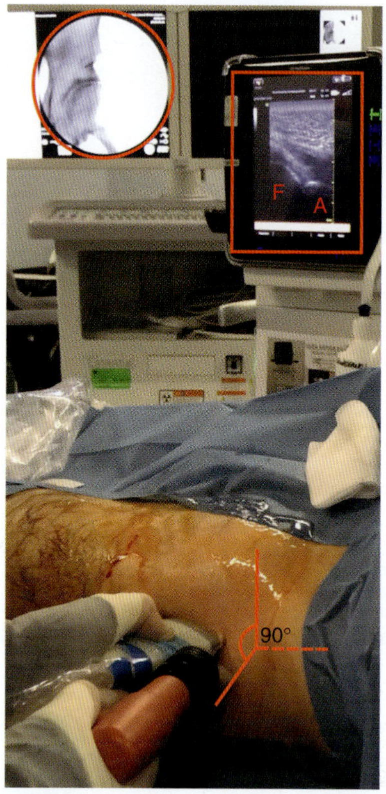

• **Fig. 34.27** Ultrasound-guided intraosseous acetabulum infiltration, confirmed with fluoroscopy. Ultrasound guidance used to identify the femoral-acetabular joint *(square)*, and guide the bone trocar down to the level of the acetabulum. Trocar location confirmed within the acetabulum with fluoroscopy *(circle)*. Note the 90-degree anterior/posterior angle of the power driver at the anatomic midpoint.

2. Acetabulum IO Infiltration:
   a. Using the curvilinear probe, identify the femoral-acetabular joint and center the acetabulum on the ultrasound screen.
   b. Move the probe laterally and posteriorly, until the probe is approximately midline between anterior and posterior acetabulum.
   c. Using an in-plane approach, advance the 15-gauge bone access trocar down to the level of the acetabulum, approximately 1 cm superior to the articular surface.
   d. Attach the automated power driver, and advance the trocar approximately 1 to 2 cm until the trocar is firmly set within the acetabulum (Fig. 34.27).
   e. Remove the automated power driver and infiltrate 5 to 8 mL of injectate.

PEARLS AND PITFALLS

- Ultrasound-guided intraosseous (IO) injections are an advanced procedure and should be performed only after a practitioner has learned fluoroscopic-guided IO injections.
- Because of the porous nature of subchondral bone, the IO injection may flow from the subchondral bone to the articular surface.

Other Intraosseous Injections

Distal Clavicle/Acromion (Fig. 34.28)
Ankle: Distal tibia and talus (Fig. 34.29)
Metacarpal (Fig. 34.30)
Sesamoid (Fig. 34.31)
Distal fibula (Fig. 34.32)
Proximal Humeral Head (Fig. 34.33)
Glenoid (Fig. 34.34)
Metatarsal (Fig. 34.35)
Foot: Medial cuneiform (Fig. 34.36)
Wrist: Scaphoid (Fig. 34.37)

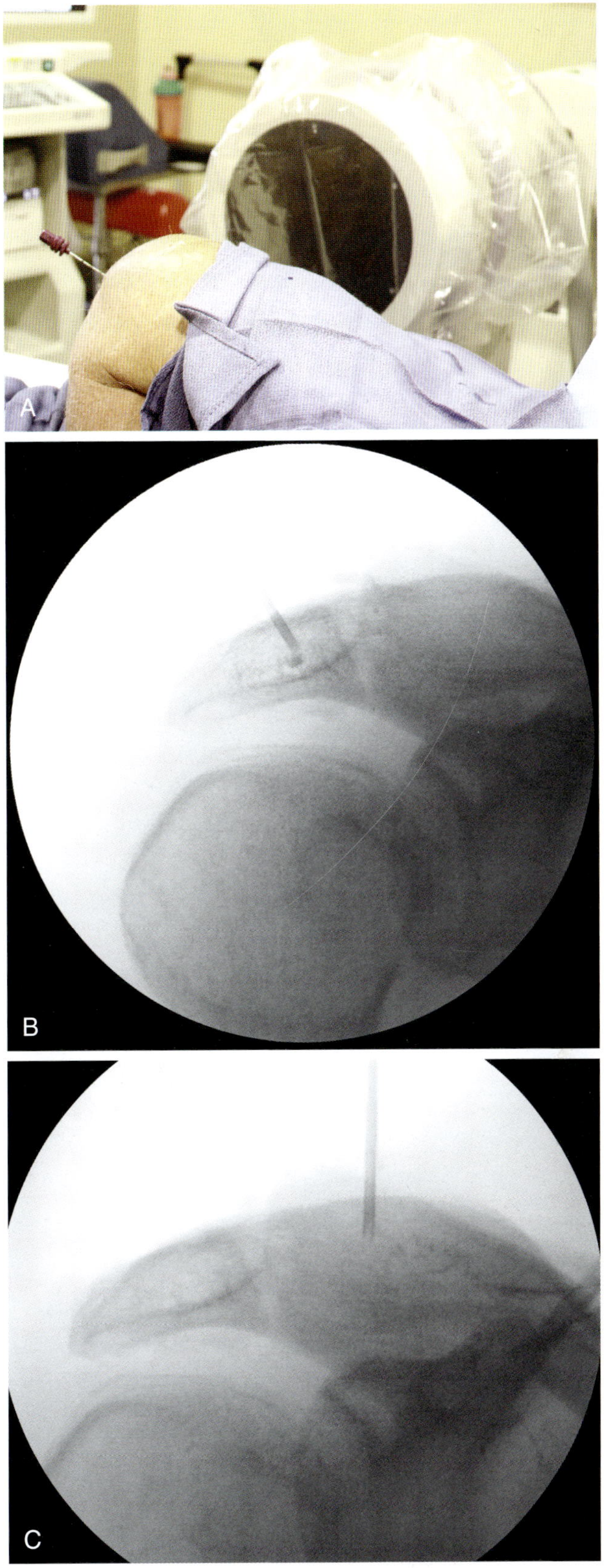

• **Fig. 34.28** (A) Acromial bone intraosseous setup; (B) acromial intraosseous injection; (C) distal clavicle intraosseous injection. (Courtesy of John Pitts.)

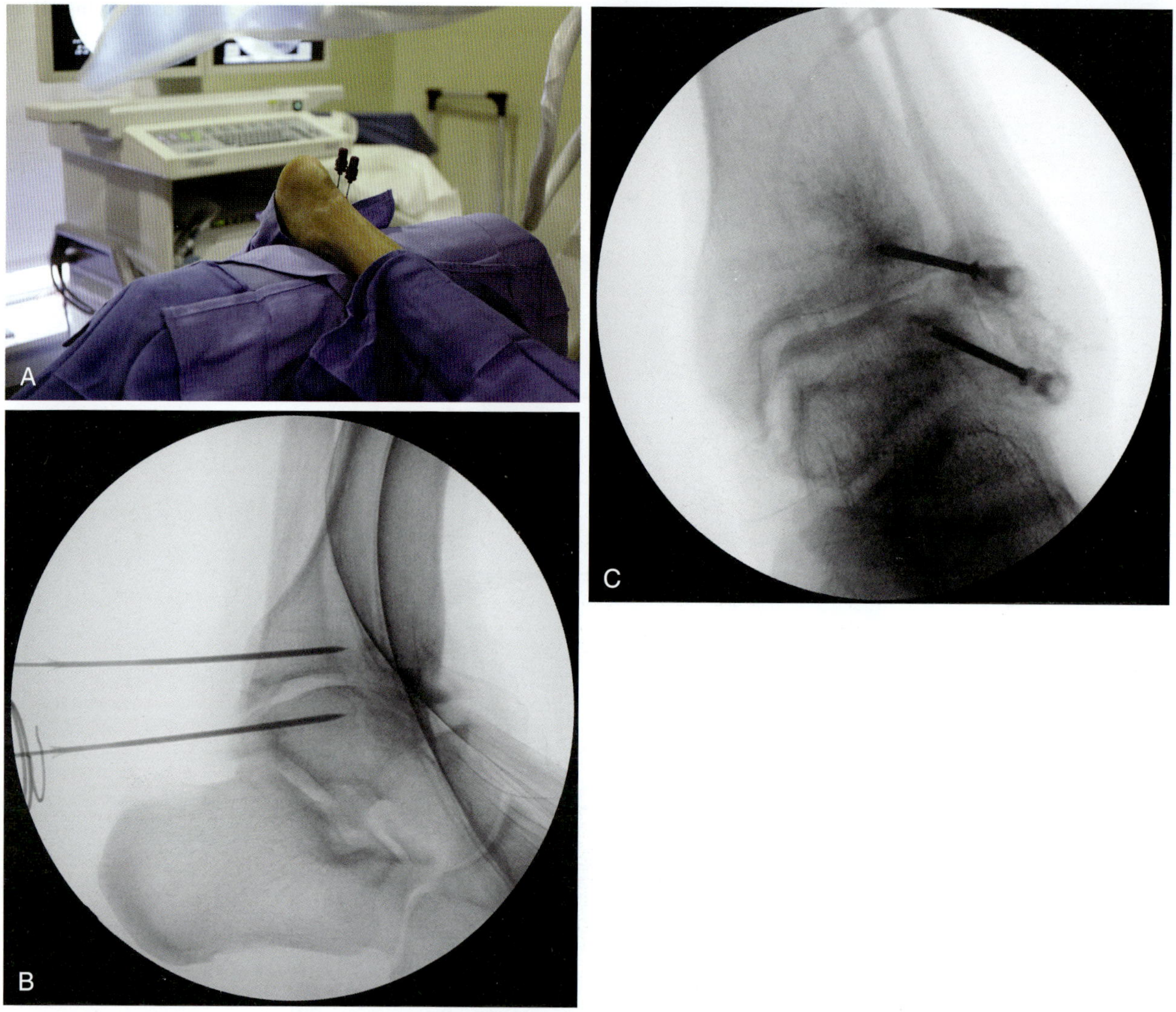

• **Fig. 34.29** (A) Setup; (B) ankle tibia and talus intraosseous needle at target (lateral); (C) ankle tibia and talus intraosseous needle at target (antero-posterior). (Courtesy of Chris Williams.)

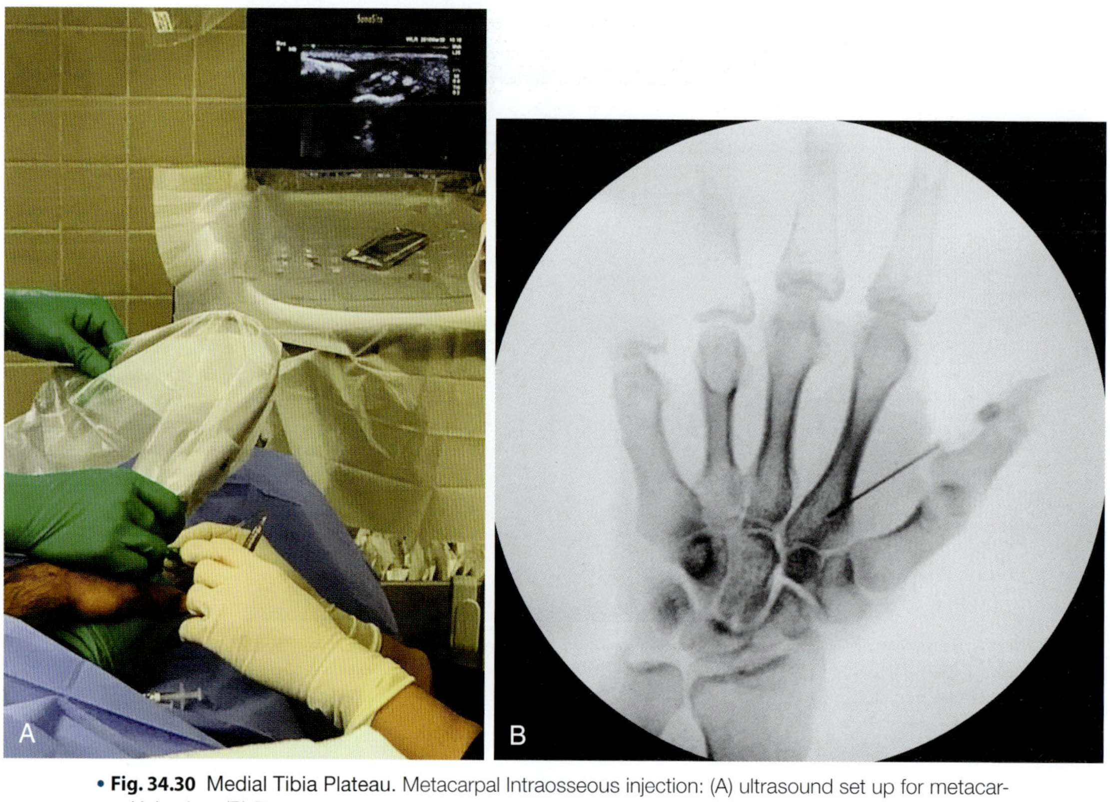

• **Fig. 34.30** Medial Tibia Plateau. Metacarpal Intraosseous injection: (A) ultrasound set up for metacarpal injection; (B) Fluoscopic image of metacarpal intraosseous injection. (Courtesy of Neil Ghodadra.)

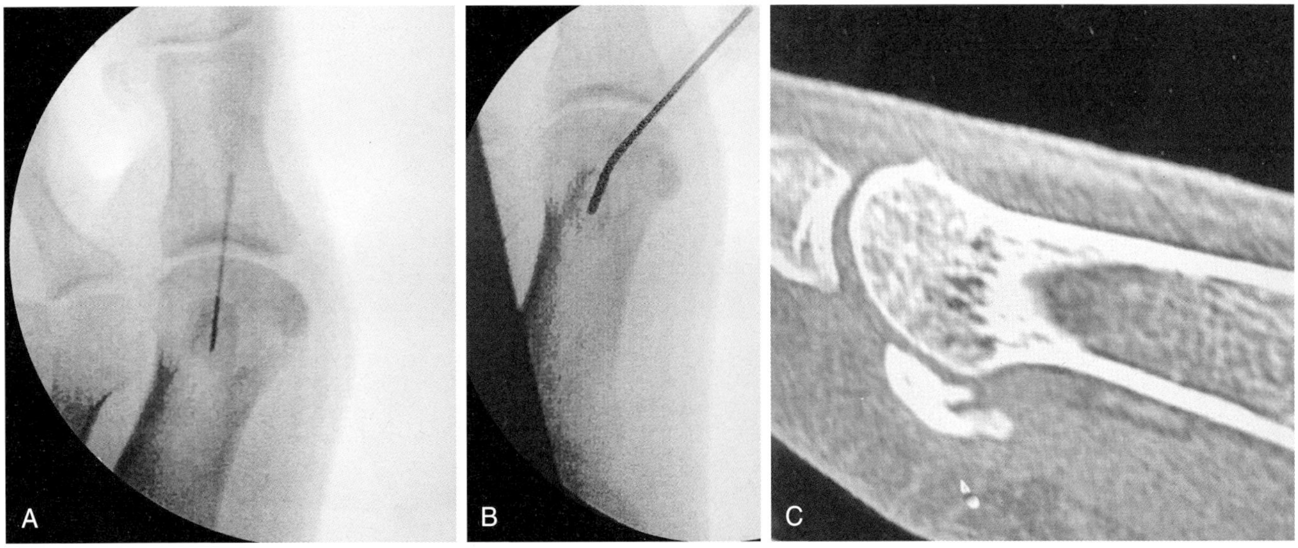

• **Fig. 34.31** Sesamoid Intraosseous. (A and B) different fluoroscopic views of sesamoid intraosseous injection. (C) MRI image of sesamoid pathology prior to intraosseous injection. (Courtesy of Steven Sampson.)

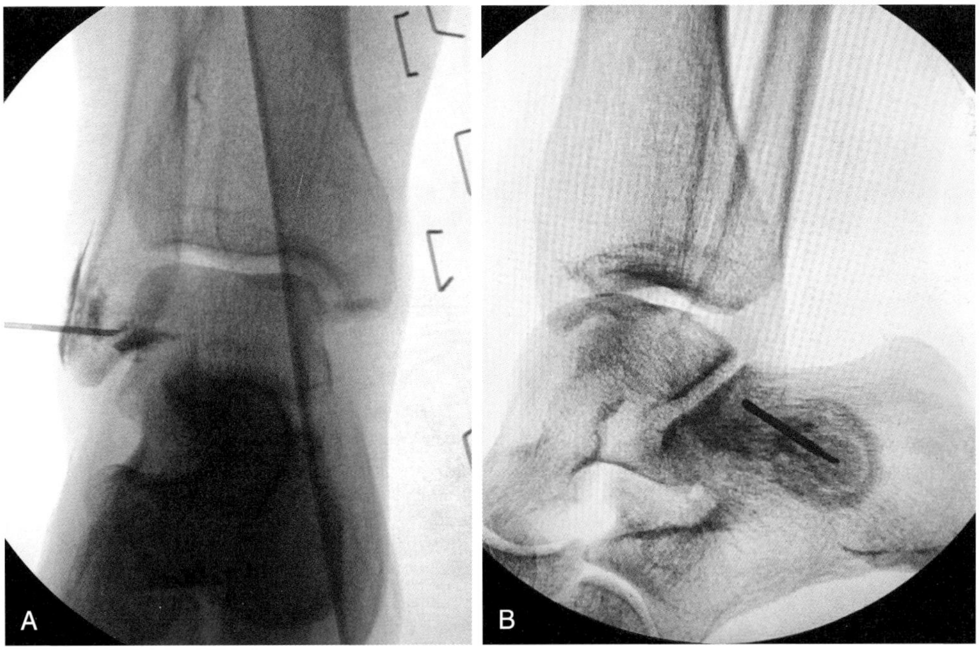

• **Fig. 34.32** Lateral Fibula Intraosseous. (A) Anteroposterior; (B) Lateral. (Courtesy of Chris Williams.)

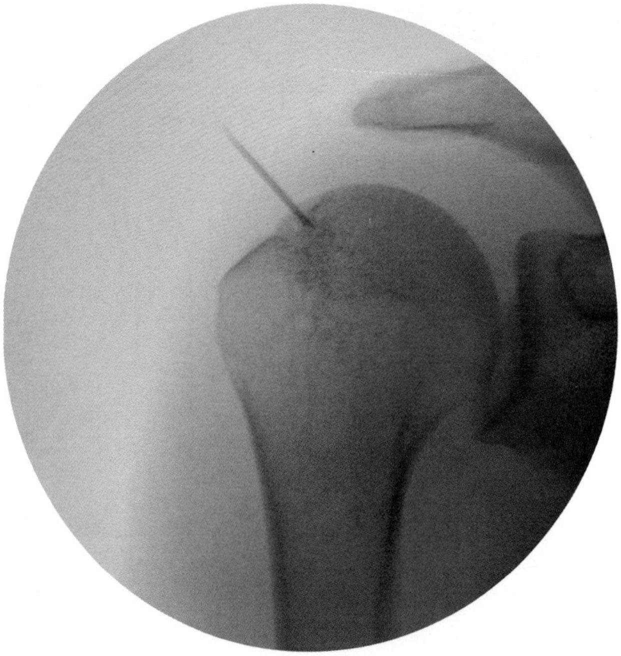

• **Fig. 34.33** Proximal Humeral Head. (Courtesy of John Pitts.)

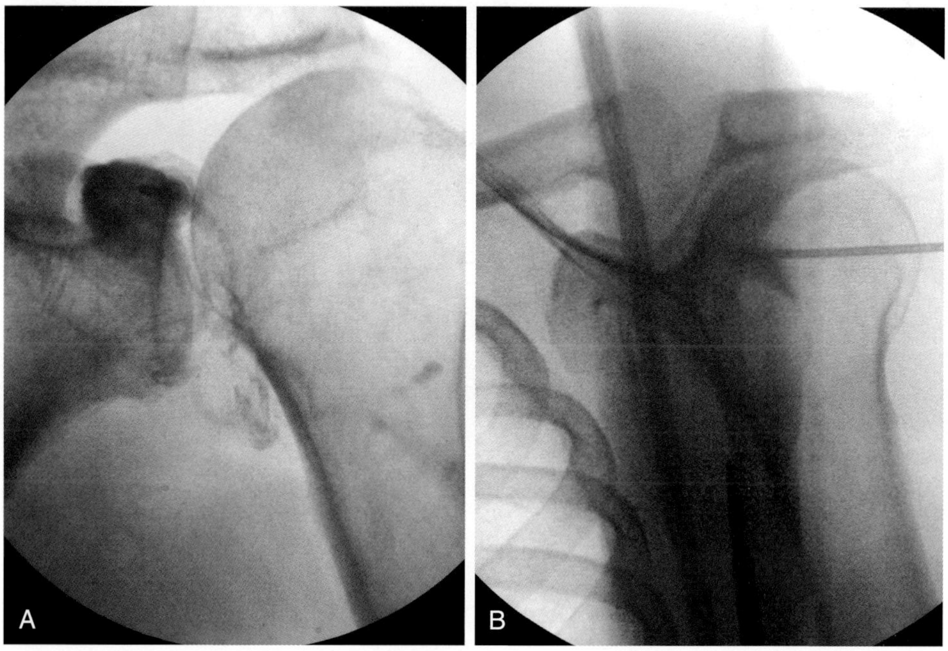

• **Fig. 34.34** Glenoid. (A) Close up fluoroscopic view of glenoid intraosseous injection; (B) anteroposterior fluoroscopic view of Humeral Head intraosseous injection. (Courtesy of Chris Williams.)

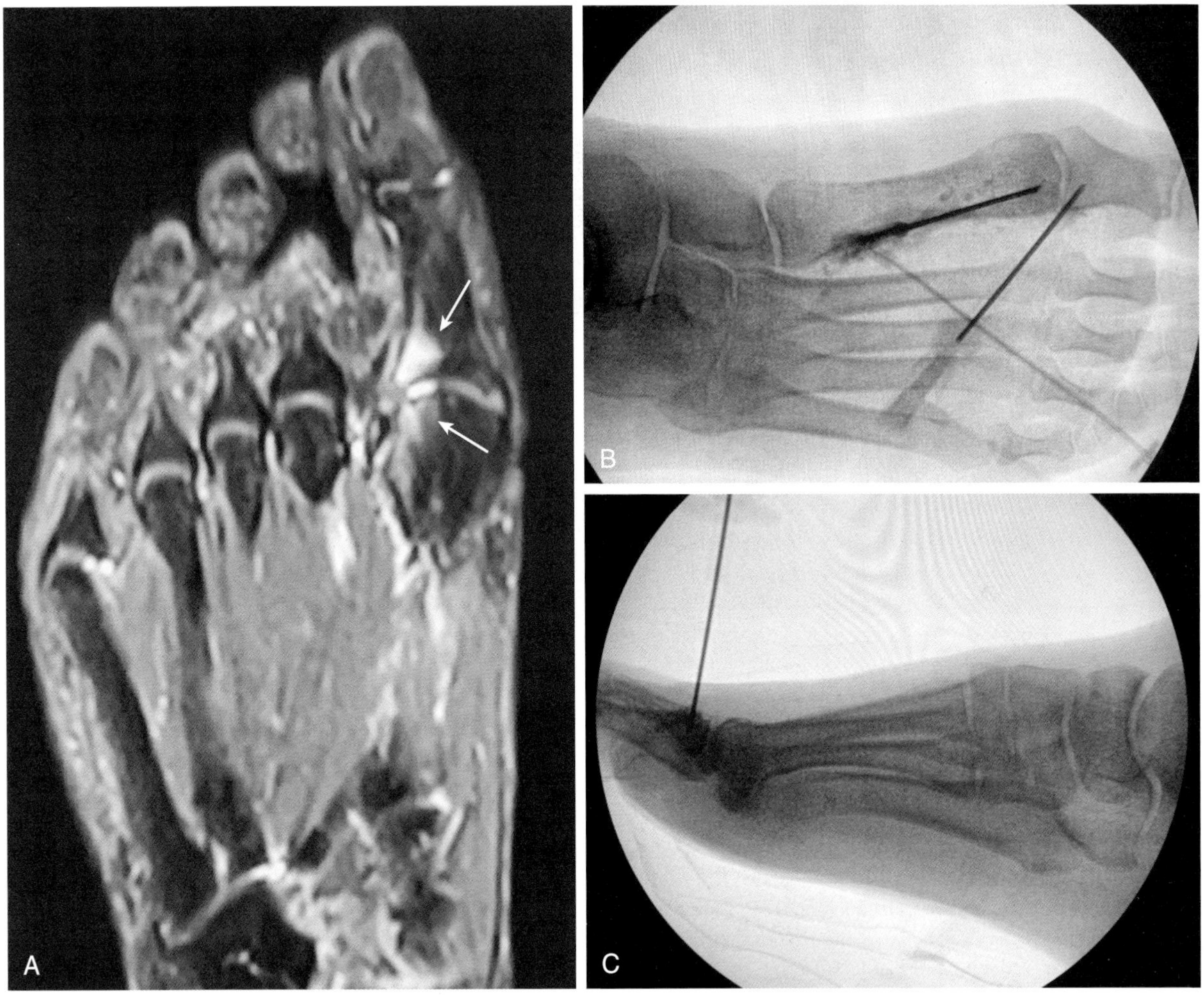

• **Fig. 34.35** Toe Magnetic Resonance Imaging. Metatarsal Intraosseous Injection: (A) MRI image showing boney edema at 1st metatarsal phalange joint; (B) Anteroposterior view of intraosseous injections to 1st metatarsal phalange joint under fluoroscopic guidance; (C) Lateral View of Fluoroscopic guidance for 1st metatarsal phalange intraosseous injection. (Courtesy of John Pitts.)

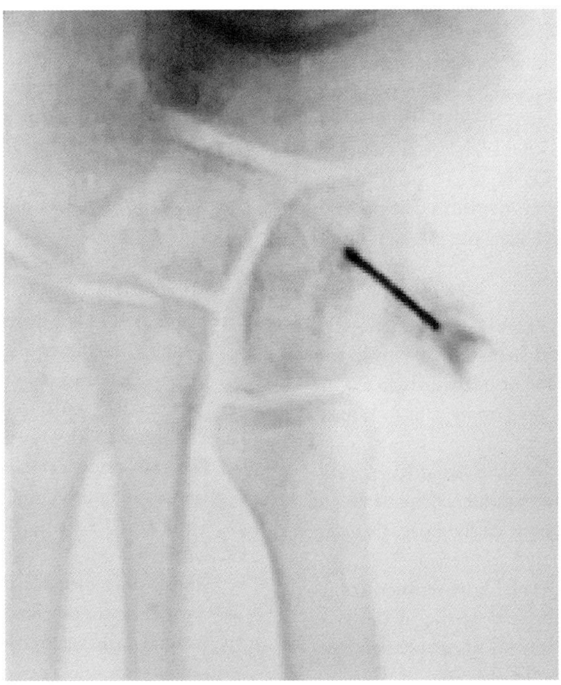

• **Fig. 34.36** Medial Cuneiform. (Courtesy of John Pitts.)

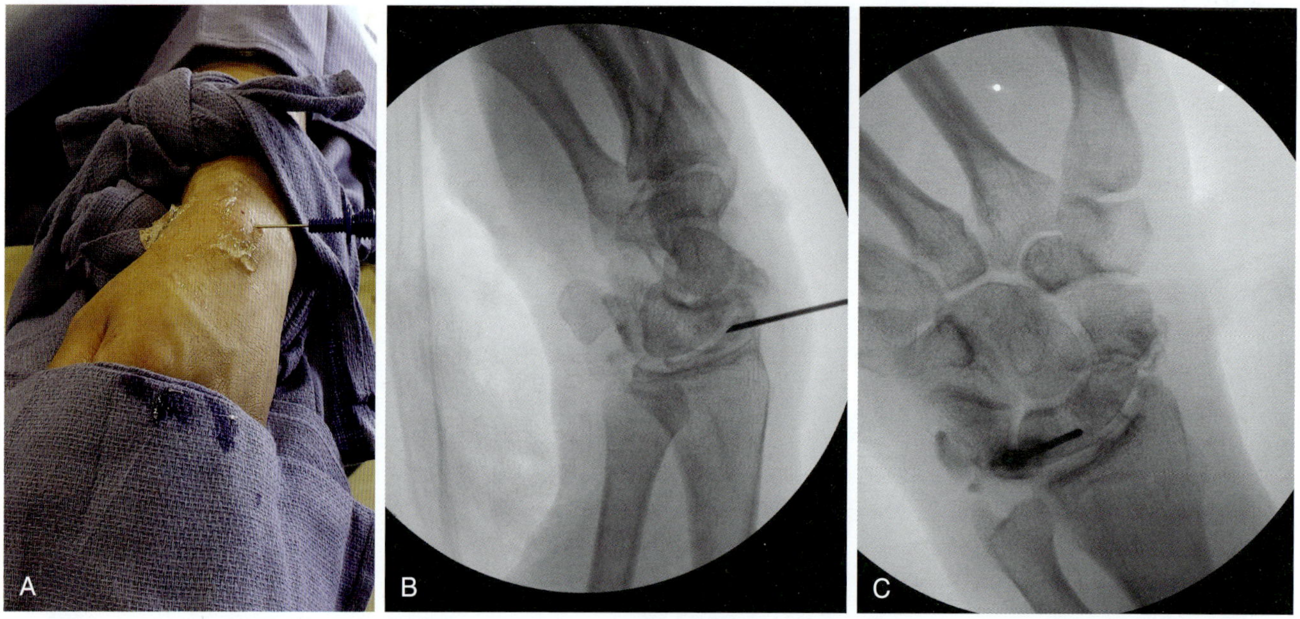

• **Fig. 34.37** (A) Proximal scaphoid intraosseous setup; (B) proximal scaphoid lateral; (C) proximal scaphoid (anteroposterior). (Courtesy of Chaz Fausel.)

References

1. Delgado D, et al. Current concepts in intraosseous platelet-rich plasma injections for knee osteoarthritis. *J Clin Orthop Trauma*. 2018.
2. Pan J, Wang B, Li W, et al. Elevated cross-talk between subchondral bone and cartilage in osteoarthritic joints. *Bone*. 2012;51:212e217.
3. Barr AJ, Campbell TM, Hopkinson D, Kingsbury SR, Bowes MA, Conaghan PG. A systematic review of the relationship between subchondral bone features, pain and structural pathology in peripheral joint osteoarthritis. *Arthritis Res Ther*. 2015;25(17):228.
4. Fiz N, Pérez JC, Guadilla J, et al. Intraosseous infiltration of platelet-rich plasma for severe hip osteoarthritis. *Arthrosc Tech*. 2017;6:e821–e825.
5. Sundaram K, Vargas-Hernandez JS, Sanchez TR, et al. Are subchondral intraosseous injections effective and safe for the treatment of knee osteoarthritis? A systematic review. *J Knee Surg*. 2019.
6. Astur DC, de Freitas EV, Cabral PB, et al. Evaluation and management of subchondral calcium phosphate injection technique to treat bone marrow lesion. *Cartilage*. 2019;10(4):395–401. https://doi.org/10.1177/1947603518770249.
7. Sánchez M, Delgado D, Pompei O, et al. Treating severe knee osteoarthritis with combination of intra-osseous and intra-articular infiltrations of platelet-rich plasma: an observational study. *Cartilage*. 2019;10(2):245–253. https://doi.org/10.1177/1947603518756462.
8. Hernigou P, Auregan JC, Dubory A, Flouzat-Lachaniette CH, Chevallier N, Rouard H. Subchondral stem cell therapy versus contralateral total knee arthroplasty for osteoarthritis following secondary osteonecrosis of the knee. *Int Orthop*. 2018. https://doi.org/10.1007/s00264-018-3916-9.
9. Davidson K, Grimm NL, Christino, et al. Retroarticular drilling with supplemental bone marrow aspirate concentrate for the treatment of osteochondritis dissecans of the knee. *Orthop J Sports Med*. 2018;6.
10. Kasik CS, Martinkovich S, Mosier B, et al. Short-term outcomes for the biologic treatment of bone marrow edema of the knee using bone marrow aspirate concentrate and injectable demineralized bone matrix. *Arthroscopy Sports Med Rehabil*. 2019.
11. Kyle N, Kunze BS, Serino J, Chahla J, Gomoll AH, Mandelbaum B. Focal chondral and subchondral bone lesions of the knee: current evidence for the use of biologic treatment. *Operat Tech Sports Med*. 2020;28(1):150716
12. Hernigou P, Dubory A, Homma Y, et al. Cell therapy versus simultaneous contralateral decompression in symptomatic corticosteroid osteonecrosis: a thirty year follow-up prospective randomized study of one hundred and twenty five adult patients. *Int Orthop (SICOT)*. 2018;42:1639–1649. https://doi.org/10.1007/s00264-018-3941-8.
13. Hernigou P, Daltro G, Hernigou J. Hip osteonecrosis: stem cells for life or behead and arthroplasty? *Int Orthop (SICOT)*. 2018;42:1425–1428. https://doi.org/10.1007/s00264-018-4026-4.
14. Hernigou P, Guerin G, Homma Y, et al. History of concentrated or expanded mesenchymal stem cells for hip osteonecrosis: is there a target number for osteonecrosis repair? *Int Orthop*. 2018. https://doi.org/10.1007/s00264-018-4000-1.
15. Andriolo L, Merli G, Tobar C, Altamura SA, Kon E, Filardo G. Regenerative therapies increase survivorship of avascular necrosis of the femoral head: a systematic review and meta-analysis. *Int Orthop*. 2018. https://doi.org/10.1007/s00264-018-3787-0.
16. Liu L, Gao F, Sun W, et al. Investigating clinical failure of core decompression with autologous bone marrow mononuclear cells grafting for the treatment of non-traumatic osteonecrosis of the femoral head. *Int Orthop*. 2018. https://doi.org/10.1007/s00264-018-3918-7.
17. Hauzeur JP, De Maertelaer V, Baudoux E, Malaise M, Beguin Y, Gangji V. Inefficacy of autologous bone marrow concentrate in stage three osteonecrosis: a randomized controlled double-blind trial. *Int Orthop*. 2017. https://doi.org/10.1007/s00264-017-3650-8.
18. Hernigou P, Thiebaut B, Housset V, et al. Stem cell therapy in bilateral osteonecrosis: computer-assisted surgery versus conventional fluoroscopic technique on the contralateral side. *Int Orthop*. 2018. https://doi.org/10.1007/s00264-018-3953-4.
19. Lebouvier A, Poignard A, Cavet M, et al. Development of a simple procedure for the treatment of femoral head osteonecrosis with intra-osseous injection of bone marrow mesenchymal stromal cells: study of their biodistribution in the early time points after injection. *Stem Cell Res Ther*. 2015;6:68. https://doi.org/10.1186/s13287-015-0036-y.

35

Advanced and Emerging Interventional Techniques

NIDAL ELBARIDI, VIRLYN BISHOP, ORLANDO LANDRUM, MARKO BODOR, AND JOHN PITTS

Spinal Cord and Dorsal Root Ganglion Stimulation

Products available:

- Boston Scientific: Spectra Wavewriter
- Abbott: The Proclaim Elite, (recharge free system)
- Nevro: HF-10
- Medtronic
- Stimwave
- Nalu.

Spinal Cord Stimulation

KEY POINTS

Spinal cord stimulation is based on the gate control theory, an idea put forth by Patrick Wall and Ronald Melzack in 1965, stating that "control of pain may be achieved by selectively activating the large, rapidly conducting fibers."[1] Two years later, the first dorsal column stimulation, conducted by Dr. Norman Shealy, occurred.[2] Based on these early studies, spinal cord stimulator (SCS) therapy succeeded by applying electric fields to membranes, altering their electric potentials and leading to either the activation or inhibition of the neuron. SCS can increase the concentration of inhibitory neurotransmitters and inhibit the nociceptive sensorimotor reflex, a polysynaptic spinal reflex intrinsic to pain sensation.[1] It is most successful for patients with pain due to failed back surgery syndrome, complex regional pain syndrome (CRPS) types I and II, and intractable neuropathic pain.[3] In current times, about 50,000 SCSs are implanted every year.

- *Traditional spinal cord stimulation* (40 to 60 Hz)—provides repetitive electrical stimulation, which is interpreted by the brain as a paresthesia sensation over the painful body part. The SCS lead is located in the midline dorsal epidural space.
- *High-frequency stimulation* (10k Hz)—involves stimulation with increased frequency rate, which results in targeting different neuronal targets and subthreshold perception (able to have stimulation without paresthesia). *High-frequency* SCS leads are located in the midline epidural space.
- *Burst stimulation* (5 pulses 500HZ 40 times per second)—altered waveform pattern of stimulation that mimics organic nerve firing. This pattern of stimulation results in subthreshold perception and improved pain control compared to traditional stimulation.[2-8]

Many studies have indicated that SCS is a safe, successful treatment for a variety of chronic pain syndromes. In 2005, North et al.[9] conducted the first randomized, controlled trial comparing 60 participants with failed back surgery syndrome who underwent either SCS or repeat lumbar spine surgery. Significantly more individuals in the SCS group endorsed pain relief. When compared to conservative managements, SCS patients experienced greater reductions in leg pain, as well as an increase in quality of life.[10] In a similar study, Kemler et al.[11] found that SCS was superior to physical therapy for patients with CRPS. The vast collection of studies investigating the efficacy of SCS is constantly increasing, although most indicate that it is an effective, minimally invasive therapy for patients with neuropathic pain conditions.[1]

The SENZA-RCT trial,[12] a multicenter, randomized, controlled trial evaluating the safety and efficacy of 10-kHz high-frequency (HF10) therapy for the management of chronic back and leg pain, represented a major change in the traditional SCS treatment algorithm. The NEVRO system delivered electrical stimulation pulses at high frequency (10,000 Hz) as compared with traditional low-frequency SCS systems (typically around 50 Hz). Significant pain relief was seen in both low back and lower extremity pain without inducing paresthesia.

New SCS programming sequences targeting microglia and astrocytes (Medtronic DTM) are emerging as another potential stimulation technology for targeting pain signaling in the central nervous system. Microglia and astrocytes within the central nervous system (CNS) have been shown to play a significant role in the development and maintenance of neuropathic pain. Following peripheral nociceptive activation (via nerve injury, infection, or inflammation), microglia become activated and release pro-inflammatory cytokines such as TNF-a, IL-1b, and IL-6, thereby initiating the pain process. Microglia propagate the neuroinflammation by recruiting other microglia and eventually activating nearby astrocytes, which prolongs the inflammatory state and leads to chronic neuropathic pain.[13]

SCS does not eliminate or mechanically alter the source of pain but, instead, blocks the transmission of pain signals in the dorsal columns so that the patient perceives less painful stimuli. The device is programmed to provide each patient with settings that are best suited to their condition. Before a permanent stimulation system is implanted, patients undergo a trial of spinal cord stimulation (typically 5 to 7 days) with temporary lead insertion to determine if the amount of relief they receive is meaningful enough to implant a permanent system. The amount of relief provided varies from person to person and, if the trial stimulator is unsuccessful, it can easily be removed and the patient can pursue other forms of treatment.

Common Pathology

Current FDA approval is targeted for patients with various pain syndromes due to failed back surgery syndrome/post-laminectomy syndrome, CRPS types I and II, intractable neuropathic pain, visceral abdominal pain, and intractable angina pectoris.[3] Success has been reported for off-label use for the treatment of vascular, abdominal, and pelvic pain.

Dorsal Root Ganglion Stimulation

Products available:

- Abbott: Proclaim dorsal root ganglion (DRG)
- Stimwave

KEY POINTS

Similar to normal SCS, dorsal root ganglion (DRG) stimulation is based on the gate control theory, an idea put forth by Patrick Wall and Ronald Melzack in 1965 stating that "control of pain may be achieved by selectively activating the large, rapidly conducting fibers."[1] Typical SCS has multiple shortcomings, such as inability to target specific dermatomes and vulnerability to position changes. DRG stimulation, on the other hand, can directly stimulate affected nerve roots.[1] *DRG stimulation* is based on targeting a different part of the spinal cord, specifically the DRG. The application of DRG SCS results in specific stimulation/pain relief that is extremely focused in a dermatomal pattern that mimics its spinal nerve level. The SCS lead is lateral and exits neural foramen (currently limited to lower thoracic and lumbar levels).

To determine the efficacy of DRG, Timothy et al.[14] performed a randomized trial, comparing DRG and SCS stimulation in patients with CRPS. This study found that 81.2% of patients that underwent DRG were relieved of their pain at 3 months, compared to 55.7% of those who underwent traditional SCS. This finding was consistent at 12 months. Similar studies had conclusions consistent with the study by Timothy et al.,[14] finding that DRG stimulation provides sustained relief in patients with focal neuropathic pain.

Common Pathology

Similar to SCS, patients can receive DRG stimulators, which are devices that interfere with pain signaling from the DRG, an easy-to-reach structure in the spine that contains a large amount of sensory nerves. This device is used to treat pain signaling from areas that are difficult to treat through SCS, such as within the hands, groin, knee, chest, or abdomen. This method does not eliminate the source of pain but, instead, blocks the sensation so that the patient feels less of it. The device is programmed to provide each patient with settings that are best suited to their condition. In addition, patients are given a remote that they can use to control their DRG stimulator, allowing them to further personalize their settings and receive the most relief possible. Before a permanent stimulator device is placed in the body, patients can trial an external version. The amount of relief provided varies from person to person and, if the trial stimulator is unsuccessful, it can easily be removed and the patient can pursue other forms of treatment.

- Mononeuritis of Lower Extremity Unspecified (G57.90)
- Other Nerve Root and Plexus Disorder (G54.8)
- Mononeuritis of Lower Extremity RIGHT (G57.91)
- Mononeuritis of Lower Extremity LEFT (G57.92)
- Failed Back Surgery Syndrome (M96.1)
- Off label use: Abdominal pain and vascular claudication

Pertinent Anatomy

- Traditional spinal cord stimulation is performed via the interlaminar approach with resulting lead placement in the epidural space.
- Vertebral body, pedicles, and dorsal epidural space

Equipment

SCS kit, per manufacturer, varies

Patient Position:

- Prone with pillow under abdomen to reduce lumbar lordosis

Clinician Position

Standing on the side of patient

C Arm Position

- AP and lateral views are necessary to track lead advancement and final position.

Needle Position

- Needle starting point typically is placed 1.5 to 2 vertebral levels below intended level to be accessed.
  - Reason for the difference in needle origin to needle target is to keep needle tip/SCS lead located in the dorsal aspect of the epidural space.

- The interlaminar approach/access is safely done utilizing a loss of resistance syringe to identify safe entry into the epidural space.

Target

- Traditional/Burst/High frequency stimulation—needle tip final position midline in dorsal aspect of epidural space. SCS lead midline space between T7 to T9.
- DRG stimulation—needle tip slightly contralateral to midline of desired exiting foramen. Needle tip one level inferior to exiting foramen.

PEARLS AND PITFALLS

- Besides traditional radicular symptoms, spinal cord stimulation can be useful. DRG/SCS has superior pain relief of distal extremity. However, reports of injury to DRG or exiting nerve root have been reported. So, caution while placing the DRG lead is imperative (Figs. 35.1 and 35.2).
- SCS trial is the most important predictor of potential success. Trials vary from 3 to 7 days. SCS trials involve evaluating the patient's degree of pain relief.

Spine Fracture Therapies

Products available

- Medtronic:

Kyphon Balloon Kyphoplasty, Vertebroplasty, Sacroplasty for vertebral column and sacral fracture repair

Stryker: AVAflex Ballon Kyphoplasty, iVAS Balloon Kyphoplasty for vertebral augmentation and sacroplasty. Spine Jack novel system that includes implantation of a fixation expandable system at spine fracture level. Indicated for vertebral fracture expansion, fixation, stabilization, and ultimately reduction and stabilization of same level.

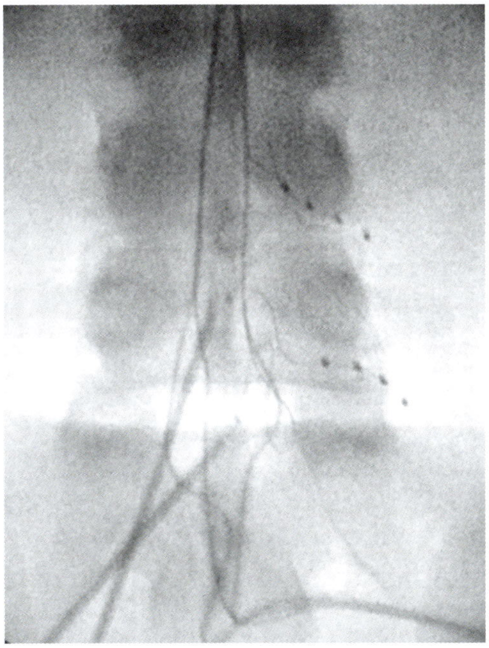

• **Fig. 35.1** Right dorsal root ganglion stimulation lead placement at L4-5 and L5-S1 on an anteroposterior fluoroscopy image.

KEY POINTS

Vertebral Augmentation (Vertebroplasty, Balloon Kyphoplasty, Spine Jack)

Vertebral compression fractures affect 26% of women over the age of 50 and 40% of women over 80 years of age. Of these individuals, more than one-third develop chronic back pain.[15] Typically, individuals with vertebral compression fractures are treated conservatively with analgesics, bed rest, external fixation, and/or rehabilitation. However, the most frequently prescribed medications are poorly tolerated by elderly patients, and bed rest can further demineralize the vertebrae, making these patients more susceptible to additional fractures. Furthermore, surgical fixation is often unsuccessful due to weakness within the osteoporotic bone. Therefore, physicians have explored other treatment options for patients with vertebral compression fractures.

Vertebroplasty is a minimally invasive procedure in which acrylic bone cement is injected into a pathologically compressed vertebral body. Studies have shown short- and long-term pain relief in 70% to 95% of patients.[16] Kyphoplasty is similar in concept to percutaneous vertebroplasty, except that an inflatable balloon is used to expand a collapsed vertebral body as close as possible to its natural height before introducing the mechanical fixation by injecting polymethylmethacrylate (PMMA), a cement-like material, into the cavity created by the balloon. In theory, the expansion of a cavity by the balloon permits infusion of bone cement into the cavity under lower pressure than the bone cement injected during vertebroplasty. Doing so can stabilize the compression fracture while realigning the endplate of the vertebral body.[15] Stabilization of the bone limits movement within the fracture, thereby relieving symptoms of pain. One of the primary reasons for choosing kyphoplasty in lieu of vertebroplasty is decreased cement leakage, which is a main complication with resulting compression of exiting spinal nerve roots or central spinal cord compression. A 2017 review article consisting of 22 studies reported 54.7% and 18.4% cement leakage for vertebroplasty and kyphoplasty, respectively.[17] Additionally, a review published in 2018 of 16 studies showed that kyphoplasty had significantly less risk of cement leakage versus vertebroplasty compared to vertebroplasty.[18] There were no significant differences in pain and functional scores.

Sacroplasty

First described in the literature in 1982, sacral insufficiency fractures (SIFs) affect 1% to 5% of patients in at-risk populations. This condition most commonly affects elderly women with osteoporosis, as well as those with pelvic radiation, steroid-induced osteopenia, rheumatoid arthritis, multiple myeloma, Paget disease, renal osteodystrophy, and hyperparathyroidism.[19] SIFs are thought to occur when stress is applied to sacral bones with insufficiency, with pain symptoms resulting from micromotion within the fracture site. However, there is often a delay in diagnosing individuals with SIFs due to the vagueness of symptoms and similarities to other diseases that frequently affect elderly populations.

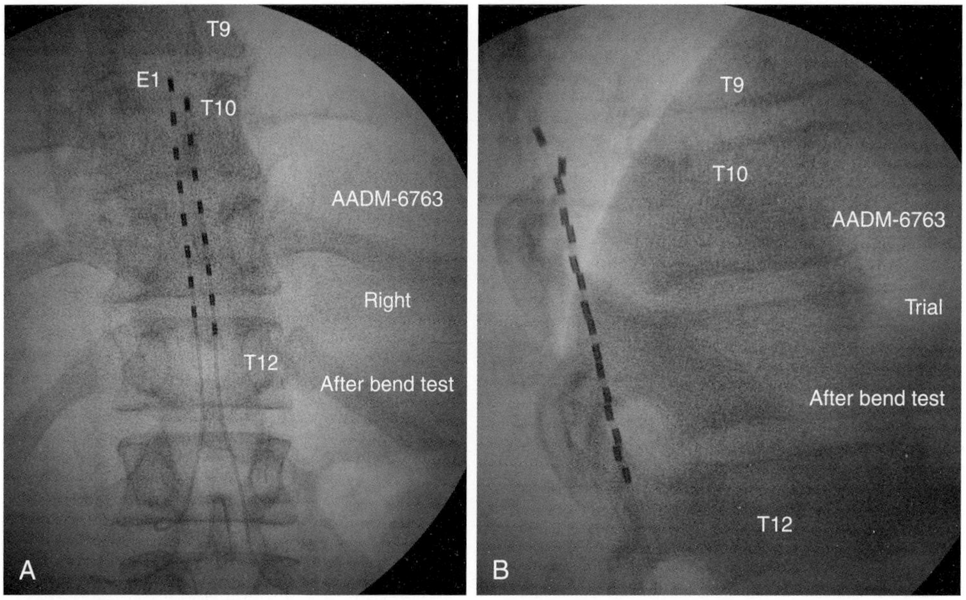

• **Fig. 35.2** (A and B) Thoracic sacral insufficiency fracture lead placement at T9 on anteroposterior and lateral fluoroscopy images.

Once diagnosed, patients are typically treated conservatively with analgesics, bed rest, external fixation, and/or rehabilitation. However, the most frequently prescribed medications are poorly tolerated by elderly patients and bed rest can further demineralize the vertebrae, making these patients more susceptible to additional fractures.[15] Therefore, physicians have explored other treatment options for patients with SIFs.

The injection of cement into the sacrum was initially used to treat painful bony metastases, expanding to SIFs in 2002.[19] During this procedure, PMMA cement is injected into the fractured sacrum with the assistance of imaging devices. This stabilizes the fracture, minimizing micromotion and relieving pain. The goal is to alleviate symptoms while increasing mobility, limiting the need for narcotics and bed rest. A study conducted by Lyders et al. looked at the efficacy of sacroplasty.

By analyzing 52 patients that underwent sacroplasties, the authors concluded that this procedure is safe and effective, providing rapid relief of pain in individuals with SIFs. Participants endorsed a 50% reduction in pain at 2 days, 80% reduction at 2 weeks, and 90% reduction at 1 year.[19] Furthermore, patients relied less on narcotic medications and endorsed improved ability to complete activities of daily living (ADLs) following the procedure. A notable complication is the unexpected extrusion of PMMA cement outside of the sacrum, resulting in neurologic sequelae, although this is rare.[19] This study did not include a control group and, therefore, it should ideally be repeated with a randomized controlled trial design. However, the results are promising, indicating that sacroplasty is an effective treatment for SIFs.

Similar to a balloon kyphoplasty, this procedure is intended to reduce pain while increasing stability for patients with the use of a biological cement. During this procedure, bone needles are inserted into the affected area with the assistance of fluoroscopy. Once in the correct position, bone cement is inserted through the needles, hardening along the fracture. Pain reduction is almost immediate, with some patients endorsing alleviation of symptoms only 30 minutes after treatment.

Pertinent Anatomy

- The vertebral body is comprised of anterior and posterior elements with the connecting element being the pedicle.
- The pedicle is both the entryway and safe zone for the procedure being done (see Fig. 13.2).

Common Pathology

- Compression fracture (with resulting pain) can occur from multiple causes (osteoporotic compression fractures, multiple myeloma, spinal tumors, hemangioma, myeloma, metastasis, and lymphoma)
- Most compression fractures occur between T9 and L4

Equipment

- Vertebral augmentation kit, per manufacturer, varies

Common Injectates

- Local anesthetics: Lidocaine 0.5%, Lidocaine 2%, Bupivacaine 0.25%
- PMMA powder/barium sulfate/tobramycin powder

Injectate Volume

- 6 to 10 mL is typical for local anesthetic injectate
- PMMA or Cortoss cement (injectate averages 2 to 3 mL per level)

Lumbar Spine

Patient Position

- Prone with abdomen on a pillow to reduce lumbar lordosis

C-Arm Position

- Appropriate vertebral body level is confirmed in the anteroposterior (AP) view by identifying the 12th rib and counting from there.
- Proceduralist will advance the needle biplanar in AP and lateral views.
- Appropriate planning for trajectory and end point being posterior ⅓ of vertebral body.

Needle Position

- Plan for trajectory by localization of local anesthetic needle under fluoroscopy at superior lateral aspect of the pedicle (respective 10 and 2 o'clock positions).
- Needle/trocar is advanced using both AP and lateral views to identify needle tip within the pedicle (NOT violating the medial pedicle body) until it passes the posterior vertebral body wall.
- Transpedicular is most common route due to its inherent safety. Prevents neural compression via cement extravasation. Guide trocar to the 10 o'clock (left side) or 2 o'clock (right side) entry to prevent medial border violation.
- Trocar needle is advanced using mallet and intermittent fluoroscopy imaging to clarify tip staying within the pedicle as it advanced

Target

- Central anterior ⅓ of vertebral body.

PEARLS AND PITFALLS

- Recommend monitored anesthesia care (MAC)
- If possible, perform a transpedicular approach, with focus on not violating medial border.
- Using blend of contrast/bone cement injected slowly to identify any extravasation into perineural structures.

Thoracic Spine[20-24]

Patient Position

- Prone

C-Arm Position

- Oblique AP view with ipsilateral pedicle 25% medial to lateral edge of the vertebral body

Needle Position

- Extrapedicular approach/intercostotransverse (thoracic)—avoids pleural and parenchymal injury. Trocar passes lateral to the transverse process and medial to the rib border. Traditional transpedicular approach is limited due to narrower pedicles and difficulty with central vertebral body endpoint.
- Parapedicular—approach to obtain more central endpoint orientation, increased risk of damage to other anatomical structures.
- Can be done with two-needle or one-needle technique, depending on need and vertebral body level.

Target

- Desired target is anterior (1/3) vertebral body, preferred contralateral vertebral body to facilitate unipedicular approach/treatment

PEARLS AND PITFALLS

- Most fractures above T2 are not operated on in an office-based setting.
- Recommend 11-gauge needle (reports of pedicle fracture with smaller 13-gauge needle, most likely secondary to challenges with needle positioning with smaller needle)
- Cement leak is the most common complication—avoided based on needle position in anterior (1/3) of vertebrae and intermittent radiographic imaging to clarify cement extravasation (Fig. 35.3).
- Second most common complication is infection—adherence to strict sterile technique with optional use of antibiotic (both intravenously and via PMMA mixture) to help decrease the risk

Cervical Spine

NOTE: This is usually not performed in office-based setting, and rarely by non-orthopedic surgeons or neurosurgeon

Patient Position

- Supine position, neck extended with towel or bolster under shoulders
- Larynx and trachea displace medially, carotid artery laterally
- Needle entry adjacent to medial border of right sternocleidomastoid muscle under direct image guidance (specifically ultrasound to assess presence of vascular structures)

C-Arm Position

- Biplanar technique with straight AP and lateral views, with neck in neutral position and cervical extension

Needle Position

- Anterolateral (cervical spine)—anterior approach into the vertebral body, avoiding blood vessels, trachea, esophagus, and neural structures. Additional ultrasonography imaging is optimal to identify a safe trocar path.

Target

- Central anterior (1/3) vertebral body.

PEARLS AND PITFALLS

- High risk procedure given the concentrated anatomy with vascular and neurologic structures in proximity.
- Cement leakage can occur between 12% to 84% of treated vertebrae, but many of those are asymptomatic.[25]

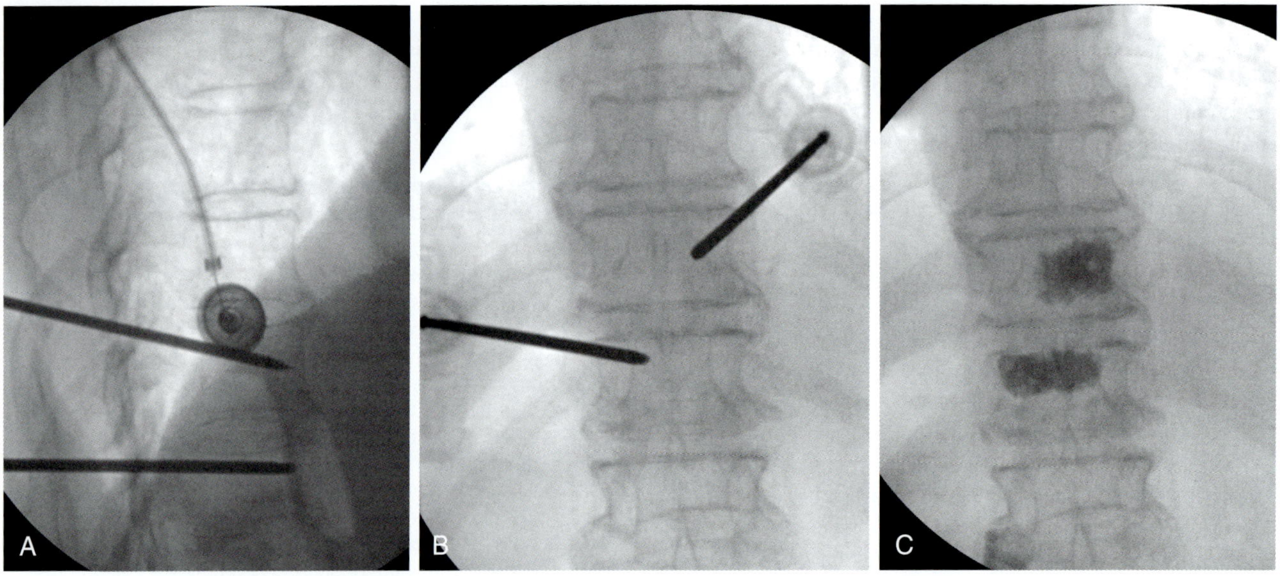

• **Fig. 35.3** (A to C) Thoracic kyphoplasty images using fluoroscopy. (A) in anteroposterior (AP) at T11 on the right and T12 on the left. (B) Lateral image of T11 and T12 with needle placement. (C) AP image with cement in T11 and T12 after needle removal.

Minimally Invasive Lumbar Decompression

Minimally Invasive Lumbar Decompression Procedure

KEY POINTS

Minimally invasive lumbar decompression (MILD) is a procedure to treat lumbar spinal stenosis (LSS) in part due to ligament flavum hypertrophy. Pain that is present in the axial spine with radicular symptoms (indicative of neurogenic claudication) is most likely to respond. Finding the greatest stenotic level on magnetic resonance imaging (MRI) with ligamentum flavum thickening (noting that both level and laterality are a must to determine targeted areas). It is an outpatient procedure performed under monitored anesthesia (i.e., MAC). It treats lumbar decompression by using a 5.1 mm gauge trocar with associated tools to remove a hypertrophied ligamentum flavum and small portions of the lamina, causing lumbar spina stenosis (LSS).

To evaluate the efficacy of MILD, scientists have compared this procedure to other common treatments for LSS, such as epidural steroid injections (ESI). In a randomized controlled study performed by Peter et al.,[26] treatment outcomes for patients with LSS and neurogenic claudication symptoms were compiled from 26 interventional pain management centers. In total, 149 MILD patients were compared to 131 patients that were treated with ESIs. They found that MILD procedures provided sustained relief, with patients endorsing significant improvements in their pain, symptoms, and physical functionality levels for up to 2 years following treatment. In addition, there were no procedure-related adverse events or spinal instability for those that underwent MILD procedures.[26] Individuals that received ESIs also endorsed alleviation of their symptoms, however, the effects were not as durable and many required repeat injections to sustain their pain relief. When compared to other spinal procedures, MILD patients are less likely to require surgical reoperation; in this study, 5.6% of MILD patients required a repeat operation at 2 years, compared to the national average of 12.5% to 16.9% for individuals that received spinal fusions and 14.4% to 26.0% for individuals that underwent interspinous process distraction.[26] This study and similar experiments indicate the MILD is successful in alleviating symptoms of LSS, providing more durable results than ESIs and other spinal operations. MILD procedure training requires attendance at a specific hands-on training course provided by the company, thus only a general explanation is presented here.

Common Pathology

LSS often leads to neurogenic claudication, which causes extremity and lower back pain that can significantly reduce an individual's quality of life. Approximately 19.4% of individuals between the ages of 60 and 69 experience LSS, making spinal surgeries common procedures within this population.[27] Usually, this condition affects both sides of the body, although symptoms can be asymmetric, with one side experiencing worse effects. About 43% of individuals with LSS experience numbness, often exacerbated by prolonged periods of standing and walking.[27] LSS is often accompanied by bulging discs, foraminal narrowing, facet hypertrophy, facet arthropathy, and degenerative disc disease. To treat this condition, many physicians offer MILD procedures, where excess bones and ligaments are removed to minimize stress on spinal nerves.

Pertinent Anatomy

- The proceduralist needs to understand and visualize on fluoroscopy the spinous processes, lamina, ligamentum flavum, and pedicles.

Common Pathology

- MILD is indicated for a thickened ligamentum flavum (2.5 mm or greater), which causes narrowing of the spinal canal.

- It is typically accompanied by neurogenic claudication, resulting in pain and numbness of the lower back, legs, and buttocks.
- It is interesting to note that other conditions may find benefit in pain relief and function due to increased canal space. Some of these conditions include bulging disc, facet hypertrophy, and foraminal narrowing.

Equipment

- C-arm fluoroscopy
- Trocar
- One sculptor/rongeur
- Tissue sculptor

Common Injectates

- Contrast for epidurogram
- Local anesthetic, with or without, corticosteroids is optional.

Injectate Volume

- 2 to 5 mL of contrast
- 2 to 5 mL of injectate

Patient Position

- Prone with abdomen on a pillow to reduce lumbar lordosis

Clinician position

- Side of patient

Fluoroscopy Position

- Posterior-anterior, lateral, and contralateral oblique view (for epidurogram)
- The fluoroscopy machine is rotated to obtain a contralateral view as the optimal working view
- Tissue removal is conducted under live fluoroscopy

Needle Position

- Epidurogram by translaminar Tuohy needle (Fig. 35.4A and B).
- Trocar will be placed just lateral to the spinous process at the lamina (Fig. 35.5A and B).
- Ligamentum flavum and boney connections are removed via bone Rongeur, then tissue sculpture, and is performed under live fluoroscopy (Fig. 35.6).
- Instruments are advanced posterior to epidurogram and should not go anterior.

Target

- Interlaminar space for hypertrophied ligamentum flavum as identified preoperatively (via MRI) and possibly intraoperatively via epidurogram. When debulking of lamina and superficial ligamentum flavum are removed, stenotic lesion improves on epidurogram.

PEARLS AND PITFALLS

- Have a clear idea of the epidural space to clarify safety margins.
- It is imperative to have an epidurogram to delineate the safety border to prevent any damage or harm to neuronal structures.
- Contralateral oblique view with aligned lamina gives target zone and placement of trocar with included tools.
- Refreshing the epidurogram allows for evaluation of tissue removal progression.
- Pre-planning and starting alignment are key to the success of the procedure.
- Alignment should be delineated on the patient by using a sterile marker and fluoroscopy to note the alignment of multiple vertebral levels based on both mid-pedicular lines and central spinous processes.

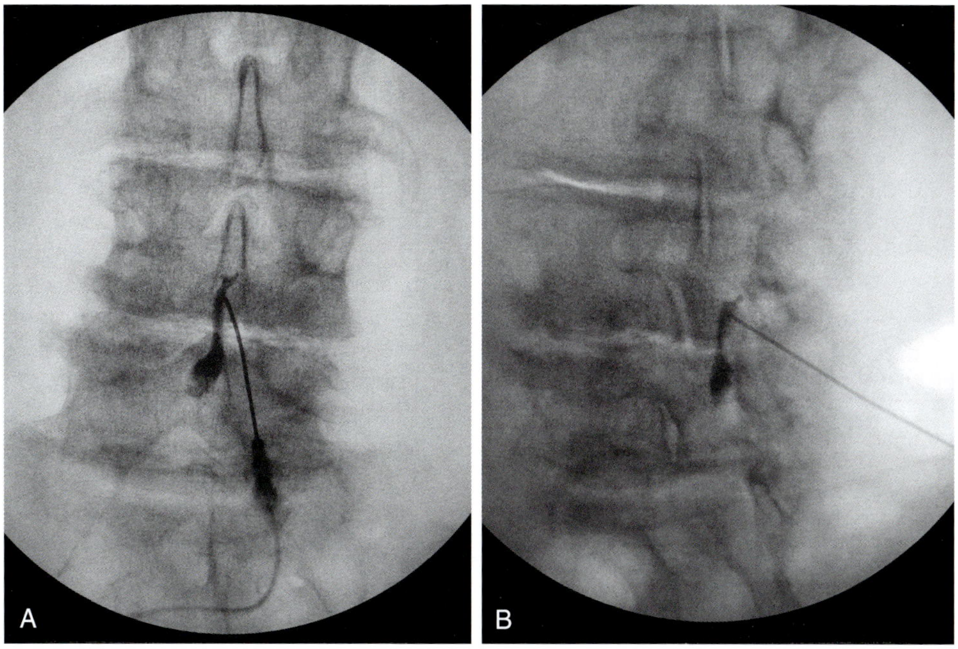

• **Fig. 35.4** (A) Epidurogram anteroposterior view. (B) Contralateral oblique view.

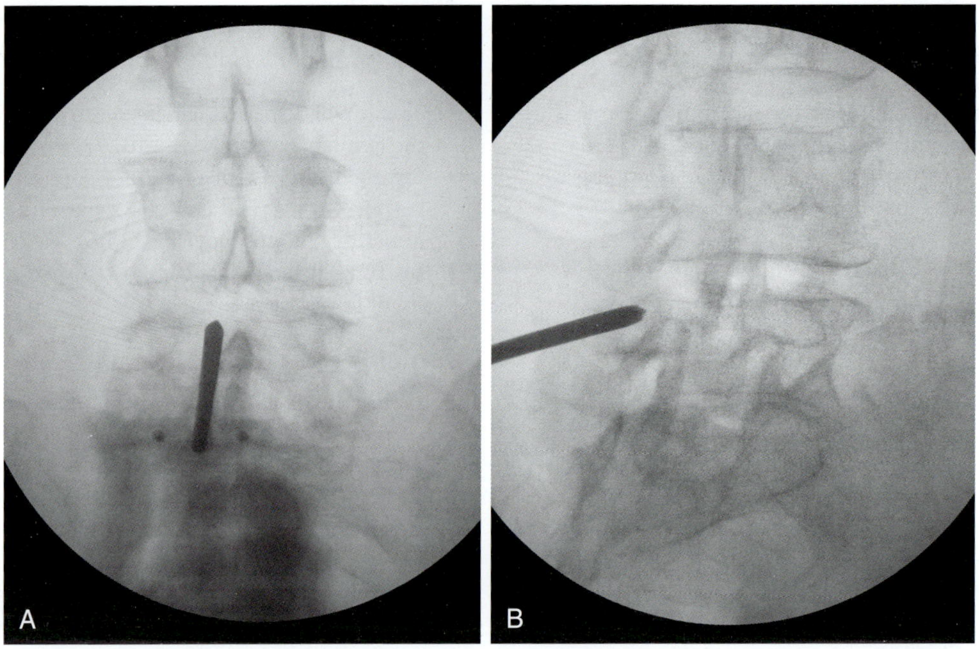

• **Fig. 35.5** (A) Trochar placement anteroposterior. (B) Contralateral oblique view.

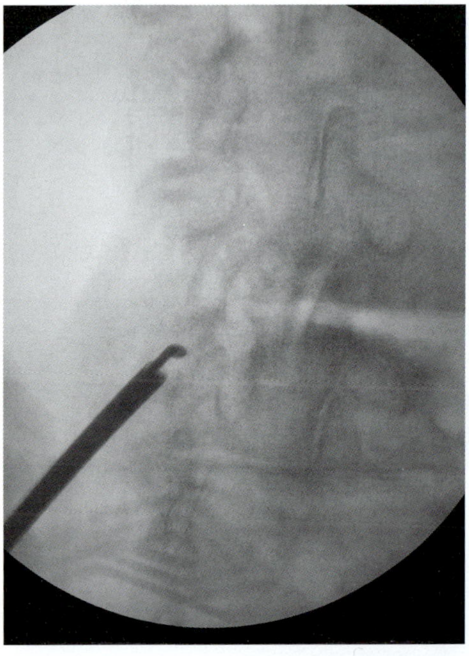

• **Fig. 35.6** Contralateral oblique view of bone Rongeur deployed.

Interspinous Spacer Implantation

Vertiflex/Superion Procedure

Background

- Within 10 years, it is estimated that 64 million older adults will be afflicted with LSS, making it the most common indication for spine surgery in individuals older than 65.[28]
- A large number of interspinous process devices (IPDs) have been recently introduced to the lumbar spine market as an alternative to conventional decompressive surgery in managing symptomatic lumbar spinal pathology.
- In the 1990s, several IDP devices displaying significant differences in design, materials, surgical techniques, and indications appeared in Europe and South America, for which there are ongoing trials of evaluation for a host of clinical indications. Kaech et al. first reported on the interspinous "U" (Coflex), suggesting that it was indicated for protection against adjacent level disc disease and restabilization of a lumbar laminectomy.[28a] Krappel et al. reported on the DIAM implant, which was indicated for a number of conditions, including degenerative disc disease, herniated nucleus pulposus, and lumbar instability.[28b] The X-Stop device (Medtronic, Tolochenaz, Switzerland) was approved by the US Food and Drug Administration (FDA) in 2005 for the treatment of neurogenic intermittent claudication (NIC) secondary to lumbar stenosis.
- Typically, patients complain about low back pain with or without pseudoradicular pain or dysesthesia. The operative "gold standard" to treat degenerative lumbar spinal disease is decompressive laminectomy, with or without fusion of the affected segment. However, some investigators began to explore novel minimally invasive approaches to stabilize the lumbar spine. Various authors suggest that advantages of IPD compared with standard surgical decompression techniques are the option of local anesthesia, preservation of bone and soft tissue, reduced risk of epidural scarring, and cerebrospinal fluid leakage, with a shorter hospital stay and rehabilitation period, as well as reversibility of the surgical procedure that does not interfere with future surgical treatment options.

- With interspinous spacer devices, the main selection criterion is that a patient's symptoms must be relieved by forward flexion of the lumbar spine.
- This phenomenon is often referred to as the "shopping cart sign" due to the improvement in walking endurance in stenotic patients when assuming a forward flexed position of lumbar spine.
- Flexion of the stenotic lumbar spine stretches the redundant ligamentum flavum and enlarges the neural foramina, thus relieving lower extremity symptoms.
- Interspinous spacer devices mechanisms of action all generally work by preserving forward flexion of the lumbar spine while increasing the central, subarticular, lateral recess, and neuroforaminal spaces by restricting dynamic narrowing of the mentioned spaces/zones of lumbar spine during extension (Gazzeri et al., 2014).
- The annual incidence of surgery for adjacent-segment disease following posterior decompression and fusion (or open posterior lateral interbody fusion or circumferential fusion) has been reported to be 2.5% per year. This means that one in four individuals will require a repeat operation within 10 years of the initial arthrodesis. There are a number of risk factors for accelerated adjacent segment disease. These include being less than 60 years of age, termination of the fusion construct at the L5 level, arthrodesis of three or more levels, and stand-alone decompression of the segment adjacent to instrumented levels.
- Spinous process fracture is the most common complication of interspinous spacer devices.
- Consequently, a patient with severe osteoporosis (defined as lumbar spine T-score <2.5 on BD DEXA scan) may represent a contraindication for interspinous device placement, because of the increased risk of fracture of the spinous process either intraoperatively or postoperatively.

KEY POINTS

- The pathoanatomic feature of NIC in lumbar degenerative diseases is the venous stasis in lumbar spine extension, causing neurologic symptoms, including motor weakness in the lower extremities, pain, tingling, and sensory deficit, which make walking for a long distance impossible (Gazzeri et al., 2015).
- Standard recommendations for the implantation of an IPD is mild to moderate central canal stenosis with NIC from spinal stenosis.
- Patients with LSS and NIC refractory to conservative treatments typically undergo posterior decompressive, laminectomy with pedicle fixation at one or more levels, or laminotomy combined with interlaminar stabilization. However, these open spine surgeries are more invasive with potentially greater risk of postoperative complications for elderly individuals as they require general anesthesia for the procedure and prolonged bed rest during recovery[29]. Considering LSS occurs most commonly in individuals that are advanced in age (over the age of 65), alternative, minimally invasive techniques are often preferred.
- Vertiflex is implanted through a minimally invasive procedure, allowing for interspinous stabilization that can treat localized stenosis in patients that cannot undergo more intensive surgeries.[29] The procedure is shorter, does not require general anesthesia, and rarely disrupts muscles and nerves within the area. In a study performed by Jason et al.,[29] 13 Vertiflex patients were compared to 73 LSS patients who underwent open surgery: 45 underwent laminectomy alone or with pedicle screw fixation and 28 received limited laminotomy combined with Coflex® implantation at one or two levels. The results indicated that Vertiflex implants are most effective, immediately and after 5 years, in alleviating symptoms for individuals with localized LSS.[29] With Vertiflex, there were no postoperative infections or hematomas, whereas six of the 45 patients that underwent laminectomy with or without pedicle screw fixation experienced cerebrospinal fluid leak. In addition, two of these individuals required a repeat surgery, six patients developed urinary retention leading to catheterization, and two subjects developed thrombophlebitis.[29]
- In a similar study performed by Bini et al.,[30] 121 patients with LSS underwent Vertiflex procedures, receiving Superion® Interspinous Spacers. Subjects endorsed a 53% decrease in extremity pain following implantation with 86% of patients confirming statistically significant reduction in pain after 1 year. In addition, 76% of patients confirmed that Vertiflex helped relieve axial pain. Sixty-four percent had improvement in their Oswestry Disability Index score, indicating that Vertiflex can significantly reduce lower back pain while improving functionality.[30] These findings, along with those from the study by Jason et al.,[29] indicate that Vertiflex is an effective procedure that is significantly safer than other spinal surgeries performed to treat LSS.
- For the 75% of spacer patients who have remained free of reoperation with an intact implant, almost 85% of patients achieved success on at least two of three ZCQ domains. Leg pain symptom amelioration remains most notable with an average improvement of 75% at 5 years over preoperative values. This suggests that the spacer continues to offer sufficient indirect decompression of neural structures in the lateral recesses and foramina to suppress claudicant and radicular symptoms[31].
- The annual incidence of surgery for adjacent-segment disease following posterior decompression and fusion (or open posterior lateral interbody fusion or circumferential fusion) has been reported to be 2.5% per year. This means that one in four individuals will require a repeat operation within 10 years of the initial arthrodesis (incidence and prevalence of surgery at segments adjacent to a previous posterior lumbar arthrodesis).[32]
- Percutaneous IPD devices, like Superion, preserve posterior stabilizing elements of the spine, which prevents excessive physiological motion at the implanted level, theoretically lowering the risk of future segmental instability.[33]

Common Pathology

- Individuals with LSS who develop NIC often have various degrees of narrowing that occurs in the central spinal canal, lateral recesses, subarticular zones, and neuroforamen. Narrowing in these various regions develops because of gradual degenerative changes, resulting in degenerative bulging discs, hypertrophy of the ligamentum flavum, and facet joint hypertrophy. Claudication pain, as well as radicular pain, may benefit from treatment with the Vertiflex procedure. LSS occurs naturally with age but can also be due to injury. NIC symptoms can occur with or without low back pain. Classic NIC symptoms are buttock, thigh and/or leg weakness, aching, cramping, and numbness in the legs, which may or may not be painful.
- With interspinous spacer devices, the main selection criterion is that a patient's symptoms must be relieved by forward flexion of the lumbar spine.
- This phenomenon is often referred to as the "shopping cart sign" due to the improvement in walking endurance in stenotic patients when assuming a forward flexed position of lumbar spine.
- Flexion of the stenotic lumbar spine stretches the redundant ligamentum flavum and enlarges the neural foramina, thus relieving lower extremity symptoms.
- Interspinous spacer devices mechanisms of action all generally work by preserving forward flexion of the lumbar spine while increasing the central, subarticular, lateral recess and neuroforaminal spaces by restricting dynamic narrowing of the mentioned spaces/zones of lumbar spine during extension (Gazzeri et al., 2014).

With the Vertiflex procedure, a small device is placed between spinous processes: thin, bony projections on the back of the spine. Unlike other procedures, such as MILD, no bone or ligaments are removed. This leads to a more rapid recovery and less trauma to muscles and other structures.

Pertinent anatomy: The superspinous and interspinous ligaments run vertically throughout the entire spine. Ventrally, they connect to the ligamentum flavum. Superiorly and inferiorly, they connect the adjacent spinous processes and are an integral contributor to spinal stability.

Equipment

- 22-gauge spinal needle
- Scalpel
- Manufacturer's kit of supplies

Technique

Patient Position

- Patient positioned in prone position on fluoroscopic table
- Pillows or commercially available gel padded positioners are used to accentuate lumbar flexion.

Procedure Description

- Fluoroscopic guidance used to identify target lumbar levels for treatment
- A 22-gauge spinal needle is inserted under AP and lateral imaging to obtain optimum trajectory and to anesthetize path of trochars in interspinous space down to level of posterior laminar line.
- A scalpel is then used to make a stab incision through skin/subcutaneous tissue and guided under AP and lateral imaging to make incision through the supraspinous ligament.
- Per manufacturer kit supplied, a trochar needle is placed to access the interspinous space along incision path and advanced with gentle malleting under lateral imaging until tip is visualized at the posterior laminar line.
- A dilator is used to open the interspinous space adequately to place a working cannula.
- Through the working cannula, a presized reamer is used to prep the interspinous space just posterior to the laminar line.
- A lever device is used to secure implant and place through the working cannula for positioning prior to deploying.
- A Superion implant is then carefully deployed by slowly opening while simultaneously using sagittal rocking motions to ensure the device's wings capture on the superior and inferior spinous processes.
- AP and lateral fluoroscopic views are obtained to confirm Superion implant deployed in appropriate AP and lateral orientations on the spinous processes prior to malleting the implant until it comes to rest along the posterior aspect of lamina (Fig. 35.7A and B).
- All deployment devices and working cannula are removed.
- Deep/subcutaneous tissues are closed with two to three subcutaneous interrupted sutures (2.0 Vicryl).
- Skin closure may be with either running subcuticular suture closure (4.0 Monocryl) or skin staples.

PEARLS AND PITFALLS

- MRI imaging that shows mild-moderate central stenosis with NIC is the "hallmark" indication for procedure, but patients with severe central stenosis, lateral recess stenosis, subarticular stenosis, and neuroforaminal stenosis also may benefit.
- It should be standard practice to order flexion and extension x-rays of lumbar spine (standing x-ray preferable) to evaluate for dynamic listhesis at level of device implantation.
- Implantation of Superion device is contraindicated if there is greater than grade I anterolisthesis or dynamic listhesis greater than 5 mm at level of stenosis
- Significant scoliosis or lateral listhesis (in which spinous processes are not sagittally aligned) are both contraindications to implantation.
- Positioning for procedure should emphasize exaggerated flexion of lumbar spine (either with pillows or commercial positioning devices) in order to facilitate placement of instruments for device insertion

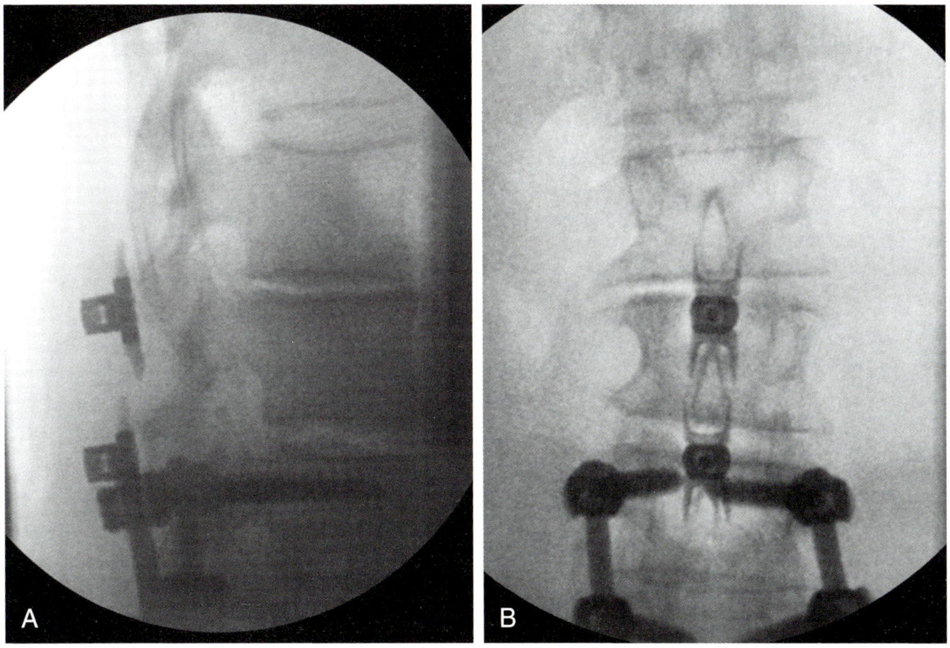

• **Fig. 35.7** (A and B) Fluoroscopy anteroposterior and lateral images of Superion device implantation.

Non-Spinal Therapies: Peripheral Nerve Stimulation

Products available:

SPR Therapeutics: Sprint peripheral nerve stimulator (PNS) system
Stimwave
Bioness: Stimrouter

KEY POINTS

Invented in the mid-1960's, peripheral nerve stimulation (PNS) interferes with chronic pain signaling from nerves located outside of the spine, thereby treating chronic pain conditions, such as peripheral nerve dysfunction, CRPS, and cranial neuralgia. Similar to normal SCS, PNS is based on gate control theory, an idea put forth by Patrick Wall and Ronald Melzack in 1965 stating that "control of pain may be achieved by selectively activating the large, rapidly conducting fibers."[1] Stimulating "gates" closes them, competitively regulating nociceptive inputs. Other theories propose that PNS prevents activation of c-fiber nociceptors, inhibits the depolarization and conduction propagation of axons, decreases hyperexcitability of dorsal horn neurons, or depletes excitatory amino acids while increasing the concentration of inhibitory transmitters.[34] When chronic pain conditions are unresponsive to conservative therapies such as medications, therapy, and nerve blocks, PNS may be considered.

To evaluate the efficacy of PNS, Mobbs et al.[35] reviewed patients with blunt or sharp nerve trauma, iatrogenic injuries from surgery, inadvertent injection of a nerve, and post-surgery for entrapment or tumor who were treated with PNS. Out of the 38 cases reviewed, 60% endorsed significant reduction of pain and improvements in their quality of life.[35] Similarly, Konstantin et al.[36] evaluated 10 patients with intractable occipital neuralgia who underwent PNS. Seventy percent of these participants expressed satisfying control of their pain and a decrease in their oral pain medication intake for an average of 22 months following the procedure. Paul et al.[37] considered 100 patients who received PNS in private practice to treat chronic craniofacial, thorax, lumbosacral, abdominal, pelvic, and groin pain conditions. On average, these individuals received a pain reduction of 4.2 ± 2.5 points on an 11-point scale. In addition, 72% of patients noted that they were using fewer analgesic medications.[37] These studies, and many more like them, indicate that PNS is a successful treatment for chronic pain conditions caused by injury to individual nerves.

Common Pathology

Similar to SCS, patients can receive PNS, devices that interfere with chronic pain signaling from nerves located outside of the spine. PNS is used to treat chronic pain due to damaged peripheral nerves, migraines, and overactive bladder. This method does not eliminate the source of pain but, instead, blocks the sensation so that the patient feels less of it. The device is programmed to provide each patient with settings that are best suited to their condition. Before a permanent stimulator device is placed in the body, patients can trial an external version. The amount of relief provided varies from person to person and, if the trial stimulator is unsuccessful, it can easily be removed and the patient can pursue other forms of treatment.

Pertinent Anatomy

- Peripheral nerve that fits pain pattern is clarified by dermatomal or cutaneous nerve distribution.
- Nerve is localized with ultrasound to clarify its location and surrounding structures.

Common Pathology

- Crush injury or surgery
- Endocrine dysregulation

- Toxins (alcohol, lead, mercury, insecticides)
- Medications (chemotherapy, antibiotics); dietary imbalances—vitamins E, B-12.[38-41]

Equipment

- Ultrasound

Implanted Flexible Percutaneous Lead References

- External battery source
- Controller

Patient position

- Pending nerve to targeted

Clinician Position

- Side of patient

Ultrasound Position

- Transducer orientation can be either long or short axis (depending on anatomy and preference)

Needle Position

- Perineural with utilization of final lead position based on imaging and amount of stimulation necessary to replicate pain pattern.

Target

- Painful peripheral nerve

PEARLS AND PITFALLS

- Ultrasound evaluation is key.
- Identification of nerve prior to lead implantation is instrumental to outcome.

Percutaneous Disc Decompression

Products available

Stryker: Dekompressor
HydroCision: Minimally invasive discectomy
PercResector
EndoResector
MicroResector

KEY POINTS

Intervertebral disc-related pain can be attributed to disc degeneration or herniation, which is often accompanied by inflammation. This condition often leads to stress on nearby nerves, resulting in referred extremity pain. With nearly 80% of individuals with lipopolysaccharide-binding protein (LBP) endorsing chronic pain, it is important to identify successful treatments in order to minimize health care expenditures. Discectomy is removal of herniated disc and there are multiple approaches to disc surgery including:

- Open discectomy: Traditional surgery involves incision with direct surgical visualization. The first open laminectomy and discectomy were performed in 1934.
- Microdiscectomy: Microdiscectomy was first pioneered in the 1970s. It involves a paramedian skin incision, followed by sequential dilators and, finally, a METRx tubular retractor with operative microscope is used to perform a smaller laminotomy and discectomy.
- Transforaminal endoscopic discectomy: Procedure that is typically muscle-sparing using the natural split between muscles of the back as opposed to cutting through them, avoiding the resulting increased recovery and altered biomechanics.[42] Most optimal indication is a lumbar disc herniation with a far lateral-to-lateral herniation. Some advantages of the technique include: shorter rehab time frame, reduced blood loss, reduced scar tissue formation, and the ability to use local anesthetic only when compared to open and microdiscectomy procedures.[43]

The road to developing percutaneous disc decompression treatments began in the 1950s, when percutaneous access to the disc was first used to perform needle biopsies of the disc. In the 1960s, this concept was expanded to treat radicular pain due to herniated discs. At that time, physicians provided treatment by injecting chymopapain percutaneously. However, this frequently led to the accidental injection of chymopapain into the subarachnoid, causing serious complications and doubt regarding the efficacy of percutaneous treatments. In the 1970s, scientists in Japan, as well as in the United States, began using endoscopic techniques to percutaneously access discs, providing a safer, more precise alternative for disc injuries.[44]

Percutaneous disc decompression has been performed for many years now, with a variety of techniques for the removal of affected disc tissue: chemonucleolysis, automated percutaneous lumbar discectomy, percutaneous laser disc decompression, and nucleoplasty.[45] A study performed by Charles et al.[45] considered the efficacy of nucleoplasty for patients with spinal stenosis. During this procedure, small amounts of nucleus pulposus are removed, allowing for inward disc retraction, thereby reducing compression of nearby nerves. Patients were evaluated at 1 week, 2 weeks, 4 weeks, 6 weeks, 6 months, and 1 year after their surgery. All subjects reported reduced pain and improved functionality at each of these intervals. In addition, they endorsed decreased usage of analgesic medications for 4 to 10 months following their nucleoplasty. From this study, the authors concluded that percutaneous disc decompression is less costly than open procedures while providing substantial relief of pain. In addition, nucleoplasty results in lower mortality rates, a shorter recovery period, and less incidental injury to the nerve root than other, open procedures to treat stenosis and disc disease. Charles et al.[45] and Alexandre et al.[46] confirmed these results, identifying 1,390 patients that endorsed alleviation of symptoms following nucleoplasty.

Many other studies have indicated similar success with other types of percutaneous disc decompression. For example, Ahn et al.[47] endorsed improvement of symptoms in 88% of his 111 laser decompression patients. Grönemeyer et al.[48] was able to eliminate or reduce back pain in 73% of patients using laser decompression. Choy et al.[49] had similar results, reporting a 78% success rate at 2-year follow-ups with 333 laser decompression patients.[44] These findings indicate that percutaneous disc decompression is a successful treatment for individuals with discogenic pain, regardless of the specific technique used.

Common Pathology

In between spinal vertebrae, there are discs, which are gel-like cushions that allow for spinal mobility, act as shock absorbers, and hold the spine together. With age or injury, these discs can begin to bulge outward, increasing inflammation and stress on nearby nerves. When this occurs with discs in the lower region of the spine, the sciatic nerve can be injured, causing sciatica. In these instances, patients usually experience pain in the legs or feet that may be alleviated by a percutaneous disc decompression. During this minimally invasive procedure, small amounts of the disc tissue are removed, relieving pressure on the nearby sciatic nerve. This treatment is most successful in patients with discs that are mildly compressed and have not ruptured. Most people that undergo percutaneous disc decompression note that their pain is relieved almost immediately following surgery.

Pertinent Anatomy

- Exiting nerve root, traversing nerve root, disc annulus, superior articulating process, vertebral endplates, sinuvertebral nerves, spinal arteries, and intervertebral veins
- Kambin's triangle:
  1. The hypotenuse is the exiting nerve root.
  2. The base is the superior border of the caudal vertebra.
  3. The height represents the superior articular process/traversing nerve root.

Common Pathology

- Herniated disc bulges with radicular symptoms

Equipment

- C-arm fluoroscopy
- Guidewire
- Curved dilator
- TESSYS endoscopic system
- Sequential size reamers
- Tissue grasper
- Bone rongeur

Patient Position

- Prone or lateral position

Clinician Position

- Side of patient

Fluoroscopy position

- AP, oblique, lateral view

Needle Position

- Needle/guided wire entry is started 11 to 16 cm lateral to midline to avoid damage to muscle planes. Needle is advanced like discogram approach.
- Sequential dilators are advanced until largest diameter is seated.
- Endoscope and tools are then advanced with correlated use of fluoroscopy and endoscope during treatment process.

Target

- Herniated disc

PEARLS AND PITFALLS

- Transforaminal endoscopic spine discectomy is an elegant procedure that can be used to treat disc herniations, which are not responsive to conservative care or basic interventional techniques.
- The most important key point is using both endoscopic and fluoroscopic views to get a robust three-dimensional picture and being cognizant of the anatomical safety boundaries.
- Fluoroscopic evaluation from AP, oblique and lateral views (in conjunction), with a solid understanding of spine anatomy on endoscope
- Having a clear understanding of Kambin's triangle
- Potential challenges, which may suggest another surgical technique/approach, include recurrent herniated disc, central or lateral recess spinal stenosis, migrated/extruded disc bulge or L5 disc bulge with high iliac crests, and spondylolisthesis.

Emerging Procedures

Cervical Anterior Longitudinal Ligament Injection

KEY POINTS

- Anterior longitudinal (ALL) ligament injuries are likely often missed in evaluating cervical pain and instability.
- ALL injuries usually occur concomitantly with other cervical injuries. Patients may have a component of extension-based exacerbation of symptoms or feeling of instability.
- ALL injury causes minor cervical destabilization, so surgery is not commonly indicated for these injuries.
- Since this problem is underdiagnosed and surgery is not often indicated, if conservative measures fail, there are not many options for care in those with chronic problems.
- Videofluoroscopy or digital motion x-ray can provide a high degree of diagnostic accuracy for identifying vertebral instability in patients with chronic pain stemming from whiplash injuries.
- Anterior widening of the vertebral body space or retrolisthesis in extension is suggestive of ALL laxity.[50]

Pertinent Anatomy

- The ALL is a thick ligamentous band traveling along the anterior vertebral bodies and discs from the atlas to the sacral.
- It resists spinal hyper extension.

Common Pathology

- The ALL can be injured with whiplash injuries with the C5-6 band being the most susceptible.[51]
- Hyperextension injury

Technique

Author has developed a technique to reliably inject the C2-C7 ALL ligament using a combination of linear ultrasound and fluoroscopic guidance. This requires great ultrasound and anatomy skills, excellent ultrasound needle visualization skills, and spatial orientation skills and should not be attempted by those just begging to perform an image-guided procedure. This is a high-risk injection procedure and this technique has not been validated or published so will not be described in detail and should not be undertaken without hands-on training. Author uses platelet-rich plasma (PRP) or bone marrow concentrate, which in other areas can improve ligament healing.

Author uses ultrasound to guide a needle under the great vessels toward the anterior vertebral body. Similar technique to a stellate ganglion block and similar technique can be used for intradiscal. Once the needle is close to the anterior vertebral body, fluoroscopy is used to obtain AP and lateral views to further place the needle accurately into the ligament. Contrast confirms ligamentous flow. The ultrasound and needle must be rotated and positioned differently to target multiple levels and is particularly tricky to inject the C2-4 ligament. Risks include great vessel and vertebral artery penetration, thyroid injury, and injury to the trachea or esophagus. The later risks are reduced by taking a right-side approach (Figs. 35.8 to 35.12).

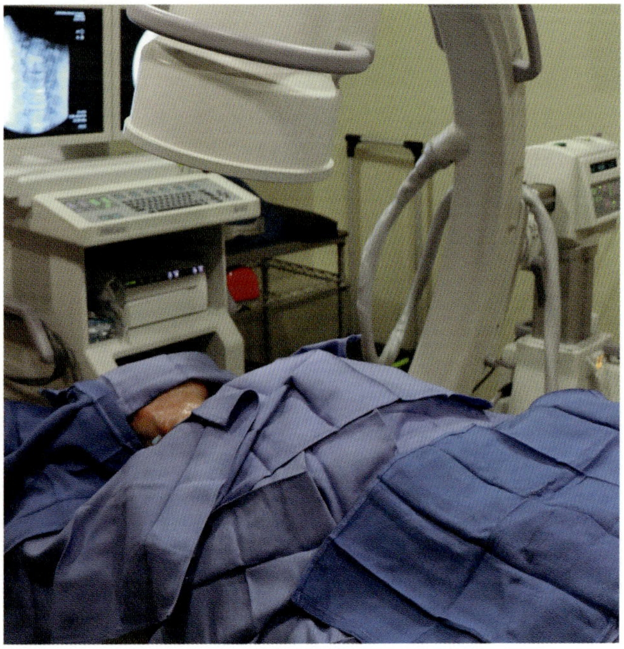

• **Fig. 35.8** EP ALL ligament injection set up.

Cervical Intradiscal Injection

KEY POINTS

This technique has been fine-tuned by the author, Marko Bodor, MD, and requires advanced interventional skills and an in-depth understanding of cervical anatomy prior to attempting.

Cervical spine discs can cause neck pain as a result of trauma or disc degeneration. Pain may radiate from the neck to the trapezius, shoulders, arms, and chest (Fig. 35.13 from Slipman CW, Plastaras C, Patel R, et al. Provocative cervical discography symptom mapping. *Spine J.* 2005;5(4):381–388). The combination of ultrasonography

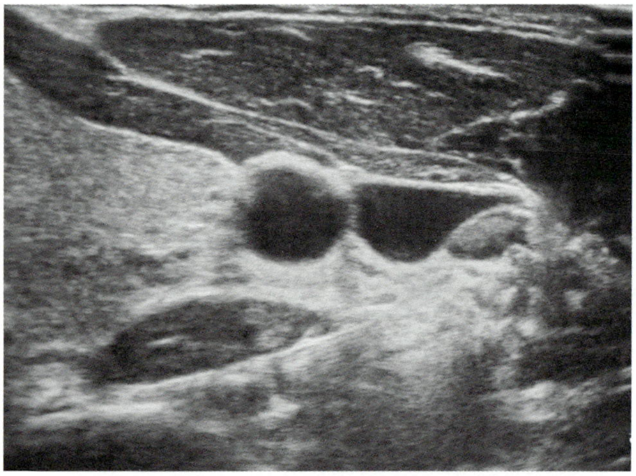

• **Fig. 35.9** EP ALL ligament ultrasound needle trajectory.

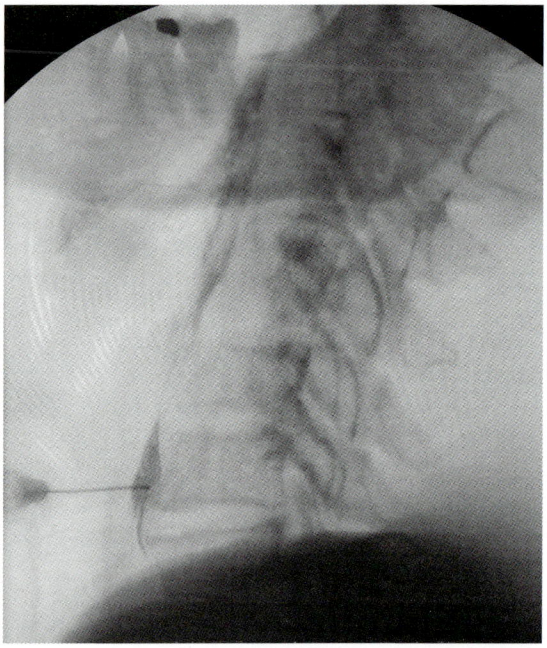

• **Fig. 35.10** EP C6 ALL ligament injection lateral fluoroscopic view confirmation with contrast.

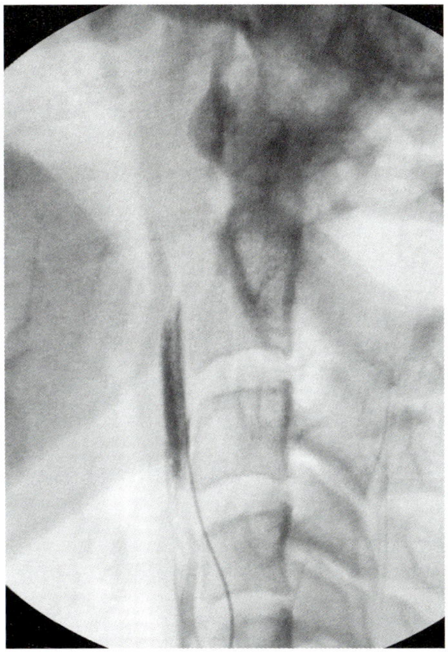

• **Fig. 35.11** EP C2-3 ALL ligament injection lateral fluoroscopic view confirmation with contrast.

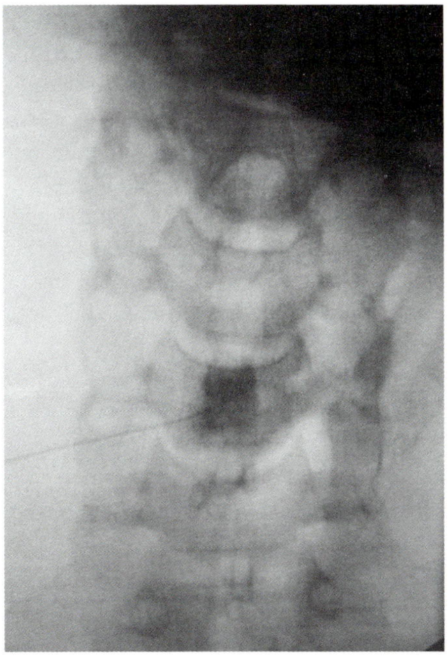

• **Fig. 35.12** EP C6 ALL ligament injection AP fluoroscopic view confirmation with contrast.

and fluoroscopy facilitates a safe and minimally invasive cervical disc injection technique while avoiding the carotid and vertebral arteries, trachea, larynx, and esophagus. The cervical discs are approximately half as high, wide, and long as the lumbar discs, thus 1/2 x 1/2 x 1/2 or ⅛ of the volume. Cervical disc procedures must be performed with the greatest degree of care, precision, and procedural experience.

Pertinent Anatomy

Cervical spine discs have a crescent-shaped anterior annulus fibrosus and a thin posterior layer of collagen (Fig. 35.14). The nucleus pulposus dehydrates and becomes fibrocartilaginous in the second and third decades.[52] The upper discs, C2-3, C3-4, and C4-5, are smaller in size than the lower discs, C5-6, C6-7 and C7-T1. The anterior longitudinal ligament, longus colli muscle, oropharynx, esophagus, and larynx lie anterior to the discs, while the posterior longitudinal ligament (PLL), meninges, and spinal cord lie posterior. Laterally, the vertebral artery is exposed between and variably below C6 in front of the transverse processes, while the carotid sheath, including the carotid artery, jugular vein, and vagus nerve, is located anterolaterally and more superficially (Figs. 35.15, 12.x). The spinal nerves and brachial plexus lie between the anterior and middle scalene muscles posterior to the carotid sheath. The lung apices and great vessels are close to the C7-T1 disc.

Common Pathology

Tears of the annulus fibrosus and defects of the fibrocartilaginous disc matrix can occur secondary to trauma or disc degeneration. Normal mature cervical discs have transverse clefts located at their posterior aspects between the uncinate processes to facilitate neck rotation. (See Fig. 35.14 from functional anatomy of the spine, Bogduk N. *Handbook of Clinical Neurology*. Vol. 136 [3rd series], Neuroimaging, Part II (Elsevier 2016).)

Equipment

High performance ultrasound machine with linear (5 to 12 MHz) and curvilinear (1 to 5 MHz) transducers, sterile covers for the transducers and controls, C-arm fluoroscope, carbon fiber imaging table, needle holder, surgical pen, #30 1" needle, #25 2" spinal needle with stylet with a smooth 10- to 15-degree curve at the distal 4 to 5 mm, 1 mL syringe.

Common Injections

Orthobiologics (PRP, bone marrow concentrate, etc.)

Injectate Volume

Averages 0.2 to 0.3 mL but can range from 0.1 to 0.5 mL

Technique

Patient Position

Supine, with the neck extended and comfortably positioned. The patient should avoid swallowing once the spinal needle is being advanced to the disc because activation of the sternohyoid muscle will cause the needle to move.

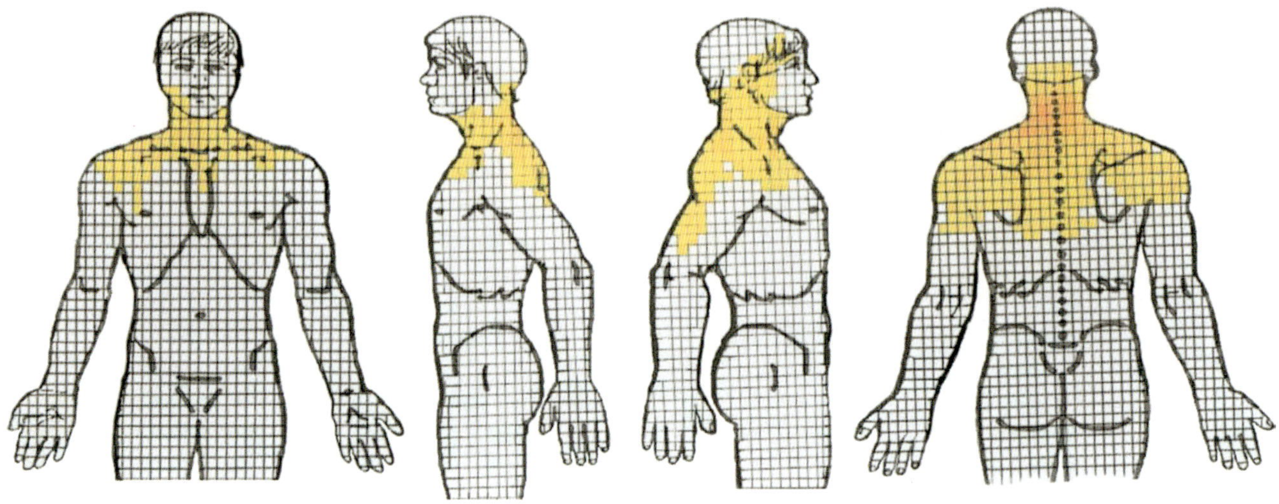

• **Fig 35.13** Composite map of C5-6 disc pain patterns obtained from 27 patients. (From Slipman CW, Plastaras C, Patel R, et al. Provocative cervical discography symptom mapping. *Spine J*. 2005;5[4]:381–388, with permission.)

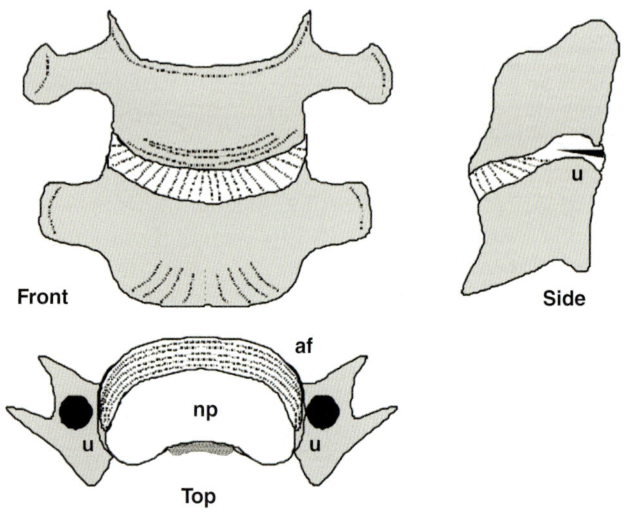

• **Fig 35.14** Cervical disc diagram showing a crescent-shaped annulus fibrosus *(af)*, fibrocartilaginous nucleus pulposus *(np)*, uncinate processes *(u)*, vertebral arteries *(solid black circles,)* and a normal posterior transverse cleft *(thin black triangle)*. (From Bogduk N. Functional anatomy of the spine. *Handbook of Clinical Neurology*, Vol. 136 (3rd series), Neuroimaging, Part II (Elsevier 2016), with permission.)

Clinician Position

Standing next to the patient's right side, C-arm monitors rostral to the patient's head and facing the physician, ultrasound machine, and monitor to the physician's left.

Transducer and C-Arm Position

Initially, an ultrasound examination of the neck is performed, assessing the carotid artery and jugular vein, thyroid gland and cartilage, vertebral artery, and esophagus or oropharynx if visibly present. Sono-assisted palpation can be performed between the carotid sheath and trachea using the examiner's little finger to assess for tenderness over each disc (Figs. 35.16 and 35.17).

The fluoroscopy C-arm is set up so it can rotate around the axis of the neck and easily obtain AP, oblique, and lateral fluoroscopic views. Starting in the AP view, the C-arm is angled caudally to obtain end-plate views of the disc being targeted, then it is rotated 20 to 30 degrees to the patient's right (Fig 35.18). The discs are typically injected from the patient's right side because the esophagus is on the left.

Using the needle holder as a pointer, potential radiographic trajectories to the disc at 10, 20 and 30 degrees C-arm rotation are identified and marked with a surgical pen. The pen marks define a line over which the ultrasound transducer is placed. Ultrasound is then used to determine an optimal trajectory toward the disc passing between the carotid sheath and thyroid cartilage or trachea. The trajectory typically passes through the thyroid gland, avoiding larger blood vessels and nodules if present. Throughout this process, it is important that the ultrasound transducer and C-arm remain at the same cranial-caudal angulation (Fig. 35.19).

Once an optimal trajectory has been determined using ultrasound (Fig. 35.20), the C-arm is rotated to match the degree of rotation of the transducer, then the transducer is removed and fluoroscopy is used to confirm that the trajectory leads to the point of entry at the lateral aspect of the disc. A typical degree of C-arm rotation is 20 to 30 degrees for the C5-6 and C6-7 discs. Greater rotation may be necessary at upper levels to bypass the thyroid cartilage.

Needle Position

Once an optimal trajectory has been determined, the skin is anesthetized using 1.0 mL of local anesthetic, then a #25 2″ spinal needle is advanced toward the disc using intermittent fluoroscopy and bevel steering (Fig. 35.21). If increased needle resistance or patient discomfort is encountered, ultrasound is used to check the position of the needle and ensure that it is not going into the larynx or trachea (Fig. 35.22). Prior to entry and in order to ensure patient safety, the

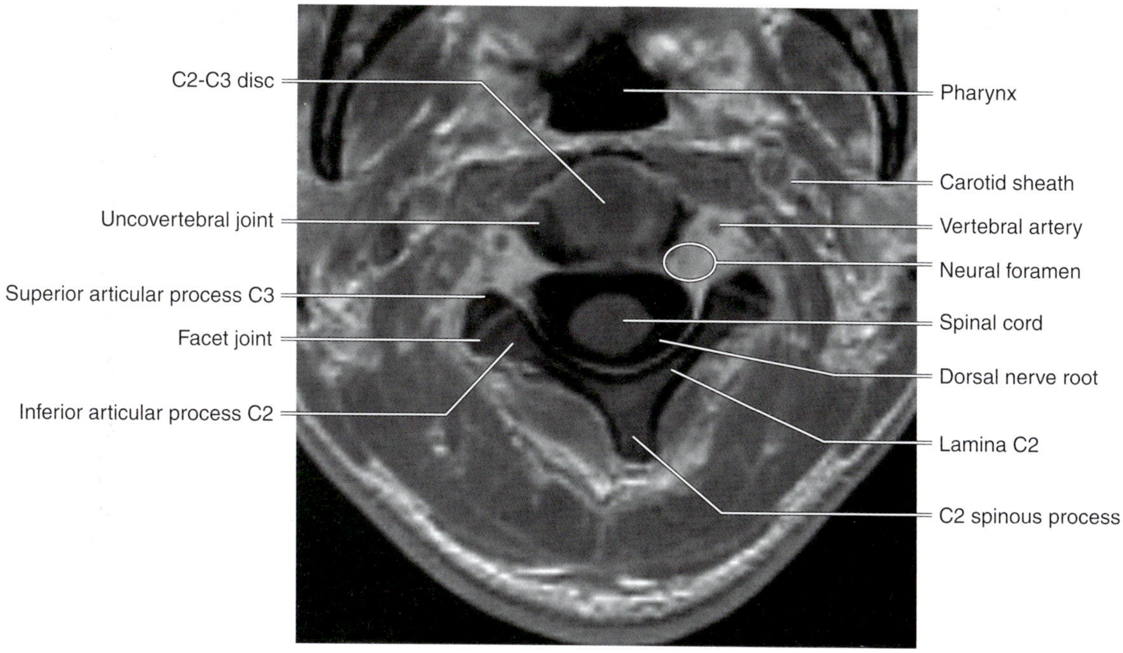

• **Fig 35.15** Axial T1-weighted gradient echo MR image of the cervical spine at C2-3. (From Osborn AG, Satzman KL, Anderson J, et al. *Imaging Anatomy: Brain and Spine.* Elsevier, Philadelphia; 2020.)

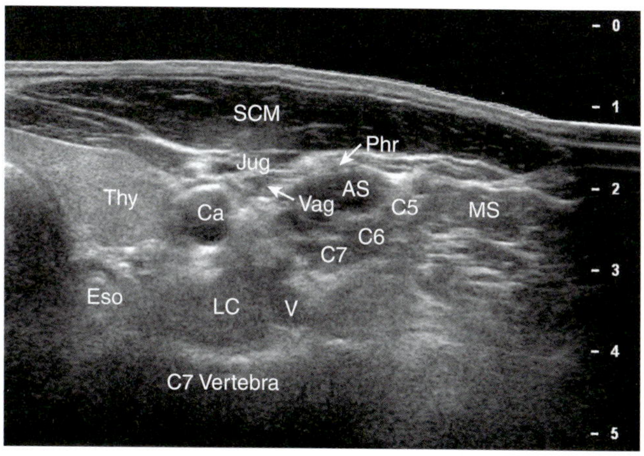

• **Fig 35.16** Axial ultrasound view of the left side of the neck at the level of the C7 vertebra (panoramic 5–12 MHz). Sternocleidomastoid muscle *(SCM)*, vagus nerve *(Vag)*, collapsed jugular vein *(Jug)*, phrenic nerve *(Phr)*, thyroid *(Thy)*, carotid artery *(Ca)*, anterior scalene *(AS)*, spinal nerves (C5, C6, C7), middle scalene *(MS)*, esophagus *(Eso)*, longus colli *(LC)*, vertebral artery *(V)*. The left side was chosen to show the esophagus, which is made more visible by having the patient swallow.

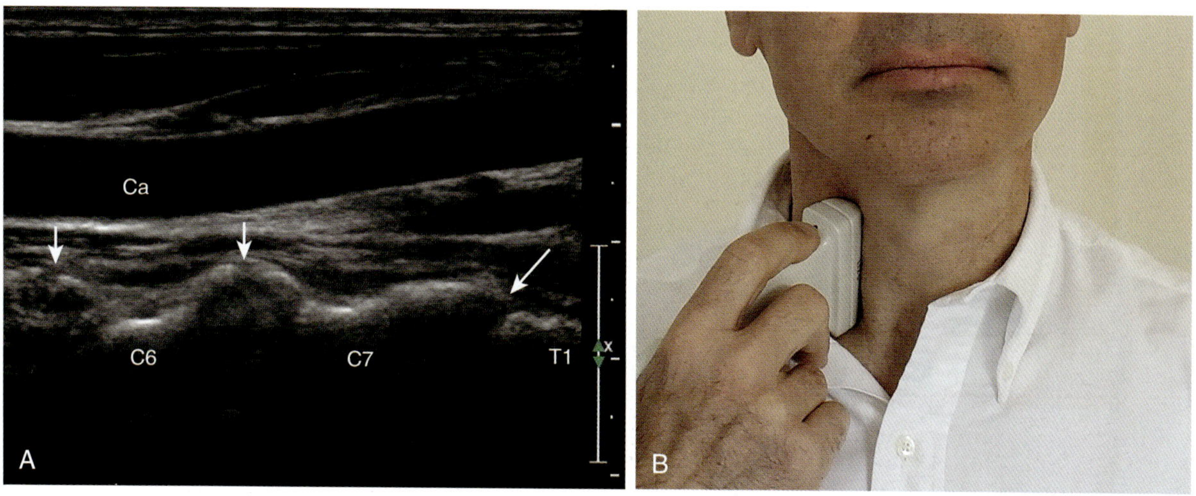

• **Fig 35.17** (A) Longitudinal ultrasound view of the cervical spine through the carotid sheath in a 60-year-old male: carotid artery *(Ca)*, anterior aspects of vertebrae (C6, C7, T1), discs *(arrows)*; (B) Transducer location on neck.

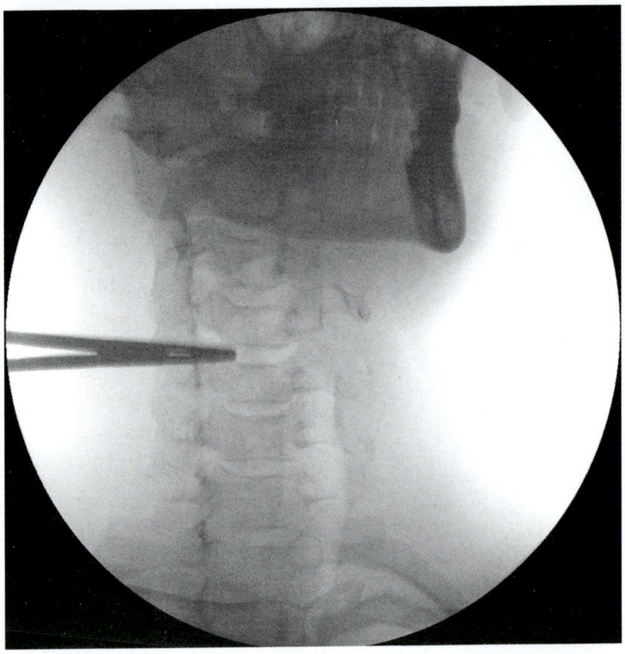

• **Fig 35.18** Fluoroscopic view of the cervical spine with 20 degrees angulation and 30 degrees rotation. The needle holder marks a potential trajectory to the C4-5 disc, which will need to be confirmed with ultrasonography.

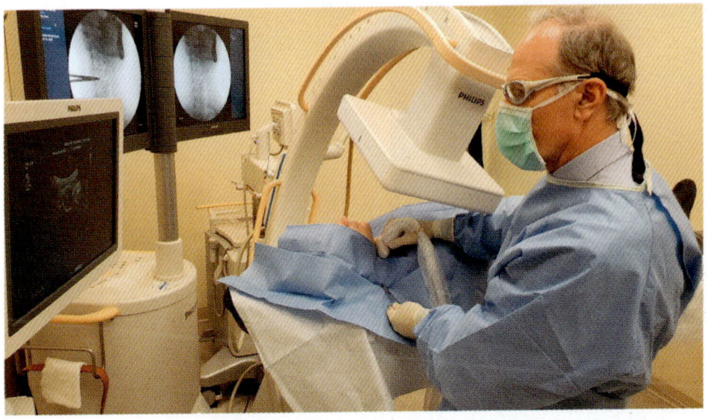

• **Fig 35.19** Operative setting for cervical disc injection. The physician has a good view of the monitors and is using ultrasound to determine the best possible trajectory to the C4-5 disc. The ultrasound transducer and C-arm are aligned.

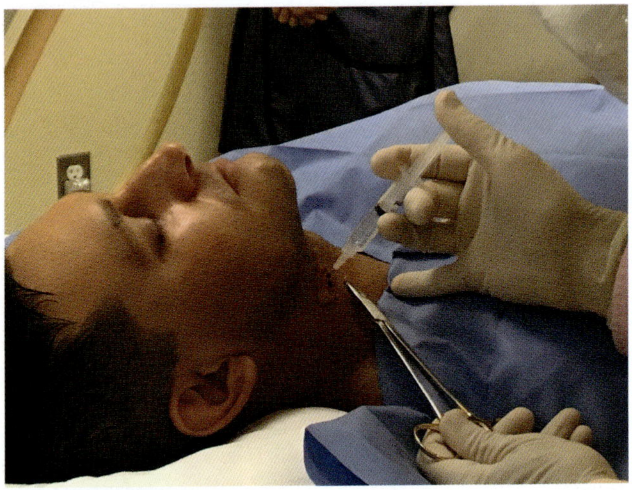

• **Fig 35.20** An optimal trajectory to the disc has been determined using fluoroscopy and ultrasonography. The skin is being anesthetized prior to insertion of the spinal needle. The pen marks denote possible fluoroscopic trajectories to the C4-5 disc. The middle trajectory was chosen on the basis of ultrasonography.

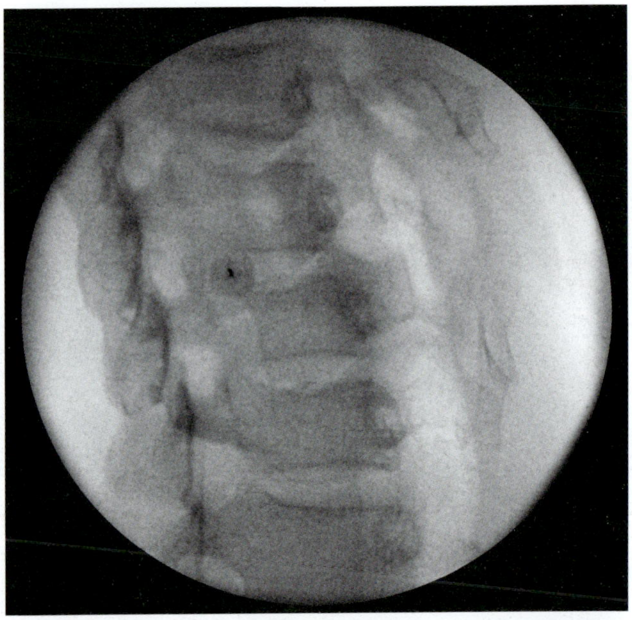

• **Fig 35.21** The needle has been inserted and is aimed at the C4-5 disc.

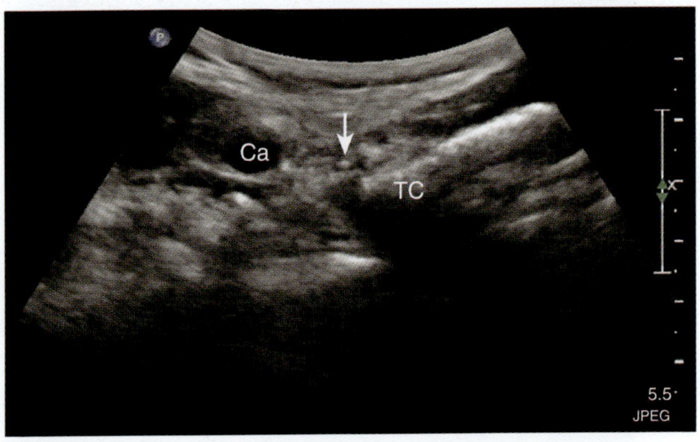

• **Fig 35.22** Ultrasound view of the needle *(arrow)* seen in the short-axis passing by the carotid artery *(Ca)* and thyroid cartilage is on its way to the C4-5 disc.

needle can be directed to touch an adjacent vertebra before advancement into the disc. Once the tip of the needle enters the disc, intermittent AP and lateral views are used to guide placement, which often requires taking full advantage of the needle's curve (Fig. 35.23). Final advancement is done in the lateral view to ensure that the needle does not penetrate beyond the disc (Figs. 35.24 to 35.26).

Target

The target for entry into the disc is the lateral aspect of the disc at or slightly lateral to the inflection point of the curve of the uncinate process. Final placement is at the center of the disc as confirmed on AP and lateral fluoroscopic views.

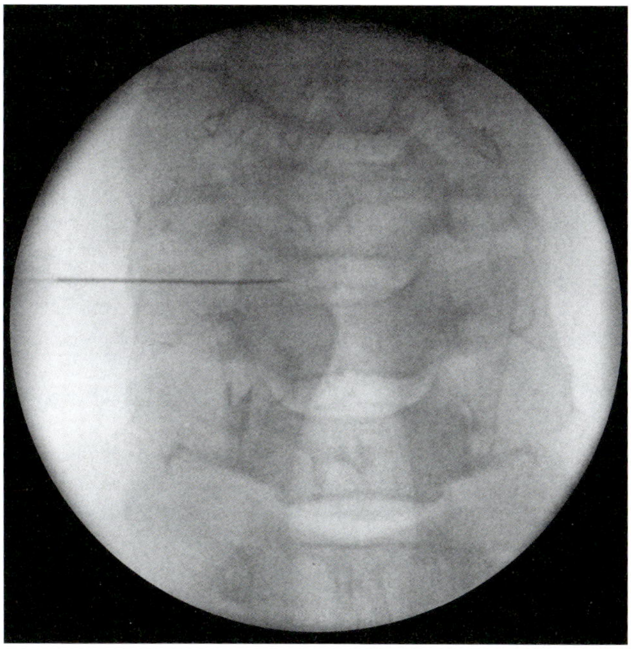

• **Fig 35.23** Anteroposterior *(AP)* fluoroscopic view of the needle as it enters the C4-5 disc.

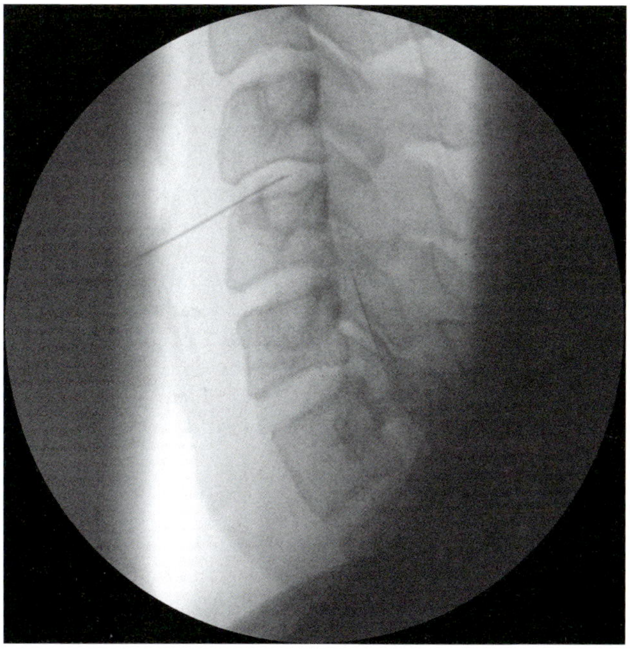

• **Fig 35.24** Lateral fluoroscopic view of the needle in final position in the C4-5 disc. The needle has been advanced a few millimeters deeper than usual in order to reach a posterior disc tear.

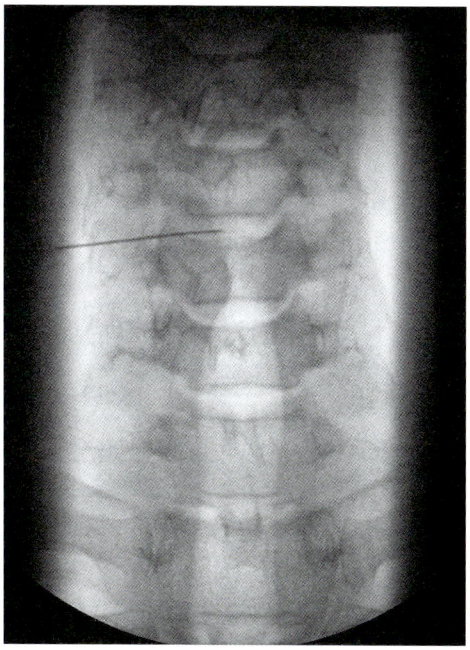

• **Fig 35.25** Anteroposterior fluoroscopy view of the needle in final position in the C4-5 disc.

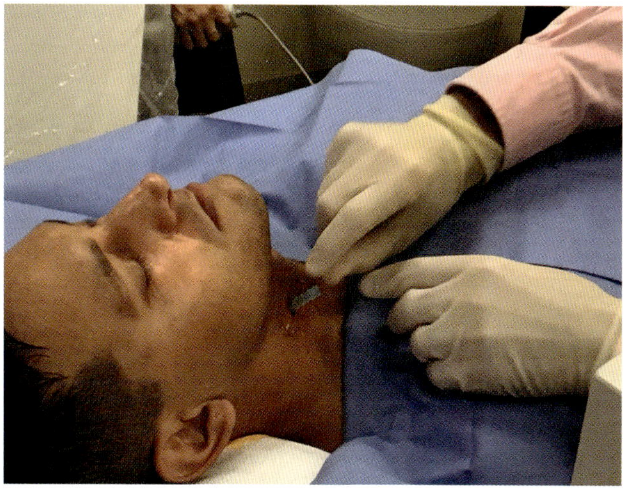

• **Fig 35.26** Photograph of the needle in final position in the C4-5 disc.

PEARLS AND PITFALLS

Cervical disc access requires precise ultrasound and fluoroscopy skills and a good rapport between the patient and the physician to facilitate relaxation and minimize movement. MR images need to be reviewed prior to each procedure to assess for relative contraindications such as spinal stenosis or anatomical variants along the intended needle trajectory. If there is concern that the needle might pass through the esophagus or oropharynx, the patient can swallow a small amount of barium sulfate suspension beforehand to outline these structures on fluoroscopy. There is normally slightly more resistance to injection of a cervical disc than a lumbar disc, but too much resistance may require slight repositioning of the needle to improve compliance. Use of a 1 ml syringe facilitates precise delivery of injectate. An increase in disc height is often seen immediately following injection. In some cases, such as status post thyroidectomy or at C2-3,[a] there may not be enough space to pass a needle between the carotid sheath and thyroid cartilage, and a trajectory through the anterior scalene may be considered, being careful to avoid the phrenic nerve or any variant intramuscular spinal nerves.

[a]We have successfully used the described technique for injections of the C3-4 through C7-T1 discs, but have not yet had the opportunity to do C2-3.

References

1. Sdrulla AD, Guan Y, Raja SN. Spinal cord stimulation: clinical efficacy and potential mechanisms. *Pain Pract.* 2018;18(8):1048–1067.
2. Shealy CN, Taslitz N, Mortimer JT, Becker DP. *Anesth Analg.* 1967;46(3):299–305. Electrical inhibition of pain: experimental evaluation.
3. Caylor J, Reddy R, Yin S, et al. Spinal cord stimulation in chronic pain: evidence and theory for mechanisms of action. *Bioelectron Med.* 2019;5:12.
4. Koeze AC de C Williams t, Reimant S. Spinal cord stimulation and the relief of chronic pain T H. *J Neurol Neurosurg Psychiatry.* 1987;50:1424–1429.
5. Vannemreddy P, Slavin KV.*J Pain Res.* 2016;9:481-492. https://doi.org/10.2147/JPR.S108884. eCollection 2016
6. Verrills P, Sinclair C, Barnard A. A review of spinal cord stimulation systems for chronic pain. *Pain Physician.* 2007;10(2):305–311.
7. Vallejo R, Kramer J, Benyamin R. Neuromodulation of the cervical spinal cord in the treatment of chronic intractable neck and upper extremity pain: a case series and review of the literature. 8 *Arthrosc Tech.* 2019;19(10):e1125–e1129. https://doi.org/10.1016/j.eats.2019.05.032. eCollection 2019 Oct.
8. Kasapovic A, Rommelspacher Y, Gathen M, et al. High-frequency spinal cord stimulation for the treatment of chronic low back and leg pain: implantation technique of percutaneous leads and implantable pulse generator
9. North RB, David HK, Farrokh F, Steven AP. Spinal cord stimulation versus repeated lumbosacral spine surgery for chronic pain: a randomized, controlled trial. *Neurosurgery.* 2005;56(1):98–106; discussion 106-7. https://doi.org/10.1227/01.neu.0000144839.65524.e0.
10. Kumar K, Rod ST, Line J, et al. Spinal cord stimulation versus conventional medical management for neuropathic pain: a multicentre randomised controlled trial in patients with failed back surgery syndrome. *Pain.* 2007;132(1–2):179–188.
11. Kemler MA, Barendse GA, van Kleef M, et al. Spinal cord stimulation in patients with chronic reflex sympathetic dystrophy. *N Engl J Med.* 2000;343(9):618–624.
12. Kapural et al. *Anesthesiology* 2015;123:851-860
13. Vallejo et al. *Anes Anesthesiol.* 2015;123:851-860.
14. Timothy RD, Robert ML, Jeffery K, et al. Dorsal root ganglion stimulation yielded higher treatment success rate for complex regional pain syndrome and causalgia at 3 and 12 months: a randomized comparative trial. *Pain.* 2017;158(4):669–681.
15. Yu C-W, Ming-Kai H, Chen L-H, et al. Percutaneous balloon kyphoplasty for the treatment of vertebral compression fractures. *BMC Surg.* 2014;14:3.
16. Mehbod A, Aunoble S, Le Huec JC. *Eur Spine J.* 2003;12 (suppl 2): S155–S162. Epub 2003 Sep 19.
17. Zhan Y, Jiang J, Liao H, Tan H, Yang K. Risk factors for cement leakage after vertebroplasty or kyphoplasty: a meta-analysis of published evidence. *World Neurosurg.* 2017;101:633–642. https://doi.org/10.1016/j.wneu.2017.01.124.
18. Wang B, Zhao CP, Song LX, Zhu L. Balloon kyphoplasty versus percutaneous vertebroplasty for osteoporotic vertebral compression fracture: a meta-analysis and systematic review. *J Orthop Surg Res.* 2018;13(1):264. Published 2018 Oct 22. https://doi.org/10.1186/s13018-018-0952-5.
19. Lyders EM, Whitlow CT, Baker MD, Morris PP. Imaging and treatment of sacral insufficiency fractures. *Am J Neuroradiol. February.* 2010;31(2):201–210.
20. Zhang S, Wang GJ, Wang Q, Yang J, Xu S, Yang CH. A mysterious risk factor for bone cement leakage into the spinal canal through the Batson vein during percutaneous kyphoplasty: a case control study. *BMC Musculoskelet Disord.* 2019;20(1):423. https://doi.org/10.1186/s12891-019-2807-6.
21. Ryu KS, Park CK, Kim MK, et al. Single balloon kyphoplasty using far lateral extrapedicular approach: technical note and preliminary results [J]. *J Spinal Disord Tech.* 2007;20:392–398.
22. Kallmes DF, Schweickert PA, Marx WF, Mary E. Jensen (see figure 35.1). August 2002 vertebroplasty in the mid- and upper thoracic spine. *AJNR Am J Neuroradiol.* 23:1117–1120,
23. Sun G, Jin P, Li M, et al. Percutaneous vertebroplasty for treatment of osteolytic metastases of the C2 vertebral body using anterolateral and posterolateral approach. *Technol Cancer Res Treat.* 2010;9(4):417–422.
24. Sun G, Wang LJ, Jin P, Liu XW, Li M. Vertebroplasty for treatment of osteolytic metastases at C2 using an anterolateral approach. *Pain Physician.* 2013;16(4):E427–E434.
25. Health Quality Ontario. Vertebral augmentation involving vertebroplasty or kyphoplasty for cancer-related vertebral compression fractures: a systematic review. *Ont Health Technol Assess Ser.* 2016;16(11):1–202. Published 2016 May 1.
26. Peter SS, Timothy BC, Go S, et al. MLong-term safety and efficacy of minimally invasive lumbar decompression procedure for the treatment of lumbar spinal stenosis with neurogenic claudication. *Reg Anesth Pain Med.* 2018;43(7):789–794.
27. Wu L, Ricardo C. *Lumbar Spinal Stenosis.* Reasure Island (FL): StatPearls Publishing; 2019.
28. Nunley et al, *Clin Interv Aging.* 2017; 12: 1409–141. https://www.ncbi.nlm.nih.gov/pubmed/28919727

28a. Kaech DL, Fernandez C, Lombardi-Weber D. The Interspinous 'U': a new restabilization device for the lumbar spine. In: Kaech DL, Jinkins JR, eds. *Spinal restabilization procedures.* Amsterdam: Elsevier; 2002:355–362.

28b. Krappel FA. Long-term results, status of studies and differential indication regarding the DIAM implant. *Der Orthopade*. 2010 Jun;39(6):585–594. https://doi.org/10.1007/s00132-009-1592-6. PMID: 20464369.
29. Jason H, Michelle G, Robert EJ. The use of Vertiflex® interspinous spacer device in patients with lumbar spinal stenosis and concurrent medical comorbidities. *Cureus*. 2019;11(8):e5374.
30. Walter B, Larry EM, Jon EB. Minimally invasive treatment of moderate lumbar spinal stenosis with the Superion® interspinous spacer. *Open Orthop J*. 2011;5:361–367.
31. Nunley et al, *Clin Interv Aging*. 2017;12:1409 -141.
32. Sears WR, Sergides IG, Kazemi N, Smith M, White GJ, *Osburg B Spine J*. 2011;11(1):11-20
33. Goyal A, Goel VK, Mehta A, Dick D, Chinthakunta SR, Ferrara L. Cyclic loads do not compromise functionality of the interspinous spacer or cause damage to the spinal segment: an in vitro analysis. *Crit Rev Neurobiol*. 2008;18:289–302.
34. Raghavendra N, Ratan K, Banik. Current innovations in peripheral nerve stimulation. *Pain Res Treat*. 2018;2018:9091216.
35. Mobbs RJ, Nair S, Blum P. Peripheral nerve stimulation for the treatment of chronic pain. *J Clin Neurosci*. 2007;14(3):216–221; discussion 222-3.
36. Konstantin VS, Hrachya N, Wess C. Peripheral neurostimulation for treatment of intractable occipital neuralgia. *Neurosurgery*. 2006;58(1):112–119; discussion 112-9.
37. Paul V, David V, Bruce M, Adele B. Peripheral nerve field stimulation for chronic pain: 100 cases and review of the literature. *Pain Med*. 2011;12(9):1395–1405.
38. Ilfeld BM. Continuous peripheral nerve blocks: an update of the published evidence and comparison with novel, alternative analgesic modalities. *Anesth Analg*. 2017;124(1):308–335.
39. Timothy RD, Sameer J, Corey H, Krishnan C. Neurostimulation for intractable chronic pain. *Brain Sci*. 2019;9(2):23.
40. Slavin KV. Peripheral nerve stimulation for neuropathic pain. *Neurotherapeutics*. 2008;5(1):100–106.
41. Krishnan C, Andrew N, Paul JC, Kayode W. Review of recent advances in Peripheral Nerve Stimulation (PNS). *Curr Pain Headache Rep*. 2016;20(11):60.
42. Gabriele PJ, Gina MF, Albert ET. A retrospective evaluation of the clinical success of transforaminal endoscopic discectomy with foraminotomy in geriatric patients retrospective study). *Pain Physician*. 2013;16:225–229.
43. Pan M, Li Q, Li S, et al. Percutaneous endoscopic lumbar discectomy: indications and complications. *Pain Physician*. 2020;23(1):49–56.
44. Vijay S, Richard D. Percutaneous lumbar disc decompression. *Pain Physician*. 2006;9(2):139–146.
45. Charles P, Jose R, Christian S. Percutaneous disc decompression for the treatment of lumbar spinal stenosis. *Pain Physician*. 2003;6(4):509–512.
46. Alexandre A, Corò L, Azuelos A, Pellone M. Percutaneous nucleoplasty for discoradicular conflict. *Acta Neurochir Suppl*. 2005;92:83–86.
47. Ahn Y, Lee SH, Lee SC, Shin SW, Chung SE. Factors predicting excellent outcome of percutaneous cervical discectomy: analysis of 111 consecutive cases. *Neuroradiology*. 2004;46(5):378–384.
48. Grönemeyer DHW, Buschkamp H, Braun M, Schirp s, Weinsheimer PA, Gevargez A. Image-guided percutaneous laser disk decompression for herniated lumbar disks: a 4-year follow-up in 200 patients. *J Clin Laser Med Surg*. 2003;21(3):131–138.
49. Choy DS, Ascher PW, Ranu HS. Percutaneous laser disc decompression. A new therapeutic modality. *Spine (Phila Pa 1976)*. 1992; 17(8):949–956.
50. Freeman MD, Katz EA, Rosa SL, Gatterman BG, Strömmer EMF, Leith WM. Diagnostic accuracy of videofluoroscopy for symptomatic cervical spine injury following whiplash trauma. *Int J Environ Res Public Health*. 2020;17(5):1693. Published 2020 Mar 5. https://doi.org/10.3390/ijerph17051693.
51. Stemper BD, Yoganandan N, Pintar FA, Rao RD. Anterior longitudinal ligament injuries in whiplash may lead to cervical instability. *Med Eng Phys*. 2006;28(6):515–524. https://doi.org/10.1016/j.medengphy.2005.09.011.
52. Oda J, Tanaka H, Tsuzuki N. Intervertebral disc changes with aging of human cervical vertebra. From the neonate to the eighties. *Spine (Phila Pa 1976)*. 1988;13(11):1205–1211.

36

Needle Arthroscopy of the Knee, Shoulder, and Hip

DON BUFORD, BRICE W. BLATZ, AND NICOLA HYDE

Needle Arthroscopy—Background

Arthroscopy is a surgical procedure in which a video imaging device is placed into a joint to allow visualization and assessment of the joint space. With additional instrumentation, surgery can be performed without making large incisions or a large dissection to open up the joint. Masaki Watanabe, a Japanese surgeon, is generally credited with being the first to use arthroscopy for knee evaluation and surgery in the late 1950s.[1] In 1964, Robert W. Jackson met Watanabe in Japan and brought this revolutionary surgical technique back to North America.[2]

Arthroscopy provides a magnified direct view of intra-articular anatomy with minimal potential complications and is the gold standard for intra-articular joint evaluation. Arthroscopy is used to guide surgical intervention for most intra-articular orthopedic pathology. Orthopedic surgeons in the United States receive 4 years of residency training on arthroscopic surgical procedures.[3] In 2013, the average orthopedic surgery resident completed over 300 diagnostic and surgical arthroscopy procedures prior to graduation.[4] The Arthroscopy Association of North America (AANA) requires a minimum of 50 arthroscopic procedures a year for active membership.[5] To obtain the sports medicine subspecialty certification from the American Board of Orthopedic Surgery, a 1-year sports medicine surgical fellowship and a minimum of 75 arthroscopies must be completed in the year prior to application.[6] Despite significant arthroscopic surgery training at the resident and fellowship levels, even experienced arthroscopists will experience a learning curve when using needle arthroscopy in the office under local anesthesia.

Traditionally, large-joint arthroscopy has been performed with an arthroscope 4 mm in diameter and 30 or 70 degrees of visual offset. Technologic advances have led to the introduction of small-diameter disposable needle arthroscopes that can be used in the office setting under local anesthesia. Imaging can be done on a portable tablet and even combined with diagnostic ultrasound imaging on the same tablet.[7] Instrumentation has been further refined to allow for surgical procedures to be done in an operating room or procedure room with the disposable needle arthroscope as the only imaging modality.[7–9] These advances have lowered the per-procedure instrument cost of diagnostic arthroscopy to as little as $500.[7–9]

With the advent of needle arthroscopy, the number of physicians interested in using diagnostic joint arthroscopy has increased, largely because hospital surgical privileges, residency training, and surgical malpractice insurance are currently not required. Physicians who have shown interest in needle arthroscopy include physiatrists, rheumatologists, and interventional radiologists. In the office, needle arthroscopy is used both for diagnosis and as a delivery system for injecting intra-articular structures or the joint itself. As a result, there is an increased demand for postdoctoral needle arthroscopy training for nonsurgeons and for needle arthroscopy protocols that promote the safe and effective evaluation of joint pathology. In-office needle arthroscopy has been evaluated over more than 1400 cases and found to pose lower surgical risks than traditional arthroscopy.[10]

We recommend that physicians in specialties where training and scope of practice do not include arthroscopic surgical procedures get advice from their state medical licensing boards and national board certifying organizations for any requirements and consensus on the use of needle arthroscopy in their specialties. Clinicians using needle arthroscopy should make sure that they have malpractice coverage for surgical procedures, both for their own protection and their patients' protection.

In-office needle arthroscopy has a diagnostic accuracy equivalent to that of magnetic resonance imaging (MRI) or traditional arthroscopy when used to evaluate intra-articular nonligamentous pathology.[11] In-office needle arthroscopy used as a diagnostic tool also involves potential financial savings compared with MRI and traditional arthroscopy.[12]

Patient evaluation—including history, physical, and relevant imaging—is always done prior to considering needle arthroscopy. Often an in-office needle arthroscopy substitutes for an MRI scan, especially if the primary clinical concern is an intra-articular derangement. We do not feel that ordering an MRI scan prior to needle arthroscopy is routinely necessary unless there is clinical concern for intraosseous, subchondral, popliteal, or extracapsular pathology. We do obtain plain radiographs prior to needle arthroscopy to evaluate joint alignment and stability as well as bony anatomy and pathology.

Our review of needle arthroscopy indications and techniques is agnostic with regard to any particular needle arthroscopy system.

Indications for Needle Arthroscopy

Common indications for using needle arthroscopy in the knee:

1. Diagnosing meniscal tears
2. Diagnosing chondral pathology
3. Diagnosing anterior and posterior cruciate ligament pathology
4. Evaluating prior intra-articular procedures
5. Guiding intra-articular injections.
6. Identifying loose bodies
7. Diagnosing patellofemoral tracking abnormalities
8. Staging osteoarthritis of the knee joint
9. Patients unable to get an MRI scan

Common indications for using needle arthroscopy in the shoulder:

1. Diagnosing labral pathology
2. Diagnosing articular-sided rotator cuff pathology
3. Diagnosing superior labrum, biceps tendon anchor pathology (SLAP lesions)
4. Diagnosing humeral head and glenoid bone loss
5. Evaluating prior intra-articular procedures
6. Guiding intra-articular injections
7. Identifying loose bodies
8. Staging osteoarthritis of the glenohumeral joint
9. Patients unable to get an MRI scan

Common indications for using needle arthroscopy in the hip:

1. Diagnosing labral pathology
2. Diagnosing femoroacetabular impingement and CAM lesions
3. Diagnosis hip joint synovitis
4. Staging osteoarthritis of the hip joint
5. Guiding intra-articular injections
6. Evaluating prior intra-articular procedures
7. Diagnosing loose bodies
8. Patients unable to get an MRI scan

Needle Arthroscopy Technique

Preparation

Clinicians should obtain preoperative informed consent prior to initiating needle arthroscopy. We typically do not give pre- or post-procedure antibiotics because there are no significant data suggesting that the extremely low infection rates associated with needle arthroscopy would be lowered further with antibiotic medications. If a patient is on anticoagulation, the clinician should decide on its appropriate management prior to the procedure. In our practice, we do not alter the patient's anticoagulation regimen since the bore of the arthroscope is not significantly larger than the bore of a 14- to 18-gauge needle. We do not typically give patients preoperative pain medications or benzodiazepines, although that may be a consideration in some clinical situations. Prior to beginning the procedure, we follow the Joint Commission Universal Protocol for Preventing Wrong Site, Wrong Procedure, and Wrong Person Surgery.[13]

The surgical site is always isolated and draped, and sterile technique is observed. The skin is prepped with an effective surgical prep such as povidone-iodine (Betadine) or chlorhexidine. Procedural anesthesia is usually obtained with a choice of lidocaine 1% to 2% and/or bupivacaine (Marcaine) 0.25%. The addition of epinephrine may be considered, depending on physician preference. Other local anesthetics can also be considered based on physician preference. It is important to wait 3 to 5 minutes after injecting the local anesthetic into the portal sites before proceeding with the arthroscopy. Under local anesthesia, the physician has 10 to 15 minutes of procedure time to evaluate the joint.

With all needle arthroscopy systems, normal saline is used to distend the joint. The volume of saline needed for needle arthroscopy is significantly less than the volume used in standard arthroscopy. Usually no more than 30 to 50 mL of normal saline is used in the joint. The normal saline can be injected using multiple small 10- to 30-mL syringes or with a larger bag of normal saline attached to the arthroscope with intravenous tubing and a three-way stopcock. While the joint is being injected, the inflow of saline can also be used as a diagnostic tool to see whether structures such as the labrum or meniscus are stable.

The Knee

I. Setup
  a. Tablet and ultrasound (US) (Fig. 36.1).
II. Positioning

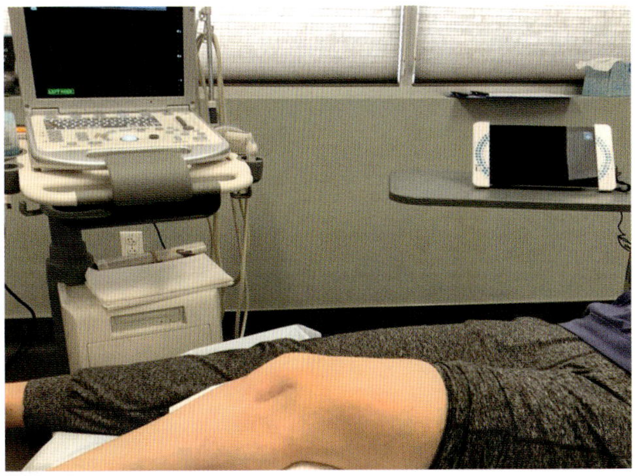

• **Fig. 36.1** Example of Patient, Ultrasound, and Tablet Positioning in Preparation for the Procedure.

a. Seated: Patient is positioned on the edge of the exam table sitting upright with legs hanging off the edge of the table.
b. Supine: Patient is positioned lying down on back with a gel or foam "bump" under the knee to create flexion.

III. Sterility
a. Layout of the Mayo stand (Fig. 36.2)
b. Drapes on the leg (Fig. 36.3)

IV. Portal placement

Suprapatellar pouch: 2 to 3 cm proximal to patella; body habitus will determine how far anterior to posterior the portal will be positioned; ultrasound makes this positioning easier and more accurate

Medial: If the medial portal is being used, it will be 1 cm down and 1.5 to 2 cm medial from the inferior pole of the patella.

Lateral: If the lateral portal is being used, it will be 1 cm down and 1 cm lateral from the inferior pole of the patella.

Note that portal placement for needle arthroscopy may differ from traditional arthroscopic portal placement.

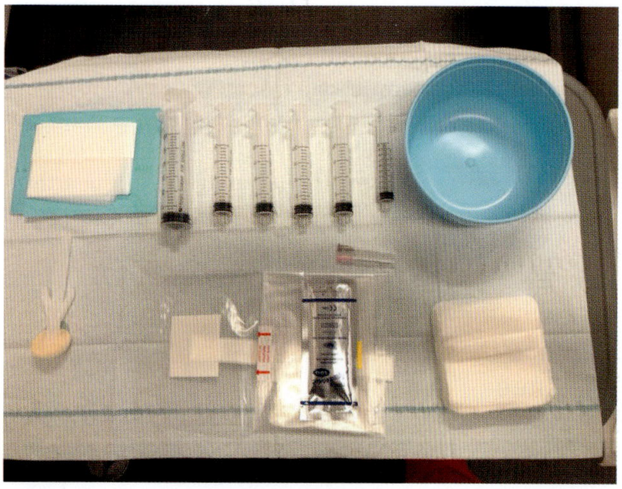

• **Fig. 36.2** Required Supplies Displayed on a Sterile-Covered Mayo Stand.

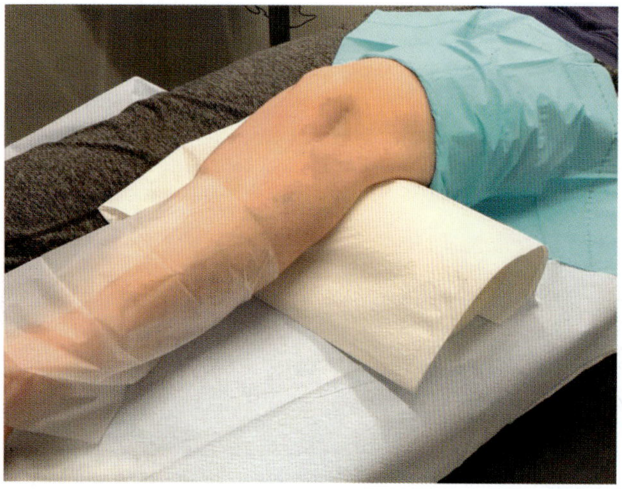

• **Fig. 36.3** Sterile Draping and Initial Positioning of the Leg.

V. US prep of procedure
a. 10 mL of 1% lidocaine, 5 mL of 0.25% Marcaine, and 1 mL of epinephrine is infiltrated into soft tissue prior to insertion of the camera into the suprapatellar pouch, lateral portal through Hoffa's fat pad, and medial portal through Hoffa's fat pad.
b. 30 mL of normal saline and 10 mL of 1% lidocaine is used to infiltrate the joint capsule.
c. Additional syringes and normal saline are kept available for extra flushing of the joint space to clear the view for the camera.
d. Suprapatellar pouch—Authors' tip: using US, infiltrate with spinal needle directed deep to the patella in anechoic space between the quadriceps and prefemoral fat pads to ensure expansion within the capsule of the joint.
e. Optional US for the medial portal (Fig. 36.4).
f. Optional US for the lateral portal (Fig. 36.5).

VI. Procedure (Most needle arthroscopy devices have a 0 degree scope; thus visualization will differ compared with a traditional arthroscopic camera.)

If further visualization is required during the procedure, the physician can perform additional manipulation by flexing the leg and/or applying varus or valgus force.

a. Placement in suprapatellar pouch (US recommended)
Be sure to be proximal enough in the pouch to allow for the full range of the camera and needle (Fig. 36.6).
i. Patellar–trochlear articulation
ii. Lateral gutter
iii. Medial gutter.
b. Placement in lateral portal (aim toward medial femoral notch/medial joint space)—US optional
i. Medial meniscus (valgus stress can be applied to the knee to open the medial space)

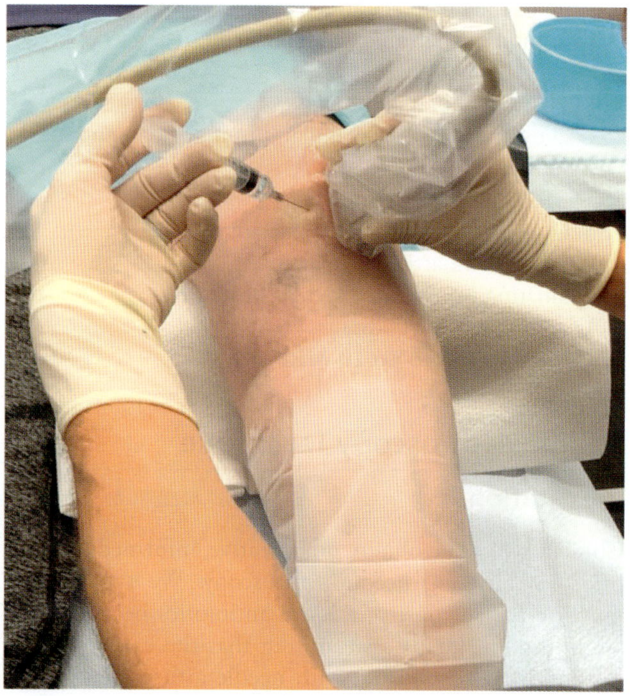

• **Fig. 36.4** Utilization of Ultrasound (Optional) for Infiltration of the Medial Portal.

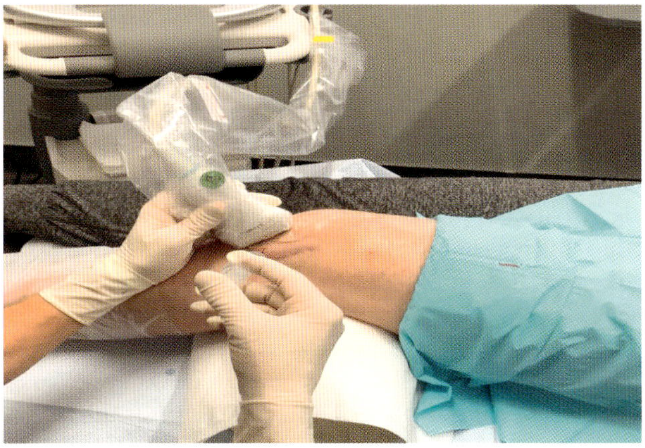

• **Fig. 36.5** Utilization of Ultrasound (Optional) for Infiltration of the Lateral Portal.

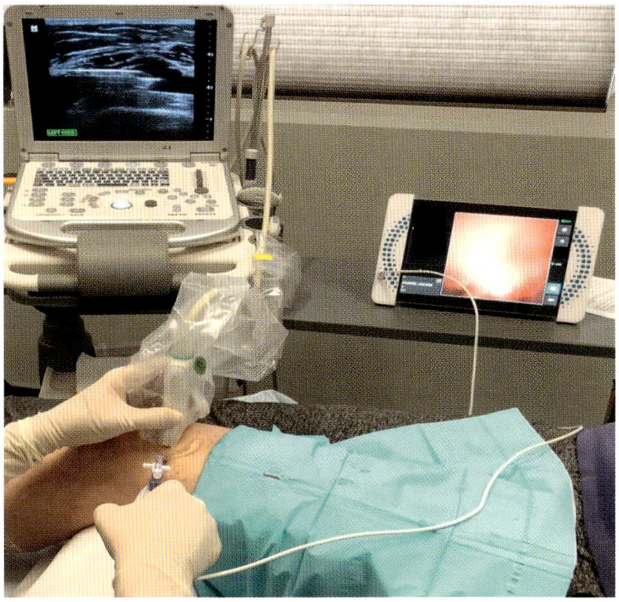

• **Fig. 36.6** Utilization of Ultrasound for Delivery of the Needle Arthroscope Into the Suprapatellar Pouch. Note in-plane visualization of needle on ultrasound image.

ii. Medial femoral condyle
iii. Medial tibial plateau
iv. Anterior cruciate ligament (ACL)/posterior cruciate ligament (PCL)

c. Placement in medial portal (aim toward lateral femoral notch/lateral joint space)—US optional
i. Lateral meniscus (The lateral meniscus may be visualized by placing the knee in a "figure four" to open the lateral compartment.) (Fig. 36.7)
ii. Lateral femoral condyle
iii. Lateral tibial plateau
iv. ACL/PCL

VII. Post-procedure
a. Use US to aspirate as much of the utilized intra-articular normal saline as possible.
b. Clean and dress the wounds with simple adhesive bandages.
c. Compress with elastic bandage or compression sleeve.

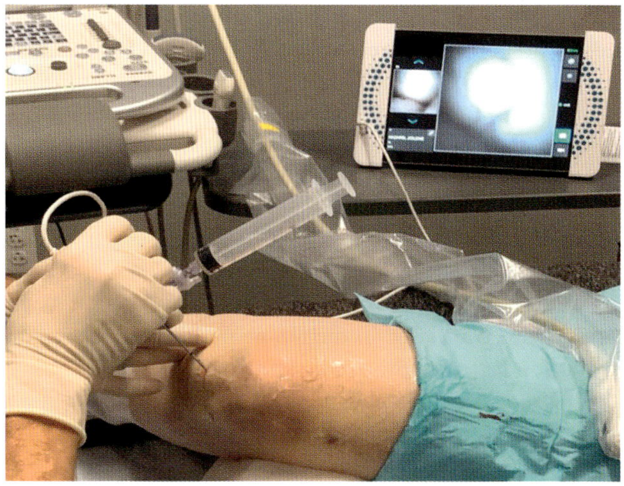

• **Fig. 36.7** Adjustment of leg into "figure four" position to allow for opening of the lateral joint space, leading to improved visualization of the structures within this compartment.

The Shoulder

Patients can be positioned either seated or in the lateral decubitus position. With the seated position, it is helpful to have an assistant available to help with positioning of the shoulder for dynamic evaluation. The physician is positioned behind the patient, since the initial portal is the posterior arthroscopy portal. In the lateral decubitus position, it is helpful to have an assistant available to abduct the shoulder. In the lateral decubitus position, an abduction bolster can also be helpful to abduct the shoulder and mimic the positioning of the arm in traditional shoulder arthroscopy with a shoulder holder.

The posterior shoulder is isolated and draped. If the physician anticipates evaluating the joint from an anterior rotator interval portal, the anterior shoulder should be prepped and draped as well before starting the procedure. Using the local anesthetic mixture previously described, we inject 10 to 15 mL into the posterior portal site and along the needle arthroscope path into the joint. The remaining 15 mL can be injected into the glenohumeral joint.

The primary shoulder portal to be used is the posterior portal. Its location is approximately 2 cm inferior and 1 cm medial to the posterolateral edge of the acromion. Locating the proper placement with US guidance simplifies the procedure and minimizes patient discomfort. With US guidance, a 22-gauge spinal needle or the needle arthroscope is inserted via a posterior off-axis technique to minimize the distance to the joint and mimic the posterior portal used in shoulder arthroscopy.

The needle arthroscope is used to visualize shoulder anatomy just as with the traditional arthroscope. Normal saline is used sparingly to allow visualization. We recommend using a diagnostic protocol that mimics the typical shoulder diagnostic evaluation.[14] A spinal needle can be placed through the rotator interval and used as a probe while watching from the posterior portal. However, it is rare that we have found the need to use an anterior portal in our needle arthroscopy of the shoulder joint.

A Band-Aid or Steri-Strip is used to cover the portal site. Patients do not need to use a sling or change their activity level after the procedure.

The Hip

Patients are positioned in the supine position. Unlike traditional hip arthroscopy, needle arthroscopy of the hip does not require special tables or traction. Typically, the mid-anterolateral portal for hip arthroscopy is used for diagnostic needle arthroscopy. The mid-anterior hip portal can be identified via surface landmarks using previously described techniques.[15] We prefer to use US to visualize the mid-anterior hip portal, simplifying insertion of a 22-gauge spinal needle and placement of the needle arthroscope into the joint. US guidance is also helpful in situations where bony landmarks are difficult to identify, and it eliminates the need for fluoroscopy.

The hip region is draped and prepped. Using the previously described local anesthetic mixture, we inject 10 to 15 mL at the site of the mid-anterior portal and along the path of the needle arthroscope into the hip joint. The remaining 10 to 15 mL can be injected into the hip joint.

The needle arthroscope is used to visualize hip anatomy just as with the traditional arthroscope. We usually have 30 mL of normal saline available to insufflate the joint, although this is used sparingly. As in other joints, normal saline inflow can also serve as a diagnostic tool to see if the labrum or chondral surfaces are stable. Having an assistant available to internally and externally rotate the hip and to flex the hip will maximize visualization of the femoral head and joint. At the end of the procedure, the saline is aspirated from the joint.

A Band-Aid or Steri-Strip is used to cover the portal site. Patients do not need to change their weight-bearing status or activity level after the procedure.

Potential Complications

Certain disadvantages and safety concerns deserve comment. Unlike surgical arthroscopy, needle arthroscopy does not allow for continuous irrigation of the joint. Consequently, needle arthroscopy of joints containing an obscuring hemarthrosis may be less diagnostically accurate. Additionally, bone pathology deep to the articular surface—such as marrow edema, sclerosis, or subchondral cysts—would not be appreciated using needle arthroscopy. As with any minimally invasive manipulation of a joint, needle arthroscopy can place the patient at risk for joint infection, bleeding, or damage to nearby structures. However, prior studies evaluating the utility of needle arthroscopy have reported no procedure- or device-related complications.

Conclusion

Needle arthroscopy has proven safety and utility as a diagnostic tool for intra-articular pathology in the knee, shoulder, and hip. The ability to convert diagnostic arthroscopy into a point-of-care, same-day imaging modality benefits patients and clinicians. Clinicians will be able to make better decisions sooner, which will hopefully lead to better patient care. When all of the costs associated with MRI scans and traditional surgical arthroscopy are considered, in-office needle arthroscopy presents distinct advantages in terms of ease, cost, safety, and efficacy. As an imaging modality, needle arthroscopy can also be used to guide surgical procedures, replacing the traditional larger arthroscope in many situations. With its many orthopedic indications, needle arthroscopy is an excellent imaging modality that represents a technologic advancement in arthroscopy.

References

1. DeMaio M. Giants of orthopaedic surgery: Masaki Watanabe MD. *Clin Orthop Relat Res*. 2013;471(8):2443–2448. https://doi.org/10.1007/s11999-013-3052-1.
2. Jackson RW. The introduction of arthroscopy to North America. *Clin Orthop Relat Res*. 2000;374:183–186. https://doi.org/10.1097/00003086-200005000-00016.
3. Kanu O, et al. Do orthopaedic resident and fellow case logs accurately reflect surgical case volume? *J Surg Edu*. 2018;75(4):1052–1057.
4. Hinds RM, et al. Trends in arthroscopic procedures performed during orthopaedic residency: an analysis of accreditation council for graduate medical education case log data. *Arthroscopy: J Arthros Relat Surg*. 2016;32(4):645–650.
5. Arthroscopy Association of North America. (2019). http://www.aana.org.
6. American Board of Orthopedic Surgery. (2019). https://www.abos.org/subspecialties/orthopaedic-sports-medicine/.
7. Trice Medical. *The mi-eye2/mi-Ultra*™; 2019. http://www.tricemedical.com.
8. *ArthrexInc. The Nanoscope*™ *System*; 2019. http://www.arthrex.com.
9. Visionscope Technologies, LLC. *The Visionscope*™; 2019. http://www.visionscope-tech.com.
10. McMillan S, et al. Risks and complications associated with intra-articular arthroscopy of the knee and shoulder in an office setting. *Orthopaed J Sport Med*. 2019;7(9): 2325967119869846.
11. Gill TJ, et al. A prospective, blinded, multicenter clinical trial to compare the efficacy, accuracy, and safety of in-office diagnostic arthroscopy with magnetic resonance imaging and surgical diagnostic arthroscopy". *Arthroscopy: J Arthrosc Relat Surg*. 2018;34(8):2429–2435.
12. McMillan S, et al. In-office diagnostic needle arthroscopy: understanding the potential value for the US healthcare system. *Am J Orthop*. 2017;46(5):252–256.
13. The Joint Commission. (2019). https://www.jointcommission.org/en/standards/universal-protocol/.
14. Buford Jr D, Snyder SJ. Diagnostic shoulder arthroscopy: the 23-point arthroscopic evaluation with normal anatomivariants and pathology. *Atlas of Shoulder Arthroscopy*. CRC Press; 2003:82–91.
15. Bond JL, et al. The 23-point arthroscopic examination of the hip: basic setup, portal placement, and surgical technique. *Arthroscopy: J Arthrosc Relat Surg*. 2009;25(4):416–429.

37 Rehabilitation Principles for Interventional Orthopedics and Orthobiologics

WALTER I. SUSSMAN, KEN MAUTNER, AND ABBY PERONE

Background

KEY POINTS

- The effects of prehabilitation in preparation for and rehabilitation after interventional orthopedic procedures have received little attention in the literature.
- Exercise is a cornerstone of management prior to and following many orthopedic and surgical procedures.

Preprocedural Considerations

Prehabilitation is the practice of training and enhancing the patient's functional capacity to prepare for a major procedure. Postoperative inactivity can lead to a decline in function, and the objective of prehabilitation is to help the patient withstand the stress of this inactivity.[1]

In total hip and knee arthroplasty, preoperative functional status is a significant predictor of postoperative function.[2–5] In fact, in one study, baseline pain and function was the single best predictor of pain and function at 6 months after a total hip or knee replacement.[3] Patients may not report a perceived benefit from prehabilitation programs,[2,4] but studies have shown functional benefit.[2] Even a 3-week preoperative strengthening program can increase lower extremity muscle strength prior to surgery and improve the immediate postoperative course.[2] The significant strength gains achieved in the 3- to 6-week preoperative period suggest that the benefit of these short prehabilitation strength training programs is increased neuromuscular coordination and not necessarily strength.[6,7] Although there maybe short-term benefits to prehabilitation after arthroplasty, the longer-term benefits are unclear.[8]

The literature on prehabilitation is more limited in other areas of orthopedics, but prehabilitation has been studied in anterior cruciate ligament (ACL) tears. Preoperative quadriceps strength is a significant predictor of knee function even 2 years after ACL reconstruction,[9] and the enhancement of quadriceps strength and function preoperatively has been shown to improve surgical outcomes.[10–13] In spinal surgery, prehabilitation showed no statistically significant difference in pain or disability, but patients reported feeling more prepared for surgery.[14] These principles have not been studied in interventional orthopedics, but it is reasonable to believe that preconditioning could also have a beneficial effect after the varied procedures outlined in this text.

Nutrition plays a role in healing, has been studied in the trauma literature[15–17] and is a concern in chronic wound management.[18] Proper nutrition is an essential parameter in musculoskeletal health, including the prevention and treatment of diseases.[19] This is likely underrecognized in elderly patients, and older adults may not have the same physiologic reserves of younger adults.[20] Malnutrition is a risk factor for wound chronicity.[21] Given the prolonged would healing process, nutrition should be considered as part of the presurgical or preprocedural assessment. Diagnostic markers of malnutrition remain elusive.[22] The focus should be on basic nutrition and a healthy diet, including adequate calories and protein supplies to support the increased energy demands of collagen synthesis, angiogenesis, fibroblast proliferation, tissue remodeling, and wound contraction during the healing process.[23] Protein deficiency has been associated with impaired fibroblast proliferation and collagen synthesis.[22] Adequate hydration can help to promote tissue perfusion, oxygenation, and waste removal,[24] and macro- and micronutrients may assist in enhancing the healing process.[22] In the literature on wound healing, there is evidence for supplementing vitamins A and C and—if there is a deficiency—supplementing arginine, glutamine, and zinc.[22] But the literature on orthobiologics is limited.

Malnutrition can take different forms; in addition to specific nutrient deficits, it can include inadequate intake and overconsumption.[25] There is evidence that obesity and associated disorders can affect stem cell function. Obesity and diabetes have been associated with abnormal cytokine signaling, impaired tissue repair, and delayed wound closure.[26] In rodent models of type 2 diabetes, endogenous mesenchymal stem cells (MSCs) were less effective at mobilizing to a site of injury than those in the nondiabetic controls,[27] and high levels of glucose were associated with the reduced growth of mesenchymal progenitor cells.[28] High glucose concentrations have been shown to reduce the osteogenic and chondrogenic potential of adipose-derived mesenchymal stem cells (ADSCs),[29] and ADSCs had a reduced differentiation potential and a lower capacity for spontaneous or therapeutic repair in patients who were obese and had metabolic syndrome.[30] In contrast, caloric restriction is known to reduce inflammation and has been shown to increase the proliferation of MSCs in mouse models[31,32]; moreover, the restriction of glucose improved the self-renewal and antisenescence abilities of MSCs.[33] Although the role of obesity or calorie restriction on clinical outcomes in orthobiologics is unclear, the literature suggests that calorie restriction may improve stem cell function.

Education has also been shown to have a positive impact on the outcomes of total knee and hip arthroplasty.[34,35] Being able to counsel patients regarding the expected postprocedural course can help them to prepare for the procedure. In theory, it could also affect the outcome after any interventional procedure. The following section outlines the expected postprocedure course of many orthobiologic procedures.

Postprocedural Considerations Basic Science

The healing potential following orthobiologic injections will vary depending on the tissue type (e.g., tendon, ligament, muscle, bone), underlying pathology (e.g., tendinopathy vs. tear), and anatomic location (e.g., Achilles vs. rotator cuff). In general, healing of tendon, ligament, muscle, and bone injuries follows the normal wound-healing cascade—a complex series of events that is typically divided into three phases: inflammatory, proliferative and maturation or remodeling. Some authors may describe a fourth phase, that of hemostasis, which is characterized by vasoconstriction and the formation of a blood clot immediately after an injury (Fig. 37.1).

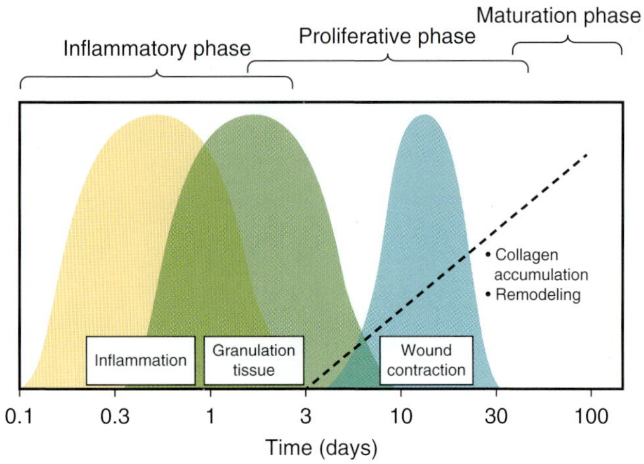

• **Fig. 37.1** Phases of Wound Healing. (Repoduced from Kumar V, Abbas A, Fausto N. Tissue renewal and repair: regeneration, healing, and fibrosis. In: *Robbins and Cotran Pathologic Basis of Disease*. 7th ed. Philadelphia, PA: Elsevier Saunders; 2005:87–118.)

There is limited evidence-based literature on the role of rehabilitation following orthobiologic or regenerative procedures.[36,37] Although rehabilitation is often encouraged for the management of many orthopedic conditions to improve range of motion (ROM), strength, and functional activities, it may play a more specific role after orthobiologic procedures. The objective of many regenerative procedures is to trigger a healing response and stimulate the body's own repair mechanism. Animal models of injury and repair are the primary means of understanding the fundamental process of healing in tendon, ligament, and muscle tissue. In a study by Virchenko and Aspenberg, rats with iatrogenically injured Achilles tendons were injected with platelet-rich plasma (PRP). Half of them received an intramuscular injection of botulinum toxin A (Botox) into the calf muscles to unloaded the tendon and had no effect from the PRP injection at 14 days compared with the control rats, who were not treated with botulinum toxin and did show neotendon development.[38] The failure of the rats treated with botulinum toxin to develop neotendons suggests that mechanical stimulation is important in the early phases of tendon regeneration. Ambrosio et al., in a mouse model, demonstrated that stem cell transplantation into injured skeletal muscle proliferated and terminally differentiated toward a myogenic lineage with daily treadmill running, whereas the transplanted stem cells failed to divide rapidly in the absence of loading.[39] Clinical studies have also supported the role of rehabilitation. In a pilot study of PRP for chronic patellar tendinopathy, Kon et al. found that subjects who did not follow the postprocedural stretching and strengthening program had poorer outcomes.[40]

Further insight is needed into the molecular and cellular response to therapeutic exercises and stress after regenerative therapies. Based science studies showing that the effects of PRP are lost when tendons are unloaded mechanically, and one conclusion is that tendon healing may require a combination of biologic and mechanical factors. The term *mechanotransduction* is often used to describe the physiologic responses by which cells convert mechanical stimuli into structural adaptations.[41–43] Mechanical stimuli or loads on a tendon are sensed by various cell surface receptors, integrins, stretch-activated ion channels, and other mechanisms, triggering cell–cell communication and changes in cellular biology within the cell nuclei.[44] Eccentric exercises, with slow lengthening of the muscle-tendon unit while under load, have been shown

TABLE 37.1 General Principles of Rehabilitation Prescription.

When rehabilitation after a regenerative procedure is being initiated, the following considerations, which align with the phases of the healing cascade, should be considered with each phase:

- Restrictions
  - Which movements and activities are to be avoided during the phase
- Appropriate therapeutic exercise
  - Appropriate exercises define the type and category of exercises for each phase
  - For example, early phases may consider partial or non–weight bearing, whereas later phases invite diverse planes of movement under varying loads
- Benchmarks to progress to next phase
  - Benchmarks are objective goals to determine preparedness to transition to the next phase of rehabilitation
  - For example, for a hip bone augmentation (see Table 37.6), patients may transition from phase I to phase II when they can "walk full weight bearing 50 ft with minimal pain"
- Pain vs. time
  - The phases are not governed by the anticipated rate of healing but are ultimately dictated by the patient's subjective pain and function
  - For a patient to complete a phase and transition to the next, the tasks of the current phase should be completed

to stimulate a cellular response, including the activation and proliferation of satellite stem cells.[45] Heavy-slow resistance (HSR) training in which each repetition is performed slowly for more than 6 seconds for both the eccentric and concentric phases has shown similar results to eccentric strengthening in long-term pain reduction. HSR has demonstrated normalization of tendon fibril morphology.[46] There is also interest in low-load resistance training with blood flow restriction (BFR), and recent studies have shown increased muscle proteins synthesis and proliferation of myogenic stem cells after BFR training.[47,48]

There are many translational questions about how to apply these principles to orthobiologic procedures. The topic of tissue repair and rehabilitation is vast, and this chapter is by no means exhaustive. The goal is to understand the basic tenets of the healing process to help clinicians design rehabilitation programs, taking into consideration the patient and his or her pathology (e.g., mechanism of injury, tissue injured, severity, age of patient), the treatment (e.g., intra-articular vs. intraosseous or intratendinous vs. paratendinous), and the different phases of healing (Table 37.1).

Rehabilitation recommendations can vary depending on the tissue treated. For example, tendons require loading in an earlier phase of rehabilitation in order to help support the development of tensile strength. Overall, the literature suggests that mechanical stress on the tendon is needed to optimize outcomes.[36] In contrast, osseous healing may require even longer periods of unloading and protected weight bearing. The severity of pathology should also be considered. For example, strengthening exercises after the injection of PRP may be started later in high-grade partial tendon tears as compared with tendinopathy.

Guidance following a procedure must also be tailored to the injectate or treatment. For example, rehabilitation following an injection around a tendon (e.g., a high-volume injection between the Achilles tendon and the Kegar fat pad) will have a different expected postprocedural course than an intratendinous procedure (e.g., PRP injected into the Achilles tendon). Likewise, an intra-articular knee injection of cortisone will have a different course than an autologous cellular injection.

Phases of Rehabilitation and The Healing Cascade

Phase I of Healing—The Inflammatory Phase (0 to 5 Days)

The inflammatory phase is the initial response to tissue damage and generally occurs within the first 5 days after injury.[49–52] This phase is initially characterized by hemostasis and "walling off" of the injured site, increased vascular permeability, and an influx of inflammatory cells. Platelets are among the first cells to respond to an injury; they form a hemostatic plug and secrete chemokines (e.g., epidermal growth factor [EGF], fibronectin, fibrinogen, histamine, platelet-derived growth factor [PDGF], serotonin, and von Willebrand factor). These factors recruit macrophages to the healing site, resulting in the scavenging of debris and in phagocytosis to debride the wound bed. Fibroblasts also migrate to the wound in this phase, initiating the formation of granulation tissue and the transition into the proliferative phase.[49] The specific cellular events will differ depending on the anatomy and physiology of the given tissue.[53]

During this phase, patients may experience varying degrees of pain, swelling, redness, and limited ROM. Some patients' symptoms are due primarily to laxity of the ligaments; if such individuals are treated, the initial swelling may sometimes actually cause a temporary improvement in perceived in stability and a reduction in symptoms, both of which dissipate once the swelling has gone down.

Phase II of Healing—The Repair Phase (5 to 21 Days)

The proliferative (granulation) phase is characterized by "rebuilding" of the local tissue, and generally lasts for several weeks after injury.[50–52] Granulation tissue formation, collagen deposition, and angiogenesis create an extracellular matrix and network of blood vessels to supply the area. Neovascularization helps to supply the wound bed with nutrients.[49] Macrophages continue to supply growth factors, and fibroblasts differentiate and produce collagen, depositing and remodeling the extracellular matrix.[49]

Initially, migrating fibroblasts will begin to synthesize collagen around day 5, but by the fourth week, there is a noticeable increase in the intrinsic proliferation of fibroblasts from the endotenon. Initially the collagen fibers are randomly oriented, but as the tissue starts to mature, the collagen fibers are increasingly oriented along the direction of force through the tendon, increasing the tensile strength of the tendon. By week 5, tenocytes become the main cell type.[54]

During this phase patients should feel a decrease in the initial postinjury/procedural pain. Preprocedural symptoms may persist, slowly improve, or wax and wane.

Phase III of Healing—The Maturation Phase (21 Days to 12 Months)

The maturation or remodeling phase starts 3 weeks after an injury and lasts up to 12 months or longer, with collagen deposition by fibroblasts continuing for this entire period.[51] Increased stability is acquired during the remodeling phase and is stimulated by continued use of the tendon. Mechanical stress influences cell signaling and behavior; it contributes to remodeling of the collagen matrix and increases the tensile strength of the tissue.[55] As the maturation process continues, the collage fibers continue to be reabsorbed and synthesized along the direction of force and cross-linking of the collagen fibrils occurs, increasing the tendons' tensile strength. Along with this, there is increased deposition of type I collagen in preference to type III collagen.[54,56] The tensile strength is estimated to reach its maximum at 3 months[57,58] but never fully returns to its preinjury strength.[59] During this period, patients are usually noticing a consistent improvement in symptoms, although their condition will still often wax and wane as tissue transitions from granulation tissue to scar formation.

Tissue-Specific Considerations

Tendons and Ligaments

Healing of tendons and ligaments follows the three phases of wound healing that have already been detailed. In the initial phase, blood clot and granulation tissue fill the gap between the tendon and ligament fibers. In tendons, fibroblasts and tenocytes in the epitenon and paratenon are recruited and proliferate, bridging the injured gap and forming a stable scar. In the early stages, the matrix is composed of increasing amounts of type III collagen.[60] After 10 weeks, a higher proportion of collagen type I is synthesized and type III collagen decreases, forming scarlike tendon tissue, a process that will continue for years.[61,62]

Muscles

Muscle strains that cause a rupture of the myofibers also go through the three phases of healing. Satellite cells begin to proliferate and form new myoblasts, which fuse into myotubes within a couple of days.[63] Similar to tendons and ligaments, fibroblasts produce collagen and form scar tissue to bridge the gap between muscle fibers.[64]

Cartilage

Articular cartilage has poor intrinsic healing capacity and generally does not heal or heals only partially under certain conditions.[65] In most cases, surgical or biologic interventions are necessary to induce a repair response. Treatments include debridement, microfracture, and autologous tissue transplantation (e.g., autologous chondrocytes or MSCs). Little is known about the histologic effects of cartilage healing after these procedures. In vitro studies have demonstrated that mechanical stress can stimulate the differentiation of MSCs into chondrocytes, extracellular matrix synthesis, and cytokine secretion,[66] whereas excessive stress may cause cell death and matrix degeneration.[67]

Bone

Injured bone (e.g., fractured or necrotic bone) is resorbed and replaced by new bone following the three phases of healing. Macrophages and osteoclasts remove injured calcified bone, and osteoblasts fill the fracture gap, forming granulation tissue. Delayed bone formation and nonunion have been attributed to variations in the local inflammatory environment as well as the recruitment of muscle-derived stromal cells and osteogenesis early in the healing process.[68] Bone repair follows two phases of healing: (1) the initial cartilaginous soft callus, followed by (2) remodeling and formation of a bony hard callus. Initially, the soft callus is formed when adjacent soft tissue and periosteum bridge the fracture site, stabilizing the fracture.[69] Osteons travel along the cortical bone (by the Haversian system); they bridge the fracture gap,[70,71] and osteoblasts synthesize woven bone, resulting in a hard callus.[68,72,73] This irregular woven bone callus remodels over months to years through continuous osteoclast resorption, while osteoblasts replace the matrix with lamellar bone to bring the bone back to its original shape, size, and strength/stability.[74]

Overview of Rehabilitation Guidelines per Phase of Healing

The objective of many traditional orthopedic injections, such as corticosteroids or ketorolac injections, is to address inflammation. The objective of orthobiologic procedures in interventional orthopedics is different, and the aim is to reduce pain and improve function. This is often achieved by stimulating a healing response by delivering growth factors to the target tissue (e.g., PRP, autologous stem cells) or controlled microtrauma to convert a chronic injury into an acute injury with healing potential (e.g., prolotherapy, percutaneous needle tenotomy, Tenex ultrasonic debridement).

The literature on rehabilitation after orthobiologic or interventional orthopedic procedures is limited, and many of the rehabilitation protocols that have been proposed constitute attempts to translate these would-be healing principles into clinical practice.[44,75–78] There is some variability in the duration and overlap of the phases of wound healing described in the literature,[49–52] and progression through the rehabilitation process should be informed by clinical progress through the program, and individualized, reflecting the type of tissue undergoing recovery (e.g., tendon, bone, ligament, muscle), severity of the underlying pathology, the patient's preprocedural fitness level, her or his physical abilities, and any existing comorbidities.

Rehabilitation in the Inflammatory Phase of Healing (0 to 5 Days)

The goal of rehabilitation in the inflammatory phase is typically one of protection, and care typically focuses on managing pain and postprocedural swelling. Management may vary, depending on the procedure, and tissue type (i.e. tendons, ligament and bone/cartilage) but is typically achieved with immobilization or bracing, ice, elevation, medications, and gentle ROM exercises to activate the vasomotor pump.[75]

Immobilization/Bracing

In most cases, protected weight bearing is recommended for pain control in the first 1 to 3 days. Most randomized controlled or prospective studies on orthobiologic procedures have prescribe a period of absolute or relative rest during the acute inflammatory phase, although no prospective studies have specifically studied these rehabilitation protocols.[36] Immobilization should not be prescribed owing to a concern that the administered orthobiologic may disperse to other locations with movement. In a cadaveric model, Achilles tendons that were injected with blue dye to simulate a PRP injection were manipulated through 100 cycles of ankle dorsiflexion and plantarflexion, resulting in no significant difference in the spread of the dye compared with control specimens that were kept in a prone resting position for 15 minutes after the injection.[79] This suggests that early motion does not increase the spread or clearance of PRP from the target site.

Limitation of joint motion can help to reduce pain in the associated area, and weight-bearing restriction or bracing can be used for this objective. Avoiding any pain-provoking activities is a common recommendation, but recommendations have varied across the literature, from avoiding all physical activity to limiting only repetitive movements. Crutches, a controlled-ankle-motion walking boot, or unloader braces can be used to limit motion or decrease stress on a joint, bone, or tendon/ligament after treatment. Any period of immobilization should be limited and guided clinically. In most randomized controlled or prospective studies that detailed postprocedure protocols, patients were usually instructed to restrict weight bearing or to immobilize the joint for 3 days to 2 weeks.[36] However, there is a concern that immobilization may have a negative impact on tendon healing. In animal models, loading the tendon resulted in neotendon development after a PRP injection versus when the tendon was unloading, there were no beneficial results.[38] Prolonged immobilization has been associated with joint contractures and functional impairment, and early gentle active ROM is considered safe.[75]

Pain Management

Postprocedural pain can vary among patients and procedures. For example, intra-articular injections are often less painful than intratendinous or intraosseous injections. Periprocedural nerve blocks, when possible, can help with acute postprocedural pain management. Longer-acting anesthetics, such as ropivacaine, can extend the efficacy of these blocks. Alternative approaches to pain management and analgesia include cryotherapy and nonsteroidal antiinflammatory drugs (NSAIDs).

There are different methods of cryotherapy, including the use of crushed ice, ice bags, chemical or gel packs, and commercially available cryotherapy devices that provide the continuous circulation of ice water. However, there is evidence that some of these methods are more effective than others.[80–82] There is some debate on the issue of limiting cryotherapy in the acute phase after an orthobiologic procedure.[36,83] Cryotherapy has been shown to be effective for managing pain in certain situations[84] and is often accepted as an integral part of the treatment of acute soft tissue injuries despite the lack of a robust evidence base.[85] In one review of regenerative procedures for tendinopathy, 20% of prospective randomized controlled studies prescribed cryotherapy for pain management.[36] The theoretical concern is that cryotherapy may reduce blood flow, which is important for healing. However, the literature is limited and the effect of cryotherapy depends on a number of factors, including the temperature of the cooling device, the depth of the subcutaneous tissue, and the frequency and duration of treatment.[81,86–88] Studies have shown that cryotherapy can temporarily decrease microcirculatory perfusion when measured at a depth of 2 to 8 mm,[89,90] but they disagree on whether this decrease in blood flow persists following active cooling.[90,91] There is limited literature on how the superficial effects of cooling affect the perfusion of deeper structures, and skin temperature has been shown to be a poor predictor of intramuscular temperature and may be a poor predictor of perfusion to deeper structures.[92] In one study of cryotherapy on the microcirculation of the midportion Achilles tendon, the authors showed reduced blood flow within the first minute of cryotherapy and return of capillary blood flow during recovery.[91] Another theoretical concern is that cryotherapy may decrease platelet activation, but in vitro studies have shown that the temperature did not affect platelet adhesion when tested at 0 and 37°C.[93]

The limitation of NSAIDs before and after an orthobiologic procedure is widely accepted across the literature. NSAIDs have been shown to inhibit platelet function and reduce the release of growth factors.[94–96] In a study using a rat animal model of a surgically repaired rotator cuff tendon, even initiating NSAIDs in the proliferative stage of healing decreased the biomechanical strength of the repaired tendon.[97]

Non-NSAID pain medications and prescription narcotics are often prescribed for the first 72 hours. Over-the-counter acetaminophen is often acceptable for pain control after most procedures and does not demonstrate any antiinflammatory activity.[96] Narcotics can be used for breakthrough pain following opioid-risk mitigation strategies, including patient education about opioids, clear instructions about when to use opioids (e.g., for moderate or severe pain only), and prescribing short-acting opioids at the lowest dose necessary. In geriatric patients, doses should be decreased by at least 50% if there is concern for cognitive impairment, risk of falls, respiratory dysfunction, or renal insufficiency.[98]

Rehabilitation in the Proliferative Phase of Healing (5 Days to 6 Weeks)

The objective of rehabilitation in the proliferative phase is to gradually increase activity. There is no consensus on the optimal timing of a stretching or strengthening program, and most published study protocols do not specify the type of strengthening recommended.[36] Rehabilitation in this phase is progressive and is typically governed by patient's tolerance. A good guideline is to limit any activity that increases the patient's pain to greater than a 3/10 during or after that activity.

Intraosseous, intraarticular, axial and injections of tendons and/or ligaments may all require different periods of rest and activity modification.[99,100] The literature on tendon healing clearly suggests that early controlled loading influences the early phases of tendon healing after regenerative injection or microtrauma (needle tenotomy)[38,101] and that appropriate mechanical loading induces the differentiation of tendon stem cells (TSCs) into tenocytes.[102] However, excessive loading can induce the differentiation of TSCs into adipocytes, chondrocytes, and osteocytes.[102] Concerns about heterotopic ossification after PRP[103], in theory may stem from the failure of rehabilitation rather than the orthobiologic injection.

Stretching

In the literature, the timing of a stretching program has ranged from 24 hours postprocedure to 1 week.[36] Studies have been performed to determine if dynamic stretching (DS), static stretching (SS), or proprioceptive neuromuscular facilitation (PNF) were superior; however, there is no consensus on the best form of stretching in early phases of healing. The literature on DS, SS, or PNF in sport shows a small to moderate effect on performance and a similar improvement in ROM with all of the stretching approaches. There is no overall effect on injuries prevention with SS and PNF, but no data is available for DS on injury prevention.[104] For tendinopathies specifically, it is inferred that static stretching is the "safest" form of stretching due to its slow and steady nature.[75,104]

Strengthening

Strengthening during the proliferative phase has also been evaluated after regenerative procedures in tendinopathy.[40] This is typically started at 2 weeks in most published postprocedure protocols,[44,75–78] but timing varies across the literature.[36] For joint injections, the strengthening program likely can be start sooner than with tendons or ligaments. Most recommendations are to have a progressive strengthening program. This is based on the progression of healing in tendons, where initially newly synthesized collagen fibers are oriented randomly, but as the proliferative phase progresses, the collagen fibers are increasingly oriented along the direction of force, thus increasing the tensile strength of the tendon.[54]

The safest type of contraction in this phase of healing may be isometric, since joint motion is limited. Isometric contractions can decrease blood flow to the active tissues, but the effect is likely temporary.[75] Isometric exercises have also been shown to be effective for short-term pain relief, and the authors typically will initially start with isometric strengthening exercises after a regenerative procedure.[105,106]

Eccentric contraction or heavy slow resistance training may be the most beneficial type of exercise for long-term pain reduction and functional improvement in tendinopathy, but it has not specifically been studied after regenerative injections.[107] Limited literature guides the ideal timing to initiate eccentric strengthening. There is some concern that if eccentric strengthening is started too soon, it may have a hypovascular effect that attenuates the healing cascade,[83] and it has been suggested that eccentric exercises should be reserved for the late proliferative or remodeling phase.[75] There is also limited literature on open-chain versus closed-chain exercises after regenerative procedures.[36,75]

Rehabilitation in the Remodeling Phase of Healing (6 Weeks to 12 Months)

The goal of rehabilitation in the remodeling, or maturation, phase is the safe return to higher-level activities and sport. At this stage, patients should have completed the early rehabilitation protocols and have full ROM across the joint. Eccentric strengthening should be started in this phase, if not initiated earlier during the late proliferative stage, and proprioceptive exercises should be added to the rehabilitation program.[75]

The literature is limited to guide return-to-play decisions; the timing should be individualized to the athlete. Initially, there should be a focus on the reintroduction of functional activities specific to the athlete's sport. Patients with lower extremity injuries can start jogging and progress activity as tolerated as long as the pain does not increase greater than a 3/10 on numeric rating scale. Sport-specific movements and activities should be included in a controlled setting before progressing to a practice or game/competition setting.

Conclusion

Postprocedure recommendations are based on the underlying physiology of the healing cascade and the relative time frames at each stage of healing. Suggested rehabilitation protocols are general guidelines (Table 37.1). Ultimately the rehabilitation protocols will have to be individualized to best benefit each particular patient in terms of the specific injury and treatment. Table 37.2 provides examples of protocols for knee, intra-articular (Table 37.3), rotator cuff intratendinous (Table 37.4), ACL intraligament (Table 37.5), and hip intraosseous (Table 37.6) orthobiologic procedures.

TABLE 37.2 General Postprocedural Recommendations per Phase of Healing.

Phase of Healing	Time Frame	Restrictions/Rehabilitation
Phase I: Inflammatory phase	Days 0–5	• Relative rest. • Avoid excessive loading/stress and consider NWB or protected WB. • Consider bracing to minimize ROM and provide protection. • Avoid NSAIDs; use alternative pain management.
Phase II	Day 5 to week 6	Early proliferative phase (day 4 through week 2) • Full WB plus/minus protection. • Active ROM. • Initiate gentle stretching program. • Avoid NSAIDs; use alternative pain management (e.g., acetaminophen, curcumin, narcotics, limited cryotherapy, heat, laser therapy). Late proliferative phase (day 4 through week 2) • Full WB without protective device. • Stretching program, adding "dynamic" stretching. • Continue activity, passive ROM can be started. • Progressive strengthening program, starting with high-repetition isometrics and progressing to eccentric exercises closer to the end of this phase. • Avoid NSAIDs; use alternative pain management.
Phase III	Week 7 and after	Weeks 7–12 • Proprioceptive training and sport-specific exercises. Week 12 • Return to sport/activity.

NSAID, Nonsteroidal antiinflammatory drug; *NWB*, non–weight bearing; *ROM*, range of motion; *WB*, weight bearing.

TABLE 37.3 Medial or Lateral Compartment Osteoarthritis of the Knee (Example: Intra-Articular Rehabilitation).

	Restrictions	Therapeutic Goals/Exercises
Phase I (days 0–5)	• WBAT. • PWB or unloader bracing of joint if experiencing moderate to severe pain. • Avoid NSAIDs.	• Daily activities as tolerated. • Gentle active ROM as tolerated. • Wound monitoring. • Pain management.
Early phase II (day 5 to week 2)	• WBAT. • Avoid excessive loading of the joint. • Unloader brace with WB activity if recommended by physician. • Avoid NSAIDs. • Avoid any activity that causes >3/10 pain during or after the activity.	• Activities as tolerated. • Continue active ROM. • Enhance blood perfusion through modalities (infrared heat, moist heat, ultrasound, etc.). • Begin isometric low-grade closed-chain program (e.g., start body weight partial squats and lunges). • Begin core activating exercises and postural therapy. • Can start swimming and/or pool therapy and biking (low resistance) on flat terrain.

Continued

TABLE 37.3 Medial or Lateral Compartment Osteoarthritis of the Knee (Example: Intra-Articular Rehabilitation).—cont'd

	Restrictions	Therapeutic Goals/Exercises
Late phase II (weeks 2–6)	• WBAT. • Unloader brace with weight-bearing activity • Avoid high-impact activities and heavy weightlifting to affected joint. • Avoid NSAIDs. • Avoid any activity that causes >3/10 pain during or after the activity.	• Continue active ROM and progress to passive ROM. • Can add resistance to closed-chain program. Start with light weight and focus on form and increasing repetition. Continue with isometric exercises and progress slowly to concentric exercises. • Can start light open kinetic chain exercises (e.g., start leg curl/extension exercises with light weight). • Incorporate core, gluteal, postural, and alignment therapies. • Continue modalities as needed • Can continue pool therapy, swimming, biking, light walking as tolerated.
Early phase III (weeks 7–12)	• Discontinue unloader brace. • Avoid any activity that causes >3/10 pain during or after the activity.	• Progress open kinetic chain exercises and functional exercise program. • Proprioception exercises, single limb stability exercises. • May resume light aerobic activities such as hiking and light agility training, and progress to jogging if able. • Can increase biking resistance. • Progress weightlifting/strength training as tolerated. • Can start to add more activities in a stepwise fashion.
Late phase III (week 13 and thereafter)	• No specific restrictions.	• Sport and activity-specific training. • Progress weightlifting/strength training. • Return to full activities as tolerated.

NSAID, Nonsteroidal antiinflammatory drug; *PWB*, partial weight bearing; *ROM*, range of motion; *WB,* weight bearing; *WBAT*, weight bearing as tolerated.

TABLE 37.4 Rotator Cuff Tear (Example: Tendon Rehabilitation).

	Restrictions	Therapeutic Goals/Exercises
Phase I (days 0–5)	• Avoid lifting, pushing, pulling. • Avoid NSAIDs. • Avoid sling or immobilization.	• Daily activities as tolerated. • Gentle active ROM as tolerated three times daily. • Wound monitoring • Pain management
Early phase II (day 5 to week 2)	• Avoid lifting >5–10 lb. • Avoid overhead activity; no overhead lifting. • Limit flexion/abduction to 90 degrees with palms up and extension to 0 degrees. • Avoid resistance exercise bands. • Avoid any activity that causes >3/10 pain during or after the activity. • Avoid NSAIDs.	• Continue active ROM (e.g., add pendulum and pulley exercises) • Enhance blood perfusion through modalities (e.g., infrared heat, moist heat, ultrasound) • Strengthen inferior traps and rhomboids (e.g., rows, extensions, abduction, triceps extensions) and forearms • Neck stabilization exercises
Late phase II (weeks 2–6)	• Avoid repetitive overhead activity, no overhead lifting. • Limit flexion/abduction to 90 degrees with palms up and extension to 0 degrees (e.g., with push-ups, keep hands shoulder width or closer). • Avoid resistance exercise bands. • Avoid any activity that causes >3/10 pain during or after the activity.	• Continue active ROM and progress to passive ROM • Begin resistance training including gentle rotator cuff strengthening. Start with isometric exercises and progress to concentric exercises. Start with low weight; focus on form and increase repetition instead of increasing weight. Progress slowly. • Continue to work on strength and flexibility, correcting poor biomechanics, asymmetry, scapular dyskinesia, and postural restoration.
Phase III (weeks 7–12)	• Can start lightweight overhead activity but avoid repetitive overhead activity. • Limit flexion/abduction to 90 degrees with palms up and extension to 0 degrees (e.g., with push-ups, keep hands at shoulder width or closer). • Avoid any activity that causes >3/10 pain during or after the activity.	• Progress strengthening exercises, adding eccentric exercises and progressing to a functional exercise program. • Proprioception exercises. • Address strength asymmetry, flexibility, poor biomechanics, and scapular dyskinesia if present. • Return to full activities as tolerated. • Can start to add more activities, including overhead, as tolerated and in a stepwise fashion.
Phase III (week 13 and thereafter)	• No strict restrictions.	• Sport- and activity-specific training • Progress weightlifting/strength training • Return to full activities as tolerated

NSAID, Nonsteroidal antiinflammatory drug; *ROM*, range of motion.

TABLE 37.5 **Anterior Cruciate Ligament (Example: Ligament Rehabilitation).**

	Restrictions	Therapeutic Goals/Exercises
Phase I (days 0–5)	• ACL or hinged knee brace (initial 4–6 weeks). • No plyometrics, cutting movements, or lateral movements. No running. • Avoid NSAIDs.	• Wound monitoring. • Pain management.
Early phase II (day 5 to week 2)	• ACL or hinged knee brace (initial 4–6 weeks). • No plyometrics, cutting movements, or lateral movements. No running. • Avoid any activity that causes >3/10 pain during or after the activity. • Avoid NSAIDs.	• Begin active ROM in knee brace. • Start stationary bike for ROM with minimal resistance. • Can start gentle isometric quad sets, hip abductor and core strengthening. • Can start elliptical in brace and swimming.
Late phase II (weeks 2–6)	• ACL or hinged knee brace (initial 4–6 weeks). Can discontinue brace if recommended by physician at 4 weeks. • No plyometrics, cutting movements, or lateral movements. No running. • Avoid any activity that causes >3/10 pain during or after the activity. • Avoid NSAIDs.	• Continue stationary bike, elliptical in brace, and swimming. • Can progress to pool jogging; chest depth, 30–45 min three to five times a week for 2 months. Can begin jogging on even terrain at 4–6 weeks if not painful. • Progress to concentric strengthening (e.g., light squats, leg presses). • Can start basic proprioceptive exercises in brace (e.g., balance board exercises).
Early phase III (weeks 7–12)	• Can discontinue brace. • Avoid any activity that causes >3/10 pain during or after the activity.	• Progress strengthening and proprioceptive exercises (e.g., ball toss on balance board). • Progress to eccentric strengthening (e.g., single leg exercises, calf raises, squats, dead lifts). • Address strength asymmetry, flexibility, poor biomechanics. • Objective ACL stability measurements at 12 weeks with Rolimeter/telos or KT 1000.
Late phase III (week 13 and thereafter)	• No strict restrictions.	• Consider repeating the MRI at 3 and 6 months. Pending results may consider repeat PRP or bone marrow concentrate. • Continue strength training, proprioceptive exercises, single-leg stability exercises, landing mechanics, neuromuscular control therapies. • Progress to return to full sport at 3–9 months with physician clearance after reviewing MRI, checking objective stability, and demonstrating correct neuromuscular control. • Should demonstrate correct form (good knee, hip, pelvic, and trunk stability) with step down, drop jump, lateral shuffle, deceleration, triple jump, and side step-cut tests before return to cutting sports. • Once the patient returns to sport, recommend the Santa Monica Sports Medicine PEP (Prevent Injury and Enhance Performance) program

ACL, Anterior cruciate ligament; *MRI*, magnetic resonance imaging; *NSAID*, nonsteroidal antiinflammatory drug; *ROM*, range of motion.

TABLE 37.6 Hip Intraosseous (Example: Intraosseous Rehabilitation).

	Restrictions	Therapeutic Goals/Exercises
Phase I (days 0–5)	• Limit WB activity as possible for 1 week. PWB with crutches (first 3–5 days), then WBAT. • Avoid NSAIDs.	• Gentle active ROM as tolerated. • Wound monitoring. • Pain management. • Prevention of DVT: leg elevation while lying, ankle pumps, (optional—compression socks when upright).
Early phase II (day 5 to week 2)	• WBAT. • Once off crutches, walking no more than 30 min at a time. • Avoid any activity that causes >3/10 pain during or after the activity. • Avoid NSAIDs.	• Continue active ROM. • Can start stationary bike for ROM. If there is access to a pool, can start walking (chest depth, 30–45 min three to five times a week). • Core stability exercises. • Enhance blood perfusion through modalities (infrared heat, moist heat, ultrasound, etc.). • Can consider hyperbaric oxygen,[108–110] PEMF therapy, and/or low-intensity pulsed ultrasound if AVN or nonunion fracture treatment.
Late phase II (weeks 2–6)	• WBAT. • Avoid high-impact activities and heavy weightlifting to affected joint. • Avoid NSAIDs. • Avoid any activity that causes >3/10 pain during or after the activity.	• Start isometric low-grade closed-chain program (e.g., start body weight partial [mini] squats and lunges). Add pelvic alignment exercises, hip abduction strengthening, and core stabilization (e.g., plank, supine bridge) with therapist. Progress to concentric exercises. • If there is access to a pool can start jogging in pool (chest depth, 30–45 min three to five times a week) or add elliptical. • Start proprioceptive exercises. • Biking with low resistance.
Early phase III (weeks 7–12)	• Avoid any activity that causes >3/10 pain during or after the activity.	• Start open kinetic chain exercises and functional exercise program. • Progress proprioception exercises • Address strength asymmetry, flexibility, poor biomechanics. • May start low- to moderate-impact activity at 2 months and progress to biking with resistance, then jogging if able. • Progress weightlifting/strength training as tolerated.
Late phase III (week 13 and thereafter)	• No specific restrictions.	• Sport and activity-specific training. • Progress to running if able. • Progress weightlifting/strength training. • Return to full activities as tolerated.

AVN, Avascular necrosis; *DVT*, deep venous thrombosis; *NSAID*, nonsteroidal antiinflammatory drug; *PEMF*, pulsed electromagnetic field; *PWB*, partial weight bearing; *ROM*, range of motion; *WB*, weight bearing; *WBAT*, weight bearing as tolerated.

References

1. Ditmyer MM, Topp R, Pifer M. Prehabilitation in preparation for orthopaedic surgery. *Orthop Nurs*. 2002;21(5):43–51; quiz 52–44.
2. Rooks DS, Huang J, Bierbaum BE, et al. Effect of preoperative exercise on measures of functional status in men and women undergoing total hip and knee arthroplasty. *Arthritis Rheum*. 2006;55(5):700–708.
3. Fortin PR, Clarke AE, Joseph L, et al. Outcomes of total hip and knee replacement: preoperative functional status predicts outcomes at six months after surgery. *Arthritis Rheum*. 1999;42(8):1722–1728.
4. D'Lima DD, Colwell Jr CW, Morris BA, Hardwick ME, Kozin F. The effect of preoperative exercise on total knee replacement outcomes. *Clin Orthop Relat Res*. 1996;(326):174–182.
5. Rodgers JA, Garvin KL, Walker CW, Morford D, Urban J, Bedard J. Preoperative physical therapy in primary total knee arthroplasty. *J Arthroplasty*. 1998;13(4):414–421.
6. American College of Sports Medicine Position Stand. The recommended quantity and quality of exercise for developing and maintaining cardiorespiratory and muscular fitness, and flexibility in healthy adults. *Med Sci Sports Exerc*. 1998;30(6):975–991.
7. Moritani T, deVries HA. Neural factors versus hypertrophy in the time course of muscle strength gain. *Am J Phys Med*. 1979;58(3):115–130.
8. Cabilan CJ, Hines S, Munday J. The effectiveness of prehabilitation or preoperative exercise for surgical patients: a systematic review. *JBI Database System Rev Implement Rep*. 2015;13(1):146–187.
9. Eitzen I, Holm I, Risberg MA. Preoperative quadriceps strength is a significant predictor of knee function two years after

anterior cruciate ligament reconstruction. *Br J Sports Med.* 2009;43(5):371–376.

10. Eitzen I, Moksnes H, Snyder-Mackler L, Risberg MA. A progressive 5-week exercise therapy program leads to significant improvement in knee function early after anterior cruciate ligament injury. *J Orthop Sports Phys Ther.* 2010;40(11):705–721.
11. Hartigan E, Axe MJ, Snyder-Mackler L. Perturbation training prior to ACL reconstruction improves gait asymmetries in non-copers. *J Orthop Res.* 2009;27(6):724–729.
12. Keays SL, Bullock-Saxton JE, Newcombe P, Bullock MI. The effectiveness of a pre-operative home-based physiotherapy programme for chronic anterior cruciate ligament deficiency. *Physiother Res Int.* 2006;11(4):204–218.
13. Shaarani SR, O'Hare C, Quinn A, Moyna N, Moran R, O'Byrne JM. Effect of prehabilitation on the outcome of anterior cruciate ligament reconstruction. *Am J Sports Med.* 2013;41(9):2117–2127.
14. Gometz A, Maislen D, Youtz C, et al. The effectiveness of prehabilitation (prehab) in both functional and economic outcomes following spinal surgery: a systematic review. *Cureus.* 2018;10(5):e2675.
15. D'Eramo AL, Sedlak C, Doheny MO, Jenkins M. Nutritional aspects of the orthopaedic trauma patient. *Orthop Nurs.* 1994;13(4):13–20; quiz 20–11.
16. Stamatos CA, Reed E. Nutritional needs of trauma patients: challenges, barriers, and solutions. *Crit Care Nurs Clin North Am.* 1994;6(3):501–514.
17. Ludwick R, Dieckman B, Snelson CM. Assessment of the geriatric orthopaedic trauma patient. *Orthop Nurs.* 1999;18(6):13–18; quiz 19–20.
18. Molnar JA, Underdown MJ, Clark WA. Nutrition and chronic wounds. *Adv Wound Care.* 2014;3(11):663–681.
19. Karpouzos A, Diamantis E, Farmaki P, Savvanis S, Troupis T. Nutritional aspects of bone health and fracture healing. *J Osteoporos.* 2017;2017:4218472.
20. Brownie S. Why are elderly individuals at risk of nutritional deficiency? *Int J Nurs Pract.* 2006;12(2):110–118.
21. Thompson C, Fuhrman MP. Nutrients and wound healing: still searching for the magic bullet. *Nutr Clin Pract.* 2005;20(3):331–347.
22. Quain AM, Khardori NM. Nutrition in wound care management: a comprehensive overview. *Wounds.* 2015;27(12):327–335.
23. Harris CL, Fraser C. Malnutrition in the institutionalized elderly: the effects on wound healing. *Ostomy Wound Manage.* 2004;50(10):54–63.
24. Dorner B, Posthauer ME, Thomas D; National Pressure Ulcer Advisory Panel. The role of nutrition in pressure ulcer prevention and treatment. *Adv Skin Wound Care.* 2009;22(5):212–221.
25. Chen CC, Schilling LS, Lyder CH. A concept analysis of malnutrition in the elderly. *J Adv Nurs.* 2001;36(1):131–142.
26. Seitz O, Schürmann C, Hermes N, et al. Wound healing in mice with high-fat diet- or ob gene-induced diabetes-obesity syndromes: a comparative study. *Exp Diabetes Res.* 2010;2010:476969.
27. Shin L, Peterson DA. Impaired therapeutic capacity of autologous stem cells in a model of type 2 diabetes. *Stem Cells Transl Med.* 2012;1(2):125–135.
28. Keats E, Khan ZA. Unique responses of stem cell-derived vascular endothelial and mesenchymal cells to high levels of glucose. *PloS One.* 2012;7(6):e38752.
29. Cramer C, Freisinger E, Jones RK, et al. Persistent high glucose concentrations alter the regenerative potential of mesenchymal stem cells. *Stem Cells Dev.* 2010;19(12):1875–1884.
30. Oñate B, Vilahur G, Ferrer-Lorente R, et al. The subcutaneous adipose tissue reservoir of functionally active stem cells is reduced in obese patients. *FASEB J.* 2012;26(10):4327–4336.
31. Cerletti M, Jang YC, Finley LW, Haigis MC, Wagers AJ. Short-term calorie restriction enhances skeletal muscle stem cell function. *Cell Stem Cell.* 2012;10(5):515–519.
32. Kim HJ, Ji BR, Kim JS, Lee HN, Ha DH, Kim CW. Proteomic analysis of proteins associated with cellular senescence by calorie restriction in mesenchymal stem cells. *In Vitro Cell Dev Biol Anim.* 2012;48(3):186–195.
33. Lo T, Ho JH, Yang MH, Lee OK. Glucose reduction prevents replicative senescence and increases mitochondrial respiration in human mesenchymal stem cells. *Cell Transplant.* 2011;20(6):813–825.
34. Daltroy LH, Morlino CI, Eaton HM, Poss R, Liang MH. Preoperative education for total hip and knee replacement patients. *Arthritis Care Res.* 1998;11(6):469–478.
35. Lin PC, Lin LC, Lin JJ. Comparing the effectiveness of different educational programs for patients with total knee arthroplasty. *Orthop Nurs.* 1997;16(5):43–49.
36. Sussman WI, Mautner K, Malanga G. The role of rehabilitation after regenerative and orthobiologic procedures for the treatment of tendinopathy: a systematic review. *Regen Med.* 2018;13(2):249–263.
37. Townsend C, Von Rickenbach KJ, Bailowitz Z, Gellhorn AC. Post-procedure protocols following platelet-rich plasma injections for tendinopathy: a systematic review. *PM R.* 2020.
38. Virchenko O, Aspenberg P. How can one platelet injection after tendon injury lead to a stronger tendon after 4 weeks? Interplay between early regeneration and mechanical stimulation. *Acta Orthopaedica.* 2006;77(5):806–812.
39. Ambrosio F, Ferrari RJ, Distefano G, et al. The synergistic effect of treadmill running on stem-cell transplantation to heal injured skeletal muscle. *Tissue Eng Part A.* 2010;16(3):839–849.
40. Kon E, Filardo G, Delcogliano M, et al. Platelet-rich plasma: new clinical application: a pilot study for treatment of jumper's knee. *Injury.* 2009;40(6):598–603.
41. Schwartz MA. Integrins and extracellular matrix in mechanotransduction. *Cold Spring Harb Perspect Biol.* 2010;2(12):a005066.
42. Thompson WR, Scott A, Loghmani MT, Ward SR, Warden SJ. Understanding mechanobiology: physical therapists as a force in mechanotherapy and musculoskeletal regenerative rehabilitation. *Phys Ther.* 2016;96(4):560–569.
43. Khan KM, Scott A. Mechanotherapy: how physical therapists' prescription of exercise promotes tissue repair. *Br J Sports Med.* 2009;43(4):247–252.
44. Head PL. Rehabilitation considerations in regenerative medicine. *Phys Med Rehabil Clin.* 2016;(4):1043–1054.
45. Valero MC, Huntsman HD, Liu J, Zou K, Boppart MD. Eccentric exercise facilitates mesenchymal stem cell appearance in skeletal muscle. *PloS One.* 2012;7(1):e29760.
46. Kongsgaard M, Qvortrup K, Larsen J, et al. Fibril morphology and tendon mechanical properties in patellar tendinopathy: effects of heavy slow resistance training. *Am J Sports Med.* 2010;38(4):749–756.
47. Nielsen JL, Aagaard P, Bech RD, et al. Proliferation of myogenic stem cells in human skeletal muscle in response to low-load resistance training with blood flow restriction. *J Physiol.* 2012;590(17):4351–4361.

48. Fujita S, Abe T, Drummond MJ, et al. Blood flow restriction during low-intensity resistance exercise increases S6K1 phosphorylation and muscle protein synthesis. *J Appl Physiol (Bethesda, Md: 1985)*. 2007;103(3):903–910.
49. Sinno H, Prakash S. Complements and the wound healing cascade: an updated review. *Plast Surg Int*. 2013;2013:146764.
50. Voleti PB, Buckley MR, Soslowsky LJ. Tendon healing: repair and regeneration. *Annu Rev Biomed Eng*. 2012;14:47–71.
51. Reinke JM, Sorg H. Wound repair and regeneration. *Eur Surg Res*. 2012;49(1):35–43.
52. Landén NX, Li D, Ståhle M. Transition from inflammation to proliferation: a critical step during wound healing. *Cell Mol Life Sci*. 2016;73(20):3861–3885.
53. Thomopoulos S, Parks WC, Rifkin DB, Derwin KA. Mechanisms of tendon injury and repair. *J Orthop Res*. 2015;33(6): 832–839.
54. Maffulli N, Moller HD, Evans CH. Tendon healing: can it be optimised? *Br J Sports Med*. 2002;36(5):315–316.
55. Del Castillo-Gonzalez F, Ramos-Alvarez JJ, Gonzalez-Perez J, Jimenez-Herranz E, Rodriguez-Fabian G. Ultrasound-guided percutaneous lavage of calcific bursitis of the medial collateral ligament of the knee: a case report and review of the literature. *Skeletal Radiol*. 2016;45(10):1419–1423.
56. Parry DA, Barnes GR, Craig AS. A comparison of the size distribution of collagen fibrils in connective tissues as a function of age and a possible relation between fibril size distribution and mechanical properties. *Proc R Soc Lond B Biol Sci*. 1978;203(1152):305–321.
57. Levenson SM, Geever EF, Crowley LV, Oates 3rd JF, Berard CW, Rosen H. The healing of rat skin wounds. *Ann Surg*. 1965;161(2):293–308.
58. Nimini ME, de Guia E, Bavetta LA. Collagen, hexosamine and tensile strength of rabbit skin during aging. *J Invest Dermatol*. 1966;47(2):156–158.
59. Miyashita H, Ochi M, Ikuta Y. Histological and biomechanical observations of the rabbit patellar tendon after removal of its central one-third. *Arch Orthop Trauma Surg*. 1997;116(8):454–462.
60. Juneja SC, Schwarz EM, O'Keefe RJ, Awad HA. Cellular and molecular factors in flexor tendon repair and adhesions: a histological and gene expression analysis. *Connect Tissue Res*. 2013;54(3):218–226.
61. Sharma P, Maffulli N. Biology of tendon injury: healing, modeling and remodeling. *J Musculoskelet Neuronal Interact*. 2006;6(2):181–190.
62. Abrahamsson SO. Matrix metabolism and healing in the flexor tendon. Experimental studies on rabbit tendon. *Scand J Plast Reconstr Surg Hand Surg Suppl*. 1991;23:1–51.
63. Rantanen J, Hurme T, Lukka R, Heino J, Kalimo H. Satellite cell proliferation and the expression of myogenin and desmin in regenerating skeletal muscle: evidence for two different populations of satellite cells. *Lab Invest*. 1995;72(3):341–347.
64. Järvinen TA, Järvinen M, Kalimo H. Regeneration of injured skeletal muscle after the injury. *Muscles Ligaments Tendons J*. 2013;3(4):337–345.
65. Hunziker EB. Articular cartilage repair: basic science and clinical progress. A review of the current status and prospects. *Osteoarthritis Cartilage*. 2002;10(6):432–463.
66. Stoddart MJ, Bara J, Alini M. Cells and secretome—towards endogenous cell re-activation for cartilage repair. *Adv Drug Deliv Rev*. 2015;84:135–145.
67. Beckett J, Jin W, Schultz M, et al. Excessive running induces cartilage degeneration in knee joints and alters gait of rats. *J Orthop Res*. 2012;30(10):1604–1610.
68. Oryan A, Monazzah S, Bigham-Sadegh A. Bone injury and fracture healing biology. *Biomed Environ Sci*. 2015;28(1):57–71.
69. Dimitriou R, Tsiridis E, Giannoudis PV. Current concepts of molecular aspects of bone healing. *Injury*. 2005;36(12): 1392–1404.
70. Isaksson H, Comas O, van Donkelaar CC, et al. Bone regeneration during distraction osteogenesis: mechano-regulation by shear strain and fluid velocity. *J Biomech*. 2007;40(9): 2002–2011.
71. Marsell R, Einhorn TA. The biology of fracture healing. *Injury*. 2011;42(6):551–555.
72. Geris L, Gerisch A, Sloten JV, Weiner R, Oosterwyck HV. Angiogenesis in bone fracture healing: a bioregulatory model. *J Theor Biol*. 2008;251(1):137–158.
73. LaStayo PC, Winters KM, Hardy M. Fracture healing: bone healing, fracture management, and current concepts related to the hand. *J Hand Ther*. 2003;16(2):81–93.
74. Pilitsis JG, Lucas DR, Rengachary SS. Bone healing and spinal fusion. *Neurosurg Focus*. 2002;13(6):e1.
75. Peck E, Mautner K. Rehabilitation after platelet-rich plasma injections for tendinopathy. In: Lana JFSD, Andrade Santana MH, Dias Belangero W, Malheiros Luzo AC, eds. *Platelet-Rich Plasma: Regenerative Medicine: Sports Medicine, Orthopedic, and Recovery of Musculoskeletal Injuries, Lecture Notes in Bioengineering*. Berlin, Germany: Springer; 2014:315–328.
76. Finnoff JT, Fowler SP, Lai JK, et al. Treatment of chronic tendinopathy with ultrasound-guided needle tenotomy and platelet-rich plasma injection. *PM R*. 2011;3(10):900–911.
77. Kaux JF, Forthomme B, Namurois MH, et al. Description of a standardized rehabilitation program based on sub-maximal eccentric following a platelet-rich plasma infiltration for jumper's knee. *Muscles Ligaments Tendons J*. 2014;4(1):85–89.
78. van Ark M, van den Akker-Scheek I, Meijer LT, Zwerver J. An exercise-based physical therapy program for patients with patellar tendinopathy after platelet-rich plasma injection. *Phys Ther Sport*. 2013;14(2):124–130.
79. Wiegerinck JI, de Jonge S, de Jonge MC, Kerkhoffs GM, Verhaar J, van Dijk CN. Comparison of postinjection protocols after intratendinous Achilles platelet-rich plasma injections: a cadaveric study. *J Foot Ankle*. 2014;53(6):712–715.
80. McMaster WC, Liddle S, Waugh TR. Laboratory evaluation of various cold therapy modalities. *Am J Sports Med*. 1978;6(5):291–294.
81. Barber FA. A comparison of crushed ice and continuous flow cold therapy. *Am J Knee Surg*. 2000;13(2):97–101; discussion 102.
82. Barber FA, McGuire DA, Click S. Continuous-flow cold therapy for outpatient anterior cruciate ligament reconstruction. *Arthroscopy*. 1998;14(2):130–135.
83. Mautner K, Malanga G, Colberg R. Optimization of ingredients, procedures and rehabilitation for platelet-rich plasma injections for chronic tendinopathy. *Pain Manag*. 2011;1(6): 523–532.
84. Block JE. Cold and compression in the management of musculoskeletal injuries and orthopedic operative procedures: a narrative review. *Open Access J Sports Med*. 2010;1:105–113.
85. MacAuley D. Do textbooks agree on their advice on ice? *Clin J Sport Med*. 2001;11(2):67–72.

86. Music M, Finderle Z, Cankar K. Cold perception and cutaneous microvascular response to local cooling at different cooling temperatures. *Microvasc Res.* 2011;81(3):319–324.
87. Bleakley C, McDonough S, MacAuley D. The use of ice in the treatment of acute soft-tissue injury: a systematic review of randomized controlled trials. *Am J Sports Med.* 2004;32(1):251–261.
88. Warren TA, McCarty EC, Richardson AL, Michener T, Spindler KP. Intra-articular knee temperature changes: ice versus cryotherapy device. *Am J Sports Med.* 2004;32(2):441–445.
89. Knobloch K, Kraemer R, Lichtenberg A, et al. Microcirculation of the ankle after Cryo/Cuff application in healthy volunteers. *Int J Sports Med.* 2006;27(3):250–255.
90. Khoshnevis S, Craik NK, Diller KR. Cold-induced vasoconstriction may persist long after cooling ends: an evaluation of multiple cryotherapy units. *Knee Surg Sports Traumatol Arthrosc.* 2015;23(9):2475–2483.
91. Knobloch K, Grasemann R, Spies M, Vogt PM. Midportion Achilles tendon microcirculation after intermittent combined cryotherapy and compression compared with cryotherapy alone: a randomized trial. *Am J Sports Med.* 2008;36(11):2128–2138.
92. Jutte LS, Merrick MA, Ingersoll CD, Edwards JE. The relationship between intramuscular temperature, skin temperature, and adipose thickness during cryotherapy and rewarming. *Arch Phys Med Rehabil.* 2001;82(6):845–850.
93. Lyman B, Rosenberg L, Karpatkin S. Biochemical and biophysical aspects of human platelet adhesion to collagen fibers. *J Clin Invest.* 1971;50(9):1854–1863.
94. Mannava S, Whitney KE, Kennedy MI, et al. The influence of naproxen on biological factors in leukocyte-rich platelet-rich plasma: a prospective comparative study. *Arthroscopy.* 2019;35(1):201–210.
95. Schippinger G, Prüller F, Divjak M, et al. Autologous platelet-rich plasma preparations: influence of nonsteroidal anti-inflammatory drugs on platelet function. *Orthop J Sports Med.* 2015;3(6):2325967115588896.
96. Jayaram P, Kennedy DJ, Yeh P, Dragoo J. Chondrotoxic effects of local anesthetics on human knee articular cartilage: a systematic review. *PM R.* 2019;11(4):379–400.
97. Chechik O, Dolkart O, Mozes G, Rak O, Alhajajra F, Maman E. Timing matters: NSAIDs interfere with the late proliferation stage of a repaired rotator cuff tendon healing in rats. *Arch Orthop Trauma Surg.* 2014;134(4):515–520.
98. Chau DL, Walker V, Pai L, Cho LM. Opiates and elderly: use and side effects. *Clin Interv Aging.* 2008;3(2):273–278.
99. Podesta LCS, Volkmer D, et al. Treatment of partial ulnar collateral ligament tears in the elbow with platelet-rich plasma. *Am J Sports Med.* 2013;41(7):1689–1694.
100. Nevalainen MT, Repo JP, Pesola M, Nyrhinen JP. Successful treatment of early talar osteonecrosis by core decompression combined with intraosseous stem cell injection: a case report. *J Orthop Case Rep.* 2018;8(1):23–26.
101. Hammerman M, Aspenberg P, Eliasson P. Microtrauma stimulates rat Achilles tendon healing via an early gene expression pattern similar to mechanical loading. *J Appl Physiol (Bethesda, Md : 1985).* 2014;116(1):54–60.
102. Zhang J, Wang JH. Platelet-rich plasma releasate promotes differentiation of tendon stem cells into active tenocytes. *Am J Sports Med.* 2010;38(12):2477–2486.
103. Poor A, Roedl J, Zoga A, Meyers W. Incidence of heterotopic ossification among NFL athletes following platelet-rich plasma (PRP) for treatment of core muscle injuries (CMI). *Orthop J Sports Med.* 2018;6:2325967118S2325960011.
104. Behm DG, Blazevich AJ, Kay AD, McHugh M. Acute effects of muscle stretching on physical performance, range of motion, and injury incidence in healthy active individuals: a systematic review. *Appl Physiol Nutr Metab.* 2016;41(1):1–11.
105. Rio E, Kidgell D, Purdam C, et al. Isometric exercise induces analgesia and reduces inhibition in patellar tendinopathy. *Br J Sports Med.* 2015;49(19):1277–1283.
106. Rio E, van Ark M, Docking S, et al. Isometric contractions are more analgesic than isotonic contractions for patellar tendon pain: an in-season randomized clinical trial. *Clin J Sport Med.* 2017;27(3):253–259.
107. Lim HY, Wong SH. Effects of isometric, eccentric, or heavy slow resistance exercises on pain and function in individuals with patellar tendinopathy: a systematic review. *Physiother Res Int.* 2018;23(4):e1721.
108. Camporesi E, Vezzani G, Zanon V, et al. Review on hyperbaric oxygen treatment in femoral head necrosis. *Undersea Hyperb Med.* 2017;44(6):497–508. https://doi.org/10.22462/11.12.2017.1.
109. Karamitros AE, Kalentzos VN, Soucacos PN. Electric stimulation and hyperbaric oxygen therapy in the treatment of nonunions. *Injury.* 2006;37(suppl 1):S63–S73. https://doi.org/10.1016/j.injury.2006.02.042.
110. Busse JW, Kaur J, Mollon B, et al. Low intensity pulsed ultrasonography for fractures: systematic review of randomised controlled trials. *BMJ.* 2009;338:b351. Published online 2009 Feb 27. https://doi.org/10.1136/bmj.b351.

38

Advanced Imaging in Interventional Orthopedics

RAHUL NAREN DESAI AND KATARZYNA IWAN

Regenerative musculoskeletal orthobiologics are a game-changing and paradigm-shifting treatment option. They require a new set of standards in terms of diagnosis, treatment regimen (moving from single joints or individual structures to treatment of the entire kinetic chain), rehabilitation protocols, and expectations. These interventions and therapeutic regimen afford physicians the ability to heal injured tissues and return them to a more normal and, in some cases, a native uninjured state. In this manner, they have also set new standards in preprocedural and postprocedural imaging.

Regenerative therapies are powerfully compelling, but consistently successful results require precision diagnosis, and delivery with the use of image guidance (Fig. 38.1). There is clear and repeatable evidence that a precisely placed image-guided injection of regenerative materials, including autologous cells, changes the tissue appearance back to a more normal morphology.[1–5]

In today's practice, there are many conventional treatment modalities that provide for improved function and reduce pain. These include palliative treatments such as corticosteroid injections, and nerve ablation. Surgeries are focused at removing the diseased tissues, whether it be a meniscus, labrum, or joint. However, the modalities all fail in regard to their ability to change the disease process of the injured tissues. Orthobiologics have shifted the perspective from palliative to restorative, further confirmed as magnetic resonance imaging (MRI) and ultrasound evidence shows return to a normal tissue morphology. Follow-up imaging allows the clinician to correlate clinical success with structural tissue improvement, further validating the source of pain and dysfunction.

Most case reports, abstracts, and white papers in orthopedic, musculoskeletal, and regenerative medicine focus heavily on pain scores and functional outcome measures such as the Oswestry Disability Index, visual analog scale (VAS) score, and Knee injury and Osteoarthritis Outcome Score (KOOS). Imaging has been used as an outcome measure to a much smaller degree, but it is a crucial and highly objective measure of outcome. Imaging is a powerful modality because it can be used in precisely defining injuries, inflammation, and dysfunction, but this does require a specific skill set by the practitioner.[6] In many instances, imaging studies are misinterpreted because of the disconnect between physical exam and diagnostic imaging interpretation. The cause for the patient's pain or dysfunction, otherwise known as the diagnosis, is present on imaging but is not interpreted as critical or important or sometimes is simply not recognized. Another reason for the disconnect is the lack of interpretation skills of the treating physician, or solely relying upon the report of the radiologist who has never seen or evaluated the patient. The pressures on the radiologists to read high volumes of cases and meet relative value units (RVU) quota further reduce the quality of imaging interpretations because the priority becomes ruling out catastrophic findings (i.e., cancer, surgical emergencies) rather than finding subtle diagnoses.[7]

The field has matured with the advent of improved point-of-care ultrasound and postinjection-limited MRI. Physicians now can reimage patients after the procedure and demonstrate healing of the tissue by delineating the morphologic difference between injured tissue versus healed tissue. This can be best accomplished with the use of MRI, ultrasound, x-ray, and computed tomography (CT) scans, which provide a detailed image of all structures and the ability to see regeneration of native tissue on a larger scale. This is a major shift in thinking compared with orthopedic and neurosurgical models, where the tissues are often severely disrupted and where postoperative imaging is less than ideal in demonstrating improvement. The tissue is often obscured by metallic artifacts; therefore the repaired tendon or tissues are poorly visualized. Artifacts may be related to screws, anchors, or even simply filings from shavers used during surgeries or arthroscopies. Postsurgical scarring involving the soft tissues, epidural space, fat pad, and other areas are also commonplace. In stark contrast, imaging in the regenerative medicine setting can demonstrate resolution of tendon tears, reformation of ruptured ligaments, healing of annular tears of discs, improved alignment of the spine, resolution of joint effusions, and even reversal of bone marrow lesions, cysts, and intraosseous edema (Figs. 38.2–38.10). Moreover, an updated imaging study prior to treatment is crucial because it focuses therapy to all the regions that

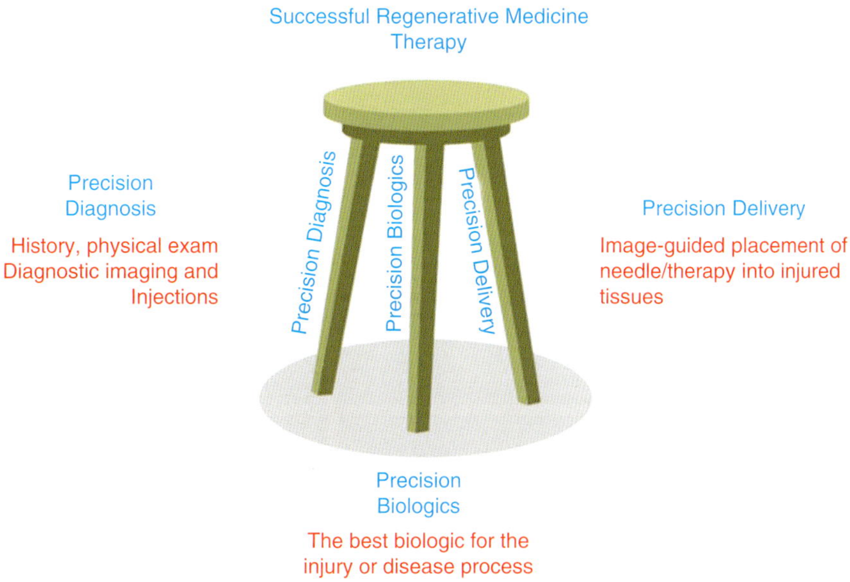

• **Fig. 38.1** Three-legged stool for successful regenerative medicine therapy comprises precision diagnosis, precision biologics, and precision delivery into injured tissues.

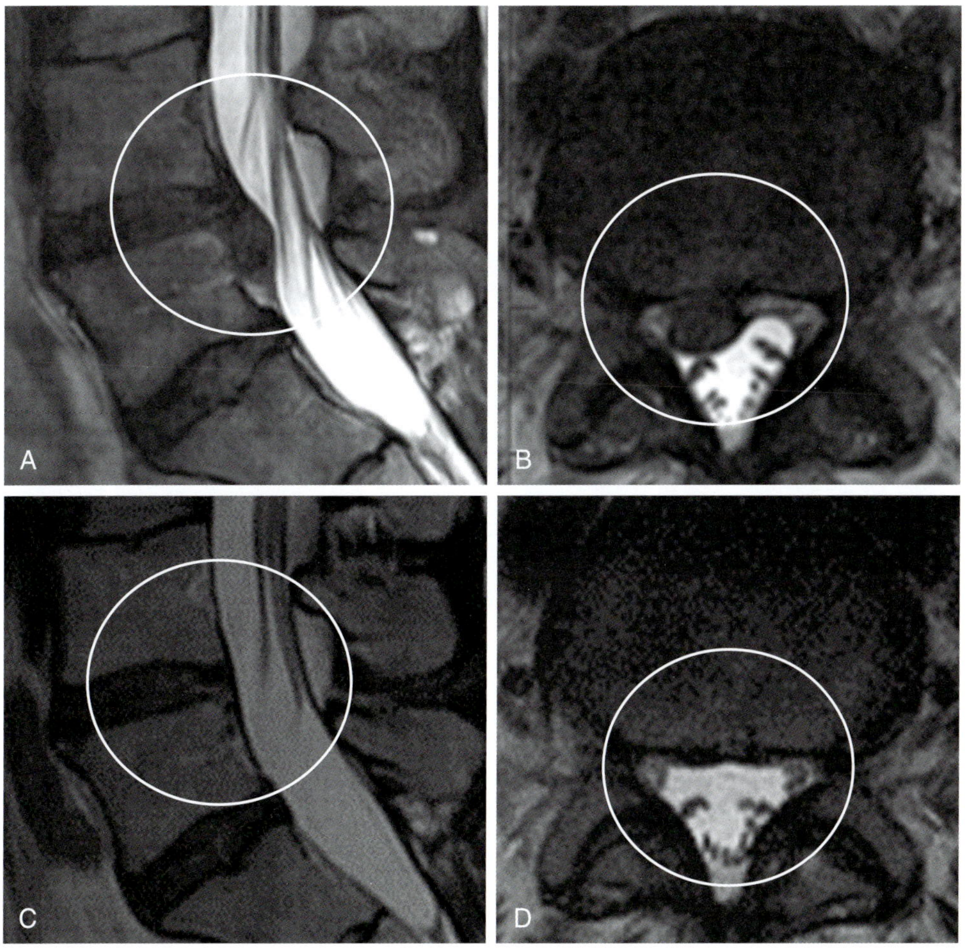

• **Fig. 38.2** Pretreatment magnetic resonance imaging (MRI) lumbar spine sagittal (A) and axial plane T2 (B) sequence demonstrates L4–L5 central, right-paracentral disc herniation with extrusion and caudal migration. Posttreatment MRI (C, D) demonstrates complete resolution of the her-niation and extrusion.

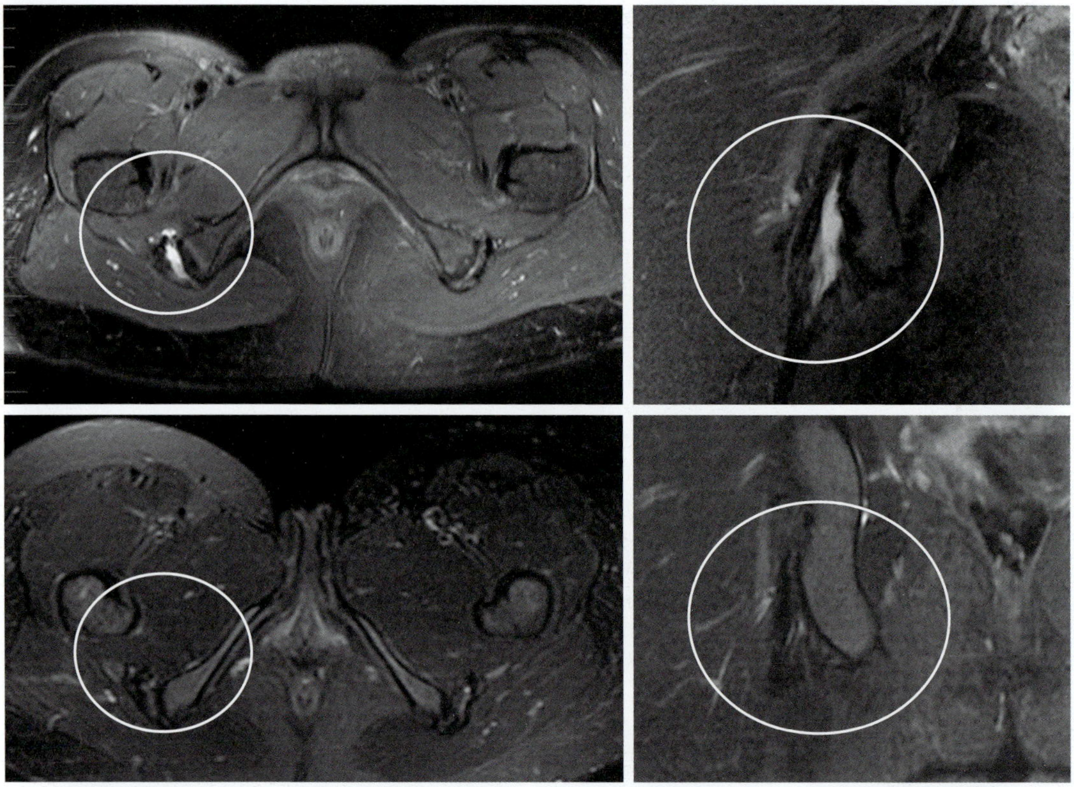

• **Fig. 38.3** *(Top images)* Pretreatment magnetic resonance imaging (MRI) of right hamstring origin demonstrates a large tear at the ischial tuberosity footprint, with fluid signal intensity filling the defect. *(Bottom images)* One-year post stem cell injection therapy demonstrates complete resolution of the defect, with normal appearing tendon origin. The patient's symptom improvement strongly correlated with these MRI findings.

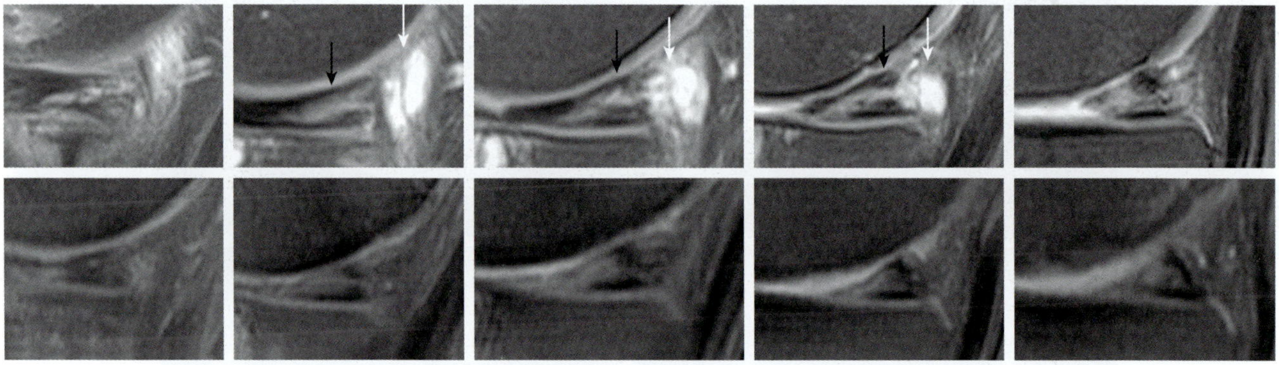

• **Fig. 38.4** *(Top images)* Pretreatment sagittal plane magnetic resonance imaging (MRI) through the posterior horn of the medial meniscus demonstrating complex horizontal tear with extension through the posterior peripheral base *(blue arrow)* and adjacent parameniscal cysts *(orange arrow)*. *(Bottom images)* Nine-month post-treatment MRI demonstrating resolution of the parameniscal cyst and coaptation and healing of the meniscal tear. Patient is symptom free and has returned to running up to 6 miles 3 to 4 times per week.

require intervention. In addition, it is most ideal to reimage the patient at approximately 3 to 6 months and 12 months after orthobiologic therapy. Practitioners should use consistent methods, imaging modalities, and imaging sequences. Local imaging centers and radiology groups are usually able to offer discounted pricing for limited sequence exams that focus on the previously injured and treated tissues. This may dramatically reduce the extent of imaging required, scan times, and costs and improve patient comfort. Imaging is beneficial in gauging the response of the injured tissue and to document the outcome, both for documentation and for research purposes. It can also dramatically improve practitioner and patient confidence that the treatments are working toward their intended outcome.

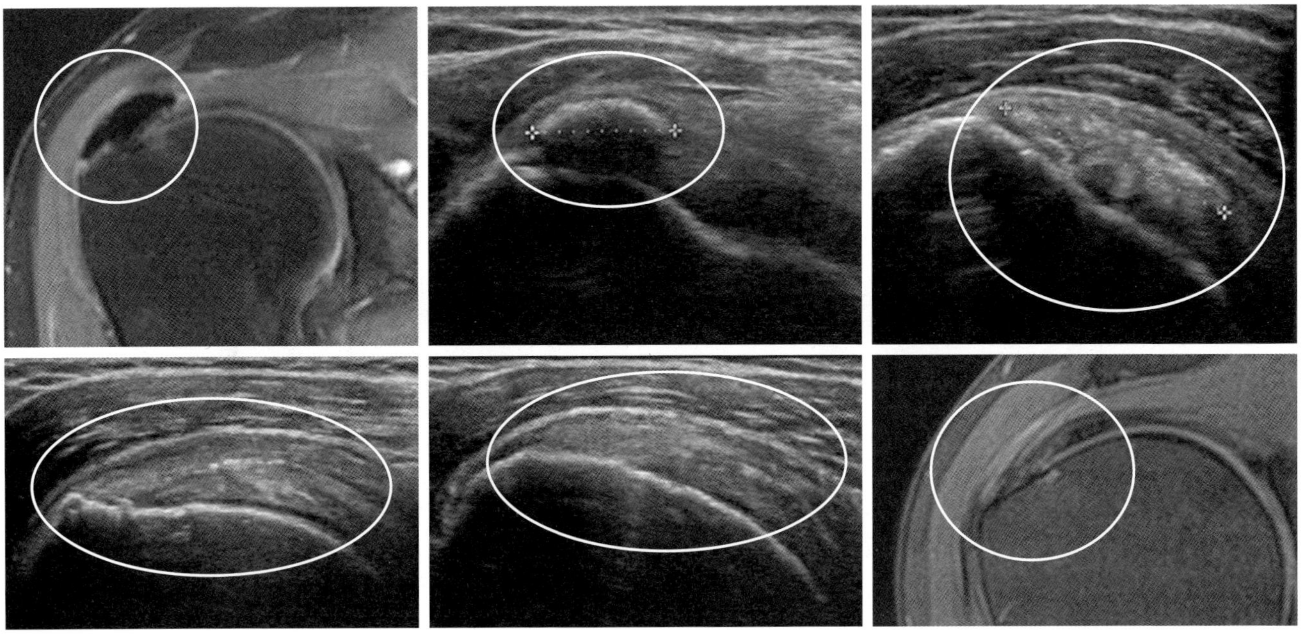

• **Fig. 38.5** Magnetic resonance imaging and ultrasound follow-up imaging of supraspinatus calcific tendinitis after tenotomy calcium debridement combined with autologous fat injection therapy

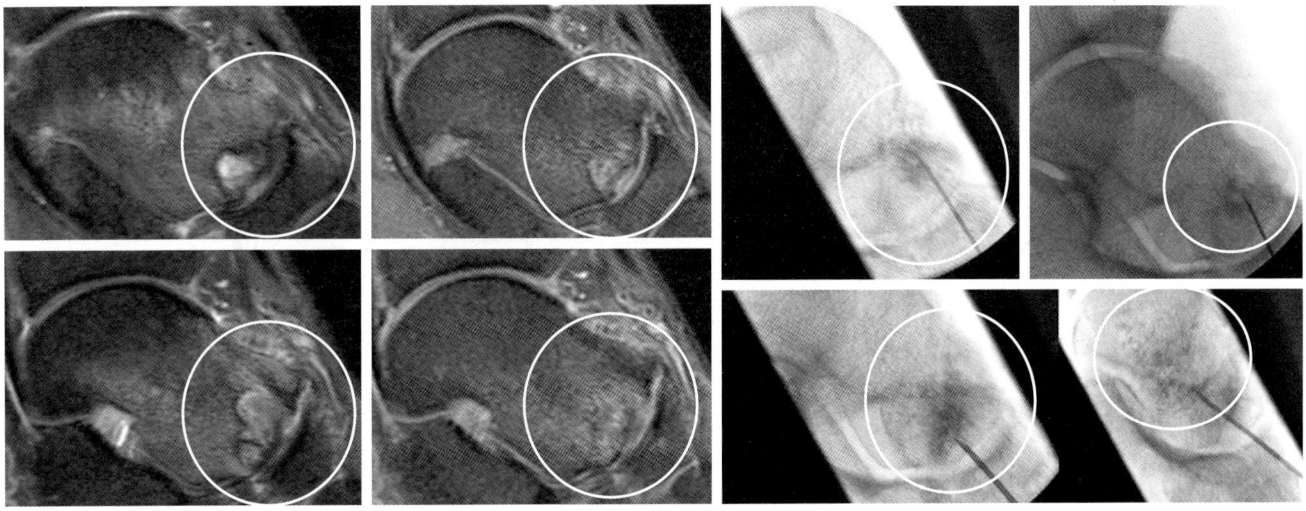

• **Fig. 38.6** *(Left images)* Magnetic resonance imaging demonstrating talonavicular arthritis, with large areas of subchondral cyst formation with sclerotic walls, and extensive marrow edema extending to the talar body. *(Right images)* Imaging post treatment at 6 months with stem cells shows dramatic improvement of the subchondral edema, normal marrow signal, and structure occupying areas of previous cystic change. The dense sclerotic walls have also resolved. *(Bottom images)* X-ray imaging demonstrates precision placement of Jamshidi needle, and contrast filling of cysts with reposition of needle into separate discrete areas of injury. Contrast is seen filling the discrete cystic regions *(top row, and right lower),* as well as flowing into the talar body with trabecular contrast depiction *(lower right image)*.

In regenerative medicine, imaging is vital for identifying injured tissues and measuring the efficacy of treatment. Imaging bridges the gap between orthobiologic therapies and outcomes, thus providing insight into healing, pathophysiology, and longitudinal restorative function. Regenerative medicine aims to enhance the body's intrinsic healing capacity, although this therapy is still not covered by most medical insurance carriers. Imaging technologies have improved significantly in recent years and provide quality images with shorter acquisition times, minimal to no radiation dose, and assessment of structural and functional improvement. In vivo imaging is a platform technology with the power to put function in its natural structural context. Modalities such as elastography ultrasound can assess tensile strength of tendons. With the drive to translate stem cell therapies into preclinical and clinical trials, early selection of the right imaging techniques is paramount to success. There are many instances in regenerative medicine where

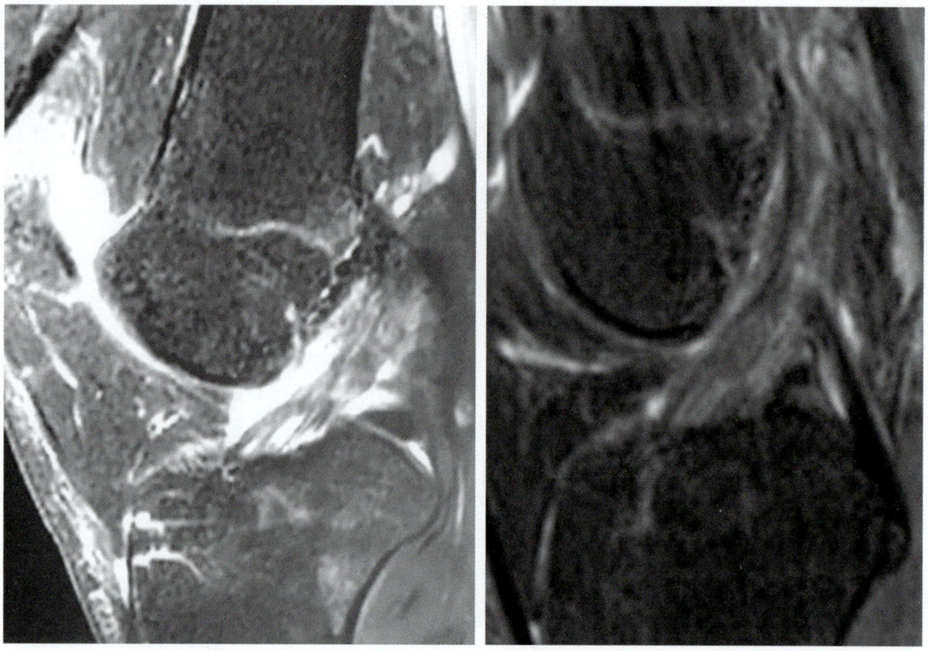

• **Fig. 38.7** (Left image) Pretreatment magnetic resonance imaging demonstrates complete rupture of anterior cruciate ligament (ACL). (Right image) Demonstrate progressive healing at 6 weeks and 3 months post treatment with bone marrow aspirate concentrate.

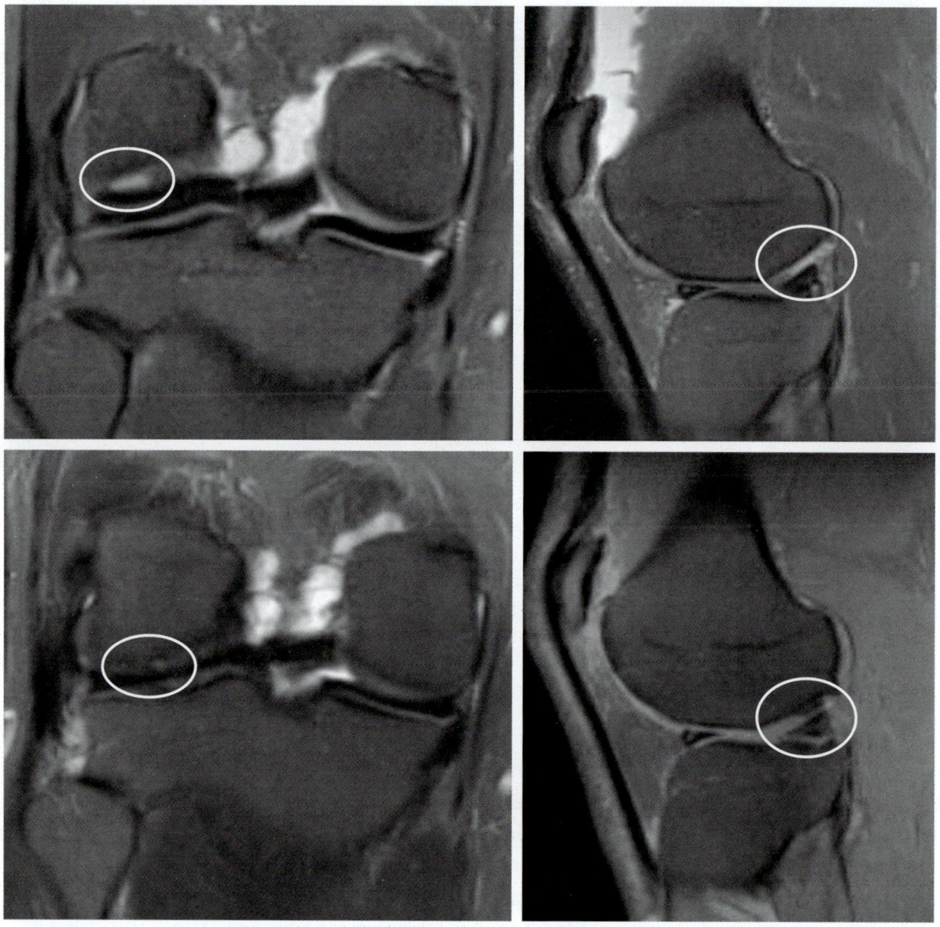

• **Fig. 38.8** (Top images) Pretreatment magnetic resonance imaging (MRI) on the top and posttreatment MRI (bottom images) taken 2 years after treatment with intra-articular and subchondral bone marrow aspirate concentrate for an osteo-chondral defect in the posterior lateral femoral condyle in a 38-year-old male with posterior lateral knee pain for 3 years.

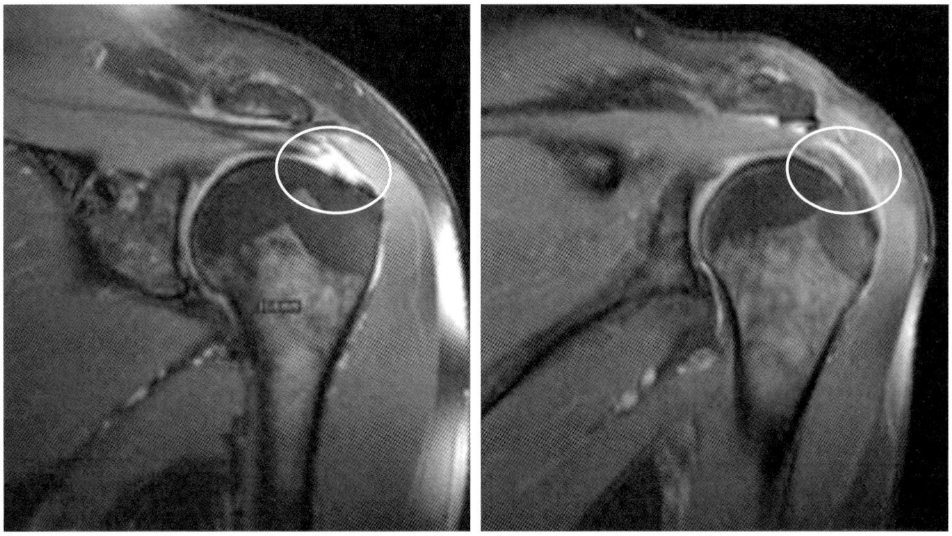

• **Fig. 38.9** The left pretreatment T2-weighted coronal image of the left shoulder of a 63-year-old female with a full-thickness rotator cuff tear measuring 1.4 cm treated with ultrasound-guided bone marrow aspirate concentrate. The posttreatment T2 coronal magnetic resonance imaging done at 2 years post treatment demonstrating significant healing and with patient-reported symptomatic improvement of 99%.

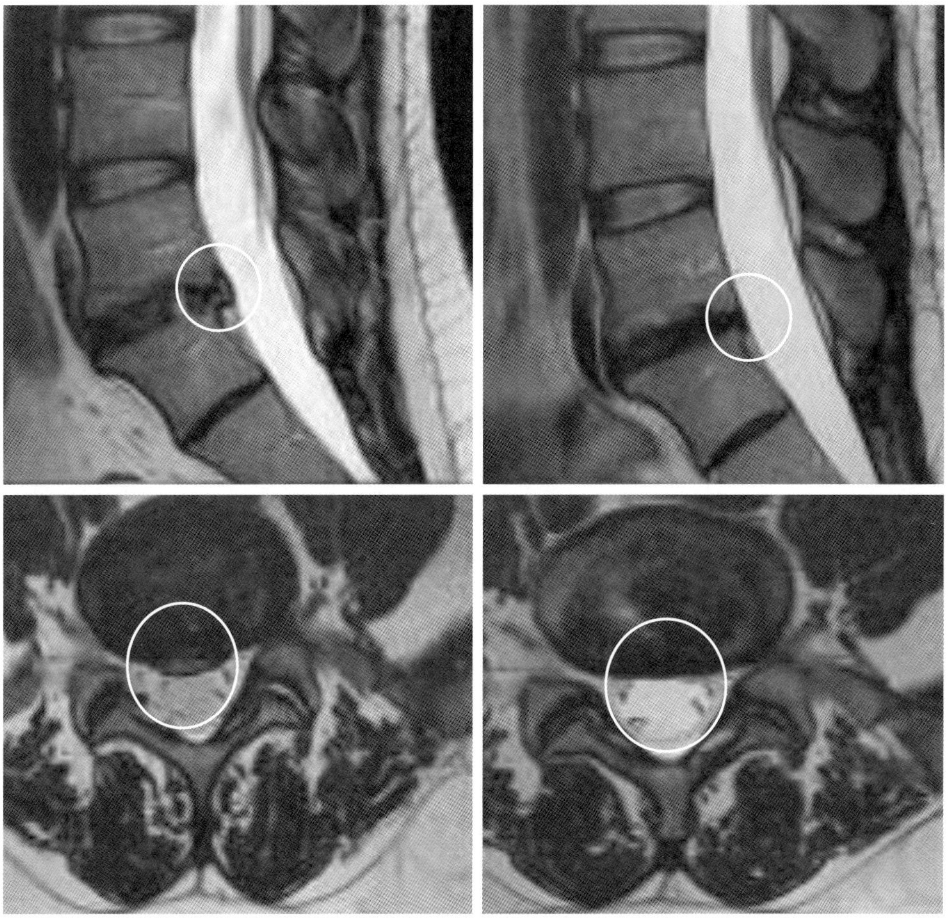

• **Fig. 38.10** *(Top images)* Pretreatment sagittal and axial T2-weighted sequence showing posterior disc bulge and annular tear at L5–S1. *(Bottom images)* The posttreatment T2 MRI images demonstrating interval improvement in disc bulge size and resolution of annular tearing.

the biologic, biochemical, and biomechanical mechanisms behind the proposed function of stem cell therapies can be elucidated by appropriate imaging.[8,9] Imaging allows providers and researchers to document objective outcome measures and further the integration of orthobiologic therapy into modern medicine.

References

1. Hurd JL, et al. Safety and efficacy of treating symptomatic, partial-thickness rotator cuff tears with fresh, uncultured, unmodified, autologous adipose-derived regenerative cells (UA-ADRCs) isolated at the point of care: a prospective, randomized, controlled first-in-human pilot study. *J Orthop Surg Res*. 2020;15(1):122. https://doi.org/10.1186/s13018-020-01631-8.
2. Lychagin A, et al. Intraosseous injections of platelet rich plasma for knee bone marrow lesions treatment: one year follow-up. *Int Orthop*. 2020 Apr 4. https://doi.org/10.1007/s00264-020-04546-5.
3. Raeissadat SA, et al. MRI changes after platelet rich plasma injection in knee osteoarthritis (randomized clinical trial). *J Pain Res*. 2020;13:65–73. https://doi.org/10.2147/JPR.S204788.
4. Buendía-López D, et al. Clinical and radiographic comparison of a single LP-PRP injection, a single hyaluronic acid injection and daily NSAID administration with a 52-week follow-up: a randomized controlled trial. *J Orthop Traumatol*. 2018;19(1):3. https://doi.org/10.1186/s10195-018-0501-3.
5. Kenmochi M, et al. Clinical outcomes following injections of leukocyte-rich platelet-rich plasma in osteoarthritis patients. *J Orthop*. 2019;18:143–149. https://doi.org/10.1016/j.jor.2019.11.041.
6. Centurion AJ, et al. Use of musculoskeletal ultrasound and regenerative therapies in soccer. *Am J Orthop (Belle Mead NJ)*. 2018;47(10). https://doi.org/10.12788/ajo.2018.0093.
7. Brady AP. Error and discrepancy in radiology: inevitable or avoidable? *Insights Imaging*. 2017;8(1):171–182. https://doi.org/10.1007/s13244-016-0534-1.
8. Leahy M, et al. Functional imaging for regenerative medicine. *Stem Cell Research & Therapy*. 2016;7(1 57). https://doi.org/10.1186/s13287-016-0315-2.
9. Li Q, et al. Advanced imaging in osteoarthritis. *Sports Health*. 2016;8(5):418–428. https://doi.org/10.1177/1941738116663922.

Index

Note: Page numbers followed by '*f*' indicate figures those followed by '*t*' indicate tables and '*b*' indicate boxes.